100,000+
Baby'Names

Bruce Lansky

D1040967

m Meadowbrook Press
Distributed by Simon & Schuster
New York

ISBN 0-88166-507-X (Meadowbrook)   ISBN 0-684-03999-0 (Simon & Schuster)
1. Names, Personal—Dictionaries. I. Title: One hundred thousand plus baby names. II. T
CS2377.L3544 2006
929.4'4—dc22

2005024101

Editorial Director: Christine Zuchora-Walske
Editors: Megan McGinnis, Angela Wiechmann
Editorial Assistants: Andrea Patch, Maureen Burns, Alicia Ester
Production Manager: Paul Woods
Graphic Design Manager: Tamara Peterson
Researchers and Translators: David Rochelero, Stephanie Owen
Researcher: Kelsey Anderson
Data Programmers: Sean Beaton, Cynthia Miller Beaton
Cover Art: Digital Vision, Corbis Images, Eyewire Images, Hemera,
        MediaFocus International

Published by Meadowbrook Press, 5451 Smetana Drive, Minnetonka, Minnesota 55343

www.meadowbrookpress.com

BOOK TRADE DISTRIBUTION by Simon and Schuster, a division of Simon and Schuster
of the Americas, New York, New York 10020

09 08 07 06   10 9 8 7 6 5 4 3

Printed in the United States of America

Contents

Acknowledgments

Bruce Lansky and Barry Sinrod. Copyright © 1998 by Meadowbrook Press.

The "Most Popular Names" lists were derived from data from the Social Security Administration. The "Popular Names around the World" lists were derived from records kept by various government agencies around the globe.

Some of the material in "Fascinating Facts about Names" comes from "The Names People Play" by Frank Remington. It originally appeared in the November 1969 issue of *Today's Health*. Used with permission.

Some of the names and occupations of persons listed in "The Name's the Game" in "Fascinating Facts about Names" are reprinted from *Remarkable Names of Real People,* compiled and annotated by John T illustrated by Pierre Le-Tan. Copyright © 1977 by John Train. Used with permission of Clarkson N. Potter

Dick Crouser's contributions to "Fascinating Facts about Names" are used with permission.

Dick Neff's contributions to "Fascinating Facts about Names" first appeared in the January 8, 1968, and April 1, 1968, issues of *Advertising Age*. Copyright © 1968 by Crain Communications, Inc. Used with permission.

Introduction

Searching for just the right name for your baby can be a pleasure if you have just the right book. Let me tell you why I think *100,000+ Baby Names* is the right book.

It contains the most names—complete with origins, meanings, variations, fascinating facts, and famous namesakes—of any book in its price range. Here you'll find the most names from major ethnic origins, such as:

- Over 11,000 American names, many of which African-American families choose for their children

- Nearly 9,000 names Hispanic families commonly use

- Over 11,000 Latin names; 9,000 Hebrew names; 7,000 Irish names; and 6,000 German names

- Nearly 19,000 English names; 11,000 Greek names; 8,000 French names; and 4,000 Arabic names

- Thousands of Scottish, Welsh, Italian, Russian, Japanese, Chinese, Scandinavian, Polish, Native American, Hawaiian, Korean, Tai, Vietnamese, Australian/Aboriginal, African, and Hindi names. Plus many more names from many more origins!

But there's more in *100,000+ Baby Names* than just pages and pages of names. Don't miss the step-by-step guide "How to Pick a Name You and Your Baby Will Love." In three simple steps, complete with easy-to-use worksheets, you can select a name that has personal meaning but is also practical. It's the perfect approach for parents who find the idea of reading over 100,000 baby names a bit overwhelming.

You'll also find over 300 fun, helpful lists that will get you brainstorming names. This includes the latest lists of the top 100 girls' and boys' names. The top 100 lists are now complete with data to help you compare rankings from the previous year's lists, so you can see which names are climbing, which are falling, and which are holding steady. To quickly see what's hot and what's not, check out the Big Gains and Big Losses lists. And to find the most popular names in the Girls' Names and Boys' Names sections, look for the special ⭐ icon. If you're expecting a double dose of joy, take a look at the lists of the most popular names for twins. Lastly, if you're interested in tracking names over the years or just looking for a timeless name, you'll love the lists of popular names over the last one hundred years, now also complete with comparison rankings from decade to decade.

Want to know what parents in Canada, Australia, Sweden, and Japan are naming their babies? Want to find that perfect name to reflect your heritage? *100,000+ Baby Names* features lists of popular names around the world as well as lists of common and interesting names from many different origins. Want to name your baby after your favorite movie star, religious figure, or locale? Check out the lists featuring names inspired by people, places, and things. These lists will get you thinking about names that have special meaning to you. In addition to the 300 fun lists, you'll find features about the names celebrities choose for their babies and for themselves, as well as a helpful Baby Name Legal Guide and hilarious Fascinating Facts about Names.

100,000+ Baby Names also has an exclusive new feature to help parents make informed choices about names. Recently, naming trends have been heading in less traditional directions. One such trend is to use traditional boys' names for girls and vice versa. Throughout the Girls' Names and Boys' Names sections, you'll find special icons highlighting names that are shared by both genders. The icons will indicate whether a shared name is used mostly for boys (BG), used mostly for girls (GB), or used about evenly by both genders (BG). Some parents want androgynous or gender-jumping names, and other parents want names with clear gender identification. Either way, the icons will help you make an informed choice.

As you browse the names with these special icons, you may be surprised to learn that certain names are shared. It's important to keep several factors in mind:

1. The data may include errors. Amanda is listed in the boys' section because records show that 1 out of every 100,000 boys are named Amanda. It's reasonable to think that some boy "Amandas" are simply recording errors, but perhaps some aren't.

2. Names have different roles in different cultures. In the U.S., Andrea is primarily a girls' name, whereas in Italy, it's often used as a boys' name (for example, opera star Andrea Bocelli).

3. This book defines a name by its spelling, not by its pronunciation or meaning. This explains why a name like Julian is listed as a shared name. Julian (pronounced "JOO-lee-en") is a form of Julius, and therefore in the Boys' Names section. Julian (pronounced "Joo-lee-ANN") is a form of Julianne, and therefore in the Girls' Names section. You could argue that these are two different names, but because this book defines a name by its spelling, it treats them as one name.

4. The gender "assignment" of names change—often in surprising ways. For years, Ashley was used often for boys. (Remember Ashley Wilkes in *Gone with the Wind*?) Twenty-five years ago, it was in the top 300 of boys' names. Today it doesn't crack the top 1000, whereas it's the eighth-most-popular name for girls. In 2000, over twice as many boys as girls were named Reese. By 2004, actress Reese Witherspoon had helped those numbers switch places—now nearly twice as many girls as boys are named Reese.

I hope you find this book fun, helpful, and easy to use as you search for just the right name that will help your baby put his or her best foot forward in life.

Bruce Lansky

How to Pick a Name You and Your Baby Will Love

The first edition of *The Best Baby Name Book in the Whole Wide World*, which I wrote back in 1978, had about 10,000 names on 120 pages. So, you could read the introductory material about "15 Things to Consider When You Name Your Baby" and browse all the main listings (and even pause to read the origins, meanings, and variations for names that appealed to you) in a few hours. It's something a couple could even do together.

100,000+ Baby Names has more than 100,000 names on 700 pages. I don't know how long it would take you and your partner to browse all the main listings and pause to read more about your favorites, but it could be a daunting task. If you're up to the challenge, go for it. You'll certainly find your favorite names and discover some new names as well.

But if the idea of wading through a sea of 100,000 names sounds overwhelming, I'd like to propose another method. The method I suggest involves generating lists of names you and your partner love and then narrowing down the lists based on how well the names might work for your baby. It's a fun, easy way to come up with a name that has special meaning but is practical as well. Let's get started.

Step 1: Make a List of Names with Special Meaning

Make a list of names to consider by writing down your answers to the following questions. (You each will make your own list.) These questions are based on the lists starting on page 6. Browse those lists to help you answer the questions and to brainstorm other questions specific to your background, preferences, and experiences.

Popular Names (pages 6–21)
What are your favorite names from the most recent Top 100 lists?
What are your favorite names from the lists of most popular names over the past 100 years?
If any of your relatives' names appear in the popularity lists from previous generations, what are your favorites?

Names around the World (pages 22–31)
What country are your parents or grandparents from? What country are you and your partner from?
If any of your relatives' names appear in the international lists, what are your favorites?
What are your favorite names that are currently popular in other countries?
What language(s) do you speak?
Where did you honeymoon?
Where do you like to vacation?
Where did you conceive?

Impressions Names Make (pages 32–38)
What might your baby's personality be like?
How might your baby look physically?
What impression would you like your baby's name to make about him/her?

Names Inspired by People, Places, and Things (pages 39–93)

Who are your favorite literary figures?
Who are your favorite historical figures?
Who are your favorite figures from religion and mythology?
Who are your favorite figures from movies and television?
Who are your favorite musicians? What are your favorite songs?
Who are your favorite sports figures?
What are your favorite natural elements and places?
What are your favorite trades?
What are your favorite pieces of pop culture?
What are your favorite other ideas for names (last names as first names, old-fashioned names, etc.)?

Once you answer these questions, turn to the Girls' Names and Boys' Names sections to find interesting spellings or variations based on the names from your list. (As you flip through the book, you might stumble across a few new names that capture your attention, too.) That will give you a long list of names to consider for the next step.

Step 2: Narrow the List Based on What Will Work Best for Your Baby

Now that you've each created a list based on personal considerations, it's time to narrow them down based on practical considerations. This way, you'll choose a name that works well for you and for your baby. You may love a particular name, but if it doesn't hold up to these basic criteria, your baby probably won't love it. It can be unpleasant going through life with a name that for whatever reason doesn't work for you.

Make enough copies of the table on the following page for each name on your list. Have your partner do the same. Rate each name on twelve factors. Example: Consider popularity for the name Jacob—if you think there might be too many Jacobs in his school, check "too popular." Consider nicknames—if you love Jake, check "appealing." Another example: Consider sound for the name Rafael—if it's music to your ears, check "pleasing." Consider its fit with your last name—if you don't think it goes so well with Abramovitz, check "doesn't fit."

When you've completed the table, add up the score by giving three points for every check in the Positive column, two points for every check in the Neutral column, and one point for every check in the Negative column. Scoring each name might help make the subjective process of selecting a name more objective to you.

(Note: If you're pinched for time, mentally complete the table for each name, keeping track of a rough score. The important part is to narrow the list to your top five boys' and girls' names.)

Name:_____

Factors	Positive	Neutral	Negative
1. Spelling	❑ easy	❑ medium	❑ hard
2. Pronunciation	❑ easy	❑ medium	❑ hard
3. Sound	❑ pleasing	❑ okay	❑ unpleasing
4. Last Name	❑ fits well	❑ fits okay	❑ doesn't fit
5. Gender ID	❑ clear	❑ neutral	❑ unclear
6. Nicknames	❑ appealing	❑ okay	❑ unappealing
7. Popularity	❑ not too popular	❑ popular	❑ too popular
8. Uniqueness	❑ not too unique	❑ unique	❑ too unique
9. Impression	❑ positive	❑ okay	❑ negative
10. Namesakes	❑ positive	❑ okay	❑ negative
11. Initials	❑ pleasing	❑ okay	❑ unpleasing
12. Meaning	❑ positive	❑ okay	❑ negative

Final Score:_____

Step 3: Make the Final Choice

List your top five boys' and girls' names in the chart below, and have your partner do the same. It's now time to share the names. If you have names in common, compare your scores; perhaps average them. If you have different names on your lists, swap names and rate them using the same table as before. In the end, you'll have a handful of names that work well for you, your partner, and your baby. Now all you have to do is make the final decision. Good luck!

Mom's Top Five Names
1._____ Mom's Score: _____ Dad's Score: _____
2._____ Mom's Score: _____ Dad's Score: _____
3._____ Mom's Score: _____ Dad's Score: _____
4._____ Mom's Score: _____ Dad's Score: _____
5._____ Mom's Score: _____ Dad's Score: _____

Dad's Top Five Names
1._____ Dad's Score: _____ Mom's Score: _____
2._____ Dad's Score: _____ Mom's Score: _____
3._____ Dad's Score: _____ Mom's Score: _____
4._____ Dad's Score: _____ Mom's Score: _____
5._____ Dad's Score: _____ Mom's Score: _____

The Most Popular Names from 1900 to 2004

The popularity of names, like the length of hemlines and the width of ties, is subject to change every year. The changes become even more noticeable when you think about the changes in name "fashions" over long periods.

Think about the names of your grandparents' generation: Margaret, Shirley, George, Harold. Very few of those names are in the current lists of top 100 names. Most names from your parents' generation—Susan, Cheryl, Gary, Ronald—don't make the current lists of top 100 names either.

It seems that every decade a new group of names rises in popularity and an old group of names declines. So, when choosing a name for your baby, it's wise to consider whether a name's popularity is rising, declining, or holding steady.

To help you assess name popularity trends, we are presenting the latest top 100 names given to baby boys and girls in the United States. The rankings are derived from a survey of new births nationwide conducted by the Social Security Administration. (Alternate spellings of each name are treated as separate names. For example, Sarah and Sara are ranked separately.) You can see from the data how the names have risen or fallen since the previous year's survey. If you're expecting two bundles of joy, don't miss the lists of most popular names for twins in the U.S. In addition, you can track popularity trends over the years with the lists of top 25 names given to girls and boys in each decade since 1900.

Enjoy the following data, but remember that the popularity issue cuts two ways: 1) Psychologists say a child with a common or popular name seems to have better odds of success in life than a child with an uncommon name. 2) A child whose name is at the top of the popularity poll may not feel as unique and special as a child whose name is less common.

Top 100 Girls' Names in 2004

2004 Rank	Name	2003 Rank	Rank Change	2004 Rank	Name	2003 Rank	Rank Change	2004 Rank	Name	2003 Rank	Rank Change	2004 Rank	Name	2003 Rank	Rank Change
1	Emily	1	-	35	Katherine	35	-	68	Sara	65	−3				
2	Emma	2	-	36	Megan	30	−6	69	Sofia	97	+28				
3	Madison	3	-	37	Alexandra	38	+1	70	Jordan	48	−22				
4	Olivia	5	+1	38	Jennifer	31	−7	71	Alexa	66	−5				
5	Hannah	4	−1	39	Destiny	37	−2	72	Rebecca	63	−9				
6	Abigail	6	-	40	Allison	46	+6	73	Gabrielle	67	−6				
7	Isabella	11	+4	41	Savannah	41	-	74	Caroline	68	−6				
8	Ashley	8	-	42	Haley	34	−8	75	Vanessa	70	−5				
9	Samantha	10	+1	43	Mackenzie	45	+2	76	Gabriella	77	+1				
10	Elizabeth	9	−1	44	Brooke	43	−1	77	Avery	89	+12				
11	Alexis	7	−4	45	Maria	42	−3	78	Marissa	95	+17				
12	Sarah	12	-	46	Nicole	40	−6	79	Ariana	85	+6				
13	Grace	13	-	47	Makayla	51	+4	80	Audrey	78	−2				
14	Alyssa	14	-	48	Trinity	56	+8	81	Jada	79	−2				
15	Sophia	20	+5	49	Kylie	52	+3	82	Autumn	75	−7				
16	Lauren	15	−1	50	Kaylee	53	+3	83	Evelyn	88	+5				
17	Brianna	17	-	51	Paige	47	−4	84	Jocelyn	87	+3				
18	Kayla	16	−2	52	Lily	69	+17	85	Maya	84	−1				
19	Natalie	23	+4	53	Faith	50	−3	86	Arianna	86	-				
20	Anna	21	+1	54	Zoe	57	+3	87	Isabel	83	−4				
21	Jessica	18	−3	55	Stephanie	49	−6	88	Amber	74	−14				
22	Taylor	19	−3	56	Jenna	54	−2	89	Melanie	93	+4				
23	Chloe	24	+1	57	Andrea	61	+4	90	Diana	108	+18				
24	Hailey	26	+2	58	Riley	72	+14	91	Danielle	82	−9				
25	Ava	39	+14	59	Katelyn	58	−1	92	Sierra	73	−19				
26	Jasmine	27	+1	60	Angelina	71	+11	93	Leslie	91	−2				
27	Sydney	25	−2	61	Kimberly	64	+3	94	Aaliyah	90	−4				
28	Victoria	22	−6	62	Madeline	60	−2	95	Erin	80	−15				
29	Ella	44	+15	63	Mary	59	−4	96	Amelia	110	+14				
30	Mia	36	+6	64	Leah	81	+17	97	Molly	100	+3				
31	Morgan	29	−2	65	Lillian	76	+11	98	Claire	92	−6				
32	Julia	33	+1	66	Michelle	62	−4	99	Bailey	98	−1				
33	Kaitlyn	32	−1	67	Amanda	55	−12	100	Melissa	96	−4				
34	Rachel	28	−6												

Top 100 Boys' Names in 2004

2004 Rank	Name	2003 Rank	Rank Change	2004 Rank	Name	2003 Rank	Rank Change	2004 Rank	Name	2003 Rank	Rank Change
1	Jacob	1	-	35	Austin	33	−2	68	Nathaniel	63	−5
2	Michael	2	-	36	Robert	35	−1	69	Ian	65	−4
3	Joshua	3	-	37	Thomas	36	−1	70	Jesus	67	−3
4	Matthew	4	-	38	Connor	43	+5	71	Carlos	66	−5
5	Ethan	6	+1	39	Evan	44	+5	72	Adrian	68	−4
6	Andrew	5	−1	40	Aidan	39	−1	73	Diego	83	+10
7	Daniel	8	+1	41	Jack	45	+4	74	Julian	77	+3
8	William	11	+3	42	Luke	46	+4	75	Cole	69	−6
9	Joseph	7	−2	43	Jordan	38	−5	76	Ashton	101	+25
10	Christopher	9	−1	44	Angel	47	+3	77	Steven	70	−7
11	Anthony	10	−1	45	Isaiah	50	+5	78	Jeremiah	90	+12
12	Ryan	13	+1	46	Isaac	48	+2	79	Timothy	76	−3
13	Nicholas	12	−1	47	Jason	42	−5	80	Chase	87	+7
14	David	14	-	48	Jackson	52	+4	81	Devin	74	−7
15	Alexander	16	+1	49	Hunter	41	−8	82	Seth	80	−2
16	Tyler	15	−1	50	Cameron	40	−10	83	Jaden	82	−1
17	James	18	+1	51	Gavin	51	-	84	Colin	88	+4
18	John	17	−1	52	Mason	54	+2	85	Cody	78	−7
19	Dylan	19	-	53	Aaron	49	−4	86	Landon	97	+11
20	Nathan	27	+7	54	Juan	55	+1	87	Carter	102	+15
21	Jonathan	22	+1	55	Kyle	53	−2	88	Hayden	84	−4
22	Brandon	21	−1	56	Charles	57	+1	89	Xavier	85	−4
23	Samuel	23	-	57	Luis	60	+3	90	Wyatt	109	+19
24	Christian	25	+1	58	Adam	59	+1	91	Dominic	81	−10
25	Benjamin	24	−1	59	Brian	58	−1	92	Richard	86	−6
26	Zachary	20	−6	60	Aiden	73	+13	93	Antonio	92	−1
27	Logan	28	+1	61	Eric	56	−5	94	Jesse	95	+1
28	Jose	30	+2	62	Jayden	75	+13	95	Blake	79	−16
29	Noah	31	+2	63	Alex	62	−1	96	Sebastian	93	−3
30	Justin	26	−4	64	Bryan	64	-	97	Miguel	94	−3
31	Elijah	37	+6	65	Sean	61	−4	98	Jake	98	-
32	Gabriel	29	−3	66	Owen	72	+6	99	Alejandro	100	+1
33	Caleb	34	+1	67	Lucas	71	+4	100	Patrick	91	−9
34	Kevin	32	−2								

Big Gains from 2003 to 2004

Girls		Boys	
Sofia	+28	Ashton	+25
Diana	+18	Wyatt	+19
Lily	+17	Carter	+15
Leah	+17	Aiden	+13
Marissa	+17	Jayden	+13
Ella	+15	Jeremiah	+12
Ava	+14	Landon	+11
Riley	+14	Diego	+10
Amelia	+14	Nathan	+7
Avery	+12	Chase	+7

Big Losses from 2003 to 2004

Girls		Boys	
Jordan	−22	Blake	−16
Sierra	−19	Cameron	−10
Erin	−15	Dominic	−10
Amber	−14	Patrick	−9
Amanda	−12	Hunter	−8
Rebecca	−9	Steven	−7
Danielle	−9	Devin	−7
Haley	−8	Cody	−7
Jennifer	−7	Zachary	−6
Autumn	−7	Cole	−6

The Most Popular Names for Twins in 2004

Twin Girls	Twin Boys	Twin Girl & Boy
Faith, Hope	Jacob, Joshua	Taylor, Tyler
Madison, Morgan	Matthew, Michael	Emma, Ethan
Mackenzie, Madison	Daniel, David	Natalie, Nathan
Hailey, Hannah	Ethan, Evan	Madison, Matthew
Anna, Emma	Alexander, Andrew	Madison, Mason
Ella, Emma	Nathan, Nicholas	Jada, Jaden
Ashley, Emily	Christian, Christopher	Brianna, Brian
Elizabeth, Katherine	Joseph, Joshua	Alexis, Alexander
Jennifer, Jessica	Andrew, Matthew	Brianna, Brandon
Abigail, Emma	Alexander, Nicholas	Emily, Matthew
Gabriella, Isabella	Isaac, Isaiah	Emma, Jacob
Hannah, Sarah	Jacob, Joseph	Zoe, Zachary
Olivia, Sophia	Jonathan, Joshua	Emily, Ethan
Haley, Hannah	Elijah, Isaiah	
Abigail, Emily	Alexander, Zachary	
Emily, Sarah	James, John	
Faith, Grace	Benjamin, Samuel	
Megan, Morgan	John, William	
Elizabeth, Emily	Joshua, Justin	
Isabella, Sophia	Joshua, Matthew	
Emma, Grace	Alexander, Benjamin	
Grace, Hannah	Hayden, Hunter	
Elizabeth, Emma	Jacob, Matthew	
Isabella, Emma	Jason, Justin	
Isabella, Olivia	Jordan, Justin	

The Most Popular Names through the Decades

Most Popular Girls' Names 2000–2004

2000s Rank	Name	1990s Rank	Rank Change
1	Emily	3	+2
2	Madison	29	+27
3	Hannah	11	+8
4	Emma	56	+52
5	Ashley	2	–3
6	Alexis	18	+12
7	Samantha	4	–3
8	Sarah	5	–3
9	Abigail	42	+33
10	Olivia	38	+28
11	Elizabeth	8	–3
12	Alyssa	21	+9
13	Jessica	1	–12
14	Grace	89	+75
15	Lauren	13	–2
16	Taylor	9	–7
17	Kayla	12	–5
18	Brianna	26	+8
19	Isabella	170	+151
20	Anna	35	+15
21	Victoria	19	–2
22	Sydney	59	+37
23	Megan	10	–13
24	Rachel	15	–9
25	Jasmine	25	—

Most Popular Boys' Names 2000–2004

2000s Rank	Name	1990s Rank	Rank Change
1	Jacob	5	+4
2	Michael	1	–1
3	Joshua	4	+1
4	Matthew	3	–1
5	Andrew	7	+2
6	Christopher	2	–4
7	Joseph	10	+3
8	Nicholas	6	–2
9	Daniel	8	–1
10	William	18	+8
11	Ethan	55	+44
12	Anthony	19	+7
13	Ryan	14	+1
14	Tyler	9	–5
15	David	12	–3
16	John	15	–1
17	Alexander	23	+6
18	James	13	–5
19	Zachary	16	–3
20	Brandon	11	–9
21	Jonathan	21	—
22	Dylan	34	+12
23	Justin	17	–6
24	Christian	32	+8
25	Samuel	33	+8

Most Popular Girls' Names
1990–1999

1990s Rank	Name	1980s Rank	Rank Change
1	Jessica	1	—
2	Ashley	4	+2
3	Emily	25	+22
4	Samantha	26	+22
5	Sarah	5	—
6	Amanda	3	−3
7	Brittany	21	+14
8	Elizabeth	9	+1
9	Taylor	200	+191
10	Megan	14	+4
11	Hannah	91	+80
12	Kayla	54	+42
13	Lauren	19	+6
14	Stephanie	6	−8
15	Rachel	16	+1
16	Jennifer	2	−14
17	Nicole	8	−9
18	Alexis	109	+91
19	Victoria	56	+37
20	Amber	12	−8
21	Alyssa	89	+68
22	Courtney	37	+15
23	Danielle	24	+1
24	Rebecca	22	−2
25	Jasmine	90	+65

Most Popular Boys' Names
1990–1999

1990s Rank	Name	1980s Rank	Rank Change
1	Michael	1	—
2	Christopher	2	—
3	Matthew	3	—
4	Joshua	4	—
5	Jacob	35	+30
6	Nicholas	19	+13
7	Andrew	13	+6
8	Daniel	7	−1
9	Tyler	47	+38
10	Joseph	10	—
11	Brandon	17	+6
12	David	5	−7
13	James	6	−7
14	Ryan	14	—
15	John	9	−6
16	Zachary	43	+27
17	Justin	12	−5
18	William	15	−3
19	Anthony	20	+1
20	Robert	8	−12
21	Jonathan	18	−3
22	Austin	95	+73
23	Alexander	50	+27
24	Kyle	30	+6
25	Kevin	23	−2

Most Popular Girls' Names
1980–1989

1980s Rank	Name	1970s Rank	Rank Change
1	Jessica	11	+10
2	Jennifer	1	−1
3	Amanda	17	+14
4	Ashley	140	+136
5	Sarah	19	+14
6	Stephanie	9	+3
7	Melissa	3	−4
8	Nicole	10	+2
9	Elizabeth	12	+3
10	Heather	8	−2
11	Tiffany	42	+31
12	Amber	65	+53
13	Michelle	4	−9
14	Megan	89	+75
15	Amy	2	−13
16	Rachel	33	+17
17	Kimberly	5	−12
18	Christina	16	−2
19	Lauren	137	+118
20	Crystal	37	+17
21	Brittany	534	+513
22	Rebecca	13	−9
23	Laura	20	−3
24	Danielle	46	+22
25	Emily	66	+41

Most Popular Boys' Names
1980–1989

1980s Rank	Name	1970s Rank	Rank Change
1	Michael	1	—
2	Christopher	2	—
3	Matthew	10	+7
4	Joshua	24	+20
5	David	4	−1
6	James	5	−1
7	Daniel	12	+5
8	Robert	8	—
9	John	6	−3
10	Joseph	11	+1
11	Jason	3	−8
12	Justin	38	+26
13	Andrew	28	+15
14	Ryan	26	+12
15	William	9	−6
16	Brian	8	−8
17	Brandon	51	+34
18	Jonathan	32	+14
19	Nicholas	52	+33
20	Anthony	22	+2
21	Eric	14	−7
22	Adam	36	+14
23	Kevin	13	−10
24	Thomas	20	−4
25	Steven	19	−6

Most Popular Girls' Names 1970–1979				Most Popular Boys' Names 1970–1979			
1970s Rank	Name	1960s Rank	Rank Change	1970s Rank	Name	1960s Rank	Rank Change
1	Jennifer	20	+19	1	Michael	1	—
2	Amy	35	+33	2	Christopher	20	+18
3	Melissa	33	+30	3	Jason	87	+84
4	Michelle	9	+5	4	David	2	−2
5	Kimberly	5	—	5	James	4	−1
6	Lisa	1	−5	6	John	3	−3
7	Angela	22	+15	7	Robert	5	−2
8	Heather	127	+119	8	Brian	16	+8
9	Stephanie	45	+36	9	William	7	−2
10	Nicole	187	+177	10	Matthew	36	+26
11	Jessica	230	+219	11	Joseph	12	+1
12	Elizabeth	17	+5	12	Daniel	19	+7
13	Rebecca	41	+28	13	Kevin	14	+1
14	Kelly	39	+25	14	Eric	111	+97
15	Mary	2	−13	15	Richard	8	−7
16	Christina	72	+56	16	Jeffrey	10	−6
17	Amanda	199	+182	17	Scott	15	−2
18	Julie	18	—	18	Mark	6	−12
19	Sarah	90	+71	19	Steven	11	−8
20	Laura	16	−4	20	Thomas	9	−11
21	Shannon	121	+100	21	Timothy	13	−8
22	Christine	27	+5	22	Anthony	22	—
23	Tammy	13	−10	23	Charles	17	−6
24	Tracy	39	+15	24	Joshua	327	+303
25	Karen	4	−21	25	Ryan	224	+199

Most Popular Girls' Names
1960–1969

1960s Rank	Name	1950s Rank	Rank Change
1	Lisa	37	+36
2	Mary	1	−1
3	Susan	4	+1
4	Karen	8	+4
5	Kimberly	90	+85
6	Patricia	3	−3
7	Linda	2	−5
8	Donna	10	+2
9	Michelle	93	+84
10	Cynthia	11	+1
11	Sandra	12	+1
12	Deborah	5	−7
13	Tammy	140	+127
14	Pamela	13	−1
15	Lori	79	+64
16	Laura	38	+22
17	Elizabeth	21	+4
18	Julie	42	+24
19	Brenda	18	−1
20	Jennifer	98	+78
21	Barbara	6	−15
22	Angela	106	+84
23	Sharon	14	−9
24	Debra	7	−17
25	Teresa	30	+5

Most Popular Boys' Names
1960–1969

1960s Rank	Name	1950s Rank	Rank Change
1	Michael	2	+1
2	David	5	+3
3	John	4	+1
4	James	1	−3
5	Robert	3	−2
6	Mark	9	+3
7	William	6	−1
8	Richard	7	−1
9	Thomas	8	−1
10	Jeffrey	24	+14
11	Steven	11	—
12	Joseph	13	+1
13	Timothy	22	+9
14	Kevin	27	+13
15	Scott	36	+21
16	Brian	34	+18
17	Charles	10	−7
18	Paul	17	−1
19	Daniel	19	—
20	Christopher	47	+27
21	Kenneth	16	−5
22	Anthony	30	+8
23	Gregory	26	+3
24	Ronald	15	−9
25	Donald	14	−11

## Most Popular Girls' Names 1950–1959				## Most Popular Boys' Names 1950–1959			
1950s Rank	Name	1940s Rank	Rank Change	1950s Rank	Name	1940s Rank	Rank Change
1	Mary	1	—	1	James	1	—
2	Linda	2	—	2	Michael	9	+7
3	Patricia	4	+1	3	Robert	2	−1
4	Susan	10	+6	4	John	3	−1
5	Deborah	68	+63	5	David	6	+1
6	Barbara	3	−3	6	William	4	−2
7	Debra	302	+295	7	Richard	5	−2
8	Karen	16	+8	8	Thomas	8	—
9	Nancy	7	−2	9	Mark	54	+45
10	Donna	17	+7	10	Charles	7	−3
11	Cynthia	47	+36	11	Steven	29	+18
12	Sandra	6	−6	12	Gary	14	+2
13	Pamela	39	+26	13	Joseph	13	—
14	Sharon	8	−6	14	Donald	12	−2
15	Kathleen	18	+3	15	Ronald	10	−5
16	Carol	5	−11	16	Kenneth	16	—
17	Diane	22	+5	17	Paul	17	—
18	Brenda	26	+8	18	Larry	11	−7
19	Cheryl	43	+24	19	Daniel	22	+3
20	Janet	21	+1	20	Stephen	25	+5
21	Elizabeth	25	+4	21	Dennis	20	−1
22	Kathy	88	+66	22	Timothy	63	+41
23	Margaret	13	−10	23	Edward	18	−5
24	Janice	23	−1	24	Jeffrey	88	+64
25	Carolyn	12	−13	25	George	15	−10

Most Popular Girls' Names
1940–1949

1940s Rank	Name	1930s Rank	Rank Change
1	Mary	1	—
2	Linda	89	+87
3	Barbara	3	—
4	Patricia	5	+1
5	Carol	11	+6
6	Sandra	48	+42
7	Nancy	9	+2
8	Sharon	83	+75
9	Judith	40	+31
10	Susan	117	+107
11	Betty	2	−9
12	Carolyn	29	+17
13	Margaret	8	−5
14	Shirley	4	−10
15	Judy	112	+97
16	Karen	138	+122
17	Donna	23	+6
18	Kathleen	72	+54
19	Joyce	12	−7
20	Dorothy	6	−14
21	Janet	26	+5
22	Diane	115	+93
23	Janice	42	+19
24	Joan	7	−17
25	Elizabeth	17	−8

Most Popular Boys' Names
1940–1949

1940s Rank	Name	1930s Rank	Rank Change
1	James	2	+1
2	Robert	1	−1
3	John	3	—
4	William	4	—
5	Richard	5	—
6	David	7	+1
7	Charles	6	−1
8	Thomas	9	+1
9	Michael	35	+26
10	Ronald	13	+3
11	Larry	30	+19
12	Donald	7	−5
13	Joseph	10	−3
14	Gary	45	+31
15	George	8	−7
16	Kenneth	15	−1
17	Paul	14	−3
18	Edward	12	−6
19	Jerry	23	+4
20	Dennis	70	+50
21	Frank	16	−5
22	Daniel	42	+20
23	Raymond	17	−6
24	Roger	41	+17
25	Stephen	105	+80

## Most Popular Girls' Names 1930–1939				## Most Popular Boys' Names 1930–1939			
1930s Rank	Name	1920s Rank	Rank Change	1930s Rank	Name	1920s Rank	Rank Change
1	Mary	1	—	1	Robert	1	—
2	Betty	4	+2	2	James	3	+1
3	Barbara	18	+15	3	John	2	−1
4	Shirley	17	+13	4	William	4	—
5	Patricia	29	+24	5	Richard	8	+3
6	Dorothy	2	−4	6	Charles	5	−1
7	Joan	60	+53	7	Donald	10	+3
8	Margaret	5	−3	8	George	6	−2
9	Nancy	62	+53	9	Thomas	11	+2
10	Helen	3	−7	10	Joseph	7	−3
11	Carol	116	+105	11	David	22	+11
12	Joyce	61	+49	12	Edward	9	−3
13	Doris	8	−5	13	Ronald	92	+79
14	Ruth	6	−8	14	Paul	14	—
15	Virginia	7	−8	15	Kenneth	19	+4
16	Marilyn	82	+66	16	Frank	12	−4
17	Elizabeth	11	−6	17	Raymond	15	−2
18	Jean	16	−2	18	Jack	17	−1
19	Frances	10	−9	19	Harold	13	−6
20	Beverly	101	+81	20	Billy	48	+28
21	Lois	22	+1	21	Gerald	44	+23
22	Alice	15	−7	22	Walter	16	−6
23	Donna	104	+81	23	Jerry	102	+79
24	Martha	23	−1	24	Joe	34	+10
25	Dolores	48	+23	25	Eugene	24	−1

Most Popular Girls' Names 1920–1929

1920s Rank	Name	1910s Rank	Rank Change
1	Mary	1	—
2	Dorothy	3	+1
3	Helen	2	−1
4	Betty	37	+33
5	Margaret	4	−1
6	Ruth	5	−1
7	Virginia	10	+3
8	Doris	32	+24
9	Mildred	6	−3
10	Frances	9	−1
11	Elizabeth	8	−3
12	Evelyn	12	—
13	Anna	7	−6
14	Marie	15	+1
15	Alice	13	−2
16	Jean	45	+29
17	Shirley	129	+112
18	Barbara	76	+58
19	Irene	17	−2
20	Marjorie	39	+19
21	Florence	14	−7
22	Lois	49	+27
23	Martha	25	−2
24	Rose	16	−8
25	Lillian	15	−10

Most Popular Boys' Names 1920–1929

1920s Rank	Name	1910s Rank	Rank Change
1	Robert	4	+3
2	John	1	−1
3	James	3	—
4	William	2	−2
5	Charles	7	+2
6	George	6	—
7	Joseph	5	−2
8	Richard	15	+7
9	Edward	8	−1
10	Donald	20	+10
11	Thomas	10	−1
12	Frank	9	−3
13	Harold	12	−1
14	Paul	14	—
15	Raymond	16	+1
16	Walter	11	−5
17	Jack	23	+6
18	Henry	13	−5
19	Kenneth	30	+11
20	Arthur	18	−2
21	Albert	17	−4
22	David	29	+7
23	Harry	19	−4
24	Eugene	39	+15
25	Ralph	21	−4

Most Popular Girls' Names 1910–1919

1910s Rank	Name	1900s Rank	Rank Change
1	Mary	1	—
2	Helen	2	—
3	Dorothy	7	+4
4	Margaret	3	−1
5	Ruth	5	—
6	Mildred	10	+4
7	Anna	4	−3
8	Elizabeth	6	−2
9	Frances	16	+7
10	Virginia	53	+43
11	Marie	8	−3
12	Evelyn	39	+27
13	Alice	11	−2
14	Florence	9	−5
15	Lillian	13	−2
16	Rose	17	+1
17	Irene	25	+8
18	Louise	27	+9
19	Edna	15	−4
20	Catherine	28	+8
21	Gladys	14	−7
22	Ethel	12	−10
23	Josephine	46	+23
24	Ruby	42	+18
25	Martha	38	+13

Most Popular Boys' Names 1910–1919

1910s Rank	Name	1900s Rank	Rank Change
1	John	1	—
2	William	2	—
3	James	3	—
4	Robert	6	+2
5	Joseph	7	+2
6	George	4	−2
7	Charles	5	−2
8	Edward	9	+1
9	Frank	8	−1
10	Thomas	10	—
11	Walter	12	+1
12	Harold	19	+7
13	Henry	11	−2
14	Paul	20	+6
15	Richard	22	+7
16	Raymond	21	+5
17	Albert	16	−1
18	Arthur	15	−3
19	Harry	13	−6
20	Donald	52	+32
21	Ralph	27	+6
22	Louis	25	+3
23	Jack	29	+6
24	Clarence	17	−7
25	Carl	26	+1

Most Popular Girls' Names
1900–1909

1900s Rank	Name	1890s Rank	Rank Change
1	Mary	1	—
2	Helen	4	+2
3	Margaret	3	—
4	Anna	2	−2
5	Ruth	6	+1
6	Elizabeth	5	−1
7	Dorothy	54	+47
8	Marie	10	+2
9	Florence	7	−2
10	Mildred	42	+32
11	Alice	24	+13
12	Ethel	8	−4
13	Lillian	16	+3
14	Gladys	43	+29
15	Edna	17	+2
16	Frances	36	+20
17	Rose	22	+5
18	Annie	19	+1
19	Grace	18	−1
20	Bertha	12	−8
21	Emma	9	−12
22	Bessie	14	−8
23	Clara	11	−12
24	Hazel	23	−1
25	Irene	44	+19

Most Popular Boys' Names
1900–1909

1900s Rank	Name	1890s Rank	Rank Change
1	John	1	—
2	William	2	—
3	James	3	—
4	George	4	—
5	Charles	5	—
6	Robert	8	+2
7	Joseph	6	−1
8	Frank	7	−1
9	Edward	9	—
10	Thomas	12	+2
11	Henry	10	−1
12	Walter	13	+1
13	Harry	11	−2
14	Willie	18	+4
15	Arthur	14	−1
16	Albert	16	—
17	Clarence	17	—
18	Fred	15	−3
19	Harold	31	+12
20	Paul	22	+2
21	Raymond	27	+6
22	Richard	26	+4
23	Roy	19	−4
24	Joe	28	+4
25	Louis	21	−4

Names around the World

Want to track popularity trends across the globe? Want to give your baby a name that reflects your heritage, language, or favorite travel destination? The following lists feature names with international flair. You'll learn the latest popular names given to baby girls and boys in several countries. Just as the U.S. popularity lists come from data compiled by the Social Security Administration, these international lists come from records kept by similar organizations across the globe. Beginning on page 26, you'll also discover a sampling of interesting names from particular cultural origins. Use those lists to get you thinking, but don't forget that there are thousands more names in the Girls' Names and Boys' Names sections with the origins you're looking for.

The Most Popular Names around the World

Most Popular Names in Austria in 2003

Girls	Boys
Sarah	Lukas
Anna	Florian
Julia	Tobias
Laura	David
Lena	Alexander
Hannah	Fabian
Lisa	Michael
Katharina	Julian
Leonie	Daniel
Vanessa	Simon

Most Popular Names in Belgium in 2003

Girls	Boys
Emma	Thomas
Laura	Lucas
Marie	Noah
Julie	Nathan
Sarah	Maxime
Manon	Hugo
Léa	Louis
Luna	Arthur
Lisa	Robbe
Charlotte	Nicolas
Camille	Simon
Louise	Alexandre
Amber	Romain
Clara	Tom
Lotte	Mohamed
Emilie	Théo
Elise	Robin
Chloé	Antoine
Océane	Milan
Eva	Wout
Jana	Senne
Pauline	Luca
Britt	Victor
Lara	Jonas
Femke	Jelle

Most Popular Names in British Columbia, Canada in 2004

Girls	Boys
Emma	Ethan
Emily	Jacob
Hannah	Matthew
Olivia	Ryan
Madison	Joshua
Sarah	Nathan
Jessica	Benjamin
Ella	Alexander
Grace	Nicholas
Sophia	Owen
Hailey	Daniel
Isabella	Liam
Abigail	Dylan
Megan	Logan
Samantha	Tyler
Lauren	Andrew
Paige	Evan
Ava	Noah
Rachel	William
Ashley	Samuel
Chloe	James
Anna	Connor
Taylor	Lucas
Julia	Adam
Mackenzie	Michael

Most Popular Names in Denmark in 2003

Girls	Boys
Emma	Mikkel
Julie	Frederik
Mathilde	Mathias
Sofia	Mads
Laura	Rasmus
Caroline	Emil
Cecilie	Oliver
Ida	Christian
Sarah	Magnus
Freja	Lucas

Most Popular Names in England/Wales in 2004

Girls	Boys
Emily	Jack
Ellie	Joshua
Jessica	Thomas
Sophie	James
Chloe	Daniel
Lucy	Samuel
Olivia	Oliver
Charlotte	William
Katie	Benjamin
Megan	Joseph
Grace	Harry
Hannah	Matthew
Amy	Lewis
Ella	Ethan
Mia	Luke
Lily	Charlie
Abigail	George
Emma	Callum
Amelia	Alexander
Molly	Mohammed
Lauren	Ryan
Millie	Dylan
Holly	Jacob
Leah	Adam
Caitlin	Ben

Most Popular Names in France in 2003

Girls	Boys
Lea	Lucas
Manon	Theo
Emma	Thomas
Chloe	Hugo
Camille	Enzo
Clara	Maxime
Oceane	Clement
Ines	Leo
Sarah	Antoine
Marie	Alexandre
Lucie	Mathis
Anais	Louis
Jade	Quentin
Lisa	Alexis
Mathilde	Romain
Julie	Tom
Laura	Nicolas
Pauline	Nathan
Eva	Baptiste
Maeva	Paul
Marine	Arthur
Lola	Matteo
Justine	Noah
Juliette	Matheo
Celia	Valentin

Most Popular Names in Germany in 2004

Girls	Boys
Marie	Maximilian
Sophie	Alexander
Maria	Paul
Anna/Anne	Leon
Leonie	Lukas/Lucas
Lea(h)	Luca
Laura	Felix
Lena	Jonas
Katharina	Tim
Johanna	David

Most Popular Names in Ireland in 2003

Girls	Boys
Emma	Sean
Sarah	Jack
Aoife	Adam
Ciara	Conor
Katie	James
Sophie	Daniel
Rachel	Michael
Chloe	Cian
Amy	David
Leah	Dylan
Niamh	Luke
Caoimhe	Ryan
Hannah	Aaron
Ella	Thomas
Lauren	Darragh
Megan	Eoin
Kate	Joshua
Rebecca	Ben

Ireland (cont.)

Girls	Boys
Jessica	Patrick
Emily	Oisin
Laura	Shane
Anna	John
Grace	Jamie
Ava	Liam
Ellen	Matthew

Most Popular Names in Japan in 2002

Girls	Boys
Misaki	Shun
Aoi	Takumi
Nanami	Shou
Miu	Ren
Riko	Shouta
Miyu	Souta
Moe	Kaito
Mitsuki	Kenta
Yuuka	Daiki
Rin	Yuu

Most Popular Names in New South Wales, Australia in 2004

Girls	Boys
Emily	Jack
Chloe	Joshua
Olivia	Lachlan
Sophie	Thomas
Jessica	William
Charlotte	James
Ella	Ethan
Isabella	Samuel
Sarah	Daniel
Emma	Ryan
Grace	Benjamin
Mia	Nicholas
Hannah	Matthew
Georgia	Luke
Jasmine	Liam
Lily	Jacob
Amelia	Alexander
Zoe	Riley
Hayley	Dylan
Ruby	Jayden
Madison	Jake
Jade	Harrison
Holly	Oliver
Maddison	Cooper
Alyssa	Max

Most Popular Names in Norway in 2004

Girls	Boys
Emma	Mathias
Julie	Markus
Thea	Martin
Ida	Kristian
Nora	Andreas
Emilie	Jonas
Maria	Tobias
Sara	Daniel
Hanna	Sander
Ingrid	Alexander
Malin	Kristoffer
Tuva	Magnus
Sofie	Adrian
Amalie	Henrik
Anna	Emil
Frida	Elias
Vilde	Fredrik
Andrea	Sebastian
Mia	Sondre
Marte	Thomas
Marie	Oliver
Karoline	Nikolai
Hedda	Jakob
Martine	Mats
Silje	Marius

Most Popular Names in Quebec, Canada in 2004

Girls	Boys
Lea	Samuel
Rosalie	William
Noemie	Alexis
Laurence	Gabriel
Jade	Jeremy
Megane	Xavier
Sarah	Felix
Audrey	Thomas
Camille	Antoine
Coralie	Olivier
Megan	Mathis
Ariane	Anthony
Florence	Nathan
Gabrielle	Zachary
Laurie	Nicolas
Oceane	Alexandre
Emilie	Justin
Juliette	Jacob
Chloe	Raphael
Amelie	Vincent

Emy	Benjamin		Natalia	Manuel
Maude	Emile		Marina	Miguel
Justine	Mathieu		Irene	Antonio
Alicia	Maxime		Carmen	Ruben
Catherine	Simon		Nuria	Juan
			Julia	Victor
			Angela	Marcos
			Sofia	Alberto
			Rocio	Marc
			Sandra	Jesus

Most Popular Names in Scotland in 2004

Girls	Boys
Emma	Lewis
Sophie	Jack
Ellie	James
Amy	Cameron
Chloe	Ryan
Katie	Liam
Erin	Jamie
Emily	Ben
Lucy	Kyle
Hannah	Callum
Rebecca	Matthew
Rachel	Daniel
Abbie	Connor
Lauren	Adam
Megan	Dylan
Aimee	Andrew
Olivia	Aidan
Caitlin	Ross
Leah	Scott
Niamh	Nathan
Sarah	Thomas
Jessica	Kieran
Holly	Alexander
Anna	Aaron
Eilidh	Joshua

Most Popular Names in Sweden in 2004

Girls	Boys
Emma	William
Maja	Filip
Ida	Oscar
Elin	Lucas
Julia	Erik
Linnéa	Emil
Hanna	Isak
Alva	Alexander
Wilma	Viktor
Klara	Anton
Ebba	Elias
Ella	Simon
Alice	Hugo
Matilda	Gustav
Moa	Albin
Amanda	Axel
Elsa	Jonathan
Sara	Linus
Emilia	Oliver
Tilda	Ludvig
Ellen	Rasmus
Saga	Max
Felicia	Adam
Tindra	Jacob
Emelie	David

Most Popular Names in Spain in 2003

Girls	Boys
Lucia	Alejandro
Maria	Daniel
Paula	Pablo
Laura	David
Marta	Javier
Andrea	Adrian
Alba	Alvaro
Sara	Sergio
Claudia	Carlos
Ana	Hugo
Nerea	Mario
Carla	Jorge
Elena	Diego
Cristina	Ivan
Ainhoa	Raul

Names from around the World

African

Girls	Boys
Afi	Afram
Adia	Axi
Adanna	Bello
Ama	Ekon
Ashanti	Enzi
Batini	Idi
Eshe	Jabari
Fayola	Kayin
Femi	Kitwana
Goma	Kosey
Halla	Kwasi
Imena	Liu
Kameke	Mansa
Kamilah	Moswen
Kia	Mzuzi
Mosi	Nwa
Pita	Nwake
Poni	Ogun
Reta	Ohin
Sharik	Okapi
Siko	Ottah
Tawia	Senwe
Thema	Ulan
Winna	Uzoma
Zina	Zareb

American

Girls	Boys
Abelina	Adarius
Akayla	Buster
Amberlyn	Caden
Betsy	Daevon
Blinda	Dantrell
Coralee	Demarius
Darilynn	Dionte
Doneshia	Jadrien
Emmylou	Jailen
Jaycee	Jamar
Jessalyn	Jareth
Johnessa	Jayce
Karolane	Lashawn
Krystalynn	Lavon
Lakiesha	Montel
Lashana	Mychal
Liza	Reno
Roshawna	Reshawn
Shaniqua	Ryker

Shantel	Tevin
Takayla	Tiger
Tenesha	Treshawn
Teralyn	Tyrees
Trixia	Woody
Tyesha	Ziggy

Arabic

Girls	Boys
Abia	Abdul
Aleah	Ahmad
Cantara	Asad
Emani	Bilal
Fatima	Fadi
Ghada	Fahaad
Habiba	Ferran
Halimah	Ghazi
Imani	Gilad
Jalila	Habib
Kalila	Hadi
Laela	Hakim
Lilith	Hassan
Maja	Imad
Marya	Ismael
Nalia	Jabir
Omaira	Jamaal
Qadira	Mohamed
Rabi	Nadim
Rasha	Omar
Rayya	Rafiq
Samira	Rahul
Shahar	Rashad
Tabina	Samír
Vega	Sayyid

Chinese

Girls	Boys
An	Chen
Bo	Cheung
Chultua	Chi
Hua	Chung
Jun	De
Lee	Dewei
Lian	Fai
Lien	Gan
Lin	Guotin
Ling	Ho
Mani	Hu
Marrim	Jin

Meiying	Keung
Nuwa	Kong
Ping	Lei
Shu	Li
Syá	Liang
Sying	On
Tao	Park
Tu	Po Sin
Ushi	Quon
Xiang	Shing
Xiu Mei	Tung
Yáng	Wing
Yen	Yu

English

Girls	Boys
Addison	Alfie
Ashley	Ashton
Beverly	Baxter
Britany	Blake
Cady	Chip
Chelsea	Cody
Ellen	Dawson
Evelyn	Edward
Hailey	Franklin
Holly	Gordon
Hope	Harry
Janet	Jamison
Jill	Jeffrey
Julie	Jeremy
Leigh	Lane
Maddie	Maxwell
Millicent	Ned
Paige	Parker
Piper	Rodney
Robin	Scott
Sally	Slade
Scarlet	Ted
Shelby	Tucker
Sigourney	Wallace
Twyla	William

French

Girls	Boys
Angelique	Adrien
Annette	Alexandre
Aubrey	Andre
Belle	Antoine
Camille	Christophe
Charlotte	Donatien
Christelle	Edouard
Cosette	François
Desiree	Gage
Estelle	Guillaume
Gabrielle	Henri
Genevieve	Jacques
Juliette	Jean
Jolie	Leroy
Lourdes	Luc
Margaux	Marc
Maribel	Marquis
Michelle	Philippe
Monique	Pierre
Nicole	Quincy
Paris	Remy
Raquel	Russel
Salina	Sebastien
Sydney	Stéphane
Yvonne	Sylvian

German

Girls	Boys
Adelaide	Adler
Amelia	Adolf
Christa	Arnold
Edda	Bernard
Elke	Claus
Elsbeth	Conrad
Emma	Derek
Frederica	Dieter
Giselle	Dustin
Gretchen	Frederick
Heidi	Fritz
Hetta	Gerald
Hilda	Harvey
Ida	Johan
Johana	Karl
Katrina	Lance
Klarise	Louis
Lisele	Milo
Lorelei	Philipp
Margret	Roger
Milia	Roland
Monika	Sigmund
Reynalda	Terrell
Velma	Ulrich
Wanda	Walter

Greek

Girls	Boys
Alexandra	Achilles
Amaryllis	Adonis
Anastasia	Alexis
Athena	Christos
Callista	Cristobal
Daphne	Damian
Delia	Darius
Delphine	Demetris
Eleanora	Elias
Eudora	Feoras
Evangelina	Gaylen
Gaea	Georgios
Helena	Julius
Hermione	Krisopher
Ianthe	Leander
Kalliope	Nicholas
Kassandra	Panos
Maia	Paris
Medea	Petros
Oceana	Rhodes
Odelia	Sebastian
Ophelia	Stefanos
Phoebe	Thanos
Rhea	Urian
Selena	Xander

Hebrew

Girls	Boys
Alia	Aaron
Anais	Abel
Becca	Ahab
Beth	Azriel
Cayla	Benjamin
Deborah	Boaz
Dinah	Caleb
Eliane	Coby
Eliza	Daniel
Hannah	Elijah
Ilisha	Emmanuel
Jana	Ira
Judith	Isaak
Kaela	Jacob
Leeza	Jeremiah
Lena	Michael
Mariam	Nathaniel
Mikala	Noah
Naomi	Oren
Rachael	Raphael
Rebecca	Reuben
Ruth	Seth
Sarah	Tobin
Tirza	Zachariah
Yael	Zachary

Irish

Girls	Boys
Aileen	Aidan
Alanna	Brenden
Blaine	Clancy
Breanna	Desmond
Brigit	Donovan
Carlin	Eagan
Colleen	Flynn
Dacia	Garret
Dierdre	Grady
Erin	Keegan
Fallon	Keenan
Ilene	Kevin
Kaitlin	Liam
Keara	Logan
Kelly	Mahon
Kyleigh	Makenzie
Maura	Nevin
Maureen	Nolan
Moira	Owen
Quincy	Phinean
Raleigh	Quinn
Reagan	Reilly
Sinead	Ryan
Sloane	Seamus
Taryn	Sedric

Latin

Girls	Boys
Allegra	Amadeus
Aurora	Antony
Beatrice	Austin
Bella	Benedict
Cecily	Bennett
Celeste	Camilo
Deana	Cecil
Felicia	Delfino
Imogene	Dominic
Josalyn	Favian
Karmen	Felix
Laurel	Griffin
Luna	Horacio
Mabel	Hugo
Madonna	Ignatius
Maren	Jerome

Maxine	Jude
Nova	Loren
Olivia	Marius
Paxton	Octavio
Persis	Oliver
Pomona	Quentin
Regina	Roman
Rose	Silas
Sabina	Valentin

Japanese

Girls	Boys
Aiko	Akemi
Aneko	Akira
Dai	Botan
Hachi	Goro
Hoshi	Hiroshi
Ishi	Isas
Jin	Joben
Keiko	Joji
Kioko	Jum
Kumiko	Kaemon
Leiko	Kentaro
Maeko	Masao
Mai	Michio
Mariko	Minoru
Masago	Naoko
Nari	Raiden
Oki	Rei
Raku	Saburo
Ran	Sen
Ruri	Takeo
Seki	Toru
Tazu	Udo
Yasu	Yasuo
Yei	Yóshi
Yoko	Yuki

Native American

Girls	Boys
Aiyana	Ahanu
Cherokee	Anoki
Dakota	Bly
Dena	Delsin
Halona	Demothi
Heta	Elan
Imala	Elsu
Izusa	Etu
Kachina	Hakan
Kanda	Huslu
Kiona	Inteus

Leotie	Istu
Magena	Iye
Netis	Jolon
Nuna	Knoton
Olathe	Lenno
Oneida	Mingan
Sakuna	Motega
Sora	Muraco
Taima	Neka
Tala	Nodin
Utina	Patwin
Wyanet	Sahale
Wyoming	Songan
Yenene	Wingi

Russian

Girls	Boys
Alena	Alexi
Annika	Christoff
Breasha	Dimitri
Duscha	Egor
Galina	Feliks
Irina	Fyodor
Karina	Gena
Katia	Gyorgy
Lelya	Igor
Liolya	Ilya
Marisha	Iosif
Masha	Ivan
Natasha	Kolya
Natalia	Leonid
Nikita	Maxim
Olena	Michail
Orlenda	Panas
Raisa	Pasha
Sasha	Pavel
Shura	Pyotr
Svetlana	Sacha
Tanya	Sergei
Valera	Valerii
Yekaterina	Viktor
Yelena	Vladimir

Scandinavian

Girls	Boys
Anneka	Anders
Birgitte	Burr
Britta	Frans
Carina	Gustaf
Elga	Hadrian
Freja	Halen

Scandinavian (cont.)

Girls	Boys
Freya	Hilmar
Gala	Kjell
Gerda	Krister
Gunda	Kristofer
Haldana	Lauris
Ingrid	Lennart
Kalle	Lunt
Karena	Mats
Karin	Mikael
Kolina	Nansen
Lena	Niklas
Lusa	Nils
Maija	Per
Malena	Reinhold
Rika	Rikard
Runa	Rolle
Ulla	Steffan
Unn	Torkel
Valma	Valter

Scottish

Girls	Boys
Aili	Adair
Ailsa	Alastair
Ainsley	Angus
Berkley	Boyd
Blair	Bret
Camden	Caelan
Connor	Cameron
Christal	Dougal
Davonna	Duncan
Elspeth	Geordan
Greer	Gregor
Isela	Henderson
Jeana	Ian
Jinny	Kennan
Keita	Kenzie
Kelsea	Lennox
Leslie	Leslie
Maisie	Macaulay
Marjie	Malcolm
Mckenzie	Morgan
Mhairie	Perth
Paisley	Ronald
Rhona	Seumas
Roslyn	Stratton
Tavie	Tavish

Spanish

Girls	Boys
Alejandra	Armando
Benita	Carlos
Clarita	Eduardo
Esmeralda	Enrique
Esperanza	Estéban
Felicia	Felipe
Gracia	Fernando
Isabel	Garcia
Jacinthe	Gerardo
Juana	Heraldo
Lola	Jose
Lucia	Jorge
Madrona	Juan
Marisol	Luis
Marquita	Marcos
Nelia	Mateo
Oleda	Pablo
Pilar	Pedro
Reina	Rafael
Rosalinda	Ramón
Rosita	Renaldo
Salvadora	Salvador
Soledad	Santiago
Toya	Tobal
Ynez	Vincinte

Vietnamese

Girls	Boys
Am	Anh
Bian	Antoan
Cai	Binh
Cam	Cadao
Hoa	Cham
Hoai	Duc
Hong	Dinh
Huong	Gia
Kim	Hai
Kima	Hieu
Lan	Hoang
Le	Huy
Mai	Lap
Nu	Minh
Nue	Nam
Ping	Ngai
Tam	Nguyen
Tao	Nien

Thanh	Phuok
Thao	Pin
Thi	Tai
Thuy	Thanh
Tuyen	Thian
Tuyet	Tuan
Xuan	Tuyen

Welsh

Girls	Boys
Bevanne	Bevan
Bronwyn	Bowen
Carys	Broderick
Deryn	Bryce
Enid	Caddock
Glynnis	Cairn
Guinevere	Davis
Gwyneth	Dylan
Idelle	Eoin
Isolde	Gareth
Linette	Gavin
Mab	Griffith
Meghan	Howell
Meredith	Jestin
Olwen	Kynan
Owena	Lewis
Rhiannon	Llewellyn
Rhonda	Lloyd
Ronelle	Maddock
Rowena	Price
Sulwen	Rhett
Teagan	Rhys
Vanora	Tristan
Wenda	Vaughn
Wynne	Wren

The Impressions Names Make

Consciously or unconsciously, we all have private pictures associated with certain names. Jackie could be sophisticated and beautiful, like Jackie Kennedy, or fat and funny, like Jackie Gleason. These pictures come from personal experience as well as from images we absorb from the mass media, and thus they may conflict in interesting ways. The name Charlton strikes many people as a sissified, passive, whiny brat—until they think of Charlton Heston. Marilyn may personify voluptuous femininity—until you think of Marilyn, your neighbor with the ratty bathrobe, curlers, and a cigarette dangling out of her mouth.

Over the years, researchers have been fascinated by this question of the "real" meanings of names and their effects. When asked to stereotype names by age, trustworthiness, attractiveness, sociability, kindness, aggressiveness, popularity, masculinity/femininity, degree of activity or passivity, etc., people actually do tend to agree on each name's characteristics.

So if people think of Mallory as cute and likeable, does that influence a girl named Mallory to become cute and likeable? Experts agree that names don't guarantee instant success or condemn people to certain failure, but they do affect self-images, influence relationships with others, and help (or hinder) success in work and school.

Robert Rosenthal's classic experiment identified what he named the Pygmalion effect: randomly selected children who'd been labeled "intellectual bloomers" actually did bloom. Here's how the Pygmalion effect works with names: Researcher S. Gray Garwood conducted a study on sixth graders in New Orleans. He found that students given names popular with teachers scored higher in skills tests, were better adjusted and more consistent in their self-perceptions, were more realistic in their evaluations of themselves, and more frequently expected that they would attain their goals—even though their goals were more ambitious than ones set by their peers. A research study in San Diego suggested that average essays by Davids, Michaels, Karens, and Lisas got better grades than average essays written by Elmers, Huberts, Adelles, and Berthas. The reason? Teachers expected kids with popular names to do better, and thus they assigned those kids higher grades in a self-fulfilling prophecy.

The Sinrod Marketing Group's International Opinion panel surveyed over 100,000 parents to discover their opinions about names. Results of this poll are presented in *The Baby Name Survey Book* by Bruce Lansky and Barry Sinrod. Their book contains the names people most often associate with hundreds of personal attributes such as intelligent, athletic, attractive, and nice (as well as dumb, klutzy, ugly, and nasty). It also contains personality profiles of over 1,700 common and unusual boys' and girls' names and includes real or fictional famous namesakes who may have influenced people's perception of each name.

What the authors found was that most names have very clear images; some even have multiple images. The following are lists of boys' and girls' names that were found to have particular image associations.

Athletic

Girls	Boys
Bailey	Alex
Billie	Ali
Bobbie	Alonso
Casey	Bart
Chris	Brian
Colleen	Buck
Dena	Chuck
Gabriella	Connor
Jackie	Cooper
Jessie	Daniel
Jill	Derek
Jody	Emmitt
Josie	Hakeem
Katie	Houston
Kelsey	Jake
Lindsay	Jock
Lola	Kareem
Martina	Kevin
Mia	Kirby
Morgan	Lynn
Natalia	Marcus
Nora	Riley
Steffi	Rod
Sue	Terry
Tammy	Trey

Beautiful/Handsome

Girls	Boys
Adrienne	Adam
Ariel	Ahmad
Aurora	Alejandro
Bella	Alonzo
Bonita	Austin
Carmen	Beau
Cassandra	Blake
Catherine	Bo
Danielle	Bryant
Ebony	Chaz
Farrah	Christopher
Genevieve	Clint
Jasmine	Damian
Jewel	David
Kendra	Demetrius
Kiera	Denzel
Lydia	Douglas
Marisa	Grant
Maya	Humphrey
Sarah	Joe
Scarlett	Jude
Simone	Kiefer
Tanya	Mitchell
Tessa	Tevin
Whitney	Vance

Blonde

Girls	Boys
Bambie	Aubrey
Barbie	Austin
Bianca	Bjorn
Blanche	Brett
Brigitte	Bud
Bunny	Chance
Candy	Chick
Daisy	Colin
Dolly	Corbin
Heidi	Dalton
Inga	Dane
Jillian	Dennis
Krystal	Dwayne
Lara	Eric
Lorna	Josh
Madonna	Keith
Marcia	Kerry
Marnie	Kipp
Olivia	Kyle
Randi	Lars
Sally	Leif
Shannon	Louis
Sheila	Martin
Tracy	Olaf
Vanna	Sven

Cute		Friendly		Funny	
Girls	**Boys**	**Girls**	**Boys**	**Girls**	**Boys**
Annie	Andrew	Bernadette	Allen	Dionne	Abbott
Becca	Antoine	Bobbie	Aubrey	Ellen	Ace
Bobbie	Antonio	Bonnie	Barrett	Erma	Allen
Cheryl	Barry	Carol	Bennie	Fanny	Archie
Christy	Benjamin	Christy	Bing	Gilda	Artie
Deanna	Chick	Dorothy	Cal	Gillian	Bennie
Debbie	Cory	Elaine	Casper	Jenny	Bobby
Dee Dee	Danny	Gwen	Cole	Julie	Carson
Emily	Eric	Joy	Dan	Lucille	Chase
Jennifer	Francisco	Kathy	Denny	Lucy	Diego
Jody	Franky	Kenya	Donovan	Maggie	Dudley
Kari	Jon	Kim	Ed	Marge	Eddie
Lacie	Kipp	Lila	Fred	Marsha	Edsel
Mallory	Linus	Marcie	Gary	Maud	Eduardo
Mandy	Louis	Millie	Hakeem	Melinda	Fletcher
Megan	Matthew	Nancy	Jeff	Mickey	Fraser
Peggy	Mike	Nikki	Jerry	Patty	Grady
Porsha	Nicholas	Opal	Jim	Paula	Jerome
Randi	Rene	Patricia	Khalil	Rosie	Keenan
Serena	Robbie	Rhoda	Rob	Roxanne	Rochester
Shannon	Rory	Rose	Russ	Sally	Rollie
Shirley	Sonny	Ruby	Sandy	Stevie	Roscoe
Stacy	Stevie	Sandy	Tony	Sunny	Sid
Tammy	Timothy	Vivian	Vinny	Sydney	Tim
Trudy	Wade	Wendy	Wally	Vivian	Vinny

Hippie	Intelligent		Nerdy	Old-Fashioned	
Girls and Boys	**Girls**	**Boys**	**Boys**	**Girls**	**Boys**
Angel	Abigail	Adlai	Arnie	Abigail	Abe
Autumn	Agatha	Alexander	Barrett	Adelaide	Amos
Baby	Alexis	Barton	Bernie	Adelle	Arthur
Breezy	Barbara	Brock	Clarence	Bea	Bertrand
Crystal	Dana	Clifford	Clifford	Charlotte	Clarence
Dawn	Daria	Colin	Creighton	Clementine	Cy
Happy	Diana	Dalton	Dexter	Cora	Cyril
Harmony	Eleanor	David	Egbert	Dinah	Dennis
Honey	Grace	Donovan	Khalil	Edith	Erasmus
Indigo	Helen	Edward	Marvin	Elsie	Erskine
Kharma	Jade	Esteban	Mortimer	Esther	Ezekiel
Love	Jillian	Fraser	Myron	Eugenia	Giuseppe
Lucky	Kate	Jefferson	Newt	Hattie	Grover
Meadow	Kaylyn	Jerome	Norman	Ida	Herbert
Misty	Laura	John	Sanford	Mamie	Herschel
Moon	Leah	Kelsey	Seymour	Martha	Jerome
Passion	Lillian	Kenneth	Sheldon	Maureen	Kermit
Rainbow	Mackenzie	Merlin	Sinclair	Meryl	Lloyd
River	Marcella	Ned	Tracy	Mildred	Sanford
Serenity	Meredith	Nelson	Truman	Meryl	Silas
Skye	Meryl	Roderick	Ulysses	Nellie	Spencer
Sparkle	Michaela	Samuel	Vern	Prudence	Stanley
Sprout	Shauna	Sebastian	Vladimir	Rosalie	Sven
Star	Shelley	Tim	Waldo	Thelma	Vic
Sunshine	Vanessa	Virgil	Xavier	Verna	Wilma

Wilma Wilfred

Quiet		Rich/Wealthy		Sexy
Girls	**Boys**	**Girls**	**Boys**	**Girls**
Bernice	Aaron	Alexis	Bartholomew	Alana
Beth	Adrian	Amanda	Bradley	Angie
Cathleen	Angel	Ariel	Brock	Bambi
Chloe	Benedict	Blair	Bryce	Brooke
Diana	Bryce	Chanel	Burke	Caresse
Donna	Carlo	Chantal	Cameron	Cari
Faith	Curtis	Chastity	Carlos	Carmen
Fawn	Cy	Chelsea	Chet	Dani
Fay	Douglas	Christina	Claybourne	Desiree
Grace	Gerald	Clara	Clinton	Donna
Jocelyn	Gideon	Crystal	Colby	Honey
Leona	Jeremiah	Darlene	Colin	Jillian
Lisa	Jermaine	Deandra	Corbin	Kirstie
Lori	Kiefer	Jewel	Dane	Kitty
Lydia	Kyle	Larissa	Dante	Kyra
Moira	Riley	Madison	Dillon	Latoya
Natalia	Robert	Marina	Frederick	Leah
Nina	Robin	Meredith	Geoffrey	Lola
Rena	Samson	Moira	Hamilton	Marilyn
Sheryl	Spencer	Porsha	Harper	Marlo
Tessa	Toby	Rachel	Montgomery	Raquel
Theresa	Tommy	Taryn	Roosevelt	Sabrina
Ursula	Tucker	Tiffany	Sterling	Sandra
Violet	Vaughn	Trisha	Winslow	Simone
Yoko	Virgil	Zsa Zsa	Winthrop	Zsa Zsa

Southern

Girls	Boys
Ada	Ashley
Alma	Beau
Annabel	Bobby
Belle	Cletus
Carolina	Clint
Charlotte	Dale
Clementine	Earl
Dixie	Jackson
Dolly	Jeb
Dottie	Jed
Ellie	Jefferson
Georgeanne	Jesse
Georgia	Jethro
Jolene	Jimmy
LeeAnn	Johnny
Luella	Lee
Mirabel	Luke
Ophelia	Luther
Patsy	Moses
Polly	Otis
Priscilla	Peyton
Rosalind	Rhett
Scarlet	Robert
Tara	Roscoe
Winona	Wade

Strong/Tough

Boys
Amos
Ben
Brandon
Brock
Bronson
Bruce
Bruno
Cain
Christopher
Clint
Cody
Coleman
Colin
Delbert
Demetrius
Duke
Jed
Judd
Kurt
Nick
Sampson
Stefan
Thor
Vince
Zeb

Sweet

Girls
Abby
Alyssa
Angela
Betsy
Candy
Cheryl
Cindy
Dana
Desiree
Elise
Ellie
Esther
Heather
Heidi
Kara
Kristi
Laura
Linda
Marjorie
Melinda
Melissa
Olivia
Rose
Shauna
Sue

Trendy		Weird		Wimpy
Girls	**Boys**	**Girls**	**Boys**	**Boys**
Alexia	Adrian	Abra	Abner	Antoine
Alia	Alec	Aida	Barton	Archibald
Britney	Angelo	Annelise	Boris	Barton
Chanel	Bradley	Athalie	Cosmo	Bernard
Char	Carson	Belicia	Earl	Bradford
Delia	Connor	Calla	Edward	Burke
Destiny	Davis	Devonna	Ferris	Cecil
Gwyneth	Dominic	Dianthe	Gaylord	Cyril
Hannah	Ellery	Elvira	Ira	Dalton
India	Garrett	Garland	Jules	Darren
Isabella	Harley	Giselle	Maynard	Duane
Jen	Harper	Happy	Mervin	Edwin
Julianna	Jefferson	Hestia	Neville	Gaylord
Keely	Kellan	Keiko	Newt	Homer
Lane	Levi	Kyrene	Nolan	Horton
Macy	Liam	Mahalia	Rod	Napoleon
Madeleine	Neil	Modesty	Roscoe	Percival
Madison	Olaf	Novia	Seth	Prescott
Morgan	Omar	Opal	Siegfried	Roosevelt
Nadia	Orlando	Poppy	Sylvester	Rupert
Natalia	Parker	Rani	Thaddeus	Ulysses
Olivia	Pierce	Sapphire	Tristan	Wesley
Paris	Remington	Tierney	Vernon	Winslow
Ricki	Simon	Twyla	Victor	Winthrop
Taylor	Warren	Velvet	Ward	Yale

Names Inspired by People, Places, and Things

What's in a name? Some parents choose names that carry special meaning. They're sports buffs who name their children after legendary athletes, bookworms who name their children after beloved characters, and nature lovers who name their children after the things they see in their favorite vistas. Then again, some people choose names not because they carry personal significance but simply because they fall in love with them. They may not be sports buffs, bookworms, or nature lovers, but they still choose names like Jordan, Bridget, and Willow.

However you approach it, here are several lists of girls' and boys' names inspired by people, places, and things. (To learn more about choosing names with special meaning, check out "How to Pick a Name You and Your Baby Will Love" on page 3.)

Literature

Authors

Female	Male
Anne (Tyler)	Ambrose (Bierce)
Barbara (Kingsolver)	Bram (Stoker)
Carolyn (Keene)	Cormac (McCarthy)
Charlotte (Brontë)	Dan (Brown)
Doris (Lessing)	Ernest (Hemingway)
Elizabeth (Barrett Browning)	George (Orwell)
Emily (Dickinson)	Henry David (Thoreau)
Harper (Lee)	Homer
Harriet (Beecher Stowe)	J. D. (Salinger)
Jane (Austen)	Jules (Verne)
Joanne Kathleen ("J. K." Rowling)	Leo (Tolstoy)
Judy (Blume)	Lewis (Carroll)
Katherine (Mansfield)	Mario (Puzo)
Louisa (May Alcott)	Nicholas (Sparks)
Lucy Maud (Montgomery)	Oscar (Wilde)
Madeleine (L'Engle)	Ray (Bradbury)
Margaret (Atwood)	Samuel (Clemens)
Marge (Piercy)	Scott (Fitzgerald)
Mary (Shelley)	Stephen (King)
Maya (Angelou)	Tennessee (Williams)
Paula (Danziger)	Tom (Clancy)
Rebecca (Wells)	Truman (Capote)
Sylvia (Plath)	Virgil
Virginia (Woolf)	Walt (Whitman)
Willa (Cather)	William (Faulkner)

Fictional Characters

Female	Male	Playwrights
Female	**Male**	**Female and Male**
Anna (Karenina)	Atticus (Finch)	Anna (Deavere Smith)
Anne (Shirley)	Billy (Coleman)	Anton (Chekhov)
Antonia (Shimerda)	Boo (Radley)	Arthur (Miller)
Bridget (Jones)	Cyrus (Trask)	August (Wilson)
Cosette (Valjean)	Edmond (Dantés)	Ben (Johnson)
Daisy (Buchanan)	Ethan (Frome)	Bertolt (Brecht)
Dorothea (Brooke)	Frodo (Baggins)	Beth (Henley)
Edna (Pontellier)	Guy (Montag)	Christopher (Marlowe)
Elizabeth (Bennet)	Harry (Potter)	Dario (Fo)
Emma (Woodhouse)	Heathcliff	Eugene (O'Neill)
Hermione (Granger)	Henry (Fleming)	George (Bernard Shaw)
Hester (Prynne)	Holden (Caulfield)	Harold (Pinter)
Isabel (Archer)	Huck (Finn)	Henrik (Ibsen)
Jane (Eyre)	Jake (Barnes)	Jean Baptiste (Poquelin Molière)
Josephine (March)	Jay (Gatsby)	Lillian (Hellman)
Juliet (Capulet)	Jean (Valjean)	Neil (Simon)
Junie (B. Jones)	John (Proctor)	Noel (Coward)
Mary (Lennox)	Odysseus	Oscar (Wilde)
Meg (Murry)	Owen (Meany)	Paula (Vogel)
Ophelia	Pip (Philip Pirrip)	Samuel (Beckett)
Phoebe (Caulfield)	Rhett (Butler)	Susan (Glaspell)
Pippi (Longstocking)	Robinson (Crusoe)	Tennessee (Willimas)
Scarlett (O'Hara)	Romeo (Montague)	Thomas Stearns ("T. S." Eliot)
Scout (Finch)	Santiago	Thornton (Wilder)
Serena (Joy)	Victor (Frankenstein)	William (Shakespeare)

Dramatic Characters

Female and Male

Abigail (Williams)

Algernon ("Algy" Moncrieff)

Bella (Kurnitz)

Blanche (DuBois)

Christine (Daaé)

Cosette (Valjean)

Edmund (Tyrone)

Eliza (Doolittle)

Emily (Webb)

George (Gibbs)

Gwendolen (Fairfax)

Henry (Higgins)

Jean (Valjean)

Jim (O'Connor)

John (Proctor)

Juliet (Capulet)

Laura (Wingfield)

Linda (Loman)

Mary (Tyrone)

Odysseus

Raoul (de Chagny)

Romeo (Montague)

Stanley (Kowalski)

Vladimir

Willy (Loman)

Shakespearean Characters

Female	Male
Adriana	Angelo
Beatrice	Antony
Cleopatra	Balthasar
Cordelia	Bertram
Emilia	Cicero
Gertrude	Claudio
Helena	Cromwell
Hermia	Duncan
Hero	Edmund
Imogen	Hamlet
Isabella	Iachimo
Juliet	Iago
Katharina	Julius (Caesar)
Lavinia	Lysander
Mariana	Malcolm
Miranda	Oberon
Olivia	Orlando
Ophelia	Othello
Paulina	Paris
Portia	Puck
Regan	Richard
Rosalind	Romeo
Titania	Titus
Ursula	Tybalt
Viola	Vincentio

Poets

Female	Male
Adrienne (Rich)	Alfred (Lord Tennyson)
Amy (Lowell)	Allen (Ginsberg)
Anne (Sexton)	Carl (Sandburg)
Christina (Rossetti)	Czeslaw (Milosz)
Denise (Levertov)	Dante (Alighieri)
Dorothy (Parker)	Dylan (Thomas)
Edna (St. Vincent Millay)	Ezra (Pound)
Elizabeth (Barrett Browning)	James (Dickey)
Emily (Dickinson)	John (Keats)
Gertrude (Stein)	Juan (Ramón Jiménez)
Gwendolyn (Brooks)	Langston (Hughes)
Jamaica (Kincaid)	Louis (Simpson)
Joy (Harjo)	Mark (Strand)
Marianne (Moore)	Matsuo (Basho)
Marilyn (Hacker)	Pablo (Neruda)
Mary (Oliver)	Percy (Bysshe Shelley)
Mary Ann ("George Eliot" Evans)	Philip (Larkin)
Maxine (Kumin)	Robert (Frost)
Maya (Angelou)	Seamus (Heaney)
Muriel (Rukeyser)	Theodore (Roethke)
Rita (Dove)	Thomas (Stearns "T. S." Eliot)
Sarah (Teasdale)	Wallace (Stevens)
Sharon (Olds)	Walt (Whitman)
Sylvia (Plath)	William (Butler Yeats)
Wislawa (Szymborska)	Yusef (Komunyakaa)

Nursery Rhyme Characters

Female and Male

Bo (Peep)
Bobby (Shaftoe)
Bonnie
Elsie (Marley)
Fred
Georgie (Porgie)
Jack
Jerry (Hall)
Jill
John (Jacob Jingleheimer Schmidt)
King Cole
Lou
MacDonald
Margery (Daw)
Mary
Michael
Nancy (Etticoat)
Peter (Piper)
Polly (Flinders)
Robin
Taffy
Tommy (Tittlemouse)
Simon
Solomon (Grundy)
Willie (Winkie)

Picture Book Characters	Comic Strip Characters	Comic Superhero Alter Egos
Female and Male	**Female and Male**	**Female and Male**
Alexander	Andy (Capp)	Arthur (Curry, "Aquaman")
Alice	Blondie (Bumstead)	Barbara (Gordon, "Bat Girl")
Arthur	Brenda (Starr)	Ben (Grim, "The Thing")
Babar	Calvin	Bruce (Wayne, "Batman")
Cinderella	Cathy	Charles (Xavier, "Professor X")
Clifford	Charlie (Brown)	Clark (Kent, "Superman")
Elmo	Dennis (Mitchell)	Diana (Prince, "Wonder Woman")
Ferdinand	Dick (Tracy)	Dick (Grayson, "Robin")
Frances	Dolly	Emma (Frost, "White Queen")
George	Elly (Patterson)	Frank (Castle, "The Punisher")
Harold	Florrie (Capp)	Hal (Jordon, "Green Lantern")
Horton	Garfield	Henry (McCoy, "Beast")
Imogene	George (Wilson)	Jean (Gray, "Phoenix")
Lilly	Hägar (the Horrible)	Logan (Howlett, "Wolverine")
Madeline	Heathcliff	Matt (Murdock, "Daredevil")
Maisy	Helga	Oliver (Queen, "Green Arrow")
Max	Hiram ("Hi" Flagston)	Peter (Parker, "Spider-Man")
Olivia	Jeffy	Reed (Richards, "Mr. Fantastic")
Paddington	Lois (Flagston)	Scott (Summers, "Cyclops")
Pat	Luann	Selina (Kyle, "Catwoman")
Peter	Michael (Doonesbury)	Steve (Rogers, "Captain America")
Ping	Odie	Susan (Richards, "Invisble Woman")
Sal	Rex (Morgan)	Tony (Stark, "Iron Man")
Tikki	Sally (Forth)	Wally (West, "Flash")
Winnie	Ziggy	Warren (Worthington III, "Archangel")

Arthurian Legend Characters	The Lord of the Rings Characters
Female and Male	**Female and Male**
Anna	Aragorn
Arthur	Arwen
Bors	Bilbo
Ector	Boromir
Emmeline	Celeborn
Gaheris	Denethor
Galahad	Elrond
Gareth	Eomer
Gawain	Eowyn
Guinevere	Faramir
Igraine	Frodo
Iseult	Galadriel
Isolde	Gandalf
Kay	Gimli
Lancelot	Gollum
Lot	Grima
Mark	Legolas
Merlin	Merry
Mordred	Pippin
Morgan (le Fey)	Rosie
Morgause	Sam
Nimue	Saruman
Percival	Sauron
Tristan	Theoden
Uther (Pendragon)	Tom

History

Harry Potter Characters

Female	Male
Alicia (Spinnet)	Albus (Dumbledore)
Angelina (Johnson)	Blaise (Zabini)
Bellatrix (Lestrange)	Cedric (Diggory)
Cho (Chang)	Colin (Creavey)
Dolores (Umbridge)	Dean (Thomas)
Fleur (Delacour)	Draco (Malfoy)
Ginny (Weasley)	Dudley (Dursley)
Hermione (Granger)	Fred (Weasley)
Katie (Bell)	George (Weasley)
Lavender (Brown)	Harry (Potter)
Lily (Potter)	James (Potter)
Luna (Lovegood)	Kingsley (Shacklebolt)
Minerva (McGonagall)	Lucius (Malfoy)
Molly (Weasley)	Neville (Longbottom)
"Moaning" Myrtle	Oliver (Wood)
Narcissa (Malfoy)	Percy (Weasley)
Nymphadora (Tonks)	Peter (Pettigrew)
Padma (Patil)	Remus (Lupin)
Pansy (Parkinson)	Ron (Weasley)
Parvati (Patil)	Rubeus (Hagrid)
Penelope (Clearwater)	Seamus (Finnigan)
Petunia (Dursley)	Severus (Snape)
Poppy (Pomfrey)	Sirius (Black)
Rita (Skeeter)	Tom (Riddle)
Sibyll (Trelawney)	Viktor (Krum)

Presidents

Male

Abraham (Lincoln)
Andrew (Jackson)
Bill (Clinton)
Calvin (Coolidge)
Chester (Arthur)
Dwight (D. Eisenhower)
Franklin (D. Roosevelt)
George (Washington)
Gerald (Ford)
Grover (Cleveland)
Harry (S. Truman)
Herbert (Hoover)
James (Madison)
Jimmy (Carter)
John (F. Kennedy)
Lyndon (B. Johnson)
Martin (Van Buren)
Millard (Fillmore)
Richard (Nixon)
Ronald (Reagan)
Rutherford (B. Hayes)
Thomas (Jefferson)
Ulysses (S. Grant)
Warren (G. Harding)
Woodrow (Wilson)

Members of First Families	Democrats	Republicans
Female and Male	**Female and Male**	**Female and Male**
Abigail (Adams)	Al (Gore)	Antonia (Novello)
Amy (Carter)	Barbara (Boxer)	Arnold (Schwarzenegger)
Barbara (Bush)	Bill (Clinton)	Barry (Goldwater)
Benjamin (Pierce)	Bob (Kerrey)	Bob (Dole)
Caroline (Kennedy)	Diane (Feinstein)	Condoleezza (Rice)
Chelsea (Clinton)	Dick (Gephardt)	Dan (Quayle)
Dolley (Madison)	George (McGovern)	Dick (Cheney)
Eleanor (Roosevelt)	Geraldine (Ferraro)	Elizabeth (Dole)
Grace (Coolidge)	Hillary (Rodham Clinton)	George (Bush)
Helen (Taft)	Hubert (Humphrey)	Gerald (Ford)
Hillary (Rodham Clinton)	Jesse (Jackson)	Henry (Kissinger)
Jacqueline (Kennedy)	Jimmy (Carter)	Jeane (Kirkpatrick)
Jeb (Bush)	John (F. Kennedy)	Laura (Bush)
Jenna (Bush)	Joseph (Lieberman)	Margaret (Chase Smith)
John (Fitzgerald Kennedy, Jr.)	Lyndon (B. Johnson)	Mary (Matalin)
Julie (Nixon)	Madeleine (Albright)	Nancy (Kassebaum)
Kermit (Roosevelt)	Michael (Dukakis)	Nelson (Rockefeller)
Laura (Bush)	Nancy (Pelosi)	Newt (Gingrich)
Martha (Washington)	Paul (Wellstone)	Patrick (Buchanan)
Mary (Todd Lincoln)	Reubin (Askew)	Richard (Nixon)
Maureen (Reagan)	Shirley (Chisholm)	Ronald (Reagan)
Nancy (Reagan)	Harry (S. Truman)	Rudy (Giuliani)
Robert (Lincoln)	Ted (Kennedy)	Rush (Limbaugh)
Rosalynn (Carter)	Tom (Daschle)	Trent (Lott)
Steven (Ford)	Walter (Mondale)	Wendell (Willkie)

Kings	Queens	British Royal Family Members
Male	**Female**	**Female and Male**
Albert	Amina	Alexander
Alexander	Anne	Alexandra
Arthur	Beatrix	Alice
Canute	Candace	Andrew
Charles	Catherine	Anne
Cormac	Charlotte	Beatrice
Cyrus	Christina	Birgitte
David	Cleopatra	Camilla
Edgar	Elizabeth	Charles
Edmund	Esther	Davina
Edward	Filippa	Diana
Ferdinand	Ingrid	Edward
Frederick	Isabella	Elizabeth
George	Jeanne	Eugenie
Harold	Juliana	Frederick
Henry	Louise	George
James	Margaret	Helen
John	Marie	Henry (Harry)
Louis	Mary	Louise
Magnus	Matilda	Michael
Malcolm	Silvia	Nicholas
Niall	Sofia	Peter
Phillip	Tamar	Philip
Richard	Victoria	Richard
William	Zenobia	William

Military Figures

Female and Male

Alexander (the Great)

Andrew (Johnson)

Attila (the Hun)

Charles (de Gaulle)

Che (Guevara)

Deborah

Douglas (MacArthur)

Dwight (D. Eisenhower)

Genghis (Khan)

George (S. Patton)

Ivan (Stepanovich Konev)

Jennie (Hodgers)

Joan (of Arc)

Julius (Caesar)

Moshe (Dayan)

Napoleon (Bonaparte)

Oliver (Cromwell)

Omar (Bradley)

Peter (the Great)

Robert (E. Lee)

Tecumseh

Ulysses (S. Grant)

William (Wallace)

Winfield (Scott)

Winston (Churchill)

Explorers

Female and Male

Amelia (Earhart)

Ann (Bancroft)

Amerigo (Vespucci)

Bartolomeu (Dias)

Christopher (Columbus)

Eric (The Red)

Ferdinand (Magellan)

Francisco (Vásquez de Coronado)

George (Everest)

Gertrude (Bell)

Harriet (Chalmers Adams)

Henry (Hudson)

Hernán (Cortés)

Hernando (de Soto)

Jacques (Cousteau)

Juan (Ponce de León)

James (Cook)

Leif (Ericsson)

Marco (Polo)

Neil (Armstrong)

Samuel (de Champlain)

Thor (Heyerdahl)

Walter (Raleigh)

William (Clark)

Zebulon (Pike)

Activists

Female and Male

Agnes ("Mother Teresa" Gonxha Bojaxhiu)

Albert (Schweitzer)

Anwar (el-Sadat)

Cesar (Chavez)

Che (Guevara)

Desmond (Tutu)

Dorothy (Day)

Elizabeth (Cady Stanton)

Frederick (Douglass)

Gloria (Steinem)

Harriet (Tubman)

Jesse (Jackson)

Jimmy (Carter)

John (Muir)

Kim (Dae-jung)

Lucy (Stone)

Malcolm (X)

Margaret (Sanger)

Martin (Luther King)

Mary (Wollstonecraft)

Nelson (Mandela)

Rachel (Carson)

Rosa (Parks)

Susan (B. Anthony)

William ("W. E. B." Du Bois)

Nobel Prize Winners	Old West Figures	Colleges and Universities
Female and Male	**Female and Male**	**Female and Male**
Agnes ("Mother Teresa" Gonxha Bojaxhiu)	Annie (Oakley)	Auburn
Albert (Einstein)	Bat (Masterson)	Berkeley
Desmond (Tutu)	Belle (Starr)	Brown
Elie (Wiesel)	Butch (Cassidy)	Bryn (Mawr)
Ernest (Hemingway)	Charles ("Black Bart" Boles)	Carleton
George (Beadle)	Clay (Allison)	Columbia
Godfrey (Hounsfield)	Cole (Younger)	Cornell
Günter (Grass)	Daniel (Boone)	Creighton
Ivan (Pavlov)	Davy (Crockett)	Drake
Jimmy (Carter)	Doc (Holliday)	Duke
Kofi (Annan)	Frank (James)	Emerson
Marie (Curie)	Harry ("Sundance Kid" Longabaugh)	Emory
Martin (Luther King)	Henry (Starr)	Kent
Mikhail (Gorbachev)	James ("Wild Bill" Hickok)	Kenyon
Milton (Friedman)	Jesse (James)	Lewis and Clark
Nadine (Gordimer)	John (Wesley Hardin)	Penn
Nelson (Mandela)	Kit (Carson)	Princeton
Niels (Bohr)	Martha Jane ("Calamity Jane" Canary)	Regis
Octavio (Paz)	Pat (Garrett)	Rhodes
Pablo (Neruda)	Roy (Bean)	Rice
Pearl (Buck)	Sally (Skull)	Sarah Lawrence
Samuel (Beckett)	Sam (Houston)	Stanford
Saul (Bellow)	Tom (Horn)	William and Mary
Seamus (Heaney)	William ("Buffalo Bill" Cody)	Xavier
Toni (Morrison)	Wyatt (Earp)	Yale

Religion and Mythology

Old Testament Figures	New Testament Figures	Biblical Women
Male	**Male**	**Female**
Abel	Agrippa	Abigail
Abraham	Andrew	Bathsheba
Adam	Annas	Deborah
Cain	Aquila	Delilah
Caleb	Gabriel	Dinah
Daniel	Herod	Eden
David	James	Elizabeth
Eli	Jesus	Esther
Elijah	John	Eve
Esau	Joseph	Hagar
Ezekiel	Judas	Hannah
Ezra	Jude	Jezebel
Isaac	Luke	Joy
Isaiah	Mark	Julia
Jacob	Matthew	Leah
Jeremiah	Nicolas	Maria
Job	Paul	Martha
Joel	Peter	Mary
Joshua	Philip	Miriam
Moses	Simon	Naomi
Nemiah	Stephen	Phoebe
Noah	Thomas	Rachel
Samson	Timothy	Rebekah
Samuel	Titus	Ruth
Solomon	Zechariah	Sarah

Saints		Popes	Christmas-Themed Names
Female	**Male**	**Male**	**Female and Male**
Agatha	Ambrose	Adrian	Angel
Agnes	Andrew	Alexander	Bell
Bernadette	Anslem	Benedict	Carol
Bridget	Anthony	Boniface	Claus
Catherine	Augustine	Celestine	Ebenezer
Cecilia	Bartholomew	Clement	Emmanuel
Clare	Benedict	Constantine	Garland
Constance	Christopher	Cornelius	Gloria
Florence	Felix	Eugene	Holly
Genevieve	Francis	Felix	Jesus
Hilary	Gregory	Gregory	Joseph
Ingrid	Ignatius	Innocent	Joy
Joan	Jerome	John Paul	King
Julia	John	Julius	Kris
Louise	Jude	Leo	Manger
Lucy	Leo	Linus	Mary
Lydia	Nicholas	Peter	Merry
Margaret	Patrick	Pius	Nicholas
Maria	Paul	Romanus	Noel
Mary	Peter	Sixtus	Peace
Monica	Sebastian	Stephan	Rudolf
Regina	Stephen	Theodore	Shepherd
Rose	Thomas	Urban	Star
Sylvia	Valentine	Valentine	Wenceslas
Teresa	Vincent	Zachary	Yule

Heavenly and Angelic Names	Jewish Figures	Muslim Figures
Female and Male	**Female and Male**	**Male**
Angel	Aaron	Adam
Angela	Akiva	Al-Yasa
Angellica	Abraham	Ayub
Angelo	Daniel	Daud
Asención	David (Ben Gurion)	Harun
Beulah	Deborah	Hud
Celeste	Esther	Ibrahim
Divinity	Golda (Meir)	Idris
Eden	Hillel	Ilyas
Faith	Isaac	Isa
Gabriel	Jacob	Ishaq
Gloria	Joseph	Ismail
Heaven	Judah (Maccabee)	Lut
Jannah	Leah	Muhammad
Lani	Maimonides	Musa
Michael	Miriam	Nuh
Nevaeh	Mordechai	Saleh
Paradise	Moses	Shoaib
Paradiso	Nachimanides	Sulayman
Raphael	Rachel	Yahya
Seraphim	Rashi	Yaqub
Seraphina	Rebecca	Yunus
Tian	Ruth	Yusuf
Trinity	Sarah	Zakariya
Zion	Yochanan (ben Zakkai)	Zulkifl

Hindu Figures	Greek Mythology Figures		Roman Mythology Figures	
Female and Male	**Female**	**Male**	**Female**	**Male**
Agni	Aphrodite	Achilles	Aurora	Aeneas
Arjuna	Artemis	Adonis	Bellona	Aesculapius
Bali	Athena	Apollo	Camilla	Amor
Brahma	Calliope	Ares	Ceres	Bacchus
Buddha	Calypso	Atlas	Clementia	Cupid
Chandra	Chloe	Dionysus	Concordia	Faunus
Devi	Daphne	Eros	Decima	Honos
Dharma	Demeter	Hades	Diana	Inuus
Indra	Echo	Hector	Fauna	Janus
Kali	Electra	Helios	Felicitas	Jove
Kama	Europa	Hercules	Flora	Jupiter
Krishna	Gaea	Hermes	Fortuna	Liber
Maya	Helen	Icarus	Hippona	Mars
Nala	Hera	Jason	Juno	Mercury
Parvati	Hestia	Midas	Juventus	Neptune
Rama	Io	Morpheus	Levana	Orcus
Ravi	Leda	Narcissus	Luna	Pluto
Sati	Medusa	Odysseus	Mania	Remus
Shiva	Nike	Orion	Minerva	Romulus
Sita	Pandora	Pan	Pax	Saturn
Surya	Penelope	Paris	Roma	Silvanus
Uma	Persephone	Perseus	Venus	Sol
Ushas	Phoebe	Poseidon	Veritas	Somnus
Vishnu	Psyche	Prometheus	Vesta	Ulysses
Yama	Rhea	Zeus	Victoria	Vulcan

Egyptian Mythology Figures	Norse Mythology Figures	African Mythology
Female and Male	**Female and Male**	**Female and Male**
Aker	Aegir	Abuk
Anouke	Astrild	Agé
Anubis	Atla	Aja
Atum	Balder	Astar
Bastet	Bragi	Buku
Bes	Edda	Deng
Buto	Forseti	Edinkira
Geb	Freya	Enekpe
Hapi	Freyr	Eshu
Hathor	Frigg	Faro
Horus	Hel	Gun
Isis	Hermod	Inkosazana
Ma'at	Hod	Kuru
Min	Idun	Loko
Neith	Loki	Mawu
Nun	Mimir	Mugasa
Nunet	Njord	Osawa
Osiris	Odin	Oshun
Ptah	Ran	Oya
Ra	Saga	Shango
Seb	Sif	Tamuno
Seth	Thor	Wele
Shu	Thrud	Woto
Sobek	Tyr	Xamaba
Thoth	Ull	Yemaja

Movies and TV

Japanese Mythology

Female and Male

Amaterasu

Amida

Benten

Bishamon

Daikoku

Dosojin

Ebisu

Fujin

Gama

Gongen

Hachiman

Hiruko

Hoderi

Inari

Isora

Jimmu

Kaminari

Kishijoten

Marisha-Ten

Onamuji

Raiden

Sengen

Susanowa

Tsuki-Yumi

Uzume

Movie Stars

Female	Male
Angelina (Jolie)	Benicio (Del Toro)
Anjelica (Huston)	Bing (Crosby)
Audrey (Hepburn)	Bruce (Willis)
Betty (Grable)	Cary (Grant)
Cameron (Diaz)	Chevy (Chase)
Catherine (Zeta-Jones)	Clark (Gable)
Cher	Clint (Eastwood)
Drew (Barrymore)	Dustin (Hoffman)
Elizabeth (Taylor)	Harrison (Ford)
Emma (Thompson)	Jack (Nicholson)
Gwyneth (Paltrow)	John (Wayne)
Halle (Berry)	Leonardo (DiCaprio)
Jodie (Foster)	Martin (Sheen)
Julia (Roberts)	Mel (Gibson)
Katharine (Hepburn)	Mickey (Rooney)
Liv (Tyler)	Orlando (Bloom)
Meg (Ryan)	Patrick (Swayze)
Meryl (Streep)	Robert (De Niro)
Michelle (Pfeiffer)	Robin (Williams)
Nicole (Kidman)	Rock (Hudson)
Penelope (Cruz)	Russell (Crowe)
Reese (Witherspoon)	Sean (Connery)
Salma (Hayek)	Spencer (Tracy)
Sandra (Bullock)	Sylvester (Stallone)
Shirley (Temple)	Tom (Cruise)

Oscar Winners

Female	Male
Angelina (Jolie)	Al (Pacino)
Anna (Paquin)	Anthony (Hopkins)
Barbara (Streisand)	Benicio (Del Toro)
Bette (Davis)	Christopher (Walken)
Charlize (Theron)	Cuba (Gooding, Jr.)
Diane (Keaton)	Daniel (Day-Lewis)
Elizabeth (Taylor)	Denzel (Washington)
Goldie (Hawn)	Dustin (Hoffman)
Halle (Berry)	Gene (Hackman)
Hilary (Swank)	Jack (Nicholson)
Jane (Fonda)	James (Stewart)
Jessica (Lange)	Jamie (Foxx)
Jodie (Foster)	Kevin (Spacey)
Julia (Roberts)	Laurence (Olivier)
Julie (Andrews)	Marlon (Brando)
Katharine (Hepburn)	Michael (Caine)
Kathy (Bates)	Morgan (Freeman)
Maggie (Smith)	Peter (Ustinov)
Marisa (Tomei)	Richard (Dreyfuss)
Meryl (Streep)	Robert (De Niro)
Sally (Fields)	Russell (Crowe)
Shirley (MacLaine)	Sidney (Poitier)
Susan (Sarandon)	Tom (Hanks)
Tatum (O'Neal)	Tommy (Lee Jones)
Whoopi (Goldberg)	Walter (Brennan)

Silver Screen Stars

Female	Male
Audrey (Hepburn)	Bing (Crosby)
Ava (Gardner)	Burt (Lancaster)
Barbara (Stanwyck)	Cary (Grant)
Bette (Davis)	Charlton (Heston)
Carole (Lombard)	Clark (Gable)
Betty (Grable)	Errol (Flynn)
Deborah (Kerr)	Frank (Sinatra)
Ginger (Rogers)	Fred (Astaire)
Grace (Kelly)	Gary (Cooper)
Greta (Garbo)	Gene (Kelly)
Ingrid (Bergman)	Gregory (Peck)
Jean (Harlow)	Henry (Fonda)
Joan (Crawford)	Humphrey (Bogart)
Judy (Garland)	James (Dean)
Katharine (Hepburn)	Jimmy (Stewart)
Lana (Turner)	John (Wayne)
Lauren (Bacall)	Laurence (Olivier)
Loretta (Young)	Marlon (Brando)
Mae (West)	Montgomery (Clift)
Marilyn (Monroe)	Orson (Welles)
Marlene (Dietrich)	Peter (O'Toole)
Natalie (Wood)	Rex (Harrison)
Rita (Hayworth)	Richard (Burton)
Veronica (Lake)	Spencer (Tracy)
Vivian (Leigh)	Walter (Brennan)

Movie Directors

Female and Male

Alfred (Hitchcock)

Clint (Eastwood)

Ethan (Coen)

Francis (Ford Coppola)

Frank (Capra)

George (Lucas)

James (Cameron)

Joel (Coen)

John (Woo)

Martin (Scorsese)

Mel (Brooks)

Michael (Moore)

Oliver (Stone)

Penny (Marshall)

Peter (Jackson)

Quentin (Tarantino)

Roman (Polanski)

Ron (Howard)

Sofia (Coppola)

Spike (Lee)

Stanley (Kubrick)

Steven (Spielberg)

Tim (Burton)

Wes (Craven)

Woody (Allen)

Movie Characters

Female	Male
Amélie (Poulain)	Atticus (Finch)
Annie (Hall)	Austin (Powers)
Bonnie (Parker)	Billy (Madison)
Bridget (Jones)	Charles (Foster Kane)
Clarice (Starling)	Forrest (Gump)
Clementine (Kruczynski)	Frodo (Baggins)
Dorothy (Gale)	George (Bailey)
Elaine (Robinson)	Hannibal (Lector)
Eliza (Doolittle)	Harry (Potter)
Ellen (Ripley)	Indiana (Jones)
Erin (Brockovich)	Jack (Sparrow)
Holly (Golightly)	Jacques (Clouseau)
Ilsa (Lund)	James (Bond)
Jean Louise ("Scout" Finch)	Jerry (Maguire)
Lara (Croft)	Judah (Ben-Hur)
Leia (Organa)	Lloyd (Dobler)
Louise (Sawyer)	Luke (Skywalker)
Marge (Gunderson)	Maximus (Decimus Meridius)
Maria (von Trapp)	Napoleon (Dynamite)
Mary (Poppins)	Neo
Norma Rae (Webster)	Norman (Bates)
Sandy (Olsson)	Rhett (Butler)
Scarlett (O'Hara)	Rick (Blaine)
Thelma (Dickerson)	Rocky (Balboa)
Trinity	Vito (Corleone)

Comedians

Female	Male
Carol (Burnett)	Adam (Sandler)
Caroline (Rhea)	Bernie (Mac)
Cheri (Oteri)	Bill (Cosby)
Ellen (DeGeneres)	Bob (Hope)
Fanny (Brice)	Cedric ("The Entertainer" Kyles)
Gilda (Radner)	Chevy (Chase)
Gracie (Allen)	Chris (Rock)
Jane (Curtain)	Dan (Aykroyd)
Janeane (Garofalo)	Dana (Carvey)
Joan (Rivers)	Dave (Chappelle)
Kathy (Griffin)	David (Letterman)
Lily (Tomlin)	Denis (Leary)
Lucille (Ball)	Drew (Carey)
Margaret (Cho)	Eddie (Murphy)
Molly (Shannon)	George (Burns)
Paula (Poundstone)	Jay (Leno)
Phyllis (Diller)	Jerry (Seinfeld)
Rita (Rudner)	Johnny (Carson)
Roseanne (Barr)	Louie (Anderson)
Rosie (O'Donnell)	Mike (Myers)
Sandra (Bernhard)	Ray (Romano)
Tina (Fey)	Rodney (Dangerfield)
Tracey (Ullman)	Steve (Martin)
Wanda (Sykes)	Tim (Allen)
Whoopi (Goldberg)	Will (Ferrell)

TV Characters

Male	Female
Al (Bundy)	Abby (Lockhart)
Alex (P. Keaton)	Ally (McBeal)
Archie (Bunker)	Buffy (Summers)
Arthur ("Fonzie" Fonzarelli)	Carmela (Soprano)
Bobby (Simone)	Carrie (Bradshaw)
Cliff (Huxtable)	Claire (Kincaid)
Cosmo (Kramer)	Daphne (Moon Crane)
Danny ("Danno" Williams)	Darlene (Conner-Healy)
Dylan (McKay)	Donna (Martin Silver)
Fox (Mulder)	Elaine (Benes)
Frasier (Crane)	Erica (Kane)
Gil (Grissom)	Felicity (Porter)
Jack (McCoy)	Fran (Fine)
Jean-Luc (Picard)	Gabrielle (Solis)
Jed (Bartlet)	Grace (Adler)
Joey (Tribbiani)	Kelly (Bundy)
John Ross ("J. R." Ewing, Jr.)	Kimberly (Shaw Mancini)
Kevin (Arnold)	Lucy (Ricardo)
Luka (Kovac)	Marcia (Brady)
Ricky (Ricardo)	Margaret ("Hot Lips"
Sam (Malone)	Houlihan)
Tony (Soprano)	Michelle (Tanner)
Vic (Mackey)	Rachel (Green)
Will (Truman)	Rebecca (Howe)
Zack (Morris)	Sydney (Bristow)
	Vanessa (Huxtable)

TV Personalities

Male	Female
Ahmad (Rashad)	Ann (Curry)
Al (Roker)	Barbara (Walters)
Alex (Trebek)	Brooke (Burke)
Bill (O'Reilly)	Connie (Chung)
Bob (Barker)	Diane (Sawyer)
Carson (Daly)	Ellen (DeGeneres)
Conan (O'Brien)	Jane (Pauley)
Dan (Rather)	Jenny (Jones)
David (Letterman)	Joan (Rivers)
Dick (Clark)	Joy (Behar)
Geraldo (Rivera)	Judy ("Judge Judy" Sheindlin)
Howard (Stern)	Kathie (Lee Gifford)
Jay (Leno)	Katie (Couric)
Jerry (Springer)	Kelly (Ripa)
Jim (Lehrer)	Leeza (Gibbons)
Johnny (Carson)	Lisa (Ling)
Larry (King)	Martha (Stewart)
Matt (Lauer)	Meredith (Vieira)
Montel (Williams)	Nancy (O'Dell)
Peter (Jennings)	Oprah (Winfrey)
Phil (McGraw)	Paige (Davis)
Regis (Philbin)	Ricki (Lake)
Simon (Cowell)	Sally (Jessy Raphaël)
Tom (Brokaw)	Star (Jones Reynolds)
Ty (Pennington)	Vanna (White)

Soap Opera Characters

Female and Male

Bo (Brady)
Carly (Corinthos)
Drucilla (Winters)
Eric (Forrester)
Erica (Kane)
Eve (Russell)
Harley (Cooper)
Hope (Brady)
Jack (Deveraux)
Jasper ("Jax" Jacks)
Laura (Spencer)
Lily (Snyder)
Luke (Spencer)
Marlena (Evans)
Nikki (Newman)
Phillip (Spaulding)
Reva (Shane)
Ridge (Forrester)
Sonny (Corinthos)
Tad (Martin)
Taylor (Hayes Forrester)
Theresa (Lopez-Fitzgerald)
Todd (Manning)
Victor (Newman)
Viki (Lord Davidson)

Disney Cartoon Characters

Male	Female
Aladdin	Alice
Bambi	Ariel
Bob (Parr)	Aurora
Buzz (Lightyear)	Belle
Chip	Boo
Christopher (Robin)	Cinderella
Dale	Daisy (Duck)
Dash (Parr)	Esmeralda
Dewey	Fauna
Donald (Duck)	Flora
Eric	Helen (Parr)
Gaston	Jane (Porter)
Hercules	Jasmine
Huey	Jessie
Ichabod (Crane)	Lilo
Jafar	Marian
Louie	Mary (Poppins)
Merlin	Megara
Mickey	Minnie
Mufasa	Mulan
Peter (Pan)	Nala
Robin (Hood)	Pocahontas
Sebastian	Ursula
Simba	Violet (Parr)
Timon	Wendy

Cartoon Characters

Female	Male
Angelica (Pickles)	Arthur
April (O'Neil)	Barney (Rubble)
Babs (Bunny)	Bart (Simpson)
Betty (Rubble)	Bobby (Hill)
Blossom	Charlie (Brown)
Daisy (Duck)	Donald (Duck)
Daphne (Blake)	Elmer (Fudd)
Daria (Morgandorffer)	Elroy (Jetson)
Dora (the Explorer)	Fred (Flintstone)
Jane (Jetson)	Garfield
Jerrica ("Jem" Benton)	George (Jetson)
Judy (Jetson)	Hank (Hill)
Kim (Possible)	Homer (Simpson)
Lil (DeVille)	Jimmy (Neutron)
Lisa (Simpson)	Johnny (Bravo)
Luanne (Platter)	Kenny (McCormick)
Lucy (Van Pelt)	Linus (Van Pelt)
Maggie (Simpson)	Marvin (Martian)
Marge (Simpson)	Pepe (Le Pew)
Peggy (Hill)	Peter (Griffin)
Petunia (Pig)	Rocky
Rainbow (Brite)	Stan (Marsh)
Sally (Brown)	Sylvester
Velma (Dinkley)	Tommy (Pickles)
Wilma (Flintstone)	Woody (Woodpecker)

Music

Pop Artists		Heavy Metal/Hard Rock Artists
Female	**Male**	**Female and Male**
Alanis (Morrisette)	Adam (Duritz)	Alice (Cooper)
Annie (Lennox)	Billy (Joel)	Angus (Young)
Avril (Lavigne)	Chris (Martin)	Axl (Rose)
Britney (Spears)	Darius (Rucker)	Bon (Scott)
Celine (Dion)	Dave (Matthews)	Chris (Cornell)
Cher	Edwin (McCain)	Courtney (Love)
Christina (Aguilera)	Elton (John)	David (Lee Roth)
Dido	Elvis (Presley)	Eddie (Van Halen)
Fiona (Apple)	Enrique (Iglesias)	Gene (Simmons)
Gloria (Estefan)	Eric (Clapton)	James (Hetfield)
Gwen (Stefani)	George (Michael)	Joe (Perry)
Janet (Jackson)	Howie (Day)	Jon (Bon Jovi)
Jessica (Simpson)	Jack (Johnson)	Kurt (Cobain)
Jewel	John (Lennon)	Layne (Staley)
Kelly (Clarkson)	Justin (Timberlake)	Lita (Ford)
Madonna	Marc (Anthony)	Marilyn (Manson)
Mandy (Moore)	Michael (Jackson)	Maynard (James Keenan)
Natalie (Imbruglia)	Nick (Lachey)	Ozzy (Osbourne)
Norah (Jones)	Paul (McCartney)	Rob (Halford)
Paula (Abdul)	Prince	Robert (Plant)
Pink	Ricky (Martin)	Scott (Weiland)
Sarah (McLachlan)	Ringo (Starr)	Sebastian (Bach)
Sheryl (Crow)	Rob (Thomas)	Steven (Tyler)
Tori (Amos)	Rod (Stewart)	Sully (Erna)
Vanessa (Carlton)	Sting	Tommy (Lee)

Classic Rock Artists	Jazz Artists	Blues Artists
Female and Male	**Female and Male**	**Female and Male**
Bob (Dylan)	Benny (Goodman)	Aaron (Thibeaux "T-Bone" Walker)
Brian (Wilson)	Billie (Holiday)	Albert (King)
Carly (Simon)	Cab (Calloway)	B. B. (King)
Carole (King)	Cassandra (Wilson)	Bessie (Smith)
Don (Henley)	Charlie (Parker)	Billie (Holiday)
George (Harrison)	Chet (Baker)	Bo (Diddley)
James (Taylor)	Dave (Koz)	Buddy (Guy)
Janis (Joplin)	David (Sanborn)	Chester ("Howlin' Wolf" Burnett)
Jerry (Garcia)	Diana (Krall)	Dinah (Washington)
Jim (Morrison)	Dizzy (Gillespie)	Elmore (James)
Jimi (Hendrix)	Duke (Ellington)	Eric (Clapton)
Jimmy (Page)	Grover (Washington, Jr.)	Huddie ("Leadbelly" Ledbetter)
Joan (Baez)	Harry (Connick, Jr.)	Jimmy (Rogers)
John (Lennon)	Herbie (Mann)	John (Lee Hooker)
Joni (Mitchell)	John (Coltrane)	Johnny (Lang)
Keith (Richards)	Louis (Armstrong)	Kevin ("Keb' Mo'" Moore)
Linda (Ronstadt)	Miles (Davis)	Muddy (Waters)
Mick (Jagger)	Norah (Jones)	Robert (Cray)
Neil (Young)	Ornette (Coleman)	Robert (Johnson)
Paul (McCartney)	Quincy (Jones)	Ruth (Brown)
Pete (Townshend)	Ray (Charles)	Sam ("Lightnin'" Hopkins)
Ringo (Starr)	Stan (Getz)	Son (House)
Robert (Plant)	William ("Count" Basie)	Stevie Ray (Vaughn)
Roger (Daltrey)	Wynton (Marsalis)	W. C. (Handy)
Stevie (Nicks)	Xavier (Cugat)	Willie (Dixon)

R&B/Soul Artists

Male	Female
Aaron (Neville)	Aaliyah
Barry (White)	Alicia (Keys)
Bill (Withers)	Aretha (Franklin)
Brian (McKnight)	Ashanti
Bobby (Brown)	Beyoncé (Knowles)
Cedric ("K-Ci" Hailey)	Brandy (Norwood)
Edwin (Starr)	Christina (Milian)
Freddie (Jackson)	Diana (Ross)
Ike (Turner)	Dionne (Warwick)
James (Brown)	Faith (Evans)
Joel ("Jo-Jo" Hailey)	Gladys (Knight)
Kenneth ("Babyface" Edmonds)	India (Arie)
Lionel (Richie)	Jennifer (Lopez)
Lou (Rawls)	Kelly (Rowland)
Luther (Vandross)	Lauryn (Hill)
Marvin (Gaye)	Macy (Gray)
Michael ("D'Angelo" Archer)	Mariah (Carey)
Otis (Redding)	Mary (J. Blige)
Percy (Sledge)	Monica (Arnold)
Ray (Charles)	Mya (Harrison)
Robert ("R. Kelly" Kelly)	Patti (LaBelle)
Ronnie (DeVoe)	Tina (Turner)
Ruben (Studdard)	Toni (Braxton)
Stevie (Wonder)	Vanessa (Williams)
Usher (Raymond)	Whitney (Houston)

Rap/Hip-Hop Artists

Female and Male

Andre ("Dr. Dre" Young)
Anthony ("Tone-Loc" Smith)
Antwan ("Big Boi" Patton)
Calvin ("Snoop Dogg" Broadus)
Carlton ("Chuck D" Ridenhour)
Christopher ("Ludacris" Bridges)
Cornell ("Nelly" Haynes, Jr.)
Curtis ("50 Cent" Jackson)
Dana ("Queen Latifah" Owens)
James ("LL Cool J" Todd Smith)
Jason ("Jam Master Jay" Mizell)
Joseph ("Run" Simmons)
Kimberly ("Lil' Kim" Jones)
Marshall ("Eminem" Mathers)
Melissa ("Missy" Elliot)
Mike ("Mike D" Diamond)
O'Shea ("Ice Cube" Jackson)
Robert ("Vanilla Ice" Van Winkle)
Sean ("P Diddy" Combs)
Shawn ("Jay-Z" Carter)
Stanley ("MC Hammer" Burrell)
Tracy ("Ice-T" Marrow)
Trevor ("Busta Rhymes" Smith, Jr.)
Tupac ("2Pac" Shakur)
William ("Flava Flav" Drayton)

Country Western Artists

Female

Alison (Krauss)
Carolyn Dawn (Johnson)
Chely (Wright)
Crystal (Gayle)
Cyndi (Thomson)
Dolly (Parton)
Faith (Hill)
Gretchen (Wilson)
Jamie (O'Neal)
Jo Dee (Messina)
Julie (Roberts)
LeAnn (Rimes)
Loretta (Lynn)
Martie (Maguire)
Martina (McBride)
Mary (Chapin Carpenter)
Mindy (McCready)
Natalie (Maines)
Patsy (Cline)
Patty (Loveless)
Reba (McEntire)
Sara (Evans)
Shania (Twain)
Tammy (Wynette)
Terri (Clark)

Male

Alan (Jackson)
Billy Ray (Cyrus)
Brad (Paisley)
Charley (Pride)
Chet (Atkins)
Clint (Black)
Darryl (Worley)
Don (Everly)
Garth (Brooks)
Gene (Autry)
George (Strait)
Hank (Williams)
Joe (Nichols)
Johnny (Cash)
Keith (Urban)
Kenny (Chesney)
Kix (Brooks)
Randy (Travis)
Ronnie (Dunn)
Tim (McGraw)
Toby (Keith)
Trace (Adkins)
Vince (Gill)
Waylon (Jennings)
Willie (Nelson)

Classical Composers and Performers

Female and Male

Andrea (Bocelli)
Antonio (Vivaldi)
Camille (Saint-Saëns)
Claude (Debussy)
Felix (Mendelssohn)
Franz (Schubert)
Frédéric (Chopin)
George (Handel)
Giacomo (Puccini)
Giuseppe (Verdi)
Igor (Stravinsky)
Johann (Sebastian Bach)
José (Carreras)
Joseph (Haydn)
Leonard (Bernstein)
Luciano (Pavarotti)
Ludwig (van Beethoven)
Maria (Callas)
Nikolay (Rimsky-Korsakov)
Plácido (Domingo)
Pyotr (Tchaikovsky)
Renata (Scotto)
Richard (Wagner)
Wolfgang (Mozart)
Yo-Yo (Ma)

Crooners

Female and Male

Al (Jolson)
Andy (Williams)
Artie (Shaw)
Bing (Crosby)
Bobby (Darin)
Cole (Porter)
Dinah (Washington)
Ella (Fitzgerald)
Frank (Sinatra)
Glenn (Miller)
Hoagy (Carmichael)
Jerry (Vale)
Mel (Tormé)
Nat ("King" Cole)
Paul (Anka)
Peggy (Lee)
Perry (Como)
Robert (Goulet)
Rosemary (Clooney)
Sammy (Davis, Jr.)
Sarah (Vaughan)
Thomas ("Fats" Waller)
Tony (Bennett)
Vic (Damone)
William ("Count" Basie)

Songs with Names in the Titles

Male	Female
"Achilles Last Stand" (Led Zeppelin)	"Alison" (Elvis Costello)
"Adam's Song" (blink-182)	"Angie" (The Rolling Stones)
"Bad, Bad Leroy Brown" (Jim Croce)	"Annie's Song" (John Denver)
"Bennie and the Jets" (Elton John)	"Beth" (Kiss)
"Billy, Don't Be a Hero" (Paper Lace)	"Billie Jean" (Michael Jackson)
"Buddy Holly" (Weezer)	"Come On Eileen" (Dexy's Midnight Runners)
"Calling Elvis" (Dire Straits)	"Georgia on My Mind" (Ray Charles)
"Daniel" (Elton John)	"Good Golly Miss Molly" (Little Richard)
"Fernando" (ABBA)	"Help Me Rhonda" (The Beach Boys)
"Galileo" (Indigo Girls)	"Jack and Diane" (John Mellencamp)
"Goodbye Earl" (Dixie Chicks)	"Janie's Got a Gun" (Aerosmith)
"Hey Joe" (Jimi Hendrix)	"Jenny from the Block" (Jennifer Lopez)
"Hey Jude" (The Beatles)	"Kathy's Song" (Simon & Garfunkel)
"James Dean" (The Eagles)	"Layla" (Derek and the Dominos)
"Jeremy" (Pearl Jam)	"Lucy in the Sky with Diamonds" (The Beatles)
"Jessie's Girl" (Rick Springfield)	"Maggie May" (Rod Stewart)
"Jim Dandy" (Black Oak Arkansas)	"Mandy" (Barry Manilow)
"Johnny B. Goode" (Chuck Berry)	"Mary Jane's Last Dance" (Tom Petty and the Heartbreakers)
"Jumpin' Jack Flash" (The Rolling Stones)	"Mustang Sally" (Wilson Pickett)
"Louie, Louie" (The Kingsmen)	"My Sharona" (The Knack)
"Me and Bobby McGee" (Janis Joplin)	"Rosalita (Come Out Tonight)" (Bruce Springsteen)
"Mickey" (Toni Basil)	"Rosanna" (Toto)
"Stan" (Eminem)	"Roxanne" (The Police)
"What's the Frequency, Kenneth?" (R.E.M.)	"Sweet Caroline" (Neil Diamond)
"You Can Call Me Al" (Paul Simon)	"Wake Up Little Susie" (The Everly Brothers)

Sports and Leisure

Musical Terms	Athletes		Baseball Players
Female and Male	**Female**	**Male**	**Male**
Allegro	Anna (Kournikova)	Andre (Agassi)	Alex (Rodriguez)
Aria	Annika (Sorenstam)	Andy (Roddick)	Babe (Ruth)
Cadence	Diana (Taurasi)	Babe (Ruth)	Barry (Bonds)
Canon	Jackie (Joyner-Kersee)	Bernie (Williams)	Catfish (Hunter)
Carol	Jennie (Finch)	Dale (Earnhardt)	Cy (Young)
Chante	Kerri (Strug)	David (Beckham)	Derek (Jeter)
Clef	Kristi (Yamaguchi)	Elvis (Stojko)	Dizzy (Dean)
Coda	Florence (Griffith Joyner)	Hulk (Hogan)	Cal (Ripken, Jr.)
Diva	Laila (Ali)	Kasey (Kahne)	Hank (Aaron)
Fermata	Lisa (Leslie)	Kobe (Bryant)	Ichiro (Suzuki)
Harmony	Marion (Jones)	Lance (Armstrong)	Jackie (Robinson)
Harp	Martina (Hingis)	Mark (Spitz)	Ken (Griffey, Jr.)
Hymn	Mary Lou (Retton)	Michael (Jordan)	Kirby (Puckett)
Lyric	Mia (Hamm)	Mike (Tyson)	Mark (McGwire)
Major	Monica (Seles)	Muhammad (Ali)	Mickey (Mantle)
Medley	Nadia (Comaneci)	Orenthal James ("O. J." Simpson)	Nolan (Ryan)
Melody	Babe (Didrikson Zaharias)	Oscar (De La Hoya)	Pete (Rose)
Musika	Oksana (Baiul)	Red (Grange)	Randy (Johnson)
Opus	Picabo (Street)	Riddick (Bowe)	Roger (Clemens)
Piano	Rebecca (Lobo)	Rocky (Balboa)	Rollie (Fingers)
Reed	Sarah (Hughes)	Scott (Hamilton)	Sammy (Sosa)
Rococo	Serena (Williams)	Tiger (Woods)	Ted (Williams)
Sonata	Sheryl (Swoopes)	Tony (Hawk)	Torii (Hunter)
Symphony	Steffi (Graf)	Wayne (Gretzky)	Wade (Boggs)
Viola	Venus (Williams)	Yao (Ming)	Willie (Mays)

Basketball Players		Football Players
Female	**Male**	**Male**
Alana (Beard)	Alonzo (Mourning)	Ahman (Green)
Alicia (Thompson)	Anfernee ("Penny" Hardaway)	Barry (Sanders)
Chantelle (Anderson)	Bill (Russell)	Bo (Jackson)
Coco (Miller)	Carmelo (Anthony)	Brett (Favre)
Dominique (Canty)	Clyde (Drexler)	Dan (Marino)
Ebony (Hoffman)	Dennis (Rodman)	Deion (Sanders)
Felicia (Ragland)	Earvin ("Magic" Johnson)	Donovan (McNabb)
Giuliana (Mendiola)	Isiah (Thomas)	Eli (Manning)
Gwen (Jackson)	Jerry (West)	Emmitt (Smith)
Jessie (Hicks)	Julius (Erving)	Frank (Gifford)
Kaayla (Chones)	Kareem (Abdul-Jabbar)	Jeremy (Shockey)
Katie (Douglas)	Karl (Malone)	Jerry (Rice)
Kiesha (Brown)	Kevin (Garnett)	Joe (Montana)
Lisa (Leslie)	Kobe (Bryant)	John (Elway)
Lucienne (Berthieu)	Larry (Bird)	Johnny (Unitas)
Michele (Van Gorp)	Latrell (Sprewell)	LaDainian (Tomlinson)
Natalie (Williams)	LeBron (James)	Michael (Vick)
Nykesha (Sales)	Michael (Jordan)	Peyton (Manning)
Olympia (Scott-Richardson)	Moses (Malone)	Priest (Holmes)
Sheryl (Swoopes)	Patrick (Ewing)	Randy (Moss)
Simone (Edwards)	Scottie (Pippen)	Ray (Lewis)
Tai (Dillard)	Shaquille (O'Neal)	Tiki (Barber)
Tamicha (Jackson)	Spud (Webb)	Troy (Aikman)
Tangela (Smith)	Wilt (Chamberlain)	William ("The Refrigerator" Perry)
Tari (Phillips)	Yao (Ming)	Woody (Hayes)

Golfers

Female	Male
Amy (Alcott)	Arnold (Palmer)
Annika (Sorenstam)	Chi Chi (Rodriguez)
Babe (Didrikson Zaharias)	Claude (Harmon)
Beth (Daniel)	Craig (Stadler)
Betsy (King)	Eldrick ("Tiger" Woods)
Betty (Jameson)	Ernie (Els)
Carol (Mann)	Gene (Littler)
Dinah (Shore)	Greg (Norman)
Donna (Caponi)	Hale (Irwin)
Dottie (Pepper)	Happy (Gilmore)
Hollis (Stacy)	Harvey (Penick)
JoAnne (Carner)	Jack (Nicklaus)
Judy (Rankin)	Jeff (Maggert)
Juli (Inkster)	Jesper (Parnevik)
Karrie (Webb)	Ken (Venturi)
Kathy (Whitworth)	Nick (Price)
Laura (Davies)	Payne (Stewart)
Louise (Suggs)	Phil (Mickelson)
Marlene (Hagge)	Raymond (Floyd)
Michelle (Wie)	Retief (Goosen)
Nancy (Lopez)	Sam (Snead)
Pat (Bradley)	Sergio (Garcia)
Patty (Berg)	Tommy (Bolt)
Sandra (Haynie)	Vijay (Singh)
Se (Ri Pak)	Walter (Hagen)

Hockey Players

Male
Bobby (Orr)
Bret (Hull)
Dominik (Hasek)
Eric (Lindros)
Gordie (Howe)
Grant (Fuhr)
Jacques (Plante)
Jarome (Iginla)
Jaromir (Jagr)
Jeremy (Roenick)
Joe (Sakic)
Mario (Lemieux)
Mark (Messier)
Martin (Brodeur)
Maurice (Richard)
Mike (Modano)
Patrick (Roy)
Paul (Coffey)
Pavel (Bure)
Peter (Forsberg)
Phil (Esposito)
Ray (Bourque)
Sergei (Fedorov)
Steve (Yzerman)
Wayne (Gretzky)

Tennis Players

Female	Male
Amanda (Coetzer)	Alex (Corretja)
Amelie (Mauresmo)	Andre (Agassi)
Anna (Kournikova)	Andy (Roddick)
Anastasia (Myskina)	Arthur (Ashe)
Billie Jean (King)	Bill (Tilden)
Chris (Evert)	Bjorn (Borg)
Elena (Dementieva)	Boris (Becker)
Gabriela (Sabatini)	Carlos (Moya)
Jennifer (Capriati)	Greg (Rusedski)
Justine (Henin-Hardenne)	Guillermo (Coria)
Kim (Clijsters)	Gustavo (Kuerten)
Lindsay (Davenport)	Ivan (Lendl)
Maria (Sharapova)	James (Blake)
Martina (Navratilova)	Jimmy (Connors)
Mary (Pierce)	John (McEnroe)
Monica (Seles)	Juan Carlos (Ferrero)
Nadia (Petrova)	Lleyton (Hewitt)
Natasha (Zvereva)	Mark (Philippoussis)
Pam (Shriver)	Michael (Chang)
Serena (Williams)	Pete (Sampras)
Steffi (Graf)	Rod (Laver)
Svetlana (Kuznetsova)	Roger (Federer)
Tatiana (Golovin)	Stefan (Edberg)
Tracy (Austin)	Todd (Woodbridge)
Venus (Williams)	Tommy (Haas)

Olympians

Female	Male
Amanda (Beard)	Alberto (Tomba)
Bonnie (Blair)	Aleksandr (Popov)
Dominique (Dawes)	Alexei (Yagudin)
Dorothy (Hamill)	Bjørn (Dæhlie)
Dot (Richardson)	Brian (Boitano)
Florence (Griffith Joyner)	Carl (Lewis)
Inge (de Bruijn)	Dan (Jansen)
Irina (Slutskaya)	Dmitri (Bilozerchev)
Jackie (Joyner-Kersee)	Elvis (Stojko)
Janet (Evans)	Eric (Heiden)
Janica (Kostelic)	Gary (Hall, Jr.)
Katarina (Witt)	Greg (Louganis)
Kerri (Strug)	Hermann (Maier)
Kristi (Yamaguchi)	Ian (Thorpe)
Larissa (Latynina)	Ingemar (Stenmark)
Mary Lou (Retton)	Ivar (Ballangrud)
Nadia (Comaneci)	Jonny (Moseley)
Nancy (Kerrigan)	Kurt (Browning)
Oksana (Baiul)	Mark (Spitz)
Olga (Korbut)	Matt (Biondi)
Peggy (Fleming)	Michael (Phelps)
Shannon (Miller)	Paul (Hamm)
Summer (Sanders)	Scott (Hamilton)
Svetlana (Boguinskaya)	Stephan (Eberharter)
Tatyana (Gutsu)	Tamas (Darnyi)

Soccer Players	Boxers	Race Car Drivers
Female and Male	**Female and Male**	**Female and Male**
Alexi (Lalas)	Christy (Martin)	A. J. (Foyt)
Anders (Svensson)	Evander (Holyfield)	Al (Unser, Jr.)
April (Heinrichs)	Fernando (Vargas)	Ashton (Lewis)
Brandi (Chastain)	Floyd (Patterson)	Bill (Elliott)
Carlos (Alberto Torres)	George (Foreman)	Bobby (Labonte)
Cristiano (Ronaldo)	Jack (Dempsey)	Dale (Earnhardt)
David (Beckham)	Jake (LaMotta)	Danica (Patrick)
Dennis (Bergkamp)	Joe (Frazier)	Darrell (Waltrip)
Diego (Maradona)	Joe (Louis)	Jeff (Gordon)
Edson ("Pele"Arantes do Nascimento)	Julio (Cesar Chavez)	Jimmie (Johnson)
Filippo (Inzaghi)	Laila (Ali)	Jimmy (Spencer)
Freddy (Adu)	Larry (Holmes)	John (Andretti)
Gabriel (Batistuta)	Lennox (Lewis)	Justin (Ashburn)
Heather (Mitts)	Leon (Spinks)	Kasey (Kahne)
Jamie (Carragher)	Marvin (Hagler)	Kenny (Irwin)
Joy (Fawcett)	Max (Schmeling)	Kevin (Harvick)
Julie (Foudy)	Mike (Tyson)	Kyle (Petty)
Kristine (Lilly)	Muhammad (Ali)	Mario (Andretti)
Landon (Donovan)	Oscar (De La Hoya)	Matt (Kenseth)
Mia (Hamm)	Riddick (Bowe)	Richard (Petty)
Michael (Owen)	Roberto (Duran)	Ricky (Rudd)
Pavel (Nedved)	Rocky (Marciano)	Rusty (Wallace)
Raul (Gonzalez Blanco)	Roy (Jones, Jr.)	Sterling (Marlin)
Roberto (Baggio)	Sonny (Liston)	Terry (Labonte)
Shannon (Boxx)	"Sugar" Ray (Leonard)	Tony (Stewart)

Nature and Places

Coaches	Sportscasters	Flowers
Female and Male	**Female and Male**	**Female**
Arnold ("Red" Auerbach)	Al (Michaels)	Angelica
Bill (Parcells)	Bob (Uecker)	Calla
Billy (Martin)	Chick (Hern)	Dahlia
Bobby (Knight)	Chris (Berman)	Daisy
Casey (Stengel)	Dan (Patrick)	Fern
Dean (Smith)	Dick (Vitale)	Flora
Don (Shula)	Frank (Gifford)	Flower
Frank (Robinson)	Greg (Gumbel)	Holly
George (Halas)	Harry (Caray)	Hyacinth
Joe (Gibbs)	Howard (Cosell)	Iris
John (Madden)	Jack (Buck)	Jasmine
Knute (Rockne)	Jim (Nantz)	Laurel
Larry (Brown)	Joe (Buck)	Lavender
Mike (Krzyzewski)	John (Madden)	Lilac
Ozzie (Guillen)	Keith (Jackson)	Lily
Pat (Summit)	Kenny (Mayne)	Marigold
Paul ("Bear" Bryant)	Lesley (Visser)	Pansy
Pete (Rose)	Linda (Cohn)	Poppy
Phil (Jackson)	Marv (Alberts)	Posy
Rick (Pitino)	Mel (Allen)	Rose
Scotty (Bowman)	Pat (Summerall)	Sage
Tom (Landry)	Peter (Gammons)	Tulip
Tommy (Lasorda)	Robin (Roberts)	Verbena
Tony (Dungy)	Terry (Bradshaw)	Vine
Vince (Lombardi)	Vin (Scully)	Violet

Rocks, Gems, Minerals	Natural Elements		Celestial Terms
Female and Male	**Female**	**Male**	**Female and Male**
Beryl	Amber	Ash	Andromeda
Clay	Autumn	Branch	Antares
Coal	Breezy	Bud	Aries
Coral	Blossom	Burr	Cassiopeia
Crystal	Briar	Canyon	Castor
Diamond	Brook	Cliff	Cloud
Esmerelda	Delta	Crag	Corona
Flint	Gale	Dale	Draco
Garnet	Hailey	Eddy	Étoile
Gemma	Heather	Field	Leo
Goldie	Ivy	Ford	Luna
Jade	Marina	Forest	Moona
Jasper	Rain	Heath	Nova
Jewel	Rainbow	Lake	Orion
Mercury	Savannah	Marsh	Pollux
Mica	Sequoia	Moss	Rigel
Opal	Sierra	Oakes	Saturn
Pearl	Skye	Thorne	Scorpio
Rock	Star	Ridge	Skye
Ruby	Summer	River	Soleil
Sandy	Sunny	Rye	Star
Sapphire	Terra	Rock	Starling
Steele	Tempest	Stone	Sunny
Stone	Willow	Storm	Ursa
Topaz	Windy	Woody	Venus

Animals	Water-Themed Names	Places	
Female and Male	**Female and Male**	**Female**	**Male**
Billy	Bay	Africa	Afton
Birdie	Brooke	Asia	Austin
Buck	Chelsea	Brooklyn	Boston
Bunny	Delmar	Cheyenne	Chad
Cat	Delta	China	Cleveland
Colt	Dewey	Dakota	Cuba
Crane	Eddy	Florence	Dakota
Cricket	Ice	Georgia	Dallas
Drake	Lake	Holland	Denver
Fawn	Marin	India	Diego
Fox	Marina	Italia	Indiana
Hawk	Marisol	Jamaica	Israel
Jaguar	Meri	Kenya	Kent
Jay	Misty	Lourdes	Laramie
Joey	Nile	Madison	London
Kitty	Oceana	Montana	Montreal
Lark	Rain	Olympia	Nevada
Newt	Rio	Paris	Orlando
Phoenix	River	Regina	Phoenix
Raven	Seabert	Savannah	Reno
Robin	Spring	Siena	Rhodes
Starling	Storm	Sydney	Rio
Tiger	Tempest	Tijuana	Sydney
Wolf	Tigris	Victoria	Tennessee
Wren	Wade	Vienna	Washington

Trades

Trade Names	Leadership Titles	Inventors
Female and Male	**Female and Male**	**Female and Male**
Baker	Baron	Alexander (Graham Bell)
Butcher	Bishop	Alfred (Nobel)
Carver	Caesar	Ann (Tsukamoto)
Chandler	Chancellor	Benjamin (Franklin)
Cooper	Deacon	Bill (Gates)
Cutler	Duke	Eli (Whitney)
Draper	Earl	Galileo (Galilei)
Fletcher	Khan	George (Pullman)
Fowler	King	Guglielmo (Marchese Marconi)
Gardner	Lord	Henry (Ford)
Hunter	Major	James (Watt)
Marshall	Marquis	Johannes (Gutenberg)
Mason	Nagid	Levi (Strauss)
Miller	Oba	Louis (Braille)
Painter	Pasha	Nikola (Tesla)
Porter	Pharaoh	Orville (Wright)
Ranger	Priest	Robert (Fulton)
Sawyer	Prince	Ruth (Handler)
Scribe	Princess	Samuel (Morse)
Shepherd	Queen	Steve (Jobs)
Slater	Rabbi	Thomas (Edison)
Smith	Shah	Tim (Berners-Lee)
Stockman	Shaman	Virginia (Apgar)
Tailor	Sharif	Wilbur (Wright)
Tanner	Sultan	Willis (Carrier)

Scientists and Mathematicians

Female	Male
Alice (Hamilton)	Abraham (Maslow)
Anna (Freud)	Albert (Einstein)
Annie (Jump Cannon)	Alexander (Fleming)
Barbara (McClintock)	Blaise (Pascal)
Caroline (Herschel)	Carl (Jung)
Christine (Ladd-Franklin)	Charles (Darwin)
Dian (Fossey)	Claudius (Ptolemy)
Dorothy (Hodgkin)	Edward (Jenner)
Elizabeth (Blackwell)	Edwin (Hubble)
Emmy (Noether)	Galileo (Galilei)
Gertrude (Elion)	Gregor (Mendel)
Grace (Hopper)	Isaac (Newton)
Hildegard (von Bingen)	Jacques (Cousteau)
Ida (Henrietta Hyde)	James (Joule)
Jane (Goodall)	Jean (Piaget)
Katherine (Blodgett)	Johannes (Kepler)
Lise (Meitner)	Jonas (Salk)
Margaret (Mead)	Louis (Pasteur)
Maria (Agnesi)	Max (Planck)
Marie (Curie)	Michael (Faraday)
Mary (Leakey)	Nicolaus (Copernicus)
Rachel (Carson)	Niels (Bohr)
Rebecca (Cole)	Robert (Oppenheimer)
Sally (Ride)	Sigmund (Freud)
Sophie (Germain)	Stephen (Hawking)

Doctors and Nurses

Female and Male

Alexander (Fleming)

Anna (Howard Shaw)

Barbara (McClintock)

Benjamin (Spock)

Clara (Barton)

Claude (Bernard)

Doogie (Howser)

Dorothea (Dix)

Edward (Jenner)

Elizabeth (Blackwell)

Florence (Nightingale)

Henry (Jekyll)

Jack (Kevorkian)

James (Kildare)

John (Dolittle)

Joseph (Lister)

Leonard (McCoy)

Louis (Pasteur)

Mary (Edwards Walker)

Michaela (Quinn)

Phil (McGraw)

Sigmund (Freud)

Victor (Frankenstein)

William (Mayo)

Yuri (Zhivago)

Artists	Dancers and Choreographers	Fashion Designers
Female and Male	**Female and Male**	**Female and Male**
Andy (Warhol)	Agnes (de Mille)	Betsey (Johnson)
Ansel (Adams)	Ann (Miller)	Bill (Blass)
Claude (Monet)	Anna (Pavlova)	Calvin (Klein)
Edgar (Degas)	Bill ("Bojangles" Robinson)	Catherine (Malandrino)
Edward (Hopper)	Bob (Fosse)	Christian (Dior)
Frida (Kahlo)	Eleanor (Powell)	Cynthia (Rowley)
Henri (Matisse)	Fred (Astaire)	Diane (von Furstenberg)
Diego (Rivera)	Gene (Kelly)	Donna (Karan)
Georgia (O'Keeffe)	Ginger (Rogers)	Ellen (Tracy)
Gustav (Klimt)	Gower (Champion)	Emilio (Pucci)
Jackson (Pollock)	Gregory (Hines)	François (Girbaud)
Jasper (Johns)	Gwen (Verdon)	Gianni (Versace)
Leonardo (da Vinci)	Irene (Castle)	Giorgio (Armani)
Marc (Chagall)	José (Greco)	Hugo (Boss)
Mary (Cassatt)	Lew (Christensen)	Jimmy (Choo)
Michelangelo (Buonarroti)	Margot (Fonteyn)	Kenneth (Cole)
Norman (Rockwell)	Michael (Kidd)	Lilly (Pulitzer)
Pablo (Picasso)	Mikhail (Baryshnikov)	Louis (Vuitton)
Paul (Cézanne)	Natalia (Makarova)	Marc (Jacobs)
Rembrandt (van Rijn)	Ruby (Keeler)	Michael (Kors)
Robert (Mapplethorpe)	Rudolf (Nureyev)	Nicole (Miller)
Roy (Lichtenstein)	Susan (Stroman)	Oscar (de la Renta)
Salvador (Dali)	Tommy (Tune)	Ralph (Lauren)
Sandro (Botticelli)	Twyla (Tharp)	Tommy (Hilfiger)
Vincent (van Gogh)	Vernon (Castle)	Vera (Wang)

Models	Chefs and Cooks	Crime Fighters
Female	**Female and Male**	**Female and Male**
Alek (Wek)	Alain (Ducasse)	Allan (Pinkerton)
Alessandra (Ambrosio)	Alfred (Portale)	Andy (Sipowicz)
Amber (Valletta)	Alice (Waters)	Barnaby (Jones)
Bridget (Hall)	Bobby (Flay)	Barney (Miller)
Brooke (Shields)	Charlie (Palmer)	Chris (Cagney)
Carolyn (Murphy)	Delia (Smith)	Dana (Scully)
Cheryl (Tiegs)	Emeril (Lagasse)	Dave (Starsky)
Christie (Brinkley)	Eric (Ripert)	Dick (Tracy)
Christy (Turlington)	Gary (Danko)	Elliot (Ness)
Cindy (Crawford)	Gordon (Ramsay)	Fox (Mulder)
Claudia (Schiffer)	Heston (Blumenthal)	Harry ("Dirty Harry" Callahan)
Elle (MacPherson)	Jacques (Pépin)	Hercule (Poirot)
Elsa (Benitez)	Jamie (Oliver)	Sonny (Crockett)
Gisele (Bundchen)	Jean-George (Vongerichten)	Jane ("Miss" Marple)
Heidi (Klum)	Joël (Robuchon)	Jill (Munroe)
Helena (Christensen)	Josefina (Howard)	Joe (Friday)
Kate (Moss)	Julia (Child)	John Edgar (Hoover)
Laetitia (Casta)	Lidia (Bastianich)	Jules (Maigret)
Linda (Evangelista)	Mario (Batali)	Kelly (Garrett)
Naomi (Campbell)	Martin (Yan)	Ken ("Hutch" Hutchinson)
Niki (Taylor)	Nigella (Lawson)	Mary Beth (Lacey)
Rebecca (Romijn)	Nobu (Matsuhisa)	Sabrina (Duncan)
Shalom (Harlow)	Rachael (Ray)	Sam (Spade)
Stephanie (Seymour)	Todd (English)	Sherlock (Holmes)
Tyra (Banks)	Wolfgang (Puck)	Thomas (Magnum)

Lawyers and Judges	Tycoons
Female and Male	**Female and Male**
Byron (White)	Andrew (Carnegie)
Charles (Whittaker)	Aristotle (Onassis)
Clarence (Darrow)	Bill (Gates)
Constance (Baker Motley)	Charles (Foster Kane)
David (Kendall)	Cornelius (Vanderbilt)
Francis (Lee Bailey)	Donald (Trump)
Hugo (Black)	Estée (Lauder)
Jacques (Vergès)	Henry (Ford)
Jane (Bolin)	Howard (Hughes)
Johnnie (Cochran)	Hugh (Hefner)
Judy (Sheindlin)	Jay (Gatsby)
Kenneth (Starr)	John (Rockefeller)
Lance (Ito)	Martha (Stewart)
Marcia (Clark)	Michael (Dell)
Morgan (Chu)	Oliver ("Daddy" Warbucks)
Oliver (Wendell Holmes)	Oprah (Winfrey)
Perry (Mason)	Ray (Kroc)
Robert (Shapiro)	Richie (Rich)
Roger (Taney)	Ross (Perot)
Ruth (Ginsburg)	Sam (Walton)
Sandra (Day O'Connor)	Steve (Jobs)
Sarah (Weddington)	Ted (Turner)
Thurgood (Marshall)	Teresa (Heinz Kerry)
Warren (Burger)	Warren (Buffet)
William (Rehnquist)	William (Randolph Hearst)

Pop Culture

Notorious Celebrity Baby Names

Female and Male

Ahmet Emuukha Rodan (son of Frank and Gail Zappa)

Apple Blythe Alison (daughter of Gwyneth Paltrow and Chris Martin)

Audio Science (son of Shannyn Sossamon and Dallas Clayton)

Coco Riley (daughter of Courteney Cox Arquette and David Arquette)

Daisy Boo (daughter of Jamie and Jools Oliver)

Dweezil (son of Frank and Gail Zappa)

Elijah Bob Patricus Guggi Q (son of Bono and Alison Stewart)

Fifi Trixiebelle (daughter of Paula Yates and Bob Geldof)

Hazel Patricia (daughter of Julia Roberts and Danny Moder)

Heavenly Hirani Tiger Lily (daughter of Paula Yates and Michael Hutchence)

Lourdes Maria Ciccone (daughter of Madonna and Carlos Leon)

Moon Unit (daughter of Frank and Gail Zappa)

Moxie CrimeFighter (daughter of Penn and Emily Jillette)

Peaches Honeyblossom (daughter of Paula Yates and Bob Geldof)

Phinnaeus Walter (son of Julia Roberts and Danny Moder)

Pilot Inspektor (son of Jason Lee and Beth Riesgraf)

Pirate Howsmon (son of Jonathan and Deven Davis)

Poppy Honey (daughter of Jamie and Jools Oliver)

Prince Michael (son of Michael Jackson and Debbie Rowe)

Prince Michael II (son of Michael Jackson)

Rocco (son of Madonna and Guy Ritchie)

Rumer Glenn (daughter of Demi Moore and Bruce Willis)

Scout LaRue (daughter of Demi Moore and Bruce Willis)

Seven Sirius (son of Andre 3000 and Erykah Badu)

Tallulah Belle (daughter of Demi Moore and Bruce Willis)

One-Name Wonders

Female and Male

Ann-Margret

Beck

Björk

Bono

Brandy

Cher

Dido

Enya

Fabio

Iman

Jewel

Liberace

Madonna

Moby

Nelly

Pelé

Prince

Roseanne

Sade

Seal

Shakira

Sinbad

Tiffany

Twiggy

Yanni

Famous People Known by Initials

Female and Male

A. A. (Milne)

A. E. (Housman)

A. J. (Foyt)

B. J. (Thomas)

C. S. (Lewis)

D. B. (Cooper)

D. H. (Lawrence)

E. E. (Cummings)

E. M. (Forster)

J. D. (Salinger)

J. K. (Rowling)

J. M. (Barrie)

J. P. (Morgan)

J. R. R. (Tolkien)

L. M. (Montgomery)

O. J. (Simpson)

P. J. (Harvey)

P. J. (O'Rourke)

P. T. (Barnum)

T. S. (Eliot)

V. C. (Andrews)

V. I. (Lennin)

W. C. (Fields)

W. E. B. (DuBois)

Y. A. (Tittle)

Brand Names

Female and Male

Avis

Chanel

Delmonte

Delta

Disney

Espn

Evian

Fanta

Godiva

Gucci

Guinness

Harley

Hennessy

Hyatt

Ikea

Jemima

Levi

Nike

Nivea

Oneida

Pepsi

Shasta

Stetson

Timberland

Velveeta

Cars

Female and Male

Audi

Avalon

Bentley

Camry

Chevy

Dakota

Diamante

Ford

Infiniti

Jaguar

Jetta

Kia

Lexus

Liberty

Lincoln

Lotus

Maverick

Maxima

Mercedes

Montero

Ram

Rover

Sedona

Sienna

Wrangler

Other Ideas for Names

Food and Beverages	Last Names as First Names
Female and Male	**Female and Male**
Alfredo	Anderson
Basil	Bradshaw
Brandy	Carter
Brie	Chavez
Candy	Chen
Chardonnay	Foster
Clementine	Gallagher
Curry	Garcia
Dill	Harper
Gin	Jackson
Ginger	Johnson
Ham	Keaton
Herb	Kennedy
Honey	Mackenzie
Kale	Madison
Margarita	Meyer
Midori	Parker
Olive	Patterson
Pepper	Ramsey
Pita	Rodriguez
Rosemary	Sanchez
Rye	Taylor
Saffron	Tennyson
Sage	Walker
Sherry	Wang

Double Names			Easily Shortened Names	
Female	**Male**		**Female**	**Male**
Anne-Marie	Aaronjames		Abigail	Andrew
Billie-Jean	Billijo		Angela	Anthony
Billie-Jo	Giancarlo		Barbara	Benjamin
Bobbi-Jo	Gianluca		Caroline	Christopher
Bobbi-Lee	Gianpaolo		Christine	Daniel
Brandy-Lynn	Jaylee		Deborah	Donald
Brooklyn	Jayquan		Elizabeth	Edward
Carolanne	Jean-Claude		Gwendolyn	Frederick
Clarabelle	Jean-Luc		Jacqueline	Gregory
Emmylou	Jean-Paul		Jennifer	Jacob
Hollyann	Jean-Sebastien		Jessica	Jeffery
Jody-Ann	Jimmyjo		Jillian	Jonathan
Julie-Anne	John-Paul		Josephine	Joseph
Katelyn	Joseluis		Katherine	Kenneth
Kellyann	Juancarlos		Lillian	Leonardo
Krystalynn	Kendarius		Margaret	Michael
Leeann	Keyshawn		Nicole	Nicholas
Mary-Kate	Markanthony		Pamela	Peter
Marylou	Michaelangelo		Rebecca	Richard
Raeann	Miguelangel		Samantha	Robert
Raelynn	Quindarius		Stephanie	Samuel
Roseanne	Rayshawn		Suzanne	Thomas
Ruthann	Tedrick		Valerie	Timothy
Saralyn	Tyquan		Victoria	Walter
Terry-Lynn	Tyshawn		Vivian	William

Names Based on Letters	Names Based on Numbers	Virtue Names
Female and Male	**Female and Male**	**Female**
Ajay	Decimus	Amity
Alpha	Deuce	Blythe
Bea	Dixie	Charity
Bebe	Nona	Chastity
Bee	Octavia	Constance
Beta	Octavious	Faith
Cee	Osen	Felicity
Ceejay	Primo	Fidelity
Dee	Quartilla	Grace
Dee Dee	Quentin	Harmony
Delta	Quincy	Honora
Elle	Quintana	Hope
Em	Reva	Innocence
Gigi	Septima	Joy
Jay	Septimus	Justice
Jaycee	Sextus	Love
Jaydee	Tan	Mercy
Kay	Tertia	Modesty
Kaycee	Tertius	Passion
Kaydee	Trent	Patience
Ojay	Trey	Prudence
Omega	Triana	Purity
Theta	Trinity	Temperance
Vijay	Una	Unity
Zeta	Uno	Verity

Names with Punctuation	Palindrome Names	Anagram Names		
Female and Male	**Female and Male**	**Female**	**Male**	**Male, Female**
'Aolani	Ada	Adria, Daria	Alec, Cale	Abe, Bea
'Aulani	Anna	Aileen, Elaine	Andrei, Darien	Aden, Edna
'Aziz	Ara	Alice, Celia	Andres, Sander	Adlar, Darla
A'lexus	Asa	Alli, Lila	Arnold, Ronald	Agni, Gina
Bre-Anne	Ava	Amy, Mya	Blake, Kaleb	Amir, Mira
D'andre	Aviva	Anise, Siena	Byron, Robyn	Amos, Soma
D'angelo	Aya	Ann, Nan	Chaz, Zach	Belamy, Maybel
D'Arcy	Aziza	April, Pilar	Darnell, Randell	Brady, Darby
D'onna	Bob	Ashanti, Tanisha	Daryn, Randy	Brion, Robin
D'quan	Davad	Ashlee, Sheela	Enzo, Zeno	Clay, Lacy
Da'shawn	Elle	Blaise, Isabel	Eric, Rice	Daly, Lyda
Da-juan	Emme	Dana, Nada	Ernest, Nester	Dashaun, Shaunda
Dan'l	Eve	Diana, Nadia	Jason, Jonas	Dylan, Lynda
Da-Ron	Hallah	Easter, Teresa	Kale, Lake	Edwyn, Wendy
Ja'lisa	Hannah	Elsa, Sela	Leo, Ole	Etta, Tate
Ja'nae	Idi	Gem, Meg	Mason, Osman	Hale, Leah
Ja'von	Iggi	Gina, Inga	Moore, Romeo	Ian, Nia
Jac-E	Lil	Hallie, Leilah	Nero, Reno	Jason, Sonja
Jo-Anna	Nan	Lena, Nela	Percy, Pryce	Karl, Lark
Mahi'ai	Natan	Leta, Teal	Roth, Thor	Kory, York
N'namdi	Nayan	Marta, Tamra	Royce, Corey	Leon, Noel
O'Shea	Olo	Mary, Myra	Ryder, Derry	Liam, Mila
O'neil	Otto	Nita, Tina	Santo, Aston	Rico, Cori
Ra'shawn	Pip	Norah, Rhona	Seaton, Easton	Ryker, Kerry
T'keyah	Viv	Sita, Tisa	Thane, Ethan	Sayid, Daisy

Rhyming Names

Female	Male	Female, Male
Addison, Madison	Aaron, Darren	Bessie, Jesse
Alyssa, Melissa	Abe, Gabe	Beth, Seth
Ann, Jan	Ace, Chase	Brandy, Randy
Anna, Hannah	Aidan, Jaiden	Cady, Brady
Candy, Mandy	Alvin, Calvin	Cleo, Leo
Carolyn, Marilyn	Barrett, Garrett	Doris, Morris
Celia, Delia	Barry, Larry	Erin, Darren
Chloe, Zoe	Brandon, Landon	Gayle, Dale
Ellen, Helen	Brian, Ryan	Grace, Chase
Erin, Karen	Cade, Jade	Gwen, Ken
Gracie, Stacie	Chance, Lance	Jeanne, Dean
Jane, Elaine	Cody, Brody	Jen, Ben
Jen, Gwen	Craig, Greg	Jodie, Cody
Kailey, Bailey	Devin, Evan	Joy, Roy
Karen, Sharon	Donald, Ronald	Kamie, Jamey
Lori, Tori	Dustin, Justin	Kate, Nate
Mae, Rae	Eric, Derek	Kay, Jay
Maura, Laura	Frank, Hank	Kim, Tim
Molly, Holly	Heath, Keith	Lori, Corey
Rhonda, Shonda	Hogan, Logan	Mandy, Andy
Sara, Kara	Jack, Mack	Mariah, Josiah
Sherry, Carrie	Jake, Blake	Mary, Harry
Stella, Bella	Jason, Mason	Millie, Billy
Valerie, Mallory	Phil, Will	Paige, Gage
Winnie, Minnie	Sean, John	Zoe, Joey

Old-Fashioned Names Now Popular

Female	Male
Abigail	Abraham
Alice	Alexander
Anna	Dominic
Ava	Elijah
Caroline	Ethan
Claire	Gabriel
Claudia	Hector
Elizabeth	Isaac
Emily	Isaiah
Emma	Ivan
Evelyn	Jasper
Grace	Julian
Hannah	Maxwell
Hazel	Nathaniel
Isabella	Noah
Katherine	Omar
Leslie	Oscar
Madeline	Owen
Margaret	Samuel
Maria	Sebastian
Olivia	Vernon
Rebecca	Vincent
Sarah	Wesley
Sofia	Xavier
Victoria	Zachary

Fun Nicknames		One-Syllable Names		Two-Syllable Names	
Female	**Male**	**Female**	**Male**	**Female**	**Male**
Anka	Binky	Ann	Blake	Anna	Ashton
Babs	Buddy	Bea	Chad	Ashley	Brian
Bertie	Chaz	Belle	Chen	Ava	Christian
Biddy	Che	Brie	Drew	Carmen	Dante
Birdie	Chip	Chai	Gabe	Carrie	David
Buffy	Danno	Cher	Hugh	Cheyenne	Dylan
Bunny	Deano	Claire	Jack	Chloe	Eric
Coco	Fonzie	Dawn	Jake	Diane	Garrett
Dodie	Fritz	Eve	John	Emma	Jacob
Fannie	Gino	Gayle	Juan	Heidi	Jesse
Fifi	Jimbo	Gwen	Lee	Jada	Jordan
Flo	Jobo	Jade	Luke	Jasmine	Joseph
Gigi	Joop	Jane	Max	Jody	Landon
Ginger	Junior	Jill	Paul	Juana	Latrell
Hattie	Kit	Kate	Pierce	Kaitlyn	Luis
Jas	Lucky	Lane	Raj	Kayla	Maddox
Kiki	Mango	Ling	Ralph	Leah	Matthew
Kitty	Paco	Lynn	Reece	Mary	Michael
Madge	Paddy	Mae	Sage	Maura	Miguel
Sissy	Pepe	Maude	Spence	Megan	Noah
Steffi	Pinky	Paige	Tad	Rachel	Owen
Stevie	Rafi	Rose	Tate	Rosa	Ryan
Tottie	Rollo	Rue	Todd	Sadie	Sanjay
Trixie	Skip	Skye	Wade	Sydney	William
Xuxa	Ziggy	Trish	Will	Zoe	Wyatt

Three-Syllable Names		Four-Syllable Names		Names of Famous Pairs
Female	**Male**	**Female**	**Male**	**Female and Male**
Aaliyah	Adrian	Alejandra	Alejandro	Adam and Eve
Andrea	Anthony	Anastasia	Antonio	Amos and Andy
Brianna	Benjamin	Angelina	Aristotle	Bert and Ernie
Claudia	Christopher	Arianna	Bartholomew	Bill and Ted
Desirae	Deondre	Carolina	Benicio	Bonnie and Clyde
Emily	Diego	Damonica	Cornelius	Brooks and Dunn
Evelyn	Dominic	Dominica	Deanthony	Cain and Abel
Gloria	Elijah	Eleanora	Demetrius	Castor and Pollux
Gwendolyn	Francisco	Elizabeth	Ebenezer	David and Goliath
Jacqueline	Gabriel	Evangeline	Ezekiel	Dick and Jane
Kimberly	Gregory	Frederica	Geronimo	Ebony and Ivory
Lakeisha	Isaiah	Gabriella	Giovanni	Hansel and Gretel
Mackenzie	Jeremy	Guadalupe	Immanuel	Jack and Jill
Madeline	Jonathan	Isabella	Indiana	Lancelot and Guenevere
Madison	Joshua	Josephina	Jebediah	Laurel and Hardy
Makayla	Julian	Julianna	Jeremiah	Laverne and Shirley
Olivia	Marcellus	Katarina	Leonardo	Lewis and Clark
Pamela	Mathias	Penelope	Macallister	Mario and Luigi
Rhiannon	Muhammad	Samuela	Napolean	Milo and Otis
Sierra	Nathaniel	Serafina	Odysseus	Romeo and Juliet
Sophia	Nicholas	Serenity	Quindarius	Romy and Michele
Stephanie	Orlando	Tatiana	Santiago	Samson and Delilah
Sylvia	Sebastian	Valentina	Thelonius	Siegfried and Roy
Tabitha	Timothy	Veronica	Valentino	Sonny and Cher
Vanessa	Tobias	Victoria	Zachariah	Thelma and Louise

Names Ending with "A"		Names Ending with "E"		Names Ending with "L"	
Female	**Male**	**Female**	**Male**	**Female**	**Male**
Alexandra	Abdula	Angie	Abe	Abigail	Abdul
Amanda	Akiva	Ashlee	Andre	Angel	Abel
Amelia	Aquila	Bette	Blake	April	Carl
Andrea	Baptista	Brooke	Blaze	Ariel	Cyrill
Brianna	Barretta	Chloe	Boone	Bell	Daniel
Carmela	Bela	Claire	Cole	Carol	Darrell
Fiona	Bubba	Gabrielle	Dale	Chantal	Denzel
Gabriella	Columbia	Grace	George	Crystal	Earl
Jana	Cuba	Jane	Ike	Ethel	Emmanuel
Julia	Dakota	Jasmine	Jade	Gail	Gabriel
Kayla	Dana	Josie	Jake	Hazel	Hershel
Kendra	Daytona	Julie	Jerome	Isabel	Jamal
Maria	Elisha	Juliette	Jesse	Jewel	Joel
Mia	Ezra	Kate	Jose	Jill	Lionel
Michaela	Garcia	Kylie	Jude	Laurel	Marshall
Pamela	Indiana	Belle	Kayne	Mabel	Maxwell
Roxanna	Joshua	Marie	Lane	Meryl	Michael
Sara	Krishna	Nicole	Lee	Muriel	Nathaniel
Selma	Luca	Paige	Louie	Nell	Neil
Sonja	Montana	Rose	Mike	Noel	Paul
Sophia	Mustafa	Sadie	Ozzie	Pearl	Phil
Tyra	Nevada	Stephanie	Pierre	Rachel	Russell
Uma	Santana	Winnie	Reece	Sheryl	Samuel
Viola	Shea	Yvonne	Vince	Sybil	Terrell
Wanda	Zacharia	Zoe	Zebedee	Val	Will

Names Ending in "N"		Names Ending with "O"		Names Ending with "R"	
Female	**Male**	**Female**	**Male**	**Female**	**Male**
Allison	Aidan	Aiko	Alberto	Amber	Alexander
Ann	Alan	Bayo	Alejandro	Blair	Arthur
Ashlyn	Ashton	Calypso	Alfonzo	Briar	Carter
Autumn	Benjamin	Cameo	Angelo	Cedar	Chandler
Caitlin	Colin	Charo	Antonio	Cher	Christopher
Carmen	Darren	Cleo	Benicio	Easter	Connor
Ellen	Donovan	Clio	Bo	Eleanor	Evander
Erin	Evan	Coco	Bruno	Ester	Homer
Fran	Flynn	Domino	Carlo	Ginger	Hunter
Gwendolyn	Hayden	Doro	Cisco	Harper	Jasper
Jillian	Holden	Echo	Eduardo	Heather	Junior
Karen	Ian	Flo	Falco	Jennifer	Oliver
Kathryn	Jordan	Gerardo	Fredo	Kashmir	Oscar
Kirsten	Justin	Indigo	Georgio	Kimber	Parker
Lauren	Keenan	Jo	Leo	Lavender	Peter
Lillian	Kevin	Juno	Marco	Pier	River
Magdalen	Llewellyn	Kameko	Mario	Pilar	Roger
Megan	Logan	Koto	Mo	Piper	Sawyer
Morgan	Marvin	Mariko	Orlando	September	Spencer
Reagan	Mason	Marlo	Pablo	Skyler	Trevor
Rosalyn	Nathan	Maryjo	Pedro	Star	Tyler
Shannon	Quentin	Orino	Sancho	Summer	Victor
Teagan	Steven	Ryo	Theo	Taylor	Walker
Vivian	Tristan	Tamiko	Waldo	Tipper	Walter
Yasmin	Warren	Yoko	Yao	Zephyr	Xavier

Names Ending with "Y"		Names Inspired by "Ann"	Names Inspired by "Elizabeth"	Names Inspired by "Jacob"
Female	**Male**	**Female**	**Female**	**Male**
Ashley	Anthony	Ana	Bess	Akiva
Audrey	Bailey	Anci	Beth	Chago
Becky	Barry	Anezka	Betsy	Coby
Bethany	Bradley	Anica	Betty	Diego
Carly	Cody	Anik	Elisa	Giacomo
Courtney	Corey	Anisha	Elise	Iago
Dorothy	Darcy	Anissa	Elizabet	Iakobos
Ebony	Farley	Anita	Elizaveta	Jack
Emily	Gary	Anja	Elizebeth	Jaco
Felicity	Gordy	Anka	Elka	Jacobi
Hailey	Hardy	Anna	Elsa	Jacobo
Jenny	Huey	Annabel	Ilse	Jacobson
Josey	Humphrey	Annah	Libby	Jacorey
Kelsey	Jeffrey	Annaliese	Liese	Jacques
Lily	Jeremey	Anne	Liesel	Jaime
Mallory	Jerry	Anneka	Lisa	Jake
Molly	Koby	Annette	Lisabeth	Jakob
Polly	Manny	Annie	Liset	James
Shelly	Ozzy	Annika	Lissie	Jock
Sidney	Randy	Anya	Liz	Kobe
Stacy	Riley	Hannah	Liza	Kuba
Tiffany	Roy	Nan	Lizabeta	Tiago
Wendy	Timothy	Nancy	Lizbeth	Yakov
Whitney	Westley	Nanette	Lizzie	Yasha
Zoey	Zachary	Nina	Yelisbeta	Yoakim

Names Inspired by "Jane"	Names Inspired by "John"	Names Inspired by "Joseph"	Names Inspired by "Katherine"
Female	**Male**	**Male**	**Female**
Chavon	Evan	Beppe	Caitlin
Ciana	Gian	Che	Cassie
Giovanna	Handel	Cheche	Cat
Jalena	Hans	Chepe	Catherine
Jan	Ian	Giuseppe	Catheryn
Jana	Ivan	Iokepa	Cathleen
Janae	Jack	Iosif	Cathy
Janelle	Jan	Jobo	Catrina
Janessa	Janek	Jody	Catriona
Janet	Jean	Joe	Ekaterina
Janica	Jens	Joeseph	Kari
Janice	Joao	Joey	Kasen
Janie	Johann	Joop	Kasia
Janiqua	John Paul	José	Katalina
Jasa	Johnson	Josef	Kate
Jasia	Jon	Jupp	Katelyn
Jean	Jonas	Osip	Kathleen
Jenine	Jonathan	Pepa	Kathlyn
Juana	Jones	Pepe	Kathryn
Maryjane	Jonny	Peppe	Kathy
Seana	Jovan	Pino	Katia
Shana	Juan	Sepp	Katie
Sinead	Sean	Yeska	Katja
Zanna	Yanni	Yosef	Katrina
Zhane	Zane	Zeusef	Kay

Names Inspired by "Margaret"	Names Inspired by "Mary"	Names Inspired by "Michael"	Names Inspired by "Peter"
Female	**Female**	**Male**	**Male**
Gita	Maija	Carmichael	Boutros
Greta	Mara	Demichael	Ferris
Gretchen	Mare	Machas	Panos
Gretl	Maren	Makel	Parnell
Madge	Mari	Mhichael	Pearson
Maggie	Maria	Micael	Peder
Maisey	Mariah	Micah	Pedro
Mamie	Marian	Michaelangelo	Peers
Maretta	Mariana	Michel	Pekelo
Margarita	Maribel	Mick	Per
Margaux	Maribeth	Mickey	Perico
Marge	Marice	Migel	Perkin
Margery	Marie	Miguel	Perry
Margie	Mariel	Mihail	Pete
Margo	Marietta	Mika	Peterson
Marguerite	Marigold	Mike	Petr
Marjorie	Marika	Mikel	Petru
Markita	Molara	Mikhail	Petter
Meg	Marilyn	Mikko	Pier
Megan	Marjorie	Miles	Pierce
Meta	Maura	Milko	Piero
Peg	Maureen	Misael	Pierre
Peggy	Miriam	Miska	Pierson
Reet	Molly	Mitchell	Pieter
Rita	Muriel	Mychael	Takis

Names Inspired by "William"

Male

Bill

Billy

Guglielmo

Guilherme

Guillaume

Guillermo

Gwilym

Liam

Uilliam

Vasyl

Vilhelm

Viljo

Welfel

Wilek

Wilhelm

Wilkins

Wilkinson

Will

Willem

Williams

Willie

Willis

Wills

Wilson

Wylie

Star Kids
What Celebrities Are Naming Their Kids

Ahmet Emuukha Rodan
son of Frank and Gail Zappa

Aidan Rose
daughter of Faith Daniels

Alaia
daughter of Stephen and Kenya Baldwin

Alexandrina Zahra Jones
daughter of David Bowie and Iman Abdulmajid

Alizeh Keshvar
daughter of Geena Davis and Reza Jarrahy

Allegra
daughter of John Leguizamo and Justine Maurer

Apple Blythe Alison
daughter of Gwyneth Paltrow and Chris Martin

Aquinnah Kathleen
daughter of Tracy Pollan and Michael J. Fox

Arpad Flynn
son of Elle Macpherson and Arpad Busson

Atherton Grace
daughter of Don and Kelley Johnson

Atticus
son of Isabella Hoffman and Daniel Baldwin

Audio Science
son of Shannyn Sossamon and Dallas Clayton

August Anna
daughter of Garth Brooks and Sandy Mahl

Aurelius Cy Andre
son of Elle Macpherson and Arpad Busson

Ava Elizabeth
daughter of Reese Witherspoon and Ryan Phillippe

Bailey
son of Tracey Gold and Roby Marshall

Bailey Jean
daughter of Melissa Etheridge and Julie Cypher

Bechet
daughter of Woody Allen and Soon-Yi Previn

Braison Chance
son of Billy Ray and Tish Cyrus

Brawley King
son of Nick Nolte and Rebecca Linger

Brooklyn Joseph
son of Victoria "Posh Spice" Adams and David Beckham

Cannon Edward
son of Larry King and Shawn Southwick-King

Carys
daughter of Catherine Zeta-Jones and Michael Douglas

Cash Anthony
son of Saul "Slash" and Perla Hudson

Casper
son of Claudia Schiffer and Matthew Vaughn

Castor
son of James and Francesca Hetfield

Coco Riley
daughter of Courteney Cox Arquette and David Arquette

Cruz
son of Victoria "Posh Spice" Adams and David Beckham

Cypress
daughter of Solé

Daisy-Boo
daughter of Jamie and Jools Oliver

Dandelion
daughter of Keith Richards and Anita Pallenberg

Darius
son of James Rubin and Christiane Amanpour

Deacon
son of Reese Witherspoon and Ryan Phillippe

Declyn Wallace
son of Cyndi Lauper and David Thornton

De'jan
daughter of Solé

Delilah Belle
daughter of Harry Hamlin and Lisa Rinna

Denim
son of Toni Braxton and Keri Lewis

Destry Allyn
daughter of Kate Capshaw and Steven Spielberg

Devo
son of Maynard James Keenan

Dexter Dean
daughter of Diane Keaton

Dhani
son of George and Olivia Harrison

Diezel
son of Toni Braxton and Keri Lewis

Diva Muffin
daughter of Frank and Gail Zappa

Dominik
daughter of Andy and Maria Victoria Garcia

Dream Sarae
daughter of Ginuwine and Solé

Dree Louise
daughter of Mariel Hemingway and Stephen Crisman

Duncan Zowie Heywood
son of David Bowie and Mary Angela Barnett

Dusti Rain
daughter of Rob "Vanilla Ice" and Laura Van Winkle

Dweezil
son of Frank and Gail Zappa

Dylan Frances
daughter of Sean and Robin Wright Penn

Elijah Bob Patricus Guggi Q
son of Alison Stewart and Bono

Eliot Pauline
son of Sting and Trudie Styler

Emerson Rose
daughter of Teri Hatcher and Jon Tenney

Enzo
son of Patricia Arquette and Paul Rossi

Esme
daughter of Samantha Morton and Charlie Creed-Miles

Fifi Trixiebelle
daughter of Paula Yates and Bob Geldof

Frances Bean
daughter of Kurt Cobain and Courtney Love

Freedom
daughter of Ving Rhames and Deborah Reed

Fushcia Katherine
daughter of Sting and Frances Tomelty

Gaia
daughter of Emma Thompson and Greg Wise

God'iss Love
daughter of Lil' Mo and Al Stone

Gracie Katherine
daughter of Faith Hill and Tim McGraw

Gulliver Flynn
son of Gary Oldman and Donya Fiorentino

Hazel Patricia
daughter of Julia Roberts and Danny Moder

Heavenly Hirani Tiger Lily
daughter of Paula Yates and Michael Hutchence

Henry Guenther Ademola Dashtu
son of Heidi Klum and Seal

Homer James Jigme
son of Richard Gere and Carey Lowell

Hopper
son of Sean Penn and Robin Wright Penn

Hudson Harden
son of Marcia Gay Harden and Thaddeus Scheel

Indianna August
daughter of Summer Phoenix and Casey Affleck

Indio
son of Deborah Falconer and Robert Downey, Jr.

Ireland Eliesse
daughter of Kim Basinger and Alec Baldwin

Jack John Christopher
son of Johnny Depp and Vanessa Paradis

Jamison
daughter of Billy Baldwin and Chynna Phillips

Jelani Asar
son of Wesley and April Snipes

Jesse James
son of Jon and Dorothea Bon Jovi

Jett
son of Kelly Preston and John Travolta

Joaquin
son of Kelly Ripa and Mark Consuelos

Julian Murray
son of Lisa Kudrow and Michel Stern

Julitta Dee
daughter of Marcia Gay Harden and Thaddeus Scheel

Kaiis Steven
son of Geena Davis and Reza Jarrahy

Kal-El
son of Nicolas Cage and Alice Kim

Karsen
daughter of Ray Liotta and Michelle Grace

Keelee Breeze
daughter of Rob "Vanilla Ice" and Laura Van Winkle

Kian William
son of Geena Davis and Reza Jarrahy

Kyd Miller
son of David Duchovny and Téa Leoni

Langley Fox
daughter of Mariel Hemingway and Stephen Crisman

Lennon
son of Patsy Kensit and Liam Gallagher

Letesha
daughter of Tracy "Ice-T" and Darlene Morrow

Lily-Rose Melody
daughter of Johnny Depp and Vanessa Paradis

Loewy
son of John Malkovich and Nicoletta Peyran

Lola Rose
daughter of Charlie Sheen and Denise Richards

Lola Simone
daughter of Chris and Malaak Rock

London Emilio
son of Saul "Slash" and Perla Hudson

Lourdes Maria Ciccone
daughter of Madonna and Carlos Leon

Lyric
daughter of Karla De Vito and Robby Benson

Maddox
son of Angelina Jolie

Madeleine West
daughter of David Duchovny and Tea Leoni

Maggie Elizabeth
daughter of Faith Hill and Tim McGraw

Magnus Paulin
son of Will Ferrell and Viveca Paulin

Makena'lei
daughter of Helen Hunt and Matthew Carnahan

Malu Valentine
daughter of David Byrne and Adelle Lutz

Manzie Tio
daughter of Woody Allen and Soon-Yi Previn

Matalin Mary
daughter of Mary Matalin and James Carville

McCanna
son of Gary Sinise and Moira Harris

McKenna Lane
daughter of Mary Lou Retton and Shannon Kelly

Memphis Eve
daughter of Alison Stewart and Bono

Milo
son of Camryn Manheim

Milo William
son of Liv Tyler and Royston Langdon

Mingus Lucien
son of Helena Christensen and Norman Reedus

Moon Unit
daughter of Frank and Gail Zappa

Moxie CrimeFighter
daughter of Penn and Emily Jillette

Najee
son of James "LL Cool J" and Simone Smith

Nala
daughter of Keenan Ivory Wayans and Daphne Polk

Natashya Lorien
daughter of Tori Amos and Mark Hawley

Nathan Thomas
son of Jon and Tracey Stewart

Nayib
son of Gloria and Emilio Estefan

Neve
daughter of Conan O'Brien and Liza Powell O'Brien

Ocean Alexander
son of Forest Whitaker

Paris
son of Blair Underwood and Desiree DeCosta

Paris Michael Katherine
daughter of Michael Jackson and Debbie Rowe

Peaches Honeyblossom
daughter of Paula Yates and Bob Geldof

Phinnaeus Walter
son of Julia Roberts and Danny Moder

Phoenix Chi
daughter of Melanie "Scary Spice" Brown and Jimmy Gulzar

Pilot Inspektor
son of Jason Lee and Beth Riesgraf

Piper Maru
daughter of Gillian Anderson and Clyde Klotz

Pirate Howsmon
son of Jonathan and Deven Davis

Pixie
daughter of Paula Yates and Bob Geldof

Poet Sienna Rose
daughter of Soleil Moon Frye and Jason Goldberg

Poppy Honey
daughter of Jamie and Jools Oliver

Presley Tanita
daughter of Tanya Tucker and Jerry Laseter

Presley Walker
son of Cindy Crawford and Rande Gerber

Prince Michael
son of Michael Jackson and Debbie Rowe

Prince Michael II (a.k.a. Blanket)
son of Michael Jackson

Puma
daughter of Erykah Badu

Rainie
daughter of Andie MacDowell and Paul Qualley

Reignbeau
daughter of Ving Rhames and Deborah Reed

Rio Kelly
son of Sean Young and Robert Lujan

Ripley
daughter of Oliver Parker and Thandie Newton

Roan
son of Sharon Stone and Phil Bronstein

Rocco
son of Madonna and Guy Ritchie

Roman Robert
son of Cate Blanchett and Andrew Upton

Rory
son of Bill Gates and Melinda French

Rumer Glenn
daughter of Demi Moore and Bruce Willis

Ryan Elizabeth
daughter of Rodney and Holly Robinson Peete

Ryder Russel
son of Kate Husdon and Chris Robinson

Saffron Sahara
daughter of Simon Le Bon and Yasmin Parvaneh

Sailor Lee
daughter of Christie Brinkley and Peter Cook

Salome Violetta
daughter of Alex Kingston and Florian Haertel

Sam J.
daughter of Charlie Sheen and Denise Richards

Saoirse Roisin
daughter of Courtney Kennedy and Paul Hill

Satchel Lewis
daughter of Spike Lee and Tonya Linette Lewis

Schuyler Frances
daughter of Tracy Pollan and Michael J. Fox

Scout LaRue
daughter of Demi Moore and Bruce Willis

Sean Preston
son of Britney Spears and Kevin Federline

Selah Louise
daughter of Lauryn Hill and Rohan Marley

Seven Sirius
son of Andre 3000 and Erykah Badu

Sindri
son of Björk and Thor Eldon

Sistine Rose
daughter of Jennifer Flavin and Sylvester Stallone

Slade Lucas Moby
son of David Brenner and Elizabeth Bryan Slater

Sonnet Noel
daughter of Forest and Keisha Whitaker

Sosie Ruth
daughter of Kyra Sedgwick and Kevin Bacon

Speck Wildhorse
son of John and Elaine Mellencamp

Story
daughter of Ginuwine and Solé

Sy'Rai
daughter of Brandy Norwood and Robert Smith

Tali
daughter of Annie Lennox and Uri Fruchtman

Tallulah Belle
daughter of Demi Moore and Bruce Willis

Taylor Mayne Pearl
daughter of Garth Brooks and Sandy Mahl

True
daughter of Forest and Keisha Whitaker

Truman Theodore
son of Rita Wilson and Tom Hanks

Tu Simone Ayer Morrow
daughter of Rob Morrow and Debbon Ayer

Vance Alexander
son of Billy Baldwin and Chyna Phillips

Weston
son of Nicolas Cage and Kristina Fulton

Willow
daughter of Will Smith and Jada Pinkett Smith

Wolfgang William
son of Eddie Van Halen and Valerie Bertinelli

Zahra Savannah
daughter of Chris and Malaak Rock

Zelda
daughter of Robin Williams and Marsha Garces Williams

Zephyr
son of Karla De Vito and Robby Benson

Zion David
son of Lauryn Hill and Rohan Marley

The Name Exchange

Historical/Political Figures
Professional Name ....Original Name

Johnny Appleseed...........................John Chapman
Sitting Bull....................................Tatanka Iyotake
Calamity Jane ....Martha Jane Burke
Butch Cassidy................................Robert LeRoy Parker
Gerald Ford ....Leslie Lynch King, Jr.
Mata Hari.....................................Margareth Geertruide Zelle
Gary Hart ....Gary Hartpence
Crazy Horse ....Tashuna-Uitco
Sundance Kid................................Harry Longbaugh
Nancy Reagan ....Anne Frances Robbins
Leon Trotsky.................................Lev Davydovich Bronstein
Woodrow Wilson ....Thomas Woodrow Wilson
Malcolm X ....Malcolm Little

Sports Figures
Professional Name ....Original Name

Kareem Abdul-Jabbar ....Ferdinand Lewis Alcindor, Jr.
Muhammad Ali ....Cassius Marcellus Clay
Andre the Giant ....Andre Roussinoff
Yogi Berra....................................Lawrence Peter Berra
Hulk Hogan ....Terry Bodello
Magic Johnson..............................Earvin Johnson
Pelé...Edson Arantes do Nascimento
Ahmad Rashad ....Bobby Moore
Tom Seaver ....George Thomas Seaver
Gene Tunney ....James Joseph Tunney
Tiger Woods ....Eldrick Woods
Cy Young ....Denton True Young

Literary Figures
Professional Name ....Original Name

Maya Angelou ....Marguerite Annie Johnson
Pearl Buck ....Pearl Comfort Sydenstricker
Truman Capote ....Truman Steckfus Pearsons
Lewis Carroll ....Charles Lutwidge Dodgson
Michael Crichton...........................John Michael Crichton
Agatha Christie ....Agatha Mary Clarissa Miller
Isak Dinesen ....Baroness Karen Blixen
Victoria Holt.................................Eleanot Burford Hibbert
Judith Krantz ....Judith Tarcher
John le Carre ....John Moore Carnwell
Toni Morrison ....Chloe Anthony Wofford
George Orwell ....Eric Arthur Blair
Satchel Paige................................Leroy Robert Paige
Anne Rice.....................................Howard Allen O'Brien
Harold Robbins ....Francis Kane

J. K. Rowling ....Joanne Kathleen Rowling
Mickey Spillane ....Frank Morrison
Danielle Steel................................Danielle Schuelein-Steel
R. L. Stine ....Robert Lawrence Stine
Dr. Seuss.....................................Theodore Seuss Geisel
J. R. R. Tolkien.............................John Ronald Reuel Tolkien
Mark Twain ....Samuel Clemens
Gore Vidal ....Eugene Luther Vidal
Nathaniel West..............................Nathaniel Wallenstein Weinstein
Tennessee Williams ....Thomas Lanier Williams

Entertainment Figures
Professional Name ....Original Name

Eddie Albert ....Edward Albert Heimberger
Alan Alda ....Alphonse D'Abruzzo
Jane Alexander..............................Jane Quigley
Jason Alexander ....Jay Scott Greenspan
Tim Allen ....Tim Allen Dick
Woody Allen ....Allen Konigsberg
Don Ameche..................................Dominic Felix Amici
Tori Amos ....Myra Ellen Amos
Julie Andrews ....Julia Vernon
Ann-Margret..................................Ann-Margret Olsson
Beatrice Arthur..............................Bernice Frankel
Ed Asner ....Yitzak Edward Asner
Fred Astaire ....Frederick Austerlitz
Lauren Bacall ....Betty Joan Perske
Anne Bancroft ....Anne Italiano
John Barrymore.............................John Blythe
Warren Beatty ....Henry Warren Beaty
Beck ....Beck Hansen
Bonnie Bedelia..............................Bonnie Culkin
Pat Benetar ....Patricia Andrejewski
Tony Bennett ....Anthony Dominick Benedetto
Jack Benny ....Joseph Kubelsky
Robbie Benson..............................Robert Segal
Ingmar Bergman ....Ernst Ingmar Bergman
Milton Berle ....Milton Berlinger
Irving Berlin ....Israel Baline
Joey Bishop...................................Joseph Abraham Gottlieb
Bjork..Björk Gudmundsdottir
Robert Blake ....Michael James Vijencio Gubitosi
Blondie...Deborah Harry
Michael Bolton ....Michael Bolotin
Jon Bon Jovi ....John Bonjiovi
Bono...Paul Hewson

Professional Name	Original Name
Sonny Bono	Salvatore Bono
Pat Boone	Charles Eugene Boone
Victor Borge	Borge Rosenbaum
Bow Wow	Shad Moss
David Bowie	David Hayward-Jones
Max Brand	Gerald Kenneth Tierney
Brandy	Brandy Norwood
Beau Bridges	Lloyd Vernet Bridges III
Charles Bronson	Charles Buchinsky
Albert Brooks	Albert Einstein
Garth Brooks	Troyal Garth Brooks
Mel Brooks	Melvin Kaminsky
Yul Brynner	Taidje Kahn, Jr.
George Burns	Nathan Birnbaum
Ellen Burstyn	Edna Rae Gillooly
Richard Burton	Richard Jenkins
Nicolas Cage	Nicholas Coppola
Michael Caine	Maurice Joseph Micklewhite
Maria Callas	Maria Anna Sophia Cecilia Kalogeropoulos
Dyan Cannon	Samile Diane Friesen
Kate Capshaw	Kathleen Sue Nail
Vikki Carr	Florencia Bisenta de Casillas Martinez Cardona
Diahann Carroll	Carol Diahann Johnson
Johnny Cash	J. R. Cash
Stockard Channing	Susan Antonia Williams Stockard
Ray Charles	Ray Charles Robinson
Charo	Maria Rosaria Pilar Martinez Molina Baeza
J. C. Chasez	Joshua Scott Chasez
Chevy Chase	Cornelius Crane Chase
Chubby Checker	Ernest Evans
Cher	Cherilyn Sarkisian LaPierre
Chyna	Joanie Laurer
Eric Clapton	Eric Clapp
Patsy Cline	Virginia Patterson Hensley
Lee J. Cobb	Leo Jacob
Perry Como	Pierino Como
Bert Convy	Bernard Whalen Patrick Convy
Alice Cooper	Vincent Damon Furnier
David Copperfield	David Kotkin
Howard Cosell	Howard William Cohen
Bob Costas	Robert Quinlan Costas
Elvis Costello	Declan Patrick McManus
Joan Crawford	Lucille Le Sueur
Bing Crosby	Harry Lillis Crosby
Tom Cruise	Thomas Cruise Mapother IV
Tony Curtis	Bernard Schwartz
Willem Dafoe	William Dafoe
D'Angelo	Michael D'Angelo Archer
Rodney Dangerfield	Jacob Cohen
Dawn	Joyce Elaine Vincent
Doris Day	Doris Kappelhoff
Sandra Dee	Alexandra Zuck
John Denver	Henry John Deutschendorf, Jr.
Bo Derek	Mary Cathleen Collins
Portia de Rossi	Amanda Rogers
Danny DeVito	Daniel Michaeli
Susan Dey	Susan Smith
Marlene Dietrich	Maria von Losch
Phyllis Diller	Phyllis Driver
Kirk Douglas	Issur Danielovitch Demsky
Mike Douglas	Michael Delaney Dowd, Jr.
Patty Duke	Anna Marie Duke
Faye Dunaway	Dorothy Faye Dunaway
Bob Dylan	Robert Zimmerman
Sheena Easton	Sheena Shirley Orr
Buddy Ebsen	Christian Ebsen, Jr.
Barbara Eden	Barbara Huffman
The Edge	David Evans
Carmen Electra	Tara Leigh Patrick
Jenna Elfman	Jenna Butala
Mama Cass Elliot	Ellen Naomi Cohen
Missy Elliott	Melissa Elliott
Elvira	Cassandra Peterson
Eminem	Marshall Mathers III
Werner Erhard	Jack Rosenberg
Dale Evans	Francis Octavia Smith
Chad Everett	Raymond Lee Cramton
Douglas Fairbanks	Julius Ullman
Morgan Fairchild	Patsy Ann McClenny
Mia Farrow	Maria de Lourdes Villiers Farrow
Farrah Fawcett	Mary Farrah Fawcett
Will Ferrell	John William Ferrell
Sally Field	Sally Mahoney
W. C. Fields	William Claude Dukenfield
Dame Margot Fonteyn	Margaret Hookham
Glenn Ford	Gwllyn Samuel Newton Ford
John Forsythe	John Freund
Jodie Foster	Alicia Christian Foster
Michael Fox	Michael Andrew Fox
Jamie Foxx	Eric Bishop
Redd Foxx	John Elroy Sanford
Anthony Franciosa	Anthony Papaleo
Connie Francis	Concetta Franconero
Carlton Fredericks	Harold Casper Frederick Kaplan

Professional Name	Original Name
Greta Garbo	Greta Gustafson
Andy Garcia	Andres Arturo Garcia-Menendez
Judy Garland	Frances Gumm
James Garner	James Baumgarner
Crystal Gayle	Brenda Gail Webb Gatzimos
Boy George	George Alan O'Dowd
Barry Gibb	Douglas Gibb
Kathie Lee Gifford	Kathie Epstein
Goldberg	Bill Goldberg
Whoopi Goldberg	Caryn Johnson
Cary Grant	Archibald Leach
Lee Grant	Lyova Haskell Rosenthal
Peter Graves	Peter Arness
Macy Gray	Natalie McIntyre
Joel Grey	Joel Katz
Charles Grodin	Charles Grodinsky
Robert Guillaume	Robert Williams
Buddy Hackett	Leonard Hacker
Geri Halliwell	Geraldine Estolle Halliwell
Halston	Roy Halston Frowick
Hammer	Stanley Kirk Hacker Burrell
Woody Harrelson	Woodrow Tracy Harrelson
Rex Harrison	Reginald Cary
Laurence Harvey	Lavrushka Skikne
Helen Hayes	Helen Brown
Marg Helgenberger	Mary Margaret Helgenberger
Margaux Hemingway	Margot Hemmingway
Audrey Hepburn	Audrey Hepburn-Ruston
Pee Wee Herman	Paul Rubenfeld
Barbara Hershey	Barbara Herzstine
William Holden	William Beedle
Billie Holiday	Eleanora Fagan
Bob Hope	Leslie Townes Hope
Harry Houdini	Ehrich Weiss
Rock Hudson	Roy Scherer, Jr.
D. L. Hughley	Darryl Lynn Hughley
Engelbert Humperdinck	Arnold Dorsey
Mary Beth Hurt	Mary Supinger
Lauren Hutton	Mary Laurence Hutton
Ice Cube	O'Shea Jackson
Billy Idol	William Broad
Don Imus	John Donald Imus, Jr.
Wolfman Jack	Robert Smith
Wyclef Jean	Nelust Wyclef Jean
Jewel	Jewel Kilcher
Elton John	Reginald Kenneth Dwight
Don Johnson	Donald Wayne
Al Jolson	Asa Yoelson
Tom Jones	Thomas Jones Woodward
Louis Jourdan	Louis Gendre
Donna Karan	Donna Faske
Boris Karloff	William Henry Pratt
Danny Kaye	David Kaminsky
Diane Keaton	Diane Hall
Michael Keaton	Michael Douglas
Alicia Keys	Alicia Augello-Cook
Chaka Khan	Yvette Stevens
Kid Rock	Robert James Ritchie
Larry King	Larry Zeiger
Ben Kingsley	Krishna Banji
Nastassia Kinski	Nastassja Naksynznki
Calvin Klein	Richard Klein
Ted Knight	Tadeus Wladyslaw Konopka
Johnny Knoxville	Phillip John Clapp
Kreskin	George Joseph Kresge Jr.
Ashton Kutcher	Christopher Ashton Kutcher
Cheryl Ladd	Cheryl Stoppelmoor
Bert Lahr	Irving Lahrheim
Ann Landers	Esther Pauline Lederer
Michael Landon	Eugene Michael Orowitz
Nathan Lane	Joseph Lane
K. D. Lang	Katherine Dawn Lang
Stan Laurel	Arthur Stanley Jefferson Laurel
Ralph Lauren	Ralph Lifshitz
Piper Laurie	Rosetta Jacobs
Jude Law	David Jude Law
Steve Lawrence	Sidney Leibowitz
Heath Ledger	Heathcliff Andrew Ledger
Bruce Lee	Lee Yuen Kam
Gypsy Rose Lee	Louise Hovick
Peggy Lee	Norma Egstrom
Spike Lee	Shelton Jackson Lee
Jay Leno	James Leno
Téa Leoni	Elizabeth Téa Pantaleoni
Huey Lewis	Hugh Cregg
Jerry Lewis	Joseph Levitch
Shari Lewis	Shari Hurwitz
Jet Li	Li Lian Jie
Liberace	Wladziu Valentino Liberace
Hal Linden	Hal Lipshitz
Meat Loaf	Marvin Lee Aday
Jack Lord	J. J. Ryan
Sophia Loren	Sophia Villani Scicolone
Peter Lorre	Laszlo Loewenstein
Courtney Love	Love Michelle Harrison
Myrna Loy	Myrna Williams
Bela Lugosi	Bela Ferenc Blasko
Loretta Lynn	Loretta Webb
Bernie Mac	Bernard Jeffery McCullough

Professional Name	Original Name
Andie MacDowell	Rosalie Anderson MacDowell
Shirley MacLaine	Shirley Beaty
Elle Macpherson	Eleanor Gow
Madonna	Madonna Louise Veronica Ciccone
Lee Majors	Harvey Lee Yeary II
Karl Malden	Mladen Sekulovich
Camryn Manheim	Debra Manheim
Jayne Mansfield	Vera Jane Palmer
Marilyn Manson	Brian Hugh Warner
Fredric March	Frederick Bickel
Penny Marshall	Carole Penny Marshall
Dean Martin	Dino Crocetti
Ricky Martin	Enrique José Martin Morales
Chico Marx	Leonard Marx
Groucho Marx	Julius Henry Marx
Harpo Marx	Arthur Marx
Zeppo Marx	Herbert Marx
Master P	Percy Miller
Walter Matthau	Walter Matuschanskayasky
Ethel Merman	Ethel Zimmermann
Paul McCartney	James Paul McCartney
A. J. McLean	Alexander James McLean
Steve McQueen	Terence Stephen McQueen
George Michael	Georgios Panayiotou
Joni Mitchell	Roberta Joan Anderson Mitchell
Jay Mohr	Jon Ferguson Mohr
Marilyn Monroe	Norma Jean Baker
Yves Montand	Ivo Livi
Demi Moore	Demetria Gene Guynes
Julianne Moore	Julie Anne Smith
Rita Moreno	Rosita Dolores Alverio
Pat Morita	Noriyuki Morita
Van Morrison	George Ivan Morrison
Zero Mostel	Samuel Joel Mostel
Ricky Nelson	Eric Hilliard Nelson
Randy Newman	Randall Stuart Newman
Thandie Newton	Thandiwe Newton
Mike Nichols	Michael Igor Peschkowsky
Stevie Nicks	Stephanie Nicks
Chuck Norris	Carlos Ray Norris
Kim Novak	Marilyn Pauline Novak
Hugh O'Brian	Hugh J. Krampe
Tony Orlando	Michael Anthony Orlando Cassavitis
Suze Orman	Suzie Orman
Ozzy Osbourne	John Michael Osbourne
Marie Osmond	Olive Marie Osmond
Peter O'Toole	Seamus O'Toole

Professional Name	Original Name
Al Pacino	Alfredo James Pacino
Jack Palance	Walter Jack Palanuik
Jane Pauley	Margaret Jane Pauley
Minnie Pearl	Sarah Ophelia Colley Cannon
Gregory Peck	Eldred Gregory Peck
Bernadette Peters	Bernadette Lazzara
Joaquin Phoenix	Joaquin Raphael Bottom
Christopher Pike	Kevin McFadden
Brad Pitt	William Bradley Pitt
Stephanie Powers	Stefania Federkiewicz
Paula Prentiss	Paula Ragusa
Priscilla Presley	Pricilla Wagner Beaulieu
Prince	Prince Rogers Nelson
William Proxmire	Edward William Proxmire
Tony Randall	Leonard Rosenberg
Robert Redford	Charles Robert Redford
Donna Reed	Donna Belle Mullenger
Della Reese	Delloreese Patricia Early
Judge Reinhold	Edward Ernest Reinhold, Jr.
Lee Remick	Ann Remick
Debbie Reynolds	Mary Frances Reynolds
Busta Rhymes	Trevor Smith
Andy Richter	Paul Andrew Richter
Edward G. Robinson	Emanuel Goldenberg
The Rock	Dwayne Douglas Johnson
Ginger Rogers	Virginia McMath
Roy Rogers	Leonard Slye
Mickey Rooney	Joe Yule, Jr.
Diana Ross	Diane Ernestine Ross
Theresa Russell	Theresa Paup
Jeri Ryan	Jeri Lynn Zimmerman
Meg Ryan	Margaret Hyra
Winona Ryder	Winona Laura Horowitz
Buffy Sainte-Marie	Beverly Sainte-Marie
Susan Saint James	Susan Miller
Soupy Sales	Milton Supman
Susan Sarandon	Susan Tomalin
Leo Sayer	Gerald Sayer
John Saxon	Carmen Orrico
Jane Seymour	Joyce Frankenberg
Shaggy	Orville Richard Burrell
Shakira	Shakira Isabel Mebarak Ripoll
Omar Sharif	Michael Shalhouz
Artie Shaw	Arthur Arshowsky
Charlie Sheen	Carlos Irwin Estevez
Martin Sheen	Ramon G. Estevez
Judith Sheindlin	Judy Blum
Brooke Shields	Christa Brooke Shields
Talia Shire	Talia Coppola

Professional Name	Original Name
Dinah Shore	Frances "Fanny" Rose Shore
Beverly Sills	Belle "Bubbles" Silverman
Neil Simon	Marvin Neil Simon
Sinbad	David Adkins
Sisqo	Mark Andrews
Ione Skye	Ione Skye Leitch
Christian Slater	Christian Hawkins
Snoop Dogg	Calvin Cordozar Broadus
Phoebe Snow	Phoebe Loeb
Leelee Sobieski	Liliane Rudabet Gloria Elsveta Sobieski
Suzanne Somers	Suzanne Mahoney
Elke Sommer	Elke Schletz
Ann Sothern	Harriet Lake
Sissy Spacek	Mary Elizabeth Spacek
Robert Stack	Robert Modini
Sylvester Stallone	Michael Sylvester Stallone
Jean Stapleton	Jeanne Murray
Ringo Starr	Richard Starkey
Cat Stevens	(Yusuf Islam) Steven Georgiou
Connie Stevens	Concetta Anne Ingolia
Jon Stewart	Jon Stuart Liebowitz
Sting	Gordon Matthew Sumner
Sly Stone	Sylvester Stone
Meryl Streep	Mary Louise Streep
Barbra Streisand	Barbara Streisand
Donna Summer	LaDonna Gaines
Max von Sydow	Carl Adolph von Sydow
Mr. T	Lawrence Tureaud
Rip Taylor	Charles Elmer, Jr.
Robert Taylor	Spangler Brugh
Danny Thomas	Amos Jacobs
Jonathan Taylor Thomas	Jonathan Weiss
Tiny Tim	Herbert Buckingham Khaury
Lily Tomlin	Mary Jean Tomlin
Rip Torn	Elmore Rual Torn, Jr.
Randy Travis	Randy Traywick
Ted Turner	Robert Edward Turner III
Tina Turner	Anna Mae Bullock
Shania Twain	Eileen Regina Twain
Twiggy	Leslie Hornby
Steven Tyler	Steven Tallarico
Rudolph Valentino	Rudolpho Alphonzo Raffaelo Pierre Filibut Guglielmo di Valentina D'Antonguolla
Rudy Vallee	Hubert Prior Vallée
Abigail Van Buren	Pauline Phillips
Christopher Walken	Ronald Walken
Nancy Walker	Ann Myrtle Swoyer
Mike Wallace	Myron Wallace
Andy Warhol	Andrew Warhola
Muddy Waters	McKinley Morganfield
John Wayne	Marion Michael Morrison
Sigourney Weaver	Susan Weaver
Raquel Welch	Raquel Tejada
Tuesday Weld	Susan Kerr Weld
Gene Wilder	Jerome Silberman
Bruce Willis	Walter Bruce Willis
August Wilson	Frederick August Kittel
Flip Wilson	Clerow Wilson
Debra Winger	Mary Debra Winger
Shelley Winters	Shirley Schrift
Reese Witherspoon	Laura Jeanne Reese Witherspoon
Stevie Wonder	Steveland Morris Hardaway
Natalie Wood	Natasha Gurdin
Jane Wyman	Sarah Jane Fulks
Tammy Wynette	Wynette Pugh
Wynonna	Christina Claire Ciminella
Ed Wynn	Isaiah Edwin Leopold
Loretta Young	Gretchen Young
Sean Young	Mary Sean Young

Baby Name Legal Guide

Shortly after your baby is born, someone on the hospital staff will ask you for information to fill out a birth certificate. If your baby is not born in a hospital, either by choice or accident, you still need to file a birth certificate. If you're on your way but don't make it to the hospital in time, the hospital will still take care of filling in the form and presenting it for your signature after you're admitted. If you plan a home birth, you will have to go to the vital statistics office and file a form there—to be certain, find out what your local laws require.

Basic facts about both parents' names, places and dates of birth, and such details about the baby as its sex, weight, length, exact time of arrival, and date of birth will be needed for a birth certificate. Questions regarding other children (if any), their ages, previous miscarriages or children's deaths, the educational levels of both parents, and so on might be asked at this time for records at your local division of vital statistics. They may not appear on the actual birth certificate, though.

The hospital staffer will type up the form and present it for the mother and doctor to sign before sending it to the vital statistics division to be recorded permanently. Once it's recorded you can request copies (needed for things like passports, some jobs, and some legal transactions).

That's what happens in the usual chain of events. But what about the technicalities and specific legal aspects of naming a child? The first thing to know is that laws that govern baby naming vary greatly throughout the country. If your choice of names is in any way unusual (such as giving your baby a hyphenated surname combining the mother's maiden name with the father's name), be sure of the law before you name the baby. And sign the official birth certificate only after it has been filled out to your satisfaction.

A few of the most commonly asked questions concerning legalities are considered here but, since state and territory laws are not uniform, even these answers cannot be definite. Your local municipal health department officials can probably lead you to the proper department or official to handle your particular situation. Contact them if you need more detailed answers to your questions.

Q. Are there any restrictions on the choice of first and middle names for a baby?

A. No, with the possible exception that the baby's names should be composed of letters, not numbers. In 1978 a district court judge refused to allow a young Minneapolis social studies teacher to legally change his name to the number 1069, calling such a change "an offense to human dignity" that would "hasten that day in which we all become lost in faceless numbers."

Freedom in choosing given names is not universal. A spokesperson for the French Consulate in Chicago confirmed that an 1813 French law still governs naming practices in France. It decrees that babies must be named after Catholic saints or "persons known in ancient history."

Q. Is a choice allowed in giving the baby its surname?

A. In former generations a baby's surname was not often considered a matter for personal decision. State regulations dictated that if the parents were married, the baby took on the father's surname. If the parents were not married, the baby's surname was that of its mother.

In the past few decades such state regulations have been changing. For example, in Florida, Hawaii, and North Carolina, federal courts have ruled those three states can no longer determine the choice of a baby's surname, leaving that decision to the parent(s).

Such court rulings represent the trend prevalent in most, if not all, states to leave the choice of babies' surnames to parents. However, to be absolutely certain, be sure to check your state's regulations on this matter.

Q. Must the baby's full name be decided upon before the birth certificate can be registered?

A. In most cases no time limit exists in which given names must be recorded. However, depending on the amount of time since the birth, the evidence required to record the name varies, ranging from a letter signed by the parent to a court order.

Q. How can a baby's name be legally changed after its birth is registered?

A. More than 50,000 Americans ask courts to change their names legally every year. Some of these changes are requested by parents for their children when the names originally chosen no longer suit them.

Changes in a minor child's given names are possible in some states without a court order, with time limits ranging from a few days after birth to any time at all. In some states a simple affidavit signed by the parents or a notarized amendment is sufficient to make a name change. Others require various documents to show proof of an established new name, such as a baptismal certificate, an insurance policy, an immunization record, or the family Bible record. For older children, school records or the school census are usually allowed.

When court procedures are necessary, they involve petitions to a county probate court, a superior court, or a district court, following state laws. Often prior newspaper publication of the intended change is required. The court then issues a "change of name" order or decree. In some states new birth certificates are issued for name changes. In others, certificates are only amended.

Informal name changes can be and often are made simply through the "common law right of choice," which allows individuals to use any names they choose. Such a change is informal, though, and is not legal in official procedures.

Q. What if a mistake is made in the baby's name on the birth certificate?

A. To repeat: the best advice of all is to avoid such an occurrence by being absolutely sure that the completely filled-out certificate is correct in every detail before signing it. If a mistake is made, it is important to handle the matter quickly. Procedures for corrections on certificates vary: sometimes signatures of the parents are sufficient, but in other cases forms must be filled out or documentary evidence supplied.

Q. What are the laws for renaming adopted children?

A. An adoption decree is a court order legally obtained through basically similar procedures in all states and territories. A child's given names are selected by the adoptive parents and the surname is chosen in accordance with whatever state or territory laws exist for surnames of biological children. Then all these names are recorded in the adoption decree. In most places an entirely new birth certificate is drawn up, although the place of birth is not usually changed. Most often, the original birth certificate is sealed with the adoption papers, and the new certificate is filed in place of the original.

Q. How may a child's name be changed by a stepfather, by foster parents, or in the case of legitimization?

A. In the case of a name change by a stepfather or by foster parents, most states require that individuals follow the appropriate procedures for adoption or for legal name change.

Changing a child's surname in the case of legitimization is virtually the same as the adoption procedure in most states and territories. Some require both an affidavit of paternity and a copy of the parents' marriage license, while others do not concern themselves with the marriage of the parents. California has no procedures whatsoever, since illegitimacy is no longer defined in that state.

Fascinating Facts about Names

New Era for Japanese Names

Naming trends change all over the world. One trend seeing a great deal of change is from Japan. Traditionally, the kanji character "ko," meaning *child*, was used as a suffix for nearly all girls' names. Now there are only four names ending in "ko" in the top 100 popular names for girls in Japan. Suffixes such as "ka" and "na" are more popular with the new generation of baby names, accounting for more than 25 percent of the top 100 list.

Mermaids and Murderers

Many names have enjoyed surges in popularity due to movies. Madison, the third-most popular girls' name, didn't appear on the naming scene until Daryl Hannah portrayed the beautiful mermaid Madison in 1984's *Splash*. But sometimes names are inspired by less positive characters. Take Samara, the name of the evil, murderous child in the horror flick *The Ring*. Before the movie premiered in 2002, Samara had barely cracked the top 1000 list. Two years later, the name had tripled in popularity.

Who Is Alan Smithee?

Alan Smithee is a prolific Hollywood director whose name has been attached to dozens of movies and TV shows. He was born in 1969, the same year he directed *Death of a Gunfighter*. How can that be, you ask? "Alan Smithee" is a pseudonym commonly used by directors who feel they have lost creative control of their movies and therefore want to distance themselves from them. (You may also know Alan's "cousin," George Spelvin, whose name appears on many a theater playbill.)

International Anonymity

"John Doe" is an anonymous, generic person in the U.S., but he has many counterparts around the globe. There's Fred Nurk (Australia), Jan Modaal (Holland), Chan Siu Ming (Hong Kong), Gyula Kovacs (Hungary), Jón Jónsson (Iceland), Mario Rossi (Italy), Juan dela Cruz (Philippines), Jan Kowalski (Poland), Juan del Pueblo (Puerto Rico), Jos Bleau (Quebec), Vasya Pupkin (Russia), Janez Novak (Slovenia), Koos van der Merwe (South Africa), and Joe Bloggs (U.K.).

"They" Said It

When you hear, "They say it's going to be a cold winter" or "They say the crime rate is rising," do you ever wonder who "they" are? Wonder no more: "They" is a good-humored inventor from Branson, Missouri. Andrew Wilson decided he would be the face behind this nameless group when he legally changed his name to They in 2004. His friends tell him, "If anyone but you changed your name to They, they would think he had a problem."

Charlize Craze

As one of Hollywood's most talented and beautiful actresses, Charlize Theron has caused a baby-naming boom in her home country of South Africa. In the U.S., the name Charlize has seen a modest rise in popularity, making it to number 625 on the Social Security Administration list, but the Oscar-winning actress recently discovered that her name is hugely popular back home. She says, "Somebody told me that now every one out of three baby girls born in South Africa is being named Charlize."

Bubba[3]

Raymond Allen Gray, Jr., of Springfield, Illinois, had gone by "Bubba" his whole life. At age thirty-nine, he decided to fully embrace his nickname, so he legally changed his first name to Bubba. He also changed his middle name to Bubba. And then he changed his last name to—you guessed it—Bubba. Bubba Bubba Bubba is taking his new moniker in stride, saying, "It's something silly to kind of poke fun with."

It's a Bird, It's a Plane, It's a Baby!

In 2003, tax authorities rejected a Swedish couple's request to name their newborn son Superman. The couple thought Superman was the perfect name because their son was born with one arm pointing upward, which resembled Superman in flight. Authorities did not allow the name, however, saying the child would be subjected to ridicule throughout life. (No telling whether those same authorities would have taken issue with Nicolas Cage's naming his son Kal-El, which is Superman's "birth" name.)

Cyber Names

Technology plays a role in nearly every facet of human life, so it's no surprise that technology would inspire names. Jon Blake Cusack and wife, Jamie, of Holland, Michigan, named their son Jon Blake Cusack Version 2.0, putting a high-tech spin on "Junior." A man in central China tried to name his son "@" but was refused because it cannot be translated into Mandarin, which is a legal requirement. Twenty-three-year-old Karin Robertson of Norfolk, Virginia, changed her name to Goveg.Com, in support of the popular website for vegetarianism. Then there's GoldenPalaceDotCom Silverman, whose parents received $15,000 for auctioning his naming rights to the online casino. As it turns out, GoldenPalaceDotCom is not as uncommon as one may think: The casino also paid $15,199 to Terri Illigan of Tennessee when she changed her name to GoldenPalace.com as a way to support her five children.

Hangover Names

Two U.K. soccer fans woke up to not only throbbing headaches but also new names the morning after a post-game bender. Jeremy Brown and his friend had legally changed their names to Crazy Horse Invincible and Spaceman Africa, respectively, while in their inebriated states. They decided to keep the names—a decision that caused some hassles: Crazy Horse had trouble booking a plane ticket to Prague because airline officials thought someone with such a name was "up to no good." (Spaceman Africa apparently had no problem booking the same flight.)

Kids Naming Kids

When Jayne and Daniel Peate, from Shropshire, England, announced they were expecting a sixth baby, their youngest felt put-out by the new addition. To ease sibling rivalry, Jayne and Daniel allowed the older children to choose their new sibling's middle name. And so they named their son Rafferty Bob Ash Chewbacca Peate, with middle names inspired by *Bob the Builder*, a *Pokemon* character, and the famous *Star Wars* wookie. (Chewbacca was a substitute for Jar Jar Binks when the family learned that each middle name could be only one word long.) The baby is affectionately known as "Chewy."

Ye Olde Names

If you think today's baby names are a little odd, consider the following names researchers in Cornwall, England, found after reviewing centuries of records: Abraham Thunderwolff, Freke Dorothy Fluck Lane, Boadicea Basher, Philadelphia Bunnyface, Faithful Cock, Susan Booze, Elizabeth Disco, Edward Evil, Fozzitt Bonds, Truth Bullock, Charity Chilly, Gentle Fudge, Obedience Ginger, and Offspring Gurney. They even found a real-life Horatio Hornblower, whose siblings were Azubia, Constantia, Jecoliah, Jedidah, Jerusha, and Erastus. The marriage records included odd pairings such

as Nicholas Bone and Priscilla Skin, Charles Swine and Jane Ham, John Mutton and Ann Veale, and Richard Dinner and Mary Cook.

How Many Names Do We Need?

Giving your children first names that start with the same letter is a popular trend. Most families need to think of only two or three such names, but coming up with double-digit number of names can be quite a task if you have a large family. The Cox family in North Carolina gave its eleven children names beginning with "Z": Zadie, Zadoc, Zeber, Zylphia, Zenobia, Zeronial, Zeslie, Zeola, Zero, Zula, and Zelbert. Jim Bob and Michelle Duggar of Arkansas used "J" names for all *sixteen* of their children: Joshua, John David, Janna, Jill, Jessa, Jinger, Joseph, Josiah, Joy-Anna, Jeremiah, Jedidiah, Jason, James, Justin, Jackson, and Johannah.

Hockeytown Baby

Nick and Sarah Arena, from Toledo, Ohio, were having trouble thinking of a baby name. After several hours of fruitless brainstorming, they took a break to watch their favorite hockey team, the Detroit Red Wings. In an instant, they both knew what to name their son. On June 6, 2002, Joe Louis Arena was born, named in homage of the stadium where the Red Wings play.

Put It All Together

On its own, Mary is a harmless, normal, beautiful name. But when combined with a middle and last name, you can get a silly moniker such as Mary Chris Smith. Other unfortunate pairings include Ivan Odor, Shanda Lear (daughter of Bill and Moya Lear of Lear Jets), Tu Morrow (daughter of actor Rob Morrow), and Ima Hogg (who, despite urban legend, did not have a sister named Ura).

Birthrights

In some tribal societies children are not considered born until they are named. Frequently the child's name consists of a statement (that is, rather than having a pool of names as Western culture does, parents in these societies name children with a phrase that describes the circumstances of the child's birth, the family's current activities, and so on). Translated, such names might be "We are glad we moved to Memphis," or "A girl at last," or "Too little rain."

Bible Studies

It's been estimated that the majority of people in the Western hemisphere have names from the Bible. Women outnumber men, yet there are 3,037 male names in the Bible and only 181 female names. The New Testament is a more popular source of names than the Old Testament.

Change of Habit

Popes traditionally choose a new name upon their election by the College of Cardinals. The practice began in 844 A.D. when a priest whose real name was Boca de Porco (Pig's Mouth) was elected. He changed his name to Sergious II.

Saint Who?

Saints' names are a common source of names in the U.S. But saints who are popular in other countries contribute very unusual, even unpronounceable, names for children born in the U.S.—like Tamjesdegerd, Borhedbesheba, and Jafkeranaegzia.

Them Bones

Praise-God Barebones had a brother named If-Christ-Had-Not-Died-For-Thee-Thou-Wouldst-Have-Been-Damned, who was called "Damned Barebones" for short.

Hello, God?

Terril William Clark is listed in the phone book under his new name—God. Now he's looking for someone to publish a book he's written. "Let's face it," he reportedly said. "The last book with my name on it was a blockbuster."

The Status Quo

The most commonly given names in English-speaking countries from about 1750 to the present are drawn from a list with only 179 entries (discounting variations in spelling). Essentially the same practice has been followed in naming children since at least the sixteenth century, though the use of middle names has increased over the years.

It's Mainly Relative

A recent study suggests that about two-thirds of the population of the U.S. is named to honor somebody. Of the people who are namesakes, about 60 percent are named after a relative and 40 percent for someone outside the family.

Once Is Enough

Ann Landers wrote about a couple who had six children, all named Eugene Jerome Dupuis, Junior. The children answered to One, Two, Three, Four, Five, and Six, respectively. Can you imagine what the IRS, the Social Security Administration, and any other institution would do with the Dupuises?

In Sickness and Health

Tonsilitis Jackson has brothers and sisters named Meningitis, Appendicitis, and Peritonitis.

The Old College Try

A couple in Louisiana named their children after colleges: Stanford, Duke, T'Lane, Harvard, Princeton, Auburn, and Cornell. The parents' names? Stanford, Sr., and Loyola.

Peace at All Costs

Harry S. Truman owed his middle name, the initial S, to a compromise his parents worked out. By using only the initial, they were able to please both his grandfathers, whose names were Shippe and Solomon.

Initials Only

A new recruit in the U.S. Army filled out all the forms he was presented with as he always had in school: R. (only) B. (only) Jones. You guessed it—from then on he was, as far as the Army cared about it, Ronly Bonly Jones, and all his records, dogtags, and discharge papers proved the point again and again.

Sticks and Stones May Break My Bones...

The nicknames children make up for each other tend to fall into four patterns: those stemming from the physical appearance of the child, those based on either real or imaginary mental traits (brains or idiocy), those based on social ranking or other relationships, and, finally, those based on plays on the child's name. Children who don't conform to the values or looks of their peers are likely to pick up more nicknames than those who do. In these ways nicknames often function as instruments of social control.

The Name's the Game

John Hotvet, of Minnetonka, Minnesota, is—of course—a veterinarian. Sometimes names and occupations get inextricably interwoven. Consider these names and professions:

Dr. Zoltan Ovary, gynecologist

Mr. A. Moron, Commissioner of Education for the Virgin Islands

Reverend Christian Church and Reverend God

Mr. Thomas Crapper of Crapper, Ltd Toilets, in London, who entitled his autobiography "Flushed with Pride"

Assorted physicians named Doctor, Docter, or Doktor

Cardinal Sin, Archbishop of Manila, the Philippines

Mr. Groaner Digger, undertaker in Houston

Mr. I. C. Shivers, iceman

Ms. Justine Tune, chorister in Westminster Choir College, Princeton, New Jersey

Ms. Lavender Sidebottom, masseuse at Elizabeth Arden's in New York City

Mssrs. Lawless and Lynch, attorneys in Jamaica, New York

Major Minor, U.S. Army

Diana Nyad, champion long-distance swimmer

Mssrs. Plummer and Leek, plumbers in Sheringham, Norfolk, England

Mr. Ronald Supena, lawyer

Mrs. Screech, singing teacher in Victoria, British Columbia

Mr. Vroom, motorcycle dealer in Port Elizabeth, South Africa

Mssrs. Wyre and Tapping, detectives in New York City

Ms. A. Forest Burns, professional forester

Dr. McNutt, head of a mental hospital, and Dr. Paul Looney, psychiatrist

Mr. Vice, arrested 820 times and convicted 421 times

Dr. Slaughter, surgeon, Dr. Needles, pediatrician, and Dr. Bonebreak, chiropractor

Time Capsule Names

Celebrities and events often inspire parents in their choices of names for children. Many people are now "dated" by their World War II names, like Pearl (Harbor), Douglas (MacArthur), Dwight (Eisenhower—whose mother named him Dwight David to avoid all nicknames, but whom everyone called Ike!), and Franklin (Roosevelt). Films and film stars contribute their share of names: Scarlett O'Hara and Rhett Butler have countless namesakes whose parents were swept away by *Gone with the Wind*. Madonna, Elvis, Prince, and virtually all other big stars have their own namesakes as well.

The UN Family

One couple took the time capsule concept to an extreme and named their triplets, born on April 5, 1979, Carter, Begin, and Sadat—to honor U.S. President Jimmy Carter, Israeli Prime Minister Menachem Begin, and Egyptian President Anwar Sadat, the three principle signers of the peace treaty signed in Washington, D.C., on March 1979.

They Add Up

Dick Crouser likes to collect unusual names. Some names tell stories, like Fanny Pistor Bodganoff (although Mr. Crouser admits that he doesn't know what a "bodgan" is); some leave messages, like Hazel Mae Call; some aren't likely to add to their owner's self-esteem, like Seldom Wright and Harley Worthit; some are mere truisms, like Wood Burns; while others announce what you might call philosophies of life, like Daily Goforth and Hazel B. Good.

Truth Stranger than Fiction

Dick Neff, columnist of *Advertising Age,* invited his readers to contribute lists of real names they had encountered that are odd and/or funny, to say the least. Among them were the following: Stanley Zigafoose, Cigar Stubbs, Ladorise Quick, Mad Laughinhouse, Lester Chester Hester, Effie Bong, Dillon C. Quattlebaum, Twila Szwrk, Harry E. Thweatt, Benjamin E. Dymshits, Elmer Ploof, Whipple Filoon, Sweetie Belle Rufus, Peculiar Smith, John Dunwrong, All Dunn, Willie Wunn, H. Whitney Clappsaddle, W. Wesley Muckenfuss, Rudolph J. Ramstack, Sarabelle Scraper Roach, James R. Stufflebeam, Shanda Lear, Arthur Crudder, Mary Crapsey, Memory Lane, Troy Mumpower, Santa Beans, Sividious Stark, Cleveland Biggerstaff, Trinkle Bott, Cleopatra Barksdale, Spring Belch, Fairy Blessing, Royal Fauntleroy Butler, Bozy Ball, Carl W. Gigl, Joy Holy, Peenie Fase, Che Che Creech, J. B. Outhouse, Katz Meow, Stephanie Snatchole, I. O. Silver, Helen Bunpain, Birdie Fawncella Feltis, Elight Starling, Farmer Slusher, Nebraska Minor, Bill Grumbles, Peter Rabbitt, Carbon Petroleum Dubbs, Kick-a-hole-in-the-soup, Wong Bong Fong, Newton Hooton, Sonia Schmeckpeeper, Lewie Wirmelskirchen, Lolita Beanblossom, Liselotte Pook, and Irmgard Quapp.

Popular Names?

In 1979, the Pennsylvania Health Department discovered these two first names among the 159,000 birth certificates issued in the state that year— Pepsi and Cola.

A Boy Named Sue

Researchers have found that boys who had peculiar first names had a higher incidence of mental problems than boys with common ones; no similar correlation was found for girls.

He Who Quacks Last

In a government check of a computer program, researchers turned up a real-life Donald Duck. It seems that programmers used his name to create a bogus G.I. to check out records—and found out he really existed. The Army Engineer won fame and a visit to the *Johnny Carson Show* as a result of this discovery.

Too-o-o-o Much

Many people dislike their own names. The most common reasons given for this dislike are that the names "sound too ugly," that they're old-fashioned, too hard to pronounce, too common, too uncommon, too long, sound too foreign, are too easy for people to joke about, and that they sound too effeminate (for men) or too masculine (for women).

What Are Parents Thinking?

It may have seemed like a good joke at the time, but did Mr. Homer Frost consider his children's future when he named them Winter Night, Jack White, Snow, Dew, Hail, and Cold (Frost)? And what was Mr. Wind thinking when he named his four children North, South, East, and West (Wind)?

For the Birds

A. Bird was the assistant manager of Britain's Royal Society for the Protection of Birds. Members of his staff were Barbara Buzzard, John Partridge, Celia Peacock, Helen Peacock, and Dorothy Rook.

Historical Irony

On July 30, 1980, *Good Morning America* announced that Richard Nixon arrested Jimmy Carter in Detroit.

Is Nothing Private Anymore?

Mr. & Mrs. Bra, a couple from South Dakota, named their two daughters Iona and Anita (Bra).

The Power of Disney

Walt Disney's popular movie *Aladdin* was released in 1992. Aladdin's love interest was named Princess Jasmine. In 1995, Jasmine was the #21 name for all girls in the U.S., the #12 name for Hispanic-American girls, and the #2 name for African-American girls.

Last But Not Least

Zachary Zzzzra has been listed in the *Guinness Book of World Records* as making "the most determined attempt to be the last personal name in a local telephone directory" in San Francisco. That happened before his place was challenged by one Vladimir Zzzzzzabakov. Zzzzra reports that he called Zzzzzzabakov and demanded to know his real name. (Zzzzra's name is really his own, he says.) Zzzzzzabakov told him it was none of his . . . business. At any rate, true to his reputation for determination, Zzzzra changed his name to regain his former—or latter?—position. When the new phone book appeared, he was relieved to find himself comfortably in the last place again, as Zachary Zzzzzzzzzra. Unknown to him, the contender, Zzzzzzabakov, had disappeared.

The End

One family that was not terribly successful in limiting its expansion has a series of children called, respectively, Finis, Addenda, Appendix, Supplement, and (last but not least) Errata.

Girls

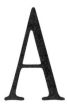

'Aolani (Hawaiian) heavenly cloud.
Aolanee, Aolaney, Aolania, Aolaniah, Aolanie,
Aolany, Aolanya

'Aulani (Hawaiian) royal messenger.
Aulanee, Aulaney, Aulania, Aulanie, Aulany,
Aulanya, Aulanyah, Lani, Lanie

A'lexus (American) a form of Alexis.

Aaleyah (Hebrew) a form of Aliya.
Aalayah, Aalayaha, Aalea, Aaleah, Aaleaha,
Aaleeyah, Aaleyiah, Aaleyyah

Aaliah (Hebrew) a form of Aliya.
Aaliaya, Aaliayah

Aalisha (Greek) a form of Alisha.
Aaleasha, Aaliesha

Aaliya (Hebrew) a form of Aliya.
Aahliyah, Aailiyah, Aailyah, Aalaiya, Aalia,
Aalieyha, Aaliyaha, Aaliyha, Aalliah, Aalliyah

Aaliyah ☀ (Hebrew) a form of Aliya.

Aalyiah (Hebrew) a form of Aliya.
Aalyah

Aaron 🅱🅲 (Hebrew) enlightened. (Arabic)
messenger. Bible: the brother of Moses and
the first high priest. See also Arin, Erin.

Aarti (Hebrew, Hindi) a form of Arti.

Aasta (Norse) love.
Aastah, Asta, Astah

Aba (Fante, Twi) born on Thursday.

Abagael, Abagail, Abbagail (Hebrew)
forms of Abigail.
Abagaile, Abagale, Abagayle, Abageal, Abagil,
Abbagael, Abbagale, Abbagayle

Abauro (Greek) tint of the sky at sunrise.

Abbey 🅶🅱 (Hebrew) a familiar form of
Abigail.
Aabbee, Abbe, Abbea, Abbee, Abbeigh, Abbye,
Abea, Abee, Abeey, Abey, Abi, Abia, Abie, Aby

Abbi, Abbie, Abby (Hebrew) familiar
forms of Abigail.

Abbigail, Abbigale, Abbigayle, Abigael,
Abigayle (Hebrew) forms of Abigail.
Abbigael, Abbigal, Abbigayl

Abbygail, Abygail (Hebrew) forms of
Abigail.
Abbygael, Abbygale, Abbygayl, Abbygayle,
Abygael, Abygaile, Abygale, Abygayl, Abygayle

Abeer (Hebrew) a short form of Abira.
Abeir, Abiir, Abir

Abegail (Hebrew) a form of Abigail.
Abegael, Abegaile, Abegale, Abegayle

Abelarda (Arabic) servant of Allah.

Abelina (American) a combination of
Abbey + Lina.
Abilana, Abilene

Abeliñe (Basque) a form of Abelina.

Abena (Akan) born on Tuesday.
Abenah, Abeni, Abina, Abinah, Abyna,
Abynah

Aberfa (Welsh) one who comes from the
mouth of the river.

Abertha (Welsh) to sacrifice.

Abia (Arabic) great.
Abbia, Abbiah, Abiah, Abya

Abiann, Abianne (American) combinations
of Abbey + Ann.
Abian

Abida (Arabic) worshiper.
Abedah, Abidah

Abidán (Hebrew) my father is judge.

Abiel (Hebrew) God is my father.

Abigail ☀ (Hebrew) father's joy. Bible: one
of the wives of King David. See also Gail.
Abaigael, Abaigeal, Abbegaele, Abbegail,
Abbegale, Abbegayle, Abbeygale, Abbiegail,
Abbiegayle, Abgail, Abgale, Abgayle, Abigaile,
Abigaill, Abigal, Abigale, Abigayil, Abigayl,
Abigel, Abigial, Abugail, Avigail

Abigaíl (Spanish) a form of Abigail.

Abinaya (American) a form of Abiann.
Abenaa, Abenaya, Abinaa, Abinaiya, Abinayan

Abira (Hebrew) my strength.
Abbira, Abeerah, Abera, Aberah, Abhira, Abirah, Abyra, Abyrah

Abiram (Hebrew) my father is great.

Abra (Hebrew) mother of many nations.
Abrah, Abree, Abri

Abria (Hebrew) a form of Abra.
Abrea, Abréa, Abreia, Abriah, Abriéa, Abrya, Abryah

Abrial (French) open; secure, protected.
Abrail, Abreal, Abreale, Abriale

Abriana, Abrianna (Italian) forms of Abra.
Abbrienna, Abbryana, Abranna, Abrannah, Abreana, Abreanna, Abreanne, Abreeana, Abreona, Abreonia, Abrianah, Abriania, Abrianiah, Abriann, Abriannah, Abrieana, Abrien, Abrienna, Abrienne, Abrietta, Abrion, Abrionée, Abrionne, Abriunna, Abryan, Abryana, Abryanah, Abryann, Abryanna, Abryannah, Abryanne, Abryona

Abrielle (French) a form of Abrial.
Aabriella, Abriel, Abriela, Abriell, Abryele, Abryell, Abryella, Abryelle

Abrienda (Spanish) opening.

Abril (French) a form of Abrial.
Abrilla, Abrille

Abundia (Latin) abundance.

Acacia (Greek) thorny. Mythology: the acacia tree symbolizes immortality and resurrection. See also Casey.
Acaciah, Acacya, Acacyah, Acasha, Acatia, Accassia, Acey, Acie, Akacia, Cacia, Caciah, Cacya, Cacyah, Casia, Kasia

Acacitlu (Nahuatl) rabbit of the water.

Acalia (Latin) Mythology: another name for Acca Larentia, the adoptive mother of Romulus and Remus.

Achcauhtli (Nahuatl) leader.

Achilla (Greek) a form of Achilles (see Boys' Names).
Achila, Achilah, Achillah, Achyla, Achylah, Achylla, Achyllah

Acima (Illyrian) praised by God.
Acimah, Acyma, Acymah

Acindina (Greek) safe.

Acquilina (Greek) a form of Aquilla.

Ada (German) a short form of Adelaide. (English) prosperous; happy. (Hebrew) a form of Adah.
Adabelle, Adan, Adaya, Adda, Auda

Adabella (Spanish) a combination of Ada and Bella.

Adah (Hebrew) ornament. (German, English) a form of Ada.
Addah

Adair **GB** (Greek) a form of Adara.
Adaire, Adare, Adayr, Adayre

Adalcira (Spanish) a combination of Ada and Alcira.

Adalene (Spanish) a form of Adalia.
Adalane, Adalena, Adalin, Adalina, Adaline, Adalinn, Adalyn, Adalynn, Adalynne, Addalyn, Addalynn

Adalgisa (German) noble hostage.

Adalia (German, Spanish) noble.
Adal, Adala, Adalah, Adalea, Adaleah, Adalee, Adalene, Adali, Adaliah, Adalie, Adall, Adalla, Adalle, Adallia, Adalliah, Adallya, Adallyah, Adaly, Adalya, Adalyah, Addal, Addala, Addaly

Adalsinda (German) noble strength.

Adaluz (Spanish) a combination of Ada and Luz.

Adama (Phoenician, Hebrew) a form of Adam (see Boys' Names).
Adamah, Adamia, Adamiah, Adamina, Adaminah, Adamya, Adamyah, Adamyna, Adamynah, Adamyne

Adamma (Ibo) child of beauty.

Adán (Spanish) a form of Adam (see Boys' Names).

Adana (Spanish) a form of Adama.
Adanah, Adania, Adaniah, Adanya

Adanna (Nigerian) her father's daughter.

Adar **GB** (Syrian) ruler. (Hebrew) noble; exalted.
Adare, Adayr

Adara (Greek) beauty. (Arabic) virgin.
Adaira, Adairah, Adaora, Adar, Adarah, Adare,
Adaria, Adarra, Adasha, Adauré, Adayra, Adayrah

Adawna (Latin) beautiful sunrise.
Adawnah

Adaya (American) a form of Ada.
Adaija, Adaijah, Adaja, Adajah, Adayah,
Adayja, Adayjah, Addiah, Adejah

Addie (Greek, German) a familiar form of
Adelaide, Adrienne.
Aday, Adde, Addee, Addey, Addi, Addia, Ade,
Adee, Adei, Adey, Adeye, Adi, Adie, Ady, Atti,
Attie, Atty

Addison BG (English) child of Adam.
Addis, Addisen, Addisson

Addolorata (Italian) a form of Dolores.

Addy GB (Greek, German) a familiar form
of Adelaide, Adrienne.

Addyson, Adyson (English) forms of Addison.
Adysen

Adela (English) a short form of Adelaide.
Adelae, Adelah, Adelista, Adella, Adelya,
Adelyah

Adelaida (German) a form of Adelaide.
Adelayda, Adelaydah, Adelka

Adelaide (German) noble and serene. See
also Ada, Adela, Adeline, Adele, Ailis, Delia,
Della, Ela, Elke, Heidi.
Adalaid, Adalaide, Adalayd, Adalayde,
Adelade, Adelaid, Adelais, Adelayd, Adelayde,
Adelei, Adelheid, Adeliade, Aley, Edelaid,
Edelaide, Laidey, Laidy

Adelais (French) a form of Adelaide.

Adelaisa (Italian) a form of Adelaida.

Adele, Adelle (English) short forms of
Adelaide, Adeline.
Adel, Adelie, Adell, Adile

Adelia (Spanish) a form of Adelaide.
Adeliah

Adelina (English) a form of Adeline.
Adalina, Adeleana, Adelena, Adeliana,
Adellena, Adellyna, Adileena, Adlena

Adelinda (Teutonic) noble; serpent.
Adelindah, Adelynda, Adelyndah

Adeline (English) a form of Adelaide.
Adaline, Adelaine, Adeleine, Adelin, Adelind,
Adelita, Adeliya, Adelyn, Adelyne, Adelynn,
Adelynne, Adlin, Adline, Adlyn, Adlynn

Adelma (Teutonic) protector of the needy.

Adelmira (Arabic) exalted.

Adelpha (Greek) sister.
Adelfa, Adelfah, Adelfe, Adelfia, Adelphah,
Adelphe, Adelphia, Adelphya, Adelphyah

Adeltruda (German) strong and noble.

Adelvina (German) ennobled by victory.

Adena (Hebrew) noble; adorned.
Adeana, Adeanah, Adeane, Adeen, Adeena,
Adeenah, Adeene, Aden, Adenah, Adene,
Adenia, Adenna

Adhara (Arabic) maiden. Astronomy: a star
in the Canis Major constellation.

Adia (Swahili) gift.
Addia, Adea, Adéa, Adiah

Adiel (Hebrew) ornament of the Lord.
(African) goat.
Adiela, Adielah, Adiele, Adiell, Adiella,
Adielle, Adyel, Adyela, Adyelah, Adyele,
Adyell, Adyella, Adyellah, Adyelle

Adien (Welsh) beautiful.

Adila (Arabic) equal.
Adeala, Adeela, Adeola, Adilah, Adileh,
Adilia, Adyla

Adilene (English) a form of Adeline.
Adilen, Adileni, Adilenne, Adlen, Adlene

Adina (Hebrew) a form of Adena. See
also Dina.
Adeana, Adiana, Adiena, Adinah, Adine,
Adinna, Adyna, Adynah, Adyne

Adira (Hebrew) strong.
Ader, Adera, Aderah, Aderra, Adhira, Adirah,
Adirana, Adyra, Adyrah

Adison BG (English) a form of Addison.
Adis, Adisa, Adisen, Adisynne

Aditi (Hindi) unbound. Religion: the
mother of the Hindu sun gods.
Aditee, Adithi, Aditie, Aditti, Adity, Adytee,
Adytey, Adyti, Adytie, Adyty

Adleigh (Hebrew) my ornament.
Adla, Adleni

Adolfa (Arabic) exalted.

Adoncia (Spanish) sweet.

Adonia (Spanish) beautiful.
Adoniah, Adonica, Adonis, Adonna, Adonnica,
Adonya, Adonyah

Adora (Latin) beloved. See also Dora.
Adorah, Adore, Adoree, Adoria, Adoriah,
Adorya, Adoryah

Adoración (Latin) the action of venerating
the magical gods.

Adra (Arabic) virgin.

Adreana, Adreanna (Latin) forms of
Adrienne.
Adrean, Adreanah, Adreane, Adreann, Adreannah,
Adreanne, Adreauna, Adreeanna, Adreen, Adreena,
Adreenah, Adreene, Adreeyana, Adrena, Adrene,
Adrenea, Adréona, Adreonia, Adreonna

Adrenilda (German) mother of the warrior.

Adria (English) a short form of Adriana,
Adrienne.
Adrea, Adreah, Adriah, Adriani, Adrya

Adriadna (Greek) she who is very holy,
who doesn't yield.

Adrian **BG** (English) a form of Adrienne.
Addrian, Adranne, Adriann

Adrián (Hispanic) from the Adriatic Sea.

Adriana, Adrianna (Italian) forms of
Adrienne.
Addrianna, Addriyanna, Adreiana, Adreinna,
Adrianah, Adriannah, Adriannea, Adriannia,
Adrionna

Adriane, Adrianne, Adrien, Adriene
(English) forms of Adrienne.

Adrielle (Hebrew) member of God's flock.
Adriel, Adrielli, Adryelle

Adrien **BG** (Greek, Latin) a form of
Adrienne.

Adrienna (Italian) a form of Adrienne. See
also Edrianna.
Adrieanna, Adrieaunna, Adriena, Adrienah,
Adrienia, Adriennah, Adrieunna, Adriyanna

Adrienne (Greek) rich. (Latin) dark. See also
Hadriane.
Adreinne, Adriayon, Adrie, Adrieanne,
Adrienn, Adrion

Adrina (English) a short form of Adriana.
Adrinah, Adrine, Adrinne

Adriyanna (American) a form of Adrienne.
Adrieyana, Adriyana, Adryan, Adryana,
Adryanah, Adryane, Adryann, Adryanna,
Adryannah, Adryanne

Adya (Hindi) Sunday.
Adia

Aelwyd (Welsh) one that comes from the
chimney.

Aerial, Aeriel (Hebrew) forms of Ariel.
Aeriale, Aeriela, Aerielah, Aeriell, Aeriella,
Aeriellah, Aerielle, Aeril, Aerile, Aeryal

Aerin (Hebrew, Arabic) a form of Aaron,
Arin.

Aerona (Welsh) berry.
Aeronah, Aeronna, Aeronnah

Afi (African) born on Friday.
Affi, Afia, Efi, Efia

Afilia (Germanic) of noble lineage.

Afina (Hebrew) young doe.
Afinah, Afynah, Aphina, Aphinah, Aphyna,
Aphynah

Afra (Hebrew) young doe. (Arabic) earth
color. See also Aphra.
Affery, Affrah, Affrey, Affrie, Afraa, Afrah,
Afria, Afriah, Afrya, Afryah

Africa (Latin, Greek) sunny; not cold.
Geography: one of the seven continents.
Affreeca, Affreecah, Affrica, Affricah, Affricka,
Affryca, Affrycah, Afreeca, Afreecah, Afric,
Africah, Africaya, Africia, Africiana, Afryca,
Afrycah, Afrycka, Afryckah, Aifric

África (Spanish) a form of Africa.

Afrika (Irish) a form of Africa.
Affreeka, Affreekah, Affryka, Affrykah,
Afreeka, Afreekah, Afrikah, Afryka, Afrykah

Afrodite (Greek) a form of Aphrodite.
Afrodita

Afton GB (English) from Afton, England.
Aftan, Aftine, Aftinn, Aftona, Aftonah, Aftone,
Aftonia, Aftoniah, Aftonie, Aftony, Aftonya,
Aftonyah, Aftonye, Aftyn

Agalia (Spanish) bright; joy.

Aganetha (Greek) a form of Agnes.

Ágape (Latin) love.

Agapita (Greek) she who is beloved and
wanted.

Agar (Hebrew) she who fled.

Ágata (Greek) friendly with everyone.

Agate (English) a semiprecious stone.

Agatha (Greek) good, kind. Literature:
Agatha Christie was a British writer of
more than seventy detective novels. See
also Gasha.
Agace, Agacia, Agafa, Agafia, Agaisha, Agasha,
Agata, Agatah, Agathia, Agathiah, Agathya,
Agathyah, Agatka, Agetha, Aggie, Ágota,
Ágotha, Agueda, Agytha, Atka

Agathe (Greek) a form of Agatha.
Agathi, Agathie, Agathy

Agdta (Spanish) a form of Ágata.

Aggie (Greek) a short form of Agatha,
Agnes.
Ag, Aggy, Agi

Agilberta (German) famous sword of combat.

Aglaia (Greek) beautiful.
Aglae, Aglaiah, Aglaya, Aglayah, Aglaye

Agnella (Greek) a form of Agnes.
Agnela, Agnelah, Agnele, Agnelia, Agneliah,
Agnelie, Agnellah, Agnelle, Agnellia, Agnelliah,
Agnellie, Agnellya, Agnellyah

Agnes (Greek) pure. See also Aneesa, Anice,
Anisha, Ina, Ines, Necha, Nessa, Nessie,
Neza, Nyusha, Una, Ynez.
Agna, Agne, Agneis, Agnés, Agnesa, Agnesca,
Agnese, Agnesina, Agness, Agnessa, Agnesse,
Agneta, Agnete, Agnetha, Agneti, Agnetis,
Agnetta, Agnette, Agnies, Agniya, Agnola,
Agnus, Aignéis, Aneska

Agnieszka (Greek) a form of Agnes.

Agrippina (Latin) born feet first.
Agripa, Agripah, Agripina, Agripinah,
Agripine, Agrippah, Agrippinah, Agrippine,
Agrypina, Agrypinah, Agrypine, Agryppina,
Agryppinah, Agryppine, Agryppyna,
Agryppynah, Agryppyne

Aguas Vivas (Spanish) living waters.

Agüeda (Greek) having many virtues.

Águeda (Spanish) a form of Ágata.

Ahava (Hebrew) beloved.
Ahavah, Ahivia, Ahuva, Ahuvah

Ahlam (Arabic) witty; one who has pleasant
dreams.

Ahliya (Hebrew) a form of Aliya.
Ahlai, Ahlaia, Ahlaya, Ahleah, Ahleeyah,
Ahley, Ahleya, Ahlia, Ahliah, Ahliyah

Ahuiliztli (Nahuatl) joy.

Ahulani (Hawaiian) heavenly shrine.
Ahulanee, Ahulaney, Ahulania, Ahulaniah,
Ahulanie, Ahulany, Ahulanya, Ahulanyah

Ai (Japanese) love; indigo blue.

Aida (Latin) helpful. (English) a form of
Ada.
Aidah, Aidee, Ayda, Aydah

Aída (Latin) a form of Aida.

Aidan BG (Latin) a form of Aida.
Adan, Aden, Adene, Aidana, Aidanah, Aidane,
Aidann, Aidanna, Aidannah, Aidanne, Aydan,
Aydana, Aydanah, Aydane, Aydann, Aydanna,
Aydannah, Aydanne

Aide (Latin, English) a short form of Aida.

Aidé (Greek) a form of Haidee.

Aiden BG (Latin) a form of Aida.

Aidia (Spanish) a form of Aida.

Aiesha (Swahili, Arabic) a form of Aisha.
Aieshah, Aieshia

Aiko (Japanese) beloved.

Ailani (Hawaiian) chief.
Aelani, Ailana

Aileen (Scottish) light bearer. (Irish) a form
of Helen. See also Eileen.
Ailean, Aileana, Aileanah, Aileane, Aileena,

Ailein, Aileina, Ailen, Ailena, Ailenah, Ailene, Aileyn, Aileyna, Aileynah, Ailin, Ailina, Ailinn, Aillen, Ailyn, Ailyna, Alean, Aleana, Aleanah, Aleane, Aylean, Ayleana, Ayleen, Ayleena, Aylein, Ayleina, Ayleyn, Ayleyna, Aylin, Aylina, Aylyn, Aylyna

Ailén (Mapuche) ember.

Aili (Scottish) a form of Alice. (Finnish) a form of Helen.
Aila, Ailee, Ailey, Ailie, Aily

Ailín, Aillén (Mapuche) transparent, very clear.

Ailis (Irish) a form of Adelaide.
Ailesh, Ailish, Ailyse, Eilis

Ailsa (Scottish) island dweller. Geography: Ailsa Craig is an island in Scotland.
Ailsah, Ailsha, Aylsa, Aylsah

Ailya (Hebrew) a form of Aliya.
Ailiyah

Aime, Aimie (Latin, French) forms of Aimee.

Aimee (Latin) a form of Amy. (French) loved.
Aimée, Aimey, Aimi, Aimia, Aimy, Aimya

Aina (Hebrew) a form of Anna.

Ainara (Basque) swallow.

Ainhoa (Basque) allusion to the Virgin Mary.

Ainoa (Basque) she who has fertile soil.

Ainona (Hebrew) a form of Aina.

Ainsley **GB** (Scottish) my own meadow.
Ainslea, Ainsleah, Ainslee, Ainslei, Ainsleigh, Ainsly, Aynslea, Aynsleah, Aynslee, Aynslei, Aynsleigh, Aynsley, Aynsli, Aynslie, Aynsly

Ainslie (Scottish) a form of Ainsley.
Ainsli

Aintzane (Spanish) glorious.

Airiana (English) a form of Ariana.
Airana, Airanna, Aireana, Aireanah, Aireanna, Aireona, Aireonna, Aireyonna, Airianna, Airianne, Airiona, Airriana, Airrion, Airryon, Airyana, Airyanna

Airiél (Hebrew) a form of Ariel.
Aieral, Aierel, Aiiryel, Aire, Aireal, Aireale, Aireel, Airel, Airele, Airelle, Airi, Airial, Airiale, Airrel

Airleas (Irish) promise.
Airlea, Airleah, Airlee, Airlei, Airleigh, Airley, Airli, Airlie, Airly, Aylie, Ayrlea, Ayrleas, Ayrlee, Ayrlei, Ayrleigh, Ayrley, Ayrli, Ayrly

Aisha (Swahili) life. (Arabic) woman. See also Asha, Asia, Iesha, Isha, Keisha, Leisha, Yiesha.
Aaisha, Aaishah, Aeisha, Aesha, Aeshah, Aeshia, Aheesha, Aiasha, Aieysha, Aiiesha, Aisa, Aischa, Aish, Aishah, Aisheh, Aiyesha, Aiysha, Aysa, Ayse, Aytza

Aishia (Swahili, Arabic) a form of Aisha.
Aishiah

Aisling (Irish) a form of Aislinn.

Aislinn, Aislynn (Irish) forms of Ashlyn.
Aishellyn, Aishlinn, Aislee, Aisley, Aislin, Aislyn, Aislynne, Ayslin, Ayslinn, Ayslyn, Ayslynn

Aisone (Basque) a form of Asunción.

Aixa (Latin, German) a form of Axelle.

Aiyana (Native American) forever flowering.
Aiyanah, Aiyhana, Aiyona, Aiyonia

Aiyanna (Native American) a form of Aiyana. (Hindi) a form of Ayanna.
Aianna, Aiyannah, Aiyonna, Aiyunna

Aja (Hindi) goat.
Ahjah, Aija, Aijah, Ajá, Ajada, Ajara, Ajaran, Ajare, Ajaree, Ajha, Ajya, Ajyah

Ajah (Hindi) a form of Aja.

Ajanae (American) a combination of the letter A + Janae.
Ajahnae, Ajahne, Ajana, Ajanaé, Ajane, Ajané, Ajanee, Ajanique, Ajena, Ajenae, Ajené

Ajee, Ajée (Punjabi, American) forms of Ajay (see Boys' Names).

Ajia (Hindi) a form of Aja.
Aijia, Ajhia, Aji, Ajiah, Ajjia

Akasha (American) a form of Akeisha.
Akasia

Akayla (American) a combination of the letter A + Kayla.
Akaela, Akaelia, Akaila, Akailah, Akala, Akaylah, Akaylia

Akeisha (American) a combination of the letter A + Keisha.
Akaesha, Akaisha, Akeecia, Akeesha, Akeishia, Akeshia, Akisha

Akela (Hawaiian) noble.
Ahkayla, Ahkeelah, Akeia, Akeiah, Akelah, Akelia, Akeliah, Akeya, Akeyah

Akeria (American) a form of Akira.
Akera, Akerah, Akeri, Akerra

Akeyla (Hawaiian) a form of Akela.
Akeylah

Aki (Japanese) born in autumn.
Akee, Akeeye, Akei, Akey, Akie, Aky

Akia (American) a combination of the letter A + Kia.
Akaja, Akeia, Akeiah, Akeya, Akeyah, Akiá, Akiah, Akiane, Akiaya, Akiea, Akiya, Akiyah, Akya, Akyan, Akyia, Akyiah

Akiko (Japanese) bright light.
Akyko

Akila (Arabic) a form of Akilah.

Akilah (Arabic) intelligent.
Aikiela, Aikilah, Akeela, Akeelah, Akeila, Akeilah, Akeiyla, Akiela, Akielah, Akilaih, Akilia, Akilka, Akilkah, Akillah, Akkila, Akyla, Akylah

Akili 🅱🅶 (Tanzanian) wisdom.
Akilea, Akileah, Akilee, Akilei, Akileigh, Akiliah, Akilie, Akily, Akylee, Akyli, Akylie

Akilina (Greek) a form of Aquilla.

Akina (Japanese) spring flower.

Akira 🅶🅱 (American) a combination of the letter A + Kira.
Akiera, Akierra, Akirah, Akire, Akiria, Akirrah, Akyra

Alaa 🅶🅱 (Arabic) a form of Aladdin (see Boys' Names).
Ala

Alaia (Basque) happy, of good cheer.

Alaina (Irish) a form of Alana.
Alain, Alainah, Alaine, Alainna, Alainnah, Allaina, Allainah, Allaine

Alair (French) a form of Hilary.
Alaira, Allaire

Alamea (Hawaiian) ripe; precious.
Alameah, Alameya, Alameyah, Alamia, Alamiah, Almya, Almyah

Alameda (Spanish) poplar tree.
Alamedah

Alana (Irish) attractive; peaceful. (Hawaiian) offering. See also Lana.
Aalaina, Alaana, Alanae, Alane, Alanea, Alania, Alawna, Aleine, Alleyna, Alleynah, Alleyne

Alanah (Irish, Hawaiian) a form of Alana.

Alandra (Spanish) a form of Alexandra, Alexandria.
Alantra, Aleandra

Alandria (Spanish) a form of Alexandra, Alexandria.
Alandrea, Aleandrea

Alani (Hawaiian) orange tree. (Irish) a form of Alana.
Alaini, Alainie, Alanea, Alanee, Alaney, Alania, Alaniah, Alanie, Alannie, Alany, Alanya, Alanyah

Alanis (Irish) beautiful; bright.
Alanisa, Alanisah, Alanise, Alaniss, Alanissa, Alanissah, Alanisse, Alannis, Alannisa, Alannisah, Alannise, Alannys, Alannysa, Alannyse, Alanys, Alanysa, Alanysah, Alanyse, Alanyss, Alanyssa, Alanyssah, Alanysse

Alanna, Alannah (Irish) forms of Alana.

Alanza (Spanish) noble and eager.

Alarice (German) ruler of all.
Alarica, Alaricah, Alaricia, Alarisa, Alarisah, Alarise, Allaryca, Allaryce, Alrica, Alricah, Alryca, Alrycah, Alryqua, Alryque

Alastrina (Scottish) defender of humankind.
Alastriana, Alastrianah, Alastriane, Alastrianna, Alastriannah, Alastrianne, Alastrinah, Alastrine, Alastryan, Alastryana, Alastryanah, Alastryane, Alastryann, Alastryanna, Alastryannah, Alastryanne, Alastryn, Alastryna, Alastrynah, Alastryne,

Alastrynia, Alastryniah, Alastrynya,
Alastrynyah

Alatea (Spanish, Greek) truth.

Alaura (American) a form of Alora.

Alaya (Hebrew) a form of Aliya.
Alayah

Alayna (Irish) a form of Alana.
Alaynah, Alayne, Alaynna, Alaynnah

Alaysha, Alaysia (American) forms of
Alicia.
Alaysh, Alayshia

Alazne (Spanish) miracle.

Alba (Latin) from Alba Longa, an ancient
city near Rome, Italy.
Albah, Albana, Albani, Albania, Albanie,
Albany, Albeni, Albina, Albinah, Albine,
Albinia, Albinka, Albyna, Albynah, Albyne,
Aubina, Aubinah, Aubine, Aubyna, Aubynah,
Aubyne, Elba

Alberta (German, French) noble and bright.
See also Auberte, Bertha, Elberta.
Albertina, Albertinah, Albertine, Albertyna,
Albertyne, Albirta, Albirtina, Albirtine,
Albirtyna, Albrette, Alburta, Alburtah,
Alburtina, Alburtinah, Alburtine, Alburtyna,
Alburtynah, Alburtyne, Albyrta, Albyrtah,
Albyrtina, Albyrtine, Albyrtyna, Albyrtynah,
Albyrtyne, Alverta, Alvertah, Alvertina,
Alvertine

Alborada (Latin) brandy-colored dawn.

Albreanna (American) a combination of
Alberta + Breanna (see Breana).
Albré, Albrea, Albreona, Albreonna, Albreyon

Alcina (Greek) strong-minded.
Alceena, Alcie, Alcinah, Alcine, Alcinia,
Alciniah, Alcyna, Alcynah, Alcyne, Alseena,
Alsina, Alsinah, Alsine, Alsinia, Alsyn,
Alsyna, Alsynah, Alsyne, Alzina, Alzinah,
Alzine, Alzyna, Alzynah, Alzyne

Alcira (German) adornment of nobility.

Alda (German) old; elder.
Aldah, Aldina, Aldine

Aldana (Spanish) a combination of Alda +
Ana.

Aldegunda (German) famous leader.

Alden **BG** (English) old; wise protector.
Aldan, Aldon, Aldyn

Aldetruda (German) strong leader.

Aldina, Aldine (Hebrew) forms of Alda.
Aldeana, Aldene, Aldona, Aldyna, Aldyne

Aldonsa, Aldonza (Spanish) nice.

Aldora (English) gift; superior.
Aldorah

Alea, Aleah (Arabic) high, exalted. (Persian)
God's being.
Aileah, Allea, Alleah, Alleea, Alleeah

Aleaha (Arabic, Persian) a form of Alea.

Aleasha (Greek) a form of Alisha.
Aleashae, Aleashea, Aleashia, Aleasia, Aleassa

Alecia (Greek) a form of Alicia.
Aalecia, Ahlasia, Aleacia, Aleacya, Aleasia,
Alecea, Aleceea, Aleceia, Aleciya, Aleciyah,
Alecy, Alecya, Aleicia, Allecia

Aleea (Arabic, Persian) a form of Alea.
(Hebrew) a form of Aliya.
Aleeah

Aleecia (Greek) a form of Alicia.
Aleeceia, Aleeciah, Aleesia, Aleesiya, Alleecia

Aleela (Swahili) she cries.
Aleala, Alealah, Aleelah, Aleighla, Aleighlah,
Aleila, Aleilah, Aleyla, Aleylah, Alila, Alile,
Alyla, Alylah

Aleena (Dutch) a form of Aleene.
Ahleena, Aleana, Aleanah, Aleeanna, Aleenah,
Aleighna, Aleighnah, Aleina, Aleinah

Aleene (Dutch) alone. See also Allene.
Aleane, Aleighn, Aleighne, Aleine, Alyn, Alyne

Aleesa (Greek) a form of Alice, Alyssa. See
also Alisa.
Aleessa

Aleesha (Greek) a form of Alisha.
Aleeshah, Aleeshia, Aleeshya

Aleeya (Hebrew) a form of Aliya.
Alee, Aleeyah, Aleiya, Aleiyah

Aleeza (Hebrew) a form of Aliza. See also
Leeza.
Aleaza, Aleazah, Aleezah, Aleiza, Aleizah,
Aleyza, Aleyzah

Alegía, Alegría, Allegría (Spanish) forms of
Allegra.

Alegria (Spanish) cheerful.
Aleggra, Alegra

Aleia, Aleigha (Arabic, Persian) forms of
Alea.
Alei, Aleiah

Aleisha (Greek) a form of Alicia, Alisha.
Aleisa

Aleja (Spanish) a form of Alejandra.

Alejandra (Spanish) a form of Alexandra.
Aleiandra, Alejanda, Alejandr, Alejandrea,
Alejandria, Alejandro

Alejandrina (Spanish) a form of Alejandra.

Aleka (Hawaiian) a form of Alice.
Aleaka, Aleakah, Aleeka, Aleekah, Aleika,
Aleikah, Alekah, Aleyka, Aleykah

Aleksa (Greek) a form of Alexa.
Aleksha

Aleksandra (Greek) a form of Alexandra.
Alecsandra, Alecxandra, Alecxandrah,
Aleczandra, Aleczandrah, Aleksandrija,
Aleksandriya, Aleksasha

Alena (Russian) a form of Helen.
Aleana, Aleanah, Aleina, Alenah, Alene,
Alenea, Aleni, Alenia, Alenka, Alenna,
Alennah, Alenya, Aliena

Aleria (Latin) eagle.
Alearia, Aleariah, Alearya, Alearyah, Aleriah,
Alerya, Aleryah

Alesha (Greek) a form of Alicia, Alisha.
Alesa, Alesah

Aleshia (Greek) a form of Alicia, Alisha.
Aleshya

Alesia, Alessia (Greek) forms of Alice,
Alicia, Alisha.
Alesiah, Alessea, Alessiah, Alesya, Alesyah,
Allesia

Alessa (Greek) a form of Alice.
Alessi, Allessa

Alessandra (Italian) a form of Alexandra.
Alesandra, Alesandrea, Alessandria,
Alessandriah, Alessandrie, Alessandryn,
Alessandryna, Alessandryne, Alissandra,
Alissondra, Allesand, Allessandra

Aleta (Greek) a form of Alida. See also Leta.
Aleata, Aleatah, Aleeta, Aleetah, Aleighta,
Aleita, Aleitah, Aletah, Aletta, Alettah, Alette,
Aleyta, Aleytah, Alletta

Aleth (Greek) a form of Alethea.

Aletha (Greek) a short form of Alethea.

Alethea (Greek) truth.
Alathea, Alatheah, Alathia, Alathiah, Aleathia,
Aleathiah, Aleathya, Aleathyah, Aleethea,
Aleetheah, Aleethia, Aleethiah, Aleethya,
Aleethyah, Aleighthea, Aleighthia, Aleighthya,
Aleithea, Aleitheah, Aleithia, Aleithiah,
Aleithya, Aleithyah, Aletea, Aletheah, Aletheia,
Aletheiah, Alethia, Alethiah, Aletia, Alithea,
Alitheah, Alithia, Alithiah, Allethea, Alythea,
Alytheah, Alythia, Alythiah, Alythya, Alythyah

Alette (Latin) wing.
Aletta, Alettah

Alex BG (Greek) a short form of Alexander,
Alexandra.
Aleix, Aleks, Alexx, Allex, Allexx

Alex Ann, Alex Anne, Alexane, Alexanne
(American) combinations of Alex + Ann.
Alex-Ann, Alex-Anne, Alexan, Alexann,
Alexanna, Alexian, Alexiana, Alexina,
Alexinah, Alexine, Alexyna, Alexynah,
Alexyne

Alexa ☆ (Greek) a short form of Alexandra.
Aleixa, Alekia, Aleksi, Alexah, Alexxa,
Allexa, Alyxa

Alexander BG (Greek) defender of
mankind. History: Alexander the Great was
the conqueror of the Greek Empire.
Al, Alec, Alecander, Alecsandar, Alecsander,
Alecxander, Alejándro, Alek, Alekos,
Aleksandar, Aleksander, Aleksei, Alekzander,
Alessander, Alessandro, Alexandar, Alexandor,
Alexandr, Alexandro, Alexandros, Alexxander,
Alexzander, Alic, Alick, Alisander, Alixander

Alexanderia (Greek) a form of Alexandria.

Alexandra ☆ GB (Greek) a form of
Alexander. History: the last czarina of

Russia. See also Lexi, Lexia, Olesia, Ritsa, Sandra, Sandrine, Sasha, Shura, Sondra, Xandra, Zandra.
Alaxandra, Alexande, Alexandera, Alexina, Alexine, Alexxandra, Alexxandrah, Alixsandra, Aljexi, Alla, Lexandra

Alexandre **BG** (Greek) a form of Alexandra.

Alexandrea (Greek) a form of Alexandria.
Alexanndrea

Alexandria (Greek) a form of Alexandra. See also Xandra, Zandra.
Alaxandria, Alecsandria, Alecxandria, Alecxandriah, Alecxandrya, Alecxandryah, Aleczandria, Aleczandriah, Aleczandrya, Aleczandryah, Alexandreia, Alexandriah, Alexandrie, Alexandriea, Alexandrieah, Alexandrya, Alexandryah, Alexanndria, Alexanndrya, Alexendria, Alexxandria, Alexxandriah, Alexxandrya, Alexxandryah, Alixandrea, Alixzandria

Alexandrine (Greek) a form of Alexandra. See also Drina.
Alecsandrina, Alejandrine, Alejandryn, Alejandryna, Alejandryne, Aleksandrina, Aleksandryne, Alexandreana, Alexandrena, Alexandrina, Alexandrinah, Alexendrine, Alexzandrina, Alexzandrinah, Alexzandrine, Alexzandryna, Alexzandrynah

Alexas, Alexes, Alexiss, Alexsis, Alexus, Alexxis, Alexxus, Alexys, Allexis, Allexus (Greek) forms of Alexis.
Alexess, Alexuss, Alexyss, Allexys

Alexcia (Greek) a form of Alexia.

Alexe (Greek) a form of Alex.

Alexi **GB** (Greek) a short form of Alexandra.
Aleksey, Aleksi, Alexey, Alexy

Alexia (Greek) a short form of Alexandria. See also Lexia.
Aleksia, Aleksiah, Aleksya, Aleksyah, Aleska, Alexea, Alexiah, Alexsia, Alexsiya, Allexia, Alyxia

Alexie (Greek) a short form of Alexandra.

Alexis ☆ **GB** (Greek) a short form of Alexandra.
Aalexis, Aalexus, Aalexxus, Aelexus, Ahlexis, Ahlexus, Alaxis, Alecsis, Alecsus, Alecxis, Aleexis, Aleksis, Aleksys, Alexias, Alexiou,

Alexiz, Alexsus, Alexsys, Alexxiz, Alexyes, Alexyis, Alixis, Alixus, Elexis, Elexus, Lexis, Lexus

Alexius (Greek) a form of Alexis.
Allexius

Alexsa (Greek) a form of Alexa.
Alexssa

Alexsandra (Greek) a form of Alexandra.
Alexsandria, Alexsandro

Alexzandra (Greek) a form of Alexandra.
Alexzand, Alexzandrah

Alexzandria (Greek) a form of Alexandria.
Alexzandrea, Alexzandriah, Alexzandrya

Aleya, Aleyah (Hebrew) forms of Aliya.
Aleayah, Aléyah, Aleyia, Aleyiah

Aleyda (Greek) she who is like Athena.

Alfie **BG** (English) a familiar form of Alfreda.
Alfi, Alfy

Alfilda (German) she who helps the elves.

Alfonsa (German) noble and eager.
Alfonsia, Alfonsina, Alfonsine, Alfonsyna, Alfonsyne

Alfreda (English) elf counselor; wise counselor. See also Effie, Elfrida, Freda, Frederica.
Alfredah, Alfredda, Alfredia, Alfreeda, Alfreida, Alfrida, Alfridah, Alfrieda, Alfryda, Alfrydah, Alfrydda, Alfryddah

Alhertina (Spanish) noble.

Ali **BG** (Greek) a familiar form of Alice, Alicia, Alisha, Alison.
Alee, Alei, Aleigh, Aley, Allea, Allee, Allei, Alleigh

Alia, Aliah, Allia, Alliah (Hebrew) forms of Aliya. See also Aaliya, Alea.
Aelia, Allea, Alleah, Alya

Alice (Greek) truthful. (German) noble. See also Aili, Aleka, Ali, Alisa, Alison, Alyce, Alysa, Elke.
Adelice, Aleece, Aleese, Alicie, Alics, Aliece, Aliese, Alla, Alleece, Alles, Allesse, Allice

Alicen, Alicyn, Alisyn, Allisyn (English) forms of Alison.

Alicia (English) a form of Alice. See also
Elicia, Licia.
Adelicia, Aelicia, Aleacia, Aleaciah, Alecea,
Aleicia, Aleiciah, Aleighcia, Aleighsia,
Aleighsya, Aleisia, Aleisiah, Aleisya, Aleisyah,
Alicea, Alicha, Alichia, Aliciah, Alician, Alicija,
Aliecia, Allicea, Ilysa

Alicja (English) a form of Alicia.
Alicya

Alida (Latin) small and winged. (Spanish)
noble. See also Aleta, Lida, Oleda.
Adelita, Aleda, Aledah, Aleida, Alidah, Alidia,
Alidiah, Alleda, Alledah, Allida, Allidah,
Alyda, Alydia, Elida, Elidia

Álida (Hebrew) a form of Hélida.

Alie, Alley, Alli, Allie, Ally, Aly (Greek)
familiar forms of Alice, Alicia, Alisha,
Alison.

Aliesha (Greek) a form of Alisha.
Alieshai, Alieshia, Alliesha

Alika (Hawaiian) truthful. (Swahili) most
beautiful.
Aleka, Alica, Alikah, Alike, Alikee, Aliki,
Aliqua, Aliquah, Alique, Alyka, Alykah,
Alyqua, Alyquah

Alima (Arabic) sea maiden; musical.
Alimah, Alyma, Alymah

Alina (Slavic) bright. (Scottish) fair. (English)
a short form of Adeline. See also Alena.
Aleana, Aleanah, Aleina, Aleinah, Aliana,
Alianna, Alinah, Alinna

Aline (Scottish) a form of Aileen, Alina.
Alianne, Alline

Alisa, Allisa (Greek) forms of Alice, Alyssa.
See also Elisa, Ilisa.
Aaliysah, Alisah, Alisea, Aliysa

Alise, Allise (Greek) forms of Alice.
Alis, Aliss, Alisse, Allis, Alliss, Allisse

Alisha (Greek) truthful. (German) noble.
(English) a form of Alicia. See also Elisha,
Ilisha, Lisha.
Aliscia, Alisea, Alishah, Alishay, Alishaye,
Alishya, Alissya, Alisyia, Alitsha, Allissia,
Alyssaya

Alishia (English) a form of Alisha.
Alishea, Alisheia, Alishiana

Alisia, Alissia (English) forms of Alisha.

Alison (English) a form of Alice. See also
Lissie.
Aleason, Aleeson, Aleighson, Aleison, Alisan,
Alisann, Alisanne, Alisen, Alisenne, Alisin,
Alision, Alisonn, Alisson, Alissun, Alissyn,
Alisun, Alles, Allesse, Alleyson, Allisan,
Allisen, Allisin, Allisine, Allisone, Allisson,
Allisun, Allsun, Alson, Alsone, Alysine, Elisan,
Elisen, Elisin, Elison, Elisun, Elisyn

Alissa, Allissa (Greek) forms of Alice,
Alyssa.
Aalissah, Alissah, Alisza, Allisah, Allissah

Alita (Spanish) a form of Alida.
Alitah, Allita, Allitah, Allitta, Allittah, Allyta,
Allytah, Alyta, Alytah

Alivia (Latin) a form of Olivia.
Alivah

Alix GB (Greek) a short form of Alexandra,
Alice.
Alixe, Alixia, Allix, Alyx

Alixandra (Greek) a form of Alexandra.
Alixandrah, Alixzandra, Alixzandrah,
Allixandra

Alixandria (Greek) a form of Alexandria.
Alixandriah, Alixandrina, Alixandrinah,
Alixandrine, Alixandriya, Alixzandria,
Alixzandriah, Alixzandrina, Alixzandryna,
Alixzandrynah, Alixzandryne, Allixandria,
Allixandrya

Aliya (Hebrew) ascender.
Aeliyah, Alieya, Alieyah, Aliyiah, Alliyha,
Alliyia

Aliyah, Alliyah (Hebrew) forms of Aliya.
Aliyyah, Alliya, Alliyyah

Aliye (Arabic) noble.
Aliyeh

Aliza (Hebrew) joyful. See also Aleeza, Eliza.
Alieza, Aliezah, Alitza, Alitzah, Alizah,
Alizee, Alyza, Alyzah

Alizabeth (Hebrew) a form of Elizabeth.
Alyzabeth

Alize (Greek, German) a form of Alice.
(Hebrew) a short form of Aliza.
Aliz

Allana, Allanah (Irish) forms of Alana.
Allanie, Allanna, Allannah, Allanne, Allauna

Allegra (Latin) cheerful.
Allegrah, Allegria, Legra

Allena (Irish) a form of Alana.
Alleyna, Alleynah

Allene (Dutch) a form of Aleene. (Scottish) a form of Aline.
Alene, Alleen

Allethea (Greek) a form of Alethea.
Allathea, Allatheah, Allathia, Allathiah, Alletheah, Allethia, Allethiah, Allethya, Allethyah, Allythea, Allytheah, Allythia, Allythiah, Allythya, Allythyah

Allicia (English) a form of Alicia.

Allisha (Greek, German, English) a form of Alisha.

Allison ★ GB (English) a form of Alison.

Allyn (Scottish) a form of Aileen, Alina. See also Aline.
Allyne, Alyne, Alynne

Allysa, Allyssa (Greek) forms of Alyssa.
Allyisa, Allysah, Allyssah

Allysen, Allyson, Alyson (English) forms of Alison.
Allysonn, Allysson, Allysun, Allysyn, Allysyne, Alysan, Alysen, Alysene, Alysin, Alysine, Alysone, Alysun, Alysyn, Alysyne, Alyzane, Alyzen, Alyzene, Alyzin, Alyzine, Alyzyn, Alyzyne

Allysha, Alycia, Alysha, Alysia (English) forms of Alicia.
Alyssha, Lycia

Alma (Arabic) learned. (Latin) soul.
Almah, Almar, Almarah

Almeda (Arabic) ambitious.
Allmeda, Allmedah, Allmeta, Almea, Almedah, Almeta, Almetah, Almetta, Almettah, Almida, Almidah, Almyda, Almydah

Almira (Arabic) aristocratic, princess; exalted. (Spanish) from Almeíra, Spain. See also Elmira, Mira.
Allmeera, Allmera, Allmerah, Allmeria, Allmira, Allmirah, Almeera, Almeeria, Almeira,
Almera, Almeria, Almeriah, Almirah, Almire, Almyra, Almyrah

Almita (Latin) kind.
Allmita, Almitah, Almyta, Almytah

Almodis (German) very happy, animated lady.

Almudena (Spanish) the city.

Almunda (Spanish) refers to the Virgin Mary.

Almundena, Almundina (Spanish) forms of Almunda.

Alodía (Basque) free land.

Alodie (English) rich. See also Elodie.
Alodea, Alodee, Alodey, Alodi, Alodia, Alody, Alodya, Alodyah, Alodye

Aloha (Hawaiian) loving, kindhearted, charitable.
Alohah, Alohi

Aloisa (German) famous warrior.
Aloisia, Aloysa, Aloysia

Aloise (Spanish) a form of Aloisa.

Aloma (Latin) a short form of Paloma.

Alonda (Spanish) a form of Alexandra.

Alondra (Spanish) a form of Alexandra.
Allandra

Alonna (Irish) a form of Alana.
Allona, Allonah, Alona, Alonah, Alonnah, Alonya, Alonyah

Alonsa (English) a form of Alonza.

Alonza BG (English) noble and eager.

Alora (American) a combination of the letter A + Lora.
Alorah, Alorha, Alorie, Aloura, Alouria

Alpha (Greek) first-born. Linguistics: the first letter of the Greek alphabet.
Alfa, Alfah, Alfia, Alfiah, Alfya, Alfyah, Alphah, Alphia, Alphiah, Alphya, Alphyah

Alta (Latin) high; tall.
Allta, Altah, Altana, Altanna, Altea, Alto

Altagracia (Spanish) refers to the high grace of the Virgin Mary.

Altair BG (Greek) star. (Arabic) flying eagle.
Altaira, Altaire, Altayr, Altayra, Altayrah,
Altayre

Altamira (Spanish) place with a beautiful
view.

Althea (Greek) wholesome; healer. History:
Althea Gibson was the first African
American to win a major tennis title. See
also Thea.
Altha, Altheah, Altheda, Althedah, Altheya,
Althia, Althiah, Althya, Althyah, Elthea,
Eltheya, Elthia

Aluminé (Mapuche) she who shines.

Alva BG (Latin, Spanish) white; light
skinned. See also Elva.
Alvah, Alvana, Alvanna, Alvannah

Alvarita (Spanish) speaker of truth.

Alvera (Latin) honest.
Alverah, Alveria, Alveriah, Alverya, Alveryah,
Alvira, Alvirah, Alvyra, Alvyrah

Alvina (English) friend to all; noble friend;
friend to elves. See also Elva, Vina.
Alveana, Alveanah, Alveane, Alveanea, Alveen,
Alveena, Alveenah, Alveene, Alveenia, Alvena,
Alvenah, Alvenea, Alvie, Alvinae, Alvinah,
Alvincia, Alvine, Alvinea, Alvinesha, Alvinia,
Alvinna, Alvinnah, Alvita, Alvona, Alvyna,
Alvynah, Alvyne, Alwin, Alwina, Alwyn

Alyah (Hebrew) a form of Aliya.
Allya, Allyah, Alya, Alyya, Alyyah

Alyce, Alyse, Alysse (Greek) forms of Alice.
Allyce, Allys, Allyse, Allyss, Alys, Alyss

Alyiah (Hebrew) a form of Aliya.
Alyia

Alyna (Dutch) a form of Aleene. (Slavic,
Scottish, English) a form of Alina.
Alynah, Alyona

Alysa (Greek) a form of Alyssa.
Alysah

Alyshia (English) a form of Alicia.

Alyssa ☀ (Greek) rational. Botany: alyssum
is a flowering herb. See also Alice, Alisa,
Elissa.
Ahlyssa, Alyesa, Alyessa, Alyissa, Alyssah,
Ilyssa, Lyssa, Lyssah

Alyssia (Greek) a form of Alyssa.

Alyx (Greek) a form of Alex.

Alyxandra (Greek) a form of Alexandra.
Alyxandrah, Alyxzandra, Alyxzandrah

Alyxandria (Greek) a form of Alexandria.
Alyxandrea, Alyxandriah, Alyxandrya,
Alyxandryah, Alyxzandria, Alyxzandriah,
Alyxzandrya, Alyxzandryah

Alyxis (Greek) a form of Alexis.

Alzena (Arabic) woman.
Alsena, Alsenah, Alxena, Alxenah, Alxina,
Alxinah, Alxyna, Alxynah, Alzenah, Alzina,
Alzinah, Alzyna, Alzynah

Am (Vietnamese) lunar; female.

Ama (African) born on Saturday.
Amah

Amabel (Latin) lovable. See also Bel, Mabel.
Amabela, Amabelah, Amabele, Amabell,
Amabella, Amabellah, Amabelle, Ambela,
Ambelah, Ambele, Ambell, Ambella, Ambellah,
Amebelle, Amibel, Amibela, Amibelah,
Amibele, Amibell, Amibella, Amibellah,
Amibelle, Amybel, Amybell, Amybella,
Amybelle

Amada (Spanish) beloved.
Amadee, Amadey, Amadi, Amadie, Amadita,
Amady, Amata

Amadea (Latin) loves God.
Amadeah, Amadeya, Amadeyah, Amadia,
Amadiah, Amadya, Amadyah

Amadis (Latin) the great love, the most
beloved.

Amairani, Amairany (Greek) forms of
Amara.
Amairaine, Amairane, Amairanie

Amal GB (Hebrew) worker. (Arabic) hopeful.
Amala, Amalah, Amalla, Amallah

Amalberta (German) brilliant work.

Amalia (German) a form of Amelia.
Ahmalia, Amalea, Amaleah, Amaleta,
Amaliah, Amalija, Amalisa, Amalita,
Amalitah, Amaliya, Amalya, Amalyah,
Amalyn

Amalie (German) a form of Amelia.
Amalee, Amalei, Amaleigh, Amaley, Amali,
Amaly

Amaline (German) a form of Amelia.
Amalean, Amaleana, Amaleane, Amaleen,
Amaleena, Amaleene, Amalin, Amalina,
Amalyn, Amalyna, Amalyne, Amalynn,
Amelina, Ameline, Amilina, Amiline, Amilyn,
Amilynn, Amilynna, Amilynne, Ammalyn,
Ammalynn, Ammalynne, Ammilina, Ammiline

Amalsinda (German) the one God points
to.

Amalur, Amalure (Spanish) homeland.

Aman BG (Arabic) a short form of Amani.
Amane

Amanada (Latin) a form of Amanda.

Amancai, Amancái, Amancay (Quechua)
yellow flower streaked with red.

Amancia (Latin) lover.

Amanda ✰ GB (Latin) lovable. See also
Manda, Mandy.
Amandah, Amandalee, Amandalyn, Amande,
Amandea, Amandee, Amandey, Amandi,
Amandia, Amandiah, Amandie, Amandina,
Amandine, Amandy, Amandya, Amandyah

Amandeep BG (Punjabi) peaceful light.

Amani GB (Arabic) a form of Imani.
Aamani, Ahmani, Amanee, Amaney, Amanie,
Ammanu

Amania (Hebrew) artist of God.

Amanjot (Punjabi) a form of Amandeep.

Amanpreet BG (Punjabi) a form of
Amandeep.

Amapola (Arabic) poppy.

Amara (Greek) eternally beautiful. See also
Mara.
Amaira, Amar, Amarah, Amaria, Amariah,
Amarya, Amaryah

Amaranta (Spanish) a flower that never
fades.
Amaranth, Amarantha, Amaranthe

Amari BG (Greek) a form of Amara.
Amaree, Amarie, Amarii, Amarri

Amarilia, Amarilla, Amarinda (Greek) she
who shines.

Amarina (Australian) rain.
Amarin, Amarinah, Amarine, Amaryn,
Amarynah, Amaryne

Amaris (Hebrew) promised by God.
Amaarisah, Amarisa, Amariss, Amarissa,
Amarys, Amarysa, Amarysah, Amaryss,
Amaryssa, Amaryssah, Maris

Amarú (Quechua) snake, boa.

Amaryllis (Greek) fresh; flower.
Amarilis, Amarillis, Amaryl, Amaryla,
Amarylah, Amarylis, Amarylla, Amaryllah

Amatista (Greek) full of wine.

Amaui (Hawaiian) thrush.

Amaya (Japanese) night rain.
Amaia, Amaiah, Amayah

Amazona (Greek) Mythology: the Amazons
were a tribe of warrior women.

Ambar GB (French) a form of Amber.

Ámbar (Arabic) the aroma of an exotic perfume.

Amber ✰ GB (French) amber.
Aamber, Ahmber, Amberia, Amberise, Ambur,
Ammber, Ember

Amber-Lynn, Amberlyn, Amberlynn
(American) combinations of Amber +
Lynn.
Ambarlina, Ambarline, Amber Lynn, Amber
Lynne, Amber-Lynne, Amberlin, Amberlina,
Amberline, Amberlyne, Amberlynne,
Amburlina, Amburline

Amberlee, Amberley, Amberly
(American) familiar forms of Amber.
Ambarlea, Ambarlee, Ambarlei, Ambarleigh,
Ambarley, Ambarli, Ambarlie, Ambarly,
Amberle, Amberlea, Amberlei, Amberleigh,
Amberli, Amberlia, Amberliah, Amberlie,
Amberlly, Amberlyah, Amberlye, Amburlea,
Amburlee, Amburlei, Amburleigh, Amburley,
Amburli, Amburlia, Amburlie, Amburly,
Amburlya

Ambra (American) a form of Amber.

Ambria (American) a form of Amber.
Ambrea, Ambriah

Ambrosia (Greek) immortal.
Ambrosa, Ambrosah, Ambrosiah, Ambrosina, Ambrosine, Ambrosyn, Ambrosyna, Ambrosyne, Ambrozin, Ambrozinah, Ambrozine, Ambrozyn, Ambrozyna, Ambrozyne

Ambyr (French) a form of Amber.
Ambyre

Amedia (Spanish) a form of Amy.

Amee, Ami, Amie, Amiee (French) forms of Amy.
Amii, Amiiee, Ammee, Ammie, Ammiee

Ameena (Arabic) a form of Amina.
Ameenah

Ameera (Hebrew, Arabic) a form of Amira.
Ameerah

Amelberga (German) protected work.

Amelia ☼ (German) hard working. (Latin) a form of Emily. History: Amelia Earhart, an American aviator, was the first woman to fly solo across the Atlantic Ocean. See also Ima, Melia, Millie, Nuela, Yamelia.
Aemilia, Aimilia, Amalie, Amaline, Amaliya, Ameila, Ameilia, Amelisa, Amelita, Amella, Amylia, Amyliah, Amylya, Amylyah

Amélia (Portuguese) a form of Amelia.

Amelie, Amely (French) forms of Amelia.
Amelee, Ameleigh, Ameley, Amélie

Amelinda (American) a combination of Amelia + Linda.
Amalinda, Amalindah, Amalynda, Amalyndah, Amelindah, Amerlindah, Amilinda, Amilindah, Amilynda, Amilyndah

America (Teutonic) industrious.
Amarica, Amaricah, Amaricka, Amarickah, Amarika, Amarikah, Americah, Americana, Americka, Amerika, Amerikah, Ameriqua, Ameriquah, Amerique, Ameryca, Amerycah, Amerycka, Ameryckah, Ameryka, Amerykah, Ameryqua, Ameryque

América (Teutonic) a form of America.

Amethyst (Greek) wine; purple-violet gemstone. History: in the ancient world, the amethyst stone was believed to help prevent drunkenness.
Amathist, Amathista, Amathiste, Amathysta,

Amathyste, Amethist, Amethista, Amethiste, Amethistia, Amethysta, Amethyste, Amethystia, Amethystya, Amethystyah

Amia (Hebrew) a form of Amy.
Amio

Amiana (Latin) a form of Amina.

Amilia (Latin, German) a form of Amelia.
Amiliah, Amilisa, Amilita, Amillia, Amilya

Amilie (Latin, German) a form of Amelia.
Amilee, Amili, Amily

Amina (Arabic) trustworthy, faithful. History: the mother of the prophet Muhammad.
Aamena, Aamina, Aminda, Amindah, Aminta, Amintah

Aminah (Arabic) a form of Amina.
Aaminah

Amira (Hebrew) speech; utterance. (Arabic) princess. See also Mira.
Amyra, Amyrah

Amirah (Hebrew, Arabic) a form of Amira.

Amiram (Hebrew) my land is lifted up.

Amissa (Hebrew) truth.
Amisa, Amisah, Amise, Amisia, Amisiah, Amissah, Amiza, Amizah, Amysa, Amysah, Amysia, Amysiah, Amysya, Amysyah, Amyza, Amyzah

Amita (Hebrew) truth.
Ameeta, Ameetah, Amitah, Amitha, Amyta, Amytah

Amity (Latin) friendship.
Amitee, Amitey, Amiti, Amitie, Amytee, Amytey, Amyti, Amytie, Amyty

Amlika (Hindi) mother.
Amlikah, Amylka, Amylkah

Amma (Hindi) mother.

Amor, Amora (Spanish) love.

Amorette (Latin) beloved; loving.
Amoreta, Amoretah, Amorete, Amorett, Amoretta, Amorettah, Amorit, Amorita, Amoritah, Amoritt, Amoritta, Amoritte, Amoryt, Amoryta, Amorytah, Amoryte, Amorytt, Amorytta, Amoryttah, Amorytte

Amorie (German) industrious leader.

Amorina (Spanish) she who falls in love easily.

Amoxtli (Nahuatl) book.

Amparo (Spanish) protected.

Amrit BG (Sanskrit) nectar.

Amrita (Spanish) a form of Amorette.
Amritah, Amritta, Amritte, Amryta, Amrytah, Amryte, Amrytta, Amryttah, Amrytte

Amser (Welsh) time.

Amuillan (Mapuche) useful, helpful.

Amunet (Egyptian) Mythology: Amaunet is a guardian goddess of the pharaohs.

Amy (Latin) beloved. See also Aimee, Emma, Esmé.
Aami, Amata, Amatah, Ame, Amei, Amey, Ammy, Amye, Amylyn

An BG (Chinese) peaceful.

Ana (Hawaiian, Spanish) a form of Hannah.

Anaba (Native American) she returns from battle.
Anabah

Anabel, Anabelle, Annabell, Annabelle (English) forms of Annabel.
Anabela, Anabele, Anabell, Anna-Bell, Annahbell, Annahbelle, Annebell, Annebelle, Annibell, Annibelle, Annybell, Annybelle

Anaclara (Spanish) a combination of Ana + Carla.

Anacleta (Greek) she who has been called on; the required one.

Anahi, Anahy (Persian) short forms of Anahita.
Anahai

Anahí, Anahid (Guarani) alluding to the flower of the ceibo tree.

Anahit (Persian) a short form of Anahita.

Anahita (Persian) the immaculate one. Mythology: a water goddess.

Anai (Hawaiian, Spanish) a form of Ana.
Anaia

Anais (Hebrew) gracious.
Anaise, Anaïse, Anaiss, Anays, Anayss

Anaís (Hebrew) God has mercy.

Anakaren (English) a combination of Ana + Karen.
Annakaren

Anala (Hindi) fine.
Analah

Analaura (English) a combination of Ana + Laura.
Annalaura

Analena (Spanish) a form of Ana.

Anali (Hindi, Indian) fire, fiery.

Analía (Spanish) a combination of Ana and Lía.

Analicia (English) a form of Analisa.
Analisha, Analisia

Analiria (Spanish) native of Almeria, Spain.

Analisa, Annalisa (English) combinations of Anna + Lisa.
Analice, Analissa, Annaliesa, Annalissa, Annalyca, Annalyce, Annalysa

Analise, Annalise (English) forms of Analisa.
Analis, Annalisse, Annalys, Annalyse

Anamaria (English) a combination of Ana + Maria.
Anamarie, Anamary

Anan, Anán, Anani (Hebrew) cloudy.

Ananda (Hindi) blissful.
Anandah

Anarosa (English) a combination of Ana + Rosa.

Anastacia, Anastazia, Annastasia (Greek) forms of Anastasia.
Anastace, Anastaciah, Anastacie, Anastacya, Anastacyah, Anastaziah, Anastazya

Anastasia (Greek) resurrection. See also Nastasia, Stacey, Stacia, Stasya.
Anastascia, Anastase, Anastasee, Anastasha, Anastashia, Anastasie, Anastasija, Anastassia, Anastassya, Anastasya, Anastatia, Anastaysia, Anastice, Anestasia, Annastasija, Annastaysia, Annastazia, Annestasia, Annestassia, Annstás, Anstace, Anstice

Anat (Egyptian) Mythology: a consort of Seth.

Anatola (Greek) from the east.
Anatolah, Anatolia, Anatoliah, Anatolya, Anatolyah, Annatola, Annatolah, Annatolia, Annatoliah, Annatolya, Annatolyah

Ancarla (Spanish) a combination of Ana and Carla.

Ancelín (Latin) single woman.

Anci (Hungarian) a form of Hannah.
Annus, Annushka

Andeana (Spanish) leaving.

Andee, Andi, Andie (American) short forms of Andrea, Fernanda.
Ande, Andea, Andy

Andere (Greek) a form of Andrea.

Andra GB (Greek, Latin) a short form of Andrea.
Andrah

Andrea ☀ GB (Greek) strong; courageous. See also Ondrea.
Aindrea, Andera, Anderea, Andraia, Andraya, Andreah, Andreaka, Andreea, Andreja, Andreka, Andrel, Andrell, Andrelle, Andreo, Andressa, Andrette, Andriea, Andrieka, Andrietta, Andris, Andrya, Andryah

Andréa (French) a form of Andrea.
Andrée

Andreana, Andreanna (Greek) forms of Andrea.
Ahndrianna, Andreanah, Andreannah, Andreeana, Andreeanah, Andrena, Andreyana, Andreyonna

Andreane, Andreanne, Andree Ann, Andree Anne (Greek) combinations of Andrea + Ann.
Andrean, Andreann, Andreean, Andreeane, Andreeanne, Andrene, Andrian, Andriann, Andrianne, Andrienne, Andryane, Andryann, Andryanne

Andree (Greek) a short form of Andrea.
Andri

Andreia (Greek) a form of Andrea.

Andréia (Portuguese) a form of Andrea.

Andreina (Greek) a form of Andrea.

Andreína (Spanish) a form of Andrea.

Andresa (Spanish) a form of Andrea.

Andreya (Greek) a form of Andrea.

Andria (Greek) a form of Andrea.
Andriah

Andriana, Andrianna (Greek) forms of Andrea.
Andrianah, Andriannah, Andrina, Andrinah, Andriona, Andrionna, Andryana, Andryanah, Andryanna, Andryannah

Andromaca, Andrómana, Andrónica, Andrómaca (Greek) she who is victorious over men.

Andromeda (Greek) Mythology: the daughter of Cepheus and Cassiopeia.

Anechka (Russian) grace.

Aneesa (Greek) a form of Agnes.
Anee, Aneesah, Aneese, Aneisa

Aneesha (Greek) a form of Agnes.
Aneeshah, Aneesia, Aneisha

Aneko (Japanese) older sister.

Anel (Hawaiian) a short form of Anela.
Anelle

Anela (Hawaiian) angel.
Anelah, Anella, Anellah

Anelida (Spanish) a combination of Ana + Elida.

Anelina (Spanish) a combination of Ana + Lina.

Anémona (Greek) she who is victorious over men.

Anesha (Greek) a form of Agnes.
Ahnesha

Aneshia (Greek) a form of Agnes.
Ahnesshia

Anesia (Greek) a form of Agnes.
Ahnesia, Anessia

Anessa, Annessa (Greek) forms of Agnes.

Aneta (Spanish) a form of Anita. (French) a form of Annette.
Anetah

Anetra (American) a form of Annette.
Anetrah

Anezka (Czech) a form of Hannah.

Anfitrita (Greek) wind, breeze.

Angel BG (Greek) a short form of Angela.
Angéle, Angil, Anjel, Anjelle

Angela (Greek) angel; messenger. See also
Engel.
*Angala, Anganita, Angelanell, Angelanette,
Angelo, Angiola, Anglea, Anjella, Anjellah*

Ángela (Spanish) a form of Angela.

Angele, Angell, Angelle (Greek) short
forms of Angela.

Angelea, Angelie (Greek) forms of Angela.
Angelee, Angeleigh, Angeli

Angelena (Russian) a form of Angela.
Angalena, Angalina, Angeleana

Angeles (Spanish) a form of Angela.

Ángeles (Catalan) a form of Angeles.

Angelia (Greek) a form of Angela.
Angeleah

Angelic (Russian) a short form of Angelica.
Angalic

Angelica, Angelika, Angellica (Greek)
forms of Angela. See also Anjelica,
Engelica.
Angelici, Angelike, Angeliki, Angilica

Angélica (Spanish) a form of Angelica.

Angelicia (Russian) a form of Angelica.

Angelina ⭐ (Russian) a form of Angela.
*Angeliana, Angelinah, Angellina, Angelyna,
Anhelina, Anjelina*

Angeline, Angelyn (Russian) forms of
Angela.
*Angeleen, Angelene, Angelin, Angelyne,
Angelynn, Angelynne*

Angelique (French) a form of Angela.
*Angeliqua, Angeliquah, Angélique, Angilique,
Anjelique*

Angelisa (American) a combination of
Angela + Lisa.

Angelita (Spanish) a form of Angela.
Angellita

Angella (Greek) a form of Angela.
Angellah

Angeni (Native American) spirit.
*Angeenee, Angeeni, Angeenie, Angeeny,
Angenia, Anjeenee, Anjeeney, Anjeeni,
Anjeenia, Anjeenie, Anjeeny, Anjenee, Anjeney,
Anjenie, Anjeny*

Angie (Greek) a familiar form of Angela.
Ange, Angee, Angey, Angi, Angy, Anjee

Angustias (Latin) she who suffers from grief
or sorrow.

Anh GB (Vietnamese) peace; safety.

Ani (Hawaiian) beautiful.
Aany, Aanye, Anee, Aney, Anie, Any

Ania (Polish) a form of Hannah.
Ahnia, Aniah

Anica, Anika (Czech) familiar forms of
Anna.
*Aanika, Anaka, Aneeky, Aneka, Anekah,
Anicah, Anicka, Anikah, Anikka, Aniko,
Annaka, Anniki, Annikki, Anyca, Anycah,
Anyka, Anykah, Anyqua, Anyquah*

Anice, Anise (English) forms of Agnes.
*Anesse, Anis, Annes, Annice, Annis, Annise,
Anniss, Annisse, Annus, Annys, Annyse,
Annyss, Annysse, Anys*

Aniceta (Spanish) she who is invincible
because of her great strength.

Aniela (Polish) a form of Anna.
*Anielah, Aniella, Aniellah, Anielle, Anniela,
Annielah, Anniella, Anniellah, Annielle,
Anyel, Anyela, Anyele, Anyella, Anyellah,
Anyelle*

Anik (Czech) a short form of Anica.
Anike, Anikke

Anila (Hindi) Religion: an attendant of the
Hindu god Vishnu.
*Anilah, Anilla, Anillah, Anyla, Anylah,
Anylla, Anyllah*

Anillang (Mapuche) stable altar; decisive and
courageously noble.

Anippe (Egyptian) daughter of the Nile.

Aniqua (Czech) a form of Anica.
Aniquah

Anisa, Anisah (Arabic) friendly. See also Anissa.

Anisha, Annisha (English) forms of Agnes, Ann.
Aanisha, Aeniesha

Anisia (Greek) she who fulfills her obligations.

Anissa (English) a form of Agnes, Ann. (Arabic) a form of Anisa.
Anissah

Anita (Spanish) a form of Ann, Anna. See also Nita.
Aneeta, Aneetah, Aneethah, Anetha, Anitha, Anithah, Anitia, Anitta, Anittah, Anitte, Annita, Annitah, Annite, Annitta, Annittah, Annitte, Annyta, Annytah, Annytta, Annyttah, Annytte, Anyta, Anytah

Anitchka (Russian) a form of Anna.

Anitra (Spanish) a form of Anita.

Aniya (Russian) a form of Anya.
Aaniyah, Anaya, Aneya, Aneyah, Aniyah

Anja (Russian) a form of Anya.
Anje

Anjali (Hindi) offering with both hands. (Indian) offering with devotion.

Anjela (Greek) a form of Angela.
Anjelah

Anjelica (Greek) a form of Angela. See also Angelica.
Anjelika

Anjélica (Spanish) a form of Angelica.

Anjelita (Spanish) a form of Angela.

Anka GB (Polish) a familiar form of Hannah.
Anke

Ann, Anne (English) gracious.
Ane, Annchen, Annze, Anouche

Ann Catherine, Anne Catherine (American) combinations of Ann + Catherine.
Ann-Catherine, Anncatherine, Anne-Catherine, Annecatherine

Ann Julie, Anne Julie (American) combinations of Ann + Julie.
Ann-Julie, Anne-Julie, Annejulie, Annjulie

Ann Marie, Ann-Marie, Anne Marie, Anne-Marie, Annemarie, Annmarie (English) combinations of Ann + Marie.
Anmaree, Anmari, Anmarie, Anmary, Anmarya, Anmaryah, Annmaree, Annmari, Annmary

Ann Sophie, Anne Sophie, Anne-Sophie (American) combinations of Ann + Sophie.
Ann-Sophie

Anna ☀ (German, Italian, Czech, Swedish) gracious. Culture: Anna Pavlova was a famous Russian ballerina. See also Anica, Anissa, Nina.
Ahnna, Anah, Aniela, Annice, Annina, Annora, Anona, Anyu, Aska

Anna Maria, Annamaria (English) combinations of Anna + Maria.
Anna-Maria

Anna Marie, Anna-Marie, Annamarie (English) combinations of Anna + Marie.

Annabel (English) a combination of Anna + Bel.
Anabele, Annabal, Annahbel, Annebel, Annebele, Annibel, Annibele, Annybel, Annybele

Annabella (English) a form of Annabel.
Anabela, Anabella, Annabelah, Annabellah, Annahbella, Annebela, Annebelah, Annebella, Annebellah, Annibela, Annibelah, Annibella, Annibellah, Annybela, Annybelah, Annybella, Annybellah

Annah (German, Italian, Czech, Swedish) a form of Anna.

Annalee (Finnish) a form of Annalie.

Annalie (Finnish) a form of Hannah.
Analee, Annalea, Annaleah, Annaleigh, Annaleigha, Annali, Anneli, Annelie

Annaliese (English) a form of Analisa.

Anneka (Swedish) a form of Hannah.
Annaka, Annekah

Anneke (Czech) a form of Anik. (Swedish) a form of Anneka.

Anneliese, Annelise (English) forms of Annelisa.
Analiese, Anelise, Annelyse

Annelisa (English) a combination of Ann + Lisa.
Anelisa, Annelys, Annelysa

Annette (French) a form of Ann. See also Anetra, Nettie.
Anet, Anete, Anett, Anetta, Anette, Annet, Anneta, Annetah, Annete, Anneth, Annett, Annetta, Annettah

Annick, Annik (Russian) short forms of Annika.
Annike

Annie, Anny (English) familiar forms of Ann.
Annee, Anney, Anni

Annie Claude (American) a combination of Annie + Claude.
Annie-Claude

Annie Kim (American) a combination of Annie + Kim.
Annie-Kim

Annie Pier (American) a combination of Annie + Pier.
Annie-Pier

Annika (Russian) a form of Ann. (Swedish) a form of Anneka.
Annicka, Anniki, Annikka, Annikki, Anninka, Annushka, Anouska, Anuska

Annina (Hebrew) graceful.
Anina, Aninah, Anninah, Annyna, Annynah, Anyna, Anynah

Annisa, Annissa (Arabic) forms of Anisa. (English) a form of Anissa.
Annisah, Annissah

Annjanette (American) a combination of Ann + Janette (see Janett).
Angen, Angenett, Angenette, Anjane, Anjanetta, Anjani

Annmaria (American) a combination of Ann + Maria.
Anmaria, Anmariah, Annmariah, Annmarya, Annmaryah

Annora (Latin) honor.
Annorah, Annore, Annoria, Annoriah, Annorya, Annoryah, Anora, Anorah, Anoria, Anoriah, Anorya, Anoryah

Anona (English) pineapple.
Annona, Annonah, Annonia, Annoniah, Annonya, Annonyah, Anonah

Anouhea (Hawaiian) cool, soft fragrance.

Anouk (Dutch) a familiar form of Anna.

Anselma (German) divine protector.
Anselmah, Anzelma, Anzelmah, Selma, Zelma

Ansleigh (Scottish) a form of Ainsley.
Anslea, Ansleah, Anslee, Anslei, Ansleigh, Ansli, Anslie, Ansly

Ansley GB (Scottish) a form of Ainsley.

Antania (Greek, Latin) a form of Antonia.

Antea (Greek) a form of Anthea.

Anthea (Greek) flower.
Antha, Anthe, Antheah, Anthia, Anthiah, Anthya, Anthyah, Thia

Anthony BG (Latin) praiseworthy. (Greek) flourishing.

Antía (Galician) a form of Antonia.

Antífona (Greek) opposite of her race.

Antígona (Greek) distinguished by her brothers.

Antigua (Spanish) old.

Antionette (French) a form of Antonia.
Anntionett, Antionet, Antionett

Antoinette (French) a form of Antonia. See also Nettie, Toinette, Toni.
Anta, Antanette, Antoinella, Antoinet, Antonice, Antonieta, Antonietta

Antolina (Spanish) a form of Antonia.

Antonella (French) a form of Antoinette.

Antonette (French) a form of Antoinette.
Antonett, Antonetta

Antonia GB (Greek) flourishing. (Latin) praiseworthy. See also Toni, Tonya, Tosha.
Ansonia, Ansonya, Antinia, Antona, Antonee, Antoney, Antoni, Antoñía, Antoniah, Antonice, Antonie, Antoniya, Antonnea, Antonnia, Antonniah, Antonya, Antonyah

Antónia (Portuguese) a form of Antonia.

Antonice (Latin) a form of Antonia.
Antanise, Antonias, Antonica, Antonicah, Antonise

Antonina (Greek, Latin) a form of Antonia.
Antonine

Antoniña (Latin) she who confronts or is the adversary.

Antonique (French) a form of Antoinette.

Antonisha (Latin) a form of Antonice.
Antanisha, Antonesha, Antoneshia

Anuncia (Latin) announcer, messenger.

Anunciación (Spanish) annunciation.

Anunciada, Anunciata (Spanish) forms of Anunciación.

Anya (Russian) a form of Anna.
Annya, Annyah, Anyah

Anyssa (English) a form of Anissa.
Annysa, Annysah, Annyssa, Anysa, Anysah, Anysha, Anyssah

Anzia (Italian) one-armed.

Aparecida (Latin) appearance.

Aparicia (Latin) ghost.

Aphra (Hebrew) young doe. See also Afra.
Aphrah

Aphrodite (Greek) Mythology: the goddess of love and beauty.
Aphrodita, Aphrodyta, Aphrodytah, Aphrodyte

Apia (Latin) devout woman.

Apolinaria, Apolinia (Spanish) forms of Appollonia.

Apoline (Greek) a form of Appollonia.
Apolina, Apollina, Apollinah, Apolline, Apollyn, Apollyna, Apollynah, Apollyne, Appolina, Appolinah, Appoline, Appollina, Appollinah, Appolline, Appollyn, Appollyna, Appollynah, Appollyne

Appollonia (Greek) a form of Apollo (see Boys' Names).
Apollonia, Apolloniah, Apollonya, Apollonyah, Apolonia, Apoloniah, Apolonie, Apolonya, Apolonyah, Appolloniah, Appollonya, Appollonyah

April (Latin) opening. See also Avril.
Aprel, Aprela, Aprele, Aprella, Aprelle, Apriell, Aprielle, Aprila, Aprilah, Aprile, Aprilett, Apriletta, Aprilette, Aprili, Aprill, Aprilla, Aprillah, Aprille

Apryl (Latin) a form of April.
Apryla, Aprylah, Apryle, Aprylla, Aprylle

Apuleya (Latin) impulsive woman.

Aquene (Native American) peaceful.
Aqueen, Aqueena, Aqueene

Aquila GB (Latin, Spanish) eagle.
Acquilla, Aquil, Aquilas, Aquileo, Aquiles, Aquilino, Aquill, Aquille, Aquillino, Aquyl, Aquyla, Aquyll, Aquylla

Aquilina (Latin) a form of Aquilla.

Aquiline (Greek) a form of Aquilla.

Aquilinia (Spanish) a form of Aquilla.

Aquilla (Latin, Spanish) a form of Aquila.

Ara BG (Arabic) opinionated.
Ahraya, Aira, Arae, Arah

Arabella (Latin) beautiful altar. See also Belle, Orabella.
Arabel, Arabela, Arabelah, Arabele, Arabell, Arabellah, Arabelle

Araceli, Aracely (Latin) heavenly altar.
Aracele, Aracelia, Aracelli

Aracelis (Spanish) a form of Araceli.

Arama (Spanish) reference to the Virgin Mary.

Arán (Catalan) she is a conflicted virgin.

Arantxa (Basque) a form of Arantzazu.

Arantzazu, Aránzazu (Basque) are you among the thorns?

Aranzuru (Spanish) a form of Arantzazu.

Araseli (Latin) a form of Araceli.
Arasely

Araya (Arabic) a form of Ara.
Arayah

Arbogasta (Greek) the rich woman.

Arcadia, Arcadía (Greek) from Arcadia, a region in Greece.

Arcángela (Greek) archangel.

Arcelia (Latin) a form of Araceli.
Arceli

Archibalda (German) born free.

Arcilla (Latin) a form of Araceli.

Ardelle (Latin) warm; enthusiastic.
Ardel, Ardela, Ardelah, Ardele, Ardelia,
Ardeliah, Ardelis, Ardell, Ardella, Ardellah

Arden GB (English) valley of the eagle.
Literature: in Shakespeare, a romantic place
of refuge.
Adeana, Ardan, Ardana, Ardane, Ardean,
Ardeane, Ardeen, Ardeena, Ardeenah, Ardeene,
Ardena, Ardenah, Ardene, Ardenia, Ardin,
Ardina, Ardinah, Ardine, Ardun, Ardyn,
Ardyna, Ardynah, Ardyne

Ardi (Hebrew) a short form of Arden,
Ardice, Ardith.
Ardie

Ardice (Hebrew) a form of Ardith.
Ardis, Ardisa, Ardisah, Ardise, Ardiss, Ardissa,
Ardisse, Ardyce, Ardys, Ardyse, Ardyss, Ardyssa,
Ardysse

Ardith (Hebrew) flowering field.
Ardath, Ardyth, Ardythe

Arebela (Latin) a form of Arabella.

Areil (American) a form of Areli.
Areile

Areli, Arely (American) forms of Oralee.
Arelee, Arelis, Arelli, Arellia, Arelly

Arella (Hebrew) angel; messenger.
Arela, Arelah, Arellah, Arelle, Orella, Orelle

Aretha (Greek) virtuous. See also Oretha,
Retha.
Areata, Areatah, Areatha, Areathah, Areathia,
Areathiah, Areeta, Areetah, Areetha, Areethah,
Areethia, Areta, Aretah, Arethea, Aretheah,
Arethia, Arethiah, Aretina, Aretta, Arettah,
Arette, Arita, Aritha, Arithah, Arytha,
Arythah, Arythia, Arythiah, Arythya,
Arythyah

Aretusa (Greek) Mythology: Artheusa was
one of the Nereids.

Argel (Welsh) refuge.

Argelia (Latin) jewelry boxes full of treas-
ures.

Argenea (Latin) she who has platinum-col-
ored hair.

Argenis (Latin) a form of Argenea.

Argentina (Latin) she who shines like gold.
Geography: a country in South America.

Argimon (German) defensive army.

Argraff (Welsh) impression.

Ari BG (Hebrew) a short form of Ariel.

Aria GB (Hebrew) a form of Ariel.
Ariea, Arya, Aryah, Aryia

Ariadna (Greek) a form of Ariadne.
Ariadnah, Aryadna, Aryadnah

Ariadne (Greek) holy. Mythology: the
daughter of King Minos of Crete.

Ariah (Hebrew) a form of Aria.

Arial (Hebrew) a form of Ariel.
Ariale

Arian BG (French) a form of Ariana.
Aerian, Aerion, Arianie, Arien, Ariene, Arieon

Ariana ☆ (Greek) holy.
Aeriana, Aerianna, Aerionna, Ahreanna,
Ahriana, Ahrianna, Airiana, Arianah,
Ariannah, Ariena, Arienah, Arienna,
Ariennah, Arihana

Ariane (French) a form of Ariana.

Arianna ☆ (Greek) a form of Ariana.

Arianne (English) a form of Ariana.
Aeriann, Aerionne, Airiann, Ariann, Ariannie,
Arieann, Arienne, Arionne

Arica, Arika (Scandinavian) forms of Erica.
Aerica, Aericka, Aeryka, Aricah, Aricca,
Ariccah, Aricka, Arickah, Arikah, Arike,
Arikka, Arikkah, Ariqua, Aryca, Arycah,
Arycca, Aryccah, Arycka, Aryckah, Aryka,
Arykah, Arykka, Arykkah, Aryqua

Aricela (Latin) a form of Araceli.

Arie BG (Hebrew) a short form of Ariel.

Arieanna (Greek) a form of Ariana.
Arieana

Ariel GB (Hebrew) lioness of God.
Ahriel, Aire, Aireal, Airial, Arieal, Arrieal

Ariela, Ariella (Hebrew) forms of Ariel.
Arielah, Ariellah, Aryela, Aryelah, Aryella, Aryellah

Ariele, Ariell, Arielle, Arriel (French) forms of Ariel.
Arriele, Arriell, Arrielle

Aries GB (Greek) Mythology: Ares was the Greek god of war. (Latin) ram.
Arees, Ares, Arie, Ariez, Aryes

Arietta (Italian) short aria, melody.
Ariet, Arieta, Arietah, Ariete, Ariett, Ariettah, Ariette, Aryet, Aryeta, Aryetah, Aryete, Aryett, Aryetta, Aryettah, Aryette

Arin BG (Hebrew, Arabic) a form of Aaron. See also Erin.
Arinn, Arrin

Ariona, Arionna (Greek) forms of Ariana.

Arissa (Greek) a form of Arista.

Arista (Greek) best.
Aris, Aristana, Aristen

Arla (German) a form of Carla.

Arlais (Welsh) what comes from the temple.

Arleen (Irish) a form of Arlene.
Arleene

Arleigh (English) a form of Harley.
Arlea, Arleah, Arlee, Arley, Arlie, Arly

Arlena (Irish) a form of Arlene.
Arlana, Arlanah, Arleena, Arleina, Arlenah, Arliena, Arlienah, Arlina, Arlinah, Arlinda

Arlene (Irish) pledge. See also Erline, Lena, Lina.
Airlen, Arlein, Arleine, Arlen, Arlenis, Arleyne, Arlien, Arliene, Arlin, Arline, Arlis

Arlette (English) a form of Arlene.
Arleta, Arletah, Arlete, Arletta, Arlettah, Arletty

Arlynn (American) a combination of Arlene + Lynn.
Arlyn, Arlyne, Arlynna, Arlynne

Armada, Armida (Spanish) forms of Armide.

Armanda (Latin) noble.

Armandina (French) a form of Armide.

Armani BG (Persian) desire, goal.
Armahni, Arman, Armanee, Armanii

Armentaria (Latin) pastor of older livestock.

Armide (Latin) armed warrior.
Armid, Armidea, Armidee, Armidia, Armidiah, Armydea, Armydee, Armydia, Armydiah, Armydya

Arminda (German) a form of Armide.

Armine (Latin) noble. (German) soldier. (French) a form of Herman (see Boys' Names).
Armina, Arminah, Arminee, Arminel, Arminey, Armini, Arminie, Armyn, Armyna, Armynah, Armyne

Armonía (Spanish) balance, harmony.

Arnalda (Spanish) strong as an eagle.

Arnelle (German) eagle.
Arnel, Arnela, Arnelah, Arnele, Arnell, Arnella, Arnellah

Arnette BG (English) little eagle.
Arnet, Arneta, Arnett, Arnetta, Arnettah

Arnina (Hebrew) enlightened. (Arabic) a form of Aaron.
Aarnina, Arninah, Arnine, Arnona, Arnonah, Arnyna, Arnynah

Arnulfa (German) eagle wolf.

Aroa (German) good person.

Arriana (Greek) a form of Ariana.
Arrianna

Artaith (Welsh) storm.

Artemia (Greek) a form of Artemis.

Artemis (Greek) Mythology: the goddess of the hunt and the moon.
Artema, Artemah, Artemisa, Artemise, Artemisia, Artemys, Artemysia, Artemysya

Artha (Hindi) wealthy, prosperous.
Arthah, Arthea, Arthi

Arti (Hebrew) a form of Ardi. (Hindi) a familiar form of Artha.
Artie

Artis BG (Irish) noble; lofty hill. (Scottish) bear. (English) rock. (Icelandic) follower of Thor.
Arthelia, Arthene, Arthette, Arthurette, Arthurina, Arthurine, Artice, Artina, Artine, Artisa, Artise, Artyna, Artynah, Artyne, Artys, Artysa, Artyse

Artura (Celtic) noble.

Aryana, Aryanna (Italian) forms of Ariana.
Aryan, Aryanah, Aryane, Aryann, Aryannah, Aryanne, Aryonna

Aryel, Aryelle (Hebrew) forms of Ariel.
Aryele, Aryell

Aryn GB (Hebrew) a form of Aaron.
Aryne, Arynn, Arynne

Aryssa (Greek) a form of Arissa.

Asa BG (Japanese) born in the morning.
Asah

Ascención (Spanish) ascension.

Asela (Latin) small donkey.

Asenka (Russian) grace.

Asgre (Welsh) heart.

Asha (Arabic, Swahili) a form of Aisha, Ashia.

Ashante, Ashanté (Swahili) forms of Ashanti.

Ashanti GB (Swahili) from a tribe in West Africa.
Achante, Achanti, Asante, Ashanta, Ashantae, Ashantah, Ashantee, Ashantey, Ashantia, Ashantie, Ashaunta, Ashauntae, Ashauntee, Ashaunti, Ashauntia, Ashauntiah, Ashaunty, Ashauntya, Ashuntae, Ashunti, Ashuntie

Asheley, Ashely (English) forms of Ashley.
Ashelee, Ashelei, Asheleigh, Ashelie, Ashelley, Ashelly

Ashia (Arabic) life.
Ayshia

Ashira (Hebrew) rich.
Ashirah, Ashyra, Ashyrah

Ashlan, Ashlen, Ashlin (English) forms of Ashlyn.
Ashliann, Ashlianne, Ashline

Ashle, Ashlea, Ashlee, Ashlei, Ashleigh, Ashli, Ashlie, Ashliegh, Ashly (English) forms of Ashley.
Ashleah, Ashleeh, Ashliee, Ashlye

Ashleen (Irish) a form of Ashlyn.
Ashlean, Ashleann, Ashleene, Ashlena, Ashlenah, Ashlene, Ashlina, Ashlinah, Ashlyna

Ashley ✰ GB (English) ash-tree meadow. See also Lee.
Ahslee, Ahsleigh, Aishlee, Ashala, Ashalee, Ashalei, Ashaley, Ashla, Ashlay, Ashleay, Ashleigh, Ashleye, Ashlia, Ashliah, Ashlya, Ashlyah

Ashlyn, Ashlynn, Ashlynne (English) ash-tree pool. (Irish) vision, dream.
Ashling, Ashlyne

Ashonti (Swahili) a form of Ashanti.

Ashten GB (English) a form of Ashton.
Ashtine, Ashtynne

Ashtin GB (English) a form of Ashton.

Ashton BG (English) ash-tree settlement.

Ashtyn (English) a form of Ashton.

Ashya (Arabic) a form of Ashia.
Ashyah, Ashyia

Asia (Greek) resurrection. (English) eastern sunrise. (Swahili) a form of Aisha.
Ahsia, Aisia, Aisian, Asian, Asianae, Ayzia, Esia, Esiah, Esya, Esyah

Asiah (Greek, English, Swahili) a form of Asia.

Asiya (Arabic) one who tends to the weak, one who heals.

Asja (American) a form of Asia.

Asma (Arabic) excellent; precious.

Aspacia, Aspasia (Greek) welcome.

Aspen GB (English) aspen tree.
Aspin, Aspina, Aspine

Aspyn (English) a form of Aspen.
Aspyna, Aspyne

Assumpta (Catalan) a form of Asunción.

Assunção (Portuguese) a form of Asunción.

Astarte (Egyptian) Mythology: a consort of Seth.

Aster (English) a form of Astra.
Astar, Astera, Asteria, Astir, Astor, Astyr

Astra (Greek) star.
Asta, Astara, Astiah, Astraea, Astrah, Astrea, Astreah, Astree, Astrey, Astria, Astrya, Astryah

Astrid (Scandinavian) divine strength.
Astrad, Astread, Astred, Astreed, Astri, Astrida, Astrik, Astrod, Astrud, Astryd, Atti, Estrid

Astriz (German) a form of Astra.

Asunción (Spanish) assumption.

Asunta (Spanish) to ascend.

Asya (Greek, English, Swahili) a form of Asia.
Asyah

Atala, Atalia (Greek) young.

Atalanta (Greek) mighty huntress. Mythology: an athletic young woman who refused to marry any man who could not outrun her in a footrace. See also Lani.
Atalantah, Atalaya, Atlee

Atalía (Spanish) guard tower.

Atanasia (Spanish) one who will be reborn; immortal.

Atara (Hebrew) crown.
Atarah, Ataree, Ataria, Atariah, Atarya, Ataryah, Ateara, Atearah, Atera, Aterah

Atenea (Greek) a form of Athena.

Atgas (Welsh) hate.

Athalia (Hebrew) the Lord is mighty.
Atali, Atalie, Athalea, Athaleah, Athalee, Athalei, Athaleigh, Athaley, Athali, Athaliah, Athalie, Athaly, Athalya, Athalyah

Athena (Greek) wise. Mythology: the goddess of wisdom.
Atheana, Atheanah, Athenah, Athenais, Athene, Athenea

Athina (Greek) a form of Athena.
Atina

Ática (Greek) the city of Athens.

Atilia (Latin) woman who has difficulty walking.

Atira (Hebrew) prayer.
Atirah, Atyra, Atyrah

Atiya (Arabic) gift.

Atl (Nahuatl) water.

Atlanta (Greek) a form of Atalanta.
Atlantah, Atlante, Atlantia, Atlantiah, Atlantya, Atlantyah

Atocha (Arabic) esparto grass.

Auberte (French) a form of Alberta.
Auberta, Aubertah, Aubertha, Auberthe, Aubertina, Aubertine, Aubine, Aubirta, Aubirtah, Aubirte, Auburta, Auburte, Aubyrta, Aubyrtah, Aubyrte

Aubree, Aubri, Aubrie, Aubry (French) forms of Aubrey.
Auberi, Aubre, Aubrei, Aubreigh, Aubria, Aubriah

Aubrey GB (German) noble; bearlike. (French) blond ruler; elf ruler.
Aubary, Aubery, Aubray, Aubrea, Aubreah, Aubrette, Aubrya, Aubryah, Aubury

Aubriana, Aubrianna (English) combinations of Aubrey + Anna.
Aubreyana, Aubreyanna, Aubreyanne, Aubreyena, Aubrian, Aubrianah, Aubriane, Aubriann, Aubriannah, Aubrianne, Aubryan, Aubryana, Aubryanah, Aubryane, Aubryann, Aubryanna, Aubryannah, Aubryanne

Aubrielle (French) a form of Aubrey.

Auburn GB (Latin) reddish brown.
Abern, Aberne, Abirn, Abirne, Aburn, Aburne, Abyrn, Abyrne, Aubern, Auberne, Aubin, Aubirn, Aubirne, Aubun, Auburne, Aubyrn, Aubyrne

Aude, Audey (English) familiar forms of Audrey.
Audi, Audie

Audelina (German) a form of Audrey.

Audra (French) a form of Audrey.
Audrah

Audrea (French) a form of Audrey.
Audria, Audriah, Audriea, Audrya, Audryah

Audreanne, Audrey Ann, Audrey Anne
(English) combinations of Audrey + Ann.
Audreen, Audrey-Ann, Audrey-Anne,
Audrianne, Audrienne

Audree, Audrie, Audry (English) forms of
Audrey.
Audre, Audri

Audrey ☆ GB (English) noble strength.
Adrey, Audey, Audray, Audrin, Audriya,
Audrye

Audrey Maud, Audrey Maude (English)
combinations of Audrey + Maud.
Audrey-Maud, Audrey-Maude, Audreymaud,
Audreymaude

Audriana, Audrianna (English) combinations of Audrey + Anna.
Audreanna, Audrienna, Audryana, Audryanna

Audrina (English) a form of Audriana.

Audris (German) fortunate, wealthy.
Audrys

August BG (Latin) born in the eighth
month. A short form of Augustine.
Auguste

Augusta (Latin) a short form of Augustine.
See also Gusta.
Agusta, Augustah, Augustia, Augustus, Austina

Augustine BG (Latin) majestic. Religion:
Saint Augustine was the first archbishop of
Canterbury. See also Tina.
Agostina, Agostine, Agostyna, Agostyne,
Agustina, Augusteen, Augusteena, Augusteene,
Augustina, Augustinah, Augustyna, Augustyne

Aundrea (Greek) a form of Andrea.
Aundreah

Aura (Greek) soft breeze. (Latin) golden. See
also Ora.
Aurah, Aurea, Aureah, Auri, Auria, Auriah,
Aurya, Auryah

Aúrea (Latin) she who has blond hair.

Aurelia (Latin) golden. See also Oralia.
Auralea, Auraleah, Auralia, Aurea, Aureah,
Aureal, Aurel, Aurela, Aurelah, Aurele,
Aurelea, Aureliana, Aurella, Aurellah, Auria,
Auriah, Aurie, Aurilia, Auriola, Auriolah,
Auriolla, Auriollah, Aurita

Aurelie (Latin) a form of Aurelia.
Auralee, Auralei, Auraleigh, Auraley, Aurali,
Auraliah, Auraly, Aurelee, Aurelei, Aureli,
Aurell, Aurelle, Auriol, Aurioll, Auriolle

Auriel (Hebrew) a form of Ariel.
Aurielle

Auristela (Latin) golden star.

Aurora (Latin) dawn. Mythology: the goddess of dawn.
Aurorah, Aurore, Aurure, Ora, Ori, Orie, Rora

Aurquena, Aurquene (Spanish) present.

Auset (Egyptian) Mythology: Aset is another
name for Isis.

Austen BG (Latin) a short form of
Augustine.
Austina, Austinah, Austyna, Austynah,
Austyne, Austynn

Austin BG (Latin) a short form of Augustine.

Austyn BG (Latin) a short form of
Augustine.

Autum (American) a form of Autumn.

Autumn ☆ (Latin) autumn.
Autom

Auxiliadora (Latin) she who protects and
helps.

Ava ☆ (Greek) a form of Eva.
Avada, Avae, Avah, Ave, Aveen

Avaline (English) a form of Evelyn.
Avalean, Avaleana, Avaleanah, Avaleen,
Avaleena, Avaleenah, Avaleene, Avalina,
Avalinah, Avalyn, Avalyna, Avalynah,
Avalyne, Avelean, Aveleana, Aveleanah,
Aveleen, Aveleena, Aveleenah, Aveleene,
Avelina, Avelinah, Avelyn, Avelyna, Avelynah,
Avelyne

Avalon (Latin) island.
Avallon, Avalona, Avalonah, Avaloni,
Avalonia, Avaloniah, Avalonie, Avalony,
Avalonya, Avalonyah

Averi, Averie (English) forms of Aubrey.
Aivree, Avaree, Avarey, Avari, Avarie, Avary,
Averee, Averey, Avry

Avery ☆ BG (English) a form of Aubrey.

Aviana (Latin) a form of Avis.
Avianca, Avianna

Avis (Latin) bird.
Avais, Aveis, Aves, Avi, Avia, Aviance, Avice, Avicia, Avise, Avyce, Avys, Avyse

Aviva (Hebrew) springtime. See also Viva.
Aviv, Avivah, Avivi, Avivice, Avivie, Avivit, Avni, Avnit, Avri, Avrit, Avy, Avyva, Avyvah

Avneet (Hebrew) a form of Avner (see Boys' Names).

Avril (French) a form of April.
Avaril, Avarila, Avarile, Avarill, Avarilla, Avarille, Averil, Averila, Averilah, Averill, Averilla, Averille, Averyl, Averyla, Averyle, Averyll, Averylla, Averylle, Avra, Avri, Avrilett, Avriletta, Avrilette, Avrilia, Avrill, Avrille, Avrillia, Avryl, Avryla, Avrylah, Avryle, Avryll, Avrylla, Avryllah, Avrylle, Avryllett, Avrylletta, Avryllette, Avy

Awel (Welsh) gentle breeze.

Axelle (Latin) axe. (German) small oak tree; source of life.

Aya (Hebrew) bird; fly swiftly.
Aia, Aiah, Aiya, Aiyah

Ayah (Hebrew) a form of Aya.

Ayalga (Asturian) treasure.

Ayan (Hindi) a short form of Ayanna.

Ayana (Native American) a form of Aiyana. (Hindi) a form of Ayanna.

Ayanna (Hindi) innocent.
Ahyana, Ayana, Ayania, Ayaniah, Ayannah, Ayannica, Ayna

Ayat (Islamic) sign, revelation.

Ayelen, Aylén (Mapuche) joy.

Ayelén (Araucanian) a form of Ayelen.

Ayesha (Persian) a form of Aisha.
Ayasha, Ayeshah, Ayeshia, Ayeshiah, Ayessa, Ayisha, Ayishah, Ayshea, Ayshia, Ayshiah, Ayshya, Ayshyah

Ayinhual (Mapuche) beloved, darling; generous.

Ayinleo (Mapuche) inextinguishable love.

Ayiqueo (Mapuche) soft-spoken; pleasant.

Ayita (Cherokee) first in the dance.
Aitah

Ayla (Hebrew) oak tree.
Aylah, Aylana, Aylanah, Aylanna, Aylannah, Aylea, Aylee, Ayleen, Ayleena, Aylena, Aylene, Aylie, Aylin

Aymara (Spanish) people and language of the south Andes.

Ayme (Mapuche) significant.

Aynkan (Indigenous) older sister.

Aysha (Persian) a form of Aisha.
Ayshah, Ayshe

Aysia (English) a form of Asia. (Persian) a form of Aisha.
Aysiah, Aysian

Aza (Arabic) comfort.
Aiza, Aizha

Azalea (Greek) dry. Botany: a shrub with showy, colorful flowers that grows in dry soil.
Azaleah, Azalee, Azalei, Azaleigh, Azaley, Azali, Azalia, Azaliah, Azalie, Azaly, Azalya, Azalyah, Azelea, Azeleah, Azelia, Azeliah, Azelya, Azelyah

Azaria (Hebrew) a form of Azuriah (see Boys' Names).
Azariah

Azia (Arabic) a form of Aza.
Aizia

Aziza (Swahili) precious.
Azizah, Azize

Azucena (Arabic) admirable mother.

Azul (Arabic) color of the sky without clouds.

Azura (Persian) blue semiprecious stone.
Azora, Azorah, Azurah, Azurina, Azurine, Azuryn, Azuryna, Azurynah, Azuryne

Azure (Persian) a form of Azura.

B

Baba (African) born on Thursday.
Aba, Abah, Babah

Babe (Latin) a familiar form of Barbara.
(American) a form of Baby.

Babesne (Arabic) a form of Amparo.

Babette (French, German) a familiar form
of Barbara.
*Babet, Babeta, Babetah, Babett, Babetta,
Babettah, Babita, Babitta, Babitte, Barbet,
Barbett, Barbetta, Barbette, Barbita*

Babs (American) a familiar form of Barbara.
Bab

Baby (American) baby.
*Babby, Babe, Babea, Babee, Babey, Babi,
Babie, Bebe, Bebea, Bebee, Bebey, Bebi, Bebia,
Bebie, Beby, Bebya*

Badia (Arabic) elegant.
Badiah

Bahiti (Egyptian) fortune.

**Bailee, Baileigh, Baili, Bailie, Baillie,
Baily** (English) forms of Bailey.
*Bailea, Baileah, Bailei, Bailia, Baillee, Bailley,
Bailli, Bailly*

Bailey ⭐ GB (English) bailiff.
Baelee, Baeleigh, Baeley, Baeli, Bali, Balley

Baka (Hindi) crane.
Bakah

Bakana (Australian) guardian.
Bakanah, Bakanna, Bakannah

Bakari BG (Swahili) noble promise.
Bakarie, Bakary

Bakarne (Basque) solitude.

Bakula (Hindi) flower.
Bakulah

Balbina (Latin) stammerer.
*Balbinah, Balbine, Balbyna, Balbynah,
Balbyne*

Baldomera (Spanish) bold; famous.

Balduina (German) brave friend.

Baleigh (English) a form of Bailey.

Bambi (Italian) child.
*Bambea, Bambee, Bambia, Bambiah, Bambie,
Bamby, Bambya*

Ban (Arabic) has revealed oneself; has appeared.

Bandi BG (Punjabi) prisoner.
*Banda, Bandah, Bandee, Bandey, Bandia,
Bandiah, Bandie, Bandy, Bandya, Bandyah*

Banon (Welsh) queen.

Bao GB (Chinese) treasure.

Baptista (Latin) baptizer.
*Baptisa, Baptissa, Baptisse, Baptiste, Baptysa,
Baptysah, Baptyse, Baptyssa, Baptysta,
Batista, Battista, Bautista*

Bara, Barra (Hebrew) chosen.
Bára, Barah, Barra, Barrah

Barb (Latin) a short form of Barbara.
Barba, Barbe

Barbada (Arabic) blessing.

Barbara (Latin) stranger, foreigner. See also
Bebe, Varvara, Wava.
*Babara, Babb, Babbie, Babe, Babette, Babina,
Babs, Barbara-Ann, Barbarina, Barbarit,
Barbarita, Barbary, Barbeeleen, Barbel,
Barbera, Barbica, Barbora, Barborah, Barborka,
Barbraann, Barbro, Barùska, Basha*

Bárbara (Greek) a form of Barbara.

Barbie (American) a familiar form of Barbara.
Barbea, Barbee, Barbey, Barbi, Barby, Baubie

Barbra (American) a form of Barbara.
Barbraa, Barbro

Bardon (Hispanic) full of hair.

Bari (Irish) a form of Barrie.

Barika (Swahili) success.
Barikah, Baryka, Barykah

Barran (Irish) top of a small hill. (Russian) ram.
Baran, Barana, Baranah, Barean, Bareana, Bareane, Bareen, Bareena, Bareenah, Bareene, Barein, Bareina, Bareinah, Bareine, Bareyba, Bareyn, Bareynah, Bareyne, Barin, Barina, Barinah, Barine, Barreen, Barreena, Barreenah, Barreene, Barrin, Barrina, Barrinah, Barrine, Barryn, Barryna, Barrynah, Barryne

Barrett 🅱🅶 (German) strong as a bear.

Barrie (Irish) spear; markswoman.
Barea, Baree, Barey, Barri, Barria, Barriah, Barrya, Barryah, Barya, Baryah, Berri, Berrie, Berry

Bartola, Bartolina (Aramaic) she who tills the soil.

Bartolomea (Spanish) child of Talmaí.

Basemat (Hebrew) balm.

Basia (Hebrew) daughter of God.
Bashiah, Bashya, Bashyah, Basiah, Basya, Basyah, Bathia, Batia, Batya, Bithia, Bitya

Basiana (Spanish) acute judgment.

Basillia (Greek, Latin) royal; queenly.
Basilia, Basiliah, Basilie, Basilla, Basillah, Basillie, Basyla, Basylah, Basyle, Basyll, Basylla, Basyllah, Basylle, Bazila, Bazilah, Bazile, Bazilie, Bazill, Bazilla, Bazillah, Bazille, Bazillia, Bazilliah, Bazillie, Bazyla, Bazylah, Bazyle, Bazyll, Bazylla, Bazyllah, Bazylle

Bastet (Egyptian) Mythology: cat-headed goddess.

Bathany (Aramaic) a form of Bethany.
Bathanea, Bathaneah, Bathanee, Bathaney, Bathani, Bathania, Bathaniah, Bathanie, Bathannee, Bathanney, Bathanni, Bathannia, Bathanniah, Bathannie, Bathanny, Bathanya, Bathenee, Batheney, Batheni, Bathenia, Batheniah, Bathenie, Batheny

Bathilda (German) warrior.
Bathildah, Bathilde, Bathylda, Bathyldah, Bathylde

Bathsheba (Hebrew) daughter of the oath; seventh daughter. Bible: a wife of King David. See also Sheba.
Bathshua, Batsheva, Batshevah, Bersaba, Bethsabee, Bethsheba

Batilde (German) a form of Bathilda.

Batini (Swahili) inner thoughts.

Batoul (Arabic) virgin.

Baudilia (Teutonic) audacious and brave.

Baylea, Bayleigh, Bayli, Baylie (English) forms of Bailey.
Bayla, Bayle, Bayleah, Baylei, Baylia, Bayliah, Bayliee, Bayliegh, Bayly

Baylee 🅶🅱 (English) a form of Bailey.

Bayley 🅶🅱 (English) a form of Bailey.

Bayo (Yoruba) joy is found.
Baio

Bea (American) a short form of Beatrice.

Beata (Latin) a short form of Beatrice.
Beatah, Beatta, Beeta, Beetah, Beita, Beitah, Beyta, Beytah

Beatrice (Latin) blessed; happy; bringer of joy. See also Trish, Trixie.
Bea, Beata, Beatrica, Béatrice, Beatricia, Beatriks, Beatrisa, Beatrise, Beatrissa, Beatrix, Beatryx, Beattie, Beatty, Bebe, Bee, Beitris, Trice

Beatris, Beatriz (Latin) forms of Beatrice.
Beatriss, Beatryz

Bebe 🅱🅶 (Spanish) a form of Barbara, Beatrice.
BB, Beebee, Bibi

Becca (Hebrew) a short form of Rebecca.
Beca, Becah, Beccah, Beka, Bekah, Bekka

Becka (Hebrew) a form of Becca.
Beckah

Becky (American) a familiar form of Rebecca.
Beckey, Becki, Beckie, Beki, Bekie, Beky

Bedelia (Irish) a form of Bridget.
Bedeelia, Bedeliah, Bedelya, Bedelyah, Biddy, Bidelia

Bee 🅱🅶 (American) a short form of Beatrice.

Bega (Germanic) illustrious; brilliant.

Begoña (Basque) the place of the dominant hill.

Begonia (Spanish) begonia.

Bel (Hindi) sacred wood of apple trees. A short form of Amabel, Belinda, Isabel. See also Belle.
Bell

Bela BG (Czech) white. (Hungarian) bright.
Belah, Belau, Belia, Beliah, Biela

Belarmina (Spanish) beautiful armor.

Belen GB (Greek) arrow. (Spanish) Bethlehem.
Belina

Belicia (Spanish) dedicated to God.
Beli, Belica, Beliciah, Belicya, Belicyah, Belysia, Belysiah, Belsya, Belsyah

Belinda (Spanish) beautiful. Literature: a name coined by English poet Alexander Pope in *The Rape of the Lock*. See also Blinda, Linda.
Balina, Balinah, Balinda, Balindah, Balinde, Baline, Ballinda, Ballindah, Ballinde, Belina, Belinah, Belindah, Belinde, Belindra, Bellinda, Bellindah, Bellinde, Bellynda, Bellyndah, Bellynde, Belynda

Belisa (Latin) the most slender.

Belisaria (Greek) right-handed archer; she who shoots arrows skillfully.

Bella (Latin) beautiful.
Bellah, Bellau

Belle (French) beautiful. A short form of Arabella, Belinda, Isabel. See also Bel, Billie.
Belita, Bell, Belli, Bellina

Belva (Latin) beautiful view.
Belvia, Belviah, Belvya, Belvyah

Bena (Native American) pheasant. See also Bina.
Benah, Benea, Benna, Bennah

Benate (Basque) a form of Bernadette.

Benecia (Latin) a short form of Benedicta.
Beneciah, Benecya, Benecyah, Beneisha, Benicia, Benish, Benisha, Benishia, Bennicia, Benniciah, Bennicie, Bennicya, Bennycia, Bennyciah, Bennycya, Bennycyah

Benedicta (Latin) blessed.
Bendite, Benedetta, Benedettah, Benedictina,

Benedikta, Benedycta, Benedykta, Bengta, Benna, Bennicia, Benoîte, Binney

Benedicte (Latin) a form of Benedicta.
Bendite, Benedette, Benedictine

Benedicto (Latin) a form of Benedicta.

Benedita (Portuguese) a form of Benedicta.

Benicio (Spanish) benevolent one.

Benigna (Spanish) kind.

Benilda (German) she who fights with bears.

Benilde (Spanish) a form of Benilda.

Benita (Spanish) a form of Benedicta.
Beneta, Benetta, Benite, Benitta, Bennita, Benyta, Benytah, Benyte, Neeta

Benjamina (Spanish) a form of Benjamin (see Boys' Names).

Bennett BG (Latin) little blessed one.
Bennet, Bennetta

Benni (Latin) a familiar form of Benedicta.
Bennie, Binni, Binnie, Binny

Bennu (Egyptian) eagle.

Bente (Latin) blessed.

Berdine (German) glorious; inner light.
Berdina, Berdinah, Berdyn, Berdyna, Berdynah, Berdyne, Birdeen, Birdeena, Birdeene, Birdena, Birdene, Birdenie, Birdina, Byrdeena, Byrdeenah, Byrdeene, Byrdina, Byrdinah, Byrdine, Byrdyna, Byrdynah, Byrdyne

Berengaria (German) strong as a bear.

Berenice, Berenise (Greek) forms of Bernice.
Berenisse, Bereniz, Berenize

Berget (Irish) a form of Bridget.
Bergette, Bergit

Berit (German) glorious.
Beret, Bereta, Berete, Berett, Beretta, Berette, Biret, Bireta, Birete, Birett, Biretta, Birette, Byret, Byreta, Byrete, Byrett, Byretta, Byrette

Berkley BG (Scottish, English) birch-tree meadow.
Berkeley, Berkly

Berlynn (English) a combination of Bertha + Lynn.
Berla, Berlin, Berlinda, Berline, Berling, Berlyn, Berlyne, Berlynne

Bernabela, Bernabella (Hebrew) child of prophecy.

Bernadette (French) a form of Bernadine. See also Nadette.
Bera, Beradette, Berna, Bernadet, Bernadeta, Bernadetah, Bernadete, Bernadett, Bernadetta, Bernadettah, Bernadit, Bernadita, Bernaditah, Bernadite, Bernadyta, Bernadytah, Bernadyte, Bernarda, Bernardette, Bernedet, Bernedette, Bernessa, Berneta

Bernadine (English, German) brave as a bear.
Bernadeen, Bernadeena, Bernadeenah, Bernadeene, Bernaden, Bernadena, Bernadenah, Bernadene, Bernadin, Bernadina, Bernadinah, Bernadyn, Bernadyna, Bernadynah, Bernadyne, Bernardina, Bernardine, Berni

Berneta (French) a short form of Bernadette.
Bernatta, Bernetah, Bernete, Bernetta, Bernettah, Bernette, Bernit, Bernita, Bernitah, Bernite, Bernyt, Bernyta, Bernytah, Bernyte

Berni (English) a familiar form of Bernadine, Bernice.
Bernie, Berny

Bernice (Greek) bringer of victory. See also Bunny, Vernice.
Berenike, Bernece, Berneece, Berneese, Bernese, Bernessa, Bernica, Bernicah, Bernicia, Bernicka, Bernika, Bernikah, Bernise, Bernyc, Bernyce, Bernyse, Nixie

Berry BG (English) berry. A short form of Bernice.
Beree, Berey, Beri, Berie, Berree, Berrey, Berri, Berrie, Bery

Berta (German) a form of Berit, Bertha.

Bertha (German) bright; illustrious; brilliant ruler. A short form of Alberta. See also Birdie, Peke.
Barta, Bartha, Berth, Berthe, Bertille, Bertita, Bertrona, Bertus, Birtha, Birthe, Byrth, Byrtha, Byrthah

Berti (German, English) a familiar form of Gilberte, Bertina.
Berte, Bertie, Berty

Bertila, Bertilia (German) forms of Bertilda.

Bertilda (German) she who fights; the distinguished one.

Bertille (French) a form of Bertha.
Bertilla

Bertina (English) bright, shining.
Berteana, Berteanah, Berteena, Berteenah, Berteene, Bertinah, Bertine, Bertyna, Bertynah, Bertyne, Birteana, Birteanah, Birteena, Birteenah, Birteene, Birtinah, Birtine, Birtyna, Birtynah, Birtyne, Byrteana, Byrteanah, Byrteena, Byrteenah, Byrteene, Byrtinah, Byrtine, Byrtyna, Byrtynah, Byrtyne

Bertoaria (German) brilliant city or army.

Bertolda (German) a form of Bertha.

Berwyn BG (Welsh) white head.
Berwin, Berwina, Berwinah, Berwine, Berwyna, Berwynah, Berwyne, Berwynn, Berwynna, Berwynnah, Berwynne

Beryl (Greek) sea green jewel.
Beral, Beril, Berila, Berile, Berill, Berille, Beryle, Berylla, Berylle

Bess (Hebrew) a short form of Bessie.

Bessie (Hebrew) a familiar form of Elizabeth.
Besee, Besey, Besi, Besie, Bessee, Bessey, Bessi, Bessy, Besy

Betania (Hebrew) a form of Bethany.

Beth (Hebrew, Aramaic) house of God. A short form of Bethany, Elizabeth.
Betha, Bethe, Bethia

Bethani, Bethanie (Aramaic) forms of Bethany.
Bethanee, Bethania, Bethaniah, Bethannee, Bethannie, Bethenee, Bethenni, Bethennie, Bethni, Bethnie

Bethann (English) a combination of Beth + Ann.
Bathana, Beth-Ann, Beth-Anne, Bethan, Bethanah, Bethane, Bethanna, Bethannah,

Bethanne, Bethena, Bethina, Bethinah,
Bethine, Bethyn, Bethyna, Bethynah, Bethyne

Bethany (Aramaic) house of figs. Bible: the
site of Lazarus's resurrection.
Bathanny, Bethaney, Bethanney, Bethanny,
Betheney, Bethenney, Bethenny, Betheny,
Bethia, Bethina, Bethney, Bethny, Betthany

Bethel (Hebrew) from God's house.
Bethal, Bethall, Bethell, Bethil, Bethill, Bethol,
Betholl, Bethyl, Bethyll

Betiñe (Basque) a form of Perpetua.

Betsabe, Betsabé (Hebrew) daughter of an
oath or pact.

Betsy (American) a familiar form of
Elizabeth.
Betsee, Betsey, Betsi, Betsia, Betsie, Betsya,
Betsyah, Betsye

Bette (French) a form of Betty.
Beta, Betah, Bete, Betea, Betia, Betka, Bett,
Betta, Bettah

Bettina (American) a combination of Beth
+ Tina.
Betina, Betinah, Betine, Betti, Bettinah,
Bettine, Bettyna, Bettynah, Bettyne, Betyna,
Betynah, Betyne

Betty (Hebrew) consecrated to God.
(English) a familiar form of Elizabeth.
Betee, Betey, Beti, Betie, Bettee, Bettey, Betti,
Bettie, Betty-Jean, Betty-Jo, Betty-Lou, Bettye,
Bettyjean, Bettyjo, Bettylou, Bety, Boski, Bözsi

Betula (Hebrew) girl, maiden.
Betulah, Betulla, Betullah

Betulia (Hebrew) birch-tree garden.

Beulah (Hebrew) married. Bible: Beulah is a
name for Israel.
Beula, Beulla, Beullah

Bev (English) a short form of Beverly.

Bevanne (Welsh) child of Evan.
Bevan, Bevann, Bevany, Bevin, Bevina,
Bevine, Bevinnah, Bevyn, Bevyna, Bevyne

Beverley (English) a form of Beverly.
Beverle, Beverlea, Beverleah, Beverlee, Beverlei,
Beverleigh

Beverly GB (English) beaver field. See also
Buffy.
Bevalee, Beverlie, Beverlly, Bevlea, Bevlee,
Bevlei, Bevleigh, Bevley, Bevli, Bevlie, Bevly,
Bevlyn, Bevlynn, Bevlynne, Bevvy, Verly

Beverlyann (American) a combination of
Beverly + Ann.
Beverliann, Beverlianne, Beverlyanne

Bian (Vietnamese) hidden; secretive.
Biane, Biann, Bianne, Byan, Byane, Byann,
Byanne

Bianca (Italian) white. See also Blanca,
Vianca.
Biancca, Biancha, Biancia, Bianco, Bianey,
Bianica, Biannca, Biannqua, Binney, Byanca,
Byancah, Byanqua

Bianka (Italian) a form of Bianca.
Beyanka, Biankah, Biannka, Byancka,
Byanckah, Byanka, Byankah

Bibi (Latin) a short form of Bibiana. (Arabic)
lady. (Spanish) a form of Bebe.
BeBe, Beebee, Byby

Bibiana (Latin) lively.
Bibianah, Bibiane, Bibiann, Bibianna,
Bibiannah, Bibianne, Bibyan, Bibyana,
Bibyanah, Bibyann, Bibyanna, Bibyannah,
Bibyanne, Bybian, Bybiana, Bybianah,
Bybiane, Bybiann, Bybianna, Bybiannah,
Bybianne, Bybyan, Bybyana, Bybyanah,
Bybyane, Bybyann, Bybyanna, Bybyannah,
Bybyanne

Bibiñe (Basque) a form of Viviana.

Biblis (Latin) swallow.

Biddy (Irish) a familiar form of Bedelia.
Biddie

Bienvenida (Spanish) welcome.

Bilal (Basque) born during summertime.

Billi (English) a form of Billie.
Biley, Bili, Billey, Billye, Bily, Byley, Byli,
Bylli, Bylly, Byly

Billie GB (English) strong willed. (German,
French) a familiar form of Belle, Wilhelmina.
Bilea, Bileah, Bilee, Bilei, Bileigh, Bilie, Billea,
Billee, Bylea, Byleah, Bylee, Bylei, Byleigh,
Bylie, Byllea, Byllee, Byllei, Bylleigh, Byllie

Billie-Jean (American) a combination of Billie + Jean.
Billiejean, Billy-Jean, Billyjean

Billie-Jo (American) a combination of Billie + Jo.
Billiejo, Billy-Jo, Billyjo

Billy BG (English) a form of Billie.

Bina (Hebrew) wise; understanding. (Swahili) dancer. (Latin) a short form of Sabina. See also Bena.
Binah, Binney, Binta, Bintah, Byna, Bynah

Binney (English) a familiar form of Benedicta, Bianca, Bina.
Binnee, Binni, Binnie, Binny

Bionca (Italian) a form of Bianca.
Beonca, Beyonca, Beyonka, Bioncha, Bionica, Bionka, Bionnca

Birdie (English) bird. (German) a familiar form of Bertha.
Bird, Birde, Birdea, Birdee, Birdella, Birdena, Birdey, Birdi, Birdy, Byrd, Byrda, Byrde, Byrdey, Byrdie, Byrdy

Birgitte (Swedish) a form of Bridget.
Berget, Bergeta, Birgit, Birgita, Birgitt, Birgitta

Birkide (Basque) a form of Bridget.

Bitilda (German) a form of Bathilda.

Bjorg (Scandinavian) salvation.
Bjorga

Bladina (Latin) friendly.
Bladea, Bladeana, Bladeanah, Bladeane, Bladeen, Bladeena, Bladeene, Bladene, Bladine, Bladyn, Bladyna, Bladyne

Blaine BG (Irish) thin.
Blain, Blane

Blair BG (Scottish) plains dweller.
Blare, Blayr, Blayre

Blaire (Scottish) a form of Blair.

Blaise BG (French) one who stammers.
Blais, Blaisia, Blaiz, Blaize, Blasha, Blasia, Blayse, Blayz, Blayze, Blaza, Blaze, Blazena, Blazia

Blake BG (English) dark.
Blaik, Blaike, Blaque, Blayk, Blayke

Blakely BG (English) dark meadow.
Blaiklea, Blaiklee, Blaiklei, Blaikleigh, Blaikley, Blaikli, Blaiklie, Blaikly, Blakelea, Blakeleah, Blakelee, Blakelei, Blakeleigh, Blakeley, Blakeli, Blakelie, Blakelyn, Blakelynn, Blakesley, Blakley, Blakli, Blayklea, Blaykleah, Blayklee, Blayklei, Blaykleigh, Blaykli, Blayklie, Blaykly

Blanca (Italian) a form of Bianca.
Belanca, Belancah, Belancka, Belanckah, Belanka, Belankah, Bellanca, Bellancah, Bellancka, Bellanckah, Bellanka, Bellankah, Blancah, Blancka, Blanka, Blankah, Blannca, Blanncah, Blannka, Blannkah, Blanqua

Blanche (French) a form of Bianca.
Blanch, Blancha, Blinney

Blanda (Latin) delicate; soft.

Blandina (Latin) flattering.

Blasa (French) a form of Blaise.

Blasina, Blasona (Latin) forms of Blaise.

Blayne BG (Irish) a form of Blaine.
Blayn

Blenda (German) white; brilliant.

Blesila (Celtic) firebrand.

Blinda (American) a short form of Belinda.
Blynda

Bliss GB (English) blissful, joyful.
Blis, Blisa, Blissa, Blisse, Blys, Blysa, Blyss, Blyssa, Blysse

Blodwyn (Welsh) flower. See also Wynne.
Blodwen, Blodwin, Blodwina, Blodwinah, Blodwine, Blodwyna, Blodwynah, Blodwyne, Blodwynn, Blodwynna, Blodwynnah, Blodwynne, Blodyn

Blondelle (French) blond, fair haired.
Blondel, Blondele, Blondelia, Blondeliah, Blondell, Blondella, Blondelya, Blondelyah

Blondie (American) a familiar form of Blondelle.
Blondea, Blondee, Blondey, Blondi, Blondia, Blondiah, Blondy, Blondya

Blossom (English) flower.

Blum (Yiddish) flower.
Bluma, Blumah

Blythe GB (English) happy, cheerful.
Blithe, Blyss, Blyth

Bo BG (Chinese) precious.
Beau, Bow

Boacha (Hebrew) blessed.

Bobbette (American) a familiar form of
Roberta.
Bobbet, Bobbetta, Bobinetta, Bobinette

Bobbi (American) a familiar form of
Barbara, Roberta.
*Baubie, Bobbe, Bobbea, Bobbee, Bobbey,
Bobbie-Jean, Bobbie-Lynn, Bobbie-Sue,
Bobbisue, Bobby, Bobbye, Bobea, Bobee, Bobey,
Bobi, Bobie, Bobina, Bobine, Boby*

Bobbi-Ann, Bobbie-Ann (American) com-
binations of Bobbi + Ann.
*Bobbi-Anne, Bobbiann, Bobbianne, Bobbie-
Anne, Bobby-Ann, Bobby-Anne, Bobbyann,
Bobbyanne*

Bobbi-Jo, Bobbie-Jo (American) combinations of Bobbi + Jo.
Bobbiejo, Bobbijo, Bobby-Jo, Bobijo

Bobbi-Lee (American) a combination of
Bobbi + Lee.
*Bobbie-Lee, Bobbilee, Bobby-Leigh, Bobbylee,
Bobile*

Bobbie GB (American) a familiar form of
Barbara, Roberta.

Bodana, Bohdana (Russian) gift from God.

Bodil BG (Norwegian) mighty ruler.
Bodila, Bodilah, Bodyl, Bodyla, Bodylah

Bolivia (Spanish) Geography: Bolivia is a
country in South America.

Bolona (German) friend.

Bolonia (Italian) Geography: a form of
Bologna, an Italian city.

Bonajunta (Latin) good; united.

Bonfila, Bonfilia (Italian) good daughter.

Bonifacia (Italian) benefactor.

Bonita (Spanish) pretty.
*Bonesha, Bonetta, Bonitah, Bonitta, Bonittah,
Bonnetta, Bonnita, Bonnitah, Bonnitta,
Bonnyta, Bonnytta, Bonyta, Bonytta*

Bonnie, Bonny (English, Scottish) beautiful,
pretty. (Spanish) familiar forms of Bonita.
*Bonea, Bonee, Boney, Boni, Bonia, Boniah,
Bonie, Bonne, Bonnea, Bonnee, Bonnell,
Bonney, Bonni, Bonnia, Bonniah, Bonnin*

Bonnie-Bell (American) a combination of
Bonnie + Belle.
*Bonnebell, Bonnebelle, Bonnibela, Bonnibelah,
Bonnibele, Bonnibell, Bonnibella, Bonnibellah,
Bonnibelle, Bonniebell, Bonniebelle, Bonnybell,
Bonnybelle*

Bonosa (Spanish) willingly; with kindness.

Bova (German) brave; illustrious.

Bracken (English) fern.
Brackin, Brackyn, Braken, Brakin, Brakyn

Bradley BG (English) broad meadow.
*Bradlea, Bradleah, Bradlee, Bradlei, Bradleigh,
Bradli, Bradlia, Bradliah, Bradlie, Bradly,
Bradlya*

Brady BG (Irish) spirited.
*Bradee, Bradey, Bradi, Bradie, Braedi, Braidee,
Braidey, Braidi, Braidie, Braidy, Braydee*

Braeden BG (English) broad hill.
*Bradyn, Bradynn, Braedan, Braedean,
Braedyn, Braidan, Braiden, Braidyn, Brayden,
Braydn, Braydon*

Braelyn (American) a combination of
Braeden + Lynn.
*Braelee, Braeleigh, Braelin, Braelle, Braelon,
Braelynn, Braelynne, Brailee, Brailenn, Brailey,
Braili, Brailyn, Braylee, Brayley, Braylin,
Braylon, Braylyn, Braylynn*

Braith (Welsh) freckle.

Branca (Portuguese) white.

Branda (Hebrew) blessing.

Brande, Brandee, Brandi, Brandie
(Dutch) forms of Brandy.
*Brandea, Brandeece, Brandeese, Brandei,
Brandia, Brandice, Brandiee, Brandii, Brandily,
Brandin, Brandina, Brani, Branndie, Brendee,
Brendi*

Branden BG (English) beacon valley.
Brandan, Brandine, Brandyn

Brandis (Dutch) a form of Brandy.
Brandise, Brandiss, Brandisse

Brandon BG (English) a form of Branden.

Brandy GB (Dutch) an after-dinner drink made from distilled wine.
Bradys, Brand, Brandace, Brandaise, Brandala, Brandeli, Brandell, Brandy-Lee, Brandy-Leigh, Brandye, Brandylee, Brandysa, Brandyse, Brandyss, Brandyssa, Brandysse, Brann, Brantley, Branyell, Brendy

Brandy-Lynn (American) a combination of Brandy + Lynn.
Brandalyn, Brandalynn, Brandelyn, Brandelynn, Brandelynne, Brandilyn, Brandilynn, Brandilynne, Brandlin, Brandlyn, Brandlynn, Brandlynne, Brandolyn, Brandolynn, Brandolynne, Brandy-Lyn, Brandy-Lynne, Brandylyn, Brandylynne

Braulia (Teutonic) gleaming.

Braulio (German) ardent; one who burns.

Braxton BG (English) Brock's town.
Braxten, Braxtyn

Bre (Irish, English) a form of Bree.

Brea, Breah (Irish) short forms of Breana, Briana.
Breea, Breeah

Breahna (Irish) a form of Breana, Briana.

Breana, Bréana, Breanna, Bréanna (Irish) forms of Briana.
Bre-Anna, Breanah, Breanda, Breannah, Breannea, Breannia, Breasha, Breawna, Breila

Breann, Breanne (Irish) short forms of Briana.
Bre-Ann, Bre-Anne, Breane, Breaunne, Breiann, Breighann, Breyenne, Brieon

Breasha (Russian) a familiar form of Breana.

Breauna, Breaunna, Breunna, Briauna, Briaunna (Irish) forms of Briana.
Breeauna, Breuna

Breck BG (Irish) freckled.
Brec, Breca, Brecah, Brecka, Breckah, Brecken, Brek, Breka, Brekah

Bree (English) broth. (Irish) a short form of Breann. See also Brie.
Breay, Brey

Breean (Irish) a short form of Briana.
Breeane, Breeann, Breeanne, Breelyn, Breeon

Breeana, Breeanna (Irish) forms of Briana.
Breeanah, Breeannah

Breena (Irish) fairy palace. A form of Brina.
Breenah, Breene, Breenea, Breenia, Breeniah, Breina, Breinah

Breeze (English) light wind; carefree.
Brease, Breaz, Breaze, Brees, Breese, Breez, Briez, Brieze, Bryez, Bryeze, Bryze

Bregus (Welsh) fragile.

Breiana, Breianna (Irish) forms of Briana.
Breian, Breianah, Breiane, Breiann, Breiannah, Breianne

Breigh (Irish) a form of Bree.
Brei

Brena, Brenna (Irish) forms of Brenda.
Bren, Brenah, Brenie, Brenin, Brenn, Brennah, Brennaugh, Brenne

Brenda (Irish) little raven. (English) sword.
Brandah, Brandea, Brendah, Brendell, Brendelle, Brendette, Brendie, Brendyl, Brennda, Brenndah, Brinda, Brindah, Brinnda, Brinndah, Brynda, Bryndah, Brynnda, Brynndah

Brenda-Lee (American) a combination of Brenda + Lee.
Brendalee, Brendaleigh, Brendali, Brendaly, Brendalys, Brenlee, Brenley

Brennan BG (English) a form of Brendan (see Boys' Names).
Brennea, Brennen, Brennon, Brennyn

Breona, Bréona, Breonna, Bréonna (Irish) forms of Briana.
Breaona, Breaonah, Breeona, Breeonah, Breiona, Breionah, Breionna, Breonah, Breonie, Breonne

Breonia (Irish) a form of Breona.

Bret BG (Irish) a short form of Britany. See also Brita.
Breat, Breatte, Breta, Bretah, Bretta, Brettah, Brettea, Brettia, Brettin, Bretton

Brett BG (Irish) a short form of Britany.

Brette (Irish) a short form of Britany.

Breyana, Breyann, Breyanna (Irish) forms of Briana.
Breyan, Breyane, Breyannah, Breyanne, Breyna, Breynah

Breyona, Breyonna (Irish) forms of Briana.
Breyonah, Breyonia

Bria, Briah (Irish) short forms of Briana. See also Brea.
Brya, Bryah

Briahna (Irish) a form of Briana.

Briana (Irish) strong; virtuous, honorable.
Bhrianna, Brana, Brianni, Briannon

Brianca (Irish) a form of Briana.

Brianda (Irish) a form of Briana.
Briand

Briann, Brianne (Irish) short forms of Briana.
Briane

Brianna ⭐ (Irish) a form of Briana.

Briannah (Irish) a form of Briana.
Brianah

Briar BG (French) heather.
Brear, Brier, Bryar

Brice BG (Welsh) a form of Bryce.

Bricia (Spanish) a form of Bridget.

Bridey (Irish) a familiar form of Bridget.
Bridea, Brideah, Bridee, Bridi, Bridie, Bridy, Brydea, Brydee, Brydey, Brydi, Brydie, Brydy

Bridget (Irish) strong. See also Bedelia, Bryga, Gitta.
Berget, Birgitte, Bride, Bridey, Bridger, Bridgeta, Bridgetah, Bridgete, Bridgid, Bridgit, Bridgita, Bridgitah, Bridgite, Bridgot, Brietta, Brigada, Briget, Brydget, Brydgeta, Brydgetah, Brydgete

Bridgett, Bridgette (Irish) forms of Bridget.
Bridgetta, Bridgettah, Bridggett, Bridgitt, Bridgitta, Bridgittah, Bridgitte, Briggitte, Brigitta, Brydgett, Brydgetta, Brydgettah, Brydgette

Brie (French) a type of cheese. Geography: a region in France known for its cheese. See also Bree.
Bri, Briea, Briena, Brieon, Brietta, Briette, Bry, Brye

Brieana, Brieanna (American) combinations of Brie + Anna. See also Briana.
Brieannah

Brieann, Brieanne (American) combinations of Brie + Ann.
Brie-Ann, Brie-Anne

Briel, Brielle (French) forms of Brie.
Breael, Breaele, Breaell, Breaelle, Breel, Breell, Breelle, Briela, Brielah, Briele, Briell, Briella, Bryel, Bryela, Bryelah, Bryele, Bryell, Bryella, Bryellah, Bryelle

Brienna (Irish) a form of Briana.
Brieon, Brieona

Brienne (French) a short form of Briana.
Briene, Brienn

Brieonna (Irish) a form of Briana.

Brigette (French) a form of Bridget.
Briget, Brigett, Brigetta, Brigettee, Brigget

Brighton BG (English) bright town.
Breighton, Bright, Brightin, Bryton

Brigid (Irish) a form of Bridget.
Brigida

Brígida, Brigidia (Celtic) forms of Bridget.

Brigit, Brigitte (French) forms of Bridget.
Briggitte, Brigita

Brillana (English) from the city of Brill, England.

Brina (Latin) a short form of Sabrina. (Irish) a familiar form of Briana.
Breina, Breinah, Brin, Brinah, Brinan, Brinda, Brindi, Brindy, Briney, Brinia, Brinlee, Brinly, Brinn, Brinna, Brinnah, Brinnan

Briona, Brionna (Irish) forms of Briana.
Brionah, Brione, Brionnah, Brionne, Briony, Briunna, Bryony

Brisa (Spanish) beloved. Mythology: Briseis was the Greek name of Achilles's beloved.
Breza, Brisah, Brisha, Brishia, Brissa, Brysa, Brysah, Bryssa, Bryssah

Brisda (Celtic) a form of Bridget.

Briselda (Spanish) a form of Bridget.

Brisia, Briza (Greek) forms of Brisa.

Bristol (English) the site of the bridge; from Bristol, England.

Brita (Irish) a form of Bridget. (English) a short form of Britany.
Breata, Breatah, Breatta, Breattah, Bretta, Briet, Brieta, Briete, Briett, Brietta, Briette, Brit, Bryt, Bryta, Brytah, Bryte, Brytia

Britaney, Britani, Britanie, Brittanee, Brittaney, Brittani, Brittanie (English) forms of Britany.
Britana, Britanah, Britane, Britanee, Britania, Britanica, Britanii, Britanna, Britanni, Britannia, Britanny, Bratatani, Brittanah, Brittane, Brittanni, Brittannia, Brittannie

Britany, Brittany (English) from Britain. See also Bret.
Briteny, Britkney, Britley, Britlyn, Brittainee, Brittainey, Brittainny, Brittainy, Brittamy, Brittana, Brittania, Brittanica, Brittany-Ann, Brittanyne, Brittell, Brittlin, Brittlynn

Britin, Brittin (English) from Britain.
Breatin, Breatina, Breatinah, Breatine, Breattin, Breattina, Breattinah, Breattine, Bretin, Bretina, Bretinah, Bretine, Bretyn, Bretyna, Bretynah, Bretyne, Britan, Britann, Britia, Britina, Britinah, Britine, Briton, Brittin, Brittina, Brittine, Bryttin, Bryttina, Bryttine

British (English) from Britain.

Britnee, Britney, Britni, Britnie, Britny, Brittnay, Brittnee, Brittney, Brittni, Brittnie, Brittny (English) forms of Britany.
Bittney, Bridnee, Bridney, Britnay, Britne, Britnei, Britnye, Brittnaye, Brittne, Brittnea, Brittnei, Brittneigh, Brytnea, Brytni

Briton BG (English) a form of Britin.

Britt BG (Swedish, Latin) a short form of Britta.
Briet, Brit, Britte, Brytte

Britta (Swedish) strong. (Latin) a short form of Britany.
Brita, Brittah, Brytta, Bryttah

Brittan BG (English) a form of Britin. A short form of Britany.

Brittanny (English) a form of Britany.

Britten BG (English) a form of Britin. A short form of Britany.

Britteny (English) a form of Britany.
Britenee, Briteney, Briteni, Britenie, Briteny, Brittenay, Brittenee, Britteney, Britteni, Brittenie

Brittiany (English) a form of Britany.
Britianey, Brittiani, Brittianni

Brittin (English) a form of Britin.

Brittini, Brittiny (English) forms of Britany.
Britini, Britinie, Brittinee, Brittiney, Brittinie

Britton BG (English) a form of Britin.

Brittony (English) a form of Britany.

Briyana, Briyanna (Irish) forms of Briana.

Brodie BG (Irish) ditch; canal builder.
Brodee, Brodi, Brody

Brogan BG (Irish) a heavy work shoe.
Brogen, Broghan, Broghen

Bronnie (Welsh) a familiar form of Bronwyn.
Bron, Broney, Bronia, Broniah, Bronie, Bronnee, Bronney, Bronny, Bronya

Bronte (Greek) thunder. (Gaelic) bestower. Literature: Charlotte, Emily, and Anne Brontë were sister writers from England.
Bronté, Brontë

Bronwen (Welsh) a form of Bronwyn.

Bronwyn (Welsh) white breasted. See also Rhonwyn.
Bronwin, Bronwina, Bronwinah, Bronwine, Bronwynn, Bronwynna, Bronwynne

Brook GB (English) brook, stream.
Bhrooke, Brookee, Brookelle, Brookey, Brookia, Brookie, Brooky

Brooke ☆ GB (English) brook, stream.

Brooke-Lynn, Brookelyn, Brookelynn (American) forms of Brooklyn.
Brookelina, Brookeline, Brookellen, Brookellin, Brookellina, Brookelline, Brookellyn, Brookellyna, Brookellyne, Brookelyn, Brookelyna, Brookelyne, Brookelynn

Brooklin (American) a form of Brooklyn.
Brooklina, Brookline

Brooklyn, Brooklyne, Brooklynn, Brooklynne (American) combinations of Brook + Lynn.
Brooklen, Brooklyna

Brooks BG (English) a form of Brook.

Bruna (German) a short form of Brunhilda.
Brona

Brunela (Italian) a form of Brunhilda.

Brunhilda (German) armored warrior.
Brinhild, Brinhilda, Brinhilde, Bruna, Brunhild, Brunhildah, Brunhilde, Brunnhild, Brunnhilda, Brunnhildah, Brünnhilde, Brynhild, Brynhilda, Brynhildah, Brynhilde, Brynhyld, Brynhylda, Brynhyldah, Brynhylde, Hilda

Brunilda (German) a form of Brunhilda.

Bryana, Bryanna (Irish) forms of Briana.
Bryanah, Bryannah, Bryanni

Bryanne (Irish) a short form of Bryana.
Bryane, Bryann

Bryce BG (Welsh) alert; ambitious.

Bryga (Polish) a form of Bridget.
Brygid, Brygida, Brygitka

Brylee, Brylie (American) combinations of the letter B + Riley.
Brylei, Bryley, Bryli

Bryn GB (Latin) from the boundary line. (Welsh) mound.
Brin, Brinn, Brynee

Bryna (Latin, Irish) a form of Brina.
Brinah, Brinan, Brinna, Brinnah, Brinnan, Brynah, Brynan, Brynna, Brynnah, Brynnan

Brynn (Latin) from the boundary line. (Welsh) mound.

Brynne (Latin, Welsh) a form of Bryn.

Bryona, Bryonna (Irish) forms of Briana.
Brionie, Bryonah, Bryone, Bryonee, Bryoney, Bryoni, Bryonia, Bryony

Bryttani, Bryttany (English) forms of Britany.
Brytanee, Brytaney, Brytani, Brytania, Brytanie, Brytanny, Brytany, Bryttanee, Bryttaney, Bryttania, Bryttanie, Bryttine

Bryttni (English) a form of Britany.
Brytnee, Brytney, Brytni, Brytnie, Brytny, Bryttnee, Bryttney, Bryttnie, Bryttny, Brytton

Buena (Spanish) good.

Buenaventura (Castilian) good fortune.

Buffy (American) buffalo; from the plains.
Bufee, Bufey, Buffee, Buffey, Buffi, Buffie, Buffye, Bufi, Bufie, Bufy

Bunny (Greek) a familiar form of Bernice. (English) little rabbit. See also Bonnie.
Bunee, Buney, Buni, Bunie, Bunnea, Bunnee, Bunney, Bunni, Bunnia, Bunnie, Buny

Burgundy (French) Geography: a region of France known for its Burgundy wine.
Burgandee, Burgandey, Burgandi, Burgandie, Burgandy, Burgunde, Burgundee, Burgundey, Burgundi, Burgundie

Bushra (Arabic) good omen.

Byanna (Irish) a form of Briana.
Biana, Bianah, Bianna, Byanah, Byannah

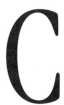

Cabeza (Spanish) head.

Cache, Cachet (French) prestigious; desirous.
Cachae, Cachea, Cachee, Cachée

Cadence (Latin) rhythm.
Cadena, Cadenah, Cadenza, Kadena, Kadenah, Kadenza, Kadenzah

Cadie, Cady (English) forms of Kady.
Cade, Cadea, Cadee, Cadey, Cadi, Cadia, Cadiah, Cadine, Cadya, Cadyah, Cadye

Cadwyn (Welsh) channel.

Cadyna (English) a form of Cadence.

Caecey (Irish) a form of Casey.
Caecea, Caecee, Caeci, Caecia, Caeciah, Caecie, Caecy, Caesea, Caesee, Caesey, Caesi, Caesie, Caesy

Caela (Hebrew) a form of Kayla.

Caeley (American) a form of Kaylee, Kelly.
*Caelea, Caeleah, Caelee, Caelei, Caeleigh,
Caeli, Caelia, Caelie, Caelly, Caely*

Caelin, Caelyn (American) forms of Kaelyn.
*Caelan, Caelean, Caeleana, Caeleanah,
Caeleane, Caeleen, Caeleena, Caeleenah,
Caeleene, Caelen, Caelena, Caelenah,
Caelene, Caelina, Caelinah, Caeline, Caelinn,
Caelyna, Caelynah, Caelyne, Caelynn*

Caethes (Welsh) slave.

Cafleen (Irish) a form of Cathleen.
*Cafflean, Caffleana, Caffleanah, Caffleane,
Caffleen, Caffleena, Caffleenah, Caffleene,
Cafflein, Caffleina, Caffleinah, Caffleine,
Cafflin, Cafflina, Cafflinah, Caffline, Cafflyn,
Cafflyna, Cafflynah, Cafflyne, Caflean,
Cafleana, Cafleanah, Cafleane, Cafleena,
Cafleenah, Cafleene, Caflein, Cafleina,
Cafleinah, Cafleine, Caflin, Caflina, Caflinah,
Cafline, Caflyn, Caflyna, Caflynah, Caflyne*

Cai 🅱🅶 (Vietnamese) feminine.
Cae, Cay, Caye

Caicey (Irish) a form of Casey.
*Caicea, Caicee, Caici, Caicia, Caiciah, Caicie,
Caicy, Caisea, Caisee, Caisey, Caisi, Caisia,
Caisiah, Caisie, Caisy*

Caila (Hebrew) a form of Kayla.

Cailee, Caileigh, Cailey (American) forms
of Kaylee, Kelly.
*Cailea, Caileah, Caili, Cailia, Cailie, Cailley,
Caillie, Caily*

Cailida (Spanish) adoring.
*Caelida, Caelidah, Cailidah, Cailidora,
Cailidorah, Callidora, Callidorah, Caylida,
Caylidah, Kailida, Kailidah, Kaylida,
Kaylidah*

Cailin, Cailyn (American) forms of Caitlin.
*Cailan, Caileen, Caileena, Caileenah,
Caileene, Cailena, Cailenah, Cailene, Cailina,
Cailine, Cailyna, Cailyne, Cailynn, Cailynne,
Calen*

**Caitlan, Caitlen, Caitlyn, Caitlynn,
Caitlynne** (Irish) forms of Caitlin, Kaitlan.
*Caitlana, Caitland, Caitlandt, Caitlane,
Caitlena, Caitlene, Caitlenn, Caitlyna,
Caitlyne*

Caitlin (Irish) pure. See also Kaitlin,
Katalina.
*Caetlan, Caetlana, Caetlane, Caetlen,
Caetlena, Caetlene, Caetlin, Caetlina,
Caetline, Caetlyn, Caetlyna, Caetlyne,
Caitleen, Caitline, Caitlinn, Caitlon*

Cala, Calla (Arabic) castle, fortress. See also
Calie, Kala.
Calah, Calan, Calana, Calia, Caliah, Callah

Calala (Spanish) a familiar form of
Chandelaria.

Calamanda (Latin) Geography: a region in
Mexico.

Calandra (Greek) lark.
*Calan, Calandre, Calandrea, Calandria,
Calandriah, Caleida, Calendra, Calendrah,
Calendre, Caylandra, Caylandrea, Caylandria,
Caylandriah, Kalandra, Kalandria*

Calantha (Greek) beautiful blossom.
*Calanthah, Calanthia, Calanthiah,
Calanthya, Calanthyah*

Caledonia (Latin) from Scotland.
*Caldona, Caldonah, Caldonia, Caldoniah,
Caldonya, Caldonyah, Caledona, Caledoniah,
Caledonya, Caledonyah*

Calee, Caleigh, Calley (American) forms
of Caeley.
Calea, Caleah, Calei, Calleigh

Calefagia (Greek) pleasant.

Caley 🅶🅱 (American) a form of Caeley.

Calfuray (Mapuche) blue violet flower.

Cali, Calli (Greek) forms of Calie. See also
Kali.
Calia, Caliah

Calida (Spanish) warm; ardent. See also
Kalida.
*Calina, Callida, Callyda, Callydah, Calyda,
Calydah*

Cálida (Spanish) a form of Calida.

Calie, Callie, Cally (Greek, Arabic) familiar
forms of Cala, Calista. See also Kalli.
*Cal, Callea, Calleah, Callee, Callei, Calli,
Callia, Calliah, Caly*

Calinda (Hindi) a form of Kalinda.
Calindah, Calinde, Callinda, Calynd,
Calynda, Calyndah, Calynde

Calínica (Greek) she who wins a great
victory.

Calíope (Greek) a form of Calliope.

Calirroe (Greek) walks with beauty.

Calista, Callista (Greek) most beautiful. See
also Kalista.
Calesta, Calestah, Calistah, Callesta, Callestah,
Callistah, Callysta, Callystah, Calysta

Calistena, Calistenia (Greek) beautiful
strength.

Calisto (Spanish, Portuguese) a form of
Calista.

Calixta, Calixto (Greek) forms of Calista.

Callan GB (German) likes to talk, chatter.
Callen, Callin, Callon, Callun, Callyn, Kallan,
Kallen, Kallin, Kallon, Kallun, Kallyn

Callidora (Greek) gift of beauty.

Calliope (Greek) beautiful voice.
Mythology: Calliope was the Muse of epic
poetry. See also Kalliope.
Calliopee

Callula (Latin) beauty; light.
Callulah, Calula, Calulah, Kallula, Kallulah,
Kalula, Kalulah

Caltha (Latin) yellow flower.

Calumina (Irish) dove.
Caluminah, Calumyna, Calumynah

Calvina (Latin) bald.
Calveana, Calveanah, Calveane, Calveania,
Calveaniah, Calveena, Calveenah, Calveenia,
Calveeniah, Calvinah, Calvine, Calvinetta,
Calvinette, Calvyna, Calvynah, Calvyne

Calyca (Greek) a form of Kalyca.
Calica, Calicah, Calicka, Calickah, Calika,
Calikah, Calycah

Calyn (Scottish) a form of Caelan (see Boys'
Names). (American) a form of Caelin.
(German) a form of Callan (see Boys'
Names).
Callyn, Caylan, Caylen, Cayley, Caylin,
Caylon, Caylyn

Calypso (Greek) concealer. Botany: a
pink orchid native to northern regions.
Mythology: the sea nymph who held
Odysseus captive for seven years.
Calipso, Caly, Lypsie, Lypsy

Cam BG (Vietnamese) sweet citrus.
Kam

Camara (American) a form of Cameron.
Camira, Camry

Camarin (Scottish) a form of Cameron.

Camberly (American) a form of Kimberly.
Camber, Camberlee, Camberleigh

Cambria (Latin) from Wales. See also Kambria.
Camberry, Cambrea, Cambree, Cambreia,
Cambriah, Cambrie, Cambrina, Cambry,
Cambrya, Cambryah

Camden BG (Scottish) winding valley.
Camdyn

Camelia, Camellia (Italian) Botany: a
camellia is an evergreen tree or shrub with
fragrant roselike flowers. See also Kamelia.
Camala, Camalia, Camallia, Camela, Cameliah,
Camelita, Camella, Camellita, Camelya,
Camelyah, Camillia, Camilliah, Chamelea,
Chameleah, Chamelia, Chameliah, Chamellia,
Chamelliah, Chamelya, Chamelyah, Chamilia,
Chamylia, Chamyliah

Cameo (Latin) gem or shell on which a
portrait is carved.
Cami, Camio, Camyo, Kameo, Kamio, Kamyo

Camera (American) a form of Cameron.
Cameri, Cameria

Cameron BG (Scottish) crooked nose. See
also Kameron.
Cameran, Camerana, Cameren, Cameria,
Cameriah, Camerie, Camerin, Camerya,
Cameryah, Cameryn, Camira, Camiran,
Camiron

Camesha (American) a form of Camisha.
Cameasha, Cameesha, Cameisha, Camesa,
Cameshaa, Cameshia, Cameshiah,
Camyeshia, Kamesha, Kameshia

Cami, Camie, Cammie, Cammy (French)
short forms of Camille. See also Kami.
Camee, Camey, Camia, Camiah, Cammi,
Cammye, Camy, Camya, Camyah

Camila, Camilla (Italian) forms of Camille.
See also Kamila, Mila.
Camilah, Camilia, Camillah, Camillia,
Camilya, Cammila, Cammilah, Cammilla,
Cammyla, Cammylah, Cammylla,
Cammyllah, Chamika, Chamila, Chamilla,
Chamylla, Chamyllah

Camille GB (French) young ceremonial
attendant. See also Millie.
Cami, Camiel, Camielle, Camil, Camile,
Camill, Cammile, Cammill, Cammille,
Cammillie, Cammilyn, Cammyl, Cammyle,
Cammyll, Cammylle, Chamelee, Chamelei,
Chameley, Chamelie, Chamelle, Chamely,
Chamille, Kamille

Camino, Camiño (Spanish) road.

Camisha (American) a combination of
Cami + Aisha.
Camiesha

Campbell BG (Latin, French) beautiful field.
(Scottish) crooked mouth.
Cambel, Cambell, Camp, Campy, Kampbell

Camri, Camrie, Camry (American) short
forms of Camryn. See also Kamri.
Camrea, Camree, Camrey

Camryn GB (American) a form of
Cameron. See also Kamryn.
Camri, Camrin, Camron, Camrynn

Camylle (French) a form of Camille.
Cammyl, Cammyle, Cammyll, Camyle,
Camyll

Cancia (Spanish) native of Anzio, Italy.

Canciana, Cancianila (Spanish) forms of
Cancia.

Canda (Greek) a form of Candace. (Spanish)
a short form of Chandelaria.

Candace (Greek) glittering white; glowing.
History: the title of the queens of ancient
Ethiopia. See also Dacey, Kandace.
Cace, Canace, Candas, Candece, Candelle,
Candiace, Candyce

Candela, Candelas (Spanish) candle; fire.

Candelaria (Spanish) a form of
Chandelaria.

Candi (American) a familiar form of
Candace, Candice, Candida. See also
Candie, Kandi. (Spanish) a familiar form of
Chandelaria.

Candice, Candis (Greek) forms of Candace.
Candes, Candias, Candies, Candise, Candiss,
Candus

Candida (Latin) bright white.
Candeea, Candi, Candia, Candide, Candita

Cándida (Latin) a form of Candida.

Candie, Candy (American) familiar forms
of Candace, Candice, Candida. See also
Candi, Kandi.
Candea, Candee, Candia, Candiah, Candya,
Candyah

Candra (Latin) glowing. See also Kandra.
Candrah, Candrea, Candria, Candriah,
Candrya, Candryah

Candyce (Greek) a form of Candace.
Candys, Candyse, Cyndyss

Canela (Latin) cinnamon.

Caniad (Welsh) a form of Carmen.

Canita (Hebrew, Latin) a form of Carmen.

Cantara (Arabic) small crossing.
Cantarah

Cantrelle (French) song.
Cantrel, Cantrela, Cantrelah, Cantrele,
Cantrella, Cantrellah, Kantrel, Kantrella,
Kantrelle

Canuta (German) of good origin.

Capitolina (Latin) she who lives with the
gods.

Capri (Italian) a short form of Caprice.
Geography: an island off the west coast of
Italy. See also Kapri.
Capree, Caprey, Capria, Capriah, Caprie,
Capry, Caprya, Capryah

Caprice (Italian) fanciful.
Cappi, Caprece, Caprecia, Capresha, Capricia,
Capriese, Caprina, Capris, Caprise, Caprisha,
Capritta

Cara, Carah (Latin) dear. (Irish) friend. See
also Karah.
Caira, Caragh, Caranda, Carrah

Caralampia (Greek) illuminated by happiness.

Caralee (Irish) a form of Cara.
Caralea, Caraleigh, Caralia, Caralie, Carely

Caralyn (English) a form of Caroline.
Caralan, Caralana, Caralanah, Caralane, Caralin, Caralina, Caralinah, Caraline, Caralynn, Caralynna, Caralynne, Carralean, Carraleana, Carraleanah, Carraleane, Carraleen, Carraleena, Carraleenah, Carraleene, Carralin, Carralina, Carralinah, Carraline, Carralyn, Carralyna, Carralynah, Carralyne

Carelyn (English) a form of Caroline.
Carrelean, Carreleana, Carreleanah, Carreleane, Carreleene, Carrelin, Carrelina, Carrelinah, Carreline, Carrelyn, Carrelyna, Carrelynah, Carrelyne

Carem (Spanish) a form of Karen.

Caren (Welsh) a form of Caron. (Italian) a form of Carina.

Carenza (Irish) a form of Karenza.
Caranza, Caranzah, Caranzia, Caranziah, Carenzah, Carenzia, Carenziah, Carenzya, Carenzyah

Caressa (French) a form of Carissa.
Carass, Carassa, Carassah, Caresa, Carese, Caresse, Charessa, Charesse, Karessa

Carey BG (Welsh) a familiar form of Cara, Caroline, Karen, Katherine. See also Carrie, Kari.
Caree, Carrey

Cari, Carie (Welsh) forms of Carey, Kari.
Caria, Cariah

Caridad, Caridade (Latin) love; affection.

Carilyn (English) a form of Caroline.
Carilean, Carileana, Carileanah, Carileane, Carileen, Carileena, Carileenah, Carileene, Carilene, Carilin, Cariline, Carrileen, Carrileena, Carrileenah, Carrileene, Carrilin, Carrilina, Carrilinah, Carriline

Carina (Italian) dear little one. (Greek) a familiar form of Cora. (Swedish) a form of Karen.
Carana, Caranah, Carena, Carenah, Carinah, Carinna, Carrina, Carrinah, Carryna, Carrynah, Caryna, Carynah

Carine (Italian) a form of Carina.
Carinne, Carrian, Carrine

Carisa, Carrisa, Carrissa (Greek) forms of Carissa.
Caris, Carisah, Carise, Carisha, Carisia, Carysa, Carysah, Charisa

Carisma (Greek) a form of Karisma.
Carismah, Carismara, Carysma, Carysmah, Carysmara

Carissa (Greek) beloved. See also Karisa.
Caressa, Cariss, Carissah, Carisse, Caryssa, Caryssah

Carita (Latin) charitable.
Caritah, Caritta, Carittah, Caryta, Carytah, Carytta, Caryttah, Karita, Karitah, Karitta, Karittah

Caritina (Latin) grace.

Carla (German) farmer. (English) strong. (Latin) a form of Carol, Caroline. See also Karla.
Carila, Carilah, Carilla, Carillah, Carlah, Carleta, Carliqua, Carlique, Carliyle, Carlonda, Carlyjo, Carlyle, Carlysle

Carlee, Carleigh, Carley, Carli, Carlie (English) forms of Carly. See also Karlee, Karley.
Carle, Carlea, Carleah, Carleh, Carlei, Carlia, Carliah

Carleen, Carlene (English) forms of Caroline. See also Karleen.
Carlaen, Carlaena, Carlane, Carlean, Carleana, Carleanah, Carleane, Carleena, Carleenah, Carleene, Carlein, Carleina, Carleine, Carlen, Carlenah, Carlenna, Carleyn, Carleyna, Carleyne, Carline, Carllen, Carlyne

Carlena (English) a form of Caroline.

Carlin BG (Irish) little champion. (Latin) a short form of Caroline.
Carlan, Carlana, Carlandra, Carlinda, Carlindah, Carline, Carllan, Carllin, Carlyn, Carrlin

Carlina (Latin, Irish) a form of Carlin.
Carlinah

Carling (Latin, Irish) a form of Carlin.

Carlisa (American) a form of Carlissa.
Carilis, Carilise, Carilyse, Carletha, Carlethe, Carlis, Carlisah, Carlise, Carlysa, Carlysah, Carlyse

Carlisha (American) a form of Carlissa.
Carleasha, Carleashah, Carleesha, Carleesia, Carleesiah, Carlesia, Carlesiah, Carlicia, Carlisia, Carlisiah

Carlissa (American) a combination of Carla + Lissa.
Carleeza, Carlisa, Carliss, Carlissah, Carlisse, Carlissia, Carlissiah, Carlista, Carlyssa, Carlyssah

Carlita (Italian) a form of Carlotta.
Carlitah

Carlotta (Italian) a form of Charlotte.
Carleta, Carletah, Carlete, Carletta, Carlettah, Carlette, Carlite, Carlot, Carlota, Carlotah, Carlote, Carlott, Carlottah, Carlotte, Carolet, Caroleta, Carolete, Carolett, Caroletta, Carolette

Carly (English) a familiar form of Caroline, Charlotte. See also Karley.
Carli, Carlie, Carlya, Carlyah, Carlye

Carlyle 🅱🅶 (English) Carla's island.
Carlyse, Carlysle

Carlyn, Carlynn (Irish) forms of Carlin.
Carllyn, Carllyna, Carllynah, Carllyne, Carlyna, Carlynah, Carlynne

Carman (Latin) a form of Carmen.

Carme (Galician) a form of Carmela.

Carmel 🅶🅱 (Hebrew) a short form of Carmela.
Carmal, Carmele, Carmelie, Carmell, Carmelle, Carmely, Carmil, Carmile, Carmill, Carmille, Carmyle, Carmylle

Carmela, Carmella (Hebrew) garden; vineyard. Bible: Mount Carmel in Israel is often thought of as paradise. See also Karmel.
Carmala, Carmalah, Carmalina, Carmalinah, Carmaline, Carmalla, Carmarit, Carmelah, Carmeli, Carmelia, Carmeliah, Carmelina, Carmeline, Carmellah, Carmellia, Carmelliah, Carmellina, Carmelya, Carmesa, Carmesha, Carmi, Carmie, Carmiel, Carmila, Carmilla, Carmillia, Carmilliah, Carmillya, Carmillyah, Carmisha, Carmyla, Carmylah, Carmylla, Carmyllia, Carmylliah, Carmyllya, Carmyllyah

Carmelit (Hebrew) a short form of Carmelita.
Carmalit, Carmellit

Carmelita (Hebrew) a form of Carmela.
Carmaletta, Carmalita, Carmelitha, Carmelitia, Carmellita, Carmellitha, Carmellitia, Leeta, Lita

Carmelo (Spanish) a form of Carmela.

Carmen 🅶🅱 (Latin) song. Religion: Nuestra Señora del Carmen—Our Lady of Mount Carmel—is one of the titles of the Virgin Mary. See also Karmen.
Carma, Carmain, Carmaina, Carmaine, Carmana, Carmanah, Carmane, Carmena, Carmencita, Carmene, Carmi, Carmia, Carmita, Carmon, Carmona

Carmina (Latin) a form of Carmine.
Carminah, Carmyna, Carmynah, Karmina, Karminah

Carmiña, Carminda (Spanish) forms of Carmen.

Carmine 🅱🅶 (Latin) song; red.
Carmin, Carmyn, Carmyne, Carmynn, Karmine, Karmyne

Carmo (Portuguese) a form of Carmela.

Carnelian (Latin) clear, reddish stone.
Carnelia, Carneliah, Carnelya, Carnelyah, Carnelyan

Carniela (Greek) a form of Karniela.
Carniela, Carniele, Carniell, Carniella, Carnielle, Carnyel, Carnyela, Carnyella, Carnyelle

Carol (German) farmer. (French) song of joy. (English) strong. See also Charlene, Kalle, Karol.
Caral, Carall, Carel, Carele, Carell, Carelle, Cariel, Caril, Carile, Carill, Caro, Carola, Carolenia, Carolinda, Caroll, Carral, Carrall, Carrel, Carrell, Carrelle, Carril, Carrill, Carrol, Carroll

Carol Ann, Carol Anne, Carolan, Carolane, Carolanne (American) combinations of Carol + Ann. Forms of Caroline.
Carolana, Carolanah, Carolann, Carolanna, Carole-Anne

Carole (English) a form of Carol.
Carolee, Karole, Karrole

Carolina (Italian) a form of Caroline. See also Karolina.
Carilena, Carlena, Caroleana, Caroleanah, Caroleena, Caroleina, Carolena, Carolinah, Carroleena, Carroleenah, Carrolena, Carrolina, Carrolinah

Caroline ✵ (French) little and strong. See also Carla, Carleen, Carlin, Karolina.
Caralyn, Carelyn, Carilyn, Carilynn, Carilynne, Caro, Carolean, Caroleane, Caroleen, Carolin, Carroleen, Carroleene, Carrolene, Carrolin, Carroline

Carolyn, Carolyne, Carolynn (English) forms of Caroline. See also Karolyn.
Carolyna, Carolynah, Carolynne, Carrolyn, Carrolyna, Carrolynah, Carrolyne, Carrolynn, Carrolynna, Carrolynnah, Carrolynne

Caron (Welsh) loving, kindhearted, charitable.
Caaran, Caaren, Caarin, Caaron, Caran, Carane, Carene, Carin, Carinn, Caronne, Carran, Carren, Carrin, Carron, Carrone, Carrun, Carun

Carona (Spanish) a form of Corona.

Carpófora (Greek) one who carries fruits.

Carra (Irish) a form of Cara.
Carrah

Carrie (English) a familiar form of Carol, Caroline. See also Carey, Kari, Karri.
Carree, Carrey, Carri, Carria, Carry, Cary

Carrigan (Irish) a form of Corrigan (see Boys' Names).
Carrigen

Carrington BG (Welsh) rocky town.

Carrola (French) a form of Carol.

Carson BG (English) child of Carr.
Carsen, Carsyn

Carter BG (English) cart driver.

Cary BG (Welsh) a form of Carey.
Carya, Caryah

Caryl (Latin) a form of Carol.
Carryl, Carryle, Carryll, Carrylle, Caryle, Caryll, Carylle

Caryn (Danish) a form of Karen.
Caaryn, Carryn, Carryna, Carrynah, Carryne, Caryna, Carynah, Caryne, Carynn

Carys (Welsh) love.
Caris, Caryse, Caryss, Carysse, Ceris, Cerys

Casandra (Greek) a form of Cassandra.
Casandera, Casandre, Casandrea, Casandrey, Casandri, Casandria, Casandrina, Casandrine, Casanndra

Casey BG (Irish) brave. (Greek) a familiar form of Acacia. See also Kasey.
Cacee, Cacy, Caecey, Caicey, Cascy, Casea, Casee, Casy, Cayse, Caysea, Caysee, Caysey, Caysy

Cashmere (Slavic) a form of Casimir.
Cash, Cashemere, Cashi, Cashmeire

Casi, Casie (Irish) forms of Casey.
Caci, Cacia, Cacie, Casci, Cascie, Casia, Cayci, Caycia, Cayciah, Caysi, Caysia, Caysiah, Caysie, Cazzi

Casiana (Latin) empty; vain.

Casidy, Cassidee, Cassidi, Cassidie (Irish) forms of Cassidy.
Casidee, Casidey, Casidi, Casidia, Casidiah, Casidie

Casiel (Latin) mother of the earth.

Casilda (Arabic) virgin carrier of the lance.

Casimir (Polish) a form of Casimira.

Casimira (Slavic) peacemaker. See also Kasimira.
Casimiera, Casimirah, Casmira, Casmirah, Casmyra, Casmyrah, Cazmira, Cazmirah, Cazmyra, Cazmyrah

Cass BG (Greek) a short form of Cassandra.
Cas, Cassa, Kas, Kass

Cassady (Irish) a form of Cassidy.
Casadea, Casadee, Casadey, Casadi, Casadia, Casadiah, Casadie, Casady, Cassaday, Cassadea, Cassadee, Cassadey, Cassadi, Cassadia, Cassadiah, Cassadie, Cassadina

Cassandra (Greek) helper of men. Mythology: a prophetess of ancient Greece whose prophesies were not believed. See also Kasandra, Krisandra, Sandra, Sandy, Zandra.
Cassander, Cassandera, Cassandri, Cassandry, Chrisandra, Chrisandrah, Crisandra, Crisandrah, Crysandra, Crysandrah

Cassandre (Greek) a form of Cassandra.

Cassaundra (Greek) a form of Cassandra.
Casaundra, Casaundre, Casaundri, Casaundria, Cassaundre, Cassaundri, Cassundra, Cassundre, Cassundri, Cassundria, Cassundrina, Cazzandra, Cazzandre, Cazzandria

Cassey, Cassi, Cassy (Greek) familiar forms of Cassandra, Catherine. See also Kassi.
Casse, Cassee, Cassii, Cassye

Cassia (Greek) a cinnamon-like spice. See also Kasia.
Casia, Casiah, Cass, Cassiah, Cassya, Cassyah, Casya, Cazia, Caziah, Cazya, Cazyah, Cazzia, Cazziah, Cazzya, Cazzyah

Cassidy GB (Irish) clever. See also Kassidy.
Casseday, Cassiddy, Cassidey, Cassidia, Cassity, Cassydi, Cassydie, Cassydy, Casydi, Casydie, Casydy, Cazidy, Cazzidy

Cassie GB (Greek) a familiar form of Cassandra, Catherine.

Cassiopeia (Greek) clever. Mythology: the wife of the Ethiopian king Cepheus; the mother of Andromeda.
Cassio

Cassondra (Greek) a form of Cassandra.
Casondra, Casondre, Casondria, Casondriah, Cassondre, Cassondri, Cassondria, Cazzondra, Cazzondre, Cazzondria

Casta (Greek) pure.

Castalia (Greek) fountain of purity.

Castel (Spanish) to the castle.

Castora (Spanish) brilliant.

Cástula (Greek) a form of Casta.

Catalín (Spanish) a form of Caitlin.

Catalina (Spanish) a form of Catherine. See also Katalina.
Cataleen, Catalena, Catalene, Catalin, Catalinah, Cataline, Catalyn, Catalyna, Catana, Catania, Catanya, Cateline, Catelini

Catalonia (Spanish) a region of Spain.

Catarina (German) a form of Catherine.
Catarena, Catarin, Catarine, Cattarina, Cattarinah, Cattarine

Catelin, Catelyn, Catelynn (Irish) forms of Caitlin.
Cateline, Catelyne

Caterina (German) a form of Catherine.
Catereana, Catereanah, Catereane, Catereena, Catereenah, Catereene, Caterin, Caterinah, Caterine, Cateryna, Caterynah, Cateryne

Catharine (Greek) a form of Catherine.
Catharen, Catharin, Catharina, Catharinah, Catharyn

Catherine GB (Greek) pure. (English) a form of Katherine.
Cairena, Cairene, Cairina, Caitrin, Cat, Cate, Cathann, Cathanne, Cathenne, Catheren, Catherene, Catheria, Catherin, Catherina, Catherinah, Catlaina, Catreeka, Catrelle, Catrice, Catricia, Catrika

Catheryn (Greek, English) a form of Catherine.
Catheryne

Cathi (Greek) a form of Cathy.
Cathie

Cathleen (Irish) a form of Catherine. See also Caitlin, Kathleen.
Caithlyn, Cathalean, Cathaleana, Cathaleanah, Cathaleane, Cathaleen, Cathaleena, Cathaleenah, Cathaleene, Cathalen, Cathalena, Cathalenah, Cathalene, Cathalin, Cathalina, Cathalinah, Cathaline, Cathalyn, Cathalyna, Cathalynah, Cathalyne, Catheleen, Catheleena, Catheleenah, Catheleene, Cathelen, Cathelena, Cathelenah, Cathelene, Cathelin, Cathelina, Cathelinah, Catheline, Cathelyn, Cathelyna, Cathelynah, Cathelyne, Cathlean, Cathleana, Cathleanah, Cathleane, Cathleena, Cathleenah, Cathleene, Cathlein, Cathleina, Cathleinah, Cathleine, Cathlen, Cathlena, Cathlenah, Cathlene, Cathleyn, Cathlin, Cathlina, Cathlinah,

Cathline, Cathlyn, Cathlyna, Cathlynah, Cathlyne, Cathlynn

Cathrine, Cathryn (Greek) forms of Catherine.
Cathrina, Cathrinah, Cathryna, Cathrynah, Cathryne, Cathrynn, Catryn

Cathy (Greek) a familiar form of Catherine, Cathleen. See also Kathi.
Catha, Cathe, Cathea, Cathee, Cathey

Catia (Russian) a form of Katia.
Cattiah

Catie (English) a form of Katie.

Catina (English) a form of Katina.
Cateana, Cateanah, Cateena, Cateenah, Cateina, Cateinah, Cateyna, Cateynah, Catinah, Catine, Catyn, Catyna, Catynah, Catyne

Catlin GB (Irish) a form of Caitlin.
Catlee, Catleen, Catleene, Catlina, Catline, Catlyn, Catlyna, Catlyne, Catlynn, Catlynne

Catriel (Hebrew) a form of Katriel.
Catriela, Catrielah, Catriele, Catriell, Catriella, Catriellah, Catrielle

Catrina (Slavic) a form of Catherine, Katrina.
Caetreana, Caetreanah, Caetreena, Caetreenah, Caetreina, Caetreinah, Caetreyna, Caetreynah, Caetrina, Caetrinah, Caetryna, Caetrynah, Caitreana, Caitreanah, Caitreena, Caitreenah, Caitreina, Caitreinah, Caitreyna, Caitreynah, Caitriana, Caitrina, Caitrinah, Caitriona, Caitryna, Caitrynah, Catreana, Catreanah, Catreane, Catreen, Catreena, Catreenah, Catreene, Catren, Catrena, Catrenah, Catrene, Catrenia, Catrin, Catrinah, Catrine, Catrinia, Catryn, Catryna, Catrynah, Catryne, Catrynia, Catrynya, Catya, Catyah, Caytreana, Caytreanah, Caytreena, Caytreenah, Caytreina, Caytreinah, Caytreyna, Caytreynah, Caytrina, Caytrinah, Caytryna, Caytrynah

Catriona (Slavic) a form of Catherine, Katrina.
Catrionah, Catrione, Catroina

Cayce (Greek, Irish) a form of Casey.
Caycea, Caycee, Caycey, Caycy

Cayetana (Spanish) native of the city of Gaeta, Italy.

Cayfutray (Mapuche) celestial waterfall from heaven.

Cayla, Caylah (Hebrew) forms of Kayla.
Caylan, Caylana, Caylanah, Caylea, Cayleah, Caylia, Cayliah

Caylee, Cayleigh, Cayley, Cayli, Caylie (American) forms of Kaylee, Kelly.
Cayle, Caylea, Cayleah, Caylei, Caylia, Cayly

Caylen, Caylin (American) forms of Caitlin.
Caylean, Cayleana, Cayleanah, Cayleane, Cayleen, Cayleena, Cayleenah, Cayleene, Caylena, Caylenah, Caylene, Caylina, Cayline, Caylyn, Caylyna, Caylyne, Caylynne

Ceaira (Irish) a form of Ciara.
Ceairah, Ceairra

Ceanna (Italian) a form of Ciana.

Ceara, Cearra (Irish) forms of Ciara.
Cearaa, Cearah, Cearie, Seara, Searah

Cecelia (Latin) a form of Cecilia. See also Sheila.
Cacelea, Caceleah, Cacelia, Cece, Ceceilia, Cecelyn, Cecette, Cescelia, Cescelie

Cecile (Latin) a form of Cecilia.
Cecilla, Cecille

Cecilia (Latin) blind. See also Cicely, Cissy, Secilia, Selia, Sissy.
Cacilia, Caciliah, Caecilia, Caeciliah, Cecil, Cecila, Cecilea, Ceciliah, Cecilija, Cecillia, Cecilya, Ceclia, Cecylia, Cecyliah, Cecylja, Cecylya, Cecylyah, Cee, Ceil, Ceila, Ceilagh, Ceileh, Ceileigh, Ceilena

Cecília (Portuguese) a form of Cecilia.

Cecily (Latin) a form of Cecilia.
Cacelee, Cacelei, Caceleigh, Caceley, Caceli, Cacilie, Caecilie, Ceceli, Cecelie, Cecely, Cecilee, Ceciley, Cecilie, Cescily, Cilley

Cedar BG (Latin) a kind of evergreen conifer.

Cedrica (English) battle chieftain.
Cadryca, Cadrycah, Cedricah

Ceferina (German) caresses like a soft wind.

Ceil (Latin) a short form of Cecilia.
Ceel, Ciel

Ceilidh (Irish) country dance.

Ceira, Ceirra (Irish) forms of Ciara.
Ceire

Celandine (Latin) an herb with yellow
flowers. (Greek) swallow.
*Celandina, Celandinah, Celandrina,
Celandrinah, Celandrine, Celandryna,
Celandrynah, Celandryne*

Celedonia (German) a form of Celidonia.

Celena (Greek) a form of Selena.
*Caleena, Calena, Celeana, Celeanah,
Celeena, Celeenah, Celenia, Cena*

Celene (Greek) a form of Celena.
*Celean, Celeane, Celeen, Celeene, Celyne,
Cylyne*

Celerina (Spanish) quick.

Celesta (Latin) a form of Celeste.
Celestah

Celeste (Latin) celestial, heavenly.
*Cele, Celeeste, Celense, Celes, Celesia,
Celesley, Celest, Celestar, Celestelle, Celestia,
Celestial, Cellest, Celleste, Seleste*

Celestina (Latin) a form of Celeste.
*Celesteana, Celesteanah, Celesteena,
Celesteenah, Celestinah, Celestinia, Celestyna,
Celestynah, Celestyne, Selestina*

Celestine GB (Latin) a form of Celeste.
*Celesteane, Celesteen, Celesteene, Celestin,
Celestyn*

Celia (Latin) a short form of Cecilia.
*Ceilia, Celea, Celeah, Celee, Celei, Celeigh,
Celey, Celi, Celiah, Celie, Cellia, Celliah,
Cellya, Cellyah, Cely*

Célia (Portuguese) a form of Celia.

Celidonia (Greek) celandine herb.

Celina (Greek) a form of Celena. See also
Selina.
*Calina, Celeana, Celeanah, Celeena,
Celeenah, Celinah, Celinda, Celinia,
Celiniah, Celinka, Celinna, Celka, Cellina,
Celyna, Celynah, Cilina, Cilinah, Cillina,
Cillinah, Cylina, Cylinah*

Celine (Greek) a form of Celena.
*Caline, Celeane, Celeene, Celin, Céline,
Cellinn, Celyn, Celyne, Ciline, Cilline*

Celmira (Arabic) brilliant one.

Celosia (Greek) dry; burning.
*Celosiah, Celosya, Celosyah, Selosia, Selosiah,
Selosya, Selosyah*

Celsa (Latin) very spiritual.

Celsey (Scandinavian, Scottish, English) a
form of Kelsey.

Cemelia (Punic) she has God present.

Cenobia (Greek) stranger.

Centehua (Nahuatl) only one.

Centola (Arabic) light of knowledge.

Cera (French) a short form of Cerise.
Cerea, Ceri, Ceria, Cerra

Cercira (Greek) Geography: native of Syrtis,
an ancient name for the gulf of the
Mediterranean Sea.

Cerella (Latin) springtime.
*Cerela, Cerelah, Cerelia, Cereliah, Cerelisa,
Cerellah, Cerelle, Cerelya, Cerelyah, Serelia,
Sereliah, Serella Serelya, Serelyah*

Ceres (Latin) Mythology: the Roman goddess of agriculture. Astronomy: the first
asteroid discovered to have an orbit
between Mars and Saturn.
Cerese, Ceress, Ceressa

Ceridwen (Welsh) poetic goddess.

Cerise (French) cherry; cherry red.
*Carisce, Carise, Carisse, Caryce, Caryse,
Cerice, Cericia, Cerissa, Cerria, Cerrice,
Cerrina, Cerrita, Cerryce, Ceryce, Ceryse,
Sherise, Sheriss, Sherisse*

Cesara, Cesaria, Cesira, Cesírea (Latin)
forms of Cesare.

Cesare (Latin) long-haired. History: Roman
emperors were given the title *Caesar*.

Cesarina (Latin) a form of Cesare.

Cesilia (Latin) a form of Cecilia.
Cesia, Cesya

Chabela (Hebrew) a form of Isabel.

Chabeli (French) a form of Chablis.
Chabelly, Chabely

Chablis (French) a dry white wine.
Geography: a region in France where wine
grapes are grown.
*Chablea, Chableah, Chablee, Chabley, Chabli,
Chablia, Chablie, Chabliss, Chably, Chablys,
Chablyss*

Chadee (French) from Chad, a country in
north-central Africa. See also Sade.
*Chadae, Chadai, Chaday, Chaddae, Chaddai,
Chadday, Chade, Chadea, Chadey, Chadi,
Chadia, Chadiah, Chadie, Chady*

Chahna (Hindi, Indian) love; light, illumina-
tion.

Chai (Hebrew) life.
*Chae, Chaela, Chaeli, Chaelia, Chaella,
Chaelle, Chaena, Chaia, Chay*

Chaka (Sanskrit) a form of Chakra. See also
Shaka.
*Chakai, Chakia, Chakiah, Chakka,
Chakkah, Chakya, Chakyah*

Chakra (Sanskrit) circle of energy.
*Chakara, Chakaria, Chakena, Chakina,
Chakira, Chakrah, Chakria, Chakriya,
Chakyra, Chakyrah, Shakra, Shakrah*

Chalchiuitl (Nahuatl) emerald.

Chalice (French) goblet.
*Chalace, Chalcia, Chalcie, Chalece, Chalicea,
Chalie, Chaliece, Chaliese, Chalis, Chalisa,
Chalise, Chalisk, Chalissa, Chalisse, Challa,
Challis, Challisa, Challise, Challiss, Challissa,
Challisse, Challyce, Challysa, Challyse,
Challysse, Chalsey, Chalyce, Chalyn, Chalyse,
Chalyssa, Chalysse*

Chalina (Spanish) a form of Rose. See also
Shalena.
*Chalin, Chalinah, Chaline, Chalini,
Challain, Challaina, Challaine, Chalyn,
Chalyna, Chalynah, Chalyne*

Chalonna (American) a combination of the
prefix Cha + Lona.
*Chalon, Chalona, Chalonah, Chalonda,
Chalone, Chalonee, Chalonn, Chalonnah,
Chalonne, Chalonnee, Chalonte, Shalon*

Chambray (French) a lightweight fabric.
Chambrae, Chambrai, Chambre, Chambree,

*Chambrée, Chambrey, Chambria, Chambrie,
Chambry, Shambrae, Shambrai, Shambre,
Shambree, Shambrée, Shambrey, Shambria,
Shambrie, Shambry*

Chamique (American) a form of Shamika.

Champagne (French) a province in eastern
France; a wine made in this province.

Chan BG (Cambodian) sweet-smelling tree.

Chana (Hebrew) a form of Hannah.
*Chanae, Chanah, Chanai, Chanay, Chanea,
Chanie, Channa, Channah*

Chance BG (English) a short form of
Chancey.

Chancey BG (English) chancellor; church
official.
Chancee, Chancie, Chancy

Chanda (Sanskrit) short tempered.
Religion: the demon defeated by the
Hindu goddess Chamunda. See also
Shanda.
*Chandah, Chandea, Chandee, Chandey,
Chandi, Chandia, Chandiah, Chandie,
Chandin, Chandy, Chandya*

Chandani (Hindi) moonlight.
*Chandanee, Chandaney, Chandania,
Chandaniah, Chandany, Chandanya,
Chandanyah*

Chandelaria (Spanish) candle.
*Candeleria, Candeleva, Candelona,
Candeloria, Canduluria, Kandelaria*

Chandelle (French) candle.
*Chandal, Chandala, Chandalah, Chandale,
Chandel, Chandela, Chandelah, Chandele,
Chandell, Chandella, Chandellah, Shandal,
Shandel, Shandela, Shandelah, Shandele,
Shandell, Shandella, Shandellah, Shandelle*

Chandi (Indian) moonlight. (Sanskrit) a
form of Chanda.

Chandler BG (Hindi) moon. (Old English)
candlemaker.
Chandlar, Chandlier, Chandlor, Chandlyr

Chandra (Sanskrit) moon. Religion: the
Hindu god of the moon. See also Shandra.
*Chandrae, Chandrah, Chandray, Chandre,
Chandrea, Chandrelle, Chandria, Chandrya*

Chanel, Channel (English) channel. See also Shanel.
Chanal, Chanall, Chanalla, Chanalle, Chaneel, Chaneil, Chanele, Channal

Chanell, Chanelle, Channelle (English) forms of Chanel.
Chanella, Channell, Shanell

Chaney BG (French) oak.
Chaynee, Cheaney, Cheney, Cheyne, Cheyney

Chanice, Chanise (American) forms of Shanice.
Chanisse, Chenice, Chenise

Channa (Hindi) chickpea.
Channah

Channing BG (English) wise. (French) canon; church official.
Chane, Chanin, Chaning, Chann, Channin, Channyn, Chanyn

Chantal, Chantale, Chantalle (French) song.
Chandal, Chantaal, Chantael, Chantala, Chantalah, Chantall, Chantasia, Chanteau, Chantle, Chantoya, Chantrill

Chantara (American) a form of Chantal.
Chantarah, Chantarai, Chantarra, Chantarrah, Chantarria, Chantarriah, Chantarrya, Chantarryah

Chante BG (French) a short form of Chantal.
Chanta, Chantae, Chantai, Chantay, Chantaye, Chantéa, Chantee, Chanti, Chaunte, Chauntea, Chauntéa, Chauntee

Chanté (French) a short form of Chantal.

Chantel, Chantele, Chantell, Chantelle (French) forms of Chantal. See also Shantel.
Chanteese, Chantela, Chantelah, Chantella, Chantellah, Chanter, Chantey, Chantez, Chantrel, Chantrell, Chantrelle, Chatell, Chontel, Chontela, Chontelah, Chontele, Chontell, Chontella, Chontellah, Chontelle

Chantia (French) a form of Chante.

Chantile (French) a form of Chantal.
Chantil, Chantila, Chantile, Chantill, Chantilla, Chantille, Chantril, Chantrill, Chantrille

Chantilly (French) fine lace. See also Shantille.
Chantiel, Chantielle, Chantil, Chantila, Chantilea, Chantileah, Chantilée, Chantilei, Chantileigh, Chantiley, Chantili, Chantilia, Chantilie, Chantill, Chantilla, Chantille, Chantillea, Chantilleah, Chantillee, Chantillei, Chantilleigh, Chantilley, Chantilli, Chantillia, Chantillie, Chantily, Chantyly

Chantrea (Cambodian) moon; moonbeam.
Chantra, Chantrey, Chantri, Chantria

Chantrice (French) singer. See also Shantrice.
Chantreese, Chantress

Chardae, Charde (Punjabi) charitable. (French) short forms of Chardonnay. See also Shardae.
Charda, Chardai, Charday, Chardea, Chardee, Chardée, Chardese, Chardey, Chardie

Chardonnay (French) a dry white wine.
Char, Chardnay, Chardney, Chardon, Chardona, Chardonae, Chardonai, Chardonay, Chardonaye, Chardonee, Chardonna, Chardonnae, Chardonnai, Chardonnee, Chardonnée, Chardonney, Shardonae, Shardonai, Shardonay, Shardonaye, Shardonnay

Charice (Greek) a form of Charis.

Charis (Greek) grace; kindness.
Charece, Chareece, Chareeze, Charese, Chari, Charie, Charise, Charish, Chariss, Charris, Charriss, Charrys, Charryss, Charys, Charyse, Charyss, Charysse

Charisma (Greek) the gift of leadership.

Charissa (Greek) a form of Charity.
Charesa, Charessa, Charisa, Charisah, Charisha, Chariss, Charissah, Charista, Charrisa, Charrisah, Charrissa, Charrissah, Charrysa, Charrysah, Charryssa, Charryssah, Charysa, Charysah, Charyssa, Charyssah

Charisse (Greek) a form of Charity.
Charese, Charesse, Charise, Charissee, Charrise, Charrisse, Charryse, Charrysse, Charysse

Charity (Latin) charity, kindness.
Chariety, Charista, Charita, Charitah, Charitas, Charitea, Charitee, Charitey,

Chariti, Charitia, Charitiah, Charitie,
Charitina, Charitine, Charityna, Charityne,
Charytey, Charytia, Charytiah, Charyty,
Charytya, Charytyah, Sharity

Charla (French, English) a short form of
Charlene, Charlotte.
Chalah, Char, Charlae, Charlai, Charlea

Charlaine (English) a form of Charlene.
Charlaina, Charlane, Charlanna, Charlayna,
Charlayne, Charlein, Charleina, Charleine,
Charleyn, Charleyna, Charleyne

Charlee, Charleigh, Charli (German,
English) forms of Charlie.
Charle, Charlea, Charleah, Charlei, Charlya

Charleen, Charline (English) forms of
Charlene.
Charleena, Charleene, Charlin, Charlina

Charlene (English) a form of Caroline. See
also Carol, Karla, Sharlene.
Charlaine, Charlean, Charleana, Charleane,
Charleesa, Charlein, Charleina, Charleine,
Charlena, Charlenae, Charlenah, Charlesena,
Charlyn, Charlyna, Charlyne, Charlynn,
Charlynne, Charlzina, Charoline

Charley BG (German, English) a form of
Charlie.

Charlie BG (German, English) strong.
Charlia, Charliah, Charyl, Chatty, Sharli,
Sharlie

Charlisa (French) a form of Charlotte.

Charlotte (French) a form of Caroline.
Literature: Charlotte Brontë was a British
novelist and poet best known for her novel
Jane Eyre. See also Karlotte, Lotte, Sharlotte,
Tottie.
Chara, Charil, Charl, Charlet, Charleta,
Charletah, Charlete, Charlett, Charletta,
Charlettah, Charlette, Charlita, Charlot,
Charlota, Charlotah, Charlote, Charlott,
Charlotta, Charlottah, Charlottie, Charlotty,
Charolet, Charolette, Charolot, Charolotte

Charly BG (German, English) a form of
Charlie.

Charmaine (French) a form of Carmen. See
also Karmaine, Sharmaine.
Charamy, Charma, Charmae, Charmagne,
Charmaigne, Charmain, Charmaina,

Charmainah, Charmalique, Charmar,
Charmara, Charmayane, Charmayn,
Charmayna, Charmaynah, Charmayne,
Charmeen, Charmeine, Charmene, Charmese,
Charmian, Charmin, Charmine, Charmion,
Charmisa, Charmon, Charmyn, Charmyne,
Charmynne

Charmane (French) a form of Charmaine.
Charman

Charnette (American) a combination of
Charo + Annette.
Charnetta, Charnita

Charnika (American) a combination of
Charo + Nika.
Charneka, Charniqua, Charnique

Charo (Spanish) a familiar form of Rosa.
Charoe, Charow

Charyanna (American) a combination of
Charo + Anna.
Charian, Charyian, Cheryn

Chase BG (French) hunter.
Chace, Chaise, Chasen, Chason, Chass,
Chasse, Chastan, Chasten, Chastin,
Chastinn, Chaston, Chasyn, Chayse

Chasidy, Chassidy (Latin) forms of
Chastity.
Chasa Dee, Chasadie, Chasady, Chasidee,
Chasidey, Chasidie, Chassedi, Chassidi,
Chasydi

Chasity (Latin) a form of Chastity.
Chasiti, Chasitie, Chasitty, Chassey, Chassie,
Chassiti, Chassity, Chassy

Chastity (Latin) pure.
Chasta, Chastady, Chastidy, Chastitea,
Chastitee, Chastitey, Chastiti, Chastitie,
Chastney, Chasty

Chauntel (French) a form of Chantal.
Chaunta, Chauntae, Chauntay, Chaunte,
Chauntell, Chauntelle, Chawntel, Chawntell,
Chawntelle, Chontelle

Chava (Hebrew) life. (Yiddish) bird.
Religion: the original name of Eve.
Chabah, Chavae, Chavah, Chavala,
Chavalah, Chavarra, Chavarria, Chave,
Chavé, Chavetta, Chavette, Chaviva, Chavvis,
Hava, Kaÿa

Chavella (Spanish) a form of Isabel.
Chavel, Chavela, Chavelah, Chavele, Chaveli, Chavelia, Chavelie, Chavell, Chavellah, Chavelle, Chavely

Chavi (Gypsy) girl.
Chavali, Chavee, Chavey, Chavia, Chaviah, Chavie, Chavy, Chavya, Chavyah

Chavon (Hebrew) a form of Jane.
Chavaughn, Chavaughna, Chavaughne, Chavawn, Chavawna, Chavawnah, Chavawne, Chavona, Chavonah, Chavonda, Chavondah, Chavondria, Chavondriah, Chavone, Chavonn, Chevaughn, Chevaughna, Chevaughne, Chevawn, Chevawna, Chevawnah, Chevawne, Chevon, Chevona, Chevonn, Shavon

Chavonne (Hebrew) a form of Chavon. (American) a combination of the prefix Cha + Yvonne.
Chavondria, Chavonna, Chavonnah, Chevonna, Chevonnah, Chevonne

Chaya (Hebrew) life; living.
Chaia, Chaiah, Chaike, Chaye, Chayka, Chayra

Chayla (English) a form of Chaylea.
Chaylah

Chaylea (English) a combination of Chaya + Lea.
Chailea, Chaileah, Chailee, Chailei, Chaileigh, Chailey, Chaili, Chailia, Chailiah, Chailie, Chaily, Chayleah, Chaylee, Chayleena, Chayleene, Chaylei, Chayleigh, Chaylena, Chaylene, Chayley, Chayli, Chaylie, Chayly

Chela, Chelo (Spanish) forms of Consuelo.

Chelby (English) a form of Shelby.

Chelci, Chelcie, Chelsee, Chelsey, Chelsi, Chelsie, Chelsy (English) forms of Chelsea.
Chelcia, Chelciah, Chellsie, Chelssey, Chelssie, Chelssy, Chelsye

Chelley (English) a form of Shelley.
Chellea, Chelleah, Chellee, Chellei, Chelleigh, Chelli, Chellie, Chelly

Chelsa (English) a form of Chelsea.
Chelsae, Chelsah

Chelse (English) a form of Chelsea.
Chelce

Chelsea (English) seaport. See also Kelsey, Shelsea.
Chelcea, Chelcee, Chelcey, Chelcy, Chelese, Chelesia, Chelli, Chellie, Chellise, Chelsay, Chelseah, Chelsei, Chelseigh, Chesea, Cheslee, Chesley, Cheslie, Chessea, Chessie

Chelsia (English) a form of Chelsea.

Chemarin (Hebrew) girl in black.
Chemarina, Chemarine, Chemaryn, Chemaryna, Chemaryne

Chenelle (English) a form of Chanel.
Chenel, Chenell

Chenetta (French) oak tree.
Chenet, Cheneta, Chenetah, Chenete, Chenett, Chenettah, Chenette

Chenoa (Native American) white dove.
Chenee, Chenika, Chenita, Chenna, Chenoah

Chepa (Hebrew) chaste.

Cher (French) beloved, dearest. (English) a short form of Cherilyn.
Chere, Sher, Shere, Sherr

Cherelle, Cherrell, Cherrelle (French) forms of Cheryl. See also Sherelle.
Charel, Charela, Charelah, Charele, Charell, Charella, Charellah, Charelle, Cherel, Cherell, Cherella, Cherille, Cherrel, Cherrela, Cherrila, Cherrile

Cherese (Greek) a form of Cherish.
Chereese, Cheresa, Cheresse

Cheri, Cherie, Cherri (French) familiar forms of Cher.
Cheree, Chérie, Cheriee, Cherree, Cherrie

Cherice, Cherise, Cherisse (French) forms of Cherish. See also Sharice, Sherice.
Cherece, Chereece, Chereese, Cheriss, Cherissa, Cherrise, Cherys, Cherysa, Cherysah, Cheryse

Cherilyn (English) a combination of Cheryl + Lynn. See also Sherylyn.
Cheralyn, Chereen, Chereena, Cherilin, Cherilina, Cherilinah, Cheriline, Cherilyna, Cherilynah, Cherilyne, Cherilynn, Cherlyn, Cherlynn, Cherralyn, Cherrilyn, Cherrylyn, Cheryl-Lyn, Cheryl-Lynn, Cheryl-Lynne,

Cherylene, Cherylin, Cheryline, Cherylyn, Cherylynn, Cherylynne

Cherish (English) dearly held, precious.
Charish, Charisha, Charishe, Charysha, Charyshah, Cheerish, Cheerisha, Cherisha, Cherishah, Cherishe, Cherrish, Cherrisha, Cherrishe, Cherysh, Cherysha, Cheryshe, Sherish

Cherita (Latin) a form of Charity.
Chereata, Chereatah, Chereeta, Chereetah, Cherida, Cherita, Cheritah, Cherrita, Cheryta, Cherytah

Cherokee GB (Native American) a tribal name.
Cherika, Cherikia, Cherkita, Cherokei, Cherokey, Cheroki, Cherokia, Cherokie, Cheroky, Cherrokee, Sherokee

Cherry (Latin) a familiar form of Charity. (French) cherry; cherry red.
Chere, Cherea, Cheree, Cherey, Cherr, Cherrea, Cherree, Cherrey, Cherreye, Cherri, Cherriann, Cherrianna, Cherrianne, Cherrie, Cherry-Ann, Cherry-Anne, Cherrye, Chery, Cherye

Cheryl (French) beloved. See also Sheryl.
Charil, Charyl, Cheral, Cheril, Cherila, Cherrelle, Cherril, Cheryl-Ann, Cheryl-Anne, Cheryl-Lee, Cheryle, Cherylee, Cheryll, Cherylle

Chesarey (American) a form of Desiree.
Chesarae

Chesna (Slavic) peaceful.
Chesnah, Chessna, Chessnah, Chezna, Cheznah, Cheznia, Chezniah, Cheznya, Cheznyah

Chesney (Slavic) a form of Chesna.
Chesnee, Chesnie, Chesny

Chessa (American) a short form of Chesarey.
Chessi, Chessie, Chessy

Chevelle (Spanish) a form of Chavella.
Chevie

Cheyann, Cheyanne (Cheyenne) forms of Cheyenne.
Cheian, Cheiann, Cheianne, Cheyan, Cheyane, Cheyeanne

Cheyanna (Cheyenne) a form of Cheyenne.
Cheyana

Cheyene (Cheyenne) a form of Cheyenne.

Cheyenna (Cheyenne) a form of Cheyenne.
Cheyeana, Cheyeanna, Cheyena

Cheyenne GB (Cheyenne) a tribal name. See also Shaianne, Sheyanne, Shian, Shyan.
Cheyeene, Cheyenn, Chi-Anna, Chianne, Chie, Chyanne

Cheyla (American) a form of Sheila.
Cheylan, Cheyleigh, Cheylo

Cheyna (American) a short form of Cheyenne.
Chey, Cheye, Cheyne, Cheynee, Cheyney, Cheynna

Chi BG (Cheyenne) a short form of Cheyenne.

Chiara (Italian) a form of Clara.
Cheara, Chiarra, Chyara

Chicahua (Nahuatl) strong.

Chika (Japanese) near and dear.
Chikah, Chikaka, Chikako, Chikara, Chikona, Chyka, Chykah

Chiku (Swahili) chatterer.

Chila (Greek) a form of Cecilia.

Chilali (Native American) snowbird.
Chilalea, Chilaleah, Chilalee, Chilalei, Chilaleigh, Chilalie, Chilaly

China (Chinese) fine porcelain. Geography: a country in eastern Asia. See also Ciana, Shina.
Chinaetta, Chinah, Chinasa, Chinda, Chine, Chinea, Chinesia, Chinita, Chinna, Chinwa, Chynna

Chinira (Swahili) God receives.
Chinara, Chinarah, Chinirah, Chynira, Chynirah

Chinue (Ibo) God's own blessing.

Chione (Egyptian) daughter of the Nile.

Chipahua (Nahuatl) clean.

Chiquita (Spanish) little one. See also Shiquita.
Chaqueta, Chaquita, Chica, Chickie, Chicky, Chikata, Chikita, Chiqueta, Chiquila, Chiquite, Chiquitha, Chiquithe, Chiquitia, Chiquitta

Chiyo (Japanese) eternal.
Chiya

Chloe ⚝ (Greek) blooming, verdant.
Mythology: another name for Demeter, the
goddess of agriculture. See also Kloe.
*Chloé, Chlöe, Chloea, Chloee, Chloey, Chloie,
Cloe*

Chloris (Greek) pale. Mythology: the only
daughter of Niobe to escape the vengeful
arrows of Apollo and Artemis. See also
Kloris, Loris.
*Chlorise, Chlorys, Chloryse, Cloris, Clorise,
Clorys, Cloryse*

Chlorissa (Greek) a form of Chloris.
Chlorisa, Chlorysa, Clorisa, Clorysa

Cho (Korean) beautiful.
Choe

Cholena (Native American) bird.
*Choleana, Choleanah, Choleane, Choleena,
Choleenah, Choleene, Choleina, Choleinah,
Choleine, Cholenah, Cholene, Choleyna,
Choleynah, Choleyne, Cholina, Cholinah,
Choline, Cholyna, Cholynah, Cholyne*

Chriki (Swahili) blessing.

Chris BG (Greek) a short form of
Christopher, Christina. See also Kris.
Chrys, Cris

Chrissa (Greek) a short form of Christina.
See also Khrissa.
*Chrisea, Chrissea, Chrysa, Chryssa, Crissa,
Cryssa*

Chrissanth (Greek) gold flower. Botany:
chrysanthemums are ornamental, showy
flowers.
*Chrisanth, Chrisantha, Chrisanthia, Chrisanthiah,
Chrisanthya, Chrisanthyah, Chrysantha,
Chrysanthe, Chrysanthia, Chrysanthiah,
Chryzanta, Chryzante, Chryzanthia,
Chryzanthiah, Chryzanthya, Chryzanthyah*

Chrissie, Chrissy (English) familiar forms of
Christina.
*Chrisee, Chrisi, Chrisie, Chrissee, Chrissey,
Chrissi, Chrisy, Chryssi, Chryssie, Chryssy,
Chrysy, Crissie, Khrissy*

Christa (German) a short form of Christina.
History: Christa McAuliffe, an American
school teacher, was the first civilian on a
U.S. space flight. See also Krista.
Christah, Christar, Christara, Crysta

Christabel (Latin, French) beautiful
Christian. See also Kristabel.
*Christabeel, Christabela, Christabelah,
Christabele, Christabell, Christabella,
Christabellah, Christabelle, Christable,
Christobel, Christobell, Christobella,
Christobelle, Chrystabel, Chrystabela,
Chrystabelah, Chrystabele, Chrystabell,
Chrystabella, Chrystabellah, Chrystabelle,
Chrystobel, Chrystobela, Chrystobelah,
Chrystobele, Chrystobell, Chrystobella,
Chrystobellah, Chrystobelle, Cristabel,
Cristabela, Cristabelah, Cristabele, Cristabell,
Cristabella, Cristabellah, Cristabelle*

Christain BG (Greek) a form of Christina.
*Christaina, Christainah, Christaine,
Christane, Christayn, Christayna,
Christaynah, Christayne*

Christal (Latin) a form of Crystal. (Scottish)
a form of Christina.
*Christalene, Christalin, Christalina,
Christaline, Christall, Christalle, Christalyn,
Christle, Chrystal*

Christan BG (Greek) a short form of
Christina. See also Kristen.
*Christana, Christanah, Christann,
Christanna, Christyne, Chrystan, Chrysten,
Chrystin, Chryston, Chrystyn*

Christel, Christelle, Chrystel (French)
forms of Christal.
Christele, Christell, Chrystelle

Christen, Christin GB (Greek) short forms
of Christina.

Christena (Greek) a form of Christina.
*Christeina, Christeinah, Christeinna,
Christeinnah*

Christene (Greek) a form of Christina.
Christein, Christeine, Christeinn, Christeinne

Christi, Christie (Greek) short forms of
Christina, Christine. See also Christy,
Cristi, Kristi, Kristy.
Christee, Christia, Chrystee, Chrysti, Chrystie

Christian BG (Greek) a form of Christina.
See also Kristian, Krystian.
Christi-Ann, Christi-Anne, Christiann,

Christianni, Christiaun, Christiean, Christien,
Christienne, Christinan, Christy-Ann,
Christy-Anne, Chrystian, Chrystiane,
Chrystiann, Chrystianne, Chrystyan,
Chrystyane, Chrystyann, Chrystyanne,
Crestian, Crestiane, Crestiann, Crestianne,
Crestienne, Crestyane, Crestyann, Crestyanne,
Cristyan, Cristyane, Cristyann, Cristyanne,
Crystian, Crystiane, Crystiann, Crystianne,
Crystyan, Crystyane, Crystyann, Crystyanne

Christiana, Christianna (Greek) forms of
Christina.
Christianah, Christiannah, Christiannia,
Christianniah, Christiena, Chrystiana,
Chrystianah, Chrystianna, Chrystiannah,
Chrystyana, Chrystyanah, Chrystyanna,
Chrystyannah, Crestiana, Crestianah,
Crestianna, Crestiannah, Crestyana,
Crestyanah, Crestyanna, Crestyannah,
Cristyana, Cristyanah, Cristyanna,
Cristyannah, Crystiana, Crystianah,
Crystyana, Crystyanah, Crystyanna,
Crystyannah

Christiane, Christianne (Greek) forms of
Christina.

Christina (Greek) Christian; anointed. See
also Khristina, Kristina, Stina, Tina.
Christeana, Christeanah, Christeena,
Christeenah, Christeina, Christeinah,
Christella, Christinaa, Christinah, Christinea,
Christinia, Christinna, Christinnah, Christna,
Christyna, Christynah, Christynna,
Chrystena, Chrystina, Chrystyna,
Chrystynah, Cristeena, Cristena

Christine (French, English) a form of
Christina. See also Khristine, Kirsten,
Kristen, Kristine.
Chrisa, Christean, Christeane, Christeen,
Christeene, Christyne, Chrystyne, Cristeen,
Cristene, Crystine

Christophe BG (Greek) a form of
Christopher.

Christopher BG (Greek) Christ-bearer.
Religion: the patron saint of travelers and
drivers.
Chrisopherson, Christapher, Christepher,
Christerpher, Christhoper, Christipher,
Christobal, Christofer, Christoff, Christoher,
Christopehr, Christoper, Christophe,

Christopherr, Christophor, Christophoros,
Christophr, Christophre, Christophyer,
Christophyr, Christorpher, Christos,
Christovao, Christpher, Christphere,
Christphor, Christpor, Christrpher,
Chrystopher, Cristobal, Cristoforo

Christy (English) a short form of Christina,
Christine. See also Christi.
Christey, Chrystey, Chrysty, Cristy

Christyn (Greek) a short form of Christina.

Chrys (English) a form of Chris.
Krys

Chrysta (German) a short form of
Christina.
Chrystah, Chrystar, Chrystara

Chrystal (Latin) a form of Christal.
Chrystal-Lynn, Chrystale, Chrystalin,
Chrystalina, Chrystaline, Chrystalla,
Chrystallina, Chrystallynn

Chrystel (French) a form of Christal.
Chrystelle

Chu Hua (Chinese) chrysanthemum.

Chumani (Lakota) dewdrops.
Chumanee, Chumany

Chun BG (Burmese) nature's renewal.

Chyann, Chyanne (Cheyenne) forms of
Cheyenne.
Chyan, Chyana, Chyane, Chyanna

Chyenne (Cheyenne) a form of Cheyenne.
Chyeana, Chyen, Chyena, Chyene, Chyenn,
Chyenna, Chyennee

Chyna, Chynna (Chinese) forms of China.
Chynah, Chynnah

Cian BG (Irish) ancient.
Ciann, Cien

Ciana, Cianna (Chinese) forms of China.
(Italian) forms of Jane.
Cianah, Ciandra

Ciara, Ciarra (Irish) black. See also Sierra.
Ceara, Chiairah, Ciaara, Ciaera, Ciaira, Ciar,
Ciarah, Ciaria, Ciarrah, Ciora, Ciorah,
Cioria, Cyara, Cyarah, Cyarra, Cyarrah

Cibeles (Greek) Mythology: another name
for the goddess Cybele.

Cicely (English) a form of Cecilia. See also Sissy.
Cicelea, Ciceleah, Cicelee, Cicelei, Ciceleigh, Ciceley, Ciceli, Cicelia, Cicelie, Ciciley, Cicilia, Cicilie, Cicily, Cile, Cilka, Cilla, Cilli, Cillie, Cilly, Siselee, Siselei, Siseleigh, Siseli, Siselie, Sisely

Cidney (French) a form of Sydney.
Cidnee, Cidni, Cidnie

Ciearra (Irish) a form of Ciara.
Cieara, Ciearria

Cielo (Latin) she who is celestial.

Cienna (Italian) a form of Ciana.

Ciera, Cierra (Irish) forms of Ciara.
Cierah, Ciere, Cieria, Cierrah, Cierre, Cierria, Cierro

Cihuaton (Nahuatl) little woman.

Cim (English) a form of Kim.

Cimberleigh (English) a form of Kimberly.

Cinderella (French, English) little cinder girl. Literature: a fairy-tale heroine.
Cindella, Cinderel, Cinderela, Cinderelah, Cinderele, Cinderellah, Cinderelle, Cynderel, Cynderela, Cynderelah, Cynderele, Cynderell, Cynderella, Cynderellah, Cynderelle, Sinderel, Sinderela, Sinderele, Sinderell, Sinderella, Sinderelle, Synderell, Synderella, Synderelle

Cindi (Greek) a form of Cindy.
Cindie

Cindy (Greek) moon. (Latin) a familiar form of Cynthia. See also Sindy.
Cindea, Cindeah, Cindee, Cindey

Cinnamon (Greek) aromatic, reddish-brown spice.
Cinamon, Cynamon, Cynnamon, Sinamon, Sinnamon, Synamon, Synnamon

Cinnia (Latin) curly haired.
Cinia, Ciniah, Cinniah, Sinia, Siniah, Sinnia, Sinniah

Cinta (Spanish) a short form of Jacinta.

Cinthia, Cinthya (Greek) forms of Cynthia.
Cinthiah, Cinthiya, Cinthyah

Cintia (Greek) a form of Cynthia.

Cíntia (Portuguese) a form of Cynthia.

Cipriana (Italian) from the island of Cyprus.
Cipres, Cipress, Cipriane, Cipriann, Ciprianna, Ciprianne, Cyprian, Cypriana, Cypriane, Cyprienne

Cipriano (Greek) born in Cyprus.

Ciprina (Spanish) blessed by the goddess of love.

Cira (Spanish) a form of Cyrilla.
Cirah, Ciria, Ciriah, Cyra, Cyrah, Cyria, Cyriah, Cyrya, Cyryah, Siria, Syria, Syrya

Circe (Greek) Mythology: a goddess who fell in love with Odysseus in Homer's *Odyssey.*

Cirenia, Cirinea (Greek) native of Cyrene, Libya.

Ciri (Greek) ladylike.

Ciriaca, Ciríaca (Greek) belonging to God.

Ciro (Spanish) sun.

Cissy (American) a familiar form of Cecilia, Cicely.
Cissey, Cissi, Cissie

Citlali (Nahuatl) star.
Citlaly

Citlalmina (Nahuatl) greatest of our heroes.

Clair (French) a form of Clara.
Claare, Klaire, Klarye

Claire ☀ (French) a form of Clair.

Clairissa (Greek) a form of Clarissa.
Clairisa, Clairisse, Claraissa

Clancy BG (Irish) redheaded fighter.
Clance, Clancee, Clancey, Clanci, Clancie, Claney, Clanse, Clansee, Clansey, Clansi, Clansie, Clansy

Clara (Latin) clear; bright. Music: Clara Schumann was a famous nineteenth-century German composer. See also Chiara, Klara.
Claara, Claarah, Claira, Clairah, Clarah, Claresta, Clarie, Clarina, Clarinda, Clarine

Clarabelle (Latin) bright and beautiful.
Clarabel, Clarabela, Clarabelah, Clarabele, Clarabell, Clarabella, Clarabellah, Clarobel, Clarobela, Clarobelah, Clarobele, Clarobell, Clarobella, Clarobellah, Clarobelle, Clarybel,

Clarybela, Clarybelah, Clarybele, Clarybell,
Clarybella, Clarybellah, Clarybelle

Clare GB (English) a form of Clara.
Clar

Clarenza (Latin) clear; victorious.
Clarensia, Clarensiah, Clarensya, Clarensyah,
Clarenzia, Clarenziah, Clarenzya,
Clarenzyah

Claribel (Latin) a form of Clarabelle.
Claribela, Claribelah, Claribele, Claribell,
Claribella, Claribellah, Claribelle

Clarice, Clarisse (Italian) forms of Clara.
Clareace, Clarease, Clareece, Clareese, Claris,
Clarise, Clariss, Claryc, Claryce, Clarys,
Claryse, Cleriese, Klarice, Klarise

Clarie (Latin) a familiar form of Clara.
Clarey, Clari, Clary

Clarinda (Latin, Spanish) bright; beautiful.
Clairinda, Clairynda, Clarindah, Clarynda,
Claryndah

Clarisa (Greek) a form of Clarissa.
Claresa, Claris, Clarisah, Clarise, Clarisia,
Clarys, Clarysa, Clarysah, Claryse

Clarissa (Greek) brilliant. (Italian) a form of
Clara. See also Klarissa.
Clarecia, Claressa, Claresta, Clariss, Clarissah,
Clarisse, Clarissia, Claritza, Clarizza,
Clarrisa, Clarrissa, Claryss, Claryssa,
Claryssah, Clarysse, Clerissa

Clarita (Spanish) a form of Clara. See also
Klarita.
Clairette, Clareata, Clareatah, Clareate,
Clareeta, Clareetah, Clareete, Claret, Clareta,
Claretah, Clarete, Clarett, Claretta, Clarettah,
Clarette, Claritah, Clarite, Claritta, Clarittah,
Claritte, Claritza, Claryt, Claryta, Clarytah,
Claryte, Clarytt, Clarytta, Claryttah, Clarytte

Claude BG (Latin, French) lame.
Claud, Claudio, Claudis, Claudius

Claudel (Latin) a form of Claude, Claudia.
Claudell, Claudelle

Claudette (French) a form of Claudia.
Clauddetta, Claudet, Claudeta, Claudetah,
Claudete, Claudett, Claudetta, Clawdet,
Clawdeta, Clawdetah, Clawdete, Clawdett,
Clawdetta, Clawdettah, Clawdette

Claudia (Latin) a form of Claude. See also
Gladys, Klaudia.
Clauda, Claudah, Claudea, Claudex,
Claudiah, Claudine

Claudía (Latin) a form of Claudia.

Claudie (Latin) a form of Claudia.
Claudee, Claudey, Claudi, Claudy

Claudine (French) a form of Claudia.
Claudan, Claudanus, Claudeen, Claudian,
Claudiana, Claudiane, Claudianus, Claudie-
Anne, Claudien, Claudin, Claudina,
Claudinah, Claudyn, Claudyna, Claudynah,
Claudyne

Clea (Greek) a form of Cleo, Clio.

Cleantha (English) glory.

Clelia (Latin) a form of Celia.

Clematis (Greek) creeping vine. Botany: a
climbing plant with colorful flowers or
decorative fruit clusters.
Clematisa, Clematise, Clematiss, Clematissa,
Clematisse, Clematys, Clematysa, Clematyse,
Clematyss, Clematyssa, Clematysse

Clemence GB (Latin) a form of Clementine.

Clementina (German) a form of
Clementine.
Clementinah, Clementyna, Clementynah

Clementine (Latin) merciful. See also
Klementine.
Clemencia, Clemencie, Clemency, Clemente,
Clementia, Clementiah, Clementina,
Clementyn, Clementyne, Clemenza, Clemette

Clemira (Arabic) brilliant princess.

Cleo BG (Greek) a short form of Cleopatra.
Chleo, Clea, Kleo

Cleodora (Greek) gift of God.

Cleofe (Greek) she who shows signs of
glory.

Cleone (Greek) famous.
Cleaona, Cleaonee, Cleaoney, Cleoni, Cleonie,
Cleonna, Cleony, Cliona

Cleopatra (Greek) her father's fame.
History: a great Egyptian queen.
Kleopatra

Cleta (Greek) illustrious.
Cletah

Cleva (English) dwells at the cliffs.

Clidia, Clidía (Greek) agitated in the sea.

Clímaca (Nahuatl) star.

Climena, Climent (Greek) impassioned by glory.

Clio (Greek) proclaimer; glorifier.
Mythology: the Muse of history.
Klio

Clío (Greek) a form of Clio.

Clitemestra (Greek) Mythology:
Clytemnestra was the daughter of
Tyndareus and Leda.

Clitia (Greek) she who likes to keep herself clean.

Clodomira (German) famous.

Clodovea, Clodoveo (Spanish) forms of Clovis.

Cloe (Greek) a form of Chloe.
Clo, Cloea, Cloee, Cloei, Cloey, Cloi, Cloie, Clowee, Clowey, Clowi, Clowie

Cloelia (Latin) a form of Celia.

Clorinda (Greek) fresh; vital.

Closinda (German) famous, notable.

Clotilda (German) heroine.
Chlotilda, Chlotilde, Clotilde, Klothilda, Klothilde

Clovis (Teutonic) famous warrior.

Coatlicue (Greek) one from the skirts of serpents.

Coaxoch (Nahuatl) serpent flower.

Cochiti (Spanish) forgotten.

Coco GB (Spanish) coconut. See also Koko.

Codi BG (English) cushion. See also Kodi.
Coady, Codea, Codee, Codey, Codia

Codie, Cody BG (English) cushion.

Coia (Catalan) a form of Misericordia.

Cointa (Egyptian) fifth.

Colbi, Colbie (English) forms of Colby.

Colby BG (English) coal town. Geography: a
region in England known for cheese-mak-
ing. See also Kolbi.
Colbea, Colbee, Colbey

Coleen (Irish) a form of Colleen.
Colean, Coleane, Coleene, Colene

Colette, Collette (Greek, French) familiar
forms of Nicole. See also Kolette.
*Coe, Coetta, Colet, Coleta, Colete, Colett,
Coletta, Colettah, Collet, Collete, Collett,
Colletta*

Colleen (Irish) girl. See also Kolina.
*Coel, Cole, Coley, Coline, Collean, Colleane,
Colleene, Collen, Collene, Collie, Collina,
Colline, Colly, Collyn, Collyne, Colyn, Colyne*

Collina (Irish) a form of Colleen.
*Coleana, Coleena, Coleenah, Colena, Colina,
Colinah, Colinda, Colleana, Colleena,
Colleenah, Collinah, Collyna, Collynah,
Colyna, Colynah*

Collipal (Mapuche) colored star.

Colman, Colmana (Latin) forms of
Colomba.

Coloma (Spanish) a form of Colomba.

Colomba (Latin) dove.

Colombia (Spanish) Geography: a country
in South America.

Colombina (Latin) a form of Colomba.

Columba BG (Latin) dove.
*Colombe, Columbe, Columbia, Columbina,
Columbinah, Columbine, Columbyna,
Columbynah, Columbyne*

Concelia (Spanish) a form of Concepción.

Concepcion (Spanish) a form of Concepción.
Concepta, Conceptia

Concepción (Spanish) refers to the
Immaculate Conception.

Concesa (Latin) award.

Conceta, Concheta (Spanish) forms of
Concetta.

Concetta (Italian) pure.
Concettina, Conchetta

Conchita (Spanish) a form of Concepción.
Chita, Concha, Conciana, Concianah,
Conciann, Concianna, Conciannah, Concianne

Concordia (Latin) harmonious. Mythology:
the goddess governing the peace after war.
Con, Concorda, Concordah, Concordiah,
Concordya, Concordyah, Cordae, Cordaye

Concordía (Latin) a form of Concordia.

Conner BG (Scottish) wise. (Irish) praised;
exalted.
Connar, Connery, Conor

Connie GB (Latin) a familiar form of
Constance.
Con, Conee, Coney, Coni, Conie, Connee,
Conney, Conni, Conny, Cony, Konnie, Konny

Connor BG (Scottish) wise. (Irish) praised;
exalted.

Consejo (Hispanic) a form of Consuelo.

Consolación (Latin) consolation.

Consorcia (Latin) association.

Constance (Latin) constant; firm. History:
Constance Motley was the first African
American woman to be appointed as a
U.S. federal judge. See also Konstance,
Kosta.
Constancia, Constancy, Constanta,
Constantia, Constantina, Constantine,
Constanza, Constynse

Constanza (Spanish) a form of Constance.
Constanz, Constanze

Consuela (Spanish) a form of Consuelo.
Consuella, Consula

Consuelo (Spanish) consolation. Religion:
Nuestra Señora del Consuelo—Our Lady of
Consolation—is a name for the Virgin Mary.
Consolata, Conzuelo, Konsuela, Konsuelo

Contessa (Italian) an Italian countess.

Cooper BG (English) barrel maker.
Coop, Couper, Kooper, Kuepper

Cora (Greek) maiden. Mythology: Kore is
another name for Persephone, the goddess

of the underworld. See also Kora.
Corah, Corra

Corabelle (American) a combination of
Cora + Belle.
Corabel, Corabela, Corabelah, Corabele,
Corabell, Corabella, Corabellah, Korabel,
Korabela, Korabelah, Korabele, Korabell,
Korabella, Korabellah

Coral (Latin) coral. See also Koral.
Coraal, Corel, Corela, Corelah, Corele, Corell,
Corella, Corellah, Corelle, Coril, Corila,
Corilah, Corill, Corilla, Corillah, Corille,
Corral, Coryl, Coryla, Corylah, Coryle,
Coryll, Corylla, Coryllah, Corylle

Coralee (American) a combination of Cora
+ Lee.
Cora-Lee, Coralea, Coraleah, Coralei,
Coraleigh, Coralena, Coralene, Coraley,
Coraline, Coraly, Coralyn, Corella, Corilee,
Koralea, Koraleah, Koralei, Koraleigh, Korali,
Koralie, Koraly

Coralie (American) a form of Coralee.
Corali, Coralia, Coraliah, Coralin, Coralina,
Coralinah, Coraline, Coralynn, Coralynne

Corazana (Spanish) a form of Corazon.

Corazon (Spanish) heart.
Corazona

Corazón (Spanish) a form of Corazon.

Corbin BG (Latin) raven.
Corbe, Corbi, Corby, Corbyn, Corbynn

Cordasha (American) a combination of
Cora + Dasha.

Cordelia (Latin) warm-hearted. (Welsh) sea
jewel. See also Delia, Della, Kordelia.
Cordae, Cordelie, Cordellia, Cordellya,
Cordett, Cordette, Cordi, Cordilia, Cordilla,
Cordula, Cordulia

Cordella (French) rope maker.
Codela, Cordel, Cordelah, Cordele, Cordell,
Cordellah, Cordelle

Cordi (Welsh) a short form of Cordelia.
Cordey, Cordia, Cordie, Cordy

Córdula (Latin) she who is out of time.

Coreen (Greek) a form of Corinne.
Coreene

Coreena (Greek) a form of Corinne.
Coreenah

Coretta (Greek) a familiar form of Cora.
See also Koretta.
Coreta, Coretah, Corete, Corett, Corettah,
Corette, Correta, Corretta, Corrette

Corey BG (Irish) from the hollow. (Greek) a
familiar form of Cora. See also Korey.
Coree, Correy, Correye, Corry

Cori GB (Irish) a form of Corey.

Coriann, Corianne (American) combina-
tions of Cori + Ann.
Corean, Coreane, Cori-Ann, Corian, Coriane,
Corri-Ann, Corri-Anne, Corrianne, Corrie-
Ann, Corrie-Anne

Corie GB (Irish) a form of Corey.

Corin BG (Greek) a form of Corinne.
Corinn

Corina, Corinna, Corrina (Greek) forms of
Corinne. See also Korina.
Coreana, Coreanah, Coriana, Corianna,
Corinah, Corinda, Corinnah, Correana,
Correanah, Correena, Correenah, Correna,
Correnah, Corrinah, Corrinna, Corrinnah,
Corryna, Corrynah, Coryna, Corynah

Corine (Greek) a form of Corinne.

Corinne (Greek) maiden.
Coren, Corinee

Corisande, Corisanda (Spanish) flower of
the heart.

Corissa (Greek) a familiar form of Cora.
Coresa, Coressa, Corisa, Corisah, Corissah,
Corysa, Corysah, Coryssa, Coryssah, Korissa

Corliss BG (English) cheerful; goodhearted.
Corlis, Corlisa, Corlisah, Corlise, Corlissa,
Corlissah, Corlisse, Corly, Corlys, Corlysa,
Corlysah, Corlyse, Corlyss, Corlyssa,
Corlyssah, Corlysse, Korliss

Cornelia (Latin) horn colored. See also
Kornelia, Nelia, Nellie.
Carna, Carniella, Corneilla, Cornela,
Cornelie, Cornella, Cornelle, Cornelya,
Cornie, Cornilear, Cornisha, Corny

Coro (Spanish) chorus.

Corona (Latin) crown.
Coronah, Coronna, Coronnah, Korona,
Koronah, Koronna, Koronnah

Corrie (Irish) a form of Corey.

Corrin GB (Greek) a form of Corinne.
Correan, Correane, Correen, Correene, Corren,
Correne, Corrinn, Corryn, Corryne

Corrine, Corrinne (Greek) forms of
Corinne.

Corsen (Welsh) red.

Cortina (American) a form of Kortina.
Cortinah, Cortine, Cortyn, Cortyna, Cortyne

Cortnee, Cortni, Cortnie (English) forms
of Courtney.
Cortnae, Cortnai, Cortnay, Cortne, Cortnea,
Cortneia, Cortny, Cortnye, Corttney

Cortney GB (English) a form of Courtney.

Cory BG (Irish) from the hollow. (Greek) a
familiar form of Cora.

Coryn, Corynn (Greek) forms of Corinne.
Coryne, Corynne

Cosette (French) a familiar form of Nicole.
Coset, Coseta, Cosetah, Cosete, Cosett,
Cosetta, Cosettah, Cossetta, Cossette, Cozette

Cosima (Greek) orderly; harmonious;
universe.
Cosimah, Cosyma, Cosymah

Coszcatl (Nahuatl) jewel.

Courtenay, Courteney (English) forms of
Courtney.
Courtaney, Courtany, Courtena, Courtene,
Courteny

Courtline, Courtlyn (English) forms of
Courtney.
Courtlin, Courtlina, Courtlinah, Courtlyna,
Courtlynah, Courtlyne, Courtlynn

Courtnee, Courtnei, Courtni, Courtnie,
Courtny (English) forms of Courtney. See
also Kortnee, Kourtnee.
Courtne, Courtnée

Courtney GB (English) from the court.
Courtnae, Courtnai, Courtnay, Courtneigh,
Courtnii, Courtoni, Courtonie, Courtony

Covadonga (Spanish) cavern of the lady. Religion: large cave that is the scene of a shrine to the Virgin Mary.

Cozamalotl (Nahuatl) rainbow.

Cragen (Welsh) shell.

Cree (Algonquin) a Native American tribe and language of central North America.

Crescencia (Latin) growth.

Crescenciana (Spanish) a form of Crescencia.

Crimilda (German) she fights wearing a helmet.

Crisana, Crisanta (Spanish) forms of Crisantema.

Crisantema (Greek) chrysanthemum, golden flower.

Crisbell (American) a combination of Crista + Belle.
Crisbel, Cristabel

Crispina (Latin) curly haired.
Crispin, Crispine, Crispyn, Crispyna, Crispynah, Crispyne

Críspula (Greek) a form of Crispina.

Crista (Italian) a form of Christa.
Cristah

Cristal (Latin) a form of Crystal.
Cristalie, Cristalle, Cristel, Cristela, Cristelia, Cristell, Cristella, Cristelle, Cristhie, Cristle

Cristan, Cristen, Cristin (Greek) forms of Christan. See also Kristin.
Cristana, Cristanah, Cristane, Criston, Cristyn, Crystan, Crysten, Crystin, Crystyn

Cristeta (Greek) a form of Crista.

Cristi, Cristy (English) familiar forms of Cristina. Forms of Christy. See also Christi, Kristi, Kristy.
Cristee, Cristey, Cristia, Cristie, Crystee, Crystey, Crysti, Crystia, Crystie, Crysty

Cristian BG (Greek) a form of Christian.
Cristiana, Cristianah, Cristiane, Cristiann, Cristianna, Cristiannah, Cristianne

Cristina (Greek) a form of Christina. See also Kristina.
Cristaina, Cristainah, Cristeana, Cristeanah, Cristeena, Cristeenah, Cristeina, Cristeinah, Cristena, Cristenah, Cristinah, Cristiona, Crystyna, Crystynah

Cristine (Greek) a form of Christine.
Cristain, Cristaine, Cristean, Cristeane, Cristeen, Cristeene, Cristein, Cristeine, Cristene, Crystyn, Crystyne

Cruz (Spanish) cross.

Cruzita (Spanish) a form of Cruz.

Crysta (Italian) a form of Christa.

Crystal (Latin) clear, brilliant glass. See also Kristal, Krystal.
Crystala, Crystale, Crystalee, Crystall, Crystalle, Crystaly, Crystela, Crystelia, Crysthelle, Crystl, Crystle, Crystol, Crystole, Crystyl

Crystalin (Latin) crystal pool. See also Krystalyn.
Cristalanna, Cristalin, Cristalina, Cristaline, Cristallina, Cristalyn, Cristalyna, Cristalyne, Cristilyn, Crystal-Lynn, Crystalina, Crystaline, Crystallynn, Crystallynne, Crystalyn, Crystalyna, Crystalyne, Crystalynn

Crystel (Latin) a form of Crystal.
Crystell, Crystella, Crystelle

Crystina (Greek) a form of Christina.
Crystin, Crystine, Crystyn, Crystyna, Crystyne

Cualli (Nahuatl) good.

Cuartila (Hispanic) a form of Quartilla.

Cucufata (Spanish) caped lady.

Cuicatl (Nahuatl) song.

Cunegunda (German) brave and famous.

Cuniberga (German) guardedly famous.

Curipán (Mapuche) brave lioness; black mountain; valorous soul.

Curran BG (Irish) heroine.
Cura, Curin, Curina, Curinna

Custodia, Custodía (Latin) guardian angel.

Cutburga (German) protector of the wise person.

Cuthberta (English) brilliant.
Cuthbertina, Cuthbirta, Cuthbirtina, Cuthburta, Cuthburtina, Cuthburtine, Cuthbyrta, Cuthbyrtina

Cuyen (Mapuche) moon.

Cybele (Greek) a form of Sybil.
Cebel, Cebela, Cebele, Cibel, Cibela, Cibele, Cibell, Cibella, Cibelle, Cybel, Cybela, Cybell, Cybella, Cybelle, Cybil, Cybill, Cybille, Cybyl, Cybyla, Cybyle, Cybyll, Cybylla, Cybylle

Cydnee, Cydney, Cydni (French) forms of Sydney.
Cydne, Cydnei, Cydnie

Cyerra (Irish) a form of Ciara.
Cyera, Cyerah, Cyerrah Cyerria, Cyra, Cyrah

Cym (Welsh) a form of Kim.

Cymreiges (Welsh) woman of Wales.

Cynara (Greek) thistle.
Cinara, Cinarah, Cynarah, Sinara, Sinarah, Synara, Synarah

Cyndee, Cyndi (Greek) forms of Cindy.
Cynda, Cyndal, Cyndale, Cyndall, Cyndel, Cyndey, Cyndia, Cyndie, Cyndle, Cyndy

Cynthia (Greek) moon. Mythology: another name for Artemis, the moon goddess. See also Hyacinth, Kynthia, Synthia.
Cyneria, Cynethia, Cynithia, Cynthea, Cynthiah, Cynthiana, Cynthiann, Cynthie, Cynthria, Cynthy, Cynthya, Cynthyah, Cyntreia

Cyntia (Greek) a form of Cynthia.

Cypress (Greek) a coniferous tree.

Cyrena (Greek) a form of Sirena.
Ciren, Cirena, Cirenah, Cirene, Cyren, Cyrenah, Cyrene, Cyrenia, Cyreniah

Cyrilla (Greek) noble.
Cerelia, Cerella, Cira, Cirah, Cirila, Cirilah, Cirilla, Cirylla, Cyrah, Cyrella, Cyrelle, Cyrila, Cyrille, Cyryll, Cyrylla, Cyrylle

Cyteria (Greek) Mythology: Cytherea is another name for Aphrodite.

Czarina (German) a Russian empress.
Tsarina

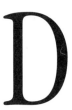

D'andra (American) a form of Deandra.

D'andrea (American) a form of Deandra.

D'asia (American) a form of Dasia.

D'ericka (American) a form of Derika.
D'erica, D'erika

D'onna (American) a form of Donna.

Da'jah (American) a form of Daja.

Dabria (Latin) Religion: one of the angelic scribes.

Dacey GB (Irish) southerner. (Greek) a familiar form of Candace.
Dacee, Dacei, Daci, Dacie, Dacy, Daicee, Daici, Daicie, Daicy, Daycee, Daycie, Daycy

Dacia (Irish) a form of Dacey.
Dacea, Daciah, Dacya, Dacyah

Dacil (Aboriginal) History: a Guanche princess from the Canary Islands.

Dae (English) day. See also Dai.

Daeja (French) a form of Déja.
Daejah, Daejia

Daelynn (American) a combination of Dae + Lynn.
Daeleen, Daelena, Daelin, Daelyn, Daelynne

Daere, Dera (Welsh) oak tree.

Daesha (American) a form of Dasha.

Daeshandra (American) a combination of Dae + Shandra.
Daeshandria, Daeshaundra, Daeshaundria, Daeshawndra, Daeshawndria, Daeshondra, Daeshondria

Daeshawna (American) a combination of Dae + Shawna.
Daeshan, Daeshaun, Daeshauna, Daeshavon, Daeshawn, Daeshawntia, Daeshon, Daeshona, Daiseana, Daiseanah, Daishaughn, Daishaughna, Daishaughnah, Daishaun, Daishauna, Daishaunah, Daishawn, Daishawna, Daishawnah, Daysean, Dayseana, Dayseanah, Dayshaughna, Dayshaughnah, Dayshaun, Dayshauna, Dayshaunah, Dayshawn, Dayshawna

Daeshonda (American) a combination of Dae + Shonda.
Daeshanda, Daeshawnda

Dafny (American) a form of Daphne.
Dafany, Daffany, Daffie, Daffy, Dafna, Dafne, Dafney, Dafnie

Dagmar (German) glorious.
Dagmara, Dagmarah, Dagmaria, Dagmariah, Dagmarya, Dagmaryah

Dagny (Scandinavian) day.
Dagna, Dagnah, Dagnana, Dagnanna, Dagne, Dagnee, Dagney, Dagnia, Dagniah, Dagnie

Dagoberta (German) radiant as the day.

Dahlia (Scandinavian) valley. Botany: a perennial flower. See also Dalia.
Dahliah, Dahlya, Dahlyah, Dahlye

Dai GB (Japanese) great. See also Dae.
Day, Daye

Daija, Daijah (French) forms of Déja.
Daijaah, Daijea, Daijha, Daijhah, Dayja

Daina (English) a form of Dana.
Dainah, Dainna

Daisey (English) a form of Daisy.

Daisha (American) a form of Dasha.
Daishae, Daishia, Daishya

Daisia (American) a form of Dasha.

Daisy (English) day's eye. Botany: a white and yellow flower.
Daisee, Daisi, Daisie, Dasee, Dasey, Dasi, Dasie, Dasy

Daiya (Polish) present.
Daia, Daiah, Daiyah, Daya, Dayah

Daja, Dajah (French) forms of Déja.
Dajae, Dajai, Daje, Dajha, Dajia

Dakayla (American) a combination of the prefix Da + Kayla.
Dakala, Dakila

Dakira (American) a combination of the prefix Da + Kira.
Dakara, Dakaria, Dakarra, Dakirah, Dakyra

Dakoda BG (Dakota) a form of Dakota.

Dakota BG (Dakota) a tribal name.
Dakkota, Dakotha, Dakotta, Dekoda, Dekodah, Dekota, Dekotah, Dekotha, Takota, Takotah

Dakotah BG (Dakota) a form of Dakota.

Dale BG (English) valley.
Dael, Daela, Dahl, Dail, Daila, Daile, Daleleana, Dalene, Dalina, Daline, Dayl

Dalena (English) a form of Dale.
Daleena, Dalenah, Dalenna, Dalennah

Dalia, Daliah (Hebrew) branch. See also Dahlia.
Daelia, Dailia, Daleah, Daleia, Dalialah, Daliyah

Dalila (Swahili) gentle.
Dalela, Dalida, Dalilah, Dalilia

Dalisha (American) a form of Dallas.
Dalisa, Dalishea, Dalishia, Dalishya, Dalisia, Dalissia, Dalissiah, Dalyssa

Dallas BG (Irish) wise.
Dallace, Dallus, Dallys, Dalyce, Dalys, Dalyss, Dalysse

Dallis BG (Irish) a form of Dallas.
Dalis, Dalise, Dalisse, Dallise

Dalma (Spanish) a form of Dalmacia.

Dalmacia (Latin) Geography: native of Dalmatia, a region on the Adriatic Sea.

Dalmira (Teutonic) illustrious; respected for her noble ancestry.

Dalton BG (English) town in the valley.
Dal, Dalaton, Dalltan, Dallten, Dalltin, Dallton, Dalltyn, Dalt, Daltan, Dalten, Daltin, Daltyn, Daulton, Delton

Damara (Greek) a form of Damaris.

Damaris (Greek) gentle girl. See also Maris.
*Dama, Damar, Damarius, Damary, Damarylis,
Damarys, Damarysa, Damaryss, Damaryssa,
Damarysse, Dameress, Dameressa, Dameris,
Damiris, Dammaris, Dammeris, Damris,
Damriss, Damrissa, Demara, Demaras,
Demaris, Demariss, Demarissa, Demarys,
Demarysa, Demarysah, Demaryse, Demaryss,
Demaryssa, Demaryssah, Demarysse*

Damasia (Spanish) a form of Dalmacia.

Damesha (Spanish) a form of Damita.
Dameshia, Damesia, Damesiah

Damia (Greek) a short form of Damiana.
Damiah, Damya, Damyah

Damiana (Greek) tamer, soother.
*Daimenia, Daimiona, Damianah, Damiane,
Damiann, Damianna, Damiannae,
Damiannah, Damianne, Damien, Damienne,
Damiona, Damon, Damyana, Damyanah,
Damyann, Damyanna, Damyannah,
Damyanne, Demion*

Damica (French) friendly.
*Damee, Dameeca, Dameecah, Dameeka,
Dameka, Damekah, Damicah, Damicia,
Damicka, Damie, Damieka, Damika,
Damikah, Damyka, Demeeca, Demeecah,
Demeeka, Demeka, Demekah, Demica,
Demicah, Demicka, Demika, Demikah,
Demyca, Demycah, Demycka, Demyka,
Demykah*

Damira (Hebrew) long live the world.

Damita (Spanish) small noblewoman.
*Dameeta, Dameetah, Dametia, Dametiah,
Dametra, Dametrah, Damitah, Damyta,
Damytah*

Damonica (American) a combination of the
prefix Da + Monica.
*Damonec, Damoneke, Damonik, Damonika,
Damonique*

Damzel (French) lady, maiden.
*Damzela, Damzele, Damzell, Damzella,
Damzellah, Damzelle*

Dana 🇬🇧 (English) from Denmark; bright as
day.
*Daena, Daenah, Danaia, Danan, Danarra,
Dane, Danean, Daneana*

Danae (Greek) Mythology: the mother of
Perseus.
*Danaë, Danai, Danay, Danayla, Danays,
Danea, Danee, Dannae, Denee*

Dánae (Greek) a form of Danae.

Danah (English) a form of Dana.

Danalyn (American) a combination of Dana
+ Lynn.
Danalee, Donaleen

Danas (Spanish) a form of Dana.

Danasia (American) a form of Danessa.

Daneil (Hebrew) a form of Danielle.
*Daneal, Daneala, Daneale, Daneel, Daneela,
Daneila, Daneille*

Daneisha (American) a form of Danessa.

Danella (American) a form of Danielle.
*Danala, Danalah, Danayla, Danela, Danelia,
Dannala, Dannalah, Donella, Donnella*

Danelle (Hebrew) a form of Danielle.
*Danael, Danale, Danalle, Danel, Danele,
Danell, Donelle, Donnelle*

Danesha (American) a form of Danessa.

Daneshia (American) a form of Danessa.

Danessa (American) a combination of
Danielle + Vanessa. See also Donesha.
*Danesa, Danesah, Danessah, Danessia,
Daniesa, Danisa, Danisah, Danissa,
Danissah, Danissia, Danissiah, Danysa,
Danysah, Danyssa, Danyssah*

Danessia (American) a form of Danessa.
Danesia, Danieshia, Danisia, Danissia

Danette (American) a form of Danielle.
*Danetra, Danett, Danetta, Donnita, Donnite,
Donnyta, Donnytta, Donnytte*

Dani, Danni (Hebrew) familiar forms of
Danielle.
*Danee, Daney, Danie, Danne, Dannee,
Danney, Dannie, Dannii, Danny, Dannye,
Dany*

Dania, Danya (Hebrew) short forms of
Danielle.
Daniah, Danja, Dannia, Danyae

Danica, Danika (Slavic) morning star. (Hebrew) forms of Danielle.
Daneca, Daneeca, Daneecah, Daneeka, Daneekah, Danicah, Danicka, Danieka, Danikah, Danikia, Danikiah, Danikla, Danneeka, Donica, Donika, Donnaica, Donnica, Donnicka, Donnika, Donnike

Danice (American) a combination of Danielle + Janice.
Danis, Danisa, Danisah, Danise, Daniss, Danissa, Danissah, Danisse, Danyce, Danys, Danysa, Danysah, Danyse, Donice

Daniel BG (Hebrew, French) a form of Danielle.
Danniel, Danniele, Danniell

Daniela (Italian) a form of Danielle.
Daniala, Danialla, Daniellah, Danijela, Dannilla, Danyela

Danielan (Spanish) a form of Danielle.

Daniele GB (Hebrew, French) a form of Danielle.

Daniell, Dannielle (Hebrew, French) forms of Danielle.

Daniella (English) a form of Dana, Danielle.
Danka, Danniella, Danyella

Danielle ☆ GB (Hebrew, French) God is my judge.
Daneen, Daneil, Daneille, Danial, Danialle, Danielan, Danielka, Danilka, Danille, Danniele, Donniella

Daniesha (American) a form of Danessa.

Danille (American) a form of Danielle.
Danila, Danile, Danilla, Dannille

Daniqua (Hebrew, Slavic) a form of Danica.
Daniquah

Danisha (American) a form of Danessa.
Danishia

Danit (Hebrew) a form of Danielle.
Danett, Danis, Daniss, Danitra, Danitrea, Danitria, Danitza, Daniz

Danita (Hebrew) a form of Danielle.

Danna, Dannah (American) short forms of Danella. (Hebrew) forms of Dana.

Dannica (Hebrew, Slavic) a form of Danica.
Dannika, Dannikah

Danyale, Danyell, Danyelle (American) forms of Danielle.
Daniyel, Danyae, Danyail, Danyaile, Danyal, Danyea, Danyele, Danyiel, Danyielle, Danyle, Donnyale, Donnyell, Donyale, Donyell

Danyel GB (American) a form of Danielle.

Danyka (American) a form of Danica.
Danyca, Danycah, Danycka, Danykah, Danyqua, Danyquah

Daphne (Greek) laurel tree.
Dafnee, Dafney, Dafni, Dafnie, Dafny, Daphane, Daphaney, Daphanie, Daphany, Dapheney, Daphna, Daphni, Daphnie, Daphnique, Daphnit, Daphny

Daphnee, Daphney (Greek) forms of Daphne.

Dara GB (Hebrew) compassionate.
Dahra, Dahrah, Daira, Dairah, Daraka, Daralea, Daralee, Daraleigh, Daraley, Daralie, Daravie, Darda, Darja, Darra

Darah, Darrah (Hebrew) forms of Dara.

Daralis (English) beloved.
Daralisa, Daralisah, Daralise, Daralysa, Daralyse

Darbi (Irish, Scandinavian) a form of Darby.
Darbia, Darbiah, Darbie

Darby GB (Irish) free. (Scandinavian) deer estate.
Darb, Darbe, Darbea, Darbee, Darbra, Darbye

Darcelle (French) a form of Darcy.
Darcel, Darcela, Darcelah, Darcele, Darcell, Darcella, Darcellah, Darselle

Darci, Darcie (Irish, French) forms of Darcy.
Darcia, Darciah

Darcy GB (Irish) dark. (French) fortress.
Darcea, Darcee, Darcey, Darsea, Darsee, Darsey, Darsi, Darsie, Darsy

Daria (Greek) wealthy.
Dari, Dariya, Darria, Darriah

Daría (Greek) a form of Daria.

Darian BG (Greek) a form of Daron.
Dariann, Dariyan, Dariyanne, Darriane,
Darriann, Darrianne

Dariane, Darianne (Greek) forms of
Daron.

Darianna (Greek) a form of Daron.
Dariana, Darriana, Darrianna, Driana

Darice (Persian) queen, ruler.
Dareece, Darees, Dareese, Daricia, Dariciah,
Darisa, Darissa, Darycia, Darys, Darysa,
Darysah, Daryse, Darysia, Darysiah,
Darysya, Darysyah

Dariel BG (French) a form of Daryl.
Dariela, Darielah, Dariele, Dariell, Dariella,
Dariellah, Darriel, Daryel, Daryelah, Daryele,
Daryell, Daryella, Daryellah, Daryelle

Darielle, Darrielle (French) forms of Daryl.

Darien BG (Greek) a form of Daron.
Dariene, Darriene

Darienne (Greek) a form of Daron.

Darilynn (American) a form of Darlene.
Daralin, Daralina, Daralinah, Daraline,
Daralyn, Daralyna, Daralyne, Daralynn,
Daralynne, Darelin, Darileana, Darileanah,
Darileen, Darileena, Darileenah, Darilin,
Darilina, Darilinah, Dariline, Darilyn,
Darilyna, Darilynah, Darilyne, Darilynne,
Darylin, Darylina, Darylinah, Daryline,
Darylyn, Darylyna, Darylynah, Darylyne,
Darylynn, Darylynne

Darion BG (Irish) a form of Daron.
Dariona, Darione, Darionna, Darionne,
Darriona, Darrionna

Darla (English) a short form of Darlene.
Darlah, Darlecia, Darli, Darlice, Darlie,
Darlis, Darly, Darlys

Darlene (French) little darling. See also
Daryl.
Darlean, Darlee, Darleen, Darleena,
Darleenah, Darleene, Darlen, Darlena,
Darlenah, Darlenia, Darlenne, Darletha

Darlin, Darlyn (French) forms of Darlene.
Darlina, Darlinah, Darline, Darling, Darlyna,
Darlynah, Darlyne, Darlynn, Darlynne

Darnee (Irish) a familiar form of Darnelle.

Darneisha (American) a form of Darnelle.
Darneishia, Darniesha, Darrenisha

Darnelle BG (English) hidden place.
Darnel, Darnela, Darnelah, Darnele, Darnell,
Darnella, Darnellah, Darnetta, Darnette,
Darnice, Darniece, Darnita, Darnyell,
Darnyella, Darnyelle

Darnesha (American) a form of Darnelle.
Darneshea, Darneshia, Darnesia

Darnisha (American) a form of Darnelle.
Darnishia, Darnisia

Daron BG (Irish) a form of Daryn.
Darona, Daronah, Darron

Daronica (American) a form of Daron.
Daronicah, Daronice, Daronicka, Daronickah,
Daronik, Daronika, Daronikah, Daroniqua,
Daronique, Daronyca, Daronycah, Daronycka,
Daronyckah, Daronyka, Daronykah,
Daronyqua

Darrian BG (Greek) a form of Daron.

Darrien BG (Greek) a form of Daron.

Darrion BG (Irish) a form of Daron.

Darselle (French) a form of Darcelle.
Darsel, Darsell, Darsella

Daru (Hindi) pine tree.
Daroo, Darua, Darue

Darya (Greek) a form of Daria.
Darrya, Darryah, Daryah, Daryia

Daryan (Greek, Irish) a form of Daryn.

Daryl BG (English) beloved. (French) a short
form of Darlene.
Darel, Darela, Darelah, Darell, Darellah,
Darelle, Daril, Darila, Darile, Darill, Darilla,
Darillah, Darille, Darilynn, Darrel, Darrell,
Darrelle, Darreshia, Darril, Darrila, Darrilah,
Darrile, Darrill, Darrilla, Darrille, Darryl,
Darryla, Darryle, Darryll, Darrylla, Darrylle,
Daryla, Daryle, Daryll, Darylla, Daryllah,
Darylle

Daryn BG (Greek) gifts. (Irish) great.
Darin, Darina, Darinah, Daryna, Darynah,
Daryne, Darynn, Darynne

Dasha (Russian) a form of Dorothy.
Dashae, Dashah, Dashenka

Dashawn BG (American) a short form of Dashawna.
Dasean, Dashaughn, Dashaun

Dashawna (American) a combination of the prefix Da + Shawna.
Daseana, Daseanah, Dashaughna, Dashaughnah, Dashauna, Dashaunah, Dashawnah, Dashawnna, Dashell, Dayshana, Dayshawnna, Dayshona

Dashay (American) a familiar form of Dashawna.

Dashia (Russian) a form of Dorothy.
Dashiah

Dashiki (Swahili) loose-fitting shirt worn in Africa.
Dasheka, Dashi, Dashika, Dashka, Desheka, Deshiki

Dashonda (American) a combination of the prefix Da + Shonda.
Dashawnda, Dishante

Dasia (Russian) a form of Dasha.
Dasiah, Daysha

Davalinda (American) a combination of Davida + Linda.
Davalindah, Davalinde, Davelinda, Davilinda, Davylinda

Davalynda (American) a form of Davalinda.
Davelynda, Davilynda, Davylinda, Davylindah, Davylynda

Davalynn (American) a combination of Davida + Lynn.
Davalin, Davalyn, Davalynne, Davelin, Davelyn, Davelynn, Davelynne, Davilin, Davilyn, Davilynn, Davilynne, Dayleen, Devlyn

David BG (Hebrew) beloved. Bible: the second king of Israel.

Davida (Hebrew) a form of David. See also Vida.
Daveda, Daveta, Davetta, Davette, Davika

Davina (Scottish) a form of Davida. See also Vina.
Dava, Davannah, Davean, Davee, Daveen, Daveena, Davene, Daveon, Davey, Davi, Daviana, Davie, Davin, Davinder, Davine, Davineen, Davinia, Davinna, Davria, Devean, Deveen, Devene

Davisha (American) a combination of the prefix Da + Aisha.
Daveisha, Davesia, Davis, Davisa

Davita (Scottish) a form of Davina.

Davon BG (Scottish, English) a short form of Davonna.
Davonne

Davonna (Scottish, English) a form of Davina, Devonna.
Davion, Daviona, Davionna, Davona, Davonah, Davonda, Davondah, Davone, Davonia, Davonnah, Davonnia

Dawn (English) sunrise, dawn.
Dawin, Dawina, Dawne, Dawnee, Dawnetta, Dawnisha, Dawnlin, Dawnlina, Dawnline, Dawnlyna, Dawnlyne, Dawnlynn, Dawnn, Dawnrae

Dawna (English) a form of Dawn.
Dawana, Dawanah, Dawandra, Dawandrea, Dawanna, Dawannah, Dawnah, Dawnna, Dawnnah, Dawnya

Dawnetta (American) a form of Dawn.
Dawnet, Dawneta, Dawnete, Dawnett, Dawnette

Dawnisha (American) a form of Dawn.
Dawnesha, Dawni, Dawniell, Dawnielle, Dawnishia, Dawnisia, Dawniss, Dawnita, Dawnnisha, Dawnysha, Dawnysia

Dawnyelle (American) a combination of Dawn + Danielle.
Dawnele, Dawnell, Dawnella, Dawnelle, Dawnyel, Dawnyell, Dawnyella

Dayana, Dayanna (Latin) forms of Diana.
Dayanara, Dayani, Dayanne, Dayanni, Deyanaira, Dyani, Dyia

Dayanira, Deyanira (Greek) she stirs up great passions.

Dayla (English) a form of Dale.
Daylea, Daylee

Daylan BG (English) a form of Dale.
Daylen, Daylon

Dayle (English) a form of Dale.

Daylin BG (English) a form of Dale.

Dayna (Scandinavian) a form of Dana.
Daynah, Dayne, Daynna, Deyna

Daysha (American) a form of Dasha.
Daysa, Dayshalie, Daysia, Deisha

Daysi (English) a form of Daisy.
Daysee, Daysey, Daysia, Daysie, Daysy

Dayton BG (English) day town; bright, sunny town.
Daytonia

Daytona BG (English) day town; bright, sunny town.

De'ja, Deja, Dejá, Dejah, Déjah (French) forms of Déja.
Deejay, Dejae, Dejai, Dejay, Dejaya

Deana (Latin) divine. (English) valley.
Deahana, Deahanah, Deanah, Deane, Deaniel, Deaniela, Deanielah, Deaniele, Deaniell, Deaniellah, Deanielle, Deanisha, Deeana

Deandra GB (American) a combination of Dee + Andrea.
Dandrea, Deandrah, Deandre, Deandré, Deandree, Deanndra, Deeandra, Deyaneira, Diondria, Dyandra

Deandrea GB (American) a form of Deandra.
Deandreia, Deandria, Deandriah, Deandrya, Deandryah

Deangela (Italian) a combination of the prefix De + Angela.
Deangala, Deangalique, Deangle

Deann, Deanne (Latin) forms of Diane.
Deahanne, Deane, Déanne, Dee-Ann, Deeann, Deeanne

Deanna, Déanna (Latin) forms of Deana, Diana.
Deaana, Deahanna, Deahannah, Deannah, Deannia

Deasia, Déasia (American) forms of Dasia.

Deaundra (American) a form of Deandra.
Deaundria

Debbie, Debby (Hebrew) familiar forms of Deborah.
Debbea, Debbee, Debbey, Debbi, Debea, Debee, Debey, Debi, Debie, Deby

Debora (Hebrew) a form of Deborah.
Debbora

Débora, Déborah, Dèbora (Hebrew) forms of Deborah.

Deborah (Hebrew) bee. Bible: a great Hebrew prophetess.
Deb, Debbera, Debberah, Debborah, Debera, Deberah, Debor, Deboran, Deborha, Deborrah, Debrena, Debrina, Debroah, Dobra

Debra (American) a form of Deborah.
Debbra, Debbrah, Debrah, Debrea, Debria

December (Latin) born in the twelfth month.

Decia (Latin) tenth child.

Dedra (American) a form of Deirdre.
Deadra, Deadrah, Dedrah

Dedriana (American) a combination of Dedra + Adriana.
Dedranae

Dee (Welsh) black, dark.
De, Dea, Deah, Dede, Dedie, Dee Dee, Deea, Deedee, Didi

Deeanna (Latin) a form of Deana, Diana.

Deedra (American) a form of Deirdre.
Deeddra, Deedrah, Deedrea, Deedri, Deedrie

Deena (American) a form of Deana, Dena, Dinah.
Deenah, Deenna, Deennah

Deianeira (Greek) Mythology: Deianira was the wife of the Greek hero Heracles.
Daeanaira, Daeanairah, Daeianeira, Daeianeirah, Daianaira, Daianairah, Dayanaira, Dayanairah, Deianaira, Deianairah, Deianeirah

Deidamia (Greek) she who is patient in battle.

Deidra, Deidre (Irish) forms of Deirdre.
Deidrah, Deidrea, Deidrie, Diedre, Dydree, Dydri, Dydrie, Dydry

Deifila, Deifilia (Greek) from the face of Zeus; loved by God.

Deina (Spanish) religious holiday.

Deirdre (Irish) sorrowful; wanderer.
Deerdra, Deerdrah, Deerdre, Deirdree, Didi, Dierdra, Dierdre, Diérdre, Dierdrie, Dyerdre

Deisy (English) a form of Daisy.
Deisi, Deissy

Deitra (Greek) a short form of Demetria.
Deatra, Deatrah, Deetra, Deetrah, Deitrah, Detria, Deytra, Deytrah

Déja (French) before.

Dejanae (French) a form of Déja.
Dajahnae, Dajona, Dejana, Dejanah, Dejanai, Dejanay, Dejane, Dejanea, Dejanee, Dejanna, Dejannaye, Dejena, Dejonae

Dejanelle (French) a form of Déja.
Dejanel, Dejanela, Dejanelah, Dejanele, Dejanell, Dejanella, Dejanellah, Dejonelle

Dejanira (Greek) destroyer of men.

Dejon **BG** (French) a form of Déja.
Daijon, Dajan, Dejone, Dejonee, Dejonna

Deka (Somali) pleasing.
Dekah

Delacey, Delacy (American) combinations of the prefix De + Lacey.
Delaceya

Delaina (German) a form of Delana.
Delainah

Delaine (Irish) a short form of Delainey.

Delainey (Irish) a form of Delaney.
Delainee, Delaini, Delainie, Delainy

Delana (German) noble protector.
Dalaina, Dalainah, Dalaine, Dalanah, Dalanna, Dalannah, Dalayna, Dalaynah, Dalina, Dalinah, Dalinda, Dalinna, Delanah, Delania, Delanna, Delannah, Delanya, Deleina, Deleinah, Delena, Delenya, Deleyna, Deleynah, Dellaina

Delaney **GB** (Irish) descendant of the challenger. (English) a form of Adeline.
Dalanee, Dalaney, Dalania, Dalene, Daleney, Daline, Del, Delane, Delanee, Delany, Delayne, Delayney, Deleine, Deleyne, Dellanee, Dellaney, Dellany

Delanie (Irish) a form of Delaney.
Delani, Delaynie, Deleani, Dellani, Dellanie

Delayna (German) a form of Delana.
Delaynah

Deleena (French) dear; small.
Deleana, Deleanah, Deleane, Deleenah, Deleene, Delyna, Delynah, Delyne

Delfia (Spanish) dolphin. Religion: refers to the thirteenth-century French Saint Delphine.

Delfina (Spanish) dolphin. (Greek) a form of Delphine.
Delfeena, Delfi, Delfie, Delfin, Delfinah, Delfine, Delfyn, Delfyna, Delfynah, Delfyne

Delia (Greek) visible; from Delos, Greece. (German, Welsh) a short form of Adelaide, Cordelia. Mythology: a festival of Apollo held in ancient Greece.
Dehlia, Delea, Deleah, Deli, Deliah, Deliana, Delianne, Delinda, Dellia, Delliah, Dellya, Dellyah, Delya, Delyah

Dèlia (Catalan) a form of Delia.

Delicia (English) delightful.
Delecia, Delesha, Delica, Delice, Delight, Delighta, Delisia, Delisiah, Deliz, Deliza, Delizah, Delize, Delizia, Delya, Delys, Delyse, Delysia, Delysiah, Delysya, Delysyah, Doleesha

Delicias (Spanish) delights.

Delilah (Hebrew) brooder. Bible: the companion of Samson. See also Lila.
Dalialah, Daliliah, Delila, Delilia, Delilla, Delyla, Delylla

Delina (French) a form of Deleena.
Delinah, Deline

Delisa (English) a form of Delicia.
Delisah, Delise

Delisha (English) a form of Delicia.
Delishia

Della (English) a short form of Adelaide, Cordelia, Delaney.
Del, Dela, Dell, Delle, Delli, Dellie, Dells

Delmar **BG** (Latin) sea.
Delma, Delmah, Delmara, Delmarah, Delmare, Delmaria, Delmariah, Delmarya, Delmaryah

Delmira (Spanish) a form of Dalmira.

Delores, Deloris (Spanish) forms of Dolores.
Delora, Delorah, Delore, Deloree, Delorey, Deloria, Deloriah, Delories, Deloriesa, Delorise, Deloriss, Delorissa, Delorissah, Delorisse, Delorita, Delorite, Deloritta, Delorys, Deloryse, Deloryss, Deloryta, Delorytta, Deloryttah, Delsie

Delphine (Greek) from Delphi, Greece. See also Delfina.
Delpha, Delphe, Delphi, Delphia, Delphiah, Delphie, Delphina, Delphinah, Delphinia, Delphiniah, Delphinie, Delphy, Delphyna, Delphynah, Delphyne, Delvina, Delvinah, Delvine, Delvinia, Delviniah, Delvyna, Delvynah, Delvyne, Delvynia, Delvyniah, Delvynya, Delvynyah, Dolphina, Dolphinah, Dolphine, Dolphyn, Dolphyna, Dolphynah, Dolphyne

Delsie (English) a familiar form of Delores.
Delcea, Delcee, Delsa, Delsea, Delsee, Delsey, Delsi, Delsia, Delsy, Delza

Delta (Greek) door. Linguistics: the fourth letter in the Greek alphabet. Geography: a triangular land mass at the mouth of a river.
Deltah, Deltar, Deltare, Deltaria, Deltarya, Deltaryah, Delte, Deltora, Deltoria, Deltra

Delwyn (English) proud friend; friend from the valley.
Delwin

Demetra (Greek) a short form of Demetria.
Demetrah

Demetria (Greek) cover of the earth. Mythology: Demeter was the Greek goddess of the harvest.
Deitra, Demeetra, Demeetrah, Demeta, Demeteria, Demetriana, Demetrianna, Demetrias, Demetrice, Demetriona, Demetris, Demetrish, Demetrius, Dymeetra, Dymeetrah, Dymetra, Dymetrah, Dymitra, Dymitrah, Dymitria, Dymitriah, Dymytria, Dymytriah, Dymytrya, Dymytryah

Demi (French) half. (Greek) a short form of Demetria.
Demee, Demey, Demia, Demiah, Demie, Demii, Demmee, Demmey, Demmi, Demmie, Demmy, Demy

Demitria (Greek) a form of Demetria.
Demita, Demitah, Demitra, Demitrah

Demofila (Greek) friend of the village.

Dena (English, Native American) valley. (Hebrew) a form of Dinah. See also Deana.
Deane, Deeyn, Denah, Dene, Denea, Deney, Denna

Denae (Hebrew) a form of Dena.
Denaé, Denai, Denay, Denee, Deneé

Deneisha (American) a form of Denisha.
Deneichia, Deneishea

Denesha (American) a form of Denisha.
Deneshia

Deni (French) a short form of Denise.
Denee, Deney, Denie, Dennee, Denney, Denni, Dennie, Denny, Deny, Dinnie, Dinny

Denica, Denika (Slavic) forms of Danica.
Denicah, Denikah, Denikia

Denice (French) a form of Denise.
Denicy

Denis BG (French) a form of Denise.

Denisa (Spanish) a form of Denise.

Denise (French) Mythology: follower of Dionysus, the god of wine.
Danice, Danise, Denece, Denese, Deni, Deniece, Deniese, Denize, Denyce, Denys, Denyse, Dineece, Dineese, Dinice, Dinise, Dinyce, Dinyse, Dynice, Dynise, Dynyce, Dynyse

Denisha (American) a form of Denise.
Deneesha, Deniesha, Denishia

Denisse (French) a form of Denise.
Denesse, Deniss, Denissa, Denyss

Denita (Hebrew) a form of Danita.

Denver BG (English) green valley. Geography: the capital of Colorado.
Denvor

Deodata (Latin) delivered to God.

Deogracias (Latin) born by the grace of God.

Deon BG (English) a short form of Deona.

Deona, Deonna (English) forms of Dena.
Deonah, Deonne

Deondra GB (American, Greek, English) a form of Deandra, Deona, Diona.

Deonilde (German) she who fights.

Derfuta (Latin) she who flees.

Derian BG (Greek) a form of Daryn.
Derrian

Derica, Derrica, Derricka (German) forms of Derika.
Dericah, Dericka, Derricah

Derifa (Arabic) graceful.

Derika (German) ruler of the people.
Dereka, Derekah, Derekia, Derekiah, Derekya, Derekyah, Derikah, Deriqua, Deriquah, Derique, Derrika, Derrikah, Derriqua, Derryca, Derrycah, Derrycka, Derryka, Derryqua

Derry BG (Irish) redhead.
Deree, Derey, Deri, Derie, Derree, Derrey, Derri, Derrie, Dery

Derwen (Welsh) oak tree.

Deryn (Welsh) bird.
Deran, Derana, Deranah, Derane, Deren, Derena, Derenah, Derene, Derien, Derienne, Derin, Derina, Derinah, Derine, Derion, Deron, Derona, Deronah, Derone, Derran, Derrana, Derranah, Derrane, Derren, Derrin, Derrina, Derrinah, Derrine, Derrion, Derriona, Derryn, Derryna, Derrynah, Derryne, Deryna, Derynah, Deryne

Desarae, Desaray (French) forms of Desiree.
Desara, Desarah, Desarai, Desaraie, Desare, Desaré, Desarea, Desaree, Desarey, Desaria, Desarie, Desary

Desdemona, Desdémona (Greek) unfortunate; unhappy.

Deserae, Deseray, Deseree (French) forms of Desiree.
Desera, Deserah, Deserai, Deseraia, Deseraie, Desere, Deseret, Deserey, Deseri, Deseria, Deserie, Deserrae, Deserrai, Deserray, Deserré, Dessirae

Desgracias (Latin) a form of Deogracias.

Deshawn BG (American) a short form of Deshawna.
Deshan, Deshane, Deshaun

Deshawna (American) a combination of the prefix De + Shawna.
Desheania, Deshona, Deshonna

Deshawnda (American) a combination of the prefix De + Shawnda.
Deshanda, Deshandra, Deshaundra, Deshawndra, Deshonda

Deshay (American) a familiar form of Deshawna.

Desi BG (French) a short form of Desiree.
Desea, Desee, Desey, Desie, Désir, Desira, Desy, Dezi, Dezia, Dezzia, Dezzie

Desideria (French) a form of Desirae.

Desirae, Desiray, Desirea, Desireé, Desirée, Desiree' (French) forms of Desiree.

Desire (French) a form of Desiree.

Desiree (French) desired, longed for.
Desira, Desirah, Desirai, Desireah, Désirée, Desirey, Desiri, Desray, Desree, Dessie, Dessirae, Dessire, Dessiree, Desyrae, Desyrai, Desyray

Despina (Greek) a form of Despoina.

Despoina (Greek) mistress, lady.

Dessa (Greek) wanderer. (French) a form of Desiree.
Desa, Desah, Dessah

Desta (Ethiopian) happy. (French) a short form of Destiny.
Destah, Desti, Destie, Desty

Destanee, Destaney, Destani, Destanie, Destany (French) forms of Destiny.
Destania, Destannee, Destanney, Destanni, Destannia, Destannie, Destanny

Desteny (French) a form of Destiny.
Destenee, Desteni, Destenia, Destenie

Destin BG (French) a short form of Destiny.

Destina (Spanish) a form of Destiny.

Destine, Destinee, Destinée, Destiney, Destini, Destinie (French) forms of Destiny.
Destiana, Destinnee, Destinni, Destinnia, Destinnie, Destnie

Destiny ✻ (French) fate.
Desnine, Desta, Desteney, Destinia, Destiniah, Destinny, Destonie, Dezstany

Destyne, Destynee, Destyni (French) forms of Destiny.
Desty, Destyn, Destynia, Destyniah, Destynie, Destyny, Destynya, Destynyah

Deva (Hindi) divine.
Deava, Deavah, Deeva, Deevah, Devah, Diva, Divah, Dyva, Dyvah

Devan BG (Irish) a form of Devin.
Devana, Devane, Devanee, Devaney, Devani, Devania, Devanie, Devann, Devanna, Devannae, Devanne, Devany

Devera (Spanish) task.

Devi (Hindi) goddess. Religion: the Hindu goddess of power and destruction.

Devika (Sanskrit) little goddess.

Devin BG (Irish) poet.
Deaven, Deven, Devena, Devene, Devenja, Devenje, Deveny, Deveyn, Deveyna, Deveyne, Devyna, Devyne, Devynee, Devyney, Devyni, Devynia, Devyniah, Devyny, Devynya, Devynyah

Devina (Scottish, Irish, Latin) a form of Davina, Devin, Divina.
Deveena, Devinae, Devinah, Devinia, Deviniah, Devinie, Devinna

Devinne (Irish) a form of Devin.
Devine, Devinn, Devinna

Devon BG (English) a short form of Devonna. (Irish) a form of Devin.
Devion, Devione, Devionne, Devone, Devoni, Devonn, Devonne

Devona (English) a form of Devonna.
Devonah, Devonda

Devonna (English) from Devonshire.
Devondra, Devonia, Devonnah, Divona, Divonah, Divonna, Divonnah, Dyvona, Dyvonah, Dyvonna, Dyvonnah

Devora (Hebrew) a form of Deborah.
Deva, Devorah, Devra, Devrah, Dyvora, Dyvorah

Devota (Latin) devoted to God.

Devyn BG (Irish) a form of Devin.
Deveyn, Devyne, Devynne

Devynn (Irish) a form of Devin.

Dextra (Latin) adroit, skillful.
Dekstra, Dextrah, Dextria

Deysi (English) a form of Daisy.
Deysia, Deysy

Dezarae, Dezaray, Dezaree (French) forms of Desiree.
Dezaraee, Dezarai, Dezare, Dezarey, Dezerai, Dezeray, Dezere, Dezerea, Dezeree, Dezerie, Dezorae, Dezorai, Dezoray, Dezra, Dezrae, Dezrai, Dezray, Dezyrae, Dezzirae, Dezzrae, Dezzrai, Dezzray

Dezirae, Deziray, Deziree (French) forms of Desiree.
Dezirea, Dezirée

Dhara (Indian) earth.

Di (Latin) a short form of Diana, Diane.
Dy

Dia (Latin) a short form of Diana, Diane.

Día (Spanish) day.

Díamantina (Latin) unconquerable.

Diamon (Latin) a short form of Diamond.

Diamond GB (Latin) precious gem.
Diamantina, Diamantra, Diamonda, Diamondah, Diamonde, Diamonia, Diamonte, Diamontina, Dimond, Dimonda, Dimondah, Dimonde

Diamonique (American, Latin) a form of Damonica, Diamond.
Diamoniqua

Diana ✻ (Latin) divine. Mythology: the goddess of the hunt, the moon, and fertility. See also Deann, Deanna, Dyana.
Daiana, Daianna, Diaana, Diaanah, Dianah, Dianalyn, Dianarose, Dianatris, Dianca, Dianelis, Diania, Dianiah, Dianiella, Dianielle, Dianita, Dianya, Dianyah, Dianys, Didi, Dihana, Dihanah, Dihanna

Díana (Greek) a form of Diana.

Diandra (American, Latin) a form of Deandra, Diana.
Diandre, Diandrea

Diane, Dianne (Latin) short forms of Diana.
Deane, Deeane, Deeanne, Diaan, Diaane, Diahann, Dian, Diani, Dianie, Diann, Dihan, Dihane, Dihann, Dihanne

Dianna (Latin) a form of Diana.
Diahanna, Diannah

Dianora, Díanora (Italian) forms of Diana.

Diantha (Greek) divine flower.
Diandre, Dianthah, Dianthe, Dyantha, Dyanthah, Dyanthe, Dyanthia, Dyanthiah, Dyanthya, Dyanthyah

Dicra (Welsh) slowly.

Diedra (Irish) a form of Deirdre.
Didra, Diedre

Diega (Spanish) supplanter.

Diella (Latin) she who adores God.

Difyr (Welsh) fun.

Digna (Latin) worthy.

Dil, Dill (Welsh) sincere.

Dillan **BG** (Irish) loyal, faithful.
Dillon, Dillyn

Dillian **BG** (Latin) worshipped.
Dilliana, Dilliane, Dillianna, Dilliannah, Dillianne, Dylian, Dyliana, Dylianah, Dyliane, Dyllian, Dylliana, Dylliane, Dylliann, Dyllianna, Dylliannah, Dyllianne, Dylyan, Dylyana, Dylyanah, Dylyane, Dylyann, Dylyanna, Dylyannah, Dylyanne

Dilly (Welsh) a form of Dil.

Dilys (Welsh) perfect; true. See also Dyllis.
Dilis, Dilisa, Dilisah, Dilise, Dillis, Dillisa, Dillisah, Dillise, Dillys, Dilysa, Dilysah, Dilyse, Dylys

Dimitra (Greek) a form of Demetria.

Dimna (Irish) convenient.

Dina (Hebrew) a form of Dinah.
Dinna

Dinah (Hebrew) vindicated. Bible: a daughter of Jacob and Leah.
Dinnah, Dyna, Dynah, Dynna, Dynnah

Dinesha (American) a form of Danessa.

Dinka (Swahili) people.
Dinkah, Dynka, Dynkah

Dinora (Hebrew) avenged or vindicated.

Dinorah (Aramaic) she who personifies light.

Diomira (Spanish) a form of Teodomira.

Diona, Dionna (Greek) forms of Dionne.
Deonia, Deonyia, Dionah, Dyona, Dyonah

Diondra (Greek) a form of Dionne.
Diondrea

Dionis, Dionisa, Dionisia (Spanish) from Dionysus, god of wine.

Dionne **GB** (Greek) divine queen. Mythology: Dione was the mother of Aphrodite, the goddess of love.
Deonne, Dion, Dione, Dionee, Dioney, Dioni, Dionie, Dionis, Dionte, Diony, Dyon, Dyone, Dyonee, Dyoney, Dyoni, Dyonie, Dyony

Dior (French) golden.
Diora, Diorah, Diore, Diorra, Diorrah, Diorre, Dyor, Dyora, Dyorah, Dyorra, Dyorrah, Dyorre

Dirce (Greek) fruit of the pine.

Dita (Spanish) a form of Edith.
Ditah, Ditka, Ditta, Dyta, Dytah

Divinia (Latin) divine.
Diveena, Divina, Divinah, Divine, Diviniah, Diviniea, Dyveena, Dyvina, Dyvinah, Dyvinia, Dyvyna, Dyvynah, Dyvynia, Dyvyniah, Dyvynya

Divya (Latin) a form of Divinia.

Dixie (French) tenth. (English) wall; dike. Geography: a nickname for the American South.
Dix, Dixee, Dixey, Dixi, Dixy, Dyxee, Dyxey, Dyxi, Dyxie, Dyxy

Diya (Hindi) dazzling personality.

Diza (Hebrew) joyful.
Ditza, Ditzah, Dizah, Dyza, Dyzah

Djanira (Portuguese) a form of Dayanira.

Doanne (English) low, rolling hills.
Doan, Doana, Doanah, Doann, Doanna, Doannah, Doean, Doeana, Doeanah, Doeane, Doeann, Doeanna, Doeannah, Doeanne

Docila (Latin) gentle; docile.
Docilah, Docile, Docilla, Docillah, Docille, Docyl, Docyla, Docylah, Docyle, Docyll, Docylla, Docyllah, Docylle

Dodie (Hebrew) beloved. (Greek) a familiar form of Dorothy.
Doda, Dode, Dodea, Dodee, Dodey, Dodi, Dodia, Dodiah, Dody, Dodya, Dodyah

Dolly (American) a short form of Dolores, Dorothy.
Dol, Dolea, Doleah, Dolee, Dolei, Doleigh, Doley, Doli, Dolia, Doliah, Dolie, Doll, Dollea, Dolleah, Dollee, Dollei, Dolleigh, Dolley, Dolli, Dollie, Dollina, Doly

Dolores (Spanish) sorrowful. Religion: Nuestra Señora de los Dolores—Our Lady of Sorrows—is a name for the Virgin Mary. See also Lola.
Deloria, Dolorcitas, Dolorita, Doloritas

Domana (Latin) domestic.

Domanique (French) a form of Dominica.

Domenica (Latin) a form of Dominica.
Domeneka, Domenicah, Domenicka, Domenika

Doménica, Domínica (Latin) forms of Dominica.

Domenique (French) a form of Dominica.
Domeneque, Domeniqua, Domeniquah

Domicia (Greek) she who loves her house.

Domiciana (Spanish) a form of Domicia.

Domilia (Latin) related to the house.

Dominica, Dominika (Latin) belonging to the Lord. See also Mika.
Domineca, Domineka, Dominga, Domini, Dominia, Dominiah, Dominicah, Dominick, Dominicka, Dominikah, Dominixe, Domino, Dominyika, Domka, Domnica, Domnicah, Domnicka, Domnika, Domonica, Domonice, Domonika

Dominique GB (French) a form of Dominica.
Domineque, Dominiqua, Dominiquah, Domino, Dominoque, Dominuque, Domique

Domino (English) a short form of Dominica.
Domina, Dominah, Domyna, Domynah, Domyno

Dominque BG (French) a short form of Dominique.

Domitila (Latin) a form of Domicia.

Domnina (Latin) lord, master.

Domonique (French) a form of Dominique.
Domminique, Domoniqua, Domoniquah

Dona (English) world leader; proud ruler. (Italian) a form of Donna.
Donae, Donah, Donalda, Donaldina, Donelda, Donellia, Doni

Doña (Italian) a form of Donna.
Donail, Donalea, Donalisa, Donay

Donata (Latin) gift.
Donatha, Donathia, Donathiah, Donathya, Donathyah, Donato, Donatta, Donetta, Donette, Donita, Donnette, Donnita, Donte

Donatila (Latin) a form of Donata.

Doncia (Spanish) sweet.

Dondi (American) a familiar form of Donna.
Dondra, Dondrea, Dondria

Doneisha (American) a form of Danessa.
Donasha, Donashay, Doneishia

Donesha (American) a form of Danessa.

Doneshia (American) a form of Danessa.
Donneshia

Donetsi (Basque) a form of Benita.

Donia (Italian) a form of Donna.
Doni, Donie, Donise, Donitrae

Donielle (American) a form of Danielle.
Doniel, Doniele, Doniell, Donniel, Donniela, Donniele, Donniell, Donnielle, Donnyel, Donnyele, Donnyell, Donnyelle, Donyel, Donyele, Donyell, Donyelle

Donina (Latin) a form of Dorothy.

Donisha, Donnisha (American) forms of Danessa.
Donisa, Donishia, Donnisa, Donnise, Donnissa, Donnisse.

Donna (Italian) lady.
Dondi, Donnae, Donnah, Donnai, Donnalee, Donnalen, Donnay, Donnaya, Donne, Donnell, Donni, Donnie, Donny, Dontia

Donniella (American) a form of Danielle.
Donella, Doniela, Doniella, Donnella, Donniellah, Donnyela, Donnyella, Donyela, Donyelah, Donyella, Donyellah

Donosa (Latin) she who has grace and charm.

Donvina (Latin) vigorous.

Donya (Italian) a form of Donna.

Dora (Greek) gift. A short form of Adora, Eudora, Pandora, Theodora.
Dorah, Doralia, Doraliah, Doralie, Doralisa, Doraly, Doralynn, Doran, Dorana, Dorchen, Dorece, Doreece, Dorelia, Dorella, Dorelle, Doresha, Doressa, Doretta, Dorielle, Dorika, Doriley, Dorilis, Dorion, Dorita, Doro

Dorabella (English) a combination of Dora + Bella.
Dorabel, Dorabela, Dorabelah, Dorabele, Dorabell, Dorabellah, Dorabelle

Doralynn (English) a combination of Dora + Lynn.
Doralin, Doralina, Doraline, Doralyn, Doralyna, Doralynah, Doralyne, Doralynne, Dorlin

Dorbeta (Spanish) reference to the Virgin Mary.

Dorcas (Greek) gazelle. Bible: New Testament translation of the name Tabitha.

Doreen (Irish) moody, sullen. (French) golden. (Greek) a form of Dora.
Doreana, Doreanah, Doreena, Doreenah, Doreene, Dorena, Dorenah, Dorene, Dorin, Dorine, Doryn, Doryna, Dorynah, Doryne

Dores (Portuguese, Galician) a form of Dolores.

Doretta (American) a form of Dora, Dorothy.
Doret, Doreta, Doretah, Dorete, Doretha, Dorett, Dorettah, Dorette, Dorettie, Dorita, Doritah, Doritta, Dorittah, Doryta, Dorytah, Dorytta, Doryttah

Dori, Dory (American) familiar forms of Dora, Doria, Doris, Dorothy.
Dore, Dorey, Dorie, Dorree, Dorri, Dorrie, Dorry

Doria (Greek) a form of Dorian.
Doriah, Dorria, Dorrya, Dorryah, Dorya, Doryah

Dorian BG (Greek) from Doris, Greece.
Dorean, Doreane, Doriana, Doriann, Dorianna, Dorina, Dorinah, Dorriane

Doriane, Dorianne (Greek) from Doris, Greece.

Dorila (Greek) a form of Teodora.

Dorinda (Spanish) a form of Dora.
Dorindah, Dorynda, Doryndah

Doris (Greek) sea. Mythology: wife of Nereus and mother of the Nereids or sea nymphs.
Doreece, Doreese, Dorice, Dorisa, Dorise, Dorreece, Dorreese, Dorris, Dorrise, Dorrys, Dorryse, Dorys

Doroteia (Spanish) a form of Dorothy.

Dorotéia (Portuguese) a form of Dorothy.

Dorothea (Greek) a form of Dorothy. See also Thea.
Dorathia, Dorathya, Dorethea, Dorofia, Dorotea, Doroteya, Dorotha, Dorothia, Dorotthea, Dorottia, Dorottya, Dorthea, Dorthia, Doryfia, Doryfya

Dorothee (Greek) a form of Dorothy.

Dorothy (Greek) gift of God. See also Dasha, Dodie, Lolotea, Theodora.
Dasya, Do, Doa, Doe, Doortje, Dorathee, Dorathey, Dorathi, Dorathie, Dorathy, Dordei, Dordi, Dorefee, Dorethie, Doretta, Dorifey, Dorika, Doritha, Dorka, Dorle, Dorlisa, Doro, Dorofey, Dorolice, Dorosia, Dorota, Dorothey, Dorothi, Dorothie, Dorottya, Dorte, Dortha, Dorthy, Doryfey, Dosi, Dossie, Dosya

Dorrit (Greek) dwelling. (Hebrew) generation.
Dorit, Dorita, Dorite, Doritt, Doritte, Dorrite, Doryt, Doryte, Dorytt, Dorytte

Dottie, Dotty (Greek) familiar forms of Dorothy.
Dot, Dotea, Dotee, Dotey, Doti, Dotie, Dott, Dottea, Dottee, Dottey, Dotti, Doty

Dreama (English) dreamer.
Dreamah, Dreamar, Dreamara, Dreamare, Dreamaria, Dreamariah, Dreamarya, Dreamaryah, Dreema, Dreemah, Dreemar, Dreemara, Dreemarah, Dreemare, Dreemaria, Dreemariah, Dreemarya, Dreemaryah

Drew BG (Greek) courageous; strong. (Latin) a short form of Drusilla.
Drewa, Drewee, Drewia, Drewie, Drewy

Drina (Spanish) a form of Alexandrine.
Dreena, Drena, Drinah, Drinka, Dryna, Drynah

Drucilla (Latin) a form of Drusilla.
Drucela, Drucella, Drucill, Drucillah, Drucyla, Drucylah, Drucyle, Drucylla, Drucyllah, Drucylle, Druscila

Drue BG (Greek) a form of Drew.
Dru

Drusi (Latin) a short form of Drusilla.
Drucey, Druci, Drucie, Drucy, Drusey, Drusie, Drusy

Drusilla (Latin) descendant of Drusus, the strong one. See also Drew.
Drewcela, Drewcella, Drewcila, Drewcilla, Drewcyla, Drewcylah, Drewcylla, Drewcyllah, Drewsila, Drewsilah, Drewsilla, Drewsillah, Drewsyla, Drewsylah, Drewsylla, Drewsyllah, Druscilla, Druscille, Drusila, Drusilah, Drusillah, Drusille, Drusyla, Drusylah, Drusyle, Drusylla, Drusyllah, Drusylle

Drysi (Russian) one who comes from Demeter.

Duena (Spanish) chaperon.
Duenah, Duenna, Duennah

Dueña (Spanish) owner.

Dula (Greek) slave.

Dulce (Latin) sweet.
Delcina, Delcine, Douce, Douci, Doucie,

Dulcea, Dulcee, Dulcey, Dulci, Dulcia, Dulciana, Dulciane, Dulciann, Dulcianna, Dulcianne, Dulcibel, Dulcibela, Dulcibell, Dulcibella, Dulcibelle, Dulcie, Dulcy, Dulse, Dulsea, Dulsee, Dulsey, Dulsi, Dulsie, Dulsy

Dulcina, Dulcinia (Spanish) forms of Dulcinea.

Dulcinea (Spanish) sweet. Literature: Don Quixote's love interest.
Dulcine, Dulcinia

Duna (German) hill.

Dunia (Hebrew, Arabic) life.

Duquine, Duquinea (Spanish) forms of Dulcinea.

Durene (Latin) enduring.
Durean, Dureana, Dureanah, Dureane, Dureen, Dureena, Dureenah, Dureene, Durena, Durenah, Durin, Durina, Durinah, Durine, Duryn, Duryna, Durynah, Duryne

Duscha (Russian) soul; sweetheart; term of endearment.
Duschah, Dusha, Dushenka

Dusti (English) a familiar form of Dustin.
Dustea, Dustee, Dustey, Dustie

Dustin BG (German) valiant fighter. (English) brown rock quarry.
Dust, Dustain, Dustan, Dusten, Dustion, Duston, Dustyn, Dustynn

Dustine (German) a form of Dustin.
Dustean, Dusteana, Dusteanah, Dusteane, Dusteena, Dusteenah, Dusteene, Dustina, Dustinah, Dustyna, Dustynah, Dustyne

Dusty BG (English) a familiar form of Dustin.

Dyamond (Latin) a form of Diamond.
Dyamin, Dyamon, Dyamonda, Dyamondah, Dyamonde, Dyamone

Dyana, Dyanna (Latin) forms of Diana.
Dyaan, Dyaana, Dyaanah, Dyan, Dyanah, Dyane, Dyann, Dyanne, Dyhan, Dyhana, Dyhane, Dyhann, Dyhanna, Dyhanne

Dyani (Native American) deer.
Dianee, Dianey, Diani, Dianie, Diany, Dyanee, Dyaney, Dyanie, Dyany

Dylan **BG** (Welsh) sea.
Dylaan, Dylane, Dylanee, Dylanie, Dylann, Dylen, Dylin, Dyllan, Dylynn

Dylana (Welsh) a form of Dylan.
Dylaina, Dylanna

Dyllis (Welsh) sincere. See also Dilys.
Dylis, Dylissa, Dylissah, Dyllys, Dyllysa, Dyllyse, Dylys, Dylysa, Dylysah, Dylyse, Dylyss, Dylyssa, Dylyssah

Dymond (Latin) a form of Diamond.
Dymin, Dymon, Dymonda, Dymondah, Dymonde, Dymone, Dymonn, Dymont, Dymonte

Dympna (Irish) convenient.

Dynasty (Latin) powerful ruler.
Dynastee, Dynasti, Dynastie

Dyshawna (American) a combination of the prefix Dy + Shawna.
Dyshanta, Dyshawn, Dyshonda, Dyshonna

E

Eadda (English) wealthy; successful.
Eada, Eadah, Eaddah

Eadmund (English) a form of Edmunda.

Eadwine (English) a form of Edwina.

Earlene (Irish) pledge. (English) noblewoman.
Earla, Earlean, Earlecia, Earleen, Earleena, Earlena, Earlina, Earlinah, Earlinda, Earline, Earlyn, Earlyna, Earlynah, Earlyne

Earna (English) eagle.

Earnestyna (English) a form of Ernestina.

Eartha (English) earthy.
Earthah, Earthia, Earthiah, Earthya, Earthyah, Ertha, Erthah

Earwyn, Earwyna (English) forms of Erwina.

Easter (English) Easter time. History: a name for a child born on Easter.
Eastan, Eastera, Easterina, Easterine, Easteryn, Easteryna, Easteryne, Eastlyn, Easton

Eastre (Germanic) a form of Easter.

Eathelin, Eathelyn (English) noble waterfall.

Eavan (Irish) fair.
Eavana, Eavanah, Eavane

Ebe (Greek) youthful like a flower.

Eber (German) wild boar.

Ebone, Eboné, Ebonee, Eboney, Eboni, Ebonie (Greek) forms of Ebony.
Ebonne, Ebonnee, Ebonni, Ebonnie

Ebony (Greek) a hard, dark wood.
Abonee, Abony, Eban, Ebanee, Ebanie, Ebany, Ebbony, Ebeni, Ebonea, Ebonique, Ebonisha, Ebonye, Ebonyi

Ebrill (Welsh) born in April.

Echidna (Egyptian) wild boar.

Echo (Greek) repeated sound. Mythology: the nymph who pined for the love of Narcissus until only her voice remained.
Echoe, Ecko, Eco, Ekko, Ekkoe

Eda (Irish, English) a short form of Edana, Edith.
Edah

Edana (Irish) ardent; flame.
Edan, Edanah, Edanna

Edda (German) a form of Hedda.
Eddah

Eddy **BG** (American) a familiar form of Edwina.
Eady, Eddee, Eddey, Eddi, Eddie, Edee, Edey, Edi, Edie, Edy

Edelburga, Edilburga (English) noble protector.

Edelia, Edilia (Greek) remains young.

Edeline (English) noble; kind.
Adeline, Edelin, Edelina, Edelinah, Edelyn, Edelyna, Edelynah, Edelyne, Ediline, Edilyne, Edolina, Edoline

Edelira (Spanish) a form of Edelmira.

Edelma, Edilma (Greek) forms of Edelia.

Edelmira (Teutonic) known for her noble heritage.

Eden GB (Babylonian) a plain. (Hebrew) delightful. Bible: the earthly paradise.
Eaden, Edan, Ede, Edena, Edene, Edenia, Edin, Edine, Edon, Edona, Edonah, Edone, Edyn, Edyne

Edén (Hebrew) a form of Eden.

Edesia (Latin) feast.

Edeva (English) expensive present.
Eddeva, Eddevah, Eddeve, Edevah

Edgarda (Teutonic) defends her homeland.

Edian (Hebrew) decoration for God.
Edia, Edya, Edyah, Edyan

Edie (English) a familiar form of Edith.
Eadie, Edi, Edy, Edye, Eyde, Eydie

Edilberta (German) she who comes from a long heritage.

Ediltrudis (German) strong; noble.

Edina (English) prosperous fort.
Edena, Edenah, Edinah, Edyna, Edynah

Edisa (Castilian) a form of Esther.

Edith (English) rich gift. See also Dita.
Eadith, Eda, Ede, Edetta, Edette, Edie, Edit, Edita, Edite, Editha, Edithe, Editta, Ediva, Edyta, Edyth, Edytha, Edythe

Edlen (English) noble waterfall.

Edlyn (English) prosperous; noble.
Edlin, Edlina, Edline, Edlyna, Edlyne

Edmanda (English) a form of Edmunda.

Edmunda (English) prosperous protector.
Edmona, Edmonah, Edmonda, Edmondah, Edmondea, Edmondee, Edmondey, Edmuna, Edmunah, Edmundea, Edmundey

Edna (Hebrew) rejuvenation. Religion: the wife of Enoch, according to the Book of Enoch.
Adna, Adnisha, Ednah, Edneisha, Edneshia, Ednisha, Ednita, Edona

Edrea (English) a short form of Edrice, Edrianna.
Edra, Edrah, Edreah, Edria, Edriah, Edrya, Edryah

Edrianna (Greek) a form of Adrienne.
Edrena, Edriana, Edrina

Edrice (English) prosperous ruler.
Edrica, Edricah, Edricia, Edriciah, Edris, Edriss, Edrissa, Edrisse, Edryca, Edrycah, Edrycia, Edryciah, Edrycya, Edrycyah, Edrys, Edryss, Edryssa, Edrysse

Eduarda, Eduardo (English) forms of Edwardina.

Edurne (Basque) snow.

Eduviges (Teutonic) fighting woman.

Eduvigis, Eduvijis (German) victorious fighter.

Eduvixes (German) battle.

Edvina (German) a form of Edwina.

Edwardina (English) prosperous guardian.
Edwardinah, Edwardine, Edwardyna, Edwardynah, Edwardyne

Edwina (English) prosperous friend. See also Winnie.
Eddwina, Eddwinah, Eddwine, Eddwyn, Eddwyna, Eddwynah, Eddwyne, Eddy, Edween, Edweena, Edweenah, Edweene, Edwena, Edwinah, Edwine, Edwinna, Edwinnah, Edwinne, Edwyn, Edwyna, Edwynah, Edwyne, Edwynn

Effia (Ghanaian) born on Friday.

Effie (Greek) spoken well of. (English) a short form of Alfreda, Euphemia.
Efea, Efee, Effea, Effee, Effi, Effia, Effy, Efi, Efie, Efy, Ephie

Efigenia (Greek) a form of Eugenia.

Efigênia (Portuguese) a form of Eugenia.

Efrata (Hebrew) honored.
Efratah

Efrona (Hebrew) songbird.
Efronah, Efronna, Efronnah

Egberta (English) bright sword.
Egbertah, Egberte, Egbirt, Egbirte, Egburt, Egburte, Egbyrt, Egbyrte

Egbertina, Egbertine, Egbertyne (English) forms of Egberta.

Egda (Greek) shield bearer.

Egeria (Greek) she who gives encouragement.

Egida (Spanish) a form of Eladia.

Egidia (Greek) a form of Eladía.

Eglantina (French) wild rose.

Egle (Greek) she who possesses splendor and shine.

Eider (Basque) beautiful.

Eileen (Irish) a form of Helen. See also Aileen, Ilene.
Eilean, Eileana, Eileane, Eileena, Eileenah, Eileene, Eilena, Eilene, Eiley, Eilie, Eilieh, Eilina, Eiline, Eilleen, Eillen, Eilyn, Eleane, Eleen, Eleene, Elene, Elin, Elyn, Elyna, Eylean, Eyleana, Eyleen, Eyleena, Eylein, Eyleina, Eyleyn, Eyleyna, Eylin, Eylina, Eylyn, Eylyna

Eira (Welsh) snow.
Eir, Eirah, Eyr, Eyra, Eyrah

Eirene (Greek) a form of Irene.
Eereen, Eereena, Eereene, Eireen, Eireena, Eirena, Ereen, Ereena, Ereene, Erena, Eyren, Eyrena, Eyrene

Eiru (Indigenous) bee.

Eirween (Welsh) white snow.
Eirwena, Eirwenah, Eirwene, Eyrwen, Irwen, Irwena, Irwenah, Irwene

Ekaterina (Russian) a form of Katherine.
Ekaterine, Ekaterini

Ela (Polish) a form of Adelaide.
Elah, Ellah

Eladia (Greek) native of Elade, Greece.

Eladía (Greek) warrior with a shield of goat skin.

Elaina (French) a form of Helen.
Elainah, Elainea, Elainia, Elainna

Elaine (French) a form of Helen. See also Laine, Lainey.
Eilane, Elain, Elaini, Elane, Elani, Elanie, Elanit, Elauna, Elayn, Elayne, Ellaine

Elana (Greek) a short form of Eleanor. See also Ilana, Lana.
Elan, Elanah, Elanee, Elaney, Elania, Elanie, Elanna, Elannah, Elanne, Elanni, Ellana, Ellanah, Ellann, Ellanna, Ellannah

Elanora (Australian) from the shore.
Elanorah, Elanore, Ellanora, Ellanorah, Ellanore, Ellanorra, Ellanorrah, Ellanorre

Elata (Latin) elevated.

Elayna (French) a form of Elaina.
Elaynah, Elayne, Elayni

Elberta (English) a form of Alberta.
Elbertah, Elberte, Elbertha, Elberthina, Elberthine, Elbertina, Elbertine, Elbirta, Elbirtah, Elburta, Elburtah, Elbyrta, Elbyrtah, Ellberta, Ellbertah, Ellberte, Ellbirta, Ellbirtah, Ellburta, Ellburtah, Ellbyrta, Ellbyrtah

Elbertyna (Greek) one who comes from Greece.

Elcira (Teutonic) noble adornment.

Elda (German) she who battles.

Eldora (Spanish) golden, gilded.
Eldorah, Eldoree, Eldorey, Eldori, Eldoria, Eldorie, Eldory, Elldora, Elldorah

Eldrida (English) wise counselor.
Eldridah, Eldryda, Eldrydah, Eldryde

Eleadora (Spanish) a form of Eleodora.

Eleanor (Greek) light. History: Anna Eleanor Roosevelt was a U.S. delegate to the United Nations, a writer, and the thirty-second First Lady of the United States. See also Elana, Ella, Ellen, Helen, Leanore, Lena, Lenore, Leonor, Leora, Nellie, Nora, Noreen.
Alienor, Elanor, Elenor, Elenore, Eleonor, Eleonore, Elianore, Elladine, Elleanor, Elleanore, Ellenor, Elliner, Ellynor, Ellynore, Elna, Elnore, Elynor, Elynore

Eleanora (Greek) a form of Eleanor. See also Lena.
Alienora, Elenora, Elenorah, Eleonora, Elianora, Elinora, Elleanora, Ellenora, Ellenorah, Ellynora, Elyenora, Elynora, Elynorah

Eleanore (Greek) a form of Eleanor.

Electa (Greek) a form of Electra.

Electra (Greek) shining; brilliant. Mythology: the daughter of Agamemnon, leader of the Greeks in the Trojan War.
Electrah, Elektra, Elektrah

Eleebana (Australian) beautiful.
Elebana, Elebanah, Elebanna, Elebannah,
Eleebanna, Eleebannah

Elena (Greek) a form of Eleanor. (Italian) a
form of Helen.
Eleana, Eleen, Eleena, Elen, Elenah, Elene,
Elenitsa, Elenka, Elenna, Elenoa, Elenola,
Lena

Eleni (Greek) a familiar form of Eleanor.
Elenee, Elenie, Eleny

Eleodora, Eliodora (Greek) she who came
from the sun.

Eleora (Hebrew) the Lord is my light.
Eleorah, Eliora, Eliorah, Elioria, Elioriah,
Eliorya, Elioryah, Elira, Elora

Elesha (Greek, Hebrew) a form of Elisha.
Eleshia, Ellesha

Elethea, Elethia (English) healer.

Eletta (English) elf; mischievous.
Eleta, Eletah, Elete, Elett, Elettah, Elette,
Elletta, Ellette

Eleuia (Nahuatl) wish.

Eleusipa (Greek) she who arrives on horseback.

Eleuteria (Greek) liberty.

Eleutería, Eleuterio (Spanish) forms of
Eleuteria.

Elexis, Elexus (Greek) forms of Alexis.
Elexas, Elexes, Elexess, Elexeya, Elexia,
Elexiah, Elexius, Elexsus, Elexxus, Elexys

Élfega (German) brightness in the heights.

Elfelda (Spanish) tall; powerful.

Elfida, Élfida (Greek) daughter of the wind.

Élfreda (Greek) she who the geniuses protect.

Elfrida (German) peaceful. See also Freda.
Elfrea, Elfreda, Elfredah, Elfredda, Elfrede,
Elfreeda, Elfreyda, Elfride, Elfrieda, Elfriede,
Elfryda, Elfrydah

Elga (Norwegian) pious. (German) a form
of Helga.
Elgah, Elgar, Elgara, Elgiva

Eli 🅱🅶 (Hebrew) uplifted. See also Elli.
Ele, Elee, Elei, Eleigh, Eley, Elie, Ely

Elia 🅶🅱 (Hebrew) a short form of Eliana.
Eliah

Eliana (Hebrew) my God has answered me.
See also Iliana.
Elianah, Elianna, Eliannah, Elliana, Ellianah,
Ellianna, Elliannah, Ellyana, Ellyanah,
Elyana, Elyanah, Elyanna, Elyannah, Liana,
Liane

Eliane, Elianne (Hebrew) forms of Eliana.
Elliane, Ellianne, Ellyane, Ellyanne, Elyanne

Elicia (Hebrew) a form of Elisha. See also
Alicia.
Elecia, Eleecia, Eleesia, Elica, Elicea, Eliceah,
Elicet, Elichia, Eliciah, Eliscia, Ellecia,
Elleecia, Elleeciah, Ellesia, Ellicia, Elliciah

Elida (Latin) a form of Alida.
Elidee, Elidia, Elidy

Élida (Greek) Geography: the Olympic city
in ancient Greece.

Elide (Latin) a form of Elida.

Eligia (Italian, Spanish) chosen one.

Elijah 🅱🅶 (Hebrew) the Lord is my God.
Bible: a great Hebrew prophet.
Elia, Elian, Elija, Elijha, Elijiah, Elijio,
Elijsha, Elijuah, Elijuo, Eliya, Eliyah, Ellija,
Ellijah, Ellyjah

Elili (Tamil) beautiful.

Elimena (Latin) stranger.

Elina (Greek, Italian) a form of Elena.
(English) a form of Ellen.
Elinah, Elinda

Elinor (Greek) a form of Eleanor.
Elinore, Ellinor, Ellinore

Elionor (Greek) a form of Helen.

Elisa, Ellisa (Spanish, Italian, English) short
forms of Elizabeth. See also Alisa, Ilisa, Lisa.
Elecea, Eleesa, Elesa, Elesia, Elisah, Elisya,
Elleesa, Ellisia, Ellissa, Ellissia, Ellissya,
Ellisya

Elisabet (Hebrew) a form of Elizabeth.
Elisabeta, Elisabete, Elisabetta, Elisabette,

Elisebet, Elisebeta, Elisebete, Elisebett, Elisebetta, Elisebette

Elisabeth (Hebrew) a form of Elizabeth.
Elisabethe, Elisabith, Elisebeth, Elisheba, Elishebah, Ellisabeth, Elsabeth, Elysabeth

Elise (French, English) a short form of Elizabeth, Elysia. See also Ilise, Liese, Liset, Lissie.
Eilis, Eilise, Eleese, Elese, Elice, Elis, Élise, Elisee, Elisie, Elisse, Elizé, Elleece, Elleese, Ellice, Ellise, Ellyce, Ellyse, Ellyze, Elyce, Elyci, Elyze

Elisea (Hebrew) God is salvation; protect my health.

Elisenda (Hebrew) a form of Elisa.

Elisha BG (Hebrew) consecrated to God. (Greek) a form of Alisha. See also Ilisha, Lisha.
Eleacia, Eleasha, Eleesha, Eleeshia, Eleisha, Eleticia, Elishah, Elishia, Elishiah, Elishua, Eliska, Ellisha, Ellishah, Ellishia, Ellishiah, Elsha

Elisheva (Hebrew) a form of Elisabeth.
Elishevah

Elisia (Hebrew) a form of Elisha.
Elissia

Elissa (Greek, English) a form of Elizabeth. A short form of Melissa. See also Alissa, Alyssa, Lissa.
Elissah, Ellissa, Ilissa, Ilyssa

Elita (Latin, French) chosen. See also Lida, Lita.
Eleata, Eleatah, Eleeta, Eleetah, Eleita, Eleitah, Elitah, Elitia, Elitie, Ellita, Ellitia, Ellitie, Ellyt, Ellyta, Ellytah, Ellyte, Elyt, Elyta, Elytah, Elyte, Ilida, Ilita, Litia

Eliza (Hebrew) a short form of Elizabeth. See also Aliza.
Eliz, Elizah, Elizaida, Elizalina, Elize, Elizea, Elizeah, Elizza, Elizzah, Elliza, Ellizah, Ellizza, Ellizzah, Ellyza, Ellyzah, Elyza, Elyzah, Elyzza, Elyzzah

Elizabet (Hebrew) a form of Elizabeth.
Elizabeta, Elizabete, Elizabett, Elizabetta, Elizabette, Elizebet, Elizebeta, Elizebete, Elizebett, Ellizebet, Ellizebeta, Ellizebete, Ellysabet, Ellysabeta, Ellysabete, Ellysabett,

Ellysabetta, Ellysabette, Ellysebet, Ellysebeta, Ellysebete, Ellysebett, Ellysebetta, Ellysebette, Elsabet, Elsabete, Elsabett, Elysabet, Elysabeta, Elysabete, Elysabett

Elizabeth ⭐ GB (Hebrew) consecrated to God. Bible: the mother of John the Baptist. See also Bess, Beth, Betsy, Betty, Elsa, Ilse, Libby, Liese, Liesel, Lisa, Lisbeth, Liset, Lissa, Lissie, Liz, Liza, Lizabeta, Lizabeth, Lizbeth, Lizina, Lizzie, Veta, Yelisabeta, Zizi.
Alizabeth, Eliabeth, Elizabea, Elizabee, Ellizabeth, Elschen, Elysabeth, Elzbieta, Elzsébet, Helsa, Ilizzabet, Lusa

Elizaveta (Polish, English) a form of Elizabeth.
Elisavet, Elisaveta, Elisavetta, Elisveta, Elizavet, Elizavetta, Elizveta, Elsveta, Elzveta

Elizebeth (Hebrew) a form of Elizabeth.
Ellizebeth

Elka (Polish) a form of Elizabeth.
Elkah, Ilka, Ilkah

Elke (German) a form of Adelaide, Alice.
Elkee, Elkey, Elki, Elkie, Elky, Ilki

Ella ⭐ (English) elfin; beautiful fairy-woman. (Greek) a short form of Eleanor.
Ela, Elah, Ellah, Ellamae, Ellia

Elle (Greek) a short form of Eleanor. (French) she.
El, Ele, Ell

Ellen (English) a form of Eleanor, Helen.
Elen, Elene, Elenee, Elenie, Eleny, Elin, Eline, Ellan, Ellene, Ellin, Ellon

Ellena (Greek, Italian) a form of Elena. (English) a form of Ellen.
Ellenah

Ellery BG (English) elder-tree island.
Elari, Elarie, Elery, Ellari, Ellarie, Ellary, Ellerey, Elleri, Ellerie

Ellfreda (German) a form of Alfreda.

Elli, Ellie, Elly (English) short forms of Eleanor, Ella, Ellen. See also Eli.
Ellea, Elleah, Ellee, Ellei, Elleigh, Elley, Ellia, Elliah, Ellya

Ellice (English) a form of Elise.
Ellecia, Ellyce, Elyce

Ellis 🅱️🅶 (English) a form of Elias (see Boys' Names).
Elis, Ellys, Elys

Ellison 🅶🅱️ (English) child of Ellis.
Elison, Ellson, Ellyson, Elson, Elyson

Ellyn (English) a form of Ellen.
Ellyna, Ellynah, Ellyne, Ellynn, Ellynne, Elyn

Elma (Turkish) sweet fruit.
Ellma, Ellmah, Ellmar, Elmah, Elmar

Elmina (English) noble.
Almina, Alminah, Almyna, Almynah, Elminah, Elmyna, Elmynah

Elmira (Arabic, Spanish) a form of Almira.
Ellmara, Ellmarah, Elmara, Elmarah, Elmear, Elmeara, Elmearah, Elmeera, Elmeerah, Elmeira, Elmeirah, Elmera, Elmerah, Elmeria, Elmirah, Elmiria, Elmiriah, Elmyra, Elmyrah, Elmyria, Elmyriah, Elmyrya, Elmyryah

Elnora (American) a combination of Ella + Nora.

Elodie (English) a form of Alodie.
Elodea, Elodee, Elodey, Elodi, Elodia, Elodiah, Elody, Elodya, Elodyah, Elodye

Eloina (French) a form of Eloisa.

Eloína (Latin) predestined.

Eloisa (French) a form of Eloise.
Eloisia, Elouisa, Elouisah, Eloysa

Eloísa (Spanish) a form of Eloise.

Eloise (French) a form of Louise.
Elois, Elouise

Elora (American) a short form of Elnora.
Ellora, Elloree, Elorah, Elorie

Eloxochitl (Nahuatl) magnolia.

Elpidia, Elpidía (Greek) waits with faith.

Elsa (German) noble. (Hebrew) a short form of Elizabeth. See also Ilse.
Elcea, Ellsa, Ellsah, Ellse, Ellsea, Ellsia, Elsah, Else, Elsia, Elsje

Elsbeth (German) a form of Elizabeth.
Elsbet, Elsbeth, Elzbet, Elzbieta

Elsie (German) a familiar form of Elsa, Helsa.
Elcee, Elcey, Ellcee, Ellcey, Ellci, Ellcia, Ellcie,

Ellcy, Ellsee, Ellsey, Ellsi, Ellsia, Ellsie, Ellsy, Elsey, Elsi, Elsy

Elspeth (Scottish) a form of Elizabeth.
Elspet, Elspie

Elva (English) elfin. See also Alva, Alvina.
Elvah, Elvie

Elvera (Latin, Spanish, German) a form of Elvira.
Elverah

Elvia (English) a form of Elva.
Elviah, Elvya, Elvyah

Elvie (English) a form of Elva.
Elvea, Elvee, Elvey, Elvi, Elvy

Elvina (English) a form of Alvina.
Elveana, Elveanah, Elvena, Elvenah, Elvenea, Elvinah, Elvine, Elvinea, Elvinia, Elvinna, Elvinnia, Elvyna, Elvynah, Elvyne, Elvynia, Elvyniah, Elvynie, Elvynna, Elvynnah, Elvyny, Elvynya, Elvynyah, Elvynye

Elvira (Latin) white; blond. (German) closed up. (Spanish) elfin. Geography: the town in Spain that hosted a Catholic synod in 300 A.D.
Elvara, Elvarah, Elvirah, Elvire, Elvyra, Elvyrah, Elwira, Elwirah, Elwyra, Elwyrah, Vira

Elvisa (Teutonic) a form of Eloise.

Elvita (Spanish) truth.

Elycia (Hebrew) a form of Elisha.
Ellycia

Elysa (Spanish, Italian, English) a form of Elisa.
Ellysa, Elyssia, Elyssya, Elysya

Elyse (French, English) a form of Elise. (Latin) a form of Elysia.
Ellyse, Elyce, Elys, Elysee, Elysse

Elysha (Hebrew) a form of Elisha.
Ellysha, Ellyshah, Ellyshia, Ellyshiah, Ellyshya, Ellyshyah, Elyshia

Elysia (Greek) sweet; blissful. Mythology: Elysium was the dwelling place of happy souls.
Elishia, Ellysia, Ellysiah, Elysiah, Elysya, Elysyah, Ilysha, Ilysia

Elyssa (Greek, English) a form of Elissa. (Latin) a form of Elysia.
Ellyssa, Elyssah

Ema (German) a form of Emma.
Emah

Emalee, Emaleigh, Emalie, Emaly (American) forms of Emily.
Emaili, Emaily, Emalea, Emali, Emalia

Eman **BG** (Arabic) a short form of Emani.

Emani (Arabic) a form of Iman.
Emane, Emaneé, Emanie, Emann

Emanuelle (Hebrew) a form of Emmanuelle.
Emanual, Emanuel, Emanuela, Emanuele, Emanuell, Emanuella, Emanuellah

Emari (German) a form of Emery.
Emarri

Ember (French) a form of Amber.
Emberlee, Emberly

Emelia (Latin) a form of Amelia.

Emelie, Emely (Latin) forms of Emily.
Emeli, Emelita, Emellie, Emelly

Emelinda (Teutonic) a form of Emily.

Emeline (French) a form of Emily.
Emelin, Emelina

Emerald (French) bright green gemstone.
Emelda, Emeldah, Emmarald, Emmerald

Emeralda (Spanish) a form of Emerald.

Emerenciana (Latin) she who will be rewarded.

Emerita (Latin) a form of Emerenciana.

Emérita (Latin) veteran; licensed.

Emery **BG** (German) industrious leader.
Emeri, Emerie, Emerre

Emesta (Spanish) serious.

Emeteria (Greek) half lion.

Emie, Emmie (German) forms of Emmy.
Emi, Emiy, Emmi

Emile **BG** (English) a form of Emily.
Emilea, Emilei, Émilie, Emiliee, Emillee, Emillie, Emmélie, Emmilee, Emmilei,

Emmileigh, Emmiley, Emmili, Emmilie, Emmilly, Emmilye

Emilee, Emileigh, Emiley, Emili, Emilie, Emilly, Emmily (English) forms of Emily.

Emilia (Italian) a form of Amelia, Emily.
Emila, Emilea, Emileah, Emiliah, Emilya, Emilyah, Emmilea, Emmileah, Emmilia, Emmilya

Emilse (German) a combination of Emily + Ilse.

Emily ✨ **GB** (Latin) flatterer. (German) industrious. See also Amelia, Emma, Millie.
Eimile, Émilie, Emilis, Emilye, Emmaley, Emmaly, Emmélie, Emyle

Emilyann (American) a combination of Emily + Ann.
Emileane, Emileann, Emileanna, Emileanne, Emiliana, Emiliann, Emilianna, Emilianne, Emillyane, Emillyann, Emillyanna, Emillyanne, Emliana, Emliann, Emlianna, Emlianne

Emilyn (American) a form of Emmalynn.
Emilynn, Emilynne

Emma ✨ (German) a short form of Emily. See also Amy.
Em, Emmah

Emmalee, Emmalie (American) combinations of Emma + Lee. Forms of Emily.
Emalea, Emalee, Emilee, Emmalea, Emmaleah, Emmalei, Emmaleigh, Emmaley, Emmali, Emmalia, Emmaliah, Emmaliese, Emmaly, Emmalya, Emmalye, Emmalyse

Emmaline (French) a form of Emily.
Emalin, Emalina, Emaline, Emilienne, Emilina, Emiline, Emillin, Emillina, Emilline, Emmalene, Emmalin, Emmalina, Emmelin, Emmilin, Emmilina, Emmiline, Emmilyn, Emmilyna, Emmilyne, Emmylin, Emmylina, Emmyline, Emylin, Emylina, Emyline

Emmalynn (American) a combination of Emma + Lynn.
Emalyn, Emalyna, Emalyne, Emelyn, Emelyna, Emelyne, Emelynne, Emlyn, Emlynn, Emlynne, Emmalyn, Emmalynne, Emylyn, Emylyna, Emylyne

Emmanuelle (Hebrew) God is with us.
Emmanuela, Emmanuele, Emmanuell,
Emmanuella, Emmanuellah

Emmeline (French) a form of Emmaline.
Emmelina

Emmy, Emy (German) familiar forms of
Emma.
Emmey, Emmye

Emmylou (American) a combination of
Emmy + Lou.
Emiloo, Emilou, Emilu, Emlou, Emmalou,
Emmelou, Emmiloo, Emmilou, Emmilu,
Emmyloo, Emmylu, Emylou, Emylu

Emna (Teutonic) a form of Emma.

Emory 🅱🅶 (German) a form of Emery.
Amory, Emmo, Emmori, Emmorie, Emmory,
Emorye

Emperatriz (Latin) empress.

Emylee (American) a form of Emily.

Ena, Enna (Irish) forms of Helen.
Enah

Enara (Basque) swallow.

Enat (Irish) little.

Encarna, Encarnita (Spanish) forms of
Encarnación.

Encarnación (Latin) incarnation of Jesus in
his mother, Mary.

Enchantra (English) enchanting.
Enchantrah, Enchantria, Enchantrya,
Enchantryah

Endora (Hebrew) fountain.
Endorah, Endorra, Endorrah

Enedina (Greek) warm; indulgent.

Engel (Greek) a form of Angel.
Engele, Engell, Engelle, Enjel, Enjele, Enjell,
Enjelle

Engela (Greek) a form of Angela.
Engelah, Engella, Engellah, Enjela, Enjelah,
Enjella

Engelica (Greek) a form of Angelica.
Engelika, Engeliqua, Engeliquah, Engelique,
Engelyca, Engelycka, Enjelliqua, Enjellique,
Enjellyca, Enjellycah, Enjellycka, Enjellyka,

Enjellykah, Enjellyqua, Enjellyquah,
Enjellyque

Engracia (Spanish) graceful.
Engrace, Engracee, Engraciah, Engracya,
Engrasia, Engrasiah, Engrasya

Enid (Welsh) life; spirit.
Enida, Ennid, Ennida, Ennyd, Ennyda,
Enyd, Enyda, Enydah

Enimia (Greek) well dressed.

Ennata (Greek) ninth.

Enrica (Spanish) a form of Henrietta. See
also Rica.
Enricah, Enrichetta, Enricka, Enrickah,
Enrieta, Enrietta, Enriette, Enrika, Enrikah,
Enrikka, Enrikkah, Enrikke, Enriqua,
Enrique, Enriqueta, Enriquetta, Enriquette,
Enryca, Enrycah, Enryka, Enrykah

Enricua (Spanish) ruler.

Enya (Scottish) jewel; blazing.
Enia, Eniah, Enyah

Enye (Hebrew) grace.

Epifana, Epifanía (Spanish) forms of
Epiphany.

Epiphany (Greek) manifestation. Religion: a
Christian feast on January 6 celebrating the
manifestation of Jesus' divine nature to the
Magi. See also Theophania.
Ephana, Epifanee, Epifaney, Epifani, Epifania,
Epifanie, Epiphanee, Epiphaney, Epiphani,
Epiphania, Epiphanie, Epyfanee, Epyfaney,
Epyfani, Epyfania, Epyfanie, Epyfany,
Epyphanee, Epyphaney, Epyphani,
Epyphania, Epyphanie, Epyphany

Eppie (English) a familiar form of
Euphemia.
Eppy

Erasma (Greek) lovable.
Erasmah

Ercilia, Ercilla (Greek) delicate; gentle.

Erda (Anglo-Saxon) Mythology: an earth
goddess after which the planet Earth is
named.

Erea (Galician) a form of Irene.

Erela (Hebrew) angel.
Elelah, Erell, Erella, Erellah

Erendira, Eréndira, Erendiria (Spanish) one with a smile.

Eres (Welsh) beautiful.

Erica (Scandinavian) ruler of all. (English) brave ruler. See also Arica, Rica, Ricki.
Ericah, Ericca, Ericha, Eriqua, Erique, Errica, Eryca, Erycah

Érica (German) a form of Erica.

Ericka (Scandinavian) a form of Erica.
Erickah, Erricka

Erika, Erikka (Scandinavian) forms of Erica.
Erikaa, Erikah, Errika, Eryka, Erykah, Erykka, Eyrika

Erin ✰ GB (Irish) peace. History: another name for Ireland. See also Arin.
Earin, Earrin, Eran, Erana, Eren, Erena, Erenah, Erene, Ereni, Erenia, Ereniah, Eri, Erian, Erina, Erine, Erinete, Erinett, Erinetta

Erinn, Errin (Irish) forms of Erin.
Erinna, Erinnah, Erinne

Erline (Irish) a form of Arlene.
Erla, Erlana, Erlean, Erleana, Erleanah, Erleane, Erleen, Erleena, Erleene, Erlene, Erlenne, Erlin, Erlina, Erlinda, Erlisha, Erlyn, Erlyna, Erlynah, Erlyne

Erma (Latin) a short form of Ermine, Hermina. See also Irma.
Ermelinda

Ermenburga (German) strong city.

Ermengarda (German) where strength dwells.

Ermengardis (German) strong garden.

Ermenilda (German) powerful warrior.

Ermerinda (Latin) a form of Erma.

Ermine (Latin) a form of Hermina.
Ermin, Ermina, Erminda, Erminia, Erminie

Ermitana (Greek) sparsely populated place.

Erna (English) a short form of Ernestine.

Ernestina (English) a form of Ernestine.
Ernesta, Ernesztina

Ernestine (English) earnest, sincere.
Erna, Ernaline, Ernesia

Ernesto (Germanic) a form of Ernestine.

Erosina (Greek) erotic lady.

Erundina (Latin) like a swallow.

Erwina, Erwyna (English) sea friend.

Eryn, Erynn (Irish) forms of Erin.
Eiryn, Eryna, Eryne, Erynna, Erynnah, Erynne

Escama, Escame (Spanish) forms of Escarna.

Escarna, Escarne, Eskarne (Spanish) merciful.

Escolástica (Latin) she who knows much and teaches.

Eshe (Swahili) life.
Eisha, Esha, Eshah

Esmé (French) a familiar form of Esmeralda. A form of Amy.
Esma, Esmae, Esmah, Esmai, Esmay, Esme, Esmëe, Esmei, Esmey

Esmerada (Latin) shining; standing out.

Esmeralda (Greek, Spanish) a form of Emerald.
Esmaralda, Esmerelda, Esmerilda, Esmiralda, Ezmerelda, Ezmirilda

Esperanza (Spanish) hope. See also Speranza.
Esparanza, Espe, Esperance, Esperans, Esperansa, Esperanta, Esperanz, Esperenza

Essence (Latin) life; existence.
Essa, Essenc, Essencee, Essences, Essenes, Essense, Essynce

Essie (English) a short form of Estelle, Esther.
Essa, Essey, Essy

Estaquia (Spanish) possessor of a head of wheat.

Estebana (Spanish) a form of Stephanie.

Estee (English) a short form of Estelle, Esther.
Esta, Estée, Estey, Esti, Estie, Esty

Estefani, Estefany (Spanish) forms of Stephanie.
Estefane, Estefanie

Estefaní, Estéfani, Estéfany (Spanish) forms of Stephanie.

Estefania (Spanish) a form of Stephanie.
Estafania, Estefana

Estefanía (Greek) a form of Stephanie.

Estela, Estella (French) forms of Estelle.
Estelah, Esteleta, Estelita, Estellah, Estellita, Esthella

Estelinda (Teutonic) she who is noble and protects the village.

Estelle (French) a form of Esther. See also Stella, Trella.
Estel, Estele, Esteley, Estelin, Estelina, Esteline, Estell, Estellin, Estellina, Estelline, Esthel, Esthela, Esthele, Esthell, Esthelle

Estephanie, Estephany (Spanish) forms of Stephanie.
Estephani, Estephania

Ester (Persian) a form of Esther.
Estera, Esterre

Éster, Ésther (Spanish) forms of Esther.

Esterina (Greek) strong and vital.

Estervina (German) friend from the east.

Esteva, Estevana (Greek) forms of Stephanie.

Esther (Persian) star. Bible: the Jewish captive whom Ahasuerus made his queen. See also Hester.
Estar, Esthur, Eszter, Eszti

Estíbalitz (Basque) sweet as honey.

Estíbaliz (Castilian) a form of Estíbalitz.

Estila (Latin) column.

Estrada (Latin) road.

Estralita (Spanish) a form of Estrella.

Estrella (French) star.
Estrela, Estrelah, Estrele, Estrelinha, Estrell, Estrelle, Estrelleta, Estrellita, Estrelyta, Estrelytah, Estrilita, Estrilyta, Estrylita, Estrylyta

Etaina (Celtic) she who shines.

Etapalli (Nahuatl) wing.

Etel (Spanish) a short form of Etelvina.

Etelburga (English) a form of Edelburga.

Etelinda (German) noble one who protects her village.

Etelreda (German) noble advice.

Etelvina (German) loyal and noble friend.

Eteria (Greek) pure air.

Eternity (Latin) eternity.

Ethana (Hebrew) strong; firm.
Ethanah, Ethena, Ethenah

Ethel (English) noble.
Ethela, Ethelah, Ethelda, Ethelin, Ethelina, Etheline, Ethella, Ethelle, Ethelyn, Ethelyna, Ethelyne, Ethelynn, Ethelynna, Ethelynne, Ethyl

Etienne 🅱🅶 (French) a form of Stephan (see Boys' Names).
Ètienne

Etilka (Hebrew) noble.

Étoile (French) star.
Etoila, Etoilah, Etoyla, Etoylah, Etoyle

Etta (German) little. (English) a short form of Henrietta.
Etka, Etke, Ettah, Etti, Ettie, Etty, Ety, Itke, Itta

Euda (German) childhood.

Eudocia, Eudosia, Eudoxia (Greek) famous; knowledgeable.

Eudora (Greek) honored gift. See also Dora.
Eudorah, Eudore

Eufonia (Greek) she who has a beautiful voice.

Eufrasia (Greek) she who is full of joy.

Eufrosina (Greek) joyful thought.

Eugena (Greek) a form of Eugenia.

Eugenia (Greek) born to nobility. See also Gina, Yevgenia.
Eugeena, Eugeenah, Eugeenia, Eugeeniah, Eugeniah, Eugenina, Eugina, Eugyna,

Eugynah, Eugynia, Eugyniah, Eujania,
Eujaniah, Eujanya, Eujanyah, Evgenia,
Evgeniah, Evgenya, Evgenyah

Eugênia (Portuguese) a form of Eugenia.

Eugenie (Greek) a form of Eugenia.
Eugeenee, Eugeeney, Eugeeni, Eugeenie,
Eugenee, Eugeney, Eugeni, Eugénie, Eugine,
Eugynie, Eugyny, Eujanee, Eujaney, Eujani,
Eujanie, Eujany

Eulalia (Greek) well-spoken. See also Ula.
Eula, Eulah, Eulalea, Eulalee, Eulalie,
Eulalya, Eulalyah, Eulia, Euliah, Eulya,
Eulyah

Eulália (Portuguese) a form of Eulalia.

Eulampia (Greek) brilliant.

Eulogia (Greek) a form of Eulalia.

Eumelia (Greek) she who sings well.

Eun (Korean) silver.
Euna, Eunah

Eunice (Greek) happy; victorious. Bible: the
mother of Saint Timothy. See also Unice.
Euna, Eunique, Eunise, Euniss, Eunisse,
Eunys, Eunysa, Eunysah, Eunyse

Eunomia (Greek) good order.

Euphemia (Greek) spoken well of, in good
repute. History: a fourth-century Christian
martyr. See also Phemie.
Effam, Eppie, Eufemia, Eufemiah, Euphan,
Euphemie, Euphemy, Euphemya, Euphemyah,
Euphie

Euporia (Greek) she who has a beautiful
voice.

Eurídice (Greek) a form of Eurydice.

Eurneid (Russian) child of Clydno.

Eurosia (Greek) eloquent.

Eurydice (Greek) wide, broad. Mythology:
the wife of Orpheus.
Euridice, Euridyce, Eurydyce

Eusebia (Greek) respectful; pious.

Eustacia (Greek) productive. (Latin) stable;
calm. See also Stacey.
Eustaciah, Eustacya, Eustasia, Eustasiah,
Eustasya, Eustasyah

Eustaquia (Greek) well-built.

Eustolia (Greek) agile.

Eustoquia (Greek) good mother.

Eutalia (Greek) abundant.

Euterpe (Greek) walks with grace.

Eutimia (Spanish) benevolent.

Eutiquia (Greek) she who entertains.

Eutropia (Greek) good character.

Euxenia (Greek) from a good family name.

Eva (Greek) a short form of Evangelina.
(Hebrew) a form of Eve. See also Ava,
Chava.
Éva, Evah, Evalea, Evaleah, Evalee, Evalei,
Evaleigh, Evaley, Evali, Evalia, Evalie, Evaly,
Evike, Evva, Ewa, Ewah

Evaline (French) a form of Evelyn.
Evalean, Evaleana, Evaleanah, Evaleane,
Evaleen, Evaleena, Evaleenah, Evaleene,
Evalene, Evalin, Evalina, Evalyn, Evalyna,
Evalynah, Evalyne, Evalynn, Evalynne

Evan BG (Irish) young warrior. (English) a
form of John (see Boys' Names).
Eoin, Ev, Evaine, Evann, Evans, Even, Evens,
Evin, Evon, Evun, Ewan, Ewen

Evangelina (Greek) bearer of good news.
Evangeleana, Evangeleanah, Evangeleena,
Evangelia, Evangelica, Evangeliqua, Evangelique,
Evangelista, Evangelyna, Evangelynah

Evangeline (Greek) a form of Evangelina.
Evangeleane, Evangeleene, Evangelene,
Evangelyn, Evangelyne, Evangelynn

Evania (Greek, Irish) a form of Evan.
Evana, Evanah, Evania, Evaniah, Evanja,
Evanjah, Evanka, Evanna, Evannah, Evanne,
Evannja, Evannjah, Evanny, Evannya, Evany,
Evanya, Evanyah, Eveania, Evvanne,
Evvunea, Evyan

Evanthe (Greek) flower.
Evantha

Evarista (Greek) excellent one.

Eve (Hebrew) life. Bible: the first woman
created by God. (French) a short form of
Evonne. See also Hava, Naeva, Vica, Yeva.
Eav, Eave, Evita, Evuska, Evyn

Eve Marie (English) a combination of Eve + Marie.
Eve-Marie

Evelia (Hebrew) a form of Eve.

Evelin, Eveline, Evelyne (English) forms of Evelyn.
Evelean, Eveleane, Eveleen, Eveleene, Evelen, Evelene

Evelina (English) a form of Evelyn.
Eveleanah, Eveleeana, Eveleena, Eveleenah, Evelena, Evelenah, Evelinah, Evelyna, Evelynah, Ewalina

Evelyn ★ GB (English) hazelnut. See also Avaline.
Evaline, Eveleen, Evelene, Evelynn, Evelynne, Evline

Everett BG (German) courageous as a boar.

Everilda (German) a form of Everett.

Evette (French) a form of Yvette. A familiar form of Evonne. See also Ivette.
Evet, Evete, Evett

Evie (Hungarian) a form of Eve.
Evee, Evey, Evi, Evicka, Evike, Evka, Evuska, Evvee, Evvey, Evvi, Evvia, Evvie, Evvy, Evvya, Evy, Ewa

Evita (Spanish) a form of Eve.
Eveta, Evetah, Evetta, Evettah, Evitta, Evyta, Evytta

Evline (English) a form of Evelyn.
Evleen, Evlene, Evlin, Evlina, Evlyn, Evlynn, Evlynne

Evodia (Greek) she who wishes others a good trip.

Evonne (French) a form of Yvonne. See also Ivonne.
Evanne, Evenie, Evenne, Eveny, Evona, Evonah, Evone, Evoni, Evonn, Evonna, Evonnie, Evonny, Evony, Evyn, Evynn, Eyona, Eyvone

Exal (Spanish) a short form of Exaltación.

Exaltación (Spanish) exalted, lifted up.

Expedita (Greek) ready to fight.

Expósita (Latin) exposed.

Exuperancia (Latin) abundant.

Exuperia (Latin) a form of Exuperancia.

Eyén (Aboriginal) break of day.

Eyota BG (Native American) great.
Eyotah

Ezmeralda (Spanish) a form of Esmeralda.

Ezrela (Hebrew) reaffirming faith.
Esrela, Esrelah, Esrele, Esrell, Esrella, Esrellah, Esrelle, Ezrelah, Ezrele, Ezrella, Ezrellah, Ezrelle

Ezri (Hebrew) helper; strong.
Ezra, Ezrah, Ezria, Ezriah, Ezrya, Ezryah

Eztli (Nahuatl) blood.

F

Fabia (Latin) bean grower.
Fabiah, Fabra, Fabria, Fabya, Fabyah

Fabiana (Latin) a form of Fabia.
Fabianah, Fabianna, Fabiannah, Fabienna, Fabiennah, Fabyana, Fabyanah, Fabyanna, Fabyannah

Fabienne (Latin) a form of Fabia.
Fabian, Fabiann, Fabianne, Fabiene, Fabienn, Fabyan, Fabyane, Fabyann, Fabyanne

Fabiola (Latin) a form of Fabia.
Fabiolah, Fabiole, Fabyola

Fabricia (Latin) a form of Fabrizia.

Fabrienne (French) little blacksmith; apprentice.
Fabreanne, Fabrian, Fabriana, Fabrianah, Fabriann, Fabrianna, Fabriannah, Fabrianne, Fabrien, Fabriena, Fabrienah, Fabrienn, Fabrienna, Fabriennah, Fabryan, Fabryana, Fabryanah, Fabryane, Fabryann, Fabryanna, Fabryannah, Fabryanne, Fabryen, Fabryena, Fabryenah, Fabryene, Fabryenn, Fabryenna, Fabryennah, Fabryenne

Fabrizia (Italian) craftswoman.
Fabriziah, Fabrizya, Fabrizyah, Fabryzia, Fabryziah, Fabryzya, Fabryzyah

Facunda (Latin) eloquent speaker.

Fadila (Arabic) generous.
Fadilah, Fadyla, Fadylah

Faina (English) happy.
Fainah, Faine, Fayin, Fayina, Fayinah,
Fayine, Fayna, Faynah, Fayne, Feana,
Feanah, Fenna

Fairlee (English) from a yellow meadow.
Faileah, Fairlea, Fairlei, Fairleigh, Fairley,
Fairli, Fairlia, Fairliah, Fairlie, Fairly, Fairlya,
Fayrlea, Fayrleah, Fayrlee, Fayrlei, Fayrleigh,
Fayrley, Fayrli, Fayrlia, Fayrliah, Fayrlie,
Fayrly, Fayrlya

Faith ☆ (English) faithful; fidelity. See also
Faye, Fidelity.
Faeth, Faethe, Faithe

Faiza, Faizah (Arabic) victorious.
Fayza, Fayzah

Falda (Icelandic) folded wings.
Faida, Faldah, Fayda, Faydah

Falicia (Latin) a form of Felicia.
Falecia, Faleshia

Faline (Latin) catlike.
Falean, Faleana, Faleanah, Faleane, Faleen,
Faleena, Faleenah, Faleene, Falena, Falene,
Falin, Falina, Falinah, Falinia, Faliniah,
Fallin, Fallina, Fallinah, Falline, Faylina,
Fayline, Faylyn, Faylynn, Faylynne, Felenia,
Felina, Felinah, Feline, Felinia, Feliniah,
Felyn, Felyna, Felynah, Felyne

Falisha (Latin) a form of Felicia.
Faleisha, Falesha, Falleshia

Fallon (Irish) grandchild of the ruler.
Fallan, Fallann, Fallanna, Fallannah,
Fallanne, Fallen, Fallenn, Fallenna, Fallennah,
Fallenne, Fallona, Fallonah, Fallone, Fallonia,
Falloniah, Fallonne, Fallonya, Fallonyah

Falon (Irish) a form of Fallon.
Falan, Falen, Phalon

Falviana (Spanish) a form of Flavia.

Falyn (Irish) a form of Fallon.
Fallyn, Fallyne, Falyna, Falynah, Falyne,
Falynn, Falynne

Fanchone (French) freedom.
Fanchon, Fanchona, Fanchonah

Fancy (French) betrothed. (English) whimsi-
cal; decorative.
Fancee, Fanchette, Fanci, Fancia, Fancie

Fannie, Fanny (American) familiar forms of
Frances.
Fan, Fanette, Fani, Fania, Fannee, Fanney,
Fanni, Fannia

Fantasia (Greek) imagination.
Fantasy, Fantasya, Fantaysia, Fantazia, Fiantasi

Fany (American) a form of Fannie.
Fanya

Faqueza (Spanish) weakness.

Farah, Farrah (English) beautiful; pleasant.
Fara, Faria, Fariah, Farra, Farria, Farriah,
Farrya, Farryah, Farya, Faryah, Fayre

Faren, Farren (English) wanderer.
Faran, Farana, Farane, Fare, Farin, Farine,
Faron, Faronah, Farrahn, Farran, Farrand,
Farrin, Farron, Farryn, Faryn, Feran, Ferin,
Feron, Ferran, Ferren, Ferrin, Ferron, Ferryn

Faría (Hebrew) pharaoh.

Farica (German) peaceful ruler.
Faricah, Faricka, Farika, Farikah, Fariqua,
Fariquah, Farique, Faryca, Farycah, Farycka,
Faryka, Faryqua, Faryquah, Faryque

Farida (Arabic) unique.

Fariha (Muslim, Arabic) happy, joyful, cheerful, glad.
Farihah

Fatema (Arabic) a form of Fatima.

Fátim, Fátima (Arabic) forms of Fatima.

Fatima (Arabic) daughter of the prophet.
History: the daughter of Muhammad.
Fathma, Fatime, Fattim, Fatyma, Fatymah

Fatimah (Arabic) a form of Fatima.

Fatma, Fatme (Arabic) short forms of
Fatima.
Fatmah

Faustine (Latin) lucky, fortunate.
Fausta, Faustah, Faustean, Fausteana,
Fausteanah, Fausteane, Fausteen, Fausteena,
Fausteenah, Fausteene, Faustin, Faustina,
Faustinah, Faustyn, Faustyna, Faustynah,
Faustyne

Favia (Latin) a form of Fabia.

Faviola (Latin) a form of Fabia.
Faviana, Faviolha

Fawn (French) young deer.
Faun, Faune, Fawne

Fawna (French) a form of Fawn.
Fauna, Faunah, Faunia, Fauniah, Fauny,
Faunya, Faunyah, Fawnah, Fawnia, Fawniah,
Fawnna, Fawny, Fawnya, Fawnyah

Faxon BG (German) long-haired.
Faxan, Faxana, Faxanah, Faxane, Faxann,
Faxanna, Faxannah, Faxanne, Faxen, Faxin,
Faxina, Faxinah, Faxine, Faxyn, Faxyna,
Faxynah, Faxyne

Fay (French, English) a form of Faye.

Fayana (French) a form of Faye.
Fayanah, Fayann, Fayanna, Fayannah,
Fayanne

Faye (French) fairy; elf. (English) a form of
Faith.
Fae, Fai, Faie, Faya, Fayah, Fayana, Fayette,
Fei, Fey, Feya, Feyah, Feye

Fayette (French) a form of Faye.
Fayet, Fayett, Fayetta, Fayettah

Fayola (Nigerian) lucky.
Faiola, Faiolah, Fayla, Fayolah, Feyla

Fayre (English) fair; light haired.
Fair, Faira, Faire, Fairey, Fairy, Faree, Farey,
Fari, Farie, Fary, Farye, Fayree, Fayrey, Fayri,
Fayrie, Fayry

Fayruz (Arabic) Turkish woman.

Faythe (English) a form of Faith.
Fayeth, Fayethe, Fayth

Fe (Latin) trust; belief.

Febe (Greek) a form of Phoebe.
Feba, Febo, Feebe, Feebea, Feebee, Fibee

Febronia (Latin) sacrifice of atonement.

Fedra (Greek) splendid one.

Feena (Irish) small fawn.
Feana, Feanah, Feenah

Felberta (English) brilliant.

Felecia (Latin) a form of Felicia.
Flecia

Felecidade (Portuguese) a form of Felicity.

Felica (Spanish) a short form of Felicia.
Falica, Falisa, Felisca, Felissa, Feliza

Felice (Latin) a short form of Felicia.
Felece, Felicie, Felis, Felise, Felize, Felyc,
Felyce, Felycie, Felycye, Felys, Felyse, Felysie,
Felysse, Felysye

Felicia (Latin) fortunate; happy. See also
Lecia, Phylicia.
Fela, Feliciah, Feliciana, Felicidad, Felicija,
Felicitas, Felicya, Felisea, Felisia, Felisiah,
Felissya, Felita, Felixia, Felizia, Felka, Fellcia,
Felycia, Felyciah, Felycya, Felycyah, Felysia,
Felysiah, Felyssia, Felysya, Felysyah, Filicia,
Filiciah, Fleasia, Fleichia, Fleishia, Flichia

Feliciana (Italian, Spanish) a form of Felicia.
Felicianna, Felicijanna, Feliciona, Felicyanna,
Felicyanne, Felisiana

Felicidade (Latin) a form of Felicity.

Felicísima (Spanish) a form of Felicity.

Felicitas (Italian) a form of Felicia.
Felicita, Felicitah, Felicyta, Felicytah, Felicytas,
Felisita, Felycita, Felycitah, Felycyta,
Felycytah, Felycytas

Felícitas (Spanish) a form of Felicity.

Felicity (English) a form of Felicia.
Falicitee, Falicitey, Faliciti, Falicitia, Falicitie,
Falicity, Félicité, Felicitee, Felicitey, Feliciti,
Felicitia, Felicitie, Felisity, Felycytee, Felycytey,
Felycyti, Felycytie, Felycyty

Felícula (Latin) kitty.

Felisa (Latin) a form of Felicia.

Felisha (Latin) a form of Felicia.
Feleasha, Feleisha, Felesha, Felishia, Fellishia,
Felysha, Flisha

Femi (French) woman. (Nigerian) love me.
Femia, Femiah, Femie, Femmi, Femmie,
Femy, Femya, Femyah

Fenella (Irish) a form of Fionnula.
Fenel, Fenell, Fenellah, Fenelle, Fennal,
Fennall, Fennalla, Fennallah, Fennella,
Fennelle, Finel, Finell, Finella, Finellah,
Finelle, Finnal, Finnala, Finnall, Finnalla,
Finnallah, Finnalle, Fynela, Fynelah, Fynele,
Fynell, Fynella, Fynelle, Fynnela, Fynnelah,

Fynnele, Fynnell, Fynnella, Fynnellah,
Fynnelle

Fenna (Irish) fair-haired.
Fena, Fenah, Fennah, Fina, Finah, Finna,
Finnah, Fyna, Fynah, Fynna, Fynnah

Feodora (Greek) gift of God.
Fedora, Fedorah, Fedoria, Fedorra, Fedorrah

Fermina (Spanish) strong.

Fern (English) fern. (German) a short form
of Fernanda.
Ferna, Fernah, Ferne, Ferni, Firn, Firne,
Furn, Furne, Fyrn, Fyrne

Fernanda (German) daring, adventurous.
See also Andee, Nan.
Ferdie, Ferdinanda, Ferdinandah, Ferdinande,
Fernandah, Fernande, Fernandette,
Fernandina, Fernandinah, Fernandine,
Fernandyn, Fernandyna, Fernandyne, Nanda

Fernley (English) from the fern meadow.
Ferlea, Fernleah, Fernlee, Fernlei, Fernleigh,
Fernli, Fernlie, Fernly

Feronia (Latin) Mythology: goddess of freedom.

Fiala (Czech) violet flower.
Fialah, Fyala, Fyalah

Fidelia (Latin) a form of Fidelity.
Fidea, Fideah, Fidel, Fidela, Fidelah, Fidele,
Fideliah, Fidelina, Fidell, Fidella, Fidellah,
Fidelle, Fydea, Fydeah, Fydel, Fydela, Fydelah,
Fydele, Fydell, Fydella, Fydellah, Fydelle

Fidelity (Latin) faithful, true. See also Faith.
Fidelia, Fidelita, Fidelitee, Fidelitey, Fideliti,
Fidelitie, Fydelitee, Fydelitey, Fydeliti,
Fydelitie, Fydelity

Fidencia (Latin) a form of Fidelity.

Fifi GB (French) a familiar form of Josephine.
Fe-Fe, Fee-Fee, Feef, Feefee, Fefe, Fefi, Fefie,
Fefy, Fiffi, Fiffy, Fifina, Fifinah, Fifine, Fy-Fy,
Fyfy, Phiphi, Phyphy

Filadelfia (Greek) a form of Filia.

Filandra (Greek) she who loves humankind.

Filemona (Greek) a form of Philomena.

Filia (Greek) friend.
Filiah, Filya, Fylia, Fyliah, Fylya, Fylyah

Filiberta (Greek) brilliant.

Filippa (Italian) a form of Philippa.
Felipa, Felipe, Felippa, Filipa, Filipina,
Filippina, Filpina

Filis (Greek) adorned with leaves.

Filma (German) veiled.
Filmah, Filmar, Filmaria, Filmarya, Fylma,
Fylmah, Fylmara, Fylmaria, Fylmarya

Filomena (Italian) a form of Philomena.
Fila, Filah, Filemon, Filomenah, Filomene,
Filomina, Filominah, Filomyna, Filomyne,
Fylomena, Fylomenah, Fylomina, Fylomine,
Fylomyna, Fylomyne

Filotea (Greek) she who loves God.

Fiona (Irish) fair, white.
Feeona, Feeonah, Feeoni, Feeonie, Feeony,
Feona, Feonah, Feonia, Feoniah, Fionah,
Fionna, Fionnah, Fionne, Fionnea, Fionneah,
Fionnee, Fionni, Fionnia, Fionniah, Fyona,
Fyonah, Fyoni, Fyonia, Fyoniah, Fyonie,
Fyony, Fyonya, Fyonyah, Phiona, Phionah,
Phyona, Phyonah

Fionnula (Irish) white shouldered. See also
Nola, Nuala.
Fenella, Fenula, Finnula, Finnulah, Finnule,
Finola, Finolah, Finonnula, Finula, Fionnuala,
Fionnualah, Fionnulah, Fionula, Fynola, Fynolah

Fiorel (Latin) a form of Flora.

Fiorela (Italian) a form of Flora.

Fiorella (Italian) little flower.
Fiorelle

Fira (English) fiery.
Firah, Fyra, Fyrah

Flair (English) style; verve.
Flaira, Flaire, Flare, Flayr, Flayra, Flayre

Flaminia (Latin) one who belongs to a religious order.

Flanna (Irish) a short form of Flannery.
Flan, Flana, Flanah, Flann, Flannah

Flannery (Irish) redhead. Literature:
Flannery O'Connor was a renowned
American writer.
Flanneree, Flannerey, Flanneri, Flannerie

Flavia (Latin) blond, golden haired.
Flavere, Flaviah, Flavianna, Flavianne, Flaviar, Flavien, Flavienne, Flaviere, Flavio, Flavya, Flavyah, Flavyere, Flawia, Flawya, Flawyah, Fulvia

Flávia (Portuguese) a form of Flavia.

Flaviana (Italian) a form of Flavia.

Flavie (Latin) a form of Flavia.
Flavi

Flérida (Greek) exuberant lady.

Fleta (English) swift, fast.
Fleata, Fleatah, Fleeta, Fleetah, Fletah, Flita, Flitah, Flyta, Flytah

Fleur (French) flower.
Fleure, Fleuree

Fleurette (French) a form of Fleur.
Fleuret, Fleurett, Fleuretta, Fleurettah, Floretta, Florettah, Florette, Flouretta, Flourette

Fliora (Irish) a form of Flora.
Fliorah

Flo (American) a short form of Florence.
Flow

Flor (Latin) a short form of Florence.
Flore

Flora (Latin) flower. A short form of Florence. See also Lore.
Fiora, Fiore, Fiorenza, Flaura, Flaurah, Flauria, Flauriah, Flaury, Flaurya, Flauryah, Fliora, Florah, Florelle, Florey, Floria, Florica

Floralia (Greek) a form of Flora.

Floramaría (Spanish) flower of Mary.

Floreal (French) flowers. History: the eighth month in the old French calendar.

Florelle (Latin) a form of Flora.
Florel, Florell, Florella, Florellah

Florence (Latin) blooming; flowery; prosperous. History: Florence Nightingale, a British nurse, is considered the founder of modern nursing. See also Florida.
Fiorenza, Fiorenze, Flarance, Flarence, Florance, Florancia, Floranciah, Florancie, Floren, Florena, Florencia, Florenciah, Florencija, Florency, Florencya, Florendra, Florene, Florentia, Florentina, Florentyna, Florenza, Florina, Florine

Flores (Spanish) a form of Flora.

Floria (Basque) a form of Flora.
Floriah, Florria, Florya, Floryah

Florian BG (Latin) flowering, blooming.
Florann, Floren, Floriana, Florianna, Florianne, Florin, Florinah, Florine, Floryn, Floryna, Florynah, Floryne

Florida (Spanish) a form of Florence.
Floridah, Floridia, Floridiah, Florind, Florinda, Florindah, Florinde, Florita, Floryda, Florydah, Florynd, Florynda, Floryndah, Florynde

Florie (English) a familiar form of Florence.
Flore, Floree, Florey, Flori, Florri, Florrie, Florry, Flory

Florimel (Greek) sweet nectar.
Florimela, Florimele, Florimell, Florimella, Florimelle, Florymel, Florymela, Florymele, Florymell, Florymella, Florymelle

Florinia (Latin) a form of Florence.

Floris (English) a form of Florence.
Florisa, Florisah, Florise, Floriss, Florissa, Florissah, Florisse, Florys, Florysa, Florysah, Floryse, Floryss, Floryssa, Floryssah, Florysse

Florisel (Spanish) a form of Flora.

Flossie (English) a familiar form of Florence.
Floss, Flossi, Flossy

Flyta (English) rapid.

Fola (Yoruba) honorable.
Floah

Foluke BG (Yoruba) given to God.
Foluc, Foluck, Foluk

Fonda (Latin) foundation. (Spanish) inn.
Fondah, Fondea, Fonta, Fontah

Fontanna (French) fountain.
Fontain, Fontaina, Fontainah, Fontaine, Fontana, Fontanah, Fontane, Fontannah, Fontanne, Fontayn, Fontayna, Fontaynah, Fontayne

Forrest BG (French) forest; forester.
Forest, Forreste, Forrestt, Forrie

Fortuna (Latin) fortune; fortunate.
Fortoona, Fortunah, Fortunata, Fortunate,
Fortune, Fortunia, Fortuniah, Fortunya,
Fortunyah

Fosette (French) dimpled.
Foset, Foseta, Fosetah, Fosete, Fosett, Fosetta

Fotina (Greek) light. See also Photina.
Fotin, Fotine, Fotinia, Fotiniah, Fotinya,
Fotinyah, Fotyna, Fotyne, Fotynia, Fotyniah,
Fotynya, Fotynyah

Fran GB (Latin) a short form of Frances.
Frain, Frann, Frayn

Frances (Latin) free; from France. See also
Paquita.
France, Francena, Francess, Francesta

Francesca, Franceska (Italian) forms of
Frances.
Francessca, Francesta

Franchesca, Francheska (Italian) forms of
Francesca.
Cheka, Chekka, Chesca, Cheska, Francheca,
Francheka, Franchelle, Franchesa, Franchessca,
Franchesska

Franchette (French) a form of Frances.
Franceta, Francetta, Francette, Francheta,
Franchetah, Franchete, Franchett, Franchetta,
Franchettah, Franzet, Franzeta, Franzetah,
Franzete, Franzett, Franzetta, Franzettah,
Franzette

Franci (Hungarian) a familiar form of
Francine.
Francee, Francey, Francia, Francie, Francy,
Francya, Francye

Francine (French) a form of Frances.
Franceen, Franceine, Franceline, Francene,
Francenia, Francin, Francina, Francyn,
Francyna, Francyne, Fransin, Fransina,
Fransinah, Fransine, Fransyn, Fransyna,
Fransynah, Fransyne, Franzin, Franzina,
Franzinah, Franzine, Franzyn, Franzyna,
Franzynah, Franzyne

Francis BG (Latin) a form of Frances.
Francise, Francys, Franis, Franise, Franiss,
Franisse, Franncia, Frantis, Frantisa, Frantise,
Frantiss, Frantissa, Frantisse

Francisca (Italian) a form of Frances.
Franciska, Franciszka, Frantiska, Franziska,
Franzyska

Francoise, Françoise (French) forms of
Frances.

Franki (American) a familiar form of
Frances.
Franca, Francah, Francka, Francki, Franka,
Frankah, Franke, Frankee, Frankey, Frankia,
Frankiah, Franky, Frankyah, Frankye

Frankie BG (American) a familiar form of
Frances.

Frannie, Franny (English) familiar forms of
Frances.
Frani, Frania, Franney, Franni, Frany

Franqueira (German) open space.

Franzea (Spanish) a form of Frances.
Franzia, Franziah, Franzya, Franzyah,
Frazea

Freda (German) a short form of Alfreda,
Elfrida, Frederica, Sigfreda.
Fraida, Fraidah, Frayda, Frayde, Fraydina,
Fraydine, Fraydyna, Fraydyne, Fredah, Fredda,
Fredra, Freeda, Freedah, Freeha

Freddi (English) a familiar form of
Frederica, Winifred.
Fredda, Freddah, Freddee, Freddey, Freddia,
Freddy, Fredee, Fredey, Fredi, Fredia, Frediah,
Fredie, Fredy, Fredya, Fredyah, Frici

Freddie BG (English) a familiar form of
Frederica, Winifred.

Fredella (English) a form of Frederica.
Fredel, Fredela, Fredelah, Fredele, Fredell,
Fredellah, Fredelle

Frederica (German) peaceful ruler. See also
Alfreda, Rica, Ricki.
Federica, Feriga, Fredalena, Fredaline,
Frederina, Frederine, Fredith, Fredora,
Fredreca, Fredrica, Fredricah, Fredricia,
Fryderica

Frederika (German) a form of Frederica.
Fredericka, Frederickina, Fredreka, Fredrika,
Fryderika, Fryderikah, Fryderyka

Frederike (German) a form of Frederica.
Fredericke, Frederyc, Frederyck, Frederyk,
Fridrike, Friederike

Frederique GB (French) a form of Frederica.
Frederiqua, Frederiquah, Frédérique, Fredriqua, Fredriquah, Fredrique, Frideryqua, Frideryquah, Frideryque, Fryderiqua, Fryderiquah, Fryderique, Rike

Fredesvinda (German) strength of the country.

Fredricka (German) a short form of Frederika.

Freedom (English) freedom.

Freida (German) a form of Frida.
Freia, Freiah, Freidah, Freide, Freyda, Freydah

Freira (Spanish) sister.

Freja (Scandinavian) a form of Freya.
Fraja, Fray, Fraya, Frayah, Frehah, Freia, Freiah

Frescura (Spanish) freshness.

Freya (Scandinavian) noblewoman. Mythology: the Norse goddess of love.
Frey, Freyah

Freyra (Slavic) a form of Freya.

Frida (German) a short form of Alfreda, Elfrida, Frederica, Sigfreda.
Fridah, Frideborg, Frieda, Friedah, Fryda, Frydah, Frydda, Fryddah

Frine, Friné (Greek) female toad.

Fritzi (German) a familiar form of Frederica.
Friezi, Fritze, Fritzee, Fritzey, Fritzie, Fritzinn, Fritzline, Fritzy, Frytzee, Frytzey, Frytzi, Frytzie, Frytzy

Frodina (German) wise friend.
Frodinah, Frodine, Frodyn, Frodyna, Frodynah, Frodyne

Froilana (Greek) rapid.

Fronde (Latin) leafy branch.

Fronya (Latin) forehead.
Fronia, Froniah, Fronyah

Fructuosa (Spanish) fruitful.

Fuensanta (Spanish) holy fountain.

Fukayna (Egyptian) intelligent.

Fulgencia (Spanish) she who excels because of her great kindness.

Fulla (German) full.
Fula, Fulah, Fullah

Fusca (Latin) dark.

Futura (Latin) future.
Futurah, Future, Futuria, Futuriah, Futurya, Futuryah

Fynballa (Irish) fair.
Finabala, Finbalah, Finballa, Finballah, Fynbala, Fynbalah, Fynballah

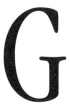

Gabele (French) a short form of Gabrielle.
Gabal, Gabala, Gabalah, Gabale, Gaball, Gaballa, Gaballah, Gaballe, Gabel, Gabela, Gabelah, Gabell, Gabella, Gabellah, Gabelle, Gable

Gabina (Latin) she who is a native of Gabio, an ancient city near Rome.

Gabor (Hungarian) God is my strength.
Gabora, Gaborah, Gabore

Gabriel BG (French) a form of Gabrielle.
Gabbriel, Gabbryel, Gabreal, Gabreale, Gabreil, Gabrial, Gabryel

Gabriela (Italian) a form of Gabrielle.
Gabriala, Gabrialla, Gabrielah, Gabrielia, Gabriellah, Gabriellia, Gabriello, Gabrila, Gabrilla, Gabryela, Gabryella, Gabryiela

Gabriele GB (French) a form of Gabrielle.

Gabriell GB (French) a form of Gabrielle.

Gabriella ☆ (Italian) a form of Gabriela.

Gabrielle ☆ GB (French) devoted to God.
Gabbrielle, Gabielle, Gabrealle, Gabriana, Gabrille, Gabrina, Gabriolett, Gabrioletta, Gabriolette, Gabriylle, Gabryell, Gabryelle, Gavriella

Gaby (French) a familiar form of Gabrielle.
Gabb, Gabbea, Gabbee, Gabbey, Gabbi,
Gabbie, Gabby, Gabey, Gabi, Gabie, Gavi,
Gavy

Gada (Hebrew) lucky.
Gadah

Gaea (Greek) planet Earth. Mythology: the
Greek goddess of Earth.
Gaeah, Gaia, Gaiah, Gaiea, Gaya, Gayah

Gaetana (Italian) from Gaeta. Geography:
Gaeta is a city in southern Italy.
Gaetan, Gaetanah, Gaétane, Gaetanna,
Gaetanne, Gaitana, Gaitanah, Gaitann,
Gaitanna, Gaitanne, Gaytana, Gaytane,
Gaytanna, Gaytanne

Gagandeep BG (Sikh) sky's light.
Gagandip, Gagnadeep, Gagndeep

Gage BG (French) promise.
Gaeg, Gaege, Gaig, Gaige, Gayg, Gayge

Gail (English) merry, lively. (Hebrew) a short
form of Abigail.
Gael, Gaela, Gaell, Gaella, Gaelle, Gaila,
Gaile, Gale, Gaylia

Gailine (English) a form of Gail.
Gailean, Gaileana, Gaileane, Gaileena,
Gailina, Gailyn, Gailyna, Gailyne, Gayleen,
Gayleena, Gaylina, Gayline, Gaylyn,
Gaylyna, Gaylynah, Gaylyne

Gala (Norwegian) singer.
Galah, Galla, Gallah

Galatea (Greek) Mythology: Galatea was a
statue of a beautiful woman carved by
Pygmalion, who fell in love with her and
persuaded the goddess Aphrodite to bring
the statue to life.
Galanthe, Galanthea, Galatee, Galatey,
Galati, Galatia, Galatiah, Galatie, Galaty,
Galatya, Galatyah

Galaxy (Latin) universe; the Milky Way.
Galaxee, Galaxey, Galaxi, Galaxia, Galaxiah

Galen BG (Greek) healer; calm. (Irish) little
and lively.
Gaelen, Gaellen, Galane, Galean, Galeane,
Galeene, Galene, Gallane, Galleene, Gallen,
Gallene, Galyn, Galyne, Gaylaine, Gayleen,
Gaylen, Gaylene, Gaylyn

Galena (Greek) healer; calm.
Galana, Galanah, Galenah, Gallana,
Gallanah, Gallena, Gallenah

Galenia (Greek) a form of Galena.

Gali (Hebrew) hill; fountain; spring.
Gailee, Galea, Galeah, Galee, Galei, Galeigh,
Galey, Galice, Galie, Gallea, Galleah, Gallee,
Gallei, Galleigh, Galley, Galli, Gallie, Gally,
Galy

Galilah (Hebrew) important; exalted.

Galilea (Hebrew) from Galilee.

Galina (Russian) a form of Helen.
Gailya, Galaina, Galainah, Galaine, Galayna,
Galaynah, Galayne, Galeana, Galeena,
Galeenah, Galenka, Galia, Galiah, Galiana,
Galianah, Galiane, Galiena, Galinah, Galine,
Galinka, Gallin, Gallina, Gallinah, Galline,
Gallyn, Gallyna, Gallynah, Gallyne, Galochka,
Galya, Galyah, Galyna, Galynah

Gamela (Scandinavian) elder.
Gamala, Gamalah, Gamale, Gamelah, Gamele

Gamila (Arabic) beautiful.

Ganesa (Hindi) fortunate. Religion:
Ganesha was the Hindu god of wisdom.
Ganesah, Ganessa, Ganessah

Ganya BG (Hebrew) garden of the Lord.
(Zulu) clever.
Gana, Gani, Gania, Ganiah, Ganice, Ganit,
Ganyah

Garabina, Garabine, Garbina, Garbine
(Spanish) purification.

Garaitz (Basque) victory.

García (Latin) she who demonstrates her
charm and grace.

Gardenia (English) Botany: a sweet-smelling
flower.
Deeni, Denia, Gardeen, Gardeena, Gardeene,
Garden, Gardena, Gardene, Gardin, Gardina,
Gardine, Gardinia, Gardyn, Gardyna, Gardyne

Garland BG (French) wreath of flowers.
Garlan, Garlana, Garlanah, Garlane, Garleen,
Garleena, Garleenah, Garleene, Garlena,
Garlenah, Garlene, Garlind, Garlinda,
Garlindah, Garlinde, Garlyn, Garlynd,
Garlynda, Garlyndah, Garlynde

Garnet 🅱🅶 (English) dark red gem.
Garneta, Garnetah, Garnete, Garnett,
Garnetta, Garnettah, Garnette

Garoa (Basque) fern.

Garyn (English) spear carrier.
Garan, Garana, Garane, Garen, Garin,
Garina, Garine, Garra, Garran, Garrana,
Garrane, Garrin, Garrina, Garrine, Garryn,
Garyna, Garyne, Garynna, Garynne

Gasha (Russian) a familiar form of Agatha.
Gashah, Gashka

Gaspara (Spanish) treasure.

Gasparina (Persian) treasure.

Gaudencia (Spanish) happy, content.

Gavriella (Hebrew) a form of Gabrielle.
Gavila, Gavilla, Gavra, Gavrel, Gavrela,
Gavrelah, Gavrelia, Gavreliah, Gavrell,
Gavrella, Gavrellah, Gavrelle, Gavrid,
Gavrieela, Gavriela, Gavrielle, Gavrila,
Gavrilla, Gavrille, Gavryl, Gavryla, Gavryle,
Gavryll, Gavrylla, Gavrylle

Gay (French) merry.
Gae, Gai, Gaie, Gaye

Gayla (English) a form of Gail.

Gayle (English) a form of Gail.
Gayel, Gayell, Gayella, Gayelle, Gayl

Gaylia (English) a form of Gail.
Gaelia, Gaeliah, Gailia, Gailiah, Gayliah

Gayna (English) a familiar form of
Guinevere.
Gaena, Gaenah, Gaina, Gainah, Gaynah,
Gayner, Gaynor

Gea (Greek) a form of Gaea.

Geanna (Italian) a form of Giana.
Geannah, Geona, Geonna

Gechina (Basque) grace.

Geela (Hebrew) joyful.
Gela, Gila

Geena (American) a form of Gena.
Geana, Geanah, Geania, Geeana, Geeanna,
Geenia

Gelasia (Greek) smiling lady.

Gelya (Russian) angelic.

Gema, Gemma (Latin, Italian) jewel, pre-
cious stone. See also Jemma.
Gem, Gemah, Gemee, Gemey, Gemia,
Gemiah, Gemie, Gemmah, Gemmee,
Gemmey, Gemmi, Gemmia, Gemmiah,
Gemmie, Gemmy, Gemy

Gemini (Greek) twin.
Gemelle, Gemina, Geminia, Geminine,
Gemmina

Geminiana (Latin) a form of Gemini.

Gen (Japanese) spring. A short form of
names beginning with "Gen."
Genn

Gena 🅶🅱 (French) a form of Gina. A short
form of Geneva, Genevieve, Iphigenia.
Genae, Genah, Genai, Genea, Geneja

Geneen (Scottish) a form of Jeanine.
Geanine, Geannine, Genene, Genine, Gineen,
Ginene

Genell (American) a form of Jenell.

Generosa (Spanish) generous.

Genesis 🅶🅱 (Latin) origin; birth.
Genes, Genese, Genesha, Genesia, Genesiss,
Genessa, Genesse, Genessie, Genicis, Genises,
Genysis, Yenesis

Genessis (Latin) a form of Genesis.

Geneva (French) juniper tree. A short form
of Genevieve. Geography: a city in
Switzerland. See also Jeneva.
Geneeva, Geneevah, Geneieve, Geneiva,
Geneive, Genevah, Geneve, Genevia,
Geneviah, Genneeva, Genneevah, Ginneeva,
Ginneevah, Ginneva, Ginnevah, Gyniva,
Gynniva, Gynnivah, Gynnyva, Gynnyvah

Genevieve (German, French) a form of
Guinevere. See also Gwendolyn.
Genaveeve, Genaveve, Genavie, Genavieve,
Genavive, Geneveve, Genevie, Geneviéve,
Genevievre, Genevive, Genivive, Genvieve,
Gineveve, Ginevieve, Ginevive, Guinevieve,
Guinivive, Guynieve, Guyniviv, Guynivive,
Gwenevieve, Gwenivive, Gwiniviev,
Gwinivieve, Gwynivive, Gynevieve, Janavieve,
Jenevieve, Jennavieve

Genevra (French, Welsh) a form of Guinevere.
Genever, Genevera, Genevrah, Genovera, Ginevra, Ginevrah

Genice (American) a form of Janice.
Genece, Geneice, Genesa, Genesee, Genessia, Genis, Genise

Genie (French) a familiar form of Gena.
Geni, Genia

Genita (American) a form of Janita.
Genet, Geneta

Genna (English) a form of Jenna.
Gennae, Gennai, Gennay, Genni, Gennie, Genny

Gennifer (American) a form of Jennifer.
Genifer

Genovieve (French) a form of Genevieve.
Genoveva, Genoveve, Genovive, Genowica

Gentil (Latin) kind.

Gentry BG (English) a form of Gent (see Boys' Names).

Georgeann, Georgeanne (English) combinations of Georgia + Ann.
Georgann, Georganne, Georgean, Georgiann, Georgianne, Georgieann, Georgyan, Georgyann, Georgyanne

Georgeanna (English) a combination of Georgia + Anna.
Georgana, Georganna, Georgeana, Georgeannah, Georgeannia, Georgyana, Georgyanah, Georgyanna, Georgyannah, Giorgianna

Georgene (English) a familiar form of Georgia.
Georgeene, Georgienne, Georgine, Georgyn, Georgyne, Jeorgine, Jeorjine, Jeorjyne

Georgette (French) a form of Georgia.
Georget, Georgeta, Georgete, Georgett, Georgetta, Georjetta

Georgia (Greek) farmer. Art: Georgia O'Keeffe was an American painter known especially for her paintings of flowers. Geography: a southern American state; a country in Eastern Europe. See also Jirina, Jorja.
Giorgia

Georgiana, Georgianna (English) forms of Georgeanna.
Georgiannah, Georgionna

Georgie (English) a familiar form of Georgeanne, Georgia, Georgiana.
Georgi, Georgy, Giorgi

Georgina (English) a form of Georgia.
Georgeena, Georgeenah, Georgeina, Georgena, Georgenah, Georgenia, Georgiena, Georgienna, Georginah, Georgine, Georgyna, Georgynah, Giorgina, Jeorgina, Jeorginah, Jeorjina, Jeorjinah, Jeorjyna, Jorgina

Geovanna (Italian) a form of Giovanna.
Geovana, Geovonna

Geralda (German) a short form of Geraldine.
Giralda, Giraldah, Gyralda, Gyraldah

Geraldine (German) mighty with a spear. See also Dena, Jeraldine.
Geralda, Geraldeen, Geraldeena, Geraldeenah, Geraldeene, Geraldina, Geraldyna, Geraldyne, Gerhardine, Gerianna, Gerianne, Gerlina, Gerlinda, Gerrianne, Gerrilee

Geralyn (American) a combination of Geraldine + Lynn.
Geralin, Geralina, Geraline, Geralisha, Geralyna, Geralyne, Geralynn, Gerilyn, Gerrilyn

Geranio (Greek) she is as beautiful as a geranium.

Gerarda (English) brave spearwoman.
Gerardine, Gerardo

Gerásima (Greek) prize.

Gerda (Norwegian) protector. (German) a familiar form of Gertrude.
Gerdah, Gerta

Geri, Gerri (American) familiar forms of Geraldine. See also Jeri.
Geree, Gerey, Gerie, Gerree, Gerrey, Gerrie, Gerry, Gery

Germaine BG (French) from Germany. See also Jermaine.
Germain, Germaina, Germainah, Germana, Germane, Germanee, Germani, Germanie, Germaya, Germayn, Germayna, Germaynah, Germayne, Germine, Germini, Germinie, Germyn, Germyna, Germyne

Gertie (German) a familiar form of Gertrude.
Gert, Gertey, Gerti, Gerty

Gertrude (German) beloved warrior. See also Trudy.
Geertrud, Geertruda, Geertrude, Geertrudi, Geertrudie, Geertrudy, Geitruda, Gerruda, Gerrudah, Gertina, Gertraud, Gertraude, Gertrud, Gertruda, Gertrudah, Gertrudia, Gertrudis, Gertruide, Gertruyd, Gertruyde, Girtrud, Girtruda, Girtrude, Gyrtrud, Gyrtruda, Gyrtrude

Gertrudes (Spanish) a form of Gertrude.

Gervaise BG (French) skilled with a spear.
Gervayse, Gervis

Gervasi (Spanish) a form of Gervaise.

Gervasia (German) a form of Gervaise.

Gessica (Italian) a form of Jessica.
Gesica, Gesika, Gesikah, Gess, Gesse, Gessika, Gessikah, Gessy, Gessyca, Gessyka, Gesyca, Gesyka

Geva (Hebrew) hill.
Gevah

Gezana, Gezane (Spanish) reference to the incarnation of Jesus.

Ghada (Arabic) young; tender.
Gada, Gadah, Ghadah

Ghita (Italian) pearly.
Ghyta, Gyta

Gia GB (Italian) a short form of Giana.
Giah, Gya, Gyah

Giacinta (Italian) a form of Hyacinth.
Giacynta, Giacyntah, Gyacinta, Gyacynta

Giacobba (Hebrew) supplanter, substitute.
Giacoba, Giacobah, Giacobbah, Gyacoba, Gyacobba, Gyacobbah

Giana, Gianna (Italian) short forms of Giovanna. See also Jianna, Johana.
Gian, Gianah, Gianel, Gianela, Gianele, Gianell, Gianella, Gianelle, Gianet, Gianeta, Gianete, Gianett, Gianetta, Gianette, Gianina, Gianinna, Giannah, Gianne, Giannee, Giannella, Giannetta, Gianni, Giannie, Giannina, Gianny, Gianoula, Gyan, Gyana, Gyanah, Gyann, Gyanna, Gyannah

Gianira (Greek) nymph from the sea.

Gibitruda (German) she who gives strength.

Gidget (English) giddy.
Gydget

Gigi (French) a familiar form of Gilberte.
G.G., Geegee, Geygey, Giggi, Gygy, Jeejee, Jeyjey, Jiji

Gilana (Hebrew) joyful.
Gila, Gilah, Gilanah, Gilane, Gilania, Gilanie, Gilena, Gilenia, Gyla, Gylah, Gylan, Gylana, Gylanah, Gylane

Gilberte (German) brilliant; pledge; trustworthy. See also Berti.
Gilberta, Gilbertia, Gilbertina, Gilbertine, Gilbertyna, Gilbertyne, Gilbirt, Gilbirta, Gilbirte, Gilbirtia, Gilbirtina, Gilbirtine, Gilburta, Gilburte, Gilburtia, Gilburtina, Gilburtine, Gilburtyna, Gilbyrta, Gilbyrte, Gilbyrtia, Gilbyrtina, Gilbyrtyna, Gylberta, Gylbertah, Gylberte, Gylbertina, Gylbertyna, Gylbirta, Gylbirte, Gylbirtia, Gylbirtina, Gylbirtine, Gylbirtyna, Gylburta, Gylburte, Gylburtia, Gylburtina, Gylburtyna, Gylbyrta, Gylbyrte, Gylbyrtia, Gylbyrtina, Gylbyrtyna

Gilda (English) covered with gold.
Gildah, Gilde, Gildi, Gildie, Gildy, Guilda, Guildah, Guylda, Guyldah, Gylda, Gyldah

Gill (Latin, German) a short form of Gilberte, Gillian.
Gili, Gilli, Gillie, Gilly, Gyl, Gyll

Gillian (Latin) a form of Jillian.
Gilian, Giliana, Gilianah, Giliane, Gilleann, Gilleanna, Gilleanne, Gilliana, Gillianah, Gilliane, Gilliann, Gillianna, Gillianne, Gillien, Gillyan, Gillyana, Gillyanah, Gillyane, Gillyann, Gillyanna, Gillyannah, Gillyanne, Gylian, Gyliana, Gylianah, Gyliane, Gyliann, Gylianna, Gyliannah, Gylianne, Gyllian, Gylliana, Gyllianah, Gylliane, Gylliann, Gyllianna, Gylliannah, Gyllianne, Gyllyan, Gyllyana, Gyllyanah, Gyllyane, Lian

Gimena (Spanish) a form of Jimena.

Gin (Japanese) silver. A short form of names beginning with "Gin."
Gean, Geane, Geen, Gyn, Gynn

Gina (Italian) a short form of Angelina, Eugenia, Regina, Virginia. See also Jina.
Geenah, Ginah, Ginai, Ginna, Gyna, Gynah

Ginebra (Celtic) white as foam.

Gines (Greek) she who engenders life.

Ginesa (Spanish) white.

Ginette (English) a form of Genevieve.
Ginata, Ginatah, Ginett, Ginetta, Ginnetta, Ginnette

Ginger (Latin) flower; spice. A familiar form of Virginia.
Ginja, Ginjah, Ginjar, Ginjer, Gynger, Gynjer

Ginia (Latin) a familiar form of Virginia.
Ginea, Gineah, Giniah, Gynia, Gyniah, Gynya, Gynyah

Ginnifer (English) white; smooth; soft. (Welsh) a form of Jennifer.
Ginifer, Gynifer, Gyniffer

Ginny (English) a familiar form of Ginger, Virginia. See also Jin, Jinny.
Gini, Ginnee, Ginney, Ginni, Ginnie, Giny, Gionni, Gionny, Gyni, Gynie, Gynni, Gynnie, Gynny

Gioconda (Latin) she who engenders life.

Giordana (Italian) a form of Jordana.
Giadana, Giadanah, Giadanna, Giadannah, Giodana, Giodanah, Giodanna, Giodannah, Giordanah, Giordanna, Giordannah, Gyodana, Gyodanah, Gyodanna, Gyodannah, Gyordana, Gyordanah, Gyordanna, Gyordannah

Giorgianna (English) a form of Georgeanna.

Giorsala (Scottish) graceful.
Giorsal, Giorsalah, Gyorsal, Gyorsala, Gyorsalah

Giovanna (Italian) a form of Jane.
Giavana, Giavanah, Giavanna, Giavannah, Giavonna, Giovana, Giovanah, Giovannah, Giovanne, Giovannica, Giovona, Giovonah, Giovonna, Giovonnah, Givonnie, Gyovana, Gyovanah, Gyovanna, Gyovannah, Jeveny

Giovanni BG (Italian) a form of Giovanna.

Gisa (Hebrew) carved stone.
Gazit, Gisah, Gissa, Gysa, Gysah

Gisal (Welsh) a form of Giselle.

Gisel, Gisell, Gissel, Gisselle (German) forms of Giselle.
Gisele, Gisele, Gissell

Gisela (German) a form of Giselle.
Giselah, Giselda, Giselia, Gisella, Gisellah, Gissela, Gissella, Gysela, Gysella

Giselle (German) pledge; hostage. See also Jizelle.
Geséle, Ghisele, Giseli, Gizela, Gysel, Gysele, Gysell, Gyselle

Gita (Yiddish) good. (Polish) a short form of Margaret.
Gitah, Gitka, Gyta, Gytah

Gitana (Spanish) gypsy; wanderer.
Gitanna, Gytana, Gytanna

Gitel (Hebrew) good.
Gitela, Gitelah, Gitele, Gitell, Gitella, Gitelle, Gytel, Gytell, Gytella, Gytellah, Gytelle

Githa (Greek) good. (English) gift.
Githah, Gytha, Gythah

Gitta (Irish) a short form of Bridget.
Getta, Gittah

Giulana (Italian) a form of Guilia.
Giulianna, Giulliana

Giulia (Italian) a form of Julia.
Guila, Guiliana, Guilietta, Guiliette

Giunia (Latin) she who was born in June.

Giuseppina (Italian) a form of Josephine.

Giustina (Italian) a form of Justine.
Giustine, Gustina, Gustinah, Gustine, Gustyn, Gustyna, Gustynah, Gustyne

Gizela (Czech) a form of Giselle.
Gizella, Gizi, Giziki, Gizus, Gyzela, Gyzelah, Gyzella

Gizelle (Czech) a form of Giselle.
Gizel, Gizele, Gizell, Gyzel, Gyzele, Gyzell, Gyzelle

Gladis (Irish) a form of Gladys.
Gladi, Gladiz

Gladys (Latin) small sword. (Irish) princess. (Welsh) a form of Claudia.
Glad, Gladdys, Gladness, Gladuse, Gladwys, Glady, Gladyss, Gleddis, Gleddys

Glafira (Greek) fine, elegant.

Glauca (Greek) green.

Glaucia (Portuguese) brave gift.

Gleda (English) happy.

Glenda (Welsh) a form of Glenna.
Glanda, Glendah, Glennda, Glenndah, Glynda

Glenna (Irish) valley, glen. See also Glynnis.
Glenetta, Glenina, Glenine, Glenn, Glenne, Glennesha, Glennia, Glennie, Glenora, Gleny, Glyn, Glynna

Glennesha (American) a form of Glenna.
Gleneesha, Gleneisha, Glenesha, Glenicia, Glenisha, Glenneesha, Glennisha, Glennishia, Glynesha, Glynisha

Gliceria (Greek) sweet.

Gloria (Latin) glory. History: Gloria Steinem, a leading American feminist, founded *Ms.* magazine.
Glorea, Gloresha, Gloriah, Gloribel, Gloriela, Gloriella, Glorielle, Gloris, Glorisha, Glorvina, Glorya, Gloryah

Gloriann, Glorianne (American) combinations of Gloria + Ann.
Glorian, Gloriana, Gloriane, Glorianna, Glorien, Gloriena, Gloriene, Glorienn, Glorienna, Glorienne, Gloryan, Gloryana, Gloryane, Gloryann, Gloryanna, Gloryanne, Gloryen, Gloryena, Gloryene, Gloryenn, Gloryenna, Gloryenne

Glory (Latin) a form of Gloria.
Glore, Gloree, Glorey, Glori, Glorie, Glorye

Glosinda (German) sweet glory.

Glynnis (Welsh) a form of Glenna.
Glenice, Glenis, Glenise, Glennis, Glennys, Glenwys, Glenys, Glenyse, Glenyss, Glinnis, Glinys, Glynice, Glynis, Glyniss, Glynitra, Glynnys, Glynys, Glynyss

Godalupe (Spanish) reference to the Virgin Mary.

Godgifu (English) a form of Godiva.

Godiva (English) God's present.
Godivah, Godyva, Godyvah

Godoberta (German) brightness of God.

Golda (English) gold. History: Golda Meir was a Russian-born politician who served as prime minister of Israel.
Goldah, Goldarina, Goldia, Goldiah, Goldine, Goldya, Goldyah

Goldie (English) a familiar form of Golda.
Goldea, Goldee, Goldey, Goldi, Goldy

Goldine (English) a form of Golda.
Goldeena, Goldeene, Golden, Goldena, Goldene, Goldina, Goldinah, Goldyn, Goldyna, Goldynah, Goldyne

Goma (Swahili) joyful dance.
Gomah

Gontilda (German) famous warrior.

Gorane (Spanish) holy cross.

Goratze (Basque) a form of Exaltación.

Gorawén (Welsh) happiness.

Gorgonia (Greek) Mythology: Gorgons were monsters who turned people to stone.

Gotzone (Spanish) angel.

Graça (Portuguese) a form of Grace.

Grace ☆ (Latin) graceful.
Engracia, Graca, Gracelia, Gracella, Gracia, Gracinha, Graciosa, Graice, Graise, Grase, Gratia, Greice, Greyce, Greyse

Graceann, Graceanne (English) combinations of Grace + Ann.
Graceanna, Graciana, Gracianna

Gracelyn, Gracelynn, Gracelynne (English) combinations of Grace + Lynn.
Gracelin, Gracelinn, Gracelinne, Gracelyne

Gracen, Gracyn (English) short forms of Graceanne.
Gracin

Gracia (Spanish) a form of Grace.
Gracea, Graciah, Graicia, Graiciah, Graisia, Graisiah, Grasia, Grasiah, Graycia, Grayciah, Graysia, Graysiah, Grazia, Graziah

Gracie (English) a familiar form of Grace.
Gracee, Gracey, Graci, Gracy, Graecie, Graysie

Graciela (Spanish) a form of Grace.
Graciella, Gracielle

Gracilia (Latin) graceful; slender.

Grant BG (English) great; giving.

Gratiana (Hebrew) graceful.
Gratian, Gratiane, Gratiann, Gratianna, Gratianne, Gratyan, Gratyana, Gratyane, Gratyann, Gratyanna, Gratyanne

Grayce (Latin) a form of Grace.

Grayson BG (English) bailiff's child.
Graison, Graisyn, Grasien, Grasyn, Gray, Graysen

Graziella (Italian) a form of Grace.
Graziel, Graziela, Graziele, Graziell, Grazielle, Graziosa, Grazyna

Grecia (Latin) a form of Grace.

Greekria (Spanish) a form of Greekrina.

Greekriana (Spanish) a form of Greekria.

Greekrina (Latin) vigilant watchperson.

Greer (Scottish) vigilant.
Grear, Grier, Gryer

Greta, Gretta (German) short forms of Gretchen, Margaret.
Grata, Gratah, Greata, Greatah, Greeta, Greetah, Gretah, Grete, Gretha, Grethe, Grette, Grieta, Gryta, Grytta

Gretchen (German) a form of Margaret.
Gretchan, Gretchin, Gretchon, Gretchun, Gretchyn

Gretel (German) a form of Margaret.
Greatal, Greatel, Gretal, Gretall, Gretell, Grethal, Grethel, Gretil, Gretill, Grettal, Gretyl, Gretyll

Gricelda (German) a form of Griselda.
Gricelle

Grimalda (Latin) happiness.

Grise (Welsh) a form of Griselda.

Grisel (German) a short form of Griselda.
Grisell, Griselle, Grissel, Grissele, Grissell, Grizel, Grizella, Grizelle

Grisela (Spanish) a form of Griselda.

Griselda (German) gray woman warrior. See also Selda, Zelda.
Griseldis, Griseldys, Griselys, Grishild,

Grishilda, Grishilde, Grisselda, Grissely, Grizelda, Gryselda, Gryzelda

Guadalupe GB (Arabic) river of black stones. See also Lupe.
Guadalup, Guadelupe, Guadlupe, Guadulupe, Gudalupe

Gualberta (German) brilliant power.

Gualteria (German) a form of Walter (see Boys' Names).

Gudelia, Gúdula (Latin) God.

Gudrun (Scandinavian) battler. See also Runa.
Gudren, Gudrin, Gudrina, Gudrine, Gudrinn, Gudrinna, Gudrinne, Gudruna

Güendolina (English) a form of Gwendolyn.

Guía (Spanish) guide.

Guillelmina (Italian, Spanish) a form of Guillermina.

Guillerma (Spanish) a short form of Guillermina.
Guilla

Guillermina (Spanish) a form of Wilhelmina.

Guinevere (French, Welsh) white wave; white phantom. Literature: the wife of King Arthur. See also Gayna, Genevra, Jennifer, Winifred, Wynne.
Guenevere, Guenna, Guinievre, Guinivere, Guinna, Gwenevere, Gwenivere, Gwenora, Gwenore, Gwynivere, Gwynnevere

Guioma (Spanish) a form of Guiomar.

Guiomar (German) famous in combat.

Gunda (Norwegian) female warrior.
Gundah, Gundala, Gunta

Gundelina (Teutonic) she who helps in battle.

Gundelinda (German) pious one in the battle.

Gundenes (German) famous.

Gundenia (German) fighter.

Gurit (Hebrew) innocent baby.
Gurita, Gurite, Guryta, Guryte

Gurleen (Sikh) follower of the guru.

Gurley (Australian) willow.
Gurlea, Gurleah, Gurlee, Gurlei, Gurleigh, Gurli, Gurlie, Gurly

Gurpreet BG (Punjabi) religion.
Gurprit

Gusta (Latin) a short form of Augusta.
Gus, Gussi, Gussie, Gussy

Gustava (Scandinavian) staff of the Goths.

Gustey (English) windy.
Gustea, Gustee, Gusti, Gustie, Gusty

Gwen (Welsh) a short form of Guinevere, Gwendolyn.
Gwenesha, Gweness, Gwenessa, Gweneta, Gwenetta, Gwenette, Gweni, Gwenisha, Gwenishia, Gwenita, Gwenite, Gwenitta, Gwenitte, Gwenn, Gwenna, Gwenneta, Gwennete, Gwennetta, Gwennette, Gwennie, Gwenny

Gwenda (Welsh) a familiar form of Gwendolyn.
Gwinda, Gwynda, Gwynedd

Gwendolyn (Welsh) white wave; white browed; new moon. Literature: Gwendoloena was the wife of Merlin, the magician. See also Genevieve, Gwyneth, Wendy.
Guendolen, Gwendalee, Gwendalin, Gwendaline, Gwendalyn, Gwendalynn, Gwendela, Gwendelyn, Gwendelynn, Gwendilyn, Gwendolen, Gwendolene, Gwendolin, Gwendolina, Gwendoline, Gwendolyne, Gwendolynn, Gwendolynne, Gwendylan, Gwindolin, Gwindolina, Gwindoline, Gwindolyn, Gwindolyna, Gwindolyne, Gwyndolin, Gwyndolina, Gwyndoline, Gwyndolyn, Gwyndolyna, Gwyndolyne, Gwynndolen

Gwyn GB (Welsh) a short form of Gwyneth.
Gwin, Gwine, Gwineta, Gwinete, Gwinisha, Gwinita, Gwinite, Gwinitta, Gwinitte Gwinn, Gwinne, Gwynn, Gwynne

Gwyneth (Welsh) a form of Gwendolyn. See also Winnie, Wynne.
Gweneth, Gwenetta, Gwenette, Gwenith, Gwenneth, Gwennyth, Gwenyth, Gwineth, Gwinneth, Gwynaeth, Gwynneth

Gypsy (English) wanderer.
Gipsea, Gipsee, Gipsey, Gipsi, Gipsie, Gipsy, Gypsea, Gypsee, Gypsey, Gypsi, Gypsie, Jipsi

H

Habiba (Arabic) beloved.
Habibah, Habibeh

Hachi (Japanese) eight; good luck. (Native American) river.
Hachee, Hachie, Hachiko, Hachiyo, Hachy

Hada, Hadda (Hebrew) she who radiates joy.

Hadara (Hebrew) adorned with beauty.
Hadarah, Hadaria, Hadariah, Hadarya, Hadaryah

Hadasa (Hebrew) a form of Hadassah.

Hadassah (Hebrew) myrtle tree.
Hadas, Hadasah, Hadassa, Haddasa, Haddasah

Hadaza (Guanche) distracted; lost.

Hadeel (Arabic) a form of Hadil.

Hadil (Arabic) cooing of pigeons.

Hadiya (Swahili) gift.
Hadaya, Hadia, Hadiyah, Hadiyyah, Hadya, Hadyea

Hadley GB (English) field of heather.
Hadlea, Hadleah, Hadlee, Hadlei, Hadleigh, Hadli, Hadlie, Hadly

Hadriane (Greek, Latin) a form of Adrienne.
Hadriana, Hadrianna, Hadrianne, Hadriene, Hadrienne

Hae (Korean) ocean.

Haeley (English) a form of Hayley.
Haelee, Haeleigh, Haeli, Haelie, Haelleigh, Haelli, Haellie, Haely

Hafsa (Muslim) cub; young lioness.
Hafsah, Hafza

Hafwen (Welsh) pleasant summer.
Hafwena, Hafwenah, Hafwene, Hafwin,

Hafwina, Hafwinah, Hafwine, Hafwyn, Hafwyna, Hafwynah, Hafwyne

Hágale (Greek) beautiful.

Hagar GB (Hebrew) forsaken; stranger. Bible: Sarah's handmaiden, the mother of Ishmael.
Hagara, Hagarah, Hagaria, Hagariah, Hagarya, Hagaryah, Haggar

Haidee (Greek) modest.
Hady, Hadyee, Haide, Haidea, Haideah, Haidey, Haidi, Haidia, Haidy, Haydee, Haydey, Haydy

Haidée, Haydée (Greek) forms of Haidee.

Haiden BG (English) heather-covered hill.
Haden, Hadyn, Haeden, Haidn, Haidyn

Haile, Hailee, Haileigh, Haili, Hailie, Haily (English) forms of Hayley.
Haiely, Hailea, Haileah, Hailei, Hailia, Haille, Haillee, Hailley, Hailli, Haillie, Hailly

Hailey ✰ GB (English) a form of Haile.

Haizea (Basque) wind.

Hajar (Hebrew) a form of Hagar.
Hajara, Hajarah, Hajaria, Hajariah, Hajarya, Hajaryah

Hala (African) a form of Halla.
Halah, Halya, Halyah

Haldana (Norwegian) half Danish.
Haldanah, Haldania, Haldaniah, Haldanna, Haldannah, Haldannya, Haldannyah, Haldanya, Haldanyah

Halee, Haleigh, Halie, Hallee, Halli, Hallie (Scandinavian) forms of Haley.
Hale, Haleh, Halei, Haliegh, Hallea, Halleah, Hallei, Halleigh, Hallia, Halliah, Hally, Hallya, Hallyah, Hallye, Haly, Halye

Haley ✰ GB (Scandinavian) heroine. See also Hayley.

Hali GB (Scandinavian) a form of Haley.

Halia (Hawaiian) in loving memory.
Halea, Haleaah, Haleah, Haleea, Haleeah, Haleia, Haleiah, Haliah, Halya, Halyah

Haliaka (Hawaiian) leader.
Haliakah, Halyaka, Halyakah

Halima (Arabic) a form of Halimah.
Halime

Halimah (Arabic) gentle; patient.
Haleema, Haleemah, Halyma, Halymah

Halimeda (Greek) loves the sea.
Halimedah, Halymeda, Halymedah

Halina (Hawaiian) likeness. (Russian) a form of Helen.
Haleen, Haleena, Halena, Halinah, Haline, Halinka, Halyn, Halyna, Halynah, Halyne

Halla (African) unexpected gift.
Hallah, Hallia, Halliah, Hallya, Hallyah

Halle (African) a form of Halla. (Scandinavian) a form of Haley.

Halley GB (Scandinavian) a form of Haley.

Halona (Native American) fortunate.
Hallona, Hallonah, Halonah, Haloona, Haona

Halsey GB (English) Hall's island.
Halsea, Halsie

Hama (Japanese) shore.

Hana, Hanah (Japanese) flower. (Arabic) happiness. (Slavic) forms of Hannah.
Hanae, Hanicka, Hanka

Hanako (Japanese) flower child.

Hanan GB (Japanese, Arabic, Slavic) a form of Hana.
Hanin

Haneen (Japanese, Arabic, Slavic) a form of Hana.

Hanele (Hebrew) compassionate.
Hanal, Hanall, Hanalla, Hanalle, Hanel, Hanela, Hanelah, Hanell, Hanella, Hanelle, Hannel, Hannell, Hannella, Hannelle

Hania (Hebrew) resting place.
Haniah, Haniya, Hanja, Hannia, Hanniah, Hanya, Hanyah

Hanifa (Arabic) true believer.
Haneefa, Hanifa, Hanyfa, Hanyfah

Hanna GB (Hebrew) a form of Hannah.
Honna

Hannah ☀ **GB** (Hebrew) gracious. Bible: the mother of Samuel. See also Anci, Anezka, Ania, Anka, Ann, Anna, Annalie, Anneka, Chana, Nina, Nusi.
Hanneke, Hannele, Hannon, Honnah

Hanni (Hebrew) a familiar form of Hannah.
Hani, Hanita, Hanitah, Hanne, Hannie, Hanny

Happy (English) happy.
Happea, Happee, Happey, Happi, Happie

Haquicah (Egyptian) honest.

Hara **GB** (Hindi) tawny. Religion: another name for the Hindu god Shiva, the destroyer.
Harah

Haralda (Scandinavian) army ruler.
Harelda, Hareldah, Heralda, Heraldah

Harjot **BG** (Sikh) God's light.

Harlee, Harleigh, Harli, Harlie (English) forms of Harley.
Harlea, Harleah, Harlei

Harleen, Harlene (English) forms of Harley.
Harlean, Harleana, Harleanah, Harleane, Harleena, Harleenah, Harleene, Harlein, Harleina, Harleinah, Harleine, Harlena, Harlenah, Harleyn, Harleyna, Harleynah, Harleyne, Harlin, Harlina, Harlinah, Harline, Harlyn, Harlyna, Harlynah, Harlyne

Harley **BG** (English) meadow of the hare. See also Arleigh.
Harleey, Harlene, Harly

Harleyann (English) a combination of Harley + Ann.
Harlann, Harlanna, Harlanne, Harleyanna, Harleyanne, Harliann, Harlianna, Harlianne

Harmony (Latin) harmonious.
Harmene, Harmeni, Harmon, Harmone, Harmonee, Harmonei, Harmoney, Harmoni, Harmonia, Harmoniah, Harmonie, Harmonya, Harmonyah

Harper **GB** (English) harp player.
Harp, Harpo

Harpreet **GB** (Punjabi) devoted to God.
Harprit

Harriet (French) ruler of the household. (English) a form of Henrietta. Literature: Harriet Beecher Stowe was an American writer noted for her novel *Uncle Tom's Cabin*.
Harietta, Hariette, Hariot, Hariott, Harri, Harrie, Harriett, Harrietta, Harriette, Harriot, Harriott, Harryet, Harryeta, Harryetah, Harryete, Harryett, Harryetta, Harryettah, Harryette, Haryet, Haryeta, Haryetah, Haryete, Haryett, Haryetta, Haryettah, Haryette

Haru (Japanese) spring.

Hasana (Swahili) she arrived first. Culture: a name used for the first-born female twin. See also Huseina.
Hasanna, Hasna, Hassana, Hassna, Hassona

Hasia (Hebrew) protected by God.
Hasiah, Hasya, Hasyah

Hasina (Swahili) good.
Haseena, Hasena, Hasinah, Hassina, Hasyn, Hasyna, Hasynah, Hasyne

Hateya (Moquelumnan) footprints.
Hateia, Hateiah, Hateyah

Hathor (Egyptian) goddess of the sky.
Hathora, Hathorah, Hathore

Hattie (English) a familiar form of Harriet, Henrietta.
Hatti, Hatty, Hetti, Hettie, Hetty

Haukea (Hawaiian) snow.
Haukia, Haukiah, Haukya, Haukyah

Hausu (Moquelumnan) like a bear yawning upon awakening.

Hava (Hebrew) a form of Chava. See also Eve.
Havah, Havvah

Haven **GB** (English) a form of Heaven.
Havan, Havana, Havanna, Havannah, Havyn

Haviva (Hebrew) beloved.
Havalee, Havelah, Havi

Haya (Arabic) humble, modest.
Haia, Haiah, Hayah

Hayat (Arabic) life.

Hayden **BG** (English) a form of Haiden.
Hayde, Haydin, Haydn, Haydon

Hayfa (Arabic) shapely.
Haifa, Haifah, Hayfah

Hayle, Haylea, Haylee, Hayleigh, Hayli, Haylie (English) forms of Hayley.
Hayleah, Haylei, Haylia, Hayliah, Haylle, Hayllie

Hayley (English) hay meadow. See also Haley.
Hayly

Hazel (English) hazelnut tree; commanding authority.
Haize, Haizela, Haizelah, Haizell, Haizella, Haizellah, Haizelle, Hayzal, Hayzala, Hayzalah, Hayzale, Hayzall, Hayzalla, Hayzallah, Hayzalle, Hazal, Hazaline, Hazall, Hazalla, Hazallah, Hazalle, Haze, Hazeline, Hazell, Hazella, Hazelle, Hazen, Hazyl, Hazzal, Hazzel, Hazzell, Hazzella, Hazzellah, Hazzelle, Heyzal, Heyzel

Heather (English) flowering heather.
Heath, Heathar, Heatherlee, Heatherly, Hethar, Hether

Heaven (English) place of beauty and happiness. Bible: where God and angels are said to dwell.
Heavan, Heavin, Heavon, Heavyn, Hevean, Heven, Hevin

Heavenly (English) a form of Heaven.
Heavenlea, Heavenleah, Heavenlee, Heavenlei, Heavenleigh, Heavenley, Heavenli, Heavenlie

Heba (Greek) a form of Hebe.
Hebah

Hebe (Greek) Mythology: the Greek goddess of youth and spring.
Hebee, Hebey, Hebi, Hebia, Hebie, Heby

Hecuba (Greek) Mythology: wife of Priam, king of Troy.

Hedda (German) battler. See also Edda, Hedy.
Heda, Hedah, Hedaya, Heddah, Hedia, Hedu

Hedwig BG (German) warrior.
Hedvick, Hedvig, Hedvige, Hedvika, Hedviga, Hedwyg, Hedwyga, Hendvig, Hendvyg, Jadviga

Hedy (Greek) delightful; sweet. (German) a familiar form of Hedda.
Heddee, Heddey, Heddi, Heddie, Heddy, Hede, Hedee, Hedey, Hedi, Hedie

Heidi, Heidy (German) short forms of Adelaide.
Heida, Heide, Heidea, Heidee, Heidey, Heidie, Heydy, Hidea, Hidee, Hidey, Hidi, Hidie, Hidy, Hiede, Hiedi, Hydi

Helah (Hebrew) rust.

Helaina (Greek) a form of Helena.
Halaina, Halainah, Helainah

Helaku BG (Native American) sunny day.
Helakoo

Helana (Greek) a form of Helena.
Helanah, Helania

Helda (German) a form of Hedda.

Helen (Greek) light. See also Aileen, Aili, Alena, Eileen, Elaina, Elaine, Eleanor, Ellen, Galina, Ila, Ilene, Ilona, Jelena, Leanore, Leena, Lelya, Lenci, Lene, Liolya, Nellie, Nitsa, Olena, Onella, Yalena, Yelena.
Elana, Ena, Halina, Hela, Helan, Hele, Helean, Heleen, Helin, Helon, Helyn, Holain

Helena (Greek) a form of Helen. See also Ilena.
Halayna, Halaynah, Halena, Halina, Helayna, Helaynah, Heleana, Heleanah, Heleena, Heleenah, Helenah, Helenia, Helenka, Helenna, Helina, Helinah, Hellaina, Hellana, Hellanah, Hellanna, Hellena, Hellenna, Helona, Helonna, Helyna, Helynah

Helene (French) a form of Helen.
Halaine, Halayn, Halayne, Helain, Helaine, Helane, Helanie, Helayn, Helayne, Heleen, Heleine, Hélène, Helenor, Heline, Hellain, Hellaine, Hellenor

Helga (German) pious. (Scandinavian) a form of Olga. See also Elga.
Helgah

Heli (Spanish) a short form of Heliana.

Helia, Heliena (Greek) sun.

Heliana (Greek) she who offers herself to God.

Helice (Greek) spiral.
Helicia, Heliciah, Helyce, Helycia, Helyciah, Helycya, Helycyah

Hélida (Hebrew) of God.

Heliodora (Greek) gift from the sun.

Helki BG (Native American) touched.
Helkee, Helkey, Helkie, Helky

Hellen (Greek) a form of Helen.
Hellan, Helle, Helli, Hellin, Hellon, Hellyn

Helma (German) a short form of
Wilhelmina.
*Halma, Halmah, Helmah, Helme, Helmi,
Helmine, Hilma, Hilmah, Hylma, Hylmah*

Heloísa (Spanish) a form of Heloise.

Heloise (French) a form of Louise.
*Heloisa, Heloisah, Héloïse, Heloysa, Heloysah,
Heloyse, Hlois*

Helsa (Danish) a form of Elizabeth.
*Helsah, Helse, Helsey, Helsi, Helsia, Helsiah,
Helsie, Helsy, Helsya, Helsyah*

Heltu (Moquelumnan) like a bear reaching
out.
Heltoo

Helvecia (Latin) happy friend. History:
Helvetians were ancient inhabitants of
Switzerland.

Helvia (Latin) blond hair.

Henar (Spanish) hay field.

Hendrika (Dutch) a form of Henrietta.
*Hendrica, Hendrinka, Hendrinkah, Henrica,
Henrika, Henryka, Henrykah*

Henedina (Greek) indulgent.

Henimia (Greek) well-dressed.

Henna (English) a familiar form of
Henrietta.
*Hena, Henaa, Henah, Heni, Henia, Henka,
Hennah, Henny, Henya*

Henrietta (English) ruler of the household.
See also Enrica, Etta, Yetta.
*Heneretta, Hennrietta, Henretta, Henrie,
Henrieta, Henrique, Henriquetta, Henriquette,
Henriquieta, Henriquiette, Henryet, Henryeta,
Henryetah, Henryete, Henryett, Henryetta,
Henryettah*

Henriette (French) a form of Henrietta.
Hennriette, Henriete, Henryette

Henriqua (Spanish) a form of Henrietta.

Hera (Greek) queen; jealous. Mythology: the
queen of heaven and the wife of Zeus.
Herah, Heria, Heriah, Herya, Heryah

Heraclia (Greek) a form of Hera.

Herberta (German) glorious soldier.
*Herbertah, Herbertia, Herbertiah, Herbirta,
Herbirtah, Herbirtia, Herburta, Herburtah,
Herburtia, Herbyrta, Herbyrtah*

Hercilia, Hersilia (Greek) she who is delicate and kind.

Herculana (Greek) a form of Hercules (see
Boys' Names).

Herena, Herenia (Greek) forms of Irene.

Heresvida (German) numerous troops.

Heriberta (German) a form of Herberta.

Heriberto (Spanish) ruler.

Herlinda (German) pleasant, sweet.

Hermelinda (German) shield of strength.

Hermenegilda (Spanish) she who offers
sacrifices to God.

Hermenexilda (German) warrior.

Hermia (Greek) messenger.

Hermilda (German) battle of force.

Hermina (Latin) noble. (German) soldier.
See also Erma, Ermine, Irma.
*Herma, Hermalina, Hermia, Herminah,
Hermine, Herminna*

Herminda (Greek) a form of Hermia.

Herminia (Latin, German) a form of
Hermina.
Hermenia, Herminiah

Hermínia (Portuguese) a form of
Hermione.

Hermione (Greek) earthy.
*Hermion, Hermiona, Hermoine, Hermyon,
Hermyona, Hermyonah, Hermyone*

Hermisenda (Germanic) path of strength.

Hermosa (Spanish) beautiful.
Hermosah

Hernanda (Spanish) bold voyager.

Hertha (English) child of the earth.
Heartha, Hearthah, Hearthea, Heartheah, Hearthia, Hearthiah, Hearthya, Hearthyah, Herta, Hertah, Herthah, Herthia, Herthiah, Herthya, Herthyah, Hirtha

Herundina (Latin) like a swallow.

Hester (Dutch) a form of Esther.
Hessi, Hessie, Hessye, Hestar, Hestarr, Hesther

Hestia (Persian) star. Mythology: the Greek goddess of the hearth and home.
Hestea, Hesti, Hestiah, Hestie, Hesty, Hestya, Hestyah

Heta (Native American) racer.
Hetah

Hetta (German) a form of Hedda. (English) a familiar form of Henrietta.

Hettie (German) a familiar form of Henrietta, Hester.
Hetti, Hetty

Hialeah (Cherokee) lovely meadow.
Hialea, Hialee, Hialei, Hialeigh, Hiali, Hialie, Hialy, Hyalea, Hyaleah, Hyalee, Hyalei, Hyaleigh, Hyali, Hyalie, Hyaly

Hiawatha BG (Iroquoian) creator of rivers. History: the Onondagan leader who organized the Iroquois confederacy.
Hiawathah, Hyawatha, Hyawathah

Hiba (Arabic) a form of Hibah.

Hibah GB (Arabic) gift.
Hyba, Hybah

Hibernia (Latin) comes from Ireland.
Hibernina, Hiberninah, Hibernine, Hibernya, Hibernyah, Hibernyna, Hybernyah, Hybernyne

Hibiscus (Latin) Botany: tropical trees or shrubs with large, showy, colorful flowers.
Hibyscus, Hybyscus

Hidalgo (Spanish) noble one.

Higinia (Greek) she who enjoys good health.

Hilary GB (Greek) cheerful, merry. See also Alair.
Hilaire, Hilarea, Hilaree, Hilarey, Hilari, Hilaria, Hilarie, Hilery, Hiliary, Hillarea, Hillaree, Hillarey, Hillari, Hillarie, Hilleary,
Hilleree, Hilleri, Hillerie, Hillery, Hillianne, Hilliary, Hillory, Hylarea, Hylaree, Hylarey, Hylari, Hylarie, Hylary, Hyllarea, Hyllaree, Hyllarey, Hyllari, Hyllarie, Hyllary

Hilda (German) a short form of Brunhilda, Hildegarde.
Hildah, Hilde, Hildee, Hildey, Hildi, Hildia, Hildie, Hildur, Hildy, Hillda, Hilldah, Hilldee, Hilldey, Hilldi, Hilldia, Hilldie, Hilldy, Hulda, Hylda, Hyldah, Hyldea, Hyldee, Hyldey, Hyldi, Hyldie, Hyldy, Hylldea, Hylldee, Hylldey, Hylldi, Hylldie, Hylldy

Hildebranda (German) battle sword.

Hildegarda (German) a form of Hildegarde.

Hildegarde (German) fortress.
Hildaagard, Hildaagarde, Hildagard, Hildagarde, Hildegard, Hildegaurd, Hildegaurda, Hildegaurde, Hildred, Hyldaagard, Hyldaagarde, Hyldaaguard, Hyldaaguarde, Hyldagard, Hyldagarde, Hyldegard, Hyldegarde, Hyldeguard, Hyldeguarde

Hildegunda (German) heroic fighter.

Hildelita, Hildeliva (Latin) warrior.

Hildemarca (German) noble warrior.

Hildemare (German) splendid.
Hildemar, Hildemara, Hyldemar, Hyldemara, Hyldemare

Hillary (Greek) cheerful, merry.

Hilma (German) protected.
Hilmah, Hylma, Hylmah

Hilmer (German) famous warrior.

Hiltruda, Hiltrudes, Hiltrudis (German) strong warrior.

Himana (Greek) membrane.

Hinda (Hebrew) hind; doe.
Hindah, Hindey, Hindie, Hindy, Hynda, Hyndah

Hipatia (Greek) best.

Hipólita (Greek) horsewoman.

Hiriko (Japanese) generous.
Hiroko, Hiryko, Hyriko, Hyroko, Hyryko

Hisa (Japanese) long lasting.
Hisae, Hisah, Hisako, Hisay, Hisayo, Hysa, Hysah

Hiti (Eskimo) hyena.
Hitty

Hoa (Vietnamese) flower; peace.
Ho, Hoah, Hoai

Hoda (Muslim, Arabic) a form of Huda.

Hogolina (Teutonic) great intelligence.

Hola (Hopi) seed-filled club.
Holah, Holla, Hollah

Holain (Greek) a form of Helen.
Holaina, Holainah, Holaine, Holana, Holanah, Holane, Holayn, Holayna, Holaynah, Holayne

Holda (Hebrew) hidden.

Holland GB (French) Geography: A popular name for the Netherlands.
Holand, Hollan

Hollee, Holley, Holli, Hollie (English) forms of Holly.
Holle

Hollis BG (English) near the holly bushes.
Holice, Holisa, Holisah, Holise, Holiss, Holissa, Holissah, Holisse, Hollice, Hollise, Hollyce, Hollys, Hollysa, Hollysah, Hollyse, Hollyss, Hollyssa, Hollyssah, Hollysse, Holyce, Holys, Holysa, Holysah, Holyse, Holyss, Holyssa, Holyssah, Holysse

Holly (English) holly tree.
Holea, Holeah, Holee, Holei, Holeigh, Holey, Holi, Holie, Hollea, Holleah, Hollei, Holleigh, Hollye, Holy

Hollyann (English) a combination of Holly + Ann.
Holliann, Hollianna, Hollianne, Hollyanne

Hollyn (English) a short form of Hollyann.
Holeena, Holin, Hollina, Hollynn

Hombelina, Humbelina (German) boss, leader.

Homera (German) woman who cannot see.

Honbria (English) sweet.

Honesta (Latin) honest.
Honest, Honestah, Honestia

Honesty (Latin) honesty.
Honestee, Honestey, Honesti, Honestie

Honey (English) sweet. (Latin) a familiar form of Honora.
Honalee, Honea, Honeah, Honee, Honi, Honia, Honiah, Honie, Honnea, Honnee, Honney, Honni, Honnie, Honny, Hony, Hunea, Hunee, Huney, Huni, Hunie, Hunnee, Hunney, Hunni, Hunnie, Hunny

Hong (Vietnamese) pink.
Hoong

Honora (Latin) honorable. See also Nora, Onora.
Honner, Honnor, Honnour, Honor, Honorah, Honorata, Honore, Honoree, Honori, Honoria, Honoriah, Honorie, Honorina, Honorine, Honour, Honoura, Honourah, Honoure, Honouria, Honouriah, Honoury, Honourya, Honouryah

Honoratas (Spanish) a form of Honora.

Honovi BG (Native American) strong.
Honovee, Honovey, Honovie, Honovy

Hope (English) hope.

Hopi (Hopi) peaceful.
Hopee, Hopey, Hopie, Hopy

Horatia (Latin) keeper of the hours.
Horacia, Horaciah, Horacya, Horacyah, Horatya, Horatyah

Hortense (Latin) gardener. See also Ortensia.
Hortencia, Hortensia, Hortensiah, Hortensya, Hortensyah

Hosanna (Latin) a shout of praise or adoration derived from the Hebrew phrase "Save now!"

Hoshi (Japanese) star.
Hoshee, Hoshey, Hoshie, Hoshiko, Hoshiyo, Hoshy

Howi BG (Moquelumnan) turtledove.
Howee, Howey, Howie, Howy

Hua (Chinese) flower.

Huanquyi (Mapuche) announcer, she who shouted.

Huata (Moquelumnan) basket carrier.
Huatah

Huberta (German) bright mind; bright
spirit.
*Hubertah, Hubertia, Hubertiah, Hubertya,
Hubertyah, Hughbirta, Hughbirtah,
Hughbirtia, Hughbirtiah, Hughbirtya,
Hughbirtyah, Hughburta, Hughburtah,
Hughburtia, Hughburtiah, Hughburtya,
Hughburtyah, Hughbyrta, Hughbyrtah,
Hughbyrtia, Hughbyrtiah, Hughbyrtya,
Hughbyrtyah*

Huda (Muslim, Arabic) to lead upon the
right path.

Huette (German) bright mind; bright spirit.
*Huet, Hueta, Huetah, Huete, Huett, Huetta,
Huettah, Hugeta, Hugetah, Hugetta, Hughet,
Hugheta, Hughetah, Hughete, Hughett,
Hughetta, Hughettah, Hughette, Huguette,
Huit, Huita, Huitah, Huitt, Huitta, Huittah,
Huitte, Huyet, Huyeta, Huyetah, Huyete,
Huyett, Huyetta, Huyette*

Huilen, Huillen, Hullen (Araucanian)
spring.

Humildad (Latin) a form of Humilia.

Humilia (Polish) humble.
*Humiliah, Humillia, Humilliah, Humylia,
Humyliah, Humylya, Humylyah*

Humiliana (Italian) a form of Humilia.

Hunter BG (English) hunter.
Hunta, Huntah, Huntar, Huntter

Huong (Vietnamese) flower.

Huseina (Swahili) a form of Hasana.

Hyacinth (Greek) Botany: a plant with col-
orful, fragrant flowers. See also Cynthia,
Giacinta, Jacinda.
*Hyacintha, Hyacinthe, Hyacinthia, Hyacinthie,
Hycinth, Hycynth*

Hydi, Hydeia (German) forms of Heidi.
*Hyde, Hydea, Hydee, Hydey, Hydia, Hydie,
Hydiea, Hydy*

Hye (Korean) graceful.

I

Ia (Greek) voice; shout.

Iafa (Hebrew) strong and beautiful.

Ian BG (Hebrew) God is gracious.
Iaian, Iain, Iana, Iann, Ianna, Iannel, Iyana

Ianina (Hebrew) a form of Juana.

Ianira (Greek) enchantress.
Ianirah, Ianyra, Ianyrah

Ianthe (Greek) violet flower.
*Iantha, Ianthia, Ianthina, Ianthine, Ianthya,
Ianthyah, Ianthyna*

Iara (Tupi) lady.

Iberia (Latin) she who is a native of Iberia.

Ibi (Indigenous) earth.

Icess (Egyptian) a form of Isis.
Ices, Icesis, Icesse, Icey, Icia, Icis, Icy

Ichtaca (Nahuatl) secret.

Icía (Galician) a form of Cecilia.

Iciar (Basque) name of the Virgin Mary.

Icnoyotl (Nahuatl) friendship.

Ida (German) hard working. (English) pros-
perous.
*Idah, Idaia, Idaly, Idamae, Idania, Idarina,
Idarine, Idaya, Idda, Ide, Idelle, Idetta, Idette,
Idys, Iida, Iidda, Yda, Ydah*

Idabelle (English) a combination of Ida +
Belle.
*Idabel, Idabela, Idabelah, Idabele, Idabell,
Idabella, Idabellah*

Idalia (Greek) sun.
Idaliah, Idalya, Idalyah

Idalina (English) a combination of Ida +
Lina.
*Idaleen, Idaleena, Idaleene, Idalena, Idalene,
Idaline*

Idalis (English) a form of Ida.
 Idalesse, Idalise, Idaliz, Idallas, Idallis, Idelis, Idelys, Idialis

Idara (Latin) well-organized woman.

Ideashia (American) a combination of Ida + Iesha.
 Idasha, Idaysha, Ideesha, Idesha

Idelgunda (German) combative.

Idelia (German) noble.
 Ideliah, Idelya, Idelyah

Idelina (German) a form of Idelia.

Idelle (Welsh) a form of Ida.
 Idela, Idelah, Idele, Idell, Idella, Idellah

Idil (Welsh) a form of Ida.
 Idal

Idla (English) battle.

Idoberga, Iduberga (German) woman; shelter.

Idoia (Spanish) reference to the Virgin Mary.

Idolina (Latin) idol.

Idoya (Spanish) pond. Religion: a place of worship of the Virgin Mary.

Idumea (Latin) red.

Idurre (Spanish) reference to the Virgin Mary.

Ieasha (American) a form of Iesha.
 Ieachia, Ieachya, Ieashe

Iedidá (Hebrew) loved.

Ieisha (American) a form of Iesha.
 Ieishia

Iesha (American) a form of Aisha.
 Iaisha, Ieaisha, Ieesha, Iescha, Ieshah, Ieshya, Ieshyah, Ieysha, Ieyshah, Iiesha, Iisha

Ieshia (American) a form of Iesha.
 Ieeshia, Ieshea, Iesheia

Ife (Egyptian) love.

Ifigenia (Greek) a form of Iphigenia.

Ifiginia (Spanish) a form of Iphigenia.

Ignacia (Latin) fiery, ardent.
 Ignaci, Ignaciah, Ignacie, Ignacya, Ignacyah, Ignasha, Ignashah, Ignashia, Ignashya,
 Ignashyah, Ignatia, Ignatya, Ignatyah, Ignatzia, Ignazia, Ignazya, Ignazyah, Ignezia, Ignezya, Ignezyah, Inignatia, Inignatiah, Inignatya, Inignatyah

Ignia (Latin) a short form of Ignacia.
 Igniah, Ignya, Ignyah

Igone (Spanish) ascension.

Igraine (Irish) graceful.
 Igraina, Igrainah, Igrayn, Igrayna, Igraynah, Igrayne

Ihuicatl (Nahuatl) sky.

Iiragarte (Basque) a form of Anunciación.

Ikerne (Basque) a form of Visitación.

Ikia (Hebrew) God is my salvation. (Hawaiian) a form of Isaiah (see Boys' Names).
 Ikaisha, Ikea, Ikeea, Ikeesha, Ikeeshia, Ikeia, Ikeisha, Ikeishi, Ikeishia, Ikesha, Ikeshia, Ikeya, Ikeyia, Ikiah, Ikiea, Ikiia, Ikya, Ikyah

Ila (Hungarian) a form of Helen.
 Ilah

Ilaina (Hebrew) a form of Ilana.
 Ilainah, Ilaine, Ilainee, Ilainey, Ilaini, Ilainia, Ilainie, Ileina, Ileinah, Ileinee, Ileiney, Ileini, Ileinie, Ileiny, Ileyna, Ileynah, Ileynee, Ileyney, Ileyni, Ileynie, Ileyny

Ilana (Hebrew) tree.
 Ilanah, Ilane, Ilanee, Ilaney, Ilani, Ilania, Ilanie, Ilanit, Illana, Illanah, Illane, Illanee, Illaney, Illani, Illanie, Illanna, Illannah, Illanne

Ilchahueque (Mapuche) young virginal woman.

Ilda (German) heroine in battle.

Ilde (English) battle.

Ildefonsa (German) ready for battle.

Ildegunda (German) she who knows how to battle.

Ileana (Hebrew) a form of Iliana.
 Ilea, Ileah, Ileanah, Ileanee, Ileaney, Ileani, Ileanie, Ileanna, Ileannah, Ileanne, Ileany, Illeana, Illeanah

Ilena (Greek) a form of Helena.
 Ileena, Ileenah, Ileina, Ilina, Ilinah, Ilinee,

Iliney, Ilini, Ilinie, Iliny, Ilyna, Ilynah, Ilynee, Ilyney, Ilyni, Ilynie, Ilyny

Ilene (Irish) a form of Helen. See also Aileen, Eileen.
Ilean, Ileane, Ileanne, Ileen, Ileene, Ileine, Ileyne, Iline, Illeane, Ilyne

Ilhuitl (Nahuatl) day.

Iliana (Greek) from Troy.
Ili, Ilia, Ilian, Iliani, Iliania, Ilina, Ilinah, Illian, Illiana, Illianah, Illiane, Illiani, Illianna, Illiannah, Illianne, Illyana, Illyane, Illyanna, Illyanne

Ilima (Hawaiian) flower of Oahu.
Ilimah, Ilyma, Ilymah

Ilisa (Scottish, English) a form of Alisa, Elisa.
Ilicia, Ilisah, Ilissa, Ilissah, Iliza, Illisa, Illisah, Illissa, Illissah

Ilise (German) a form of Elise.
Ilese, Ilisse, Illyse, Illysse, Ilyce, Ilyse, Ilysse

Ilisha (Hebrew) a form of Alisha, Elisha. See also Lisha.
Ileshia, Ilishia, Ilysha, Ilyshia

Ilka (Hungarian) a familiar form of Ilona.
Ilke, Ilki, Ilkie, Ilky, Milka, Milke

Ilona (Hungarian) a form of Helen.
Illona, Illonia, Illonya, Ilone, Iloni, Ilonie, Ilonka, Ilyona

Ilsa (German) a form of Ilse.

Ilse (German) a form of Elizabeth. See also Elsa.
Ilsey, Ilsie, Ilsy

Iluminada (Spanish) shining.
Ilumina, Iluminah, Ilumine, Ilumyna, Ilumynah, Ilumyne

Ilyssa (Scottish, English) a form of Ilisa.
Illysa, Illysah, Illyssa, Illyssah, Ilycia, Ilysa, Ilysah, Ilysia, Ilyssah, Ilyza

Ima (Japanese) presently. (German) a familiar form of Amelia.
Imah

Imaculada (Portuguese) a form of Inmaculada.

Imala (Native American) strong-minded.
Imalah

Iman GB (Arabic) believer.
Aman, Imana, Imanah, Imane

Imani GB (Arabic) a form of Iman.
Imahni, Imanee, Imania, Imaniah, Imanie, Imanii, Imany

Imber (Polish) ginger.
Imbera, Imberah, Imbere

Imelda (German) warrior.
Imalda, Imeldah, Irmhilde, Melda

Imena (African) dream.
Imee, Imenah, Imene

Immaculada (Spanish) a form of Inmaculada. Religion: refers to the Immaculate Conception.

Imogene (Latin) image, likeness.
Emogen, Emogena, Emogene, Emojean, Emojeana, Imagena, Imagene, Imagina, Imajean, Imogeen, Imogeene, Imogen, Imogena, Imogene, Imogenia, Imogina, Imogine, Imogyn, Imogyne, Imojean, Imojeen

Imoni (Arabic) a form of Iman.
Imonee

Imperia, Imperio (Latin) imperial ruler.

Ina (Irish) a form of Agnes.
Ena, Inanna, Inanne

Inalén (Aboriginal) to be close by.

Inari (Finnish) lake.
Inaree, Inarey, Inarie, Inary

Inca (Spanish) ruler. History: a Quechuan people from highland Peru who established an empire from northern Ecuador to central Chile before being conquered by the Spanish.
Incah, Incan, Incana, Inka, Inkah

Indalecia (Latin) compassionate lady.

Indamira, Indemira (Arabic) the guest of the princess.

India (Sanskrit) river. Geography: a country of southern Asia.
Indea, Indeah, Indee, Indeia, Indeya, Indi, Indiah, Indie, Indy

Indiana 🅱🅶 (American) Geography: a state in the north-central United States.
Indeana, Indeanah, Indeanna, Indeannah, Indian, Indianah, Indiane, Indianna, Indiannah, Indianne, Indyana, Indyanah, Indyann, Indyanna, Indyannah, Indyanne

Indíana (American) a form of Indiana.

Indigo (Latin) dark blue color.
Indego, Indiga, Indygo

Indira (Hindi) splendid. History: Indira Nehru Gandi was an Indian politician and prime minister.
Indiara, Indirah, Indra, Indre, Indria, Indyra, Indyrah

Indya (Sanskrit) a form of India.
Indieya, Indiya

Ines, Inez (Spanish) forms of Agnes. See also Ynez.
Inés, Inesa, Inesita, Inésita, Inessa

Inês (Portuguese) a form of Ines.

Inéz (Spanish) a form of Ines.

Infantita (Spanish) immaculate child.

Infiniti (Latin) a form of Infinity.

Infinity (Latin) infinity.

Inga (Scandinavian) a short form of Ingrid.
Ingaberg, Ingaborg, Ingah, Inge, Ingeberg, Ingeborg, Ingela

Ingrid (Scandinavian) hero's daughter; beautiful daughter.
Inger, Ingrede

Iniga (Latin) fiery, ardent.
Ingatia, Inigah, Inyga, Inygah

Inmaculada (Latin) immaculate.

Inoa (Hawaiian) name.
Inoah

Inocencia (Spanish) innocent.
Innocencia, Innocenciah, Innocencya, Innocencyah, Innocentia, Innocenzia, Innocenziah, Innocenzya, Innocenzyah, Inocenciah, Inocencya, Inocenzia, Inocenzya

Inoceneia, Inocenta (Spanish) forms of Inocencia.

Inti (Quechua) sunshine. Mythology: Inca sun god.

Invención (Latin) invention.

Ió, Ioes (Greek) forms of Iola.

Ioana (Romanian) a form of Joan.
Ioanah, Ioani, Ioanna, Ioannah, Ioanne

Iola (Greek) dawn; violet colored. (Welsh) worthy of the Lord.
Iolah, Iole, Iolee, Iolia

Iolana (Hawaiian) soaring like a hawk.
Iolanah, Iolane, Iolann, Iolanna, Iolannah, Iolanne

Iolanthe (English) a form of Yolanda. See also Jolanda.
Iolanda, Iolande, Iolantha

Iona (Greek) violet flower.
Ione, Ionee, Ioney, Ioni, Ionia, Ioniah, Ionie, Iony, Iyona, Iyonna

Iosune (Basque) a form of Jesus.

Iphigenia (Greek) sacrifice. Mythology: the daughter of the Greek leader Agamemnon. See also Gena.
Iphgena, Iphigeniah, Iphigenya, Iphigenyah

Ipi (Mapuche) harvester; careful.

Iquerne (Spanish) visitation.

Ira 🅱🅶 (Hebrew) watchful. (Russian) a short form of Irina.
Irah

Iracema (Tupi) from where the honey comes.

Iragarzte (Basque) annunciation.

Iraida, Iraides, Iraís (Greek) descendent of Hera.

Irakusne (Basque) a form of Estefania.

Irati (Navarro) Geography: a jungle of Navarra, Spain.

Iratze (Basque) reference to the Virgin Mary.

Irena (Russian) a form of Irene.
Ireana, Ireanah, Ireena, Ireenah, Irenah, Irenea, Irenka

Irene (Greek) peaceful. Mythology: the goddess of peace. See also Eirene, Orina, Rena, Rene, Yarina.
Irean, Ireane, Ireen, Ireene, Irén, Irien, Irine, Iryn, Iryne, Jereni

Ireny (Greek) a familiar form of Irene.
Irenee, Ireney, Ireni, Irenie, Iryni, Irynie, Iryny

Iria (English) lady.

Iridia (Latin) belonging to Iris.

Iriel (Hebrew) God is my light.

Irimia (Spanish) Geography: where the Miño River starts.

Irina (Russian) a form of Irene.
Eirena, Erena, Ira, Irana, Iranda, Iranna, Iriana, Irin, Irinah, Irinia, Irona, Iryna, Irynah, Rina

Iris (Greek) rainbow. Mythology: the goddess of the rainbow and messenger of the gods.
Irisa, Irisha, Iriss, Irissa, Irisse, Irita, Irys, Irysa, Irysah, Iryse, Iryssa, Iryssah, Irysse

Irma (Latin) a form of Erma. (German) a short form of Irmgaard.
Irmah

Irmã (Portuguese) a form of Irma.

Irma de la Paz (Spanish) peaceful Irma.

Irmgaard (German) noble.
Irmguard, Irmi

Irmine (Latin) noble.
Irmina, Irminah, Irminia, Irmyn, Irmynah, Irmyne

Irta (Russian) a form of Rita.

Irune (Basque) reference to the Holy Trinity.

Irupe, Irupé (Guarani) irupe flower.

Irvette (Irish) attractive. (Welsh) white river. (English) sea friend.
Irvet, Irveta, Irvetah, Irvete, Irvett, Irvetta, Irvettah

Isa BG (Spanish) a short form of Isabel.
Isah, Issa, Issah

Isabeau (French) a form of Isabel.

Isabel ✰ (Spanish) consecrated to God. See also Bel, Belle, Chavella, Ysabel.
Isabal, Isabeal, Isabele, Isabeli, Isabelia, Isabelita, Isabello, Isbel, Iseabal, Ishbel, Issabel, Issie, Izabel, Izabele

Isabela (Italian) a form of Isabel.
Issabella

Isabelina (Hebrew) a form of Isabel.

Isabell, Isabelle (French) forms of Isabel.
Issabell, Issabelle

Isabella ✰ (Italian) a form of Isabel.

Isadora (Latin) gift of Isis.
Isadoria, Isadoriah, Isadorya, Isadoryah, Isidora, Izadora, Izadorah, Izadore

Isaldina, Isolina (German) powerful warrior.

Isamar (Hebrew) a form of Itamar.
Isamari, Isamaria

Isaura (Greek) native of Isauria, an ancient region in Asia Minor.

Isberga (German) a form of Ismelda.

Isel (Scottish) a short form of Isela.

Isela (Scottish) a form of Isla.

Iselda (German) she who remains faithful.

Iseult (Welsh) Literature: also known as Isolde, a princess in the Arthurian legends; a heroine of medieval romance. See also Yseult.

Isha (American) a form of Aisha.
Ishae, Ishah, Ishana, Ishanaa, Ishanda, Ishanee, Ishaney, Ishani, Ishanna, Ishaun, Ishawna, Ishaya, Ishenda, Ishia, Iysha

Ishi (Japanese) rock.
Ishiko, Ishiyo, Shiko, Shiyo

Isi (Spanish) a short form of Isabel.

Isibeal (Irish) a form of Isabel.

Isis (Egyptian) supreme goddess. Mythology: the goddess of nature and fertility.
Ices, Icess, Isiss, Issis, Issisa, Issise, Issys, Isys

Isla (Scottish) Geography: the River Isla in Scotland.
Islah

Isleta (Spanish) small island.

Ismaela (Hebrew) God will hear.
Ismaila, Ismayla

Ismelda (German) she who battles with sword.

Ismena (Greek) wise.
Ismenah, Ismenia, Ismeniah, Ismenya, Ismenyah

Isobel (Spanish) a form of Isabel.
Isobell, Isobella, Isobelle, Isopel

Isoka (Benin) gift from God.
Isokah, Soka

Isolde (Welsh) fair lady. Literature: also known as Iseult, a princess in the Arthurian legends; a heroine of medieval romance.
Isault, Isolad, Isolda, Isolt, Izolde, Izolt

Isona (Spanish) a form of Isabel.

Isra (Iranian) rainbow.

Issie (Spanish) a familiar form of Isabel.
Issi, Issy, Iza

Ita (Irish) thirsty.
Itah

Italia (Italian) from Italy.
Italea, Italeah, Italee, Italei, Italeigh, Itali, Italiah, Italie, Italy, Italya, Italyah

Italina (Italian) a form of Italia.

Itamar (Hebrew) palm island.
Ithamar, Ittamar

Itatay (Guarani) hand bell.

Itati, Itatí (Guarani) white rock.

Itotia (Nahuatl) dance.

Itsaso (Basque) sea.

Itsel (Spanish) a form of Itzel.
Itesel, Itssel

Itxaro (Spanish) hope.

Itzal (Basque) shadow.

Itzayana (Spanish) a form of Itzel.

Itzel (Spanish) protected.
Itcel, Itchel, Itza, Itzallana, Itzell, Ixchel

Itziar (Basque) high area covered by pines overlooking the ocean.

Iuitl (Nahuatl) feather.

Iulene (Basque) soft.

Iva (Slavic) a short form of Ivana.
Ivah

Ivana (Slavic) God is gracious. See also Yvanna.
Ivanah, Ivania, Ivaniah, Ivanka, Ivany, Ivanya, Ivanyah

Ivanna (Slavic) a form of Ivana.
Ivannah, Ivannia, Ivanniah, Ivannya, Ivannyah

Iverem (Tiv) good fortune; blessing.

Iverna (Latin) from Ireland.
Ivernah

Iveta (French) a form of Yvette.

Ivette (French) a form of Yvette. See also Evette.
Ivet, Ivete, Iveth, Ivetha, Ivett, Ivetta

Ivey (English) a form of Ivy.
Ivee

Ivon (French) a form of Ivonne.
Ivona, Ivone

Ivón (Spanish) a form of Ivonne.

Ivonne (French) a form of Yvonne. See also Evonne.
Ivonna, Iwona, Iwonka, Iwonna, Iwonne

Ivory GB (Latin) made of ivory.
Ivoory, Ivoree, Ivorey, Ivori, Ivorie, Ivorine, Ivree

Ivria (Hebrew) from the land of Abraham.
Ivriah, Ivrit

Ivy GB (English) ivy tree.
Ivi, Ivia, Iviann, Ivianna, Ivianne, Ivie, Ivye

Ixcatzin (Nahuatl) like cotton.

Ixtli (Nahuatl) face.

Iyabo (Yoruba) mother has returned.

Iyana, Iyanna (Hebrew) forms of Ian.
Iyanah, Iyannah, Iyannia

Iyesha (American) a form of Iesha.

Izabella (Spanish) a form of Isabel.
Izabela, Izabell, Izabellah, Izabelle, Izobella

Izar, Izarra, Izarre (Basque) star.

Izarbe (Aragonese) Virgin Mary of the Pyrenees Mountains.

Izaskum (Basque) above the valley.

Izazcun, Izazkun (Spanish) reference to the Virgin Mary.

Izel (Nahuatl) unique.

Iziar (Basque) name of the Virgin Mary.

Izusa (Native American) white stone.
Izusah

Ja BG (Korean) attractive. (Hawaiian) fiery.
Jah

Ja'lisa (American) a form of Jalisa.

Ja'nae (American) a form of Janae.

Jaafar (Arabic) small stream.

Jaamini (Hindi) evening.
Jaaminee, Jaaminey, Jaaminie, Jaaminy

Jabel (Hebrew) flowing stream.

Jabrea, Jabria (American) combinations of the prefix Ja + Brea.
Jabreal, Jabree, Jabreea, Jabreena, Jabrelle, Jabreona, Jabri, Jabriah, Jabriana, Jabrie, Jabriel, Jabrielle, Jabrienna, Jabrina

Jacalyn (American) a form of Jacqueline.
Jacalean, Jacaleana, Jacaleanah, Jacaleane, Jacaleen, Jacaleena, Jacaleenah, Jacaleene, Jacalein, Jacaleina, Jacaleinah, Jacaleine, Jacaleyn, Jacaleyna, Jacaleynah, Jacaleyne, Jacalin, Jacalina, Jacalinah, Jacaline, Jacalyna, Jacalynah, Jacalyne, Jacalynn

Jacarandá (Tupi) fragrant flower.

Jacee, Jaci, Jacie (Greek) forms of Jacey.
Jacci, Jacia, Jaciah, Jaciel, Jaciela, Jaciele

Jacelyn (American) a form of Jocelyn.
Jacelean, Jaceleana, Jaceleanah, Jaceleane, Jaceleen, Jaceleena, Jaceleenah, Jaceleene, Jacelein, Jaceleina, Jaceleinah, Jaceleine, Jaceleyn, Jaceleyna, Jaceleynah, Jaceleyne, Jacelin, Jacelina, Jacelinah, Jaceline, Jacelyna, Jacelynah, Jacelyne, Jacelynn, Jacelynna, Jacelynnah, Jacelynne, Jacilin, Jacilina, Jacilinah, Jaciline, Jacilyn, Jacilyne, Jacilynn, Jacylin, Jacylina, Jacylinah, Jacyline, Jacylyn, Jacylyna, Jacylynah, Jacylyne, Jacylynn

Jacey GB (American) a combination of the initials J. + C. (Greek) a familiar form of Jacinda.
Jac-E, Jace, Jacea, Jacya, Jacyah, Jaice, Jaicee, Jaici, Jaicie

Jacinda (Greek) beautiful, attractive. (Spanish) a form of Hyacinth.
Jacenda, Jacindah, Jacinde, Jacindea, Jacindee, Jacindey, Jacindi, Jacindia, Jacindie, Jacindy, Jacinna, Jacinnia, Jacyn, Jacynda, Jacyndah, Jacyndea, Jacyndee, Jacyndi, Jacyndia, Jacyndy, Jakinda, Jasinda, Jasindah, Jasinde, Jasindea, Jasindey, Jasindi, Jasindia, Jasindy, Jasynda, Jasyndah, Jasyndea, Jasyndee, Jasyndey, Jasyndi, Jasyndia, Jasyndie, Jasyndy, Jaxina, Jaxine, Jaxyn, Jaxyna, Jaxynah, Jaxyne, Jazinda, Jazindah, Jazindea, Jazindee, Jazindia, Jazindie, Jazindy

Jacinta (Greek) a form of Jacinda.
Jacanta, Jacent, Jacenta, Jacentah, Jacente, Jacintah, Jacintia, Jacynta, Jacyntah, Jasinta, Jasintah, Jasinte, Jaxinta, Jaxintah, Jaxinte, Jazinta, Jazintah, Jazynte

Jacinthe (Spanish) a form of Jacinda.
Jacinte, Jacinth, Jacintha, Jacinthia, Jacinthy

Jackalyn (American) a form of Jacqueline.
Jackalean, Jackaleana, Jackaleanah, Jackaleane, Jackaleen, Jackaleena, Jackaleenah, Jackaleene, Jackalein, Jackaleina, Jackaleinah, Jackaleine, Jackalene, Jackaleyn, Jackaleyna, Jackaleynah, Jackaleyne, Jackalin, Jackalina, Jackalinah, Jackaline, Jackalyna, Jackalynah, Jackalyne, Jackalynn, Jackalynne

Jackeline, Jackelyn (American) forms of Jacqueline.
Jackelin, Jackelline, Jackellyn, Jackelynn, Jackelynne, Jockeline

Jacki (American) a familiar form of Jacqueline. See also Jacqui.
Jackea, Jackee, Jackey, Jackia, Jackiah, Jackielee, Jacky, Jackye

Jackie BG (American) a familiar form of Jacqueline.

Jackilyn (American) a form of Jacqueline.
Jackilean, Jackileana, Jackileanah, Jackileane, Jackileen, Jackileena, Jackileenah, Jackileene, Jackilein, Jackileina, Jackileinah, Jackileine, Jackileyn, Jackileyna, Jackileynah, Jackileyne, Jackilin, Jackilynn, Jackilynne

Jacklyn, Jacklynn (American) short forms of Jacqueline.
Jacklin, Jackline, Jacklyne, Jacklynne

Jackolyn (American) a form of Jacqueline.
Jackolin, Jackoline, Jackolynn, Jackolynne

Jackquel (French) a short form of Jacqueline.

Jackquelyn (French) a form of Jacqueline.
Jackqueline, Jackquelyna, Jackquelynah, Jackquelyne, Jackquelynn, Jackquelynna, Jackquelynnah, Jackquelynne, Jackquetta, Jackquilin, Jackquiline, Jackquilyn, Jackquilynn, Jackquilynne

Jackson BG (English) child of Jack.
Jacksen, Jacksin, Jacson, Jakson, Jaxon

Jaclyn, Jaclynn (American) short forms of Jacqueline.
Jacleen, Jaclin, Jacline, Jaclyne

Jacob BG (Hebrew) supplanter, substitute. Bible: son of Isaac, brother of Esau.

Jacobella (Italian) a form of Jacobi.
Jacobela, Jacobell

Jacobi BG (Hebrew) a form of Jacob.
Coby, Jacoba, Jacobah, Jacobea, Jacobee, Jacobella, Jacobette, Jacobia, Jacobiah, Jacobie, Jacobina, Jacobinah, Jacobine, Jacoby, Jacobya, Jacobyah, Jacobye, Jacolbi, Jacolbia, Jacolby, Jacovina, Jacovinah, Jacovine, Jacuba, Jakoba, Jakobea, Jakobee, Jakobey, Jakobi, Jakobia, Jakobiah, Jakobie, Jakoby, Jakobya, Jakubah, Jocoby, Jocolby, Jocovyn, Jocovyna, Jocovynah, Jocovyne

Jacolyn (American) a form of Jacqueline.
Jacolean, Jacoleana, Jacoleanah, Jacoleane, Jacoleen, Jacoleena, Jacoleenah, Jacoleene, Jacolein, Jacoleina, Jacoleinah, Jacoleine, Jacolin, Jacolina, Jacolinah, Jacoline, Jacolyna, Jacolynah, Jacolyne, Jacolynn, Jacolynna, Jacolynnah, Jacolynne

Jacqualine (French) a form of Jacqueline.
Jacqualin, Jacqualine, Jacqualyn, Jacqualyne, Jacqualynn

Jacqueena (French) a form of Jacqueline.
Jacqueen, Jacqueenah, Jacqueene, Jacqueenia, Jacqueeniah, Jacqueenie, Jacqueine, Jacquine, Jaqueen, Jaqueena, Jaqueenah, Jaqueene, Jaqueenia, Jaqueeniah, Jaqueenie, Jaqueeny, Jaqueenya, Jaqueenyah

Jacquelin, Jacquelyn, Jacquelyne, Jacquelynn (French) forms of Jacqueline.
Jacquelynne

Jacqueline (French) supplanter, substitute; little Jacqui.
Jacquel, Jacquelean, Jacqueleana, Jacqueleanah, Jacqueleane, Jacqueleen, Jacqueleena, Jacqueleenah, Jacqueleene, Jacquelein, Jacqueleina, Jacqueleinah, Jacqueleine, Jacquelene, Jacqueleyn, Jacqueleyna, Jacqueleynah, Jacqueleyne, Jacquelina, Jacquelinah, Jacquena, Jacquene, Jacquenetta, Jacquenette, Jacquiline, Jocqueline

Jacquetta (French) a form of Jacqueline.
Jacquette

Jacqui (French) a short form of Jacqueline. See also Jacki.
Jacquai, Jacquay, Jacqué, Jacquee, Jacqueta, Jacquete, Jacquey, Jacquie, Jacquise, Jacquita, Jakquee, Jakquei, Jakquey, Jakqui, Jakquie, Jakquy, Jaquai, Jaquay, Jaquee, Jaquei, Jaquey, Jaqui, Jaquie, Jaquiese, Jaquina, Jaquy

Jacquiline (French) a form of Jacqueline.
Jacquil, Jacquilin, Jacquilyn, Jacquilyne, Jacquilynn

Jacqulin, Jacquline, Jacqulyn (American) forms of Jacqueline.
Jacqul, Jacqulyne, Jacqulynn, Jacqulynne, Jacquoline

Jacy GB (American) a combination of the initials J. + C. (Greek) a familiar form of Jacinda.

Jacyline (French) a form of Jacqueline.
Jacylean, Jacyleana, Jacyleanah, Jacyleane, Jacyleen, Jacyleena, Jacyleenah, Jacyleene, Jacylein, Jacyleina, Jacyleinah, Jacyleine, Jacyleyn, Jacyleyna, Jacyleynah, Jacyleyne, Jacylin, Jacylina, Jacylinah, Jacylyn, Jacylyna,

Jacylynah, Jacylyne, Jacylynn, Jacylynna, Jacylynnah, Jacylynne

Jacynthe (Spanish) a form of Jacinda.
Jacynta, Jacynth, Jacyntha, Jacyntheia, Jacynthia, Jacynthy

Jada ☆ (Hebrew) wise. (Spanish) a form of Jade.
Jadae, Jadah, Jadda, Jaddah, Jadea, Jadeah

Jade GB (Spanish) jade.
Jadeann, Jadee, Jadera, Jadienne, Jaed

Jadelyn (American) a combination of Jade + Lynn.
Jadalyn, Jadelaine, Jadeline, Jadelyne, Jadelynn, Jadielin, Jadielyn

Jaden BG (Spanish) a form of Jade.
Jadeen, Jadeena, Jadena, Jadene, Jadeyn, Jadienna, Jadienne, Jadin, Jadine, Jadynn, Jaeden, Jaedine

Jadie (Spanish) a familiar form of Jade.
Jadi

Jadyn GB (Spanish) a form of Jade.

Jadzia (Spanish) a form of Jade.
Jadziah

Jae BG (Latin) jaybird. (French) a familiar form of Jacqueline.
Jaea, Jaey, Jaya

Jaeda (Spanish) a form of Jada.
Jaedah, Jaedra

Jaedyn (Spanish) a form of Jade.
Jaedynn

Jael GB (Hebrew) mountain goat; climber. See also Yael.
Jaele, Jaelea, Jaeleah, Jaelee, Jaelei, Jaeleigh, Jaeley, Jaeli, Jaelia, Jaeliah, Jaelie, Jaell, Jaelle, Jaelly, Jaely, Jahla, Jahlea, Jahlee, Jahlei, Jahleigh, Jahley, Jahli, Jahlia, Jahliah, Jahlie, Jahly, Jahlya, Jahlyah, Jailea, Jaileah, Jailee, Jailei, Jaileigh, Jailey, Jaili, Jailia, Jailiah, Jailie, Jaily

Jaela (Hebrew) a form of Jael.
Jaelah, Jaella, Jaellah, Jaelya, Jaelyah

Jaelyn, Jaelynn (American) combinations of Jae + Lynn.
Jaeleen, Jaeleena, Jaeleenah, Jaeleene, Jaelen, Jaelena, Jaelenah, Jaelene, Jaelin, Jaeline, Jaelinn, Jaelyna, Jaelynah, Jaelyne

Jaffa (Hebrew) a form of Yaffa.
Jaffice, Jaffit, Jafit, Jafra

Jaha (Swahili) dignified.
Jahaida, Jahida, Jahira, Jahitza

Jahaira (Swahili) a form of Jaha.
Jaharra, Jahayra

Jahna (American) a form of Johna.
Jahnaia, Jahnaya

Jai BG (Tai) heart. (Latin) a form of Jaye.

Jaid, Jaide (Spanish) forms of Jade.

Jaida (Hebrew, Spanish) a form of Jada.
Jaidah

Jaiden BG (Spanish) a form of Jade.
Jaidan, Jaidey, Jaidi, Jaidin, Jaidon

Jaidyn (Spanish) a form of Jade.

Jaila (Hebrew) a form of Jael.
Jailya, Jailyah

Jailene (American) a form of Jaelyn.
Jaileen, Jaileena, Jaileenah, Jaileene, Jailen, Jailena, Jailenah

Jailyn (American) a form of Jaelyn.
Jailin, Jailine, Jailyna, Jailynah, Jailyne

Jaime BG (French) I love.
Jaema, Jaemah, Jaemea, Jaemeah, Jahmea, Jaima, Jaimah, Jaimini, Jaimme, Jaimy, Jamee

Jaimee, Jaimi, Jaimie (French) forms of Jaime.
Jaemee, Jaemey, Jaemi, Jaemia, Jaemiah, Jaemie, Jaemy, Jaemya, Jaemyah, Jahmee, Jahmey, Jahmi, Jahmie, Jahmy, Jaimea, Jaimeah, Jaimey, Jaimia, Jaimiah, Jaimmie, Jaimy, Jaimya, Jaimyah

Jaimica (Spanish) a form of James.

Jaimilynn (English) a combination of Jaime + Lynn.
Jaimielin, Jaimielina, Jaimielinah, Jaimieline, Jaimielyn, Jaimielyna, Jaimielyne, Jaimielynn, Jaimielynne, Jaimilin, Jaimilina, Jaimilinah, Jaimiline, Jaimilyn, Jaimilyna, Jaimilyne, Jaimilynn, Jaimilynna, Jaimilynne, Jaymielin, Jaymielina, Jaymielinah, Jaymieline, Jaymielyn, Jaymielyna, Jaymielyne, Jaymielynn, Jaymielynne, Jaymilin, Jaymilina, Jaymilinah, Jaymiline, Jaymilyn, Jaymilyna, Jaymilyne, Jaymilynn, Jaymilynna, Jaymilynne

Jaina (Hebrew, American) a form of Janae.
Jainah

Jaione (Spanish) reference to the nativity.

Jaira (Spanish) Jehovah teaches.
Jahra, Jahrah, Jairah, Jairy, Jayra, Jayrah

Jakalyn (American) a form of Jacqueline.
*Jakalean, Jakaleana, Jakaleanah, Jakaleane,
Jakaleen, Jakaleena, Jakaleenah, Jakaleene,
Jakalein, Jakaleina, Jakaleinah, Jakaleine,
Jakaleyn, Jakaleyna, Jakaleynah, Jakaleyne,
Jakalin, Jakalina, Jakalinah, Jakaline, Jakalyna,
Jakalynah, Jakalyne, Jakalynn, Jakalynna,
Jakalynnah, Jakalynne*

Jakeisha (American) a combination of Jakki
+ Aisha.
*Jacqeesha, Jacqueisha, Jacqueysha, Jakeesha,
Jakeeshia, Jakeishia, Jakeishiah, Jakeisia,
Jakesha, Jakeshia, Jakeshiah, Jakeysha,
Jakeyshia, Jakeyshiah, Jakisha, Jakishia,
Jakishiah, Jaqueisha, Jaqueishia, Jaqueishiah,
Jaqueysha, Jaquisha, Jaquysha*

Jakelin (American) a form of Jacqueline.
Jakeline, Jakelyn, Jakelynn, Jakelynne

Jakeria (American) a form of Jacki.

Jakia (American) a form of Jacki.
*Jakiah, Jakiya, Jakiyah, Jakkea, Jakkia,
Jakkiah, Jakkya, Jakkyah*

Jakinda (Spanish) a form of Jacinda.
*Jackinda, Jackindra, Jakindah, Jakynda,
Jakyndah, Jakyndra, Jakyndrah*

Jakki (American) a form of Jacki.
*Jakala, Jakea, Jakee, Jakeela, Jakeida, Jakeita,
Jakel, Jakela, Jakelah, Jakelia, Jakeliah, Jakell,
Jakella, Jakelle, Jakena, Jakenah, Jaket, Jaketa,
Jaketah, Jakete, Jaketta, Jakettah, Jakette,
Jakeva, Jakevah, Jakevia, Jaki, Jakie, Jakita,
Jakke, Jakkee, Jakkie, Jakky, Jaky*

Jakolyn (American) a form of Jacqueline.
*Jakolean, Jakoleana, Jakoleanah, Jakoleane,
Jakoleen, Jakoleena, Jakoleenah, Jakoleene,
Jakolein, Jakoleina, Jakoleinah, Jakoleine,
Jakoleyn, Jakoleyna, Jakoleynah, Jakoleyne,
Jakolin, Jakolina, Jakolinah, Jakoline, Jakolyna,
Jakolynah, Jakolyne, Jakolynn, Jakolynna,
Jakolynnah, Jakolynne*

Jakqueline (French) a form of Jacqueline.
Jakquelean, Jakqueleana, Jakqueleanah,

*Jakqueleane, Jakqueleen, Jakqueleena,
Jakqueleenah, Jakqueleene, Jakquelein,
Jakqueleina, Jakqueleinah, Jakqueleine,
Jakqueleyn, Jakqueleyna, Jakqueleynah,
Jakqueleyne, Jakquelin, Jakquelina,
Jakquelinah, Jakquelyn, Jakquelyna,
Jakquelynah, Jakquelyne, Jakquelynn,
Jakquelynna, Jakquelynnah, Jakquelynne*

Jakyra (American) a form of Jacki.
Jakira

Jala (Iranian) brightness. (Arabic) clarity, elu-
cidation.

Jalea, Jalia (American) combinations of Jae
+ Leah.
Jaleah, Jalee, Jaleea, Jaleeya, Jaleia, Jalitza

Jalecia (American) a form of Jalisa.

Jaleesa (American) a form of Jalisa.
*Jaleasa, Jalece, Jalecea, Jaleesah, Jaleese, Jaleesia,
Jaleisa, Jaleisha, Jaleisya*

Jalen BG (American) a short form of Jalena.

Jalena (American) a combination of Jane +
Lena.
*Jalaina, Jalainah, Jalaine, Jalana, Jalanah,
Jalane, Jalani, Jalanie, Jalanna, Jalanne,
Jalayna, Jalaynah, Jalayne, Jaleana, Jaleanah,
Jaleena, Jaleenah, Jalenah, Jallena*

Jalene BG (American) a form of Jalena.
Jalean, Jaleane, Jaleen, Jaleene

Jalesa, Jalessa (American) forms of Jalisa.
Jalese, Jalesha, Jaleshia, Jalesia

Jalicia, Jalisha (American) forms of Jalisa.
Jalisia

Jalila (Arabic) great.
*Jalilah, Jalile, Jallila, Jallilah, Jallile, Jallyl,
Jallyla, Jallyle*

Jalinda (American) a combination of Jae +
Linda.
*Jaelinda, Jaelindah, Jaelynda, Jaelyndah,
Jailinda, Jailindah, Jailynda, Jailyndah,
Jaylinda, Jaylindah, Jaylynda, Jaylyndah*

Jalini (Hindi) lives next to the ocean.
Jalinee, Jaliney, Jalinie, Jaliny

Jalisa, Jalissa (American) combinations of
Jae + Lisa.
Jalise

Jaliya (American) a form of Jalea.

Jalyn GB (American) a combination of Jae + Lynn. See also Jaylyn.
Jalin, Jalina, Jalinah, Jaline, Jalyna, Jalynah, Jalyne, Jalynne

Jalynn (American) a combination of Jae + Lynn.

Jalysa (American) a form of Jalisa.
Jalyse, Jalyssa, Jalyssia

Jama (Sanskrit) daughter.
Jamah

Jamaica (Spanish) Geography: an island in the Caribbean.
Jamacia, Jameca, Jameica, Jamoka, Jemaica

Jamani (American) a form of Jami.
Jamana

Jamara (American) a form of Jamaria.

Jamaria (American) a combination of Jae + Maria.
Jamar, Jamarea, Jamaree, Jamari, Jamarie, Jameira, Jamerial

Jamecia (Spanish) a form of Jamaica.

Jamee (French) a form of Jaime.
Jamea, Jameah, Jamei, Jammee

Jameela (Arabic) a form of Jamila.
Jameelah, Jameele

Jameika (Spanish) a form of Jamaica.
Jamaika, Jamaka

Jameisha (American) a form of Jami.
Jamiesha

Jameka (Spanish) a form of Jamaica.
Jamecka, Jamekka

Jamekia (Spanish) a form of Jamaica.

Jamelia (Arabic) a form of Jamila.
Jahmelia, Jameelia, Jameeliah, Jameliah, Jamelya, Jamilya, Jamilyah

James BG (Hebrew) supplanter, substitute. (English) a form of Jacob. Bible: James the Great and James the Less were two of the Twelve Apostles.

Jamese (American) a form of Jami.
Jamesse, Jamis, Jamise

Jamesha (American) a form of Jami.
Jamesa, Jamesah, Jameshya, Jamesica, Jamesika, Jamesina, Jamesinah, Jamesine, Jamessa, Jameta, Jametta, Jamette, Jameysha, Jameyshya, Jameysina, Jameysinah, Jameysine, Jameysyna, Jameysynah, Jameysyne, Jammysha, Jamysha

Jameshia (American) a form of Jami.
Jameshyia, Jameyshia, Jameyshiah, Jameyshyah

Jamesia (American) a form of Jami.

Jamey GB (English) a form of Jami.
Jammey

Jami (Hebrew, English) a form of James.
Jamani, Jamay, Jamii, Jamy, Jamye, Jamyee, Jaymie

Jamia (English) a form of Jami.
Jamea, Jamiah, Jamiea, Jamiia, Jammea, Jammia, Jammiah, Jammiia, Jammiiah, Jaymea, Jaymeah, Jaymia, Jaymmea, Jaymmeah, Jaymmia, Jaymmiah, Jaymmya, Jaymya, Jaymyea

Jamica, Jamika (Spanish) forms of Jamaica.
Jamikah, Jamyka, Jamykah, Jemika, Jemyka

Jamie GB (Hebrew, English) a form of James.

Jamie-Lee (American) a form of Jamilee.
Jamielee

Jamie-Lynn (American) a form of Jamilynn.
Jami-Lyn, Jami-Lynn, Jami-Lynne, Jamie-Lyn, Jamie-Lynne

Jamila (Arabic) beautiful. See also Yamila.
Jahmeala, Jahmealah, Jahmeale, Jahmela, Jahmil, Jahmila, Jahmilah, Jahmill, Jahmilla, Jahmille, Jahmyla, Jahmylah, Jahmylla, Jahmyllah, Jahmylle, Jaimeala, Jaimealah, Jaimeale, Jaimila, Jaimilah, Jaimile, Jaimilla, Jaimillah, Jaimille, Jaimyla, Jaimylah, Jaimyle, Jaimylla, Jaimyllah, Jaimylle, Jameala, Jamealah, Jameale, Jameall, Jamealla, Jamealle, Jamela, Jamelah, Jamell, Jamella, Jamellah, Jamelle, Jamely, Jamiela, Jamyla, Jemila

Jamilah, Jamilla, Jamillah (Arabic) forms of Jamila.
Jamille

Jamilee (English) a combination of Jami + Lee.
Jahmilea, Jahmileah, Jahmilee, Jahmilei, Jahmileigh, Jahmili, Jahmilia, Jahmiliah, Jahmilie, Jahmily, Jaimilea, Jaimileah, Jaimilee, Jaimilei, Jaimileigh, Jaimiley, Jaimili, Jaimilia, Jaimiliah, Jaimilie, Jaimily, Jamilea, Jamileah, Jamilei, Jamileigh, Jamiley, Jamili, Jamilie, Jamily, Jaymilea, Jaymileah, Jaymilee, Jaymilei, Jaymileigh, Jaymiley, Jaymili, Jaymilia, Jaymiliah, Jaymilie, Jaymily, Jaymyly

Jamilia (Arabic) a form of Jamila.
Jamiliah, Jamillia, Jamilliah

Jamilynn (English) a combination of Jami + Lynn.
Jahmielin, Jahmielina, Jahmielinah, Jahmieline, Jahmielyn, Jahmielyna, Jahmielynah, Jahmielyne, Jahmielynn, Jahmielynne, Jahmilin, Jahmilina, Jahmilinah, Jahmiline, Jahmilyn, Jahmilyna, Jahmilyne, Jahmilynn, Jahmilynna, Jahmilynne, Jamielin, Jamielina, Jamielinah, Jamieline, Jamielyn, Jamielyna, Jamielyne, Jamielynn, Jamielynne, Jamilean, Jamileana, Jamileanah, Jamileane, Jamileen, Jamileena, Jamileenah, Jamileene, Jamilin, Jamilina, Jamilinah, Jamiline, Jamilyn, Jamilyna, Jamilynah, Jamilyne, Jamilynna, Jamilynne

Jamira (American) a form of Jamaria.

Jamisha (American) a form of Jami.
Jamisa, Jamisah, Jammesha, Jammisha

Jamison 🅱🅶 (English) child of James.
Jaemison, Jaemyson, Jaimison, Jaimyson, Jamiesen, Jamieson, Jamisen, Jamyson, Jaymison, Jaymyson

Jamiya (English) a form of Jami.
Jamiyah

Jammie (American) a form of Jami.
Jammi, Jammice, Jammii, Jammiie, Jammise

Jamonica (American) a combination of Jami + Monica.
Jamoni

Jamya (English) a form of Jami.
Jamyah

Jamylin (American) a form of Jamilynn.
Jamylin, Jamyline, Jamylyn, Jamylyne, Jamylynn, Jamylynne, Jaymylin, Jaymyline, Jaymylyn, Jaymylyne, Jaymylynn, Jaymylynne

Jan 🅱🅶 (English) a short form of Jane, Janet, Janice.
Jaan, Jandy, Jann, Janne

Jana (Hebrew) gracious, merciful. (Slavic) a form of Jane. See also Yana.
Jaana, Jaanah, Janah, Janalee, Janalisa, Janya, Janyah

Janae (American) a form of Jane. (Hebrew) a form of Jana.
Jaeena, Jaena, Janaea, Janaeh, Janah, Jannae

Janaé (American, Hebrew) a form of Janae.

Janai (American) a form of Janae.
Janaia, Janaiah, Janaira, Janaiya, Jannai, Jenai, Jenaia, Jennai

Janaki (Hindi) mother.
Janakee, Janakey, Janakie, Janaky

Janalee (American) a combination of Jana + Lee.
Janalea, Janaleah, Janalei, Janaleigh, Janaley, Janaly

Janalynn (American) a combination of Jana + Lynn.
Janalin, Janalina, Janaline, Janalyn, Janalyna, Janalyne, Janalynna, Janalynne

Janan (Arabic) heart; soul.
Jananee, Jananey, Janani, Janania, Jananiah, Jananie, Janann, Jananni, Janany

Janay, Janaye (American) forms of Jane. (Hebrew, Arabic) forms of Janna.
Jannay

Janaya (American) a form of Jane. (Hebrew, Arabic) a form of Janna.
Jananyah

Jane (Hebrew) God is gracious. See also Chavon, Jean, Joan, Juanita, Seana, Shana, Shawna, Sheena, Shona, Shunta, Sinead, Zaneta, Zanna, Zhana.
Jaane, Jaeen, Jaeene, Jaen, Jaene, Jahne, Jain, Jaine, Janka, Jasia

Janea, Janee (American) forms of Janae.
Janée

Janecia (Hebrew, English) a form of Janice.
Janeciah

Janeen (French) a form of Janine.
Janeena, Janeene

Janeisha (American) a form of Janessa.
Janiesha

Janel, Janell, Jannell, Jannelle (French)
forms of Janelle.
Jaenel, Jaenela, Jaenelah, Jaenell, Jainel, Jainela, Jainelah, Jainell, Janela, Janiel, Jannel, Janyll, Jaynel, Jaynela, Jaynelah, Jaynell

Janelle (French) a form of Jane.
Jaenele, Jaenella, Jaenellah, Jaenelle, Jainele, Jainella, Jainelle, Janele, Janelis, Janella, Janellah, Janelys, Janielle, Janille, Jannella, Jannellah, Jannellies, Jaynele, Jaynella, Jaynelle

Janelly, Janely (French) forms of Janelle.
Janelli, Janellie

Janese (Hebrew) a form of Janis. (English) a
form of Jane.
Janesey, Janess, Janesse

Janesha (American) a form of Janessa.
Janeshia, Janishia, Jannesha, Jannisha, Janysha, Jenesha, Jenisha, Jennisha

Janessa (American) a form of Jane.
Janeesa, Janesa, Janesea, Janesia, Janeska, Janessi, Janessia, Janiesa, Janisa, Janisah, Janissa, Jannesa, Jannessa, Jannisa, Jannisah, Jannissa, Jannysa, Jannysah, Janysa, Janysah, Janyssa, Janyssah, Jenesa, Jenissa, Jennisa, Jennissa

Janet (English) a form of Jane. See also
Jessie, Yanet.
Janata, Janeat, Janeata, Janeatah, Janeate, Janeet, Janeeta, Janeetah, Janeete, Janeta, Janetah, Janete, Janneta, Jannite, Janot, Janota, Janote, Janta, Jante, Janyt, Janyte, Jenet, Jenete

Janeth (English) a form of Janet.
Janetha, Janith, Janithe, Janneth

Janett, Janette, Jannet, Jannette (French)
forms of Janet.
Janeatt, Janeatte, Jannett, Jannitte, Janytte

Janetta (French) a form of Janet.
Janeattah, Janettah, Jannetta

Janey, Jani, Janie, Jany (English) familiar
forms of Jane.
Janiyh, Jaynee

Jania (Hebrew) a form of Jana. (Slavic) a
form of Jane.
Janiah

Janica (Hebrew) a form of Jane.
Janicka

Janice (Hebrew) God is gracious. (English) a
familiar form of Jane. See also Genice.
Janece, Janizzette, Jannice, Jannyc, Jannyce, Janyce, Jhanice, Jynice

Janick (Slavic) a short form of Janica.
Janyck

Janiece (Hebrew, English) a form of Janice.
Janeace, Janeece, Janeice, Janneece, Janneice, Janniece

Janik (Slavic) a short form of Janika.
Janike, Janikke, Jannik, Jannike, Janyk

Janika (Slavic) a form of Jane.
Janaca, Janeca, Janecka, Janeeca, Janeeka, Janeica, Janeika, Janeka, Janieka, Janikka, Janka, Jankia, Jannica, Jannika, Jannyca, Janyca, Janycah, Janycka, Janyka, Jonika

Janina (French) a form of Jane.
Janeana, Janena, Janinah, Jannina, Jannyna, Janyna, Janynah, Jenina, Jenyna, Jenynah

Janine (French) a form of Jane.
Janean, Janeane, Janeann, Janeanne, Janene, Jannen, Jannene, Jannine, Jannyne, Janyne, Jeneen, Jenyne

Janiqua (French) a form of Jane.
Janicqua, Janicquah, Janiquah, Janyqua, Janyquah, Jeniqua, Jeniquah, Jenyqua, Jenyquah

Janique (French) a form of Jane.
Janic, Janicque, Jannique, Janyque, Jenique, Jenyque

Janis **GB** (Hebrew, English) a form of Janice.
Janease, Janees, Janeese, Janeise, Janiese, Janisse, Jannis, Jannise, Jannisse, Jannys, Jannyse, Janys, Janyse, Janyss, Janysse, Jenesse, Jenis, Jennise, Jennisse

Janise (Hebrew, English) a form of Janice.

Janisha (American) a form of Janessa.

Janita (American) a form of Juanita. See also
Genita.
Janeata, Janeatah, Janeeta, Janeetah, Janeita,
Janeitah, Janitah, Janitra, Janitza, Janneta,
Jannita, Jannitah, Jannitta, Jannittah, Janyta,
Janytah, Janytta, Janyttah, Jaynita, Jaynite,
Jaynitta, Jaynitte, Jeneata, Jeneatah, Jeneeta,
Jeneetah, Jenita, Jenitah, Jennita, Jennitah,
Jennyta, Jenyta, Jenytah

Janna (Arabic) harvest of fruit. (Hebrew) a
short form of Johana.
Jannae, Jannai, Jannia, Janniah, Jannya,
Jannyah

Jannah (Hebrew, English) a form of Janna.

Jannali (Australian) moon.
Janali, Janalia, Janaliah, Janalie, Jannalea,
Jannaleah, Jannalee, Jannalei, Jannaleigh,
Jannaley, Jannalia, Jannaliah, Jannalie, Jannaly,
Jannalya, Jannalyah

Jannick (Slavic) a form of Janick.

Jannie (English) a familiar form of Jan, Jane.
Janney, Janni, Janny

Japonica (Latin) from Japan. Botany: an
ornamental shrub with red flowers native
to Japan.
Japonicah, Japonicka, Japonika, Japonikah,
Japonyca, Japonycah, Japonycka, Japonyka,
Japonykah

Jaquana (American) a combination of
Jacqueline + Anna.
Jaqua, Jaquai, Jaquanda, Jaquania, Jaquanna

Jaquelen, Jaquelin, Jaqueline, Jaquelyn
(French) forms of Jacqueline.
Jaquala, Jaqualin, Jaqualine, Jaquelean,
Jaqueleana, Jaqueleanah, Jaqueleane, Jaqueleen,
Jaqueleena, Jaqueleenah, Jaqueleene, Jaquelein,
Jaqueleina, Jaqueleinah, Jaqueleine, Jaqueleyn,
Jaqueleyna, Jaqueleynah, Jaqueleyne, Jaquelina,
Jaquelinah, Jaquella, Jaquelyna, Jaquelynah,
Jaquelyne, Jaquelynn, Jaquelynna, Jaquelynnah,
Jaquelynne, Jaquera, Jaqulene, Jaquonna

Jaquetta (French) a form of Jacqui.

Jaquiline (French) a form of Jacqueline.
Jaquilean, Jaquileana, Jaquileanah, Jaquileane,
Jaquileen, Jaquileena, Jaquileenah, Jaquileene,
Jaquilein, Jaquileina, Jaquileinah, Jaquileine,
Jaquileyn, Jaquileyna, Jaquileynah, Jaquileyne,

Jaquilin, Jaquilina, Jaquilinah, Jaquilyn,
Jaquilyna, Jaquilynah, Jaquilyne, Jaquilynn,
Jaquilynna, Jaquilynnah, Jaquilynne

Jaquinda (Spanish) a form of Jacinda.

Jaquita (French) a form of Jacqui.

Jardena (French, Spanish) garden. (Hebrew)
a form of Jordan.
Jardan, Jardana, Jardanah, Jardane, Jardania,
Jarden, Jardene, Jardenia, Jardin, Jardina,
Jardinah, Jardine, Jardyn, Jardyna, Jardyne,
Jardynia

Jarian (American) a combination of Jane +
Marian.

Jarita (Arabic) earthen water jug.
Jara, Jareata, Jareatah, Jareet, Jareeta, Jareetah,
Jareita, Jareitah, Jaretta, Jari, Jaria, Jariah,
Jarica, Jarida, Jarietta, Jariette, Jarika, Jarina,
Jarinah, Jaritta, Jaritte, Jaritza, Jarixa, Jarnita,
Jarnite, Jarrika, Jarrike, Jarrina, Jarrine, Jaryta,
Jarytah, Jaryte, Jarytta, Jarytte

Jarmilla (Slavic) a form of Yarmilla.
Jarmila, Jarmilah, Jarmile, Jarmill, Jarmille,
Jarmyla, Jarmylah, Jarmyle, Jarmyll, Jarmylla,
Jarmyllah, Jarmylle

Jarnila (Arabic) beautiful.
Jarnilah, Jarnile, Jarnill, Jarnilla, Jarnillah,
Jarnille, Jarnyl, Jarnyla, Jarnylah, Jarnyle,
Jarnyll, Jarnylla, Jarnyllah, Jarnylle

Jarvia (German) skilled with a spear.
Jarviah, Jarvya, Jarvyah

Jarvinia (German) intelligent; keen as a
spear.
Jarviniah, Jarvinya, Jarvinyah, Jarvynya,
Jarvynyah

Jas BG (American) a short form of Jasmine.
Jase, Jass, Jaz, Jazz, Jazze

Jasa (Polish) a form of Jane.
Jasyah, Jaysa

Jasey (Polish) a form of Jane.
Jasea

Jasia (Polish) a form of Jane.
Jaisha, Jasha, Jashae, Jashala, Jashona,
Jashonte, Jazia, Jaziah, Jazya, Jazyah, Jazzia,
Jazziah, Jazzya, Jazzyah

Jaskiran (Sikh) a form of Jaskaran (see Boys' Names).

Jasleen (Latin) a form of Jocelyn.
Jaslene, Jaslien, Jasline

Jaslyn (Latin) a form of Jocelyn.
Jaslin, Jaslynn, Jaslynne

Jasma (Persian) a short form of Jasmine.

Jasmain, Jasmaine (Persian) forms of Jasmine.
Jasmane, Jassmain, Jassmaine

Jasman (Persian) a form of Jasmine.

Jasmarie (American) a combination of Jasmine + Marie.
Jasmari

Jasmeen (Persian) a form of Jasmine.

Jasmeet BG (Persian) a form of Jasmine.
Jasmit, Jassmit

Jasmin GB (Persian) a form of Jasmine.
Jasmynn, Jasmynne, Jassmin, Jassminn, Jassmyn

Jasmina (Persian) a form of Jasmine.
Jasminah, Jasmyna, Jasmynah, Jassma, Jazmina, Jazminah, Jazmyna, Jazmynah, Jazzmina, Jazzminah, Jazzmyna, Jazzmynah, Jesmina, Jesminah, Jesmyna, Jesmynah, Jessmina, Jessminah, Jessmyna, Jessmynah, Jezmina, Jezminah, Jezzmina, Jezzminah, Jezzmyna, Jezzmynah

Jasmine ☆ (Persian) jasmine flower. See also Jessamine, Yasmin.
Jasimin, Jasmain, Jasme, Jasmen, Jasmene, Jasminne, Jasmira, Jasmon, Jassmon, Jesmin, Jesmine, Jesmyn, Jesmyne, Jessmin, Jessmine, Jessmyn, Jessmyne

Jasmyn, Jasmyne, Jassmine (Persian) forms of Jasmine.

Jasone (Basque) assumption.

Jasper BG (French) red, yellow, or brown ornamental stone.
Jaspa, Jaspah, Jaspar, Jaspera, Jaspere

Jaspreet BG (Punjabi) virtuous.
Jasparit, Jasparita, Jasparite, Jasprit, Jasprita, Jasprite, Jaspryta, Jasprytah, Jaspryte

Jassi (Persian) a familiar form of Jasmine.
Jasee, Jasi, Jasie, Jassee, Jassey, Jassie, Jassy

Jatara (American) a combination of Jane + Tara.
Jatarah, Jataria, Jatariah, Jatarra, Jatarrah, Jatarria, Jatori, Jatoria, Jatoriah, Jatorie, Jatory, Jatorya, Jatoryah

Javán (Hebrew) from Greece.

Javana (Malay) from Java.
Javanah, Javanna, Javannah, Javanne, Javannia, Jawana, Jawanna, Jawn

Javiera (Spanish) owner of a new house. See also Xaviera.
Javeera, Javeerah, Javierah, Javyra, Javyrah, Viera

Javon BG (Malay) a short form of Javana.

Javona, Javonna (Malay) forms of Javana.
Javonah, Javonda, Javone, Javoni, Javonia, Javonn, Javonnah, Javonne, Javonni, Javonnia, Javonniah, Javonya, Javonyah

Jaya (Hindi) victory.
Jaea, Jaia, Jaiah, Jayah

Jayanna (American) a combination of Jaye + Anna.
Jay-Anna, Jaye-Anna, Jayeanna

Jayce BG (American) a form of Jacey.
Jaycey, Jaycy

Jaycee, Jayci, Jaycie (American) forms of Jacey.

Jayda (Spanish) a form of Jada.
Jaydah, Jeyda

Jayde GB (Spanish) a form of Jade.
Jayd

Jaydee (American) a combination of the initials J. + D.
Jadee, Jadey, Jady, Jaydey, Jaydi, Jaydie, Jaydy

Jayden BG (Spanish) a form of Jade.
Jaydeen, Jaydene, Jaydin, Jaydn

Jaydon BG (Spanish) a form of Jayden.

Jaye BG (Latin) jaybird.
Jae, Jah, Jay

Jayla (American) a short form of Jayleen.
Jaylaa, Jaylah, Jaylea, Jayleah, Jaylei, Jayleigh, Jayley, Jayli, Jaylia, Jayliah, Jaylie, Jayly

Jaylee GB (American) a familiar form of Jaylyn.

Jayleen, Jaylene (American) forms of Jaylyn.
Jayelene, Jayleana, Jayleena, Jayleenah, Jayleene, Jaylena, Jaylenne, Jayline

Jaylen BG (American) a form of Jaylyn.
Jaylan, Jaylinn

Jaylin BG (American) a form of Jaylyn.

Jaylyn BG (American) a combination of Jaye + Lynn. See also Jalyn.
Jaylyna, Jaylynah, Jaylyne, Jaylynne

Jaylynn (American) a combination of Jaye + Lynn.

Jayme GB (English) a form of Jami.
Jayma, Jaymey, Jaymine, Jaymini, Jaymma, Jaymmi, Jaymmie, Jaymmy, Jaymy, Jaymye, Jaymyee

Jaymee, Jaymi, Jaymie (English) forms of Jami.

Jayna (Hebrew) a form of Jane.
Jaena, Jaenah, Jaina, Jainah, Jaynae, Jaynah, Jaynna, Jaynnah

Jayne (Hindi) victorious. (English) a form of Jane.
Jayn, Jaynn, Jaynne

Jaynee, Jaynie (English) familiar forms of Jayne.
Jaynay, Jayni

Jazlyn, Jazlynn, Jazzlyn (American) combinations of Jazman + Lynn.
Jazaline, Jazalyn, Jazlean, Jazleana, Jazleanah, Jazleane, Jazleen, Jazleena, Jazleenah, Jazleene, Jazlene, Jazlin, Jazlina, Jazlinah, Jazline, Jazlon, Jazlyna, Jazlynah, Jazlyne, Jazlynna, Jazlynnah, Jazlynne, Jazzalyn, Jazzleen, Jazzleena, Jazzleenah, Jazzleene, Jazzlene, Jazzlin, Jazzlina, Jazzlinah, Jazzline, Jazzlyna, Jazzlynah, Jazzlyne, Jazzlynn, Jazzlynna, Jazzlynnah, Jazzlynne

Jazman, Jazmen, Jazmin, Jazmine, Jazmyn, Jazmyne, Jazzmen, Jazzmin, Jazzmine, Jazzmyn, Jazzmyne (Persian) forms of Jasmine.
Jazmaine, Jazminn, Jazmon, Jazmynn,
Jazmynne, Jazzman, Jazzmeen, Jazzmene, Jazzmenn, Jazzmon, Jezmin, Jezmine, Jezzmin, Jezzmine, Jezzmyn, Jezzmyne

Jazmín (Arabic) a form of Jasmine.

Jazz BG (American) jazz.
Jaz, Jazee, Jazey, Jazi, Jazie, Jazy, Jazzee, Jazzey, Jazzi, Jazzie, Jazzy

Jean BG (Scottish) God is gracious. See also Kini.
Jeanann, Jeancie, Jeane, Jeaneia, Jeaneva, Jeanice, Jeanmaria, Jeanmarie, Jeann, Jeanné, Jeantelle, Jeen, Jeene

Jeana, Jeanna (Scottish) forms of Jean.
Jeanae, Jeannae, Jeannah, Jeannia, Jeena, Jeenia

Jeanelle (American) a form of Jenell.
Jeanell

Jeanetta (French) a form of Jean.
Jeanettah

Jeanette, Jeannett, Jeannette (French) forms of Jean.
Jeanet, Jeaneta, Jeanetah, Jeanete, Jeanett, Jeanetton, Jeanita, Jeannete, Jeannetta, Jeannita, Jeannot, Jinet, Jineta, Jinetah, Jinete, Jinett, Jinetta, Jinettah, Jinette, Jonet, Joneta, Jonetah, Jonete, Jonett, Jonetta, Jonettah, Jonette, Jynet, Jyneta, Jynetah, Jynete, Jynett, Jynetta, Jynettah, Jynette

Jeanie, Jeannie (Scottish) familiar forms of Jean.
Jeanee, Jeani, Jeannee, Jeanney, Jeanny, Jeany

Jeanine, Jeannine, Jenine (Scottish) forms of Jean. See also Geneen.
Jeaneane, Jeaneen, Jeanene, Jeanina, Jeannina, Jennine

Jeanne (Scottish) a form of Jean.

Jelani BG (Russian) a form of Jelena.
Jelanni

Jelena (Russian) a form of Helen. See also Yelena.
Jelaina, Jelainah, Jelaine, Jelana, Jelanah, Jelane, Jelayna, Jelaynah, Jelayne, Jelean, Jeleana, Jeleanah, Jeleane, Jeleen, Jeleena, Jeleenah, Jeleene, Jelenah, Jelene, Jelin, Jelina, Jelinah, Jeline, Jelyn, Jelyna, Jelynah, Jelyne

Jelisa (American) a combination of Jean + Lisa.
Jelesha, Jelise, Jellese, Jellice, Jelysa, Jillisa

Jelissa (American) a form of Jelisa.
Jelessa, Jelyssa, Jillissa

Jem GB (Hebrew) a short form of Jemima.
Gem, Jemee, Jemey, Jemi, Jemie, Jemm, Jemy

Jemila (Arabic) a form of Jamila.
Jemeala, Jemealah, Jemeela, Jemeelah, Jemeelia, Jemeeliah, Jemela, Jemelah, Jemelia, Jemeliah, Jemila, Jemilla, Jemillah, Jemille, Jemyl, Jemyla, Jemylah, Jemyle, Jemyll, Jemylla, Jemyllah, Jemylle

Jemima (Hebrew) dove.
Gemima, Gemimah, Jamim, Jamima, Jemimah, Jemyma, Jemymah

Jemina, Jenima (Hebrew) forms of Jemima.

Jemma (Hebrew) a short form of Jemima. (English) a form of Gema.
Jema, Jemah, Jemia, Jemiah, Jemmah, Jemmee, Jemmey, Jemmi, Jemmia, Jemmiah, Jemmie, Jemmy, Jemmya, Jemmyah

Jena, Jennah (Arabic) forms of Jenna.
Jenah, Jenal, Jenya, Jenyah

Jenae, Jenay (American, Hebrew) forms of Janae. (Arabic) forms of Jenna.
Jenai, Jenea, Jennae, Jennay, Jennaye

Jenara (Latin) dedicated to the god Janus.

Jenaya (American, Hebrew) a form of Janae. (Arabic) a form of Jenna.
Jenia, Jeniah, Jennaya

Jendaya (Zimbabwean) thankful.
Daya, Jandaiah, Jenda, Jendaia, Jendayah

Jendayi (Egyptian) a form of Jendaya.

Jeneleah (American) a combination of Jenny + Leah.
Jenalea, Jenaleah, Jenalia, Jenaliah, Jenelea, Jenelia, Jeneliah, Jenilea, Jenileah, Jenilia, Jeniliah, Jennalea, Jennaleah, Jennalia, Jennaliah, Jennelea, Jenneleah, Jennelia, Jenneliah, Jennilea, Jennileah, Jennilia, Jenniliah, Jennylea, Jennyleah, Jennylia, Jennyliah, Jenylea, Jenyleah, Jenylia, Jenyliah

Jenell, Jenelle, Jennelle (American) combinations of Jenny + Nell.
Genell, Jenall, Jenalle, Jenel, Jenela, Jenelah, Jenele, Jenella, Jenellah, Jenille, Jennel, Jennele, Jennell, Jennella, Jennielle, Jennille, Jinelle, Jinnell

Jenessa (American) a form of Jenisa.
Jenesa, Jenese, Jenesia, Jenessia, Jennesa, Jennese, Jennessa, Jinessa

Jenette (French) a form of Jean.
Jeneta, Jenetah, Jenett, Jenetta, Jenettah, Jennet, Jennett, Jennetta, Jennette, Jennita

Jeneva (French) a form of Geneva.
Janeva, Jeaneva, Jenava, Jenavah, Jenevah, Jenevia, Jeneviah, Jenniva, Jennivah

Jeni, Jenni, Jennie (Welsh) familiar forms of Jennifer. See also Jenny.
Jenee, Jenie, Jenne, Jenné, Jennee, Jenney, Jennia, Jenniah, Jennier, Jennita, Jennora

Jenica, Jenika, Jennica, Jennicah (Romanian) forms of Jane.
Jeneca, Jenicah, Jenicka, Jenickah, Jenikah, Jenikka, Jeniqua, Jeniquah, Jenique, Jennicka, Jennickah, Jennika, Jennikah, Jenniqua, Jenniquah, Jennique, Jennyca, Jennycah, Jennycka, Jennyckah, Jennyka, Jennykah, Jennyqua, Jennyquah, Jenyca, Jenycah, Jenyka

Jenice, Jenise (Hebrew) forms of Janice.
Jenicee, Jenicy, Jenisse, Jennyce, Jennyse

Jenifer, Jeniffer, Jenniffer (Welsh) forms of Jennifer.
Jenifar, Jenipher

Jenilee, Jennilee (American) combinations of Jeni + Lee. See also Jenny Lee.
Jenelee, Jenelei, Jeneleigh, Jeneley, Jeneli, Jenelie, Jenelly, Jenely, Jenilei, Jenileigh, Jeniley, Jenili, Jenilie, Jenily, Jennelee, Jennelei, Jenneleigh, Jennely, Jennielee, Jennilee, Jennilei, Jennileigh, Jenniley, Jennili, Jennilie, Jennily, Jinnalee

Jenisa (American) a combination of Jennifer + Nisa.
Jenisha, Jenissa, Jenisse, Jennisa, Jennise, Jennisha, Jennissa, Jennisse, Jennysa, Jennyssa, Jenysa, Jenyse, Jenyssa, Jenysse

Jenka (Czech) a form of Jane.

Jenna ⁂ (Arabic) small bird. (Welsh) a short form of Jennifer. See also Gen.
Janah, Jennae, Jennai, Jennat, Jennay, Jennaya, Jennaye, Jhenna

Jenna-Lee, Jennalee (American) combinations of Jenna + Lee.
Jenalee, Jenalei, Jenaleigh, Jenaley, Jenali, Jenalie, Jenaly, Jenna-Leigh, Jennalei, Jennaleigh

Jennafer (Welsh) a form of Jennifer.
Jenafar, Jenafer, Jennafar

Jennifer ⁂ GB (Welsh) white wave; white phantom. A form of Guinevere. See also Gennifer, Ginnifer, Yenifer.
Jen, Jenefar, Jenefer, Jeneffar, Jeneffer, Jennefar, Jennefer, Jennifar, Jenniferanne, Jenniferlee, Jenniffe, Jenniffier, Jennifier, Jenniphe, Jennipher

Jennilyn, Jennilynn (American) combinations of Jeni + Lynn.
Jenalin, Jenalyn, Jenelyn, Jenilyn, Jennalin, Jennaline, Jennalyn, Jennalyne, Jennalynn, Jennalynne, Jennilin, Jenniline, Jennilyne, Jennilynne

Jenny (Welsh) a familiar form of Jennifer. See also Jeni.
Jenney, Jennya, Jennyah, Jeny, Jenya, Jenyah

Jenny Lee (American) a combination of Jenny + Lee. See also Jenilee.
Jennylee, Jennylei, Jennyleigh, Jennyley, Jennyli, Jennylie, Jennyly, Jenylee, Jenylei, Jenyleigh, Jenyley, Jenyli, Jenylie, Jenyly

Jennyfer (Welsh) a form of Jennifer.
Jennyfar, Jenyfar, Jenyfer

Jensen GB (Scandinavian) a form of Janson (see Boys' Names).
Jensan, Jensin, Jenson, Jensyn

Jensine (Welsh) a form of Jeni.

Jeraldine (English) a form of Geraldine.
Jeraldeen, Jeraldeena, Jeraldena, Jeraldene, Jeraldin, Jeraldina, Jeraldinah, Jeraldyn, Jeraldyna, Jeraldynah, Jeraldyne, Jeralee

Jeremia (Hebrew) God will uplift.
Jeramia, Jeramiah, Jeramya, Jeramyah, Jeremiah, Jeremya, Jeremyah

Jereni (Russian) a form of Irene.
Jerena, Jerenae, Jerenee, Jerenia, Jereniah, Jerenie, Jereny, Jerenya, Jerenyah, Jerina

Jeri, Jerri, Jerrie (American) short forms of Jeraldine. See also Geri.
Jera, Jerae, JeRae, Jeree, Jerey, Jerie, Jeriel, Jerilee, Jerinda, Jerra, Jerrah, Jerrece, Jerree, Jerrey, Jerriann, Jerrilee, Jerrine, Jerry, Jerrylea, Jerrylee, Jerryne, Jery, Jerzy

Jerica, Jericka, Jerika, Jerrica, Jerrika (American) combinations of Jeri + Erica.
Jereca, Jerecka, Jericah, Jerice, Jerikah, Jeriqua, Jeriquah, Jerreka, Jerricah, Jerricca, Jerrice, Jerricha, Jerricka, Jerrieka, Jeryca, Jerycah, Jerycka, Jeryka, Jerykah, Jeryqua, Jeryquah

Jerilyn (American) a combination of Jeri + Lynn.
Jeralin, Jeralina, Jeralinah, Jeraline, Jeralyn, Jeralyna, Jeralynah, Jeralyne, Jeralynn, Jeralynne, Jerelin, Jereline, Jerelyn, Jerelyne, Jerelynn, Jerelynne, Jerilin, Jerilina, Jerilinah, Jeriline, Jerilyna, Jerilynah, Jerilyne, Jerilynn, Jerilynna, Jerilynnah, Jerilynne, Jerrilin, Jerriline, Jerrilyn, Jerrilyne, Jerrilynn, Jerrilynne, Jerylin, Jerylina, Jerylinah, Jeryline, Jerylyn, Jerylyna, Jerylynah, Jerylyne

Jermaine BG (French) a form of Germaine.
Jerma, Jermain, Jermaina, Jermainah, Jerman, Jermanay, Jermanaye, Jermane, Jermanee, Jermani, Jermanique, Jermany, Jermayn, Jermayna, Jermaynah, Jermayne, Jermecia, Jermia, Jermice, Jermicia, Jermila

Jermeka (French) a form of Jermaine.
Jermika

Jeroma (Latin) holy.
Geroma, Geromah, Jeromah, Jerometta, Jeromette, Jeromima, Jeromyma

Jerónima (Greek) a form of Jeroma.

Jerusalem (Hebrew) vision of peace. Geography: Jerusalem is a holy city in Israel.

Jerusalén (Spanish) a form of Jerusalem.

Jerusha (Hebrew) inheritance.
Jerushah, Yerusha

Jesenia, Jessenia (Arabic) flower.
Jescenia, Jesceniah, Jescenya, Jescenyah, Jeseniah, Jesenya, Jesenyah, Jessennia, Jessenya

Jesi, Jessye (Hebrew) forms of Jessie.
Jese, Jessee

Jesica, Jesika, Jessicca, Jessika (Hebrew) forms of Jessica.
Jesicah, Jesicca, Jesikah, Jessikkah, Jessikah

Jésica (Slavic) a form of Jessica.

Jessa (American) a short form of Jessalyn, Jessamine, Jessica.
Jesa, Jesha, Jessah

Jessalyn (American) a combination of Jessica + Lynn.
Jesalin, Jesaline, Jesalyn, Jesalyne, Jesalynn, Jesalynne, Jessalin, Jessalina, Jessalinah, Jessaline, Jessalyna, Jessalynah, Jessalyne, Jessalynn, Jessalynne, Jesselin, Jesseline, Jesselyn, Jesselyne, Jesselynn, Jesselynne

Jessamine (French) a form of Jasmine.
Jesamin, Jesamina, Jesaminah, Jesamine, Jesamon, Jesamona, Jesamone, Jesamyn, Jesamyna, Jesamynah, Jesamyne, Jessamin, Jessamina, Jessaminah, Jessamon, Jessamona, Jessamonah, Jessamone, Jessamy, Jessamya, Jessamyah, Jessamyn, Jessamyna, Jessamynah, Jessamyne, Jessemin, Jessemina, Jesseminah, Jessemine, Jessimin, Jessimine, Jessmin, Jessmina, Jessminah, Jessmine, Jessmon, Jessmona, Jessmonah, Jessmone, Jessmy, Jessmyn, Jessmyna, Jessmynah, Jessmyne

Jesse BG (Hebrew) a form of Jessie.

Jesseca (Hebrew) a form of Jessica.
Jessecah, Jesseeca, Jesseeka, Jesseka, Jessekah

Jessi GB (Hebrew) a form of Jessie.

Jessica ☆ GB (Hebrew) wealthy. Literature: a name perhaps invented by Shakespeare for a character in his play *The Merchant of Venice*. See also Gessica, Yesica.
Jesicka, Jessaca, Jessca, Jesscia, Jessia, Jessiah, Jessicia, Jessicka, Jessieka, Jessiqua, Jessiquah, Jessique, Jezeca, Jezecah, Jezecka, Jezeka, Jezekah, Jezica, Jezicah, Jezicka, Jezika, Jezikah, Jeziqua, Jeziquah, Jezyca, Jezycah, Jezycka, Jezyka, Jisica, Jisicah, Jisicka, Jisika, Jisikah, Jisiqua, Jisiquah, Jysica, Jysicah, Jysicka, Jysika, Jyssica, Jyssicah, Jyssicka, Jyssika, Jyssikah, Jyssiqua, Jyssiquah, Jyssyca, Jyssycka, Jyssyka, Jyssykah, Jysyka, Jysykah, Jysyqua, Jysyquah

Jessica-Lynn (American) a combination of Jessica + Lynn.
Jessica-Lyn, Jessica-Lynne, Jessicalyn, Jessicalynn, Jessicalynne

Jessie BG (Hebrew) a short form of Jessica. (Scottish) a form of Janet.
Jescie, Jesea, Jesee, Jesey, Jesie, Jess, Jessé, Jessea, Jessee, Jessey, Jessia, Jessiah, Jessiya, Jesy

Jessilyn (American) a form of Jessalyn.
Jesilin, Jesiline, Jesilyn, Jesilyne, Jesilynn, Jesilynne, Jessilynn

Jesslyn (American) a short form of Jessalyn.
Jesslin, Jesslynn, Jesslynne

Jessy BG (Hebrew) a short form of Jessica. (Scottish) a form of Janet.

Jessyca, Jessyka (Hebrew) forms of Jessica.
Jessycka, Jessyqua, Jessyquah

Jesus BG (Hebrew) God is my salvation. A form of Joshua. Bible: son of Mary and Joseph, believed by Christians to be the Son of God.

Jesusa (Spanish) a form of Jesus.

Jésusa (Spanish) a form of Jesus.
Jesusita, Jesusyta

Jetta (English) jet black mineral. (American) a familiar form of Jevette.
Jeta, Jetah, Jetia, Jetiah, Jetje, Jett, Jettah, Jette, Jetti, Jettia, Jettiah, Jettie, Jetty, Jettya, Jettyah

Jevette (American) a combination of Jean + Yvette.
Jeva, Jeveta, Jevetta

Jewel (French) precious gem.
Jewal, Jewele, Jewelei, Jeweleigh, Jeweli, Jewelie, Jewely, Juel, Juela, Juele

Jewelana (American) a combination of Jewel + Anna.
Jewelanah, Jewelann, Jeweliana, Jeweliann, Juelana, Juelanah, Julana, Julanah

Jewell (French) a form of Jewel.
Jewella, Jewelle, Jewellea, Jewelleah, Jewellee, Jewellene, Jewellie

Jezabel (Hebrew) a form of Jezebel.
*Jesabel, Jesabela, Jesabelah, Jesabele, Jesabell,
Jesabella, Jesabellah, Jesabelle, Jessabel,
Jessabela, Jessabelah, Jessabele, Jessabell,
Jessabella, Jessabellah, Jessabelle, Jezabela,
Jezabelah, Jezabele, Jezabell, Jezabella,
Jezabellah, Jezabelle*

Jezebel (Hebrew) unexalted; impure. Bible:
the wife of King Ahab.
*Jesibel, Jessebel, Jessebela, Jessebelah, Jessebele,
Jessebell, Jessebella, Jessebellah, Jessebelle, Jez,
Jezebela, Jezebelah, Jezebele, Jezebell,
Jezebella, Jezebellah, Jezebelle*

Jianna (Italian) a form of Giana.
*Jiana, Jianah, Jianina, Jianine, Jiannah, Jianni,
Jiannini, Jyana, Jyanah, Jyanna, Jyannah*

Jibon (Hindi) life.
*Jibona, Jibonah, Jibone, Jybon, Jybona,
Jybonah, Jybone*

Jill (English) a short form of Jillian.
Jil, Jyl, Jyll

Jillaine (Latin) a form of Jillian.
*Jilain, Jilaina, Jilaine, Jilane, Jilayne, Jillain,
Jillaina, Jillane, Jillayn, Jillayna, Jillayne,
Jylain, Jylaina, Jylaine, Jylan, Jylane, Jyllain,
Jyllaina, Jyllaine, Jyllane, Jyllanne, Jyllayn,
Jyllayna, Jyllayne*

Jillanna (Latin) a form of Jillian.
*Jilan, Jilana, Jillana, Jillann, Jillannah,
Jillanne, Jylana, Jyllana, Jyllanah, Jyllann,
Jyllanna, Jyllannah*

Jilleen (Irish) a form of Jillian.
*Jileen, Jilene, Jiline, Jillene, Jillenne, Jilline,
Jillyn*

Jilli (Australian) today.
*Jilea, Jileah, Jilee, Jilei, Jileigh, Jili, Jilie, Jillea,
Jilleah, Jillee, Jillei, Jilleigh, Jilley, Jillie, Jilly,
Jily, Jylea, Jyleah, Jylee, Jylei, Jyleigh, Jyley,
Jyli, Jylie, Jyllea, Jylleah, Jyllee, Jyllei, Jylleigh,
Jylli, Jyllie, Jylly, Jyly*

Jillian (Latin) youthful. See also Gillian.
*Jilian, Jiliana, Jilianah, Jiliane, Jiliann,
Jilianna, Jiliannah, Jilianne, Jilienna, Jilienne,
Jillaine, Jillanna, Jilleen, Jilliana, Jillianah,
Jilliane, Jilliann, Jillianna, Jilliannah, Jillianne,
Jillien, Jillienne, Jillion, Jilliyn, Jillyan, Jillyana,
Jillyanah, Jillyane, Jillyann, Jillyanna,
Jillyannah, Jillyanne, Jilyan, Jilyana, Jilyanah,*

*Jilyane, Jilyann, Jilyanna, Jilyannah, Jilyanne,
Jyllian*

Jimena (Hebrew, American) a form of Jimi.

Jimi 🅑🅖 (Hebrew) supplanter, substitute.
*Jimae, Jimaria, Jimee, Jimella, Jimey, Jimia,
Jimiah, Jimie, Jimiyah, Jimmee, Jimmeka,
Jimmet, Jimmey, Jimmi, Jimmia, Jimmie,
Jimmy, Jimy, Jymee, Jymey, Jymi, Jymie,
Jymmee, Jymmey, Jymmi, Jymmie, Jymmy,
Jymy*

Jimisha (American) a combination of Jimi +
Aisha.
Jimica, Jimicia, Jimmicia, Jimysha

Jin 🅑🅖 (Japanese) tender. (American) a short
form of Ginny, Jinny.
Jyn

Jina 🅖🅑 (Swahili) baby with a name. (Italian)
a form of Gina.
*Jinae, Jinah, Jinan, Jinda, Jinna, Jinnae,
Jinnah, Jyna, Jynah, Jynna, Jynnah*

Jinny (Scottish) a familiar form of Jenny.
(American) a familiar form of Virginia. See
also Ginny.
*Jinee, Jiney, Jini, Jinie, Jinnee, Jinney, Jinni,
Jinnie, Jiny, Jynee, Jyney, Jyni, Jynie, Jynnee,
Jynney, Jynni, Jynnie, Jynny, Jyny*

Jira (African) related by blood.

Jirakee (Australian) waterfall, cascade.
*Jirakei, Jirakey, Jiraki, Jirakie, Jiraky, Jyrakee,
Jyrakei, Jyrakey, Jyraki, Jyrakie, Jyraky*

Jirina (Czech) a form of Georgia.
*Jirah, Jireana, Jireanah, Jireena, Jireenah, Jireh,
Jirinah, Jiryna, Jirynah, Jyreana, Jyreanah,
Jyreena, Jyreenah, Jyrina, Jyrinah, Jyryna,
Jyrynah*

Jizelle (American) a form of Giselle.
*Jessel, Jezel, Jezela, Jezelah, Jezele, Jezell,
Jezella, Jezellah, Jezelle, Jisel, Jisela, Jisele,
Jisell, Jisella, Jiselle, Jissel, Jissell, Jissella,
Jisselle, Jizel, Jizela, Jizele, Jizell, Jizella,
Joselle, Jyzel, Jyzela, Jyzele, Jyzell, Jyzella,
Jyzelle*

Jo 🅖🅑 (American) a short form of Joana,
Jolene, Josephine.
Joangie, Joe, Joee, Joetta, Joette, Joh

Joan GB (Hebrew) God is gracious. History: Joan of Arc was a fifteenth-century heroine and resistance fighter. See also Ioana, Jane, Jean, Juanita, Siobhan.
Joaneil, Joanmarie, Joannanette, Joayn, Joen, Joenn, Jonni

Joana, Joanna (English) forms of Joan. See also Yoana.
Janka, Jhoana, Jo-Ana, Jo-Anie, Jo-Anna, Jo-Annie, Joahna, Joanah, Joananna, Joandra, Joanka, Joannah, Joayna, Joeana, Joeanah, Joeanna, Joeannah, Joena, Joenah, Joenna, Joennah

Joanie, Joannie, Joanny, Joany (Hebrew) familiar forms of Joan.
Joanee, Joaney, Joani, Joanney, Joanni, Joenie

Joann, Joanne (English) forms of Joan.
Jo-Ann, Jo-Anne, Joanann, Joananne, Joane, Joayne, Joeane, Joeann, Joeanne, Joenn, Joenne

Joaquina (Hebrew) God will establish.
Joaquinah, Joaquine, Joaquyn, Joaquyna, Joaquynah, Joaquyne

Joba (Hebrew) a form of Joby.

Jobeth (English) a combination of Jo + Beth.
Jobetha, Jobethe, Joebeth, Joebetha, Joebethe, Johbeth, Johbetha, Johbethe

Jobina (Hebrew) a form of Joby.
Jobeana, Jobeanah, Jobeena, Jobeenah, Jobin, Jobinah, Jobine, Jobyna, Jobynah, Jobyne

Joby BG (Hebrew) afflicted. (English) a familiar form of Jobeth.
Jobea, Jobee, Jobey, Jobi, Jobie, Jobina, Jobita, Jobitt, Jobitta, Jobitte, Jobrina, Jobya, Jobye

Jocacia (American) a combination of Joy + Acacia.

Jocelin, Joceline, Jocelyne, Jocelynn (Latin) forms of Jocelyn.
Jocelina, Jocelinah, Jocelinn, Jocelynne

Jocelín, Joselín (Latin) forms of Jocelyn.

Jocelyn ⚝ GB (Latin) joyous. See also Yocelin, Yoselin.
Jocalin, Jocalina, Jocaline, Jocalyn, Jocelle, Joci, Jocia, Jocilyn, Jocilynn, Jocinta, Joscelin, Josilin, Jossalin

Joclyn (Latin) a short form of Jocelyn.
Joclynn, Joclynne

Jocosa, Jocose (Latin) jubilant.

Jodee, Jodi, Jodie (American) familiar forms of Judith.
Jode, Jodea, Jodele, Jodell, Jodelle, Jodevea, Jodey, Jodi-Lee, Jodi-Lynn, Jodia, Jodiee, Jodilee, Jodilynn, Joedee, Joedey, Joedi, Joedie, Joedy, Johdea, Johdee, Johdey, Johdi, Johdie, Johdy, Jowdee, Jowdey, Jowdi, Jowdie, Jowdy

Jodiann (American) a combination of Jodi (see Jodee) + Ann.
Jodene, Jodi-Ann, Jodi-Anna, Jodi-Anne, Jodianna, Jodianne, Jodine, Jody-Ann, Jody-Anna, Jody-Anne, Jodyann, Jodyanna, Jodyanne, Jodyne

Jody BG (American) a familiar form of Judith.

Joelle (Hebrew) God is willing.
Joela, Joelah, Joele, Joelee, Joeli, Joelia, Joelie, Joell, Joella, Joellah, Joëlle, Joelli, Joelly, Joely, Jowel, Jowela, Jowelah, Jowele, Jowell, Jowella, Jowellah, Jowelle, Joyelle

Joelynn (American) a combination of Joelle + Lynn.
Joelean, Joeleana, Joeleanah, Joeleane, Joeleen, Joeleena, Joeleenah, Joeleene, Joelena, Joelenah, Joelene, Joelin, Joelina, Joelinah, Joeline, Joellen, Joellena, Joellenah, Joellene, Joellyn, Joelyn, Joelyne

Joey BG (American) a familiar form of Jo.

Johana, Johanna, Johannah (German) forms of Joana. See also Giana.
Johan, Johanah, Johanka, Johann, Johonna, Joyhanna, Joyhannah

Johanie, Johannie, Johanny (Hebrew) forms of Joanie.
Johane, Johani, Johanni, Johany

Johanne (German) a short form of Johana. A form of Joann.

Johna, Johnna (American) forms of Joana, Johana.
Jhona, Jhonna, Johnda, Joncie, Jonda, Jondrea, Jutta

Johnae (American) a form of Janae.

Johnesha (American) a form of Johnnessa.
Johnecia

Johnetta (American) a form of Jonita.
Johnette, Jonetta, Jonette

Johnisha (American) a form of Johnnessa.

Johnnessa (American) a combination of Johna + Nessa.
Jahnessa, Johneatha, Johnetra, Johnishi, Johnnise, Jonyssa

Johnnie BG (Hebrew) a form of Joanie.
Johni, Johnie, Johnni, Johnnie-Lynn, Johnnielynn, Johnny

Joi, Joie (Latin) forms of Joy.
Joia, Joiah

Jokia (Swahili) beautiful robe.
Jokiah, Jokya, Jokyah

Jolan (Hungarian) violet blossom.
Jola, Jolán, Jolana, Jolanah, Jolane, Jolanee, Jolaney, Jolani, Jolania, Jolaniah, Jolanie, Jolany, Jolanya, Jolanyah

Jolanda (Greek) a form of Yolanda. See also Iolanthe.
Joland, Jolande, Jolander, Jolanka, Jolánta, Jolante, Jolantha, Jolanthe

Jolee (French) a form of Jolie.
Jole, Jolea, Joleah, Jolei, Joleigh, Joley, Jollea, Jolleah, Jollee, Jollei, Jolleigh

Joleen, Joline (English) forms of Jolene.
Jolean, Joleane, Joleene, Jolin, Jolinn, Jolleen, Jolleene, Jollene, Jollin, Jolline

Jolena (Hebrew) a form of Jolene.
Jolaina, Jolana, Jolanna, Jolanta, Joleana, Joleanah, Joleena, Joleenah, Jolenna, Jolina, Jolinah, Jolinda, Jolinna, Jolleena, Jollina, Jollinah, Jollyna, Jollynah, Jolyana, Jolyanna, Jolyannah, Jolyna, Jolynah

Jolene (Hebrew) God will add, God will increase. (English) a form of Josephine.
Jolaine, Jolane, Jolanne, Jolayne, Jole, Joléne, Jolenne, Jolleane, Jollyn, Jollyne, Jolyne

Jolie (French) pretty.
Joli, Jolibeth, Jolli, Jollie, Jolly, Joly, Jolye

Jolisa (American) a combination of Jo + Lisa.
Joleesa, Joleisha, Joleishia, Jolieasa, Jolise, Jolisha, Jolisia, Jolissa, Jolysa, Jolyssa

Jolyane (English) a form of Jolene.
Jolyanne

Jolyn, Jolynn (American) combinations of Jo + Lynn.
Jolyna, Jolynah, Jolyne, Jolynne

Jona (Hebrew) a short form of Jonina.
Jonah, Jonai, Jonia, Joniah, Jonnah

Jonae (American, Hebrew) a form of Janae. A form of Jona.

Jonatha (Hebrew) a form of Jonathan.
Johnasha, Johnasia

Jonathan BG (Hebrew) gift of God. Bible: the son of King Saul who became a loyal friend of David.

Jonell, Jonelle (American) combinations of Joan + Elle.
Jahnel, Jahnell, Jahnelle, Joanel, Joanela, Joanele, Joanelle, Joannel, Johnel, Johnela, Johnele, Johnell, Johnella, Johnelle, Jonel, Jonela, Jonelah, Jonele, Jonella, Jonilla, Jonille, Jonyelle, Jynell, Jynelle

Jonesha (American) a form of Jonatha.
Joneisha, Jonesa, Joneshia, Jonessa, Jonneisha, Jonnesha, Jonnessia

Joni (American) a familiar form of Joan.
Jonann, Joncee, Joncey, Jonci, Joncie, Jone, Jonee, Joney, Joni-Lee, Jonice, Jonie, Jonilee, Jony

Jonika (American) a form of Janika.
Johnica, Johnique, Johnnica, Johnnika, Johnquia, Joneeka, Joneika, Jonica, Jonicah, Joniqua, Jonique

Jonina (Hebrew) dove. See also Yonina.
Jona, Joneen, Joneena, Joneene, Joninah, Jonine, Jonnina, Jonyna, Jonynah

Jonisha (American) a form of Jonatha.
Jonis, Jonisa, Jonise, Jonishah, Jonishia

Jonita (Hebrew) a form of Jonina. See also Yonita.
Johnita, Johnittia, Jonatee, Jonatey, Jonati, Jonatia, Jonatie, Joneata, Joneatah, Joneeta, Joneetah, Jonit, Jonitae, Jonitah, Jonite, Jonnita, Jonyta, Jonytah

Jonna (American) a form of Joana, Johana.

Jonni, Jonnie (American) familiar forms of Joan.
Jonny

Jonquil (Latin, English) Botany: an ornamental plant with fragrant yellow flowers.
Jonquelle, Jonquie, Jonquila, Jonquile, Jonquill, Jonquilla, Jonquille, Jonquyl, Jonquyla, Jonquylah, Jonquyle, Jonquyll, Jonquylla, Jonquyllah, Jonquylle

Jontel (American) a form of Johna.
Jonta, Jontae, Jontaé, Jontai, Jontaia, Jontaya, Jontaye, Jontela, Jontele, Jontell, Jontella, Jontelle, Jontia, Jontiah, Jontila, Jontrice

Jora GB (Hebrew) autumn rain.
Jorah, Jorai, Joria, Joriah

Jordain, Jordane (Hebrew) forms of Jordan.
Jordaine, Jordayn, Jordayne

Jordan ⭐ BG (Hebrew) descending. See also Jardena.
Jordea, Jordee, Jordi, Jordian, Jordie

Jordana, Jordanna (Hebrew) forms of Jordan. See also Giordana, Yordana.
Jorda, Jordah, Jordaina, Jordannah, Jordayna, Jordena, Jordenna, Jordina, Jordinna, Jordona, Jordonna, Jordyna, Jordynna, Jourdana, Jourdanna

Jordann, Jordanne, Jordyne, Jordynn (Hebrew) forms of Jordan.
Jordene, Jordenn, Jordenne, Jordine, Jordinn, Jordinne, Jordone, Jordonne, Jordynne

Jorden BG (Hebrew) a form of Jordan.

Jordin, Jordyn GB (Hebrew) forms of Jordan.

Jordon BG (Hebrew) a form of Jordan.

Jorgelina (Greek) she who works well in the countryside.

Jori, Jorie (Hebrew) familiar forms of Jordan.
Jorea, Joree, Jorée, Jorey, Jorin, Jorina, Jorine, Jorita, Jorre, Jorrey, Jorri, Jorrian, Jorrie, Jorry

Joriann (American) a combination of Jori + Ann.
Jori-Ann, Jori-Anna, Jori-Anne, Jorian,

Joriana, Jorianah, Joriane, Jorianna, Joriannah, Jorianne, Jorriann, Jorrianna, Jorrianne, Jorryann, Jorryanna, Jorryanne, Joryana, Joryanah, Joryane, Joryann, Joryanna, Joryanne

Jorja (American) a form of Georgia.
Jeorgi, Jeorgia, Jorga, Jorgah, Jorgan, Jorgana, Jorgane, Jorgi, Jorgia, Jorgiah, Jorgie, Jorgina, Jorgine, Jorjan, Jorjana, Jorjanah, Jorjane, Jorji, Jorjia, Jorjiah, Jorjina, Jorjiya, Jorjiyah

Jory BG (Hebrew) a familiar form of Jordan.

Josafata (Hebrew) God will judge.

Josalyn, Jossalin (Latin) forms of Jocelyn.
Josalene, Josalin, Josalina, Josalinah, Josalind, Josaline, Josalynn, Joshalyne Jossalina, Jossalinah, Jossaline, Jossalyn, Jossalynn, Jossalynne

Joscelin, Joscelyn (Latin) forms of Jocelyn.
Josceline, Joscelyne, Joscelynn, Joscelynne

Jose BG (Spanish) a form of Joseph.

Josee, Josée (American) familiar forms of Josephine.
Joesee, Josse, Jossee, Jozee

Josefina (Spanish) a form of Josephine.
Josaffina, Josaffine, Josefa, Josefena, Joseffa, Josefine, Jozafin, Jozafina, Jozafine, Jozefa, Jozefin, Jozefina, Jozefinah, Jozefine

Joselin, Joseline, Joselyn, Joselyne, Josselyn (Latin) forms of Jocelyn.
Joselina, Joselinah, Joselinne, Joselynn, Joselynne, Joshely, Josselen, Josselin, Josseline, Jossellen, Jossellin, Jossellyn, Josselyne, Josselynn, Josselynne

Joselle (American) a form of Jizelle.
Joesell, Joesella, Joeselle, Josel, Josela, Josele, Josell, Josella, Jozelle

Joseph BG (Hebrew) God will add, God will increase. Bible: in the Old Testament, the son of Jacob who came to rule Egypt; in the New Testament, the husband of Mary.

Josepha (German) a form of Josephine.
Josephah, Jozepha

Josephina (French) a form of Josephine.
Fina, Josaphina, Josephena, Josephyna

Josephine (French) a form of Joseph. See also Fifi, Giuseppina, Pepita, Yosepha.
Josaphine, Josephene, Josephin, Josephiney, Josephyn, Josephyne, Jozephine, Sefa

Josette (French) a familiar form of Josephine.
Joesetta, Joesette, Joset, Joseta, Josetah, Josete, Josett, Josetta, Josettah, Joshet, Josheta, Joshetah, Joshete, Joshett, Joshetta, Joshettah, Joshette, Josit, Josita, Jositah, Josite, Jositt, Jositta, Josittah, Jositte, Josyt, Josyta, Josytah, Josyte, Josytt, Josytta, Josyttah, Josytte, Jozet, Jozeta, Jozetah, Jozete, Jozett, Jozetta, Jozettah, Jozette

Josey ☝ (Hebrew) a familiar form of Josephine.
Joesey, Josia, Josiah, Josy, Josye

Joshann (American) a combination of Joshlyn + Ann.
Joshan, Joshana, Joshanah, Joshanna, Joshannah, Joshanne

Joshelle (American) a combination of Joshlyn + Elle.
Joshel, Joshela, Joshelah, Joshele, Joshell, Joshella, Joshellah

Joshlyn (Latin) a form of Jocelyn. (Hebrew) a form of Joshua.
Joshalin, Joshalina, Joshalinah, Joshaline, Joshalyn, Joshalynn, Joshalynne, Joshlean, Joshleana, Joshleanah, Joshleane, Joshleen, Joshleena, Joshleenah, Joshleene, Joshlene, Joshlin, Joshlina, Joshlinah, Joshline, Joshlyna, Joshlynah, Joshlyne, Joshlynn, Joshlynna, Joshlynnah, Joshlynne

Joshua ☝ (Hebrew) God is my salvation. Bible: led the Israelites into the Promised Land.

Josi, Josie, Jossie (Hebrew) familiar forms of Josephine.

Josiane, Josiann, Josianne (American) combinations of Josie (see Josi) + Ann.
Josian, Josiana, Josianna, Josie-Ann, Josieann, Josina, Josinah, Josine, Josinee, Josyn, Josyna, Josyne, Jozan, Jozana, Jozane, Jozian, Joziana, Joziane, Joziann, Jozianna, Jozianne, Jozyn, Jozyna, Jozyne

Josilin, Josilyn (Latin) forms of Jocelyn.
Josielin, Josielina, Josieline, Josiline, Josilyne, Josilynn, Josilynne

Joslin, Joslyn, Joslynn (Latin) short forms of Jocelyn.
Joslina, Joslinah, Josline, Joslyne, Joslynne, Josslyn, Josslyne, Josslynn, Josslynne

Jossline (Latin) a form of Jocelyn.
Josslin

Josune (Spanish) a form of Jesus.

Jourdan ☝ (Hebrew) a form of Jordan.
Jourdain, Jourdann, Jourdanne, Jourden, Jourdian, Jourdon, Jourdyn

Journey (English) journey.

Jovana (Latin) a form of Jovanna.
Jovanah, Jovane, Jovania, Jovaniah

Jovanna (Latin) majestic. (Italian) a form of Giovanna. Mythology: Jove, also known as Jupiter, was the supreme Roman god.
Jeovana, Jeovanna, Jouvan, Jovado, Joval, Jovan, Jovann, Jovannah, Jovannia, Jovanniah, Jovannie, Jovena, Jovenah, Jovenia, Joveniah, Joviana, Jovina, Jovon, Jovona, Jovonah, Jovonda, Jovone, Jovonia, Jovonn, Jovonna, Jovonnah, Jovonne, Jowan, Jowana, Jowanna

Jovannie (Italian) a familiar form of Jovanna.
Jovanee, Jovaney, Jovani, Jovanie, Jovanne, Jovannee, Jovanni, Jovanny, Jovany, Jovonnie

Jovi (Latin) a short form of Jovita.
Jovee, Jovey, Jovia, Joviah, Jovie, Jovy, Jovya, Jovyah

Joviana (Latin) a form of Jovanna.
Jovian, Jovianah, Joviane, Joviann, Jovianna, Joviannah, Jovianne, Jovyan, Jovyana, Jovyanah, Jovyane, Jovyann, Jovyanna, Jovyannah, Jovyanne

Jovina (Latin) a form of Jovanna.
Jovinah, Jovine, Jovyn, Jovyna, Jovynah, Jovyne

Jovita (Latin) jovial.
Joveda, Jovet, Joveta, Jovete, Jovett, Jovetta, Jovette, Jovi, Jovida, Jovidah, Jovit, Jovitah, Jovite, Jovitt, Jovitta, Jovitte, Jovyta, Jovytah, Jovyte, Jovytt, Jovytta, Jovyttah, Jovytte

Joxepa (Hebrew) a form of Josefina.

Joy (Latin) joyous.
Joye, Joyeeta, Joyella, Joyous, Joyvina

Joya (Latin) a form of Joy.
Joyah, Joyia

Joyann, Joyanne (American) combinations of Joy + Ann.
Joian, Joiana, Joianah, Joiane, Joiann, Joianna, Joiannah, Joianne, Joyan, Joyana, Joyanah, Joyane, Joyanna, Joyannah

Joyce (Latin) joyous. A short form of Joycelyn.
Joice, Joise, Joycee, Joycey, Joycia, Joyciah, Joycie, Joyse, Joysel

Joycelyn (American) a form of Jocelyn.
Joycalin, Joycalina, Joycalinah, Joycaline, Joycalyn, Joycalyna, Joycalynah, Joycalyne, Joycelin, Joycelina, Joycelinah, Joyceline, Joycelyna, Joycelynah, Joycelyne, Joycelynn, Joycelynne, Joysalin, Joysalina, Joysalinah, Joysaline, Joysalyn

Joyceta (Spanish) a form of Joyce.

Joylyn (American) a combination of Joy + Lynn.
Joialin, Joialine, Joialyn, Joialyna, Joialyne, Joilin, Joilina, Joilinah, Joiline, Joilyn, Joilyna, Joilynah, Joilyne, Joy-Lynn, Joyleen, Joylene, Joylin, Joylina, Joylinah, Joyline, Joylyna, Joylynah, Joylyne, Joylynn, Joylynne

Jozephine (French) a form of Josephine.
Jozaphin, Jozaphina, Jozaphinah, Jozaphine, Jozaphyn, Jozaphyna, Jozaphynah, Jozaphyne, Jozephin, Jozephina, Jozephinah, Jozephyn, Jozephyna, Jozephynah, Jozephyne

Jozie (Hebrew) a familiar form of Josephine.
Joze, Jozee, Jozée, Jozey, Jozi, Jozy, Jozze, Jozzee, Jozzey, Jozzi, Jozzie, Jozzy

Juana (Spanish) a short form of Juanita.
Juanah, Juanell, Juaney, Juanika, Juanit, Juanna, Juannah, Juannia

Juana del Pilar (Spanish) Juana of the pillar.

Juandalyn (Spanish) a form of Juanita.
Jualinn, Juandalin, Juandalina, Juandaline, Juandalyna, Juandalyne, Juandalynn, Juandalynne

Juaneta (Spanish) a form of Juana.

Juanita (Spanish) a form of Jane, Joan. See also Kwanita, Nita, Waneta, Wanika.
Juaneice, Juanequa, Juanesha, Juanice, Juanicia, Juaniqua, Juanisha, Juanishia

Jubilee (Latin) joyful celebration.
Jubilea, Jubileah, Jubilei, Jubileigh, Jubili, Jubilia, Jubiliah, Jubilie, Jubily, Jubilya, Jubilyah, Jubylea, Jubyleah, Jubylee, Jubylei, Jubyleigh, Jubyley, Jubyli, Jubylia, Jubyliah, Jubylie, Jubyly

Juci (Hungarian) a form of Judy.
Jucee, Jucey, Jucia, Juciah, Jucie, Jucika, Jucy, Jucya, Jucyah

Jucunda (Latin) pleasant.

Judine (Hebrew) a form of Judith.
Judeen, Judeena, Judeenah, Judena, Judene, Judin, Judina, Judinah, Judyn, Judyna, Judynah, Judyne

Judith (Hebrew) praised. Mythology: the slayer of Holofernes, according to ancient Jewish legend. See also Yehudit, Yudita.
Giuditta, Ioudith, Jude, Judett, Judetta, Judette, Judine, Judit, Judita, Judite, Juditha, Judithe, Juditt, Juditta, Juditte, Judyta, Judytt, Judytta, Judytte, Jutka

Judy (Hebrew) a familiar form of Judith.
Judea, Judee, Judey, Judi, Judie, Judye

Judyann (American) a combination of Judy + Ann.
Judana, Judane, Judiana, Judiane, Judiann, Judianna, Judiannah, Judianne, Judyanna, Judyanne

Jula (Polish) a form of Julia.
Jewlah, Juela, Juelah, Julah, Julca, Julcia, Julea, Juleah, Juliska, Julka

Julee (English) a form of Julie.

Julene (Basque) a form of Julia. See also Yulene.
Julean, Juleana, Juleanah, Juleane, Juleen, Juleena, Juleenah, Juleene, Julena, Julenah, Julenia, Juleniah, Julina, Juline, Julinka, Juliska, Jullean, Julleana, Julleanah, Julleane, Julleen, Julleena, Julleenah, Julleene, Jullena, Jullene, Jullin, Jullina, Jullinah, Julline, Jullyna, Jullynah, Jullyne, Julyna, Julynah, Julyne

Julia ☀ (Latin) youthful. See also Giulia, Jill, Jillian, Sulia, Yulia.
Iulia, Jewelea, Jeweleah, Jewelia, Jeweliah, Jewelya, Jewlya, Jewlyah, Juelea, Jueleah, Jula, Julea, Juleah, Juliah, Julica, Juliea, Julija, Julita, Juliya, Julka, Julya

Julian BG (English) a form of Julia. See also Julie Ann.
Jewelian, Jeweliane, Jeweliann, Jewelianne, Jewliane, Jewliann, Jewlianne, Julean, Juleann, Julijanne, Juline, Julyan, Julyane, Julyann, Julyanne

Juliana (Czech, Spanish) a form of Julia.
Jeweliana, Jewelianah, Jewelianna, Jeweliannah, Jewliana, Jewlianah, Jewlianna, Jewliannah, Julianah, Juliannah, Julieana, Julieanah, Juliena, Julienna, Juliennah, Julijana, Julijanah, Julijanna, Julijannah, Julina, Julinah, Julliana, Jullianna, Julyana, Julyanah, Julyanna, Julyannah, Yuliana

Juliane, Juliann, Julianne (English) forms of Julia.

Julianna (Hungarian) a form of Julia. See also Juliana.

Julie (English) a form of Julia.
Jewelee, Jewelei, Jeweleigh, Jeweli, Jewelie, Jewlie, Juel, Juelee, Juelei, Jueleigh, Jueli, Juelie, Juely, Jule, Julei, Juleigh, Julene, Juli, Julie-Lynn, Julie-Mae, Julle, Jullee, Julli, Jullie, Jully, July

Julie Ann, Julie Anne, Julieann (American) combinations of Julie + Ann. See also Julian.
Julie-Ann, Julie-Anne, Juliean, Julieane, Julieanne

Julieanna (American) a form of Juliana.
Julie Anna, Julie-Anna

Julienne (English) a form of Julia.
Julien, Juliene, Julienn

Juliet, Juliette (French) forms of Julia.
Jewelett, Jeweletta, Jewelette, Jeweliet, Jeweliete, Jeweliett, Jeweliette, Jewelyet, Jewelyete, Jewelyett, Jewelyette, Jolet, Jolete, Juelet, Juelete, Juelett, Juelette, Juleate, Juliete, Juliett, Jullet, Julliet, Julliete, Julliett, Julliette, Julyet, Julyete, Julyett, Julyette

Julieta (French) a form of Julia.
Guilietta, Jewelieta, Jewelietta, Jewelyeta, Jewelyetta, Juleata, Juleatah, Julietah, Julietta, Juliettah, Jullieta, Jullietah, Jullietta, Julyeta, Julyetah, Julyetta, Julyettah

Julisa, Julissa (Latin) forms of Julia.
Julis, Julisha, Julysa, Julyssa

Julita (Spanish) a form of Julia.
Joleta, Joletah, Jueleta, Jueletah, Jueletta, Juelettah, Juleet, Juleeta, Juleetah, Juleete, Julet, Juleta, Juletah, Julett, Juletta, Julette, Julit, Julitah, Julite, Julitt, Julitta, Julittah, Julitte, Julyta

Jullian BG (English) a form of Julia.

Jumaris (American) a combination of Julie + Maris.

Jun BG (Chinese) truthful.

June (Latin) born in the sixth month.
Juin, Juine, Juna, Junel, Junell, Junella, Junelle, Junett, Junetta, Junette, Juney, Juniet, Junieta, Juniett, Junietta, Juniette, Junill, Junilla, Junille, Junina, Junine, Junita, Junn, Junula

Junee (Latin) a familiar form of June.
Junea, Juney, Juni, Junia, Juniah, Junie, Juny

Juno (Latin) queen. Mythology: the supreme Roman goddess.

Jupita (Latin) Mythology: Jupiter is the supreme Roman god and the husband of Juno. Astronomy: Jupiter is the largest planet in the solar system and the fifth planet from the sun.
Jupitah, Jupitor, Jupyta, Jupytah, Jupyter, Jupytor

Jurisa (Slavic) storm.
Jurisah, Jurissa, Jurissah, Jurysa, Jurysah, Juryssa, Juryssah

Jurnee (American) a form of Journey.

Justa (Latin) a short form of Justina, Justine.
Justah, Juste, Justea, Justi, Justie, Justy

Justice GB (Latin) a form of Justin.
Justys, Justyse

Justin BG (Latin) just, righteous.

Justina (Italian) a form of Justine. See also Giustina.
Jestena, Justeana, Justeanah, Justeena,

Justeenah, Justeina, Justeinah, Justeyna,
Justeynah, Justinah, Justinna

Justine **GB** (Latin) a form of Justin.
Jestine, Justean, Justeane, Justeen, Justeene,
Justein, Justeine, Justeyn, Justeyne

Justiniana (Spanish) a form of Justine.

Justis **BG** (Latin) a form of Justice.
Justiss, Justisse

Justise, Justyce (Latin) forms of Justice.

Justus **BG** (Latin) a form of Justice.

Justyna (Italian) a form of Justine.
Justynah

Justyne (Latin) a form of Justine.
Justyn, Justynn, Justynne

Juvencia (Latin) a form of Juventina.

Juventa (Greek) a form of Juventina.

Juventina (Latin) youth.

Jyllian (Latin) a form of Jillian.
Jylian, Jyliana, Jylianah, Jyliane, Jyliann,
Jylianna, Jyliannah, Jylianne, Jylliana,
Jyllianah, Jylliane, Jylliann, Jyllianna,
Jylliannah, Jyllianne, Jyllyan, Jyllyana,
Jyllyanah, Jyllyane, Jyllyann, Jyllyanna,
Jyllyannah, Jyllyanne

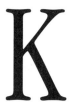

Ka'la (Arabic) a form of Kala.

Kacee, Kaci, Kacie (Irish, American) forms of Kacey.

Kacey **GB** (Irish) brave. (American) a form of Casey. A combination of the initials K. + C.
Kace, Kaecee, Kaecey, Kaeci, Kaecie, Kaecy,
Kaicee, Kaicey, Kaici, Kaicie, Kaicy, Kasci

Kachina (Native American) sacred dancer.
Kachin, Kachinah, Kachine, Kachinee,
Kachiney, Kachyn, Kachyna, Kachynah,
Kachyne

Kacia (Greek) a short form of Acacia.
Kacya, Kaecea, Kaecia, Kaeciah, Kaesea,
Kaesia, Kaesiah, Kaicea, Kaicia, Kaiciah,
Kaisea, Kaisia, Kaisiah, Kasea, Kasya,
Kaycia, Kaysea, Kaysia

Kacy **GB** (Irish) brave. (American) a form of Casey. A combination of the initials K. + C.

Kadedra (American) a combination of Kady + Dedra.
Kadeadra, Kadedrah, Kadedria

Kadee, Kadi, Kadie (English) forms of Kady.
Kaddia, Kaddiah, Kaddie, Kadia, Kadiah

Kadeejah (Arabic) a form of Kadijah.
Kadeeja

Kadeesha (American) a form of Kadesha.
Kadeeshia, Kadeesia, Kadeesiah, Kadeezia

Kadeidra (American) a form of Kadedra.
Kadeedra, Kadeidre, Kadeidria

Kadeija (Arabic) a form of Kadijah.
Kadeijah

Kadeisha (American) a form of Kadesha.

Kadeja, Kadejah (Arabic) forms of Kadijah.
Kadejá, Kadejia

Kadelyn (American) a combination of Kady + Lynn.

Kadesha (American) a combination of Kady + Aisha.
Kadesa, Kadessa, Kadiesha, Kadieshia,
Kadysha, Kadyshia

Kadeshia (American) a form of Kadesha.
Kadesheia

Kadesia (American) a form of Kadesha.
Kadezia

Kadija (Arabic) a form of Kadijah.

Kadijah (Arabic) trustworthy.
Kadajah

Kadisha (American) a form of Kadesha.
Kadishia, Kadisia

Kady (English) a form of Katy. A combination of the initials K. + D. See also Cadie.
K. D., Kaddy, Kade, Kadea, Kadey, Kadya,
Kadyn, Kaidi, Kaidy

Kae (Greek, Teutonic, Latin) a form of Kay.

Kaedé (Japanese) maple leaf.

Kaela (Hebrew, Arabic) beloved, sweetheart. A short form of Kalila, Kelila.
Kaelah, Kaelea, Kaeleah

Kaelee, Kaeleigh, Kaeley, Kaeli, Kaelie, Kaely (American) forms of Kaela.
Kaelei, Kaelia, Kaeliah, Kaelii, Kaelly, Kaelye

Kaelen 🅱🅶 (American) a form of Kaelyn.
Kaelean, Kaeleana, Kaeleane, Kaeleen, Kaeleena, Kaeleene, Kaelein, Kaeleina, Kaeleine, Kaelene, Kaelina, Kaeline, Kaelinn, Kaelynne

Kaelin 🅱🅶 (American) a form of Kaelyn.

Kaelyn (American) a combination of Kae + Lynn. See also Caelin, Kaylyn.
Kaelan, Kaeleyn, Kaeleyna, Kaeleyne, Kaelyna, Kaelyne

Kaelynn (American) a form of Kaelyn.

Kaetlyn (Irish) a form of Kaitlin.
Kaetlin, Kaetlynn, Kaetlynne

Kaferine (Greek) a form of Katherine.
Kaferin, Kaferina, Kaferinah, Kaferyn, Kaferyna, Kaferynah, Kaferyne, Kafferin, Kafferina, Kafferinah, Kafferine, Kafferyn, Kafferyna, Kafferynah, Kafferyne

Kafleen (Irish) a form of Kathleen.
Kafflean, Kaffleana, Kaffleanah, Kaffleane, Kaffleen, Kaffleena, Kaffleenah, Kaffleene, Kafflein, Kaffleina, Kaffleinah, Kaffleine, Kafflin, Kafflina, Kafflinah, Kaffline, Kafflyn, Kafflyna, Kafflynah, Kafflyne, Kaflean, Kafleana, Kafleanah, Kafleane, Kafleena, Kafleenah, Kafleene, Kaflein, Kafleina, Kafleinah, Kafleine, Kaflin, Kaflina, Kaflinah, Kafline, Kaflyn, Kaflyna, Kaflynah, Kaflyne

Kagami (Japanese) mirror.
Kagamee

Kahla (Arabic) a form of Kala.
Kahlah, Kahlea, Kahleah

Kahli (American) a form of Kalee.
Kahlee, Kahlei, Kahleigh, Kahley, Kahlie, Kahly

Kahsha (Native American) fur robe.
Kashae, Kashia

Kai 🅱🅶 (Hawaiian) sea. (Hopi, Navajo) willow tree.
Kae, Kaie

Kaia (Greek) earth.
Kaiah

Kaija (Greek) a form of Kaia.

Kaila (Hebrew) laurel; crown.
Kailea, Kaileah, Kailia, Kailiah

Kailah (Hebrew) a form of Kaila.

Kailani (Hawaiian) sky. See also Kalani.
Kaelana, Kaelanah, Kaelanea, Kaelanee, Kaelaney, Kaelani, Kaelania, Kaelaniah, Kaelanie, Kaelany, Kaelanya, Kailana, Kailanah, Kailanea, Kailanee, Kailaney, Kailania, Kailaniah, Kailanie, Kailany, Kailanya

Kaile, Kailee, Kaileigh, Kailey, Kailie, Kaily (American) familiar forms of Kaila. Forms of Kaylee.
Kaileh, Kailei, Kailia, Kailiah, Kailli, Kaillie, Kailya

Kaileen (American) a form of Kaitlin.
Kaileena, Kaileene

Kailen 🅶🅱 (American) a form of Kaitlin.
Kailan, Kailean, Kaileana, Kaileane, Kailein, Kaileina, Kaileine, Kailena, Kailene, Kaileyne, Kailina, Kailine, Kailon, Kailyna, Kailyne, Kailynne

Kaili 🅶🅱 (American) a familiar form of Kaila. A form of Kaylee.

Kaimana (Hawaiian) diamond.
Kaemana, Kaemanah, Kaemane, Kaiman, Kaimanah, Kaimane, Kayman, Kaymana, Kaymanah, Kaymane

Kaimi (Hawaiian) seeker.

Kaira (Greek) a form of Kairos. (Greek, Danish) a form of Kara.
Kairra

Kairos (Greek) opportunity.

Kaisa (Swedish) pure.
Kaisah, Kaysa, Kaysah

Kaisha (American) a short form of Kaishawn.

Kaishawn (American) a combination of Kai + Shawna.
Kaeshun, Kaishala, Kaishon

Kaitlan, Kaitlen, Kaitlinn, Kaitlyne, Kaitlynn, Kaitlynne (Irish) forms of Kaitlin.
Kaitlinne, Kaitlyna, Kaitlynah

Kaitland (Irish) a form of Caitlin.
Kaitlind

Kaitlin (Irish) pure. See also Caitlin, Katelin.
Kaitelynne, Kaitleen, Kaitlina, Kaitlinah, Kaitline, Kaitlon

Kaitlyn ☆ (Irish) a form of Kaitlin.

Kaiya (Japanese) forgiveness. (Aboriginal) a type of spear.
Kaiyah, Kaiyia

Kala **GB** (Arabic) a short form of Kalila. A form of Cala.

Kalah, Kalla (Arabic) forms of Kala.
Kallah

Kalama **BG** (Hawaiian) torch.

Kalan **BG** (American) a form of Kaelyn, Kaylyn. (Hawaiian) a short form of Kalani. (Slavic) a form of Kallan.

Kalani **GB** (Hawaiian) chieftain; sky. See also Kailani.
Kalana, Kalanah, Kalanea, Kalanee, Kalaney, Kalania, Kalaniah, Kalanie, Kalona, Kalonah, Kalonea, Kalonee, Kaloney, Kaloni, Kalonia, Kaloniah, Kalonie, Kalony

Kalare (Latin, Basque) bright; clear.

Kalasia (Tongan) graceful.
Kalasiah, Kalasya, Kalasyah

Kalauni (Tongan) crown.
Kalaunea, Kalaunee, Kalauney, Kalaunia, Kalauniah, Kalaunie, Kalauny, Kalaunya

Kalea **GB** (Hawaiian) bright; clear.
Kahlea, Kahleah, Kailea, Kaileah, Kaleah, Kaleeia, Kaleia, Kallea, Kalleah, Khalea, Khaleah

Kalee, Kalei, Kaleigh, Kaley, Kalie, Kalley, Kally, Kaly (American) forms of Calee, Kaylee. (Sanskrit, Hawaiian) forms of Kali. (Greek) forms of Kalli. (Arabic) famil-iar forms of Kalila.
Kallee, Kalleigh, Kallye

Kaleen, Kalene (Hawaiian) short forms of Kalena.

Kaleena (Hawaiian) a form of Kalena. (Slavic) a form of Kalina.

Kalei (Hawaiian) flower wreath.
Kahlei, Kailei, Kallei, Kaylei, Khalei

Kalen **BG** (Slavic) a form of Kallan.
Kallen

Kalena (Hawaiian) pure. See also Kalina.
Kalenea, Kalenna

Kalere (Swahili) short woman.
Kaleer

Kali **GB** (Hindi) the black one. (Hawaiian) hesitating. Religion: a form of the Hindu goddess Devi. See also Cali.

Kalia, Kaliah (Hawaiian) forms of Kalea.
Kaliea, Kalieya, Kalya

Kalid (Arabic) a form of Khalida.

Kalida (Spanish) a form of Calida.
Kalidah, Kallida, Kallidah, Kallyda, Kallydah, Kalyda, Kalydah

Kalifa (Somali) chaste; holy.
Califa, Califah, Kalifah

Kalila (Arabic) beloved, sweetheart. See also Kaela.
Calila, Calilah, Kahlila, Kaleela, Kalilla, Kallila, Kaylil, Kaylila, Kylila, Kylilah, Kylillah

Kalin **BG** (Slavic, Hawaiian) a short form of Kalina. (American) a form of Kaelyn, Kaylyn.

Kalina (Slavic) flower. (Hawaiian) a form of Karen. See also Kalena.
Kalinah, Kaline, Kalinna, Kalyna, Kalynah, Kalynna

Kalinda (Hindi) sun. See also Calinda.
Kaleenda, Kalindah, Kalindi, Kalindie, Kalindy, Kalynd, Kalynda, Kalynde, Kalyndi

Kalisa (American) a combination of Kate + Lisa.
Kalise, Kalysa, Kalyssa

Kalisha (American) a combination of Kate + Aisha.
Kaleesha, Kaleisha, Kalishia

Kaliska (Moquelumnan) coyote chasing deer.
Kaliskah, Kalyska, Kalyskah

Kalissa (American) a form of Kalisa.

Kalista, Kallista (Greek) forms of Calista.
*Kalesta, Kalistah, Kallesta, Kallistar,
Kallistara, Kallistarah, Kallistarr, Kallistarra,
Kallistarrah, Kallysta, Kaysta*

Kallan (Slavic) stream, river.
Kalahn, Kalan, Kallin, Kallon, Kallyn, Kalon

Kalle BG (Finnish) a form of Carol.
Kaille, Kaylle

Kalli, Kallie (Greek) forms of Calie. Familiar forms of Kalista, Kalliope, Kalliyan.
Kalle, Kallee, Kallita, Kally

Kalliope (Greek) a form of Calliope.
Kalliopee, Kallyope

Kalliyan (Cambodian) best.

Kallolee (Hindi) happy.
*Kallolea, Kalloleah, Kallolei, Kalloleigh,
Kalloley, Kalloli, Kallolie, Kalloly*

Kaloni (Tongan) fragrant; perfume.
*Kalona, Kalonah, Kalonee, Kaloney, Kalonia,
Kaloniah, Kalonie, Kalony, Kalonya,
Kalonyah*

Kalonice (Greek) beauty's victory.

Kaltha (English) marigold, yellow flower.

Kaluwa (Swahili) forgotten one.
Kalua

Kalyca (Greek) rosebud. See also Calyca.
*Kalica, Kalicah, Kalika, Kaly, Kalycah,
Kalyka, Kalykah*

Kalyn GB (American) a form of Kaylyn.
*Kalin, Kallen, Kallin, Kallon, Kallyn, Kalyne,
Kalynne*

Kalynn (American) a form of Kaylyn.

Kama (Sanskrit) loved one. Religion: the Hindu god of love.
Kamah, Kamma, Kammah

Kamala (Hindi) lotus.
Kamalah, Kammala

Kamalei (Hawaiian) beloved child.
Kamalea, Kamaleah, Kamaleigh

Kamali (Rhodesian) spirit guide; protector.
Kamaley, Kamalie, Kamaly

Kamalynn, Kamalynne (American) combinations of Kama + Lynn.
*Kamlean, Kamleana, Kamleanah, Kamleane,
Kamleen, Kamleena, Kamleenah, Kamleene,
Kamlin, Kamlina, Kamlinah, Kamline,
Kamlyn, Kamlyna, Kamlynah, Kamlyne,
Kammalean, Kammaleana, Kammaleanah,
Kammaleane, Kammaleen, Kammaleena,
Kammaleenah, Kammaleene, Kammalin,
Kammalina, Kammalinah, Kammaline,
Kammalyn, Kammalyna, Kammalynah,
Kammalyne, Kammalynn*

Kamara (Swahili) a short form of Kamaria.

Kamari BG (Swahili) a short form of Kamaria.
Kamaree, Kamarie

Kamaria (Swahili) moonlight.
*Kamar, Kamarae, Kamariah, Kamariya,
Kamariyah, Kamarya, Kamaryah*

Kamata (Moquelumnan) gambler.

Kamballa (Australian) young woman.
Kambala, Kambalah, Kamballah

Kambria (Latin) a form of Cambria.
Kambra, Kambrie, Kambriea, Kambry

Kamea (Hawaiian) one and only; precious.
*Camea, Cameah, Kameah, Kamee, Kameo,
Kammia, Kammiah, Kamya, Kamyah*

Kameke (Swahili) blind.

Kameko (Japanese) turtle child. Mythology: the turtle symbolizes longevity.
Kameeko, Kamiko, Kamyko

Kameli (Hawaiian) honey.
Kamely

Kamelia (Italian) a form of Camelia.
*Kameliah, Kamellia, Kamelya, Kamelyah,
Kamilia, Kamillia, Kamilliah, Kamillya,
Kamilya, Kamylia, Kamyliah*

Kameron BG (American) a form of Cameron.
Kameran, Kamerona, Kameronia

Kameryn (American) a form of Cameron.

Kami GB (Japanese) divine aura. (Italian, North African) a short form of Kamila, Kamilah. See also Cami.
Kamey, Kammi, Kammie, Kammy, Kammye, Kamy

Kamie (Italian, North African, Japanese) a form of Kami.

Kamila (Slavic) a form of Camila. See also Millie.
Kameela, Kamela, Kamella, Kamilka, Kamilla, Kamillah, Kamma, Kammilla, Kamyla, Kamylla, Kamylle

Kamilah (North African) perfect.
Kameela, Kameelah, Kamillah, Kammilah, Kamylah, Kamyllah

Kamille (Slavic) a short form of Kamila.
Kamil, Kamile, Kamyl, Kamyle, Kamyll

Kamiya (Hawaiian) a form of Kamea.
Kamia, Kamiah, Kamiyah

Kamri (American) a short form of Kameron. See also Camri.
Kamree, Kamrey, Kamrie

Kamry (American) a form of Kamri.
Kamrye

Kamryn GB (American) a short form of Kameron. See also Camryn.
Kamren, Kamrin, Kamron, Kamrynn

Kanani (Hawaiian) beautiful.
Kana, Kanae, Kanan, Kanana, Kananah, Kananea, Kananee, Kanania, Kananiah, Kananie, Kanany, Kananya, Kananyah

Kanda (Native American) magical power.

Kandace, Kandice (Greek) glittering white; glowing. (American) forms of Candace, Candice.
Kandas, Kandess, Kandus

Kandi (American) a familiar form of Kandace. See also Candi.
Kandea, Kandee, Kandey, Kandhi, Kandia, Kandiah, Kandie, Kandy, Kandya, Kandyah,
Kendi, Kendie, Kendy, Kenndi, Kenndie, Kenndy

Kandis, Kandyce (Greek, American) forms of Kandace.
Kandise, Kandiss, Kandys, Kandyse

Kandra (American) a form of Kendra. See also Candra.
Kandrah, Kandrea, Kandree, Kandria, Kandriah, Kandrya, Kandryah

Kane BG (Japanese) two right hands.

Kaneesha (American) a form of Keneisha.

Kaneisha (American) a form of Keneisha.
Kaneasha, Kanecia, Kaneysha, Kaniece

Kaneli (Tongan) canary yellow.
Kanelea, Kaneleah, Kanelee, Kanelei, Kaneleigh, Kanelia, Kaneliah, Kanelie, Kanely, Kanelya

Kanene (Swahili) a little important thing.

Kanesha (American) a form of Keneisha.
Kanesah, Kaneshea, Kaneshia, Kanessa

Kani (Hawaiian) sound.
Canee, Caney, Cani, Canie, Cany, Kanee, Kanie, Kany

Kanika (Mwera) black cloth.
Kanica, Kanicka

Kanisha (American) a form of Keneisha.
Kanishia

Kaniva (Tongan) Milky Way, universe, galaxy.
Kanivah, Kanyva, Kanyvah

Kaniya (Hindi, Tai) a form of Kanya.
Kanea, Kania, Kaniah

Kannitha (Cambodian) angel.

Kanoa BG (Hawaiian) free.

Kanya GB (Hindi) virgin. (Tai) young lady. Religion: a form of the Hindu goddess Devi.
Kanja, Kanjah, Kanyah, Kanyia

Kapri (American) a form of Capri.
Kapre, Kapree, Kapria, Kaprice, Kapricia, Kaprisha, Kaprisia

Kapua (Hawaiian) blossom.

Kapuki (Swahili) first-born daughter.

Kara (Greek, Danish) pure.

Karah (Greek, Danish) a form of Kara. (Irish, Italian) a form of Cara.

Karalana (English) a combination of Kara + Lana.
Karalain, Karalaina, Karalainah, Karalaine, Karalanah, Karalane, Karalayn, Karalayna, Karalaynah, Karalayne

Karalee (English) a combination of Kara + Lee.
Karalea, Karaleah, Karalei, Karaleigh, Karaley, Karali, Karalia, Karaliah, Karalie, Karaly, Karralea, Karraleah, Karralee, Karralei, Karraleigh, Karraley, Karrali, Karralie, Karraly

Karalyn (English) a form of Karalynn. (American) a form of Karolyn.
Karalyna

Karalynn (English) a combination of Kara + Lynn.
Karalin, Karaline, Karalyne, Karalynne

Kareela (Australian) southern wind.
Kareala, Karealah, Karealla, Kareallah, Karela, Karelah, Karella, Karellah

Kareema (Arabic) a form of Karimah.
Kareemah

Kareen (Scandinavian) a short form of Karena. A form of Karin.
Karean, Kareane, Kareene, Karene, Karrane, Karreen, Karrene

Kareena (Scandinavian) a form of Karena.
Kareenah, Karreena

Karel BG (American) a form of Carol.
Karell

Karelle (American) a form of Carol.

Karely (American) a familiar form of Karel.
Kareli

Karen (Greek) pure. See also Carey, Carina, Caryn.
Kaaran, Kaaren, Kaarun, Karaina, Karan, Karna, Karon, Karran, Karren, Karrun

Karena (Scandinavian) a form of Karen.
Kareana, Kareina, Karenah, Karrana, Karranah, Karrena, Karrenah

Karenza (Cornish) loving, affectionate. See also Carenza.
Karansa, Karansah, Karansia, Karansiah, Karanza, Karanzah, Karanzia, Karanziah, Karanzya, Karanzyah, Karensa, Karensah, Karensia, Karensiah, Karenzah, Karenzia, Karenziah, Karenzya, Karenzyah, Kerensa

Karessa (French) a form of Caressa.

Karey GB (Greek, Danish) a form of Kari.

Kari (Greek) pure. (Danish) a form of Caroline, Katherine. See also Carey, Cari, Carrie, Karri.
Karee

Karia (Greek, Danish) a form of Kari.
Kariah

Kariane, Kariann, Karianne (American) combinations of Kari + Ann.
Karian, Kariana, Karianna

Karida (Arabic) untouched, pure.
Kareeda, Karidah, Karinda, Karita, Karyda, Karydah, Karynda, Karyndah

Karie, Kary (Greek, Danish) forms of Kari.

Karilyn, Karilynn (American) combinations of Kari + Lynn.
Kareelin, Kareeline, Kareelinn, Kareelyn, Kareelyne, Kareelynn, Kareelynne, Karilin, Kariline, Karilinn, Karilyne, Karilynne, Karylin, Karyline, Karylinn, Karylyn, Karylyne, Karylynn, Karylynne

Karima (Arabic) a form of Karimah.

Karimah (Arabic) generous.
Karim, Karime, Karyma, Karymah

Karin (Scandinavian) a form of Karen.
Kaarin, Karinne, Karrin, Karrine

Karina (Russian) a form of Karen.
Kaarina, Karinna, Karrina, Karrinah

Karine (Russian) a form of Karen.
Karrine, Karryne, Karyne

Karis (Greek) graceful.
Kares, Karese, Karess, Karesse, Karice, Karise, Kariss, Karisse, Karris, Karys, Karyse, Karyss, Karysse

Karisa, Karissa, Karrisa (Greek) forms of Carissa.
Karesa, Karesah, Karessa, Karessah, Karisah,

Karisha, Karissah, Karissimia, Kariza, Karrissa, Kerisa

Karishma (American) a form of Karisma.

Karisma (Greek) divinely favored. See also Carisma.
Karismah, Karismara, Karysma, Karysmah, Karysmara

Karla (German) a form of Carla. (Slavic) a short form of Karoline.
Karila, Karilla, Karle, Karlea, Karleah, Karlicka, Karlinka, Karlisha, Karlisia, Karlitha, Karlla, Karlon

Karlee, Karleigh, Karli, Karlie (American) forms of Karley. See also Carli.
Karlia, Karliah

Karleen, Karlene (American) forms of Karla. See also Carleen.
Karlean, Karleane, Karleene, Karlein, Karleine, Karlen, Karleyn, Karleyne, Karlign, Karlin, Karline, Karlyan

Karlena (American) a form of Karleen.
Karleana, Karleanah, Karleena, Karleenah, Karleina, Karleinah, Karlenah, Karleyna, Karleynah, Karlina, Karlinah, Karlinna, Karlyna, Karlynah

Karley, Karly (Latin) little and strong. (American) forms of Carly.
Karlea, Karleah, Karlei, Karlya, Karlyah, Karlye

Karlotte (American) a form of Charlotte.
Karletta, Karlette, Karlita, Karlotta

Karlyn (American) a form of Karla.
Karlyne, Karlynn, Karlynne

Karma (Hindi) fate, destiny; action.
Carma, Carmah, Karmah, Karmana

Karmaine (French) a form of Charmaine.
Karmain, Karmaina, Karmane, Karmayn, Karmayna, Karmayne, Karmein, Karmeina, Karmeine, Karmeyn, Karmeyna, Karmeyne, Kharmain, Kharmaina, Kharmaine, Kharmayn, Kharmayna, Kharmayne, Kharmein, Kharmeina, Kharmeine, Kharmeyn, Kharmeyna, Kharmeyne

Karmel BG (Hebrew) a form of Carmela.
Karmeita, Karmela, Karmelah, Karmele, Karmelina, Karmell, Karmella, Karmellah,

Karmelle, Karmellia, Karmelliah, Karmellya, Karmellyah, Karmiella, Karmielle, Karmyla

Karmen (Latin) song.
Karman, Karmencita, Karmin, Karmita, Karmon, Karmyn, Karmyna, Karmynah

Karmiti (Bantu) tree.
Karmitee, Karmitey, Karmitie, Karmity, Karmytee, Karmytey, Karmyti, Karmytie, Karmyty

Karniela (Greek) cornel tree. (Latin) horn colored. See also Carniela.
Karniel, Karnielah, Karniele, Karniella, Karnielle, Karnis, Karnyel, Karnyela, Karnyele, Karnyell, Karnyella, Karnyelle

Karol BG (Slavic) a form of Carol.
Karilla, Karily, Karola, Karole, Karoly, Karrol, Karyl, Karyla, Karyle, Karyll, Karylle, Kerril

Karol Ann, Karolane, Karolann, Karolanne (American) combinations of Karol + Ann.
Karol-Anne, Karolan

Karolina (Slavic) a form of Carolina.
Karalena, Karilena, Karilina, Karolainah, Karolayna, Karolaynah, Karoleena, Karolena, Karolinah, Karolinka, Karrolena

Karoline (Slavic) a form of Caroline.
Karaleen, Karalene, Karalin, Karaline, Karileen, Karilene, Karilin, Kariline, Karlen, Karling, Karolin, Karroleen, Karrolene, Karrolin, Karroline

Karoll (Slavic) a form of Carol.

Karolyn (American) a form of Carolyn.
Karilyn, Karilyna, Karilynn, Karilynne, Karolyna, Karolynah, Karolyne, Karolynn, Karolynne, Karrolyn, Karrolyna, Karrolynn, Karrolynne

Karon BG (American) a form of Karen.
Kaaron, Karona, Karonah, Karone, Karonia, Karoniah, Karonie, Karony, Karonya, Karonyah, Karron, Kerron

Karra (Greek, Danish) a form of Kara.

Karrah (Greek, Danish, Irish, Italian) a form of Karah.

Karri, Karrie (American) forms of Carrie. See also Kari.
Karree, Karrey, Karry

Karsen BG (English) child of Kar. A form of Carson.

Karson BG (English) child of Kar. A form of Carson.

Karsyn (English) child of Kar. A form of Carson.

Karuna (Hindi) merciful.

Karyn (American) a form of Karen.
Kaaryn, Karryn, Karryne, Karyne, Karynn, Kerrynn, Kerrynne

Karyna (American) a form of Karina.
Karryna, Karrynah, Karynah, Karynna

Karyssa (Greek) a form of Carissa.
Karysa, Karysah, Karyssah

Kasa (Hopi) fur robe.

Kasandra, Kassandra, Kassandre (Greek) forms of Cassandra.
Kasander, Kasandrah, Kasandre, Kasandria, Kasandrina, Kasandrine, Kasoundra, Kassandr, Kassandrah, Kassandré, Kassandria, Kassandriah, Kassundra, Kassundre, Kassundria, Kassundriah, Kazandra, Kazandrah, Kazandria, Kazandriah, Kazzandra, Kazzandrah, Kazzandre, Kazzandria, Kazzandriah, Kazzandrya, Kazzandryah

Kasaundra, Kassaundra (Greek) forms of Kasandra.
Kasaundrah, Kassaundre, Kassaundria, Kassaundriah

Kasen BG (Danish) a form of Katherine.
Kasena, Kasenah, Kasene, Kasin

Kasey GB (Irish) brave. (American) a form of Casey, Kacey.
Kaesee, Kaesey, Kaesi, Kaesie, Kaesy, Kaisee, Kaisey, Kaisi, Kaisie, Kaisy, Kasci, Kascy, Kasee, Kassee, Kasy

Kasha (Native American) a form of Kahsha. (American) a form of Kashawna.
Kashae

Kashawna (American) a combination of Kate + Shawna.
Kashana, Kashanna, Kashauna, Kashawn, Kasheana, Kasheanna, Kasheena, Kashena, Kashonda, Kashonna

Kashmere (Sanskrit) a form of Kashmir.

Kashmir (Sanskrit) Geography: a region located between India and Pakistan.
Cashmere, Kashmear, Kashmia, Kashmira, Kasmir, Kasmira, Kazmir, Kazmira

Kasi (Hindi) from the holy city.

Kasia (Polish) a form of Katherine. See also Cassia.
Kashia, Kasiah, Kasian, Kasienka, Kasja, Kaska, Kassa, Kassya, Kassyah, Kasya, Kasyah, Kazia, Kaziah, Kazya, Kazyah, Kazzia, Kazziah, Kazzya, Kazzyah

Kasidy (Irish) a form of Kassidy.

Kasie (Irish, American) a form of Kasey. (Hindi) a form of Kasi.

Kasimira (Slavic) a form of Casimira.
Kasimera, Kasimerah, Kasimiera, Kasimirah, Kasmira, Kasmirah, Kasmiria, Kasmiriah, Kasmirya, Kasmiryah, Kasmyra, Kasmyrah, Kazmira, Kazmirah, Kazmiria, Kazmiriah, Kazmyra, Kazmyrah, Kazmyria, Kazmyriah, Kazmyrya, Kazmyryah, Kazzmira, Kazzmirah, Kazzmiria, Kazzmiriah, Kazzmirya, Kazzmiryah, Kazzmyra, Kazzmyrah, Kazzmyrya, Kazzmyryah

Kasinda (Umbundu) our last baby.

Kasondra, Kassondra (Greek) forms of Cassandra.
Kassondrah, Kassondria

Kassey (American) a form of Kassi. (Irish, American) a form of Kasey.

Kassi, Kassie, Kassy (American) familiar forms of Kasandra, Kassidy. See also Cassey.
Kassee, Kasy, Kazi, Kazie, Kazy, Kazzi, Kazzie, Kazzy

Kassia (Polish) a form of Kasia. (American) a form of Kassi.
Kassiah

Kassidee, Kassidi (Irish, American) forms of Kassidy.
Kasidee

Kassidy GB (Irish) clever. (American) a form of Cassidy.
Kasadee, Kasadey, Kasadi, Kasadia, Kasadie, Kasady, Kasidey, Kasidi, Kasidia, Kasidie, Kassadea, Kassadee, Kassadey, Kassadi,

Kassadia, Kassadiah, Kassadie, Kassadina, Kassady, Kassadya, Kasseday, Kassedee, Kassiddy, Kassidea, Kassidey, Kassidia, Kassidiah, Kassidie, Kassity, Kassydee, Kassydi, Kassydia, Kassydie, Kassydy, Kasydee, Kasydey, Kasydi, Kasydie, Kasydy, Kazadea, Kazadee, Kazadey, Kazadi, Kazadia, Kazadiah, Kazadie, Kazady, Kazadya, Kazidy, Kazydy, Kazzadea, Kazzadee, Kazzadey, Kazzadi, Kazzadia, Kazzadiah, Kazzadie, Kazzady

Katalina (Irish) a form of Caitlin. See also Catalina.
Kataleen, Kataleena, Katalena, Katalin, Katalinah, Kataline, Katalyn, Katalynn

Katarina (Czech) a form of Katherine.
Kata, Katarain, Kataraina, Katarainah, Kataraine, Katareena, Katarena, Katarin, Katarinah, Katarine, Katarinna, Katarinne, Katarrina, Kataryn, Kataryna, Katarynah, Kataryne, Katinka, Katrika, Katrinka

Katarzyna (Czech) a form of Katherine.

Kate (Greek) pure. (English) a short form of Katherine.
Kait, Kata, Katica, Katka, Kayt

Kate-Lynn (American) a combination of Kate + Lynn.
Kate Lyn, Kate Lynn, Kate Lynne, Kate-Lyn, Kate-Lynne

Katee, Katey (English) familiar forms of Kate, Katherine. See also Katie.

Kateland (Irish) a form of Caitlin.
Katelind

Katelee (American) a combination of Kate + Lee.
Katelea, Kateleah, Katelei, Kateleigh, Kateley, Kateli, Katelia, Kateliah, Katelie, Kately

Katelin (Irish) a form of Caitlin. See also Kaitlin.
Kaetlin, Katalin, Katelan, Kateleen, Katelen, Katelene, Kateline, Katelinn, Katelun, Katelyna, Katelynah, Katewin, Katewina, Katewinah, Katewine, Katewyn, Katewyna, Katewynah, Katewyne

Katelyn ☆ (Irish) a form of Katelin.
Katelyne, Katelynn, Katelynne

Katerina (Slavic) a form of Katherine.
Katenka, Katereana, Katereanah, Katereena, Katereenah, Katerinah, Katerini, Katerinia, Kateriniah, Katerinka, Kateriny

Katerine (Slavic) a form of Katherine.
Kateren

Katharina (Greek) a form of Katharine.
Katharinah, Katharyna, Katharynah

Katharine, Katharyn (Greek) forms of Katherine.
Katharaine, Katharin, Katharyne

Katherin, Katheryn, Katheryne (Greek) forms of Katherine.

Katherina (Greek) a form of Katherine.
Katherinah, Katheryna, Katherynah

Katherine ☆ (Greek) pure. See also Carey, Catherine, Ekaterina, Kara, Karen, Kari, Kasia, Katerina, Yekaterina.
Ekaterina, Ekatrinna, Kasen, Kat, Katchen, Kathann, Kathanne, Kathereen, Katheren, Katherene, Katherenne, Kathyrine, Katlaina, Katoka, Katreeka, Katreen

Kathi, Kathy (English) familiar forms of Katherine, Kathleen. See also Cathi, Cathy.
Kaethe, Katha, Kathe, Kathee, Kathey, Kathie, Katka, Katla, Kató

Kathia, Kathya (English) forms of Kathi.
Kathiah, Kathye

Kathleen (Irish) a form of Katherine. See also Cathleen.
Katheleen, Kathelene, Kathileen, Kathlean, Kathleena, Kathleenah, Kathleene, Kathlein, Kathleina, Kathleinah, Kathleine, Kathlene, Kathlina, Kathlinah, Kathline, Katleen

Kathlyn (Irish) a form of Kathleen.
Kathlin, Kathlyna, Kathlynah, Kathlyne, Kathlynn

Kathrin, Kathrine (Greek) forms of Katherine.
Kathran, Kathreen, Kathren, Kathrene, Kathron, Kathrun, Kathryn

Kathrina (Danish) a form of Katherine.
Kathreena, Kathrinah, Kathryna, Kathrynah

Kathryn, Kathryne, Kathrynn (English) forms of Katherine.
Kathren, Kathrynne

Kati (Estonian) a familiar form of Kate.

Katia, Katya (Russian) forms of Katherine.
Cattiah, Kãtia, Katiah, Katinka, Katiya, Kattia, Kattiah, Katyah

Katie (English) a familiar form of Kate. See also Katy.
Kaaitea, Kaitee, Kaitey, Kaitie

Katie-Lynn (American) a combination of Katie + Lynn.
Katie Lyn, Katie Lynn, Katie Lynne, Katie-Lyn, Katie-Lynne, Katy Lyn, Katy Lynn, Katy Lynne, Katy-Lyn, Katy-Lynn, Katy-Lynne

Katilyn (Irish) a form of Katlyn.
Katilin, Katilynn

Katina (English, Russian) a form of Katherine.
Kateana, Kateanah, Kateena, Kateenah, Kateina, Kateinah, Kateyna, Kateynah, Katinah, Katine, Katyn, Katyna, Katynah, Katyne

Katixa (Basque) a form of Catalina.

Katja (Estonian) a form of Kate.
Kaatje, Katye

Katlin, Katlyne, Katlynn (Greek, Irish) forms of Katlyn.
Katlina, Katline, Katlyna, Katlynd, Katlynne

Katlyn (Greek) pure. (Irish) a form of Katelin.
Kaatlain, Katland

Katreen, Katrin, Katrine (English) forms of Katherine.
Katreene, Katren, Katrene, Katrian, Katriane, Katriann, Katrianne, Katrien, Katrinne, Katryn, Katryne

Katrena (German) a form of Katrina.
Katrenah

Katrice (German) a form of Katrina.
Katricia

Katriel GB (Hebrew) God is my crown. See also Catriel.
Katrelle, Katri, Katrie, Katriela, Katrielah, Katriele, Katriell, Katriella, Katriellah, Katrielle, Katry, Katryel, Katryela, Katryelah, Katryele, Katryell, Katryella, Katryellah, Katryelle

Katrina (German) a form of Katherine. See also Catrina, Trina.
Kaetreana, Kaetreanah, Kaetreena, Kaetreenah, Kaetreina, Kaetreinah, Kaetreyna, Kaetreynah, Kaetrina, Kaetrinah, Kaetryna, Kaetrynah, Kaitreana, Kaitreanah, Kaitreena, Kaitreenah, Kaitreina, Kaitreinah, Kaitreyna, Kaitreynah, Kaitrina, Kaitrinah, Kaitryna, Kaitrynah, Katreana, Katreanah, Katreena, Katreenah, Katreina, Katreinah, Katreyna, Katreynah, Katri, Katriana, Katrianah, Katrianna, Katriannah, Katrien, Katriena, Katrienah, Katrinah, Katrinia, Katrinna, Katrinnah, Katriona, Kattrina, Kattryna, Katus, Kaytreana, Kaytreanah, Kaytreena, Kaytreenah, Kaytreina, Kaytreinah, Kaytreyna, Kaytreynah, Kaytrina, Kaytrinah, Kaytryna, Kaytrynah

Katrinelle (American) a combination of Katrina + Elle.
Katrinal, Katrinel, Katrinela, Katrinele, Katrinell, Katrinella, Katrynel, Katrynela, Katrynele, Katrynell, Katrynella, Katrynelle

Katryna (German) a form of Katrina.
Katrynah

Kattie, Katty (English) familiar forms of Kate.
Katti

Katy (English) a familiar form of Kate. See also Cadie, Katie.

Kaulana (Hawaiian) famous.
Kahuna, Kaula, Kauna

Kaveri (Hindi) Geography: a sacred river in India.

Kavindra (Hindi) poet.

Kavita (Indian) a poem.

Kawena (Hawaiian) glow.
Kawana, Kawona

Kay GB (Greek) rejoicer. (Teutonic) a fortified place. (Latin) merry. A short form of Katherine.
Caye, Kaye

Kaya (Hopi) wise child. (Japanese) resting place.
Kaea, Kaja, Kayah, Kayia

Kayanna (American) a combination of Kay + Anna.
Kay Anna

Kayce, Kaycee, Kayci, Kaycie, Kaysie (American) combinations of the initials K. + C.
Kaycey, Kaycy, Kaysci, Kaysee, Kaysey, Kaysi, Kaysii, Kaysy

Kaydee (American) a combination of the initials K. + D. See also Katie.
Kayda, Kayde, Kaydey, Kaydi, Kaydie, Kaydy

Kayden BG (American) a form of Kaydee.

Kayla ⚝ (Arabic, Hebrew) laurel; crown. A form of Kaela, Kaila. See also Cayla.
Kaelea, Kaylea

Kaylah (Arabic, Hebrew) a form of Kayla.

Kaylan GB (Hebrew) a form of Kayleen.
Kayland, Kaylann, Kaylean, Kayleana, Kayleanna, Kaylenn

Kaylani (Hawaiian) a form of Kailani, Keilana.
Kaylana, Kaylanah, Kaylanea, Kaylanee, Kaylaney, Kaylania, Kaylaniah, Kaylanie, Kaylany, Kaylanya

Kayle GB (American) a form of Kaylee.

Kaylea (Hawaiian) a form of Kalea. (Arabic, Hebrew) a form of Kayla.
Kayleah

Kaylee ⚝ (American) a form of Kayla. See also Caeley, Kalee.
Kaylei, Kayly, Kaylya, Keylea, Keyleah, Keylee, Keylei, Keyleigh, Keyley, Keyli, Keylia, Keyliah, Keylie, Keyly

Kayleen, Kaylene (Hebrew) beloved, sweetheart. Forms of Kayla.
Kaylean, Kayleane, Kayleene, Kaylein, Kayleine

Kayleigh, Kayley, Kayli, Kaylie (American) forms of Kaylee.

Kaylen GB (Hebrew) a form of Kayleen.

Kaylena (Hebrew) a form of Kayleen.
Kayleana, Kayleena, Kayleina

Kaylia (Arabic, Hebrew) a form of Kayla. (American) a form of Kaylee.
Kayliah

Kaylin GB (American) a form of Kaylyn.
Kaylina, Kayline

Kaylon BG (American) a form of Kaylyn.

Kaylyn, Kaylynn, Kaylynne (American) combinations of Kay + Lynn. See also Kaelyn.
Kaylyna, Kaylyne

Kayte, Kaytie (English) forms of Katy.
Kaytee

Kaytlin, Kaytlyn (Irish) forms of Kaitlin.
Kaytlan, Kaytlann, Kaytlen, Kaytlyne, Kaytlynn, Kaytlynne

Kc BG (American) a combination of the initials K. + C.
K. C.

KC BG (American) a combination of the initials K. + C.

Keagan BG (Irish) a form of Keegan.
Keagean, Keagen, Keaghan, Keagyn

Keaira, Keairra (Irish) forms of Keara.
Keair, Keairah, Keairre, Keairrea

Keala (Hawaiian) path.
Kealah, Kealea, Kealeah, Kealee, Kealei, Kealeigh, Keali, Kealia, Kealiah, Kealie, Kealy, Kealya

Keana, Keanna (German) bold; sharp. (Irish) beautiful.
Keanah, Keanne, Keenan, Keeyana, Keeyanah, Keeyanna

Keandra (American) a form of Kenda.
Keandrah, Keandre, Keandrea, Keandria, Kedeana, Kedia

Keanu BG (German, Irish) a form of Keana.

Keara (Irish) dark; black.
Kearah, Kearia

Kearra (Irish) a form of Keara.

Kearsten, Kearstin, Kearston (Greek) forms of Kirsten.
Kearstyn

Keasha (African) a form of Keisha.
Keashia

Keaton BG (English) where hawks fly.
Keatan, Keaten, Keatin, Keatton, Keatun, Keatyn, Keetan, Keeten, Keetin, Keeton, Keetun, Keetyn, Keitan, Keiten, Keiton, Keitun, Keityn, Keytan, Keyten, Keytin, Keyton, Keytun, Keytyn

Kecia (American) a form of Keshia.

Keegan BG (Irish) little; fiery.
Kaegan, Kagan, Keegen, Keeghan, Keegin, Keegon, Keegun, Kegan, Keigan

Keeley GB (Irish) a form of Kelly.
Kealee, Kealey, Keali, Kealie, Keallie, Kealy, Keela, Keelah, Keelan, Keele, Keelea, Keeleah, Keelee, Keelei, Keeleigh, Keeli, Keelia, Keeliah, Keelie, Keellie, Keelya, Keelyah, Keelye, Kiela, Kiele, Kieley, Kielly, Kiely

Keelin, Keelyn (Irish) forms of Kellyn.
Kealyn, Keilan, Kielyn

Keely (Irish) a form of Kelly.

Keena (Irish) brave.
Keenah, Keenya, Keina, Keinah, Keyna, Keynah, Kina

Keera (Irish) a form of Keara. (Persian, Latin) a form of Kira. (Greek) a form of Kyra.
Keerra

Keesha (American) a form of Keisha.
Keesa, Keeshae, Keeshana, Keeshanne, Keeshawna, Keeshia, Keeshiah, Keeshonna, Keeshy, Keeshya, Keeshyah

Kei (Japanese) reverent.

Keiana, Keianna (Irish) forms of Keana. (American) forms of Kiana.
Keiann, Keiannah

Keiara, Keiarra (Irish) forms of Keara.
Keiarah

Keiki (Hawaiian) child.
Keikana, Keikann, Keikanna, Keikanne, Keyki, Kiki

Keiko (Japanese) happy child.
Keyko

Keila, Keilah (Arabic, Hebrew) forms of Kayla.

Keilana (Hawaiian) gloriously calm.
Kealaina, Kealainah, Kealana, Kealanah,

Kealanna, Kealannah, Keelaina, Keelainah, Keelana, Keelanah, Keelayna, Keelaynah, Keilaina, Keilainah, Keilanah, Keilanna, Keilannah, Keilayna, Keilaynah, Keylaina, Keylainah, Keylana, Keylanah, Keylayna, Keylaynah

Keilani (Hawaiian) glorious chief.
Kealaine, Kealainee, Kealane, Kealanee, Kealanne, Kealannee, Keelane, Keelanee, Keelayn, Keelayne, Keelaynee, Keilaine, Keilainee, Keilan, Keilane, Keilanee, Keilanne, Keilannee, Keilany, Keilayn, Keilayne, Keilaynee, Kelana, Kelanah, Kelane, Kelani, Kelanie, Keylaine, Keylainee, Keylane, Keylanee, Keylayn, Keylayne, Keylaynee

Keily (Irish) a form of Keeley, Kiley.
Keighla, Keighlea, Keighlee, Keighlei, Keighleigh, Keighley, Keighli, Keighlia, Keighliah, Keighlie, Keighly, Keilea, Keileah, Keilee, Keilei, Keileigh, Keiley, Keili, Keilia, Keiliah, Keilie, Keilley, Keilly, Keilya

Keiona, Keionna (Irish) forms of Keana.

Keiosha (American) a form of Keesha.

Keira, Keirra (Irish) forms of Keara.
Keirrah

Keirsten, Keirstin, Keirstyn (Greek) forms of Kirsten.
Keirstan, Keirstein, Keirston, Keirstynne

Keisha (African) favorite.
Keishah, Keishaun, Keishauna, Keishawn, Keishia, Keishiah, Keishya, Keishyah, Keschia

Keita (Scottish) woods; enclosed place.
Keiti

Kekona (Hawaiian) second-born child.

Kela (Arabic, Hebrew) a form of Kayla.
Kelah

Kelby BG (German) farm by the spring.
Kelbea, Kelbee, Kelbey, Kelbi, Kelbie

Kelcee, Kelci, Kelcie, Kelcy (Scottish) forms of Kelsey.
Kelce, Kelcea, Kelcia, Kellcea, Kellcee, Kellcey, Kellci, Kellcia, Kellciah, Kellcie, Kellcy

Kelcey GB (Scottish) a form of Kelsey.

Kele BG (Hopi) sparrow hawk.
Kelea, Keleah

Kelemon (Welsh) child of Kei.

Keli GB (Irish) a form of Kelly.
*Kelee, Kelei, Keleigh, Keley, Kelie, Kellei,
Kellisa*

Kelia (Irish) a form of Kelly.
Keliah, Kellea, Kelleah, Kellia, Kelliah

Kelila (Hebrew) crown, laurel. See also
Kaela, Kayla, Kalila.
Kelilah, Kelula, Kelulah

Kellan BG (Irish) a form of Kellyn.
Kelleen, Kellene

Kellee, Kelleigh, Kelli, Kellie (Irish) forms
of Kelly.

Kellen BG (Irish) a form of Kellyn.

Kelley GB (Irish) a form of Kelly.

**Kellsey, Kellsie, Kelsea, Kelsee, Kelsei,
Kelsi, Kelsie, Kelsy** (Scandinavian,
Scottish, English) forms of Kelsey.
*Kellsea, Kellsee, Kellsei, Kellsia, Kellsiah,
Kellsy, Kelsae, Kelsay, Kelsye*

Kelly GB (Irish) brave warrior. See also
Caeley.
Kellye, Kely, Kelya

Kelly Ann, Kelly Anne, Kellyanne (Irish)
combinations of Kelly + Ann.
Kelliann, Kellianne, Kellyann

Kellyn, Kellynn (Irish) combinations of
Kelly + Lynn.
Kellina, Kellinah, Kelline, Kellynne

Kelsa (Scandinavian, Scottish, English) a
short form of Kelsey.
Kelse

Kelsey GB (Scandinavian, Scottish) ship
island. (English) a form of Chelsea.
Kelda

Kemberly (English) a form of Kimberly.
*Kemberlea, Kemberleah, Kemberlee, Kemberlei,
Kemberleigh, Kemberli, Kemberlia,
Kemberliah, Kemberlie, Kemberly*

Kena, Kenna (Irish) short forms of
Kennice.
Kenah, Kennah

Kenadee, Kenadi, Kennadi, Kennady
(Irish) forms of Kennedy.
Kennadee, Kennadie

Kenda (English) water baby. (Dakota) magical power.
Kendah, Kennda

Kendahl (English) a form of Kendall.
*Kendala, Kendalah, Kendale, Kendalie,
Kendalla, Kendallah, Kendalle, Kendela,
Kendelah, Kendele, Kendella, Kendellah,
Kendelle*

Kendal GB (English) a form of Kendall.

Kendall GB (English) ruler of the valley.
*Kendera, Kendia, Kendil, Kinda, Kindal,
Kindall, Kindi, Kindle, Kynda, Kyndel*

Kendalyn (American) a form of Kendellyn.
Kendalin, Kendalynn

Kendel BG (English) a form of Kendall.

Kendell BG (English) a form of Kendall.

Kendellyn (American) a combination of
Kendall + Lynn.
*Kendelan, Kendelana, Kendelanah,
Kendelane, Kendelin, Kendelina, Kendelinah,
Kendeline, Kendellan, Kendellana,
Kendellanah, Kendellane, Kendellyna,
Kendellynah, Kendellyne, Kendelyn,
Kendelyna, Kendelynah, Kendelyne*

Kendra (English) a form of Kenda.
Kendrah, Kendre, Kenndra, Kentra, Kentrae

Kendria (English) a form of Kenda.
*Kendrea, Kendreah, Kendriah, Kendrya,
Kendryah*

Kendyl, Kendyll (English) forms of Kendall.
Kendyle

Kenedi, Kennedi, Kennedie (Irish) forms
of Kennedy.
Kenedee, Kenedey, Kenedie, Kenedy

Keneisha (American) a combination of the
prefix Ken + Aisha.
*Keneesha, Kenneisha, Kennysha, Kenysha,
Kenyshah, Kineisha*

Kenenza (English) a form of Kennice.
Kenza

Kenesha (American) a form of Keneisha.
Keneshia, Kennesha, Kenneshia

Kenia, Kennia (Hebrew) forms of Kenya.
Keniah, Keniya, Kenja, Kenjah

Kenise (English) a form of Kennice.
Kenisa, Kenissa, Kenissah, Kennis, Kennisa, Kennisah, Kennise, Kenniss, Kennissa, Kennissah, Kennisse, Kenys, Kenysa, Kenysah, Kenyse, Kenyss, Kenyssa, Kenyssah, Kenysse

Kenisha, Kennisha (American) forms of Keneisha.
Kenishah, Kenishia

Kenley BG (English) royal meadow.
Kenlea, Kenlee, Kenleigh, Kenli, Kenlie, Kenly, Kennlea, Kennlee, Kennleigh, Kennley, Kennli, Kennlie, Kennly

Kennedy GB (Irish) helmeted chief. History: John F. Kennedy was the thirty-fifth U.S. president.
Kenidee, Kenidi, Kenidie, Kenidy, Kennedee, Kennedey, Kennidee, Kennidi, Kennidy, Kynnedi

Kenni (English) a familiar form of Kennice.
Kenee, Keni, Kenne, Kennee, Kenney, Kennie, Kenny, Kennye

Kennice (English) beautiful.
Kanice, Keneese, Kenenza, Kenese

Kenya GB (Hebrew) animal horn. Geography: a country in Africa.
Keenya, Kenyah, Kenyia

Kenyana (Hebrew) a form of Kenya.

Kenyata (American) a form of Kenya.
Kenyatah, Kenyatte, Kenyattia

Kenyatta GB (American) a form of Kenyata.

Kenyetta (American) a form of Kenya.
Kenyette

Kenzi (Scottish, Irish) a form of Kenzie.

Kenzie GB (Scottish) light skinned. (Irish) a short form of Mackenzie.
Kenzea, Kenzee, Kenzey, Kenzia, Kenzy

Keona, Keonna (Irish) forms of Keana.
Keeyona, Keeyonna, Keoana, Keonnah

Keondra (American) a form of Kenda.
Keonda, Keondre, Keondria

Keoni BG (Irish) a form of Keana.
Keonia, Keonni, Keonnia

Keosha (American) a short form of Keneisha.
Keoshae, Keoshi, Keoshia, Keosia

Kera, Kerra (Hindi) short forms of Kerani.
Kerah

Kerani (Hindi) sacred bells. See also Rani.
Kerana, Keranee, Keraney, Kerania, Keraniah, Keranie, Kerany, Keranya, Keranyah

Keren (Hebrew) animal's horn.
Keran, Keron, Kerran, Kerre, Kerren, Kerron, Keryn, Kieren, Kierin, Kieron, Kieryn

Kerensa (Cornish) a form of Karenza.
Kerensah, Kerenza, Kerenzah

Keri, Kerri, Kerrie (Irish) forms of Kerry.

Keriann, Kerrianne (Irish) combinations of Keri + Ann.
Kerian, Keriana, Kerianah, Keriane, Kerianna, Keriannah, Kerriane, Kerriann, Kerrianne, Kerryann, Kerryanna, Kerryannah, Kerryanne, Keryan, Keryana, Keryanah, Keryane, Keryann, Keryanna, Keryannah, Keryanne

Kerielle, Kerrielle (American) combinations of Keri + Elle.
Keriel, Keriela, Kerielah, Keriele, Keriell, Keriella, Keriellah, Kerriel, Kerriela, Kerrielah, Kerriele, Kerriell, Kerriella, Kerriellah, Kerryell, Kerryella, Kerryellah, Kerryelle, Keryel, Keryela, Keryelah, Keryele, Keryell, Keryella, Keryellah, Keryelle

Kerrin (Hebrew) a form of Keren.
Kerin

Kerry GB (Irish) dark haired. Geography: a county in Ireland.
Keary, Keiry, Keree, Kerey, Kery

Kersten, Kerstin, Kerstyn (Scandinavian) forms of Kirsten.
Kerstain, Kerstaine, Kerstan, Kerstane, Kerste, Kerstean, Kersteane, Kersteen, Kersteene, Kerstein, Kerstene, Kerstie, Kerstien, Kerstine, Kerston, Kerstyne, Kerstynn

Kerstina (Scandinavian) a form of Kristina.
Kerstaina, Kerstainah, Kerstana, Kerstanah, Kersteana, Kersteanah, Kersteena, Kersteenah,

Kerstena, Kerstenah, Kerstinah, Kerstyna, Kerstynah, Kurstaina, Kurstainah, Kursteana, Kursteanah, Kursteena, Kursteenah, Kurstina, Kurstinah, Kurstyna, Kurstynah

Kesare (Latin) long haired. (Russian) a form of Caesar (see Boys' Names).

Kesha (American) a form of Keisha.
Keshah, Keshal, Keshala

Keshara (American) a form of Keisha.

Keshawna (American) a form of Keisha.
Keshan, Keshana, Keshawn, Keshawnna

Keshet (Hebrew) rainbow.
Kesetta, Kesettah, Kesette, Kesheta, Keshetah, Keshete, Keshett, Keshetta, Keshettah, Keshette

Keshia (American) a form of Keisha. A short form of Keneisha.
Keshea

Kesi (Swahili) born during difficult times.
Kesee, Kesey, Kesie, Kesy

Kesia (African) favorite.
Kesiah, Kessia, Kessiah, Kessya, Kessyah

Kesley (Scandinavian, Scottish) a form of Kelsey.
Kesly

Kessie (Ashanti) chubby baby.
Kess, Kessa, Kesse, Kessey, Kessi

Ketifa (Arabic) flower.
Ketifah, Kettifa, Kettifah, Kettyfa, Kettyfah, Ketyfa, Ketyfah

Ketina (Hebrew) girl.
Keteena, Keteenah, Ketinah, Ketyna, Ketynah

Kevina (Irish) a form of Kevyn.
Kevinah

Kevyn BG (Irish) beautiful.
Keva, Kevan, Keven, Kevern, Keverna, Kevernah, Kevia, Keviana, Kevine, Kevinna, Kevion, Kevionna, Kevirn, Kevirna, Kevirnah, Kevirne, Kevon, Kevona, Kevone, Kevonia, Kevonna, Kevonne, Kevonya, Kevynn, Kevyrn, Kevyrna, Kevyrnah, Kevyrne

Keyana, Keyanna (American) forms of Kiana.
Keya, Keyanah, Keyanda, Keyannah

Keyandra (American) a form of Kiana.

Keyara, Keyarra (Irish) forms of Kiara.
Keyarah, Keyari

Keyera, Keyerra (Irish) forms of Kiara.
Keyeira, Keyerah

Keyla (Arabic, Hebrew) a form of Kayla.
Keylah

Keyona, Keyonna (American) forms of Kiana.
Keyonnie

Keyonda (American) a form of Kiana.

Keyondra (American) a form of Kiana.

Keyonia (American) a form of Kiana.
Keyonnia

Keyosha (American) a form of Keisha.
Keyoshia

Keysha (American) a form of Keisha.
Keyshah, Keyshana, Keyshanna, Keyshawn, Keyshawna, Keyshia, Keyshiah, Keyshla, Keyshona, Keyshonna, Keyshya, Keyshyah

Kezia (Hebrew) a form of Keziah.
Kezzia

Keziah (Hebrew) cinnamon-like spice. Bible: one of the daughters of Job.
Kazia, Kaziah, Ketzi, Ketzia, Ketziah, Ketzya, Ketzyah, Kezi, Kezya, Kezyah, Kezziah, Kizia, Kiziah, Kizzia, Kizziah, Kyzia, Kyziah, Kyzzia, Kyzziah, Kyzzya, Kyzzyah

Khadeeja (Arabic) a form of Khadijah.
Khadeejah

Khadeja, Khadejah (Arabic) forms of Khadijah.
Khadejha

Khadija (Arabic) a form of Khadijah.

Khadijah (Arabic) trustworthy. History: Muhammed's first wife.
Khadaja, Khadajah, Khadije, Khadijia, Khadijiah

Khalia, Khaliah (Arabic) forms of Khalida.

Khalida (Arabic) immortal, everlasting.
Khali, Khalidda, Khalita

Khalilah (Arabic) a form of Kalila.
Khalila, Khalillah

Khaliyah (Arabic) a form of Khalida.

Khayla (Arabic, Hebrew) a form of Kayla.

Khepri (Egyptian) emerging sun.

Khiana (American) a form of Kiana.
Khianah, Khianna

Khimberly (English) a form of Kimberly.
*Khimberlea, Khimberleah, Khimberlee,
Khimberlei, Khimberleigh, Khimberley,
Khimberli, Khimberlia, Khimberliah,
Khimberlie, Khymberlea, Khymberleah,
Khymberlee, Khymberlei, Khymberleigh,
Khymberley, Khymberli, Khymberlia,
Khymberliah, Khymberlie, Khymberly*

Khrisha (American, Czech) a form of
Khrissa.
Krisia, Krysha

Khrissa (American) a form of Chrissa.
(Czech) a form of Krista.
Khrishia, Khryssa, Kryssa

Khristina (Russian, Scandinavian) a form of
Kristina, Christina.
*Khristeana, Khristeanah, Khristeena,
Khristeenah, Khristeina, Khristeinah,
Khristinah, Khristya, Khristyana, Khristyna,
Khristynah, Khrystyna, Khrystynah*

Khristine (Scandinavian) a form of
Christine.
*Khristean, Khristeane, Khristeen, Khristeene,
Khristein, Khristeine, Khristeyn, Khristeyne,
Khristyne, Khrystean, Khrysteane, Khrysteen,
Khrysteene, Khrystein, Khrysteine, Khrysteyn,
Khrysteyne, Khrystyne, Khrystynne*

Ki 🅱🅶 (Korean) arisen.

Kia (African) season's beginning. (American)
a short form of Kiana.

Kiah (African, American) a form of Kia.

Kiahna (American) a form of Kiana.

Kiaira (Irish) a form of Kiara.

Kiana (American) a combination of the prefix Ki + Ana.
Kianah, Kiandria, Kiane, Kianne

Kiandra (American) a form of Kiana.

Kiani (American) a form of Kiana.
Kiania, Kianni

Kianna (American) a form of Kiana.
Kiannah

Kiara (Irish) little and dark.

Kiaria (Japanese) fortunate.
Kichi

Kiarra (Irish) a form of Kiara. (Japanese) a
form of Kiaria.

Kiauna (American) a form of Kiana.
Kiaundra

Kieanna (American) a form of Kiana.

Kieara (Irish) a form of Kiara.
Kiearah, Kiearra

Kiele 🅶🅱 (Hawaiian) gardenia; fragrant blos-
som.
*Kiela, Kielea, Kieleah, Kielee, Kielei, Kieleigh,
Kieley, Kieli, Kielia, Kieliah, Kielie, Kielli,
Kielly, Kiely*

Kiera, Kierra (Irish) forms of Kerry.
Kierea

Kieran 🅱🅶 (Irish) little and dark; little Keir.
A form of Kerry. (Hindi) a form of Kiran.
*Kierana, Kieranah, Kierane, Kieranna, Kieren,
Kieron*

Kiersten, Kierstin, Kierston, Kierstyn
(Scandinavian) forms of Kirsten.
Kierstan, Kierstynn

Kiesha (American) a form of Keisha.

Kigva (Welsh) Mythology: wife of
Partholon's son.

Kiki 🅶🅱 (Spanish) a familiar form of names
ending in "queta."
Kikee, Kikey, Kikie, Kiky

Kiku (Japanese) chrysanthemum.
Kiko

Kilee (Irish) a form of Kiley.
Killee

Kiley 🅶🅱 (Irish) attractive; from the straits.
See also Kylie.
*Kielea, Kieleah, Kielee, Kielei, Kieleigh,
Kieley, Kieli, Kielia, Kieliah, Kielie, Kiely,
Kilea, Kileah, Kilei, Kileigh, Kili, Kilie,
Killey, Killi, Killie, Killy, Kily*

Kilia (Hawaiian) heaven.
Kiliah, Killea, Killeah, Killia, Killiah, Kylia, Kyliah, Kylya, Kylyah

Kim GB (Vietnamese) needle. (English) a short form of Kimberly.
Kem, Khim, Khime, Khimm, Khym, Khyme, Khymm, Kima, Kimette, Kimm

Kimalina (American) a combination of Kim + Lina.
Kimalinah, Kimaline, Kimalyn, Kimalyna, Kimalynah, Kimalyne, Kymalyn, Kymalyna, Kymalynah, Kymalyne

Kimana (Shoshone) butterfly.
Kiman, Kimanah, Kimane, Kimann, Kimanna, Kimannah, Kimanne, Kymana, Kymanah, Kymane, Kymanna, Kymannah, Kymanne

Kimani BG (Shoshone) a form of Kimana.

Kimbalee (English) a form of Kimberly.
Kimbalea, Kimbaleah, Kimbalei, Kimbaleigh, Kymbalea, Kymbaleah, Kymbalee, Kymbalei, Kymbaleigh, Kymbali, Kymbalia, Kymbaliah, Kymbalie, Kymballea, Kymballeah, Kymballee, Kymballei, Kymballeigh, Kymballie

Kimber (English) a short form of Kimberly.
Kimbra

Kimberlee, Kimberley, Kimberli, Kimberlie (English) forms of Kimberly.
Kimberlea, Kimberleah, Kimberlei, Kimberleigh, Kimberlia, Kimberliah, Kimbley

Kimberlin, Kimberlyn, Kimberlynn (English) forms of Kimberly.
Kemberlin, Kemberlina, Kemberlinah, Kemberline, Kemberlyn, Kemberlyna, Kemberlynah, Kemberlyne, Khimberlin, Khimberlina, Khimberlinah, Khimberline, Khimberlyn, Khimberlyna, Khimberlynah, Khimberlyne, Kimbalina, Kimbalinah, Kimbaline, Kimbalyn, Kimbalyna, Kimbalynah, Kimbalyne, Kimberlina, Kimberlinah, Kimberline, Kimberlyna, Kimberlynah, Kimberlyne, Kymbalin, Kymbalina, Kymbalinah, Kymbaline

Kimberly ⭐ (English) chief, ruler.
Cymberly, Cymbre, Kimba, Kimbalee, Kimbely, Kimberely, Kimbery, Kimbria, Kimbrie, Kimbry

Kimi (Japanese) righteous.
Kimee, Kimey, Kimia, Kimie, Kimiyo, Kimmi, Kimy

Kimiko (Japanese) righteous child.
Kimik, Kimika, Kimyko, Kymyko

Kimmie, Kimmy (English) familiar forms of Kimberly.
Kimme, Kimmee, Kimmey, Kimmi

Kina (Hawaiian) from China. (Irish) wise.
Kinah, Kyna, Kynah

Kindra (English) a form of Kendra.

Kineisha (American) a form of Keneisha.
Kineesha, Kinesha, Kineshia, Kinisha, Kinishia

Kineta (Greek) energetic.
Kinet, Kinetah, Kinete, Kinett, Kinetta, Kinettah, Kinette, Kynet, Kyneta, Kynetah, Kynete, Kynett, Kynetta, Kynettah, Kynette

Kini GB (Hawaiian) a form of Jean.
Kina

Kinsey GB (English) offspring; relative.
Kinsee

Kinsley (American) a form of Kinsey.
Kinslee, Kinslie, Kinslyn

Kinza (American) a form of Kinsey.

Kinzie (Scottish, Irish) a form of Kenzie. (English) a form of Kinsey.
Kinze, Kinzee, Kinzey, Kinzi, Kinzie, Kinzy

Kioko (Japanese) happy child.
Kioka, Kiyo, Kiyoko

Kiona (Native American) brown hills.
Kionah, Kioni, Kiowa, Kiowah, Kyona, Kyonah, Kyowa, Kyowah

Kionna (Native American) a form of Kiona.

Kip BG (English) pointed hill.
Kipp, Kyp, Kypp

Kipa (Indigenous) young girl.

Kira (Persian) sun. (Latin) light. See also Kyra.
Kirah, Kiria, Kiro, Kirra, Kirrah, Kirri, Kirrie

Kiran GB (Hindi) ray of light.
Kearan, Kearen, Kearin, Kearon, Keeran, Keerana, Keeranah, Keerane, Keeren, Keerin, Keeron, Keiran, Keiren, Keirin, Keiron, Keiryn, Kirana, Kiranah, Kirane, Kirran, Kirrana, Kirranah, Kirrane, Kyran, Kyrana, Kyranah, Kyrane, Kyren, Kyrin, Kyron, Kyryn

Kiranjit (Hindi) a form of Kiran.

Kiranjot (Hindi) a form of Kiran.

Kirby BG (Scandinavian) church village. (English) cottage by the water.
Kerbea, Kerbee, Kerbey, Kerbi, Kerbie, Kerby, Kirbea, Kirbee, Kirbey, Kirbi, Kirbie, Kyrbea, Kyrbee, Kyrbey, Kyrbi, Kyrbie, Kyrby

Kiri (Cambodian) mountain. (Maori) tree bark.
Kirea, Kiree, Kirey, Kirie, Kiry

Kiriann, Kirianne (American) combinations of Kiri + Ann.
Kirian, Kiriana, Kirianah, Kiriane, Kirianna, Kiriannah, Kyrian, Kyriana, Kyrianah, Kyriane, Kyriann, Kyrianna, Kyriannah, Kyrianne, Kyryan, Kyryana, Kyryanah, Kyryane, Kyryann, Kyryanna, Kyryannah, Kyryanne

Kirilina (American) a combination of Kiri + Lina.
Kirilin, Kirilinah, Kiriline, Kirilyn, Kirilyna, Kirilynah, Kirilyne, Kyrilin, Kyrilina, Kyrilinah, Kyriline, Kyrilyn, Kyrilyna, Kyrilynah, Kyryline, Kyrylyn, Kyrylyna, Kyrylinah, Kyryline, Kyrylyn, Kyrylyna, Kyrylynah, Kyrylyne

Kirima (Eskimo) hill.

Kirsi (Hindi) amaranth blossoms.
Kirsie

Kirsta (Scandinavian) a form of Kirsten.
Kirstai, Kirste

Kirstan, Kirstin, Kirstyn (Greek, Scandinavian) forms of Kirsten.
Kirstine, Kirstyne, Kirstynn

Kirsten (Greek) Christian; anointed. (Scandinavian) a form of Christine.
Karsten, Karstin, Karstina, Karstinah, Karstine, Kirstain, Kirstaine, Kirstane, Kirsteen, Kirstene, Kirsteni, Kirstien, Kirston, Kirstone, Kjersten, Kurstain, Kurstaine,

Kurstean, Kursteane, Kursteen, Kursteene, Kursten, Kurstin, Kurstine, Kurstyn, Kurstyne

Kirsti, Kirstie, Kirsty (Greek, Scandinavian) familiar forms of Kirsten.
Kerstea, Kerstee, Kerstey, Kersti, Kerstia, Kerstiah, Kerstie, Kersty, Kirstea, Kirstee, Kirstey, Kirstia, Kirstiah, Kirstya, Kirstye, Kjersti, Kurstea, Kurstee, Kurstey, Kursti, Kurstia, Kurstiah, Kurstie, Kursty, Kyrstea, Kyrstee, Kyrstey, Kyrsti, Kyrstie, Kyrsty

Kirstina (Scandinavian) a form of Kristina.
Kirstaina, Kirstainah, Kirstana, Kirstanah, Kirstinah, Kirstona, Kirstonah, Kirstyna, Kirstynah

Kisa (Russian) kitten.
Kisah, Kiska, Kiza, Kysa, Kysah, Kyssa, Kyssah

Kisha (African) a form of Keisha. (Russian) a form of Kisa.
Kishanda

Kishi (Japanese) long and happy life.
Kishee, Kishey, Kishie, Kishy

Kismet (Arabic) lot, fate; fortune.
Kismeta, Kismetah, Kismete, Kismett, Kismetta, Kismettah, Kismette, Kissmet, Kissmeta, Kissmetah, Kissmete, Kissmett, Kissmetta, Kissmettah, Kissmette, Kysmet, Kysmeta, Kysmetah, Kysmete, Kysmett, Kysmetta, Kysmettah, Kysmette, Kyssmet, Kyssmeta, Kyssmetah, Kyssmete, Kyssmett, Kyssmetta, Kyssmettah, Kyssmette

Kissa (Ugandan) born after twins.
Kissah, Kysa, Kysah, Kyssa, Kyssah

Kita (Japanese) north.

Kitra (Hebrew) crowned.
Kitrah

Kitty (Greek) a familiar form of Katherine.
Ketter, Ketti, Ketty, Kit, Kittee, Kitteen, Kittey, Kitti, Kittie

Kiwa (Japanese) borderline.

Kiya, Kiyah (American) short forms of Kiyana.

Kiyana, Kiyanna (American) forms of Kiana.
Kiyan, Kiyani, Kiyenna

Kizzy (American) a familiar form of Keziah.
Kezi, Kezie, Kezy, Kezzee, Kezzey, Kezzi,
Kezzie, Kezzy, Kissie, Kizee, Kizey, Kizi,
Kizie, Kizy, Kizzee, Kizzey, Kizzi, Kizzie,
Kyzee, Kyzey, Kyzi, Kyzie, Kyzy, Kyzzee,
Kyzzey, Kyzzi, Kyzzie, Kyzzy

Klaire (French) a form of Clair.
Klair

Klara (Hungarian) a form of Clara.
Klaara, Klaarah, Klaare, Klára, Klarah, Klari,
Klarika

Klarise (German) a form of Klarissa.
Klarice, Kláris, Klarisse, Klaryce, Klaryse,
Klaryss

Klarissa (German) clear, bright. (Italian) a
form of Clarissa.
Klarisa, Klarisah, Klarissah, Klarisza,
Klarrisa, Klarrissa, Klarrissia, Klarysa,
Klarysah, Klaryssa, Klaryssah, Klarysse,
Kleresa

Klarita (Spanish) a form of Clarita.
Klareata, Klareatah, Klareate, Klareeta,
Klareetah, Klareete, Klaret, Klareta, Klaretah,
Klarete, Klarett, Klaretta, Klarettah, Klarette,
Klaritah, Klarite, Klaritta, Klarittah, Klaritte,
Klaryta, Klarytah, Klaryte, Klarytta,
Klaryttah, Klarytte

Klaudia (American) a form of Claudia.
Klaudiah, Klaudija, Klaudja, Klaudya,
Klaudyah

Klementine (Latin) a form of Clementine.
Klementina, Klementinah, Klementyn,
Klementyna, Klementynah, Klementyne

Kloe (American) a form of Chloe.
Khloe, Khloea, Khloee, Khloey, Khloi, Khloie,
Khloy, Kloea, Kloee, Kloey, Klohe, Kloi,
Kloie, Klowee, Klowey, Klowi, Klowie, Klowy

Kloris (Greek) a form of Chloris.
Khloris, Khlorisa, Khlorise, Khlorys, Khlorysa,
Khloryse, Klorisa, Klorise, Klorys, Klorysa,
Kloryse

Kodi BG (American) a form of Codi.
Kodea, Kodee, Kodey, Kodye, Koedi

Kodie BG (American) a form of Codi.

Kody BG (American) a form of Codi.

Koemi (Japanese) smiling.
Koemee, Koemey, Koemie, Koemy

Koffi (Swahili) born on Friday.
Kaffe, Kaffi, Koffe, Koffie

Koko (Japanese) stork. See also Coco.

Kolbi (American) a form of Colby.
Kobie, Koby, Kolbee, Kolbey, Kolbie

Kolby BG (American) a form of Colby.

Kolette (Greek, French) a form of Colette.
Kolet, Koleta, Koletah, Kolete, Kolett, Koletta,
Kolettah, Kollette

Koleyn (Australian) winter.
Kolein, Koleina, Koleine, Koleyna, Koleynah,
Koleyne

Kolfinnia (Scandinavian) white.
Kolfinia, Kolfiniah, Kolfinna, Kolfinnah,
Kolfinniah

Kolina (Swedish) a form of Katherine. See
also Colleen.
Koleena, Kolena, Koli, Kolinah, Kollena,
Kolyna, Kolynah

Kolleen (Swedish) a form of Kolina. (Irish) a
form of Colleen.
Koleen, Kolene, Kollene, Kolyn, Kolyne

Kolora (Australian) lake.
Kolorah, Kolori, Kolorie, Kolory

Komal (Hindi, Indian) delicate.
Komala

Kona BG (Hawaiian) lady. (Hindi) angular.
Koni, Konia

Konrada (German) brave counselor.
Conrada

Konstance (Latin) a form of Constance.
Konstancia, Konstancja, Konstancy,
Konstancyna, Konstantina, Konstantine,
Konstanza, Konstanze

Kontxexi (Basque) a form of Conchita.

Kora (Greek) a form of Cora.
Korah, Kore, Koressa, Korra

Koral (American) a form of Coral.
Korel, Korele, Korella, Korilla, Korral, Korrel,
Korrell, Korrelle

Kordelia (Latin, Welsh) a form of Cordelia.
Kordel, Kordellia, Kordellyah, Kordellyah,
Kordelya, Kordelyah, Kordula

Koren (Greek) a form of Karen, Kora,
Korin.

Koretta (Greek) a familiar form of Kora.
See also Coretta.
Koret, Koreta, Koretah, Korete, Korett,
Korette, Korretta

Korey BG (American) a familiar form of
Korina. See also Corey, Cori.
Koree, Koria, Korrie, Korry

Kori, Korie GB (American) familiar forms
of Korina.

Korin, Korine, Korinne, Korrin, Koryn
(Greek) short forms of Korina.
Korane, Koranne, Korean, Koreane, Koreen,
Koreene, Koreine, Korene, Koreyne, Koriane,
Korianne, Korinn, Korrine, Korrinne, Korryn,
Korrynne, Koryne, Korynn, Korynne

Korina (Greek) a form of Corina.
Korana, Koranah, Koranna, Korannah,
Koreana, Koreanah, Koreena, Koreenah,
Koreina, Koreinah, Korena, Korenah,
Koreyna, Koreynah, Koriana, Korianna,
Korinah, Korine, Korinna, Korinnah,
Korreena, Korrina, Korrinna, Koryna,
Korynah, Korynna, Korynnah

Kornelia (Latin) a form of Cornelia.
Korneliah, Kornelija, Kornelis, Kornelya,
Kornelyah, Korny

Korri (American) a familiar form of Korina.

Kortina (American) a combination of Kora
+ Tina. See also Cortina.
Kortinah, Kortine, Kortyn, Kortyna, Kortyne

Kortnee, Kortni, Kortnie (English) forms
of Courtney.
Kortnay, Kortny

Kortney GB (English) a form of Courtney.

Kory BG (American) a familiar form of
Korina.

Kosma (Greek) order; universe.
Cosma

Kosta (Latin) a short form of Constance.
Kostia, Kostiah, Kostya, Kostyah

Koto (Japanese) harp.

Kourtnee, Kourtnei, Kourtney, Kourtni,
Kourtnie (American) forms of Courtney.
Kourtnay, Kourtne, Kourtneigh, Kourtny,
Kourtynie

Krin (Indigenous) star.

Kris BG (American) a short form of
Kristine. A form of Chris.
Khris, Khriss, Khrys, Khryss, Kriss, Krys,
Kryss

Krisandra (Greek) a form of Cassandra.
Khrisandra, Khrisandrah, Khrysandra,
Khrysandrah, Krisanda, Krissandra,
Krizandra, Krizandrah, Krysandra,
Krysandrah, Kryzandra, Kryzandrah

Krishna BG (Hindi) delightful, pleasurable.
Religion: one of the human incarnations
of the Hindu god Vishnu.
Kistna, Kistnah, Krishnah, Kryshna,
Kryshnah

Krissa (American, Czech) a form of Khrissa.
Kryssa

Krissy (American) a familiar form of Kris.
Krissey, Krissi, Krissie

Krista (Czech) a form of Christina. See also
Christa.
Khrista, Khrysta, Krysta

Kristabel (Latin, French) a form of
Christabel.
Kristabela, Kristabelah, Kristabele, Kristabell,
Kristabella, Kristabellah, Kristabelle,
Krystabel, Krystabele, Krystabell, Krystabella,
Krystabelle

Kristain (Greek) a form of Kristen.
Khristein, Kristaina, Kristainah, Kristaine,
Kristayn, Kristayna, Kristaynah, Kristayne,
Kristein, Kristeine, Kristeyn, Kristeyne,
Krystein, Krysteine

Kristal, Kristel, Kristelle (Latin) forms of
Crystal. See also Krystal.
Kristale, Kristall, Kristalle, Kristele, Kristell,
Kristella, Kristill, Kristl, Kristle

Kristalyn (American) a form of Krystalyn.
Kristalina, Kristaline, Kristalyna, Kristalyne,
Kristalynn

Kristan (Greek) a form of Kristen.
Kristana, Kristanah, Kristane, Kristanna, Kristanne

Kristen GB (Greek) Christian; anointed.
(Scandinavian) a form of Christine.
Christen, Khristen, Khristin, Khristyn, Khrystin, Kristene, Kristiin

Kristena (Greek, Scandinavian) a form of Kristina.

Kristi, Kristie (Scandinavian) short forms of Kristine.
Christi, Khristee, Khristi, Khristie, Khrystee, Khrysti, Khrystie, Kristia, Krysti, Krystie

Kristian BG (Greek) Christian; anointed. A form of Christian.
Khristian, Khristiane, Khristiann, Khristianne, Khristien, Krestian, Krestiane, Krestiann, Krestianne, Kristi-Ann, Kristi-Anne, Kristiane, Kristiann, Kristianne, Kristien, Kristienne, Kristy-Ann, Kristy-Anne, Kristyan, Kristyane, Kristyann, Kristyanne

Kristiana, Kristianna (Greek) forms of Kristian.
Khristeana, Khristeanah, Khristiana, Khristianah, Khristianna, Khristiannah, Krestiana, Krestianah, Krestianna, Krestiannah, Kristianah, Kristiannah, Kristyana, Kristyanah, Kristyanna, Kristyannah

Kristin (Scandinavian) a form of Kristen.
See also Cristan.
Kristinn

Kristina (Greek) Christian; anointed.
(Scandinavian) a form of Christina. See also Cristina.
Khristina, Kristeena, Kristeenah, Kristeina, Kristeinah, Kristinah

Kristine (Scandinavian) a form of Christine.
Khristean, Khristeane, Kristeen, Kristeene, Kristein, Kristeine, Kristene, Kristyne, Kristynn, Kristynne

Kriston BG (Greek) a form of Kristen.

Kristy (American) a familiar form of Kristine, Krystal. See also Cristi, Kristi.
Khristey, Khristy, Khrystey, Khrysty, Kristey

Kristyn (Greek) a form of Kristen.
Khristyn, Khrystyn, Kristyne, Kristynn, Kristynne

Kristyna (Greek, Scandinavian) a form of Kristina.
Kristynah, Kristynna, Kristynnah

Krysta (Polish) a form of Krista.
Krystah, Krystka

Krystal (American) clear, brilliant glass.
Krystalann, Krystalanne, Krystale, Krystall, Krystalle, Krystil, Krystol, Krystyl, Krystyle, Krystyll, Krystylle

Krystalee (American) a combination of Krystal + Lee.
Kristalea, Kristaleah, Kristalee, Krystalea, Krystaleah, Krystlea, Krystleah, Krystlee, Krystlelea, Krystleleah, Krystlelee

Krystalyn, Krystalynn (American) combinations of Krystal + Lynn. See also Crystalin.
Khristalin, Khristalina, Khristaline, Khrystalin, Khrystalina, Khrystaline, Kristelina, Kristeline, Kristilyn, Kristilynn, Kristlyn, Krystaleen, Krystalene, Krystalin, Krystalina, Krystaline, Krystallyn, Krystalyna, Krystalyne, Krystalynne, Krystelina, Krysteline

Krystan, Krysten (Greek) forms of Kristen.
Krystana, Krystanah, Krystane, Krystena, Krystenah, Krystene, Krystenia, Kryston

Krystel, Krystelle (Latin) forms of Krystal.
Krystele, Krystell, Krystella

Krystian BG (Greek) a form of Christian.
Krystiann, Krystianne, Krysty-Ann, Krysty-Anne, Krystyan, Krystyane, Krystyann, Krystyanne, Krystyen

Krystiana (Greek) a form of Krystian.
Krysteana, Krysteanah, Krystianah, Krystianna, Krystiannah, Krystyana, Krystyanah, Krystyanna, Krystyannah

Krystin, Krystyn (Czech) forms of Kristin.
Krystyne, Krystynn, Krystynne

Krystina (Greek) a form of Kristina.
Krysteana, Krysteanah, Krysteena, Krysteenah, Krysteina, Krysteinah, Krystena, Krystinah

Krystine (Scandinavian) a form of Kristina. (Czech) a form of Krystin.
Krystean, Krysteane, Krysteen, Krysteene, Krystein, Krysteine, Krysteyn, Krysteyne, Kryston

Krystle (American) a form of Krystal.
Krystl, Krystyl, Krystyle, Krystyll, Krystylle

Krystyna (Greek) a form of Kristina.
Krystynah, Krystynna, Krystynnah

Kudio (Swahili) born on Monday.

Kuma (Japanese) bear. (Tongan) mouse.
Kumah

Kumari (Sanskrit) woman.
Kumaree, Kumarey, Kumaria, Kumariah, Kumarie, Kumary, Kumarya, Kumaryah

Kumberlin (Australian) sweet.
Cumberlin, Cumberlina, Cumberline, Cumberlyn, Cumberlyne, Kumberlina, Kumberline, Kumberlyn, Kumberlyne

Kumi (Japanese) braid.
Kumee, Kumie, Kumy

Kumiko (Japanese) girl with braids.

Kumuda (Sanskrit) lotus flower.

Kunani (Hawaiian) beautiful.
Kunanee, Kunaney, Kunanie, Kunany

Kuniko (Japanese) child from the country.

Kunto (Twi) third-born.

Kuri (Japanese) chestnut.
Curee, Curey, Curi, Curie, Cury, Kuree, Kurey, Kurie, Kury

Kusa (Hindi) God's grass.

Kuyen (Mapuche) moon.

Kwanita (Zuni) a form of Juanita.

Kwashi (Swahili) born on Sunday.

Kwau (Swahili) born on Thursday.

Kya (African) diamond in the sky. (American) a form of Kia.

Kyah (African, American) a form of Kya.

Kyana, Kyanna (American) forms of Kiana.
Kyanah, Kyani, Kyann, Kyannah, Kyanne, Kyanni, Kyeana, Kyeanna

Kyara (Irish) a form of Kiara.
Kiyara, Kiyera, Kiyerra, Kyarah, Kyaria, Kyarie, Kyarra

Kyera, Kyerra (Irish) forms of Kiara.

Kyla (Irish) lovely. (Yiddish) crown; laurel.
Khyla, Kyela, Kyella, Kylia

Kylah (Irish, Yiddish) a form of Kyla.

Kyle BG (Irish) attractive.
Kial, Kiele, Kiell, Kielle, Kile, Kyel, Kyele, Kyell, Kyelle

Kylea, Kylee, Kyleigh, Kyley, Kyli (West Australian Aboriginal, Irish) forms of Kylie.
Kyleah, Kyllea, Kylleah, Kyllee, Kylleigh, Kylley, Kylli

Kyleen, Kylene (Irish) forms of Kyle.

Kyler BG (English) a form of Kyle.
Kylar, Kylor

Kylie ☆ (West Australian Aboriginal) curled stick; boomerang. (Irish) a familiar form of Kyle. See also Kiley.
Kye, Kylei, Kylia, Kyliah, Kyliee, Kyliegh, Kyllei, Kyllia, Kylliah, Kyllie, Kylly, Kyly, Kylya, Kylyah

Kylynn (Irish) a form of Kyle.
Kylenn, Kylynne

Kym (Vietnamese, English) a form of Kim.
Kymm

Kymber (English) a form of Kimber.

Kymberlee, Kymberli, Kymberly (English) forms of Kimberly.
Kymberlea, Kymberleah, Kymberlei, Kymberleigh, Kymberley, Kymberlia, Kymberliah, Kymberlie

Kymberlyn (English) a form of Kimberlin.
Kymberlynn, Kymberlynne

Kyndal (English) a form of Kendall.
Kyndahl, Kyndalle, Kyndel, Kyndell, Kyndelle, Kyndle, Kyndol

Kyndall GB (English) a form of Kendall.

Kyndra (English) a form of Kendra.

Kynthia (Greek) a form of Cynthia.
Kyndi

Kyoko (Japanese) mirror.
Kyoka, Kyokah

Kyra (Greek) noble. A form of Cyrilla. See also Kira.
Kyrah, Kyria, Kyriah, Kyriann, Kyrra, Kyrrah

Kyrene (Greek) noble.
Kirena, Kirenah, Kirene, Kyrena, Kyrenah

Kyrie (Cambodian, Maori) a form of Kiri. (Greek) a familiar form of Kyra.
Kyrea, Kyree, Kyrey, Kyri, Kyry

Kyrsten, Kyrstin, Kyrstyn (Greek, Scandinavian) forms of Kirsten.
Kyersten

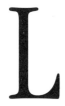

La Cienega (Spanish) the marsh.

La Reina, La-Reina (Spanish) the queen.

Labreana (American) a combination of the prefix La + Breana.
Labreanah, Labreann, Labreanna, Labreannah, Labreanne, Labrenna, Labrennah

Labrenda (American) a combination of the prefix La + Brenda.
Labrinda, Labrindah, Labrynda, Labryndah

Lace, Lacee, Laci, Lacie (Greek, Latin) forms of Lacey.

Lacey (Latin) cheerful. (Greek) a familiar form of Larissa.
Lacea, Lacia, Laciah, Laciann, Lacianne, Lacye, Laicee, Laicey, Laici, Laicia, Laiciah, Laicie, Laicy, Layce, Lece

Lachandra (American) a combination of the prefix La + Chandra.
Lachanda, Lachandah, Lachander, Lachandice, Lachandrah, Lachandrica, Lachandrice, Lachandryce

Lachlanina (Scottish) land of lakes.
Lachianina, Lachianinah, Lachlanee, Lachlani, Lachlania, Lachlanie, Lachlany, Lachyanina, Lachyaninah, Lochlanee, Lochlaney, Lochlani, Lochlanie, Lochlany

Lacole (Italian) a form of Nicole.
Lacola, Lacollah, Lacolle, Lecola, Lecole, Lecolla, Lecolle

Lacrecia (Latin) a form of Lucretia.
Lacrasha, Lacreash, Lacreasha, Lacreashia, Lacreisha, Lacresha, Lacreshah, Lacreshia, Lacreshiah, Lacresia, Lacretia, Lacretiah, Lacretya, Lacretyah, Lacricia, Lacriciah, Lacriesha, Lacrisah, Lacrisha, Lacrishia, Lacrishiah, Lacrissa, Lacrycia, Lacryciah, Lacrycya, Lacrycyah

Lacy GB (Latin) cheerful. (Greek) a familiar form of Larissa.

Lada (Russian) Mythology: the Slavic goddess of beauty.
Ladah, Ladia, Ladiah, Ladya, Ladyah

Ladaisha (American) a form of Ladasha.
Ladaisa, Ladaishea, Ladaishia

Ladan (American) a short form of Ladana.
Ladann, Ladanne

Ladana (American) a combination of the prefix La + Dana.
Ladanah, Ladanna, Ladannah

Ladanica (American) a combination of the prefix La + Danica.
Ladanicah, Ladanicka, Ladanika, Ladanikah, Ladanyca, Ladanycah, Ladanycka, Ladanyka, Ladanykah

Ladasha (American) a combination of the prefix La + Dasha.
Ladaesha, Ladaseha, Ladashah, Ladashia, Ladashiah, Ladasia, Ladassa, Ladaysha, Ladesha, Ladisha, Ladosha

Ladawna (American) a combination of the prefix La + Dawna.
Ladawn, Ladawnah, Ladawne, Ladawnee, Ladawni, Ladawnia, Ladawniah, Ladawnie, Ladawny

Ladeidra (American) a combination of the prefix La + Deidra.
Ladedra, Ladiedra

Ladivina (American) a combination of the prefix La + Divinia.
Ladivinah, Ladivine, Ladivyna, Ladivynah, Ladivyne, Ladyvyna, Ladyvynah, Ladyvyne

Ladonna (American) a combination of the prefix La + Donna.
Ladon, Ladona, Ladonah, Ladonia, Ladoniah, Ladonnah, Ladonne, Ladonnia, Ladonniah, Ladonnya, Ladonnyah, Ladonya, Ladonyah

Laela (Arabic, Hebrew) a form of Leila.
Lael, Laele, Laelea, Laeleah, Laelee, Laelei, Laeleigh, Laeley, Laeli, Laelia, Laeliah, Laelie, Laell, Laella, Laellah, Laelle, Laely, Laelya, Laelyah

Laeticia, Laetitia (Latin) forms of Leticia.
Laeticha, Laetichah, Laetichya, Laetichyah, Laeticiah, Laeticya, Laeticyah, Laetita, Laetitiah, Laetizia, Laetiziah, Laetizya, Laetycia, Laetyciah, Laetycya, Laetycyah, Laetyta, Laetytah, Laetyte, Laetytia, Laetytiah, Laitichya, Laitichyah, Laiticia, Laiticiah, Laitita, Laititah, Laititia, Laititiah, Laytitia, Laytitiah, Laytytia, Laytytiah, Laytytya, Laytytyah

Laflora (American) a combination of the prefix La + Flora.
Laflorah, Leflora, Leflorah

Lahela (Hawaiian) a form of Rachel.
Lahelah

Laia (Greek) a form of Lalia.

Laica (Greek) pure; secular.

Laila (Arabic) a form of Leila.
Lailah, Laile, Lailea, Laileah, Lailee, Lailei, Laileigh, Lailey, Laili, Lailia, Lailiah, Lailie, Lailla, Laillah, Laille, Laily, Lailya, Lailyah

Lailaka (Tongan) lilac.
Laelaka, Laelakah, Lailakah, Laylaka, Laylakah

Laina (French) a form of Laine. (English) a form of Lane.
Laena, Laenah, Lainah, Lainna, Layna, Laynah

Laine ☆☆ (French) a short form of Elaine. See also Lane.
Laen, Laene, Laenia, Laeniah, Lain, Lainia, Lainiah

Lainey (French) a familiar form of Elaine.
Laenee, Laeney, Laeni, Laenie, Laeny, Laenya, Laenyah, Lainee, Laini, Lainie, Lainy, Lainya, Lainyah

Laione (Tongan) lion.
Laeona, Laeonah, Laeone, Laiona, Laionah, Layona, Layonah, Layone

Lais (Greek) one who is friendly with everyone.

Lajessica (American) a combination of the prefix La + Jessica.
Lajesica, Lajesicah, Lajesika, Lajesikah, Lajessicah, Lajessika, Lajessikah, Lajessyca, Lajessycah, Lajessycka, Lajessyckah, Lajessyka, Lajessykah

Lajila (Hindi) shy; coy.
Lajilah, Lajilla, Lajillah

Lajuana (American) a combination of the prefix La + Juana.
Lajuanah, Lajuanna, Lajuannah, Lajunna, Lajunnah, Lawana, Lawanah, Lawanna, Lawannah, Lawanne, Lawanza, Lawanze, Laweania

Lajuliet, Lajuliette (American) combinations of the prefix La + Juliet.
Lajulieta, Lajulietah, Lajuliete, Lajuliett, Lajulietta, Lajuliettah, Lajulyet, Lajulyeta, Lajulyetah, Lajulyete, Lajulyett, Lajulyetta, Lajulyettah, Lajulyette

Laka (Hawaiian) attractive; seductive; tame. Mythology: the goddess of the hula.
Lakah

Lakaya (American) a form of Lakayla.

Lakayla (American) a combination of the prefix La + Kayla.
Lakala, Lakeila, Lakela, Lakella

Lakeisha (American) a combination of the prefix La + Keisha. See also Lekasha.
Lakaiesha, Lakaisha, Lakaysha, Lakaysia, Lakeasha, Lakeysha, Lakeyshah

Laken, Lakin, Lakyn (American) short forms of Lakendra.
Lakena, Lakine, Lakyna, Lakynn

Lakendra (American) a combination of the prefix La + Kendra.
Lakanda, Lakandah, Lakande, Lakandra, Lakedra, Laken, Lakenda, Lakendrah, Lakendrya, Lakendryah

Lakenya (American) a combination of the prefix La + Kenya.
Lakeena, Lakeenna, Lakeenya, Lakena, Lakenah, Lakenia, Lakeniah, Lakenja, Lakenyah, Lakina, Lakinja, Lakinya, Lakinyah, Lakwanya, Lekenia, Lekeniah, Lekenya, Lekenyah

Lakesha (American) a form of Lakeisha.
Lakasha, Lakeesh, Lakeesha, Lakesa

Lakeshia (American) a form of Lakeisha.
Lakashia, Lakeashia, Lakeashiah, Lakeashya, Lakeashyah, Lakecia, Lakeciah, Lakeeshia, Lakeeshiah, Lakeeshya, Lakeeshyah, Lakeishia, Lakeishiah, Lakese, Lakeseia, Lakeshiah, Lakeshya, Lakeshyah, Lakesi, Lakesia, Lakesiah, Lakeyshia, Lakezia, Lakicia, Lakieshia

Laketa (American) a combination of the prefix La + Keita.
Lakeet, Lakeeta, Lakeetah, Lakeita, Lakeitha, Lakeithia, Laketha, Laketia, Laketiah, Lakett, Laketta, Lakette, Lakieta, Lakietha, Lakyta, Lakytah, Lakyte, Lakytia, Lakytiah, Lakytta, Lakyttah, Lakytte, Lakytya, Lakytyah

Lakeya (Hindi) a form of Lakya.
Lakeyah

Lakia (Arabic) found treasure.
Lakiah, Lakiea, Lakkia

Lakiesha (American) a form of Lakeisha.

Lakisha (American) a form of Lakeisha.

Lakita (American) a form of Laketa.
Lakitia, Lakitiah, Lakitra, Lakitri, Lakitt, Lakitta, Lakitte

Lakiya (Hindi) a form of Lakya.
Lakieya

Lakkari (Australian) honeysuckle tree.
Lakaree, Lakarey, Lakari, Lakaria, Lakariah, Lakarie, Lakary, Lakkaree, Lakkarey, Lakkarie, Lakkary, Lakkarya, Lakkaryah

Lakmé (Hindi) born in milk.

Lakota BG (Dakota) a tribal name.
Lakoda, Lakohta, Lakotah

Lakresha (American) a form of Lucretia.
Lacresha, Lacreshia, Lacreshiah, Lacresia, Lacresiah, Lacretia, Lacretiah, Lacrisha, Lakreshia, Lakreshiah, Lakrisha, Lakrysha,

Lakryshah, Lekresha, Lekreshia, Lekreshiah, Lekreshya, Lekreshyah, Lekresia

Lakya (Hindi) born on Thursday.
Lakyah, Lakyia

Lala (Slavic) tulip.
Lalah, Lalla, Lallah

Lalasa (Hindi) love.
Lalassa, Lallasa

Laleh (Persian) tulip.
Lalah

Lali (Spanish) a form of Lulani.
Lalea, Laleah, Lalee, Lalei, Laleigh, Laley, Lalia, Laliah, Lalie, Laly, Lalya, Lalyah

Lalirra (Australian) chatty.
Lalira, Lalirah, Lalirrah, Lalyra, Lalyrah, Lalyrra, Lalyrrah, Lira, Lirra, Lirrah, Lyra, Lyrah, Lyrra, Lyrrah

Lalita (Greek) talkative. (Sanskrit) charming; candid.
Laleata, Laleatah, Laleate, Laleeta, Laleetah, Laleete, Laleita, Laleitah, Laleite, Lalitah, Lalite, Lalitt, Lalitta, Lalitte, Lalyta, Lalytah, Lalyte, Lalytta, Lalyttah, Lalytte

Lallie (English) babbler.
Lallea, Lalleah, Lallee, Lallei, Lalleigh, Lalley, Lalli, Lallia, Lalliah, Lally, Lallya, Lallyah

Lama (German) a short form of Lamberta.
Lamah

Lamani BG (Tongan) lemon.
Lamanee, Lamaney, Lamania, Lamaniah, Lamanie, Lamany, Lamanya, Lamanyah

Lamberta (German) bright land.
Lamberlina, Lamberline, Lamberlynn, Lamberlynne, Lambirta, Lambirtah, Lambirte, Lamburta, Lamburtah, Lamburte, Lambyrta, Lambyrtah, Lambyrte

Lamesha (American) a combination of the prefix La + Mesha.
Lamees, Lameesa, Lameesha, Lameise, Lameisha, Lameshia, Lameshiah, Lamisha, Lamishia, Lamysha, Lemesha, Lemisha, Lemysha

Lamia (German) a short form of Lamberta.
Lamiah, Lamya, Lamyah

Lamis (Arabic) soft to the touch.
Lamese, Lamisa, Lamisah, Lamise, Lamiss,
Lamissa, Lamissah, Lamisse, Lamys, Lamysa,
Lamyss, Lamyssa

Lamonica (American) a combination of the
prefix La + Monica.
Lamoni, Lamonika

Lamya (Arabic) dark lipped.
Lama

Lan (Vietnamese) flower.
Lann, Lanne

Lana (Latin) woolly. (Irish) attractive, peace-
ful. A short form of Alana, Elana.
(Hawaiian) floating; bouyant.
Lanah, Lanai, Lanaia, Lanata, Lanay,
Lanaya, Lanayah, Laneah, Laneetra

Lanae (Latin, Irish, Hawaiian) a form of
Lana.

Lanca (Latin) blessed one.

Landa (Spanish) reference to the Virgin
Mary.

Landeberta (Latin) a form of Lamberta.

Landelina (German) patriot.

Landon BG (English) open, grassy meadow.
Landan, Landen, Landin

Landra (German, Spanish) counselor.
Landrah, Landrea, Landreah, Landria,
Landriah, Landrya, Landryah

Landrada (Spanish) a form of Landra.

Landyn (English) a form of Landon,
London.
Landynne

Lane BG (English) narrow road. See also
Laine, Layne.
Lanee

Laneisha (American) a combination of the
prefix La + Keneisha.
Laneasha, Lanecia, Laneciah, Laneesha,
Laneise, Laneishia, Laneysha, Lanysha

Lanelle (French) a combination of Lane +
Elle.
Lanel, Lanela, Lanelah, Lanele, Lanell,
Lanella, Lanellah

Lanesha (American) a form of Laneisha.
Laneshe, Laneshea, Laneshia, Lanesia, Laness,
Lanessa, Lanesse

Lanette (Welsh, French) a form of Linette.

Laney (English) a familiar form of Lane.
Lannee, Lanni, Lannia, Lanniah, Lannie,
Lanny, Lany

Langley GB (English) long meadow.
Lainglea, Lainglee, Laingleigh, Laingley,
Laingli, Lainglie, Laingly, Langlea, Langlee,
Langleigh, Langli, Langlie, Langly

Lani GB (Hawaiian) sky; heaven. A short
form of 'Aulani, Atlanta, Laulani, Leilani,
Lulani.
Lanee, Lanei, Lania, Lanita, Lanney, Lanni,
Lannie, Lanny, Lany

Lanie (English) a form of Laney. (Hawaiian)
a form of Lani.

Lanisha (American) a form of Laneisha.
Lanishia

Lanna (Latin, Irish, Hawaiian) a form of
Lana.
Lannah, Lannaia, Lannaya

Lantha (Greek) purple flower.
Lanthia, Lanthiah, Lanthya, Lanthyah

Laodamia (Greek) she who leads her community.

Laodicea (Greek) she who is fair with her
community.

Laporsha (American) a combination of the
prefix La + Porsha.
Laporcha, Laporche, Laporscha, Laporsche,
Laporschia, Laporshe, Laporshia, Laportia

Laqueena (American) a combination of the
prefix La + Queenie.
Laqueen, Laqueene, Laquena, Laquenah,
Laquene, Laquenetta, Laquinna

Laquesha (American) a form of Laquisha.

Laquinta (American) a combination of the
prefix La + Quintana.
Laquanta, Laqueinta, Laquenda, Laqueneta,
Laquenete, Laquenett, Laquenetta, Laquenette,
Laquenta, Laquinda, Laquintah, Laquynta,
Laquyntah

Laquisha (American) a combination of the prefix La + Queisha.
Laquasha, Laquaysha, Laqueisha, Laquiesha

Laquita (American) a combination of the prefix La + Queta.
Laqeita, Laqueta, Laquetta, Laquia, Laquiata, Laquieta, Laquitta, Lequita

Lara (Greek) cheerful. (Latin) shining; famous. Mythology: a Roman nymph. A short form of Laraine, Larissa, Laura.
Larah, Laretta, Larette, Laria, Lariah, Larra, Larrah, Larrya, Larryah, Larya, Laryah

Larae (Greek, Latin) a form of Lara.

Laraina (Latin) a form of Lorraine.
Laraena, Laraenah, Larainah, Larana, Laranah, Laranna, Larannah, Larayna, Laraynah, Laraynna, Lareina, Lareinah, Larena, Larenah, Lareyna, Lareynah, Larraina, Larrainah, Larrayna, Larraynah, Larreina, Larreinah, Larreyna, Larreynah, Lauraina, Laurainah, Laurayna, Lauraynah, Lawraina, Lawrainah, Lawrayna, Lawraynah

Laraine (Latin) a form of Lorraine.
Laraen, Laraene, Larain, Larainee, Larane, Larann, Laranne, Larayn, Larayne, Larein, Lareine, Larene, Lareyn, Lareyne, Larrain, Larraine, Larrayn, Larrayne, Larrein, Larreine, Larreyn, Larreyne, Laurain, Lauraine, Laurainne, Laurayn, Laurayne, Laurraine, Lawrain, Lawraine, Lawrayn, Lawrayne

Laramie GB (French) tears of love. Geography: a town in Wyoming on the Overland Trail.
Laramee, Laramey, Larami, Laramy, Laremy

Laren (Latin) a form of Laraine. (Greek) a short form of Larina.
Larenn, Larrine, Laryn, Laryne

Lari (Latin) a familiar form of Lara. A short form of names starting with "Lari."
Laree, Larey, Larie, Larilia, Larrie

Larianna (American) a combination of Lari + Anna.
Larian, Lariana, Larianah, Lariane, Lariann, Lariannah, Larianne, Larrian, Larriana, Larrianah, Larriane, Larriann, Larrianna, Larriannah, Larrianne, Larryan, Larryana, Larryanah, Larryane, Larryann, Larryanna, Larryannah, Larryanne

Laricia (Latin) a form of Laura.
Lariciah, Laricya, Laricyah, Larikia, Larycia, Laryciah, Larycya, Larycyah, Larykia, Lauricia

Lariel (Hebrew) God's lioness.
Lariela, Larielah, Lariele, Lariell, Lariella, Lariellah, Larielle, Laryel, Laryela, Laryelah, Laryele, Laryell, Laryella, Laryellah, Laryelle

Larina (Greek) sea gull.
Larena, Larenah, Larenee, Larinah, Larine, Larrina, Larrinah, Laryna, Larynah

Larisa, Larrisa, Larrissa (Greek) forms of Larissa.
Lareesa, Lareese, Laresa, Laris, Larise, Larysa, Laurisa, Lorysa, Lorysah

Larisha (Greek) a form of Larissa.

Larissa (Greek) cheerful. See also Lacey.
Laressa, Larissah, Larisse

Lark (English) skylark.
Larke, Larkee, Larkey

Larlene (Irish) promise.
Larlean, Larleana, Larleanah, Larleane, Larleen, Larleena, Larleenah, Larleene, Larlin, Larlina, Larlinah, Larline, Larlyn, Larlyna, Larlynah, Larlyne

Larmina (Persian) blue sky.
Larminah, Larmine, Larmyn, Larmyna, Larmynah, Larmyne

Larnelle (Latin) high degree.
Larnel, Larnela, Larnelah, Larnele, Larnell, Larnella, Larnellah

Larunda, Laurinda, Laurita (Spanish) forms of Laura.

Laryssa (Greek) a form of Larissa.
Larryssa, Larysse, Laryssia

Lasha (American) a form of Lashae.

Lashae, Lashai, Lashay, Lashea (American) combinations of the prefix La + Shay.
Lashaye

Lashana (American) a combination of the prefix La + Shana.
Lashan, Lashanay, Lashane, Lashanee, Lashann, Lashanna, Lashanne, Lashannon, Lashona, Lashonna

Lashanda (American) a combination of the prefix La + Shanda.
Lashandra, Lashanta, Lashante

Lashaun BG (American) a short form of Lashawna.
Lasean, Laseane, Lashaughn, Lashaughne, Lashaune, Lashaunne, Lashawne, Lesean, Leseane, Leshaun, Leshaune, Leshawn, Leshawne

Lashawn BG (American) a short form of Lashawna.

Lashawna (American) a combination of the prefix La + Shawna.
Laseana, Laseanah, Lashaughna, Lashaughnah, Lashauna, Lashaunna, Lashaunnah, Lashaunta, Lashawni, Lashawnia, Lashawnie, Lashawny, Lashona, Lashonna, Leseana, Leseanah, Leshauna, Leshaunah, Leshawna, Leshawnah

Lashawnda (American) a form of Lashonda.
Lashawnd, Lashawndra

Lashaya (American) a form of Lasha.
Lashaia

Lashon GB (American) a short form of Lashawna.

Lashonda (American) a combination of the prefix La + Shonda.
Lachonda, Lashaunda, Lashaundra, Lashond, Lashonde, Lashondia, Lashonta, Lashunda, Lashundra, Lashunta, Lashunte, Leshande, Leshandra, Leshondra, Leshundra

Lashondra (American) a form of Lashonda.

Lassie (Irish) young girl.
Lasee, Lasey, Lasi, Lasie, Lass, Lasse, Lassee, Lassey, Lassi, Lassy, Lasy

Latanya (American) a combination of the prefix La + Tanya.
Latana, Latanah, Latandra, Latania, Lataniah, Latanja, Latanna, Latanua, Latonshia

Latara (American) a combination of the prefix La + Tara.
Latarah, Lataria, Latariah, Latarya, Lotara, Lotarah, Lotaria, Lotarya

Lataree (Japanese) bent branch.
Latarea, Latarey, Latari, Latarie, Latary

Latasha (American) a combination of the prefix La + Tasha.
Latacha, Latai, Lataisha, Latashah, Lataysha, Letasha

Latashia (American) a form of Latasha.
Latacia, Latasia

Latavia (American) a combination of the prefix La + Tavia.

Lateasha (American) a form of Leticia, Latisha.
Lateashya, Lateashyah

Lateefah (Arabic) pleasant. (Hebrew) pat, caress.
Lateefa, Lateifa, Lateyfa, Lateyfah, Letifa

Lateesha (American) a form of Leticia, Latisha.

Lateisha (American) a form of Leticia, Latisha.
Lateicia, Letashia, Letasiah

Latesha (American) a form of Leticia.
Lataeasha, Latecia, Latesa, Latessa, Lateysha, Latisa, Latissa, Latytia, Latytiah, Latytya, Latytyah, Leteisha, Leteshia

Lateshia (American) a form of Leticia.
Lateashia, Lateashiah

Latia (American) a combination of the prefix La + Tia.
Latea, Lateia, Lateka, Latiah, Latja, Latya, Latyah

Laticia (Latin) a form of Leticia.
Laticiah

Latifah (Arabic, Hebrew) a form of Lateefah.
Latifa, Latipha

Latika (Hindi) elegant.
Lateeka, Lateka, Latik, Latikah, Latyka, Latykah

Latina (American) a combination of the prefix La + Tina.
Latean, Lateana, Lateanah, Lateane, Lateen, Lateena, Lateenah, Lateene, Latinah, Latine, Latyna, Latynah, Latyne

Latisha (Latin) joy. (American) a combination of the prefix La + Tisha.
Laetisha, Laetysha, Latecia, Latice, Latiesha,

Latishah, Latishia, Latishya, Latissha, Latitia,
Latysha, Latyshia, Latyshiah, Latysya,
Latysyah

Latona (Latin) Mythology: the powerful
goddess who bore Apollo and Diana.
Latonah, Latonna, Latonnah, Latonne

Latonia (Latin, American) a form of
Latonya.
Latoni, Latoniah, Latonie

Latonya (American) a combination of the
prefix La + Tonya. (Latin) a form of
Latona.
Latonee, Latonyah

Latoria (American) a combination of the
prefix La + Tori.
Latoira, Latorea, Latoreah, Latoree, Latorey,
Latori, Latorio, Latorja, Latorray, Latorreia,
Latory, Latorya, Latoyra, Latoyria, Latoyrya

Latosha (American) a combination of the
prefix La + Tosha.
Latoshia, Latoshya, Latosia

Latoya (American) a combination of the
prefix La + Toya.
Latoia, Latoiya, Latoiyah, La Toya, Latoye,
Latoyia, Latoyita, Latoyo

Latrice (American) a combination of the
prefix La + Trice.
Latrece, Latreece, Latreese, Latresa, Latrese,
Latressa, Letreece, Letrice

Latricia, Latrisha (American) combinations
of the prefix La + Tricia.
Latrecia, Latreciah, Latresh, Latresha,
Latreshia, Latreshiah, Latreshya, Latrica,
Latricah, Latriciah, Latrishia, Latrishiah,
Latrysha, Latryshia, Latryshiah, Latryshya

Laudelina (Latin) deserves laud.

Laulani (Hawaiian) heavenly tree branch.
Laulanea, Laulanee, Laulaney, Laulania,
Laulaniah, Laulanie, Laulany, Laulanya,
Laulanyah

Laumalie (Tongan) lively, full of spirit.
Laumalea, Laumaleah, Laumalee, Laumalei,
Laumaleigh, Laumali, Laumalia, Laumaliah,
Laumaly

Laura GB (Latin) crowned with laurel.
Laurah, Laure, Laurella, Laurka, Lavra,
Lawra, Lawrah, Lawrea, Loura

Lauralee (American) a combination of
Laura + Lee. (German) a form of Lorelei.
Lauralea, Lauraleah, Lauralei, Lauraleigh,
Lauraley, Laurali, Lauralia, Lauraliah,
Lauralie, Lauraly, Lauralya

Lauralyn (American) a combination of
Laura + Lynn.
Lauralin, Lauralina, Lauralinah, Lauraline,
Lauralyna, Lauralyne, Lauralynn, Lauralynna,
Lauralynne, Laurelen

Lauran, Laurin (English) forms of Lauren.
Laurine

Laure (Italian) a form of Laura.
Lauré, Lawre

Laureanne (English) a short form of
Laurianna. (American) a form of Laurie
Ann.

Laurel (Latin) laurel tree.
Laural, Laurala, Lauralah, Laurale, Laurela,
Laurelah, Laurele, Laurell, Laurella, Laurellah,
Laurelle, Lawrel, Lawrela, Lawrelah, Lawrele,
Lawrell, Lawrella, Lawrellah, Lawrelle, Lorel,
Lorelle

Laurelei (German) a form of Lorelei.
(American) a form of Lauralee.
Laurelea, Laurelee, Laureleigh

Lauren ⭐ GB (English) a form of Laura.
Laureen, Laureene, Laurena, Laurenah,
Laurene, Laurenne, Laurien

Laurence GB (Latin) crowned with laurel.
Laurencia, Laurenciah, Laurens, Laurent,
Laurentana, Laurentia, Laurentiah,
Laurentina, Laurentya, Lawrencia

Lauretta (English) a form of Loretta.
Lauret, Laureta, Lauretah, Laurete, Laurett,
Laurettah, Laurette

Lauriane, Laurianne (English) short forms
of Laurianna. (American) forms of Laurie
Ann.
Laurian

Laurianna (English) a combination of Laurie + Anna.
Laurana, Lauranah, Laurane, Laurann, Lauranna, Laurannah, Lauranne, Laureana, Laureena, Laureenah, Laurenna, Laurennah, Lauriana, Laurina, Lauryna, Laurynah, Lawrana, Lawranah, Lawrena, Lawrenah, Lawrina, Lawrinah, Lawryna, Lawrynah

Laurie GB (English) a familiar form of Laura.
Lauree, Lauri, Lawree, Lawri, Lawria, Lawriah, Lawrie

Laurie Ann, Laurie Anne (American) combinations of Laurie + Ann.
Laurie-Ann, Laurie-Anne

Laurissa (Greek) a form of Larissa.
Laurissah

Laury (English) a familiar form of Laura.
Lawrey, Lawry, Lawrya, Lawryah

Lauryn (English) a familiar form of Laura.
Lauryna, Laurynah, Lauryne, Laurynn, Laurynna, Laurynnah, Laurynne

Lavani (Tongan) necklace.
Lavanea, Lavaneah, Lavanee, Lavaney, Lavania, Lavaniah, Lavany, Lavanya

Lave BG (Italian) lava. (English) lady. (Tongan) touch.
Lav

Laveda (Latin) cleansed, purified.
Lavare, Lavedah, Laveta, Lavetah, Lavete, Lavett, Lavetta, Lavette

Lavelle BG (Latin) cleansing.
Lavel, Lavela, Lavelah, Lavele, Lavell, Lavella, Lavellah

Lavena (Irish, French) joy. (Latin) a form of Lavina.
Lavana, Lavania, Lavenah, Lavenia, Laveniah, Lavenya, Lavenyah

Lavender (Latin) bluish violet, purple. Botany: a plant with clusters of pale purple flowers.
Lavenda, Lavende

Laveni (Tongan) lavender; light purple.
Lavenee, Laveney, Lavenie, Laveny

Lavenita (Tongan) lavender fragrance.
Lavenit, Lavenitah, Lavenyt, Lavenyta, Lavenytah, Lavenyte

Laverne (Latin) springtime. (French) grove of alder trees. See also Verna.
La Verne, Laverine, Lavern, Laverna, Lavernia, Laverniah, Lavernya, Lavernyah, Laveryne

Laviana (Latin) a form of Lavina.

Lavina (Latin) purified; woman of Rome. See also Vina.
Lavena, Lavinah, Lavyna, Lavynah, Lavyne

Lavinia (Latin) a form of Lavina.
Laviniah, Lavinie, Laviniya, Laviniyah, Lavyni, Lavynia, Lavyniah, Lavyny, Lavynya, Lavynyah, Levenia, Leveniah, Levinia, Leviniah, Leviniya, Leviniyah, Levynia, Levyniah, Levynya, Levynyah, Livinia, Liviniah, Lovinia, Lyvinia, Lyviniah, Lyvinya, Lyvinyah

Lavonna (American) a combination of the prefix La + Yvonne.
Lavona, Lavonah, Lavonda, Lavonde, Lavonder, Lavondria, Lavonee, Lavoney, Lavonia, Lavoniah, Lavonica, Lavonie, Lavonnah, Lavonnee, Lavonney, Lavonni, Lavonnie, Lavonny, Lavonnya, Lavonya, Lovona, Lovonah, Lovoni, Lovonia, Lovoniah, Lovonie, Lovonna, Lovonnah, Lovony, Lovonya, Lovonyah

Lavonne (American) a short form of Lavonna.
Lavon, Lavone, Lavonn, Lovon, Lovone, Lovonne

Lawan (Tai) pretty.
Lawana, Lawane, Lawanne

Lawanda (American) a combination of the prefix La + Wanda.
Lawandah, Lawinda, Lawindah, Lawonda, Lawynda, Lawyndah

Lawren (American) a form of Lauren.
Lawran, Lawrane, Lawrene, Lawrin, Lawrine, Lawryn, Lawryne

Layan (Iranian) bright; shining.

Layce (American) a form of Lacey.
Laycee, Laycey, Layci, Laycia, Laycie, Laycy, Laysa, Laysea, Laysie

Layla (Hebrew, Arabic) a form of Leila.
Laylah, Laylea, Layleah, Laylee, Laylei,
Layleigh, Layli, Laylia, Layliah, Laylie,
Laylla, Laylle, Layly, Laylya, Laylyah

Layne BG (French) a form of Laine. See also
Laine.
Layn

Layney (French) a familiar form of Elaine.
Laynee, Layni, Laynia, Layniah, Laynie,
Layny

Lazalea (Greek) eagle ruler.
Lazaleah, Lazalee, Lazalei, Lazaleigh,
Lazaley, Lazali, Lazalia, Lazaliah, Lazalie,
Lazaly, Lazalya

Le BG (Vietnamese) pearl.

Lea (Hawaiian) Mythology: the goddess of
canoe makers. (Hebrew) a form of Leah.

Lea Marie (American) a combination of Lea
+ Marie.
Lea-Marie, Leah Marie, Leah-Marie

Leah ⭐ (Hebrew) weary. Bible: the first
wife of Jacob. See also Lia.
Léa

Leala (French) faithful, loyal.
Leal, Lealia, Lealiah, Lealie, Leela, Leelah,
Leial

Lean, Leann, Leanne (English) forms of
Leeann, Lian.

Leana, Leanna, Leeanna (English) forms of
Liana.
Leeana, Leiana, Leianah, Leianna, Leiannah,
Leyana, Leyanah, Leyanna, Leyannah

Leandra (Latin) like a lioness.
Leanda, Leandrah, Leandre, Leandrea,
Leandria, Leeanda, Leeandra, Leeandrah,
Leianda, Leiandah, Leiandra, Leiandrah,
Leighandra, Leighandrah, Leyandra,
Leyandrah

Leanore (Greek) a form of Eleanor.
(English) a form of Helen.
Lanore, Lanoree, Lanorey, Lanori, Lanoriah,
Lanorie, Lanory, Lanorya, Lanoryah, Leanor,
Leanora, Leanorah

Lece (Latin) a form of Lacey.
Lecee, Lecey, Leci, Lecie, Lecy

Lecia (Latin) a short form of Felecia.
Leacia, Leaciah, Leacya, Leacyah, Leasia,
Leasiah, Leasie, Leasy, Leasya, Leasyah,
Leasye, Lesha, Leshia, Lesia, Lesiah, Lesya,
Lesyah

Leda (Greek) lady. Mythology: the queen of
Sparta and the mother of Helen of Troy.
Leada, Leadah, Ledah, Leeda, Leedah, Leida,
Leidah, Leighda, Leighdah, Leyda, Lyda,
Lydah

Ledicia (Latin) great joy.

Lee BG (Chinese) plum. (Irish) poetic.
(English) meadow. A short form of Ashley,
Leah.
Ly

Leea (American) a form of Leah.
Leeah

Leeann, Leeanne (English) combinations of
Lee + Ann. Forms of Lian.
Leane, Leean, Leian, Leiane, Leiann, Leianne,
Leyan, Leyane, Leyann, Leyanne

Leeba (Yiddish) beloved.
Leaba, Leabah, Leebah, Leiba, Leibah,
Leighba, Leighbah, Leyba, Leybah, Liba,
Libah, Lyba, Lybah

Leena (Estonian) a form of Helen. (Greek,
Latin, Arabic) a form of Lina.
Leenah, Leina, Leinah

Leesa (Hebrew, English) a form of Leeza,
Lisa.

Leesha (American) a form of Lecia.
Leecia, Leeciah, Leecy, Leecya, Leecyah, Leesia,
Leesiah

Leewan (Australian) wind.
Leawan, Leawana, Leawanah, Leewana,
Leewanah, Leighwan, Leighwana,
Leighwanah, Leiwan, Leiwana, Leiwanah,
Leywan, Leywana, Leywanah, Liwan,
Liwana, Liwanah, Lywan, Lywana, Lywanah

Leeza (Hebrew) a short form of Aleeza.
(English) a form of Lisa, Liza.
Leaza, Leazah, Leezah, Leighza, Leighzah,
Leiza, Leizah, Leyza, Leyzah

Lefitray (Mapuche) speed of sound.

Leflay (Mapuche) lethargic woman.

Legarre (Spanish) reference to the Virgin Mary.

Lei BG (Hawaiian) a familiar form of Leilani.

Leia (Hebrew) a form of Leah. (Spanish, Tamil) a form of Leya.
Leiah

Leif BG (Scandinavian) beloved.
Leaf, Leaff, Leiff, Leyf, Leyff

Leigh GB (English) a form of Lee.

Leigha (English) a form of Leah.

Leighann, Leighanne (English) forms of Leeann.
Leigh Ann, Leigh Anne, Leigh-Ann, Leigh-Anne, Leighane

Leighanna (English) a form of Liana.
Leigh Anna, Leigh-Anna, Leighana, Leighanah

Leiko (Japanese) arrogant.
Leako, Leeko, Leyko

Leila (Hebrew) dark beauty; night. (Arabic) born at night. See also Laela, Layla, Lila.
Leela, Leelah, Leilia, Leland

Leilah (Hebrew, Arabic) a form of Leila.

Leilani (Hawaiian) heavenly flower; heavenly child.
Lailanee, Lailani, Lailanie, Lailany, Lailoni, Lealanea, Lealaneah, Lealanee, Lealaney, Lealani, Lealania, Lealaniah, Lealanie, Lealany, Leelanea, Leelaneah, Leelanee, Leelaney, Leelani, Leelania, Leelaniah, Leelanie, Leelany, Lei, Leighlanea, Leighlaneah, Leighlanee, Leighlaney, Leighlani, Leighlania, Leighlaniah, Leighlanie, Leighlany, Leilanea, Leilaneah, Leilanee, Leilaney, Leilania, Leilaniah, Leilanie, Leilany, Leiloni, Leilony, Lelanea, Lelaneah, Lelanee, Lelaney, Lelani, Lelania, Lelanie, Lelany, Leylanea, Leylaneah, Leylanee, Leylaney, Leylani, Leylania, Leylaniah, Leylanie, Leylany

Leira (Basque) reference to the Virgin Mary.

Leisa (Hebrew, English) a form of Lisa.
Leisah

Leisha (American) a form of Leticia.

Lekasha (American) a form of Lakeisha.
Lekeesha, Lekesha, Lekeshia, Lekeshiah, Lekeshya, Lekesia, Lekesiah, Lekesya, Lekicia, Lekiciah, Lekisha, Lekishah, Lekysha, Lekyshia, Lekysya

Lekeisha (American) a form of Lakeisha.

Lela (French) a form of Leala. (Hebrew, Arabic) a form of Leila.
Lelah

Leli (Swiss) a form of Magdalen.
Lelee, Lelie, Lely

Lelia (Greek) fair speech. (Hebrew, Arabic) a form of Leila.
Leliah, Lelika, Lelita, Lellia, Lelliah

Lelica (Latin) talkative.

Lelya (Russian) a form of Helen.
Lellya, Lellyah, Lelyah

Lemana (Australian) oak tree.
Leaman, Leamana, Leamanah, Leemana, Leemanah, Leimana, Leimanah, Lemanah, Leymana, Leymanah

Lemuela (Hebrew) devoted to God.

Lena (Hebrew) dwelling or lodging. (Latin) temptress. (Norwegian) illustrious. (Greek) a short form of Eleanor. Music: Lena Horne, a well-known African American singer and actress.
Lenah, Lenee, Lenka, Lenna, Lennah

Lenci (Hungarian) a form of Helen.
Lencea, Lencee, Lencey, Lencia, Lencie, Lency

Lene (German) a form of Helen.
Leni, Line

Leneisha (American) a combination of the prefix Le + Keneisha.
Lenease, Lenece, Leneece, Leneese, Lenesha, Leniesha, Lenieshia, Leniesia, Leniessia, Lenisa, Lenisah, Lenise, Lenisha, Leniss, Lenissa, Lenissah, Lenisse, Lennise, Lennisha, Lenysa, Lenysah, Lenyse, Lenysha, Lenyss, Lenyssa, Lenyssah, Lenysse, Lynesha

Lenia (German) a form of Leona.
Lenayah, Lenda, Lenea, Leneen, Leney, Lenie, Lenna, Lennah, Lennea, Lennee, Lenney, Lenni, Lennie, Lenny, Leny, Lenya, Lenyah

Lenis (Latin) soft; silky.

Lenita (Latin) gentle.
Leneta, Lenett, Lenetta, Lenette, Lenitah,
Lenite, Lennett, Lennetta, Lennette

Lenora (Greek, Russian) a form of Eleanor.
Lenorah

Lenore (Greek, Russian) a form of Eleanor.
Lenor, Lenoree

Leocadia, Leocadía (Greek) shining; white.

Leocricia (Greek) she who judges her village well.

Leola (Latin) lioness.
Leolah

Leolina (Welsh) a form of Leola.
Leolinah, Leoline, Leolyn, Leolyna, Leolynah,
Leolyne

Leoma (English) brilliant.

Leona (German) brave as a lioness. See also Lona.
Leoine, Leonae, Leonah, Leone, Leonel,
Leonela, Leonelah, Leonella, Leonelle, Leonia,
Leonice, Leonicia, Leonissa, Liona

Leonarda (German) brave as a lioness.
Leonardina, Leonardine, Leonardyn,
Leonardyna, Leonardyne

Leoncia (Latin) a form of Leonarda.

Leondra (German) a form of Leonarda.
Leondrea, Leondria

Leónida (Greek) a form of Leonarda.

Leonie (German) a familiar form of Leona.
Leonee, Leoney, Leoni, Léonie, Leonni,
Leonnie, Leony

Leonila (Latin) a form of Leonarda.

Leonilda (German) fighter.

Leonna (German) a form of Leona.
Leonne

Leonor, Leonore (Greek) forms of Eleanor.
See also Nora.
Leonora, Leonorah, Léonore

Leontine (Latin) like a lioness.
Leonina, Leonine, Leontina, Leontyn,
Leontyna, Leontyne, Léontyne, Liontin,
Liontina, Liontine, Liontyna, Liontyne,
Lyontina, Lyontine, Lyontyna, Lyontyne

Leopolda (German) princess of the village.

Leora (Hebrew) light. (Greek) a familiar
form of Eleanor. See also Liora.
Leeora, Leorah, Leorit

Leotie (Native American) prairie flower.
Leotee, Leoti, Leoty

Lepati (Tongan) leopard.
Leapati, Leapatie, Leapaty, Leipati, Leipatie,
Leipaty, Lepatie, Lepaty, Leypati, Leypatie,
Leypaty

Lera (Russian) a short form of Valera.
Lerah, Leria, Leriah, Lerra, Lerrah

Lesbia (Greek) native of the Greek island of
Lesbos.

Leslee, Lesleigh, Lesli, Lesly, Leslye
(Scottish) forms of Lesley.
Lesslie, Lessly

Lesley (Scottish) gray fortress.
Leslea, Lesleah, Leslei, Lezlea, Lezleah,
Lezlee, Lezlei, Lezleigh, Lezley, Lezli, Lezlie,
Lezly

Leslie ☆ GB (Scottish) a form of Lesley.

Leta (Latin) glad. (Swahili) bringer. (Greek) a
short form of Aleta.
Leata, Leatah, Leighta, Leightah, Leita,
Leitah, Leyta, Leytah

Letha (Greek) forgetful; oblivion.
Leitha, Leithia, Lethia, Leythia, Leythiah,
Leythya, Leythyah

Leticia (Latin) joy. See also Laeticia, Latisha,
Tisha.
Lateacia, Lateaciah, Lateacya, Lateacyah,
Latycia, Latyciah, Latycya, Latycyah, Let,
Letesa, Letice, Letichia, Leticya, Letisia,
Letisiah, Letissa, Letiza, Letizah, Letizia,
Letiziah, Letizya, Letizyah, Letty, Letycia,
Letyciah, Letycya, Letycyah, Letysya, Letyza,
Letyzia, Letyziah, Letyzya, Letyzyah

Letifa (Arabic) a form of Lateefah.
Leitifa, Leitifah, Leitipha, Leitiphah, Letifah,
Letipha, Letiphah, Letyfa, Letyfah, Letypha,
Letyphah

Letisha (Latin) a form of Leticia.
Leshia, Letesha, Leteshia, Letish, Letishah,
Letishia, Letishya, Letysha, Letyshya

Letitia (Latin) a form of Leticia.
Letita, Letitah, Letiticia, Loutitia, Loutitiah, Loutitya, Loutytia, Loutytiah, Loutytya, Loutytyah

Letty (English) a familiar form of Leticia.
Letee, Letey, Leti, Letie, Letta, Lettah, Lettee, Lettey, Letti, Lettie, Lety

Levana (Hebrew) moon; white. (Latin) risen. Mythology: the goddess of newborn babies.
Lévana, Levanah, Levanna, Levannah, Levenia, Lewana, Livana

Levani (Fijian) anointed with oil.
Levanee, Levaney, Levanie, Levany

Levania (Latin) rising sun.
Leavania, Leevania, Leivania, Levannia, Levanya, Leyvania

Levia (Hebrew) joined, attached.
Leevya, Levi, Leviah, Levie, Levya, Levyah

Levina (Latin) flash of lightning.
Levene, Levinah, Livina, Livinna, Lyvina, Lyvinah, Lyvyna, Lyvynah

Levita, Levyna (English) twinkle, sparkle.

Levona (Hebrew) spice; incense.
Leavona, Leavonah, Leavonia, Leavoniah, Leavonna, Leavonnah, Leavonnia, Leavonniah, Leevona, Leevonah, Leevonia, Leevoniah, Leevonna, Leevonnia, Leevonniah, Leighvona, Leighvonah, Leighvonna, Leighvonnah, Leighvonne, Leivona, Leivonia, Leivoniah, Leivonna, Leivonnah, Leivonnia, Leivonnya, Levon, Levonah, Levonat, Levone, Levonee, Levoni, Levonia, Levoniah, Levonna, Levonnah, Levonne, Levony, Levonya, Levonyah, Leyvona, Leyvonah, Leyvone, Leyvonn, Leyvonna, Leyvonnah, Leyvonne, Livona

Lewana (Hebrew) a form of Levana.
Leawana, Leawanah, Leawanna, Leawannah, Lebhanah, Leewana, Leewanah, Leewanna, Leewannah, Leiwana, Leiwanah, Leiwanna, Leiwannah, Lewanah, Lewanna, Lewannah

Lexandra (Greek) a short form of Alexandra.
Lexa, Lexah, Lexandrah, Lexandria, Lexandriah, Lexandrya, Lexandryah, Lezandra, Lezandrah, Lezandria, Lezandriah, Lixandra, Lixandrah, Lyxandra, Lyxandrah

Lexi, Lexie, Lexy (Greek) familiar forms of Alexandra.
Leksi, Lexey

Lexia (Greek) a familiar form of Alexandra.
Leska, Lesya, Lexane, Lexiah, Lexina, Lexine

Lexis, Lexxus (Greek) short forms of Alexius, Alexis.
Laexis, Lexius, Lexsis, Lexuss, Lexxis, Lexyss

Lexus GB (Greek) a short form of Alexius, Alexis.

Leya (Spanish) loyal. (Tamil) the constellation Leo.

Leyla (Hebrew, Arabic) a form of Leila. (Spanish, Tamil) a form of Leya.
Leylah

Leyna (Estonian, Greek, Latin, Arabic) a form of Leena.
Leynah

Lia (Greek) bringer of good news. (Hebrew, Dutch, Italian) dependent. See also Leah.
Liah, Lya, Lyah

Lía (Hebrew) a form of Leah.

Liama (English) determined guardian.
Liamah, Lyama, Lyamah

Lian GB (Chinese) graceful willow. (Latin) a short form of Gillian, Lillian.
Lean, Liann, Lyan, Lyann

Liana, Lianna (Latin) youth. (French) bound, wrapped up; tree covered with vines. (English) meadow. (Hebrew) short forms of Eliana.
Lianah, Liannah, Lyana, Lyanah, Lyanna, Lyannah

Liane, Lianne (Hebrew) short forms of Eliane. (English) forms of Lian.
Lyane, Lyanne

Libby (Hebrew) a familiar form of Elizabeth.
Ibby, Lib, Libbea, Libbee, Libbey, Libbi, Libbie, Libea, Libee, Libey, Libi, Libie, Liby, Lyb, Lybbea, Lybbee, Lybbey, Lybbi, Lybbie, Lybby, Lybea, Lybee, Lybey, Lybi, Lybie, Lyby

Libera, Líbera (Latin) she who bestows abundance.

Liberada, Liberata, Liberdade (Latin)
forms of Liberty.

Liberia, Liberta (Spanish) forms of Liberty.

Libertad (Latin) she who acts in good faith.

Liberty (Latin) free.
*Libertee, Liberti, Libertie, Libirtee, Libirtey,
Libirti, Libirtie, Libirty, Librada, Liburtee,
Liburtey, Liburti, Liburtie, Liburty, Libyrtee,
Libyrtey, Libyrti, Libyrtie, Libyrty, Lybertee,
Lybertey, Lyberti, Lybertia, Lyberty, Lybertya,
Lybirtee, Lybirtey, Lybirti, Lybirtie, Lybirty,
Lyburtee, Lyburtey, Lyburti, Lyburtie, Lyburty,
Lybyrtee, Lybyrtey, Lybyrti, Lybyrtie, Lybyrty*

Libia (Latin) comes from the desert.

Libitina (Latin) she who is wanted.

Libna (Latin) whiteness.

Liboria (Latin) free.

Lican (Mapuche) flint.

Licia (Greek) a short form of Alicia.
*Licha, Liciah, Licya, Licyah, Lishia, Lisia,
Lycha, Lycia, Lycya, Lycyah*

Lida (Greek) happy. (Slavic) loved by people.
(Latin) a short form of Alida, Elita.
Leeda, Lidah, Lidochka, Lyda, Lydah

Lide (Latin, Basque) life.
Lidee, Lyde, Lydee

Lidia (Greek) a form of Lydia.
*Lidea, Lidi, Lidiah, Lidija, Lidiya, Lidka,
Lidya*

Lidía, Lídia, Lydía (Greek) forms of Lydia.

Liduvina (German) friend of the village.

Lien (Chinese) lotus.
*Liena, Lienn, Lienna, Lienne, Lyen, Lyena,
Lyenn, Lyenna, Lyenne*

Liesabet (German) a short form of
Elizabeth.
Liesbeth, Lyesabet, Lyesabeth

Liese (German) a familiar form of Elise,
Elizabeth.
Liesa, Liesah, Lieschen, Lise

Liesel (German) a familiar form of
Elizabeth.
Leasel, Leasela, Leaselah, Leasele, Leasle,

*Leesel, Leesela, Leeselah, Leesele, Leesl, Leesle,
Leezel, Leezl, Leisel, Leisela, Leiselah, Leisele,
Leisle, Leysel, Liesl, Liezel, Liezl, Lisel,
Lisela, Liselah, Lisele, Lysel, Lysela, Lyselah,
Lysele*

Liesha (Arabic) a form of Aisha.
*Liasha, Liashah, Lieshah, Lyaisha, Lyaishah,
Lyasha, Lyashah, Lyeisha, Lyeishah, Lyesha,
Lyeshah*

Ligia (Greek) clear voiced; whistling.

Lígia (Portuguese) a form of Ligia.

Lila (Arabic) night. (Hindi) free will of God.
(Persian) lilac. A short form of Dalila,
Delilah, Lillian.
Lilla, Lillah

Lilac (Sanskrit) lilac; blue purple.
Lilack, Lilak, Lylac, Lylack, Lylak

Lilah (Arabic, Hindi, Persian) a form of Lila.

Lili, Lillie (Latin, Arabic) forms of Lilly.
Lilie, Lilli

Lilí (English) a form of Alicia.

Lilia (Persian) a form of Lila.
*Lilea, Liliah, Lillea, Lilleah, Lilya, Lilyah,
Lylea, Lyleah, Lylia, Lyliah, Lyllea, Lylleah,
Lylya, Lylyah*

Lilian, Liliane (Latin) forms of Lillian.
*Liliann, Lilianne, Lilion, Lilyan, Lylian,
Lyliane, Lyliann, Lylianne, Lylion, Lylyon*

Lilián (Spanish) a form of Lillian.

Lílian (Portuguese) a form of Lillian.

Liliana, Lilliana, Lillianna (Latin) forms of
Lillian.
*Lileana, Lilianah, Lilianna, Lilliana,
Lillianah, Lilliannah, Lyliana, Lylianah,
Lylianna, Lyliannah*

Lilibeth (English) a combination of Lilly +
Beth.
*Lillibeth, Lillybeth, Lilybeth, Lylibeth,
Lyllibeth, Lyllybeth, Lylybeth*

Lilis (Hebrew) a form of Lilith.
*Lilisa, Lilise, Liliss, Lilissa, Lilisse, Lillis, Lylis,
Lylisa, Lylise, Lyliss, Lylissa, Lylisse, Lylys,
Lylysa, Lylyse, Lylyss, Lylyssa, Lylysse*

Lilit (Hebrew) patriot.

Lilith (Arabic) of the night; night demon. Mythology: the first wife of Adam, according to ancient Jewish legends.
Lillith, Lilyth, Lyllyth, Lylyth

Lillian ☀ (Latin) lily flower.
Lil, Lilas, Lileane, Lilias, Liliha, Lilja, Lilla, Lilli, Lillia, Lilliane, Lilliann, Lillianne, Liuka

Lilly (Latin, Arabic) a familiar form of Lilith, Lillian, Lillyann.
Líle, Lilea, Lilee, Lilei, Lileigh, Liley, Lilijana, Lilika, Lilike, Liliosa, Lilium, Lilka, Lille, Lillee, Lillei, Lilleigh, Lilley, Lylee, Lylei, Lyleigh, Lyley, Lyli, Lylie, Lyllee, Lyllei, Lylleigh, Lylly, Lyly

Lillyann (English) a combination of Lilly + Ann. (Latin) a form of Lillian.
Lillyan, Lillyanna, Lillyanne, Lilyan, Lilyana, Lilyann, Lilyanna, Lilyanne

Lillybelle, Lilybelle (English) combinations of Lilly + Belle.
Lilibel, Lilibela, Lilibelah, Lilibele, Lilibell, Lilibella, Lilibellah, Lillibel, Lillibela, Lillibelah, Lillibele, Lillibell, Lillibella, Lillibellah, Lillibelle, Lilybel, Lilybela, Lilybelah, Lilybele, Lilybell, Lilybella, Lilybellah, Lilybelle, Lylibel, Lylibela, Lylibelah, Lylibele, Lylibell, Lylibella, Lylibellah, Lylibelle, Lyllibel, Lyllibela, Lyllibelah, Lyllibele, Lyllibell, Lyllibella, Lyllibellah, Lyllibelle, Lyllybel, Lyllybela, Lyllybelah, Lyllybele, Lyllybell, Lyllybella, Lyllybellah, Lyllybelle, Lylybel, Lylybela, Lylybelah, Lylybele, Lylybell, Lylybella, Lylybellah, Lylybelle

Lillybet, Lilybet (English) combinations of Lilly + Elizabeth.
Lilibet, Lilibeta, Lilibetah, Lilibete, Lillibet, Lillibeta, Lillibete, Lillybeta, Lillybete, Lillybett, Lillybetta, Lillybette, Lilybet, Lilybeta, Lilybete, Lilybett, Lilybetta, Lilybette, Lylibet, Lylibeta, Lylibetah, Lylibete, Lyllibet, Lyllibeta, Lyllibete, Lyllibett, Lyllibetta, Lyllibette, Lyllybet, Lyllybeta, Lyllybete, Lyllybett, Lyllybetta, Lyllybette, Lylybet, Lylybeta, Lylybete, Lylybett, Lylybetta, Lylybette

Lilvina (Latin, German) friend of the iris.

Lily ☀ (Latin, Arabic) a form of Lilly.

Limber (Tiv) joyful.
Limba, Limbah, Limbera, Lymba, Lymbah, Lymber, Lymbera

Lin 🇬🇧 (Chinese) beautiful jade. (English) a form of Lynn.
Linley, Linn, Linne

Lina (Greek) light. (Arabic) tender. (Latin) a form of Lena.
Linah, Linna, Linnah

Linda (Spanish) pretty. See also Lynda.
Lind, Lindah, Linita

Linden 🇧🇬 (English) linden-tree hill.
Lindan, Lindin, Lindon, Lyndan, Lynden, Lyndin, Lyndon, Lyndyn

Lindsay 🇬🇧 (English) a form of Lindsey.
Lindze, Lindzee, Lindzey, Lindzy

Lindsee, Lindsi, Lindsie, Lindsy (English) forms of Lindsey.

Lindsey 🇬🇧 (English) linden-tree island; camp near the stream.
Lind, Lindsea, Lindsei, Lindsi

Lindy (Spanish) a familiar form of Linda.
Linde, Lindea, Lindee, Lindey, Lindi, Lindie

Linette (Welsh) idol. (French) bird.
Linet, Lineta, Linetah, Linete, Linett, Linetta, Linettah, Linnet, Linneta, Linnetah, Linnete, Linnett, Linnetta, Linnettah, Linnette

Ling (Chinese) delicate, dainty.

Linh (Chinese, English) a form of Lin.

Linley 🇬🇧 (English) flax meadow.
Linlea, Linleah, Linlee, Linlei, Linleigh, Linli, Linlia, Linliah, Linlie, Linly, Lynlea, Lynleah, Lynlee, Lynlei, Lynleigh, Lynley, Lynli, Lynlia, Lynliah, Lynlie, Lynly

Linnea (Scandinavian) lime tree. Botany: the national flower of Sweden.
Linae, Linea, Lineah, Linnae, Linnaea, Linneah

Linsey, Linzee, Linzy (English) forms of Lindsey.
Linsay, Linsea, Linsee, Linsi, Linsie, Linsy, Linzey, Linzi, Linzie, Linzzi

Lioba (German) beloved, valued.

Liolya (Russian) a form of Helen.
Liolia, Lioliah, Liolyah, Lyolya, Lyolyah

Liona (German) a form of Leona.
Lionah, Lione, Lionee, Lioney, Lioni, Lionia, Lioniah, Lionie, Liony, Lyona, Lyonah, Lyone, Lyonee, Lyoney, Lyoni, Lyonia, Lyoniah, Lyonie, Lyony, Lyonya, Lyonyah

Lionetta (Latin) small lioness.
Lionet, Lioneta, Lionetah, Lionete, Lionett, Lionettah, Lionette, Lyonet, Lyoneta, Lyonetah, Lyonete, Lyonett, Lyonetta, Lyonettah, Lyonette

Liora (Hebrew) light. See also Leora.
Liorah, Lyora, Lyorah

Lirit (Hebrew) poetic; lyrical, musical.
Lirita, Lirite, Lyrit, Lyrita, Lyrite

Liron BG (Hebrew) my song.
Leron, Lerone, Lirona, Lironah, Lirone, Lyron, Lyrona, Lyronah, Lyrone

Lis (French) lily.
Lys

Lisa (Hebrew) consecrated to God. (English) a short form of Elizabeth.
Leasa, Leasah, Leassa, Leassah, Liisa, Lisah, Lisenka, Liszka, Litsa

Lisa Marie (American) a combination of Lisa + Marie.
Lisa-Marie

Lisandra (Greek) a form of Lysandra.
Lisandrah, Lisandria, Lisandriah, Lissandra, Lissandrah, Lissandria, Lissandriah

Lisann, Lisanne (American) combinations of Lisa + Ann.
Lisanna, Lisannah, Lizanne

Lisavet (Hebrew) a form of Elizabeth.

Lisbet (English) a short form of Elizabeth.
Lisbeta, Lisbete, Lisbett, Lisbetta, Lisbette, Lysbet, Lysbeta, Lysbete, Lysbett, Lysbetta, Lysbette

Lisbeth (English) a short form of Elizabeth.
Lysbeth

Lise GB (German) a form of Lisa.

Liset, Lisette, Lisset, Lissette (French) forms of Lisa. (English) familiar forms of Elise, Elizabeth.
Liseta, Lisete, Lisett, Lisetta, Lisettina, Lissete, Lissett

Liseth (French, English) a form of Liset.

Lisha (Arabic) darkness before midnight. (Hebrew) a short form of Alisha, Elisha, Ilisha.
Lishah, Lishe, Lysha, Lyshah, Lyshe

Lissa (Greek) honey bee. A short form of Elissa, Elizabeth, Melissa, Millicent.
Lissah

Lissie (American) a familiar form of Alison, Elise, Elizabeth.
Lissee, Lissey, Lissi, Lissy, Lissye

Lita (Latin) a familiar form of names ending in "lita."
Leata, Leatah, Leet, Leeta, Leetah, Litah, Litia, Litiah, Litta, Lyta, Lytah, Lytia, Lytya

Litonya (Moquelumnan) darting hummingbird.
Litania, Litaniah, Litanya, Litanyah, Litonia, Litoniah, Lytania, Lytaniah, Lytanya, Lytanyah, Lytonia, Lytoniah, Lytonya, Lytonyah

Liuba (Russian) a form of Caridad.

Liv (Latin) a short form of Livia, Olivia.
Lyv

Livana (Hebrew) a form of Levana.
Livanah, Livane, Livanna, Livannah, Livanne, Livna, Livnat, Lyvan, Lyvana, Lyvanah, Lyvane, Lyvanna, Lyvannah, Lyvanne

Livia (Hebrew) crown. A familiar form of Olivia. (Latin) olive.
Levia, Livi, Liviah, Livie, Livy, Livye, Lyvi, Lyvia, Lyviah, Lyvie, Lyvy

Liviya (Hebrew) brave lioness; royal crown.
Leviya, Levya, Liviyah, Livya, Lyvya, Lyvyah

Livona (Hebrew) a form of Levona.
Livonah, Livone, Livonna, Livonnah, Livonne, Lyvona, Lyvonah, Lyvone, Lyvonna, Lyvonnah, Lyvonne

Liyah (Hebrew) a form of Leah.
Liya

Liz (English) a short form of Elizabeth.
Lizz, Lyz, Lyzz

Liza (American) a short form of Elizabeth.
Lizah, Lizela, Lizka, Lizza, Lizzah, Lyza, Lyzah, Lyzza, Lyzzah

Lizabeta (Russian) a form of Elizabeth.
Lisabeta, Lisabetah, Lisabetta, Lisabettah, Lizabetah, Lizabetta, Lizaveta, Lizonka, Lysabetta, Lysabettah, Lyzabeta, Lyzabetah, Lyzabetta, Lyzabettah

Lizabeth (English) a short form of Elizabeth. See also Lyzabeth.
Lisabet, Lisabete, Lisabeth, Lisabett, Lisabette, Lizabet, Lizabete, Lizabett, Lizabette

Lizbet (English) a short form of Elizabeth.
Lizbeta, Lizbete, Lizbett, Lizbetta, Lizbette, Lyzbet, Lyzbeta, Lyzbete

Lizbeth (English) a short form of Elizabeth.
Lyzbeth

Lizet, Lizett, Lizette, Lizzet, Lizzette
(French) forms of Liset.
Lizete

Lizeth (French) a form of Liset.
Lizzeth

Lizina (Latvian) a familiar form of Elizabeth.
Lixena, Lixenah, Lixina, Lixinah, Lixyna, Lixynah, Lizinah, Lizine, Lizyna, Lizynah, Lizyne, Lyxina, Lyxinah, Lyxine, Lyxyna, Lyxynah, Lyxyne, Lyzina, Lyzinah, Lyzine, Lyzyna, Lyzynah, Lyzyne

Lizzie, Lizzy (American) familiar forms of Elizabeth.
Lizy

Llanquipan (Mapuche) fallen branch; solitary lioness.

Llanquiray (Mapuche) fallen flower.

Lledó (Catalan) hackberry tree.

Llesenia (Spanish) Television: the female lead in a 1970s soap opera.

Llian (Welsh) linen.
Lliana, Llianah, Lliane, Lliann, Llianna, Lliannah, Llianne, Llyan, Llyana, Llyanah, Llyane, Llyann, Llyanna, Llyannah, Llyanne

Lluvia (Spanish) rain.

Locaia (Greek) white roses.

Lodema, Lodima, Lodyma (English) guide.

Logan ⓑⓖ (Irish) meadow.
Logann, Loganne, Logen, Loghan, Logun, Logyn, Logynn

Loida, Loída (Greek) example of faith and piousness.

Loila (Australian) sky.
Loilah, Loyla, Loylah

Lois (German) famous warrior.
Loease, Loise, Loiss, Loissa, Loisse, Loyce, Loys, Loyss, Loyssa, Loysse

Lokalia (Hawaiian) garland of roses.
Lokaliah, Lokalya, Lokalyah

Lola (Spanish) a familiar form of Carlotta, Dolores, Louise.
Lolah

Lolita (Spanish) sorrowful. A familiar form of Lola.
Loleata, Loleatah, Loleate, Loleeta, Loleetah, Loleete, Loleighta, Loleita, Loleitah, Loleta, Loletah, Lolit, Lolitah, Lolyta, Lolytah, Lolyte, Lulita

Lolly (English) sweet; candy. A familiar form of Laura.
Lolea, Loleah, Lolee, Lolei, Loleigh, Loli, Lolia, Loliah, Lolie, Lollea, Lolleah, Lollee, Lollei, Lolleigh, Lolley, Lolli, Lollie, Loly

Lolotea (Zuni) a form of Dorothy.
Lolotee, Loloti, Lolotia, Lolotie, Loloty

Lomasi (Native American) pretty flower.
Lomasee, Lomasey, Lomasie, Lomasy

Lona (Latin) lioness. (English) solitary. (German) a short form of Leona.

London ⓑⓖ (English) fortress of the moon. Geography: the capital of the United Kingdom.
Londen, Londun, Londyn

Loni (American) a form of Lona.
Lonea, Loneah, Lonee, Loney, Lonia, Loniah, Lonie, Lonnea, Lonnee, Lonney, Lonni, Lonnia, Lonniah, Lonnie, Lonny, Lonnya, Lony, Lonya, Lonyah

Lonlee (English) a form of Lona.
Lonlea, Lonleah, Lonlei, Lonleigh, Lonley, Lonli, Lonlia, Lonliah, Lonlie, Lonly

Lonna (Latin, German, English) a form of Lona.

Lora (Latin) crowned with laurel. (American) a form of Laura.
Lorae, Lorah, Lorra, Lorrah

Loraine (Latin) a form of Lorraine.
Loraen, Loraena, Loraenah, Loraene, Lorain, Loraina, Lorainah, Lorane, Lorann, Lorayn, Lorayna, Loraynah, Lorayne, Lorein, Loreina, Loreinah, Loreine, Loreyn, Loreyna, Loreynah, Loreyne

Lorda (Spanish) a form of Lourdes.

Lore (Basque) flower. (Latin) a short form of Flora.
Lor, Lorre

Lorea (Basque) grove; light.

Loreal (German) a form of Lorelei.

Lorelei (German) alluring. Mythology: the siren of the Rhine River who lured sailors to their deaths. See also Lurleen.
Loralea, Loraleah, Loralee, Loralei, Loraleigh, Loraley, Lorali, Loralie, Loralyn, Lorelea, Loreleah, Lorelee, Loreleigh, Loreli, Lorilea, Lorileah, Lorilee, Lorilei, Lorileigh, Loriley, Lorili, Lorilia, Loriliah, Lorilie, Lorily, Lorilyn, Lorylea, Loryleah, Lorylee, Lorylei, Loryleigh, Loryley, Loryli, Lorylie, Loryly

Loreley (German) a form of Lorelei.

Lorelle (American) a form of Laurel.
Loral, Lorala, Lorel, Lorela, Lorelah, Lorele, Lorell, Lorella, Lorellah, Loriel, Loriela, Lorielah, Loriele, Loriell, Loriella, Loriellah, Lorielle, Lorrel, Lorrela, Lorrelah, Lorrele, Lorrell, Lorrella, Lorrelle, Loryal, Loryala, Loryalah, Loryale, Loryall, Loryalla, Loryallah, Loryalle, Loryel, Loryela, Loryelah, Loryele, Loryell, Loryella, Loryellah, Loryelle

Loren GB (American) a form of Lauren.
Loran, Lorren, Lorrene, Lorrin, Lorrine, Lorryn, Lorryne, Loryne, Lorynn, Lorynne

Lorena (English) a form of Lauren.
Lorana, Loranah, Lorenah, Lorenea, Lorenia, Lorenna, Lorina, Lorinah, Lorrena, Lorrenah, Lorrina, Lorrinah, Lorryna, Lorrynah, Loryna, Lorynah, Lorynna, Lorynnah

Lorene (American) a form of Lauren.
Loreen, Lorine

Lorenza BG (Latin) a form of Laura.
Laurencia, Laurensa, Laurensah, Laurentia, Laurentina, Laurenza, Laurenzah, Lawrensa, Lawrensah, Lawrenza, Lawrenzah, Lorensa, Lorensah, Lorenzah, Lorinsa, Lorinsah, Lorinza, Lorinzah, Lorynsa, Lorynsah, Lorynza, Lorynzah

Loreto (Spanish) forest.

Loretta (English) a familiar form of Laura.
Larretta, Lawret, Lawreta, Lawretah, Lawrete, Lawrett, Lawretta, Lawrettah, Lawrette, Loret, Loreta, Loretah, Lorete, Lorett, Lorettah, Lorette, Lorit, Lorita, Loritah, Lorite, Loritta, Lorittah, Loritte, Lorreta, Lorretah, Lorrete, Lorretta, Lorrette, Lorrit, Lorrita, Lorritah, Lorritta, Lorritte, Loryt, Loryta, Lorytah, Loryte, Lorytt, Lorytta, Loryttah, Lorytte

Lori (Latin) crowned with laurel. (French) a short form of Lorraine. (American) a familiar form of Laura.
Loree, Lorey, Loria, Loriah, Lorree, Lorrey, Lorri, Lorria, Lorriah, Lorrya, Lorrye, Lorya, Loryah

Loriann, Lorianne (American) combinations of Lori + Ann.
Loreean, Loreeana, Loreeanah, Loreeane, Loreeann, Loreeanna, Loreeannah, Loreeanne, Lorian, Loriana, Lorianah, Loriane, Lorianna, Loriannah, Lorrian, Lorriana, Lorrianah, Lorriane, Lorriann, Lorrianna, Lorriannah, Lorrianne, Lorryan, Lorryana, Lorryanah, Lorryane, Lorryann, Lorryanna, Lorryannah, Lorryanne, Loryan, Loryana, Loryanah, Loryane, Loryann, Loryanna, Loryannah, Loryanne

Loric (Latin) armor.
Lorick, Lorik, Loriq, Loriqua, Lorique, Loryc, Loryck, Loryk, Loryque

Lorie, Lorrie, Lory (Latin, French, American) forms of Lori.
Lorry

Lorielle (American) a combination of Lori + Elle.
Loreel, Loriel, Loriela, Lorielah, Loriele, Loriell, Loriella, Loryel, Loryela, Loryelah, Loryele, Loryell, Loryella, Loryellah, Loryelle

Lorikeet (Australian) beautiful, colorful bird.
Lorikeat, Lorikeata, Lorikeatah, Lorikeate, Lorikeeta, Lorikeetah, Lorikeete, Loriket, Loriketa, Loriketah, Lorikete, Lorikett, Loriketta, Lorikette, Lorykeet

Lorin 🇬🇧 (American) a form of Lauren.

Lorinda (Spanish) a form of Laura.
Lorind, Lorindah, Lorinde, Lorynd, Lorynda, Loryndah, Lorynde

Loris 🇬🇧 (Latin) thong. (Dutch) clown. (Greek) a short form of Chloris.
Laurice, Laurys, Loreace, Lorease, Loreece, Loreese, Lorice, Lorise, Loriss, Lorisse, Loryce, Lorys, Loryse, Loryss, Lorysse

Lorissa (Greek, Latin, Dutch) a form of Loris. A form of Larissa.
Lorisa, Lorisah, Lorissah, Lorysa, Lorysah, Loryssa, Loryssah

Lorna (Latin) crowned with laurel. Literature: probably coined by Richard Blackmore in his novel *Lorna Doone.*
Lornah, Lorne, Lornee, Lorney, Lorrna

Lorraine (Latin) sorrowful. (French) from Lorraine, a former province of France. See also Rayna.
Loraine, Lorine, Lorraen, Lorraena, Lorraenah, Lorraene, Lorrain, Lorraina, Lorrainah, Lorrane, Lorrayn, Lorrayna, Lorraynah, Lorrayne, Lorrein, Lorreina, Lorreinah, Lorreine, Lorreyn, Lorreyna, Lorreynah, Lorreyne

Loryn (American) a form of Lauren.

Lotte (German) a short form of Charlotte.
Lota, Lotah, Lotta, Lottah, Lottchen

Lottie (German) a familiar form of Charlotte.
Lote, Lotea, Lotee, Lotey, Loti, Lotie, Lottea, Lottee, Lottey, Lotti, Lotty, Loty

Lotus (Greek) lotus.
Lottus

Lou 🇧🇬 (American) a short form of Louise, Luella.
Lu

Louam (Ethiopian) sleep well.
Louama

Louisa (English) a familiar form of Louise. Literature: Louisa May Alcott was an American writer and reformer best known for her novel *Little Women.*
Aloisa, Eloisa, Heloisa, Lawisa, Lawisah, Loeasa, Loeasah, Loeaza, Loeazah, Loisa, Loisah, Looesa, Looesah, Louisah, Louisetta, Louisian, Louisina, Louiza, Louizah, Louyza, Louyzah, Lovisa

Louise (German) famous warrior. See also Alison, Eloise, Heloise, Lois, Lola, Ludovica, Luella, Lulu.
Lawis, Lawise, Leweese, Leweez, Loeaze, Loise, Looise, Louisane, Louisette, Louisiane, Louisine, Louiz, Louize, Louyz, Louyze, Lowise, Loyce, Loyise, Luis, Luise, Luiz, Luize, Luys, Luyse, Luyz, Luyze

Lourdes 🇬🇧 (French) from Lourdes, France. Religion: a place where the Virgin Mary was said to have appeared.

Louvaine (English) Louise's vanity.
Louvain, Louvaina, Louvayn, Louvayna, Louvaynah, Louvayne, Lovanne, Luvain, Luvaina, Luvainah, Luvaine, Luvayn, Luvayna, Luvaynah, Luvayne

Love (English) love, kindness, charity.
Lovee, Lovewell, Lovey, Lovi, Lovia, Loviah, Lovie, Lovy, Lovya, Lovyah, Luv, Luvi, Luvia, Luviah, Luvvy, Luvya, Luvyah

Lovely (English) lovely.

Lovinia (Latin) a form of Lavina.
Louvinia, Louviniah, Lovena, Lovenah, Lovenia, Loveniah, Lovina, Lovinah, Loviniah, Lovinya, Lovinyah, Lovynia, Lovyniah, Lovynya, Lovynyah

Lovisa (German) a form of Louisa.
Lovesah, Lovese, Lovessa, Lovessah, Lovesse, Lovisah, Lovissa, Lovissah, Lovisse, Lovys, Lovysa, Lovysah, Lovyse, Lovyss, Lovyssa, Lovyssah, Lovysse

Lowri (Welsh) a form of Laura.

Lúa (Latin) moon.

Luann (Hebrew, German) graceful woman warrior. (Hawaiian) happy; relaxed. (American) a combination of Louise + Ann.
Louann, Louanne, Lu, Lua, Luan, Luane, Luanne, Luanni, Luannie, Luanny

Luanna (German) a form of Luann.
Lewana, Lewanna, Louana, Louanah, Louanna, Louannah, Luana, Luwana, Luwanna

Lubiana (Slavic) a form of Luvena.

Lubov (Russian) love.
Luba, Lubna, Lubochka, Lyuba, Lyubov

Luca BG (Italian) a form of Lucy.
Lucah, Lucka, Luckah, Luka, Lukah

Lucelia (Spanish) a combination of Luz + Celia.

Lucena (Spanish) a form of Lucy.

Lucerne (Latin) lamp; circle of light. Geography: the Lake of Lucerne is in Switzerland.
Lucerina, Lucerinah, Lucerine, Lucerna, Luceryn, Luceryna, Lucerynah, Luceryne

Lucero (Latin) a form of Lucerne.

Lucetta (English) a familiar form of Lucy.
Luceta, Lucetah, Lucettah

Lucette (French) a form of Lucy.
Lucet, Lucete, Lucett

Lucha (Spanish) a form of Luisa.

Luci, Lucie (French) familiar forms of Lucy.
Loucee, Louci, Loucie, Lucee

Lucia (Italian, Spanish) a form of Lucy.
Loucea, Loucia, Louciah, Lucea, Lucija, Luciya, Lucya, Lucyah, Luzia, Luziah, Luzya, Luzyah

Lucía (Latin) a form of Lucy.

Lúcia (Portuguese) a form of Lucy.

Luciana (Italian, Spanish) a form of Lucy.
Lucianah, Luciann, Lucianna, Luciannah, Lucianne

Lucienne (French) a form of Lucy.
Lucien, Luciena, Lucienah, Luciene, Lucienna, Luciennah, Lucyan, Lucyana, Lucyanah,

Lucyane, Lucyann, Lucyanna, Lucyannah, Lucyanne

Lucila (English) a form of Lucille.
Loucila, Loucilah, Loucilla, Loucillah, Lucilah, Lucilla, Lucillah, Lucyla, Lucylah, Lucylla, Lucyllah, Lusila, Lusilah, Lusilla, Lusillah, Lusyla, Lusylah, Lusylla, Lusyllah, Luzela, Luzelah, Luzella, Luzellah

Lucille (English) a familiar form of Lucy.
Loucil, Loucile, Loucill, Loucille, Lucile, Lucill, Lucyl, Lucyle, Lucyll, Lucylle, Lusil, Lusile, Lusill, Lusille, Lusyl, Lusyle, Lusyll, Lusylle, Luzel, Luzele, Luzell, Luzelle

Lucinda (Latin) a form of Lucy. See also Cindy.
Loucind, Loucinda, Loucindah, Loucinde, Loucint, Loucinta, Loucintah, Loucinte, Loucynd, Loucynda, Loucyndah, Loucynde, Loucynta, Loucyntah, Loucynte, Lousind, Lousinda, Lousindah, Lousinde, Lousynd, Lousynda, Lousyndah, Lousynde, Lousynta, Lousyntah, Lousynte, Lucida, Lucind, Lucindah, Lucinde, Lucindea, Lucinta, Lucintah, Lucintea, Lucynd, Lucynda, Lucyndah, Lucynde, Lucynta, Lucyntah, Lucynte, Lusind, Lusinda, Lusindah, Lusinde, Lusinta, Lusintah, Lusinte, Lusintea, Lusynda, Lusyndah, Lusynde, Luzinda, Luzindah, Luzinde, Luzinta, Luzintah, Luzinte, Luzintea, Luzynda, Luzyndah, Luzynde, Luzynta, Luzyntah, Luzynte, Luzyntea

Lucindee (Latin) a familiar form of Lucinda.
Lucindey, Lucindi, Lucindia, Lucindiah, Lucindie, Lucindy, Lucintee, Lucinti, Lucintia, Lucintiah, Lucintie, Lucinty, Lusintee, Lusintey, Lusinti, Lusintia, Lusintiah, Lusintie, Lusinty, Luzintee, Luzintey, Luzinti, Luzintia, Luzintiah, Luzintie, Luzyntee, Luzyntey, Luzynti, Luzyntia, Luzyntiah, Luzyntie, Luzynty

Lucine (Arabic) moon. (Basque) a form of Lucy.
Lucin, Lucina, Lucinah, Lucyn, Lucyna, Lucynah, Lucyne, Lukena, Lukene, Lusin, Lusina, Lusinah, Lusine, Lusyn, Lusyna, Lusynah, Lusyne, Luzin, Luzina, Luzinah, Luzine, Luzyn, Luzyna, Luzynah, Luzyne

Lucita (Spanish) a form of Lucy.
Luceata, Luceatah, Luceeta, Luceetah, Lucyta, Lucytah, Lusita

Lucky BG (American) fortunate.
Luckee, Luckey, Lucki, Luckia, Luckiah, Luckie, Luckya, Lukee, Lukey, Luki, Lukia, Lukiah, Lukie, Luky

Lucretia (Latin) rich; rewarded.
Lacrecia, Lucrece, Lucréce, Lucrecia, Lucreciah, Lucreecia, Lucreeciah, Lucresha, Lucreshia, Lucreshiah, Lucreshya, Lucreshyah, Lucrezia, Lucrisha, Lucrishah, Lucrishia, Lucrishiah

Lucrezia (Italian) a form of Lucretia. History: Lucrezia Borgia was the Duchess of Ferrara and a patron of learning and the arts.
Lucreziah, Lucrezya, Lucrezyah

Lucy (Latin) light; bringer of light.
Loucey, Loucy, Luca, Luce, Lucetta, Lucette, Lucika, Lucine, Lucita, Lucye, Lucyee, Luzca, Luzi, Luzy

Ludmilla (Slavic) loved by the people. See also Mila.
Ludie, Ludka, Ludmila, Ludmilah, Ludmile, Ludmyla, Ludmylah, Ludmylla, Ludmyllah, Ludmylle, Lyuda, Lyudmila

Ludovica (German) a form of Louise.
Liudvika, Ludovika, Ludwiga

Luella (English) elf. (German) a familiar form of Louise.
Loella, Loellah, Loelle, Looela, Looelah, Looele, Looella, Looellah, Looelle, Louela, Louelah, Louele, Louella, Louellah, Louelle, Ludel, Ludela, Ludelah, Ludele, Ludella, Ludellah, Ludelle, Luela, Luelah, Luele, Luell, Luellah, Luelle

Luisa (Spanish) a form of Louisa.
Luisah, Luiza, Luizah, Lujza, Lujzika, Luysa, Luysah, Luyza, Luyzah

Luísa (Germanic) a form of Luisa.

Luisina (Teutonic) a form of Luisa.

Luján (Spanish) Geography: a city in Argentina.

Lulani BG (Polynesian) highest point of heaven.
Lali, Loulanee, Loulaney, Loulani, Loulanie,

Loulany, Lulanea, Lulanee, Lulaney, Lulanie, Lulany, Lulanya, Lulanyah

Lulie (English) sleepy.
Lulea, Luleah, Lulee, Lulei, Luleigh, Luley, Luli, Lulia, Luliah, Luly

Lulu (Arabic) pearl. (English) soothing, comforting. (Native American) hare. (German) a familiar form of Louise, Luella.
Lolo, Looloo, Loulou, Lula

Lulú (French) a form of Luisa.

Luminosa (Latin) she who illuminates.

Luna (Latin) moon.
Lunah, Lune, Lunet, Luneta, Lunetah, Lunete, Lunetta, Lunettah, Lunette, Lunneta, Lunnete, Lunnett, Lunnetta, Lunnettah, Lunnette

Lundy GB (Scottish) grove by the island.
Lundea, Lundee, Lundeyn, Lundi, Lundie

Lupa (Latin) a form of Lupe.

Lupe (Latin) wolf. (Spanish) a short form of Guadalupe.
Lupee, Lupi, Luppi, Lupy

Lupine (Latin) like a wolf.
Lupina, Lupinah, Lupyna, Lupynah, Lupyne

Lupita (Latin) a form of Lupe.
Lupeata, Lupeatah, Lupeeta, Lupeetah, Lupet, Lupeta, Lupete, Lupett, Lupetta, Lupette, Lupyta, Lupytah, Lupyte

Lur (Spanish) earth.

Lurdes (Portuguese, Spanish) a form of Lourdes.

Lurleen, Lurlene (Scandinavian) war horn. (German) forms of Lorelei.
Lura, Luralin, Luralina, Luralinah, Luralyn, Luralyna, Luralynah, Luralyne, Lurana, Lurette, Lurlina, Lurlinah, Lurline, Lurlyn, Lurlyna, Lurlynah, Lurlyne

Lusa (Finnish) a form of Elizabeth.
Lusah, Lussa, Lussah

Lusela (Moquelumnan) like a bear swinging its foot when licking it.
Luselah, Lusella, Lusellah, Luselle

Lutana (Australian) moon.
Lutanah, Lutane, Lutania, Lutaniah,

Lutanna, Lutannah, Lutanne, Lutannia,
Lutannya, Lutanya

Lutgarda (German) she who protects her
village.

Lutrudis (German) strength of the village.

Luvena (Latin, English) little; beloved.
Louvena, Louvenah, Lovena, Lovina,
Luvenah, Luvenia, Luvenna, Luvennah,
Luvina

Luyu BG (Moquelumnan) like a pecking
bird.

Luz (Spanish) light. Religion: Nuestra
Señora de Luz—Our Lady of the Light—is
another name for the Virgin Mary.
Luzee, Luzi, Luzie, Luzija, Luzy

Luzmaria (Spanish) a combination of Luz +
Maria.

Luzmila (Slavic) loved by the village.

Ly (French) a short form of Lyla.

Lycoris (Greek) twilight.
Licoris

Lyda (Greek) a short form of Lydia.

Lydia (Greek) from Lydia, an ancient land in
Asia. (Arabic) strife.
Lydie, Lydië, Lydya, Lydyah

Lyla (French) island. (English) a form of Lyle
(see Boys' Names). (Arabic, Hindi, Persian)
a form of Lila.
Lylah, Lylla, Lyllah

Lynae, Lynnae (English) forms of Lynn.

Lynda (Spanish) pretty. (American) a form of
Linda.
Lyndah, Lynde, Lynnda, Lynndah

Lyndee, Lyndi, Lyndie (Spanish) familiar
forms of Lynda.
Lyndea, Lyndey, Lyndy, Lynndie, Lynndy

Lyndell (English) a form of Lynelle.
Lindal, Lindall, Lindel, Lindil, Lyndal,
Lyndall, Lyndel, Lyndella, Lyndelle, Lyndil

Lyndsay, Lyndsee, Lyndsey, Lyndsie,
Lyndsy (American) forms of Lindsey.
Lyndsaye, Lyndsea, Lyndsi, Lyndzee,
Lyndzey, Lyndzi, Lyndzie, Lyndzy, Lynndsie

Lynelle (English) pretty.
Linel, Linell, Linnell, Lynel, Lynell, Lynella,
Lynnell

Lynette (Welsh) idol. (English) a form of
Linette.
Lynet, Lyneta, Lynetah, Lynete, Lynett,
Lynetta, Lynettah

Lynlee (English) a form of Lynn.
Lynlea, Lynleah, Lynlei, Lynleigh, Lynley,
Lynli, Lynlia, Lynliah, Lynlie, Lynly

Lynn GB (English) waterfall; pool below a
waterfall. See also Lin.
Lyn, Lynlee

Lynna (Greek, Latin, Arabic) a form of Lina.
Lyna, Lynah, Lynnah

Lynne (English) waterfall; pool below a
waterfall.

Lynnea (Scandinavian) a form of Linnea.
Lynea, Lyneah, Lynneah

Lynnell (English) a form of Lynelle.
Lynnella, Lynnelle

Lynnette (Welsh, English) a form of Lynette.
Lyannette, Lynnet, Lynnett, Lynnetta,
Lynnettah

Lynsey, Lynsie, Lynzee, Lynzie (American)
forms of Lindsey.
Lynnsey, Lynnzey, Lynsy, Lynzey, Lynzi,
Lynzy

Lyonella (French) lion cub.
Lionel, Lionela, Lionell, Lionella, Lyonela,
Lyonele, Lyonelle

Lyra (Greek) lyre player.
Lira, Lirah, Lirra, Lirrah, Lyrah, Lyre, Lyrie,
Lyris, Lyrra, Lyrrah

Lyric (Greek) songlike; words of a song.
Liric, Lirick, Lirik, Lirique, Lyrica, Lyrick,
Lyrik, Lyrique, Lyryk, Lyryque

Lyris (Greek) lyre player.
Liris, Lirisa, Lirise, Liriss, Lirissa, Lirisse,
Lyrisa, Lyrisah, Lyrise, Lyriss, Lyrissa, Lyrisse,
Lyrysa, Lyrysah, Lyryssa, Lyryssah

Lysa (Hebrew, English) a form of Lisa.
Lyesa, Lyesah, Lysah

Lysandra (Greek) liberator.
Lysandrah, Lyssandra, Lyssandrah, Lytle

Lysandre (Greek) a form of Lysandra.

Lysann, Lysanne (American) combinations of Lysandra + Ann.
Lysanna, Lysannah

Lysette (French, English) a form of Liset.

Lyssa (Greek) a form of Lissa.
Lyssah

Lyzabeth (English) a short form of Elizabeth. See also Lizabeth.
Lysabet, Lysabete, Lysabeth, Lysabett, Lysabette, Lyzabet, Lyzabete, Lyzabett, Lyzabette

M

Ma Kayla (American) a form of Michaela.

Mab (Irish) joyous. (Welsh) baby. Literature: queen of the fairies.
Mabb, Mabry

Mabbina (Irish) a form of Mabel.
Mabine

Mabel (Latin) lovable. A short form of Amabel.
Mabbina, Mabella, Mabelle, Mabil, Mabill, Mable, Mabyn, Maebell, Maibel, Maibele, Maibell, Maible, Maiebell, Maybeline, Maybell, Moibeal

Mabella (English) a form of Mabel.
Mabela, Mabilla, Maebella, Maibela, Maibella, Maiebella

Mabelle (French) a form of Mabel.
Mabele, Mabell, Mabille, Maibelle, Maiebelle

Mac Kenzie (Irish) a form of Mackenzie.

Macaela (Hebrew) a form of Michaela.

Macarena (Spanish) she who carries the sword; name for the Virgin Mary.

Macaria (Greek) happy.
Macariah, Macarya, Macaryah

Macawi (Dakota) generous; motherly.
Macawee, Macawia, Macawie, Macawy

Macayla (American) a form of Michaela.
Macaila, Macala, Macalah, Macaylah, Macayle, Macayli

Macee, Macey, Maci, Macie (Polish) familiar forms of Macia.
Macye

Machaela (Hebrew) a form of Michaela.
Machael, Machaelah, Machaelie, Machaila, Machala, Macheala

Machiko (Japanese) fortunate child.
Machi, Machika, Machikah, Machyka, Machyko

Macia (Polish) a form of Miriam.
Macelia, Machia, Maciah, Macya, Macyah, Masha, Mashia, Mashiah

Maciela (Latin) very slender.

Mackayla (American) a form of Michaela.

Mackenna (American) a form of Mackenzie.
Mackena, Mackenah, Mykena, Mykenah, Mykenna, Mykennah

Mackensie, Mackenzi (American) forms of Mackenzie.
Mackensi, Mackenze, Mackenzye

Mackenzie ☆ GB (Irish) child of the wise leader. See also Kenzie.
Macenzie, Mackenzee, Mackenzey, Mackenzia, Mackinsey, Mackynze, Mykenzie

Mackenzy BG (American) a form of Mackenzie.

Mackinsey (Irish) a form of Mackenzie.
Mackinsie, Mackinze, Mackinzee, Mackinzey, Mackinzi, Mackinzie

Macra (Greek) she who grows.

Macrina, Macronia (Greek) forms of Macra.

Macuilxóchitl (Nahuatl) five flowers.

Macy GB (Polish) a familiar form of Macia.

Mada (English) a short form of Madaline, Magdalen.
Madah, Madda, Maddah, Mahda

Madalaine (English) a form of Madeline.
Madalain, Madalaina, Madalane, Madalayn, Madalayna, Madalayne, Madaleine

Madaline (English) a form of Madeline.
Madaleen, Madalene, Madalin

Madalyn, Madalynn (Greek) forms of
Madeline.
Madalyne, Madalynne

Maddie (English) a familiar form of
Madeline.
*Maddea, Maddee, Maddey, Maddi, Maddy,
Madea, Madee, Madey, Madi, Madie, Mady,
Maidie, Maydey*

**Maddisen, Maddison, Madisen,
Madisson, Madisyn** (English) forms of
Madison.
*Maddisson, Maddisyn, Madissen, Madissyn,
Madisynn, Madisynne*

Maddox BG (Welsh, English) benefactor's
child.
Madox

Madeira (Spanish) sweet wine.

Madelaine, Madeleine, Madeliene
(French) forms of Madeline.
*Madelain, Madelane, Madelayne, Madelein,
Madeleyn, Madeleyne*

Madelena (English) a form of Madeline.
*Madalana, Madalena, Madalina, Maddalena,
Maddelena, Maddelina, Madelaina,
Madeleina, Madeleyna, Madelina, Madelinah,
Madelyna*

Madelene, Madelin, Madelyn (Greek,
English) forms of Madeline.
Maddelene, Madelyne, Madelynn, Madelynne

Madeline ☆ (Greek) high tower. See also
Lena, Lina, Maud.
*Madailéin, Maddeline, Madel, Madelia,
Madella, Madelle, Madelon, Maighdlin*

Madelón (Spanish) a form of Madeline.

Madena, Madina (Greek) forms of
Madeline.

Madge (Greek) a familiar form of Madeline,
Margaret.
*Madgee, Madgey, Madgi, Madgie, Madgy,
Mage*

Madhubala (Hindi) little girl of honey.

Madia (Greek) a form of Madeline.

Madilyn, Madilynn (Greek) forms of
Madeline.
Madilen, Madiline, Madilyne

Madison ☆ GB (English) good; child of
Maud.
*Maddisan, Maddisin, Maddisun, Maddyson,
Maddysyn, Madisan, Madisin, Madissan,
Madissin, Madisun*

Madlaberta (German) brilliant work.

Madlyn (Greek, English) a form of
Madeline.
Madlen, Madlin, Madline

Madolyn (Greek) a form of Madeline.
Madoline, Madolyne, Madolynn, Madolynne

Madonna (Latin) my lady.
Maddona, Maddonah, Madona, Madonnah

Madra (Spanish) a form of Madrona.

Madrona (Spanish) mother.
Madre, Madrena

Madysen, Madyson (English) forms of
Madison.
Madysan, Madysin, Madysun, Madysyn

Mae (English) a form of May. History: Mae
Jemison was the first African American
woman in space.
Maelea, Maeleah, Maelen, Maelle, Maeona

Maegan, Maegen, Maeghan (Irish) forms
of Megan.
*Maeghen, Maeghin, Maeghon, Maeghyn,
Maegin, Maegon, Maegyn*

Maeko (Japanese) honest child.
Maemi

Maeve (Irish) joyous. Mythology: a
legendary Celtic queen. See also Mavis.
Maevi, Maevy, Maive, Mayve

Magali, Magalie, Magaly (Hebrew) from
the high tower.
Magally

Magalí (Spanish) a form of Magali.

Magan, Maghan (Greek) forms of Megan.
Maggen, Maggin

Magda (Czech, Polish, Russian) a form of
Magdalen.
Magdah, Mahda, Makda

Magdalen (Greek) high tower. Bible: Magdala was the home of Saint Mary Magdalen. See also Madeline, Malena, Marlene.
Magdala, Magdalane, Magdaleen, Magdaline, Magdalyn, Magdalyne, Magdalynn, Magdelan, Magdelane, Magdelen, Magdelene, Magdelin, Magdeline, Magdelon, Magdelone, Magdelyn, Magdelyne, Magdlen, Magola, Maighdlin, Mala, Malaine

Magdalén (Spanish) a form of Magdalen.

Magdalena (Greek) a form of Magdalen.
Magdalana, Magdaleny, Magdalina, Magdalona, Magdalonia, Magdalyna, Magdelana, Magdelena, Magdelina, Magdelona, Magdelonia, Magdelyna, Magdolna

Magdalene (Greek) a form of Magdalen.

Magen GB (Greek) a form of Megan.

Magena (Native American) coming moon.
Magenna

Maggi, Maggy (English) forms of Maggie.
Magy

Maggie (Greek) pearl. (English) a familiar form of Magdalen, Margaret.
Mag, Magee, Magey, Magge, Maggee, Maggey, Maggia, Maggiemae, Magi, Magie, Mags

Magina (Latin) magician.

Magna (Latin) great.

Magnolia (Latin) flowering tree. See also Nollie.
Magnolea, Magnoleah, Magnoliah, Magnolya, Nola

Maha (Iranian) crystal. (Arabic) wild cow; cow's eyes.

Mahal (Filipino) love.

Mahala (Arabic) fat; marrow; tender. (Native American) powerful woman.
Mahalah, Mahalar, Mahalla, Mahela, Mahila, Mahlah, Mahlaha, Mehala, Mehalah

Mahalia (American) a form of Mahala.
Mahaley, Mahaliah, Mahalie, Mahaylia, Mahelea, Maheleah, Mahelia, Mahilia, Mehalia, Mehaliah, Mehalya, Mehalyah

Maharene (Ethiopian) forgive us.

Mahayla (American) a form of Mahala.
Mahaylah

Mahesa BG (Hindi) great lord. Religion: a name for the Hindu god Shiva.
Maheesa, Mahisa, Mahissa, Mahysa, Mahyssa

Mahila (Sanskrit) woman.
Mahilah, Mahyla, Mahylah

Mahina (Hawaiian) moon glow.
Mahinah, Mahyna, Mahynah

Mahira (Hebrew) energetic.
Mahirah, Mahri, Mahyra, Mahyrah

Mahlí (Hebrew) astute.

Mahogany (Spanish) rich; strong.
Mahoganee, Mahoganey, Mahogani, Mahogania, Mahoganie

Mahogony (Spanish) a form of Mahogany.
Mahagony, Mahogney, Mahogny, Mahogonee, Mahogoney, Mahogoni, Mahogonia, Mahogonie, Mahogonya, Mohogany, Mohogony

Mahuitzic (Nahuatl) honored, glorious.

Mahuizoh (Nahuatl) glorious person.

Mai (Japanese) brightness. (Vietnamese) flower. (Navajo) coyote.
Maie

Maia (Greek) mother; nurse. (English) kinswoman; maiden. Mythology: the loveliest of the Pleiades, the seven daughters of Atlas, and the mother of Hermes. See also Maya.
Maea

Maiah (Greek, English) a form of Maia.

Maiara (Tupi) wise.

Maida (English) maiden. (Greek) a short form of Madeline.
Maeda, Maidah, Maidel, Maieda, Mayda, Maydah, Maydena, Mayeda

Maigan (American) a form of Megan.

Maija (Finnish) a form of Mary.
Maiji, Maikki

Maika (Hebrew) a familiar form of Michaela.
Maikala, Maikka, Maiko

Maili (Polynesian) gentle breeze.

Maimi (Japanese) smiling truth. See also Mamie.
Maemee, Maimee, Maimey, Maimi, Maimie, Maimy

Maira (Irish) a form of Mary.
Maairah, Maera, Maerah, Mairah, Mairia, Mairiah, Mairim, Mairin, Mairona, Mairwen, Mairwin, Mairwyn

Maire (Irish) a form of Mary.
Mair, Mayr, Mayre

Mairghread (Irish, Scottish) a form of Margaret.
Maergrethe, Maigret, Mairgret

Mairi (Irish) a form of Mary.
Mairee, Mairey, Mairie, Mairy

Maisey, Maisie (Scottish) familiar forms of Margaret.
Maesee, Maesey, Maesi, Maesie, Maesy, Maisa, Maise, Maisee, Maisi, Maizie, Mazey, Mazie, Mazy, Mazzy, Mysie, Myzie

Maisha (Arabic) walking with a proud, swinging gait.
Maisaha

Maison BG (Arabic) a form of Maysun.

Maita (Spanish) a form of Martha.
Maeta, Maetah, Maitia, Maitya, Maityah, Mayta, Maytya, Maytyah

Maitana, Maitea, Maiten, Maitena (Spanish) forms of Maite.

Maitane (English) a form of Maite.

Maite (Spanish) lovable. A combination of Maria + Teresa. A form of Maita.

Maitland GB (American) a form of Maitlyn.

Maitlyn (American) a combination of Maita + Lynn.
Maitlan, Maitlynn, Mattilyn

Maiya (Greek) a form of Maia.
Maiyah

Maja (Arabic) a short form of Majidah.
Majah, Majal, Majalisa, Majalyn, Majalyna, Majalyne, Majalynn, Majalynne

Majalí (Hebrew) astute.

Majesta (Latin) majestic.
Magestic, Magestica, Magesticah, Magestiqua, Magestique, Majestah, Majestic, Majestiqua, Majestique

Majidah (Arabic) splendid.
Majid, Majida, Majyd, Majyda, Majydah

Majorie (Greek, Scottish) a form of Marjorie.

Makaela (American) a form of Michaela.
Makaelah, Makaelee, Makaella, Makaely, Makealah

Makaila (American) a form of Michaela.
Makail, Makailah, Makailea, Makaileah, Makailee, Makailei, Makaileigh, Makailey, Makaili, Makailla, Makaillah, Makaily

Makala (Hawaiian) myrtle. (Hebrew) a form of Michaela.
Makalae, Makalah, Makalai, Makalea, Makaleah, Makalee, Makalei, Makaleigh, Makaley, Makali, Makalia, Makaliah, Makalie, Makaly, Makalya

Makana (Hawaiian) gift, present.
Makanah, Makanna, Makannah

Makani BG (Hawaiian) wind.
Makanee, Makania, Makaniah, Makanie, Makany, Makanya, Makanyah

Makara (Hindi) Astrology: another name for the zodiac sign Capricorn.
Makarah, Makarra, Makarrah

Makayla ⭐ (American) a form of Michaela.
Makaylah, Makaylla

Makaylee (American) a form of Michaela.
Makaylea, Makayleah, Makaylei, Makayleigh, Makayley, Makayli, Makaylia, Makayliah, Makaylie, Makayly

Makeda (Ethiopian) beautiful.

Makell (American) a short form of Makaela, Makala, Makayla.
Makela, Makelah, Makele, Makella, Makelle, Mekel

Makena, Makenna (American) forms of Mackenna.
Makenah, Makennah

Makensie, Makenzee, Makenzi (American) forms of Mackenzie.
Makense, Makensey, Makenze, Makenzey, Makenzy, Makenzye, Makinzey, Makynzey, Mykenzie

Makenzie GB (American) a form of Mackenzie.

Makia, Makiah (Hopi) forms of Makyah (see Boys' Names).

Makyla (American) a form of Michaela.
Makylah

Mala (Greek) a short form of Magdalen.
Malee, Mali

Malachie (Hebrew) angel of God.
Malachee, Malachey, Malachi, Malachy

Malaika (African) angel.

Malaina (French) a form of Malena.
Malainah

Malají (Hebrew) my messenger.

Malak (Hungarian) a form of Malika.

Malana (Hawaiian) bouyant, light.
Malanah, Malanna, Malannah

Malanie (Greek) a form of Melanie.
Malanee, Malaney, Malani, Malania, Malaniah, Malany

Malaya (Filipino) free.
Malaia, Malaiah, Malayaa, Malayah, Malayna

Malea, Maleah (Filipino) forms of Malaya. (Hawaiian, Zuni, Spanish) forms of Malia.

Maleeka (Hungarian) a form of Malika.

Maleena (Hebrew, English, Native American, Russian) a form of Malina.

Maleka (Hungarian) a form of Malika.

Malena (Swedish) a familiar form of Magdalen.
Malayna, Malen, Malenna, Malin, Maline, Malini, Malinna

Malerie (French) a form of Mallory.
Mallerie

Malfreda (German) peaceful worker.
Malfredah, Malfredda, Malfrida, Malfryda, Malfrydda

Malha (Hebrew) queen.

Mali (Tai) jasmine flower. (Tongan) sweet. (Hungarian) a short form of Malika.
Malee, Malei, Maleigh, Maley, Malie, Mallee, Mallei, Malleigh, Malley, Malli, Mallie, Mally, Maly

Malia (Hawaiian, Zuni) a form of Mary. (Spanish) a form of Maria.
Maleeya, Maleeyah, Maleia, Maleiah, Maleigha, Maliaka, Maliasha, Malie, Maliea, Mallea, Malleah, Malleia, Malleiah, Malleigha, Malleya, Mallia, Malliah, Mallya, Malya, Malyah

Maliah (Hawaiian, Zuni, Spanish) a form of Malia.

Malika (Hungarian) industrious. (Arabic) queen.
Malik, Malikee, Maliki, Malikia, Malky, Malyka, Malykah

Malikah (Hungarian) a form of Malika.

Malina (Hebrew) tower. (Native American) soothing. (Russian) raspberry.
Malin, Malinah, Maline, Malinna, Mallie, Malyn, Malyna, Malynah, Malyne

Malinalxochitl (Nahuatl) grass flower.

Malinda (Greek) a form of Melinda.
Malindah, Malinde, Malindea, Malindee, Malindia, Malinna, Malynda, Malyndah

Malini (Hindi) gardener.
Malinee, Malinia, Malinie, Maliny, Malyni, Malynia, Malynie, Malyny, Malynya

Malisa, Malissa (Greek) forms of Melissa.
Malisah, Mallissa

Maliyah (Hawaiian, Zuni, Spanish) a form of Malia.
Maliya

Malka (Hebrew) queen.
Malkah, Malki, Malkia, Malkiah, Malkya, Malkyah

Malki (Hebrew) a form of Malka.
Malkee, Malkeh, Malkey, Malkie, Malkiya, Malkiyah

Mallalai (Pashto) beautiful.

Malley (American) a familiar form of Mallory.
Mallee, Malli, Mallie, Mally, Maly

Mallori, Mallorie, Malori, Malorie, Malory (French) forms of Mallory.
Malloree, Malloreigh, Mallorree, Mallorri, Mallorrie, Maloree, Malorey, Melorie, Melory

Mallory GB (German) army counselor. (French) unlucky.
Malarie, Maliri, Mallari, Mallary, Mallauri, Mallery, Malley, Mallorey, Mallorrey, Mallorry, Malorym, Malree, Malrie, Mellory

Malú (Spanish) a combination of Maria + Luisa.

Maluhia (Hawaiian) peaceful.

Malulani (Hawaiian) under a peaceful sky.
Malulanea, Malulanee, Malulaney, Malulania, Malulanie, Malulany

Malva (English) a form of Melba.
Malvah, Malvi, Malvy

Malvina (Scottish) a form of Melvina. Literature: a name created by the eighteenth-century Romantic poet James Macpherson.
Malvane, Malveen, Malveena, Malveenah, Malvinah, Malvine, Malvinia, Malviniah, Malvyna, Malvynah, Malvyne, Malvynia, Malvyniah, Malvynya, Malvynyah

Malyssa (Greek) a form of Melissa.

Mamen (Hebrew) a form of Carmen.

Mamie (American) a familiar form of Margaret. See also Maimi.
Maeme, Maemey, Maemi, Maemie, Maemy, Mame, Mamee, Mami, Mammie, Mamy, Mamye, Maymee, Maymey, Maymi, Maymie, Maymy

Mamo BG (Hawaiian) saffron flower; yellow bird.

Mana (Hawaiian) psychic; sensitive.
Manah, Manna, Mannah

Manal (Hawaiian) a form of Mana.
Manali, Manalia

Manar (Arabic) guiding light.
Manara, Manayra

Manauia (Nahuatl) defend.

Manda (Spanish) woman warrior. (Latin) a short form of Amanda.
Mandah, Mandea

Mandara (Hindi) calm.
Mandarah

Mandee, Mandi, Mandie (Latin) forms of Mandy.

Mandeep BG (Punjabi) enlightened.
Manddep

Mandisa (Xhosa) sweet.
Mandisa, Mandissa, Mandissah, Mandysa, Mandysah, Mandyssa, Mandyssah

Mandy (Latin) lovable. A familiar form of Amanda, Manda, Melinda.
Mandey

Manela (Catalan) a form of Manuela.

Manette (French) a form of Mary.
Manet, Maneta, Manete, Manett, Manetta

Mangena (Hebrew) song, melody.
Mangina, Mangyna

Mani (Chinese) a mantra repeated in Tibetan Buddhist prayer to impart understanding.
Manee, Maney, Manie, Many

Manilla (Australian) meandering, winding river.
Manila, Manilah, Manillah, Manille, Manyla, Manylah, Manylla, Manyllah

Manisha (Indian) intellect.
Mohisha

Manjot BG (Indian) light of the mind.
Manjyot

Manka (Polish, Russian) a form of Mary.
Mankah

Manoela, Manoli (Hebrew) forms of Manuela.

Manola (Spanish) a form of Manuela.

Manon (French) a familiar form of Marie.
Mannon, Manona, Manone, Manyn, Manyne

Manón (Spanish) a form of María.

Manpreet GB (Punjabi) mind full of love.
Manpret, Manprit

Manque (Mapuche) condor; woman of unyielding character.

Mansi (Hopi) plucked flower.
Mancee, Mancey, Manci, Mancie, Mancy, Mansee, Mansey, Mansie, Mansy

Manuela (Spanish) a form of Emmanuelle.
Manuala, Manuel, Manuele, Manuelita, Manuell, Manuella, Manuelle

Manya (Russian) a form of Mary.
Mania, Maniah, Manyah

Mar (Spanish) sea.

Mara (Hebrew) melody. (Greek) a short form of Amara. (Slavic) a form of Mary.
Mahra, Marae, Maralina, Maraline, Marra, Marrah

Marabel (English) a form of Maribel.
Marabela, Marabelah, Marabele, Marabell, Marabella, Marabellah, Marabelle

Marah (Greek, Hebrew, Slavic) a form of Mara.

Maranda (Latin) a form of Miranda.
Marandah

Maravillas (Latin) admiration.

Maraya (Hebrew) a form of Mariah.
Marayah, Mareya

Marcedes (American) a form of Mercedes.

Marcela (Latin) a form of Marcella.
Marcele, Marcelia

Marcelen (English) a form of Marcella.
Marcelin, Marceline, Marcellin, Marcellina, Marcelline, Marcelyn, Marcilen

Marceliana (Latin) a form of Marcela.

Marcelina (English) a form of Marcella.

Marcella (Latin) martial, warlike. Mythology: Mars was the god of war.
Mairsil, Marca, Marce, Marceil, Marcello, Marcena, Marciella, Marcile, Marcilla, Marella, Marsella, Marshella, Marsial, Marsiala, Marsiale, Marsiella

Marcelle (French) a form of Marcella.
Marcell, Marcile, Marcille, Marselle, Marsielle

Marcena (Latin) a form of Marcella, Marcia.
Maracena, Marceen, Marceena, Marceenah, Marceene, Marcenah, Marcene, Marcenia, Marceyne, Marcina, Marseena, Marseenah, Marseene

Marchelle (American) a form of Marcelle.
Marchella

Marci, Marcie, Marcy (English) familiar forms of Marcella, Marcia.
Marca, Marcee, Marcey, Marcita, Marcye, Marsey, Marsi, Marsie, Marsy

Marcia (Latin) martial, warlike. See also Marquita.
Marcea, Marcena, Marchia, Marchiah, Marciale, Marcsa, Marcya, Marcyah, Marsia

Márcia (Portuguese) a form of Marcia.

Marciann (American) a combination of Marci + Ann.
Marciana, Marciane, Marcianna, Marcianne, Marcyane, Marcyanna, Marcyanne

Marcilynn (American) a combination of Marci + Lynn.
Marcelyn, Marcilin, Marciline, Marcilyn, Marcilyne, Marcilynne, Marcylen, Marcylin, Marcyline, Marcylyn, Marcylyne, Marcylynn, Marcylynne

Marcionila (Latin) a form of Marcia.

Mardella (English) meadow near a lake.
Mardela, Mardelah, Mardele, Mardell, Mardellah, Mardelle

Marden BG (English) from the meadow with a pool.
Mardana, Mardanah, Mardane, Mardena, Mardenah, Mardene

Mardi (French) born on Tuesday. (Aramaic) a familiar form of Martha.
Mardea, Mardee, Mardey, Mardie, Mardy

Mare (Irish) a form of Mary.

Mareena (Latin) a form of Marina.
Mareenah, Mareenia

Marelda (German) renowned warrior.
Mareldah, Marella, Marilda, Marildah, Marylda, Maryldah

Maren GB (Latin) sea. (Aramaic) a form of Mary. See also Marina.
Mareane, Marene, Miren, Mirene, Myren, Myrene

Marena (Latin) a form of Marina.
Marenah, Marenka

Maresa, Maressa (Latin) forms of Marisa.
Maresha, Meresa

Maretta (English) a familiar form of
Margaret.
*Maret, Mareta, Maretah, Marete, Marett,
Marettah, Marette*

Margaret (Greek) pearl. History: Margaret
Hilda Thatcher served as British prime
minister. See also Gita, Greta, Gretchen,
Gretel, Marjorie, Markita, Meg, Megan,
Peggy, Reet, Rita.
*Marga, Margalo, Marganit, Margara,
Margarett, Margarette, Margaro, Margarta,
Margat, Margeret, Margeretta, Margerette,
Margetha, Margetta, Margiad, Margisia*

Margarete (German) a form of Margaret.
Margen, Marghet

Margaretha (German) a form of Margaret.
Margareth, Margarethe

Margarit (Greek) a form of Margaret.
*Margalide, Margalit, Margalith, Margarid,
Margarite, Margaritt, Margerit*

Margarita (Italian, Spanish) a form of
Margaret.
*Malgerita, Malgherita, Margareta, Margaretta,
Margarida, Margaritis, Margaritta, Margeretta,
Margharita, Margherita, Margrieta, Margrita,
Margurita, Marguryta, Marjarita*

Margaux (French) a form of Margaret.
Margeaux

Marge (English) a short form of Margaret,
Marjorie.

Margery (English) a form of Margaret. See
also Marjorie.
*Margeree, Margerey, Margeri, Margerie,
Margori, Margorie, Margory*

Margie (English) a familiar form of Marge,
Margaret.
Margey, Margi, Margy

Margit (Hungarian) a form of Margaret.
Marget, Margette, Margita

Margo, Margot (French) forms of
Margaret.
Mago, Margaro, Margolis, Margote

Margret (German) a form of Margaret.
Margreta, Margrete, Margreth, Margrethe,

*Margrett, Margretta, Margrette, Margriet,
Margrieta*

Margryta (Lithuanian) a form of Margaret.
Margrita, Margruta, Marguta

Marguerite (French) a form of Margaret.
*Margarete, Margarite, Margerite, Marguareta,
Marguarete, Marguaretta, Marguarette,
Marguarita, Marguarite, Marguaritta,
Marguerette, Marguerita, Margueritta,
Margueritte, Margurite, Marguritte, Marguryt,
Marguryte*

Mari (Japanese) ball. (Spanish) a form of
Mary.
Maree, Marree, Marri

Maria ☆ (Hebrew) bitter; sea of bitterness.
(Italian, Spanish) a form of Mary.
*Maie, Marea, Mareah, Mariabella, Mariae,
Mariesa, Mariessa, Marrea, Marria*

María (Hebrew) a form of Maria.

María de la Concepción (Spanish) Mary of
the conception.

María de la Paz (Spanish) Mary of peace.

María de las Nieves (Spanish) Mary of the
snows.

María de las Victorias (Spanish) victorious
Mary.

María de los Angeles (Spanish) angelic
Mary.

María de los Milagros (Spanish) miraculous
Mary.

María del Mar (Spanish) Mary of the sea.

María Inmaculada (Spanish) Immaculate
Mary.

María José (Latin) a combination of María
+ José.

María Noel (Latin) a combination of María
+ Noel.

Mariaelena (Italian) a combination of Maria
+ Elena.
Maria Elena

Mariah, Marriah (Hebrew) forms of Mary.
See also Moriah.
Maraia, Marrya, Marryah

Mariam (Hebrew) a form of Miriam.
Mariame, Mariem, Meriame, Meryam

Mariama (Hebrew) a form of Mariam.

Marian GB (English) a form of Mary Ann.
Marien, Mariene, Marienn, Marienne, Marrian, Marriane, Marriann, Marrianne

Marián (Spanish) a short form of Mariana.

Mariana, Marianna (Spanish) forms of Marian.
Marianah, Mariena, Marienah, Marienna, Mariennah, Marriana, Marrianna, Maryana, Maryanna, Maryannah

Mariane, Mariann, Marianne (English) forms of Mary Ann.

Marianela (Spanish) a combination of Mariana + Estela.

Mariángeles (Spanish) a combination of María + Ángeles.

Maribel (French) beautiful. (English) a combination of Maria + Bel.
Marbelle, Mareabel, Mareabela, Mareabele, Mareabell, Mareabella, Mareabelle, Mareebel, Mareebela, Mareebelah, Mareebele, Mareebell, Mareebella, Mareebellah, Mareebelle, Mariabella, Maribela, Maribelah, Maribele, Maribell, Maribella, Maribellah, Maribelle, Maridel, Marybel, Marybela, Marybelah, Marybele, Marybell, Marybella, Marybellah, Marybelle

Maribeth (American) a form of Mary Beth.
Maribette, Mariebeth

Marica (Italian) a form of Marice. (Dutch, Slavic) a form of Marika.
Maricah

Maricarmen (American) a form of Marycarmen.

Marice (Italian) a form of Mary. See also Maris.
Maryce

Maricela (Latin) a form of Marcella.
Maricel, Mariceli, Maricelia, Maricella, Maricely

Maricruz (Spanish) a combination of María + Cruz.

Maridel (English) a form of Maribel.

Marie (French) a form of Mary.
Maree, Marrie

Marie Andree (French) a combination of Marie + Andree.

Marie Ann, Marie Anne (American) combinations of Marie + Ann.
Marie-Ann, Marie-Anne

Marie Chantal (French) a combination of Marie + Chantal.
Marie-Chantal

Marie Christi (American) a combination of Marie + Christi.
Marie Christie, Marie Christy, Marie-Christi, Marie-Christie, Marie-Christy

Marie Clair, Marie Claire (American) combinations of Marie + Clair.
Marie Clare, Marie-Clair, Marie-Claire, Marie-Clare

Marie Claude (French) a combination of Marie + Claude.
Marie-Claude

Marie Elaine (American) a combination of Marie + Elaine.
Marie-Elaine

Marie Eve, Marie-Eve (American) combinations of Marie + Eve.

Marie Frances (French) a combination of Marie + Frances.
Marie-Frances

Marie Helene (American) a combination of Marie + Helene.
Marie-Helene

Marie Jeanne (American) a combination of Marie + Jeanne.
Marie Jean, Marie-Jean, Marie-Jeanne

Marie Joelle (French) a combination of Marie + Joelle.
Marie-Joelle

Marie Josee (French) a combination of Marie + Josee.
Marie Josie, Marie-Josee, Marie-Josie

Marie Kim (American) a combination of Marie + Kim.
Marie-Kim

Marie Laurence (French) a combination of Marie + Laurence.
Marie-Laurence

Marie Lou (American) a combination of Marie + Lou.
Marie-Lou

Marie Louise (American) a combination of Marie + Louise.
Marie-Louise

Marie Maud, Marie Maude (American) combinations of Marie + Maud.
Marie-Maud, Marie-Maude

Marie Michele, Marie Michell (American) combinations of Marie + Michele.
Marie Michelle, Marie-Michele, Marie-Michell, Marie-Michelle

Marie Noelle (American) a combination of Marie + Noelle.
Marie Noel, Marie Noele, Marie-Noel, Marie-Noele, Marie-Noelle

Marie Pascale (French) a combination of Marie + Pascale.
Marie Pascal, Marie-Pascal, Marie-Pascale

Marie Philippa (French) a combination of Marie + Philippa.
Marie Philipa, Marie-Philipa, Marie-Philippa

Marie Pier, Marie Pierre, Marie-Pier (French) combinations of Marie + Pier.
Marie-Pierre

Marie Soleil (Spanish) a combination of Marie + Soleil (see Solana).
Marie-Soleil

Marie Sophie (French) a combination of Marie + Sophie.
Marie-Sophie

Mariel, Marielle (German, Dutch) forms of Mary.
Marial, Mariale, Mariall, Marialle, Marieke, Marielana, Mariele, Marieli, Marielie, Mariell, Marielsie, Mariely, Marielys, Maryal, Maryel, Maryil, Maryile, Maryille

Mariela, Mariella (German, Dutch) forms of Mary.
Mariala, Marialah, Marialla, Maryila, Maryilla

Marielena (German, Dutch) a form of Mary.

Marietta (Italian) a familiar form of Marie.
Maretta, Marette, Mariet, Marieta, Mariett, Mariette, Marriet, Marrieta, Marriete, Marrietta, Marriette

Marieve (American) a combination of Mary + Eve.

Marigold (English) Mary's gold. Botany: a plant with yellow or orange flowers.
Mareagold, Mareegold, Mariegold, Marygold

Mariha (Hebrew, Italian, Spanish) a form of Maria.

Marija (Hebrew, Italian, Spanish) a form of Maria.

Marika (Dutch, Slavic) a form of Mary.
Mareeca, Mareecah, Mareeka, Maricka, Marieka, Marieke, Marijke, Marikah, Marike, Marikia, Marikka, Mariqua, Marique, Mariska, Mariske, Marrica, Marricah, Marrika, Marrike, Maryca, Marycah, Marycka, Maryk, Maryka, Maryke, Merica, Mericah, Merika, Merikah, Meriqua, Merique

Mariko (Japanese) circle.
Mareako, Mareecko, Mareeco, Mareeko, Maricko, Marico, Marycko, Maryco, Maryko

Marilee, Marilie, Marily (American) combinations of Mary + Lee. See also Merrilee.
Marilea, Marileah, Marilei, Marileigh, Mariley, Marili, Marilia, Marrilee, Marylea, Maryleah, Marylee, Marylei, Maryleigh, Maryley, Maryli, Marylie, Maryly

Marilín (Spanish) a combination of Maria + Linda.

Marilla (Hebrew, German) a form of Mary.
Marella, Marelle, Marila, Marilah, Marillah, Maryla, Marylah, Marylla

Marilou, Marilu (American) forms of Marylou.
Mariluz

Marilú (Spanish) a combination of María + Luz.

Marilyn (Hebrew) Mary's line or descendants. See also Merilyn.
Maralin, Maralyn, Maralyne, Maralynn, Maralynne, Marelyn, Marielin, Marielina, Marieline, Marilena, Marilene, Marilin, Marilina, Mariline, Marillyn, Marolyn, Marralynn, Marrilin, Marrilyn, Merrilyn

Marilyne, Marilynn (Hebrew) forms of Marilyn.
Marilynne, Marrilynn, Marrilynne

Marin GB (Latin, Aramaic) a form of Maren.
Marinn, Maryne

Marina (Latin) sea. See also Maren.
Mareana, Mareanah, Marinae, Marinah, Marinka, Marrina, Marrinah, Marrinia, Maryna, Marynah, Marynna, Marynnah, Marynne, Mayne, Mirena, Myrena, Myrenah

Mariña (Latin) a form of Marina.

Marinda (Latin) a form of Marina.
Marindi

Marine, Maryn (Latin, Aramaic) forms of Maren.

Marinés (Spanish) a combination of María + Inés.

Marini (Swahili) healthy; pretty.
Marinee, Mariney, Marinie, Marynee, Maryney, Maryni, Marynie, Maryny

Marinna (Latin) a form of Marina.

Mariola (Italian) a form of María.

Marion GB (French) a form of Mary.
Mariun, Marrian, Marrion, Maryon, Maryonn

Marión, Mariona (Spanish) forms of Marion.

Mariposa (Spanish) butterfly.

Maris (Latin) sea. (Greek) a short form of Amaris, Damaris. See also Marice.
Maries, Marise, Mariss, Marisse, Marris, Marys, Meris, Merris

Marisa (Latin) sea.
Mariesa, Marisah

Marisabel (Spanish) a combination of María + Isabel.

Marisabela (Spanish) a combination of María + Isabela.

Marisel (Spanish) a form of Marisabel.

Marisela (Latin) a form of Marisa.
Mariseli, Marisella, Marishelle, Marissela

Marisha (Russian) a familiar form of Mary.
Mareshah, Marishah, Marishenka, Marishka, Mariska, Marrisha, Marrishah

Marisol (Spanish) sunny sea.
Marise, Marizol, Marysol, Marysola, Maryzol, Maryzola

Marissa ☀ (Latin) a form of Maris, Marisa.
Mariessa, Marissah, Marisse, Marizza, Morissa

Marit (Aramaic) lady.
Marite, Maryt, Maryte

Marita (Spanish) a form of Marisa. (Aramaic) a form of Marit.
Maritah, Marité, Maritha, Maryta

Maritsa (Arabic) a form of Maritza.
Maritsah, Maritssa

Maritxu (Basque) a familiar form of Maria.

Maritza (Arabic) blessed.
Maritzah, Marytsa, Marytsah, Marytza, Marytzah

Mariya, Mariyah (Hebrew, Italian, Spanish) forms of Maria. (Arabic) forms of Mariyan.

Mariyan (Arabic) purity.
Mariyana, Mariyanna

Mariza (Latin) a form of Marisa.

Marja (Finnish) a form of Maria.
Marjae, Marjah, Marjatta, Marjatte, Marjie

Marjan (Persian) coral. (Polish) a form of Mary.
Marjana, Marjanah, Marjane, Marjaneh, Marjanna

Marjie (Scottish) a familiar form of Marjorie.
Marje, Marjey, Marji, Marjy

Marjolaine (French) marjoram.
Marjolain, Marjolaina, Marjolayn, Marjolayna, Marjolayne

Marjorie (Greek) a familiar form of Margaret. (Scottish) a form of Mary. See also Margery.
Marjarie, Marjary, Marjerie, Marjery, Marjie, Marjoree, Marjorey, Marjori, Marjory

Markayla (American) a combination of Mary + Kayla.
Marka, Markaiah, Markaya, Markayel, Markeela

Markeisha (English) a combination of Mary + Keisha.
Markasha, Markeesha, Markeisa, Markeisia, Markeysha, Markeyshia, Markeysia, Markiesha, Markieshia, Markiesia, Markysia, Markysiah, Markysya, Markysyah

Markell BG (Latin) a form of Mark (see Boys' Names).
Markel

Markelle (Latin) a form of Mark (see Boys' Names).

Markesha (English) a form of Markeisha.

Markeshia (English) a form of Markeisha.
Markesia, Markesiah

Marketa (Czech) a form of Markita.
Markete, Marketta, Markette

Marki (Latin) a form of Markie.

Markia (Latin) a form of Markie.

Markie (Latin) martial, warlike.
Marka, Marke, Markeah, Markee, Markey, Marky, Marquee, Marquey, Marqui, Marquie, Marquy

Markisha (English) a form of Markeisha.
Markishia, Markisia

Markita (Czech) a form of Margaret.
Markeata, Markeatah, Markeda, Markeeda, Markeeta, Markieta, Markitah, Markitha, Markketta, Markkette, Markkyt, Markkyta, Markyttah, Merkate

Marla (English) a short form of Marlena, Marlene.
Marlah

Marlaina (English) a form of Marlena.
Marlainna

Marlana (English) a form of Marlena.
Marlanah, Marlania, Marlanna

Marlayna (English) a form of Marlena.

Marlee, Marleigh, Marlie, Marly (English) forms of Marlene.
Marlea, Marleah, Marli

Marleen (Greek, Slavic) a form of Marlene.
Marleene

Marlen (Greek, Slavic) a form of Marlene. See also Marlyn.
Marlenne, Marline

Marlena (German) a form of Marlene.
Marlaena, Marleana, Marleanah, Marleena, Marleenah, Marleina, Marlyna, Marlynah

Marlene (Greek) high tower. (Slavic) a form of Magdalen.
Marlaine, Marlane, Marlayne, Marlean, Marlein, Marleine

Marleny (Greek, Slavic) a familiar form of Marlene.
Marleni, Marlenie

Marley GB (English) a form of Marlene.

Marlin BG (Greek, Slavic) a form of Marlene.

Marlina (Greek, Slavic) a form of Marlena.
Marlinah, Marlinda

Marlis (English) a short form of Marlisa.
Marles, Marlise, Marliss, Marlisse, Marlys, Marlyse, Marlyss, Marlysse

Marlisa (English) a combination of Maria + Lisa.
Marlissa, Marlysa, Marlyssa

Marlo BG (English) a form of Mary.
Marlon, Marlona, Marlonah, Marlone, Marlow, Marlowe

Marlyn (Hebrew) a short form of Marilyn. (Greek, Slavic) a form of Marlene. See also Marlen.
Marlyne, Marlynn, Marlynne

Marmara (Greek) sparkling, shining.
Marmarah, Marmee

Marni, Marnie (Hebrew) short forms of Marnina.
Marna, Marnah, Marnay, Marne, Marnea, Marnee, Marney, Marnia, Marniah, Marnique, Marnja, Marny, Marnya, Marnyah, Marnye

Marnina (Hebrew) rejoice.
Marneena, Marneenah, Marninah, Marnyna

Marnisha (Hebrew) a form of Marnina.

Maroula (Greek) a form of Mary.
Maroulah, Maroulla, Maroullah

Marquesa (Spanish) she who works with a hammer.

Marquesha (American) a form of Markeisha.

Marquetta (Spanish) a form of Marcia.
Marquet, Marqueta, Marquete, Marquette

Marquilla (Spanish) bitter.

Marquis BG (French) a form of Marquise.

Marquise BG (French) noblewoman.
Makeese, Markese, Marquees, Marquese, Marquice, Marquies, Marquiese, Marquisa, Marquisee, Marquisse, Marquiste, Marquyse

Marquisha (American) a form of Marquise.
Marquiesha, Marquisia

Marquita, Marquitta (Spanish) forms of Marcia.
Marquatte, Marqueda, Marquedia, Marquee, Marqueeda, Marqueita, Marqueite, Marquia, Marquida, Marquietta, Marquiette, Marquite, Marquitia, Marquitra, Marquyta, Marquytah, Marquyte, Marquytta, Marquyttah, Marquyte

Marrisa, Marrissa (Latin) forms of Marisa.
Marrisah, Marrissia

Marsala (Italian) from Marseilles, France.
Marsal, Marsali, Marsalla, Marsallah, Marseilles, Marsela, Marselah, Marsella, Marsellah, Marselle

Marsha (English) a form of Marcia.
Marcha, Marchah, Marchia, Marchya, Marchyah, Marshah, Marshel, Marshele, Marshell, Marshelle, Marshia, Marshiah, Marshiela, Marshya, Marshyah

Marshae, Marshay (English) forms of Marsha.

Marta (English) a short form of Martha, Martina.
Martá, Martä, Martah, Marte, Marttaha, Merta, Merte

Martha (Aramaic) lady; sorrowful. Bible: a friend of Jesus. See also Mardi.
Martaha, Marth, Marthan, Marthe, Marthy, Marticka, Martita, Martus, Martuska, Masia

Marti GB (English) a familiar form of Martha, Martina.
Martie

Martia (Latin) a form of Marcia.
Martiah

Martina (Latin) martial, warlike. See also Tina.
Martaina, Martainah, Martana, Martanah, Martanna, Martannah, Martayna, Martaynah, Marteana, Marteanah, Marteena, Marteenah, Martella, Marthena, Marthina, Martinah, Martinia, Martino, Martosia, Martoya, Martricia, Martrina, Martyna, Martynah

Martine (Latin) a form of Martina.
Martain, Martaine, Martane, Martanne, Martayn, Martayne, Martean, Marteane, Marteen, Marteene, Martel, Martelle, Martene, Marthine, Martyn, Martyne, Martynne

Martiniana (Latin) a form of Martina.

Martirio (Spanish) martyrdom.

Martisha (Latin) a form of Martina.

Martiza (Arabic) blessed.
Martisa, Martisah, Martizah, Martysa, Martysah, Martyza, Martyzah

Marty BG (English) a familiar form of Martha, Martina.

Maru (Japanese) round.
Maroo

Maruca (Spanish) a form of Mary.
Mariucca, Maruja, Maruka

Maruska, Marusya (Russian) tart.

Marva (Hebrew) sweet sage.
Marvah

Marvella (French) marvelous.
Marvel, Marvela, Marvele, Marvell, Marvellah, Marvelle, Marvely, Marvetta, Marvette, Marvia, Marvil, Marvila, Marvile, Marvill, Marvilla, Marville, Marvyl, Marvyla, Marvyle, Marvyll, Marvylla, Marvylle

Marvina (English) lover of the sea.
Marvinah, Marvinia, Marviniah, Marvyna, Marvynah, Marvynia, Marvyniah, Marvynya, Marvynyah

Mary ✳ (Hebrew) bitter; sea of bitterness. Bible: the mother of Jesus. See also Maija, Malia, Maren, Mariah, Marjorie, Maura,

Maureen, Miriam, Mitzi, Moira, Molly, Muriel.
Maeree, Maerey, Maeri, Maerie, Maery, Maree, Marella, Marelle, Maricara, Mariquilla, Mariquita, Marrey, Marry, Marye, Maryla, Marynia, Mavra, Meridel, Mirja, Morag, Moya

Mary Ann, Maryan, Maryann, Maryanne
(English) combinations of Mary + Ann.
Marryann, Mary Anne, Mary-Ann, Mary-Anne, Maryane, Maryen, Maryena, Maryene, Maryenn, Maryenna, Maryenne, Meryen

Mary Beth, Marybeth (American) combinations of Mary + Beth.
Mareabeth, Mareebeth

Mary Kate, Mary-Kate, Marykate
(American) combinations of Mary + Kate.

Mary Katherine (American) a combination of Mary + Katherine.
Mary Catherine, Mary Kathryn, Mary-Catherine, Mary-Katherine, Mary-Kathryn

Mary Margaret, Mary-Margaret
(American) combinations of Mary + Margaret.

Marya (Arabic) purity; bright whiteness.

Maryah (Arabic) a form of Marya.

Maryam (Hebrew) a form of Miriam.
Maryama

Marycarmen (American) a combination of Mary + Carmen.

Maryellen (American) a combination of Mary + Ellen.
Marielen, Mariellen, Mary Ellen, Mary-Ellen, Maryelen

Maryjane (American) a combination of Mary + Jane.
Mary Jane, Mary-Jane

Maryjo (American) a combination of Mary + Jo.
Mareajo, Mareejo, Marijo, Marijoe, Marijoh, Mary Jo, Mary-Jo, Maryjoe, Maryjoh

Marylene (Hebrew) a form of Marylin.
Marylina, Maryline

Marylin (Hebrew) a form of Marilyn.
Marylinn, Marylyn, Marylyna, Marylyne, Marylynn, Marylynne

Marylou (American) a combination of Mary + Lou.
Mareelou, Mareelu, Mary Lou, Marylu

Marysa, Maryse, Maryssa (Latin) forms of Marisa.
Marrysa, Marrysah, Marryssa, Marryssah, Marysia

Masada (Hebrew) strong foundation, support.
Masadah, Massada, Massadah

Masago (Japanese) sands of time.
Massago

Masani (Luganda) gap toothed.
Masanee, Masaney, Masania, Masaniah, Masanie, Masany, Masanya, Masanyah

Masha (Russian) a form of Mary.
Mascha, Mashah, Mashenka, Mashka

Mashika (Swahili) born during the rainy season.
Mashyka, Mashykah, Masika

Masiel (English) a form of Massiel.

Mason BG (Arabic) a form of Maysun.

Massiel (Hebrew) she who comes down from the stars.

Mastidia (Greek) whip.

Matahari (Indonesian) light of the day.

Matana (Hebrew) gift.
Matanah, Matania, Mataniah, Matanna, Matannah, Matannia, Matanniah, Matanya, Matanyah, Matat

Mathena (Hebrew) gift of God.
Mathenah

Mathieu BG (French) a form of Matthew.
Mathieux, Matthieu

Mathilde (German) a form of Matilda.
Mathild, Mathilda, Mathildis

Matilda (German) powerful battler. See also Maud, Tilda, Tillie.
Máda, Mafalda, Mahaut, Maitilde, Malkin, Mat, Matelda, Matilde, Matilly, Mattilda, Mattylda, Matusha, Matyld, Matylda, Matyldah, Matylde, Metild, Metilda, Metildah, Metilde, Metyld, Metylda, Metyldah, Metylde

Matrika (Hindi) mother. Religion: a name for the Hindu goddess Shakti in the form of the letters of the alphabet.
Matrica, Matricah, Matricka, Matrickah, Matryca, Matrycah, Matrycka, Matryckah, Matryka, Matrykah

Matrona (Latin) mother.

Matsuko (Japanese) pine tree.

Mattea (Hebrew) gift of God.
Matea, Mateah, Mathea, Matheah, Mathia, Mathiah, Matia, Matteah, Matthea, Matthia, Matthiah, Mattia, Mattya, Mattyah, Matya

Matthew BG (Hebrew) gift of God. Bible: author of the Gospel of Matthew.
Mathie, Mathiew, Matthiew, Mattieu, Mattieux

Mattie (English) a familiar form of Martha, Matilda.
Matte, Mattey, Matti, Mattye

Mattison BG (English) a form of Madison.

Matty BG (English) a familiar form of Martha, Matilda.

Matusha (Spanish) a form of Matilda.
Matuja, Matuxa

Matxalen (Basque) a form of Magdalena.

Maud, Maude (English) short forms of Madeline, Matilda. See also Madison.
Maudea, Maudee, Maudey, Maudi, Maudie, Maudine, Maudlin, Maudy

Mauli BG (Tongan) a New Zealander of Pacific Island descent, also known as a Maori.
Maulea, Mauleah, Maulee, Maulei, Mauleigh, Maulia, Mauliah, Maulie, Mauly

Maura (Irish) dark. A form of Mary, Maureen. See also Moira.
Maurah, Maure, Mauree, Maurette, Mauri, Mauricette, Maurie, Maurita, Mauritia, Maury, Maurya

Maureen (French) dark. (Irish) a form of Mary. See also Morena.
Maireen, Maireena, Maireene, Mairin, Mairina, Mairine, Maurena, Maurene, Maurina, Maurine, Mauritzia, Moureen

Maurelle (French) dark; elfin.
Mauriel, Mauriell, Maurielle

Maurise (French) dark skinned; moor; marshland.
Maurisse, Maurita, Maurizia, Mauriziah, Maurizya, Maurizyah, Mauryzya, Mauryzyah

Maurissa (French) a form of Maurise.
Maurisa, Maurisah, Maurisia, Maurisiah, Maurissah

Mausi (Native American) plucked flower.
Mausee, Mausie, Mausy

Mauve (French) violet colored.
Mauv

Maverick BG (American) independent.
Maveric, Maverik, Maveryc, Maveryck, Maveryk

Mavia (Irish) happy.
Maviah, Mavie, Mavya, Mavyah

Mavis (French) thrush, songbird. See also Maeve.
Mavas, Mavies, Mavin, Mavine, Maviss, Mavon, Mavos, Mavra, Mavus, Mavys

Maxie (English) a familiar form of Maxine.
Maxi, Maxy

Máxima, Máximina (Latin) forms of Maxine.

Maxime BG (Latin) a form of Maxine.
Maxima, Maximiliane

Maximiana (Spanish) a form of Máxima.

Maximiliana (Latin) eldest of all.

Maxine (Latin) greatest.
Max, Maxa, Maxeen, Maxeena, Maxeene, Maxena, Maxene, Maxina, Maxna, Maxyn, Maxyna, Maxyne, Mazeen, Mazeena, Mazeene, Mazin, Mazina, Mazine, Mazyn, Mazyna, Mazyne

May (Latin) great. (Arabic) discerning. (English) flower; month of May. See also Mae, Maia.
Maj, Mayberry, Maybeth, Mayday, Maydee, Maydena, Maye, Mayela, Mayella, Mayetta, Mayrene

Maya ⭐ (Hindi) God's creative power. (Greek) mother; grandmother. (Latin) great. A form of Maia.
Mayam, Mya

Mayah (Hindi, Greek, Latin) a form of Maya.

Maybeline (Latin) a familiar form of Mabel.
Maebelina, Maebeline, Maibelina, Maibeline, Maibelyna, Maibelyne, Maybelina, Maybelyna, Maybelyne

Maybell (Latin) a form of Mabel.
Maybel, Maybela, Maybele, Maybella, Maybelle, Maybull, Mayebell, Mayebella, Mayebelle

Maycee (Scottish) a form of Maisey.
Maysee, Maysey, Maysi, Maysie, Maysy, Mayzie

Maygan, Maygen (Irish) forms of Megan.
Mayghan, Maygon

Maylyn (American) a combination of May + Lynn.
Mayelene, Mayleen, Maylen, Maylene, Maylin, Maylon, Maylynn, Maylynne

Mayola (Latin) a form of May.

Mayoree (Tai) beautiful.
Mayaria, Mayariah, Mayariya, Mayarya, Mayaryah, Mayree

Mayra (Australian) spring wind. (Tai) a form of Mayoree.
Mayrah

Maysa (Arabic) walks with a proud stride.

Maysun (Arabic) beautiful.
Maesun, Maisun, Mayson

Mayte (Spanish) a form of Maite.

Mazel (Hebrew) lucky.
Mazal, Mazala, Mazalah, Mazela, Mazella, Mazelle

Mc Kenna, Mckena (American) forms of Mackenna.
Mckennah, Mckinna, Mckinnah

Mc Kenzie, McKenzie BG (Irish) forms of Mackenzie.
Mckennzie, Mckensee, Mckensi, McKensi, Mckensy, Mckenze, McKenzee, Mckenzey, McKenzey, McKenzi, McKenzy, Mckenzye

Mckaela (American) a form of Michaela.

Mckaila (American) a form of Michaela.

Mckala (American) a form of Michaela.

Mckayla (American) a form of Michaela.
Mckaylah, Mckayle, Mckayleh

Mckaylee (American) a form of Michaela.
Mckayleigh, Mckayli, Mckaylia, Mckaylie

Mckell (American) a form of Makell.
Mckelle

Mckenna GB (American) a form of Mackenna.

Mckenzie GB (Irish) a form of Mackenzie.

Mckinley BG (Scottish) child of the learned ruler.
Mckinlee, Mckinleigh, Mckinlie, Mckinnley

Mckinzie (American) a form of Mackenzie.
Mckinsey, Mckinze, Mckinzea, Mckinzee, Mckinzi, Mckinzy, Mckynze, Mckynzie

Mead BG (Greek) honey wine.
Meada, Meadah, Meed, Meede

Meade (Greek) honey wine.

Meadow (English) meadow.

Meagan, Meagen (Irish) forms of Megan.
Meagain, Meagann, Meagin, Meagnah, Meagon

Meaghan (Welsh) a form of Megan.
Meaghann, Meaghen, Meaghin, Meaghon, Meaghyn, Meahgan

Meara (Irish) mirthful.
Mearah, Mearia, Meariah, Mearya, Mearyah

Mecatl (Nahuatl) rope; lineage.

Mecha (Latin) a form of Mercedes.

Mechelle (French) a form of Michelle.

Meda (Native American) prophet; priestess.
Medah

Medea (Greek) ruling. (Latin) middle. Mythology: a sorceress who helped Jason get the Golden Fleece.
Medeah, Medeia, Media, Mediah, Medya, Medyah

Medina (Arabic) History: the site of Muhammad's tomb.
Medeana, Medeanah, Medeena, Medeenah, Medinah, Medyna, Medynah

Medora (Greek) mother's gift. Literature: a character in Lord Byron's poem *The Corsair.*
Medorah

Meena (Hindi) blue semiprecious stone; bird. (Greek, German, Dutch) a form of Mena.
Meenah

Meera (Hebrew) a form of Meira.
Meerah

Meg (English) a short form of Margaret, Megan.
Megg

Megan ★ GB (Greek) pearl; great. (Irish) a form of Margaret.
Magana, Meegen, Meeghan, Meeghen, Meeghin, Meeghon, Meeghyn, Meegin, Meegon, Meegyn, Meganna, Megin, Megon, Megyn, Meigan, Meigen, Meigin, Meigon, Meigyn, Meygan, Meygen, Meygin, Meygon, Meygyn

Megane, Megann, Meganne, Megen, Meggan (Irish) forms of Megan.
Meggen

Megara (Greek) first. Mythology: Heracles's first wife.

Megean (American) a form of Megan.

Meggie, Meggy (English) familiar forms of Margaret, Megan.
Meggi

Megha (Welsh) a short form of Meghan.

Meghan, Meghann (Welsh) forms of Megan.
Meehan, Meghana, Meghane, Meghanne, Meghean, Meghen, Meghon, Meghyn, Mehgan, Mehgen

Mehadi (Hindi) flower.
Mehadee, Mehadie, Mehady

Mehira (Hebrew) speedy; energetic.
Mahira, Mahirah, Mehirah, Mehyra, Mehyrah

Mehitabel (Hebrew) benefited by trusting God.
Hetty, Hitty, Mehetabel, Mehitabelle

Mehri (Persian) kind; lovable; sunny.
Mehree, Mehrie, Mehry

Mei (Hawaiian) great. (Chinese) a short form of Meiying.
Meiko

Meira (Hebrew) light.
Meirah, Mera, Meyra, Meyrah

Meit (Burmese) affectionate.
Meita, Meyt, Meytah

Meiying (Chinese) beautiful flower.
Mei

Mejorana (Spanish) marjoram.
Mejoranah, Mejoranna, Mejorannah

Meka GB (Hebrew) a familiar form of Michaela.
Mekah

Mekayla (American) a form of Michaela.
Mekaela, Mekaila, Mekala, Mekayela, Mekaylia

Mekenzie (American) a form of Mackenzie.
Mekensie, Mekenzi

Mel BG (Portuguese, Spanish) sweet as honey.
Mell

Mela (Hindi) religious service. (Polish) a form of Melanie.
Melah, Mella, Mellah

Melaida (Spanish) a form of Melissa.

Melaina (Latin, Greek) a form of Melina.
Melainah

Melana (Russian) a form of Melanie.
Melanna, Melena, Melenah

Melaney, Melani, Melannie, Melany (Greek) forms of Melanie.
Melanney, Melanya

Melanie ★ (Greek) dark skinned.
Meila, Meilani, Meilin, Melaine, Melainie, Melane, Melanee, Melania, Mélanie, Melanka, Melasya, Melayne, Melenee, Meleney, Meleni, Melenia, Melenie, Meleny, Mellanee, Mellaney, Mellani, Mellanie, Mellany, Mellenee, Melleney, Melleni, Mellenie, Melleny, Melya, Milya

Melantha (Greek) dark flower.
Melanthe

Melba (Greek) soft; slender. (Latin) mallow flower.
Malba, Malbah, Melbah, Melva, Melvah

Mele (Hawaiian) song; poem.
Melle

Melea, Meleah (German) forms of Melia.

Melecent (English) a form of Millicent.
Melacent, Melacenta, Melacente, Melacint, Melacinte, Melecenta, Melecente, Melecint, Melecinta, Melecinte

Melecia (Greek) studious woman.

Meleni (Tongan) melon.
Melenee, Meleney, Melenia, Meleniah, Meleny, Melenya, Melenyah

Melesse (Ethiopian) eternal.
Mellesse

Melia (German) a short form of Amelia.
Melcia, Meleia, Meleisha, Meli, Meliah, Melida, Melika, Melya, Melyah, Mema, Mylia, Myliah, Mylya, Mylyah

Melibea (Greek) she who takes care of the oxen.

Melicent (English) a form of Millicent.
Meliscent, Melisent, Melissent, Mellicent, Mellisent, Melycent, Melycente, Melycint, Melycinta, Melycinte, Melycynt, Melycynta, Melycynte

Melina (Latin) canary yellow. (Greek) a short form of Melinda.
Meleana, Meleanah, Meleane, Meleena, Melena, Melenah, Meline, Melinia, Meliniah, Melinna, Melinnah, Melinne

Melinda (Greek) honey. See also Linda, Melina, Mindi.
Maillie, Melindah, Melinde, Melindee, Melinder, Melindia, Melindiah, Mellinda, Milinda, Milynda, Mylenda, Mylinda, Mylynda

Meliora (Latin) better.
Melior, Meliori, Melioria, Meliorie, Mellear, Mellor, Mellora, Mellorah, Melyor, Melyora, Melyorah

Melisa, Mellisa, Mellissa (Greek) forms of Melissa.
Melisah, Mellissah

Melisande (French) a form of Melissa, Millicent.
Lisandra, Malisande, Malissande, Malyssandre, Melesande, Melicend, Melisanda, Melisandra, Melisandre, Mélisandré, Melisenda, Melisende, Melissande, Melissandre, Mellisande, Melond, Melysanda, Melysande, Melyssandre

Melissa ⭐ (Greek) honey bee. See also Elissa, Lissa, Melisande, Millicent.
Malessa, Melesa, Melessa, Melessah, Mélisa, Melise, Melisha, Melishia, Melisia, Mélissa, Melissah, Melisse, Melissia, Meliza, Melizah, Milissa, Molissia, Mollissa

Melita (Greek) a form of Melissa. (Spanish) a short form of Carmelita.
Malita, Meleata, Meleatah, Meleatta, Meleattah, Meleeta, Meleetah, Meleetta, Meleettah, Meleta, Melitah, Melitta, Melittah, Melitza, Melletta, Melyta, Melytah, Melytta, Melyttah, Molita

Melitina (Latin) a form of Melinda.

Melitona (Greek) she who was born in Malta.

Melly (American) a familiar form of names beginning with "Mel." See also Millie.
Meli, Melie, Melli, Mellie

Melodía (Greek) a form of Melody.

Melodie (Greek) a form of Melody.

Melody (Greek) melody. See also Elodie.
Meladia, Meloda, Melodah, Melodea, Melodee, Melodey, Melodi, Melodia, Melodiah, Melodya, Melodyah, Melodyann, Melodye

Melonie (American) a form of Melanie.
Melloney, Mellonie, Mellony, Melona, Melonah, Melone, Melonee, Meloney, Meloni, Melonia, Meloniah, Melonnie, Melony, Melonya, Melonyah

Melosa (Spanish) sweet; tender.
Malosa, Malosah, Malossa, Malossah, Mellosa, Mellosah, Melosah, Melossa, Melossah

Melosia (Spanish) sweet.

Melrose (American) a combination of Melanie + Rose.
Melrosa, Melrosah

Melusina (Greek) a form of Melissa.

Melvina (Irish) armored chief. See also Malvina.
Melevine, Melva, Melveen, Melveena, Melveenah, Melveene, Melveenia, Melvena, Melvene, Melvinda, Melvine, Melvinia, Melviniah, Melvonna, Melvyna, Melvynah, Melvyne, Melvynia, Melvyniah, Melvynya, Melvynyah

Melyna (Latin, Greek) a form of Melina.
Melynah, Melynna, Melynnah

Melynda (Greek) a form of Melinda.
Melyndah, Melyne

Melyne (Greek) a short form of Melinda.
Melyn, Melynn, Melynne

Melyssa (Greek) a form of Melissa.
Melysa, Melysah, Melyssah, Melysse

Mena (German, Dutch) strong. (Greek) a short form of Philomena. History: Menes is believed to be the first king of Egypt. See also Mina.
Meana, Meanah, Meina, Meinah, Menah, Meyna, Meynah

Mendi (Basque) a form of Mary.
Menda, Mendy

Menodora (Greek) gift of Mene, the moon goddess.

Menora (Hebrew) candleholder. Religion: a menorah is a special nine-branched candleholder used during the holiday of Hanukkah.
Menorah, Minora, Minorah, Mynora, Mynorah

Meranda, Merranda (Latin) forms of Miranda.
Merana, Merandah, Merandia, Merannda

Mérane (French) a form of Mary.
Meraine, Merrane

Mercades (Latin, Spanish) a form of Mercedes.
Mercadez, Mercadie

Mercé (Spanish) a short form of Mercedes.

Mercede (Latin, Spanish) a form of Mercedes.
Merced, Merceda, Mersade

Mercedes (Latin) reward, payment. (Spanish) merciful.
Meceades, Mercedeas, Mercedees, Mercedies, Mercedis, Mersades

Mercedez (Latin, Spanish) a form of Mercedes.
Mercedeez

Merces (Latin) mercies.

Mercia (English) a form of Marcia. History: an ancient British kingdom.

Mercilla (English) a form of Mercy.
Mercillah, Mercille, Mersilla, Mersillah, Mersille

Mercuria (Greek) refers to the Greek god Mercury.

Mercy (English) compassionate, merciful. See also Merry.
Merce, Mercee, Mercey, Merci, Mercia, Merciah, Mercie, Mercina, Mercinah, Mercya, Mercyah, Mersee, Mersey, Mersi, Mersie, Mersina, Mersinah, Mersy

Meredith GB (Welsh) protector of the sea.
Meredeth, Meredif, Merediff, Meredithe, Meredy, Meredyth, Meredythe, Merrydith, Merrydithe, Merrydyth

Meri (Finnish) sea. (Irish) a short form of Meriel.
Meree, Merey, Merie, Mery

Meria (African) rebellious.

Meriah (Hebrew) a form of Mariah. (African) a form of Meria.

Meridith (Welsh) a form of Meredith.
Meridath, Merideth, Meridie, Meridithe, Meridyth, Merridie, Merridith, Merridithe, Merridyth

Meriel (Irish) shining sea.
Merial, Meriele, Meriella, Merielle, Meriol, Merrial, Merriel, Meryel, Meryela, Meryelah, Meryell, Meryella, Meryellah, Meryelle

Merilyn (English) a combination of Merry + Lynn. See also Marilyn.
Meralin, Meralina, Meraline, Meralyn, Meralyna, Meralyne, Merelan, Merelen, Merelin, Merelina, Mereline, Merelyn, Merelyna, Merelyne, Merilan, Merilen, Merilin, Merilina, Meriline, Merilyna, Merilyne, Merlyn, Merralin, Merralyn, Merrelina, Merreline, Merrelyn, Merrelynn, Merrillin, Merrillina, Merrilline, Merrilyn, Merrilynn, Merrylyn, Merrylyna, Merrylyne, Merylin, Merylina, Meryline, Merylyn, Merylyna, Merylyne

Merina (Latin) a form of Marina. (Australian) a form of Merrina.
Merinah

Merinda (Australian) beautiful.
Merindah, Merynda, Meryndah

Merisa, Merissa (Latin) forms of Marisa.
Merisah, Merisha, Merissah, Merrisa, Merrisah, Merrissa, Merrissah, Merrysa, Merrysah, Merryssa, Merryssah

Merite (Latin) deserving.
Merita, Meritah, Meritta, Merittah, Meritte, Merrita, Meryta, Merytah, Merytta

Merle BG (Latin, French) blackbird.
Mearl, Mearla, Mearle, Merl, Merla, Merlina, Merline, Merola, Murle, Myrl, Myrle, Myrleen, Myrlene, Myrline

Merpati (Indonesian) dove.
Merpatee, Merpatie, Merpaty

Merrilee (American) a combination of Merry + Lee. See also Marilee.
Merrilei, Merrileigh, Merriley, Merrili, Merrily, Merrylea, Merryleah, Merrylee, Merrylei, Merryleigh, Merryley, Merryli, Merrylia, Merrylie, Merryly, Merylea, Meryleah, Merylee, Merylei, Meryleigh, Meryley, Meryli, Merylie, Meryly

Merrina (Australian) grass seed.
Meriwa, Meriwah, Merrinah, Merriwa, Merriwah, Merryna, Merrynah, Merrywa, Merrywah, Meryn, Meryna, Merynah

Merritt BG (Latin) a form of Merite.
Merit, Meritt, Meryt, Meryte, Merytt, Merytte

Merry (English) cheerful, happy. A familiar form of Mercy, Meredith.
Merree, Merri, Merrie, Merrielle, Mery

Mertysa (English) famous.

Merudina (German) famous, notable.

Meruvina (German) famous victory.

Meryl (German) famous. (Irish) shining sea. A form of Meriel, Muriel.
Maral, Marel, Meral, Merel, Merelle, Merill, Merrall, Merrel, Merrell, Merrelle, Merril, Merrile, Merrill, Merryl, Meryle, Meryll, Mirel, Mirell, Mirelle, Mirle, Myral, Myrel, Myrelle, Myril, Myrila, Myrile, Myryl, Myryla, Myryle

Mesalina (Italian) History: Messalina was a Roman empress.

Mesha (Hindi) another name for the zodiac sign Aries.
Meshah, Meshai, Meshal

Mesi (Egyptian) water.

Meskhenet (Egyptian) destiny.

Messalina (Latin) she who has an insatiable appetite.

Messina (Latin) middle child. (African) spoiler.
Mesina, Mesinah, Messinah, Messyna, Messynah, Mesyna, Mesynah

Meta (German) a short form of Margaret.
Metah, Metta, Mettah, Mette, Metti

Metodia (Greek) methodical woman.

Metrodora (Greek) gift of the city.

Meztli (Nahuatl) moon.

Mhairie (Scottish) a form of Mary.
Mhaire, Mhairee, Mhairey, Mhairi, Mhairy, Mhari, Mhary

Mia ⭐ (Italian) mine. A familiar form of Michaela, Michelle.
Mea, Meah

Mía (Spanish) a form of Maria.

Miah (Italian) a form of Mia.

Mica (Hebrew) a form of Micah.

Micaela (Hebrew) a form of Michaela.
Micaelah, Micaele, Micaella, Miceala, Mycael, Mycaela, Mycaelah, Mycaele, Mycala, Mycalah, Mycale

Micah BG (Hebrew) a form of Michael. Bible: one of the Old Testament prophets.
Meecah

Micaiah BG (Hebrew) a form of Micah.

Micaila (Hebrew) a form of Michaela.

Micala (Hebrew) a form of Michaela.
Micalah

Micayla (Hebrew) a form of Michaela.
Micayle, Micaylee

Micha GB (Hebrew) a form of Micah.

Michael BG (Hebrew) who is like God?
Michaelann, Michaell, Michaelle, Michaelyn

Michaela, Michaella (Hebrew) forms of Michael.

Michaila (Hebrew) a form of Michaela.

Michal BG (Hebrew) a form of Michael. (Italian) a form of Michele.

Michala, Michalla (Hebrew) forms of Michaela.
Michalah, Michalann, Michale, Michalene, Michalin, Michalina, Michalisha, Michalle

Michayla (Hebrew) a form of Michaela.
Michaylah, Michayle. Micheyla

Micheala (Hebrew) a form of Michaela.
Michealia

Michel BG (Italian) a form of Michele. (French) a form of Michelle.

Michela (Hebrew) a form of Michala. (Italian) a form of Michele.
Michelia, Michely, Michelyn

Michele GB (Italian) a form of Michelle.

Michelina (Italian) a form of Michaela.
Michaelina, Michalina, Mychelina

Micheline (Italian) a form of Michelina.
Michaeline, Michaline, Michellene, Mycheline

Michell (Italian) a form of Michelle.

Michelle ☀ (French) who is like God? See also Shelley.
Machealle, Machele, Machell, Machella, Machelle, Meichelle, Meschell, Meshell, Meshelle, Michaelle, Michéle, Michella, Michellah, Michellyn, Mischel, Mischelle, Mishael, Mishaela, Mishayla, Mishel, Mishele, Mishell, Mishella, Mishellah, Mishelle, Mitchele, Mitchelle, Mychel, Mychele, Mychell, Mychella, Mychelle, Myshel, Myshele, Myshell, Myshella, Myshellah, Myshelle

Michi (Japanese) righteous way.
Miche, Michee, Michey, Michie, Michy

Michiko (Japanese) righteous child.

Mickaela (Hebrew) a form of Michaela.
Mickael

Mickala (Hebrew) a form of Michaela.
Mickalla

Mickayla (Hebrew) a form of Michaela.
Mickeel, Mickell, Mickelle

Mickenzie GB (American) a form of Mackenzie.
Mickensie, Mickenzee, Mickenzi, Mickenzy

Micki (American) a familiar form of Michaela.
Mickee, Mickeeya, Mickia, Mickie, Micky, Mickya, Miquia

Micol, Milca, Milcal (Hebrew) she who is queen.

Midori (Japanese) green.
Madorea, Madoree, Madorey, Madori, Madorie, Madory, Midorea, Midoree, Midorey, Midorie, Midory, Mydorea, Mydoree, Mydorey, Mydori, Mydorie, Mydory

Mieko (Japanese) prosperous.
Mieke, Myeko

Mielikki (Finnish) pleasing.

Miette (French) small; sweet.
Mieta, Mietah, Mietta, Miettah, Myeta, Myetah, Myett, Myetta, Myettah, Myette

Migdana (Hebrew) present.
Migdanna, Migdannah, Mygdana, Mygdanah

Migina (Omaha) new moon.
Migeana, Migeanah, Migeena, Migeenah, Miginah, Migyna, Migynah, Mygeana, Mygeanah, Mygeena, Mygeenah, Mygina, Myginah, Mygyna, Mygynah

Mignon (French) dainty, petite; graceful.
Mignona, Mignone, Minyonne, Mygnona, Mygnonah, Mygnone

Mignonette (French) flower.
Mignonetta, Mignonettah, Minnionette, Minnonette, Minyonette, Mygnonetta, Mygnonette

Miguela (Spanish) a form of Michaela.
Micquel, Miguelina, Miguelita

Mika GB (Japanese) new moon. (Russian) God's child. (Native American) wise raccoon. (Hebrew) a form of Micah. (Latin) a form of Dominica.

Mikaela (Hebrew) a form of Michaela.
Mikael, Mikaelah, Mikail, Mikalene,
Mikalovna, Mikalyn, Mikea, Mikeisha,
Mikeita, Mikeya, Mikiala, Mikiela, Mikkel

Mikah BG (Hebrew, Japanese, Russian,
Native American) a form of Mika.

Mikaila (American) a form of Michaela.

Mikal BG (Hebrew) a short form of
Michael, Michaela.

Mikala, Mikalah (Hebrew) forms of
Michaela.
Mikale, Mikalea, Mikalee, Mikaleh

Mikayla (American) a form of Michaela.
Mikayle

Mikel BG (Hebrew) a short form of
Michael, Michaela.

Mikela (Hebrew) a form of Michaela.
Mikele, Mikell, Mikella

Mikelena (Danish) a form of Michaela.
Mykelena

Mikelle (Hebrew) a short form of Michael,
Michaela.

Mikenna (American) a form of Mackenna.
Mikena, Mikenah, Mikennah

Mikenzie (American) a form of Mackenzie.
Mikenzee, Mikenzi, Mikenzy

Mikesha (American) a form of Michaela.

Mikhaela (American) a form of Michaela.
Mikhalea, Mikhelle

Mikhaila (American) a form of Michaela.
Mikhail

Mikhala (American) a form of Michaela.

Mikhayla (American) a form of Michaela.

Miki GB (Japanese) flower stem.
Mikee, Mikey, Mikie, Mikita, Mikiyo, Mikko,
Miko, Miky

Mikia (Japanese) a form of Miki.
Mikkia, Mikkiya

Mikka (Hebrew, Japanese, Russian, Native
American) a form of Mika.

Mikki (Japanese) a form of Miki.
Mikkie

Mikyla (American) a form of Michaela.

Mila (Russian) dear one. (Italian, Slavic) a
short form of Camila, Ludmilla.
Milah, Milla, Millah, Myla

Milada (Czech) my love.
Miladah, Miladi, Miladie, Milady, Mylada,
Myladah, Myladi, Myladie, Mylady

Milagres (Latin) a form of Milagros.

Milagros (Spanish) miracle.
Milagritos, Milagro, Milagrosa, Milrari,
Milrarie

Milan BG (Italian) from Milan, Italy.
Milane, Milanne

Milana (Italian) from Milan, Italy. (Russian)
a form of Melana.
Milani, Milania, Milanie, Milanka, Milanna

Milba, Milva (German) kind protector.

Milburga, Milburgues (German) pleasant
city.

Mildereda, Mildreda (German) forms of
Mildred.

Mildred (English) gentle counselor.
Mil, Milda, Mildrene, Mildrid, Mylda,
Myldred, Myldreda

Milena (Greek, Hebrew, Russian) a form of
Ludmilla, Magdalen, Melanie.
Milenah, Milène, Milenia, Milenny, Milini,
Millini, Mylena, Mylenah

Milenka (Russian) my small one.

Mileta (German) generous, merciful.
Miletah, Milett, Miletta, Milette, Milita,
Militah, Myleta, Myletah, Mylita, Mylitah,
Mylyta, Mylytah

Milgita (German) pleasant woman.

Milia (German) industrious. A short form of
Amelia, Emily.
Milea, Mileah, Miliah, Millea, Milleah,
Millia, Milliah, Millya, Milya, Milyah, Mylea,
Myleah, Mylia, Myliah, Myllia, Mylliah,
Myllya, Myllyah, Mylya, Mylyah

Miliani (Hawaiian) caress.
Milanni, Miliany, Milliani

Mililani BG (Hawaiian) heavenly caress.
Mililanee, Mililaney, Mililanie, Mililany,
Millilani, Mylilanee, Mylilaney, Mylilani,
Mylilania, Mylilaniah, Mylilanie, Mylilany,
Mylylanee, Mylylaney, Mylylani, Mylylania,
Mylylanie

Milissa (Greek) a form of Melissa.
Milessa, Milisa, Milisah, Milissah, Millisa,
Millissa, Mylisa, Mylisah, Mylisia, Mylissa,
Mylissah, Mylissia, Mylysa, Mylysah,
Mylyssa, Mylyssah

Milka (Czech) a form of Amelia.
Milica, Milicah, Milika, Milikah, Milkah,
Mylka, Mylkah

Millaray (Mapuche) golden, fragrant flower.

Millicent (English) industrious. (Greek) a
form of Melissa. See also Lissa, Melisande.
Milicent, Milicenta, Milisent, Milissent,
Milliestone, Millisent, Millisenta, Milzie,
Myllicent, Myllicenta, Myllicente, Myllycent,
Myllycenta, Myllycente, Myllysent,
Myllysenta, Myllysente, Mylycent, Mylycenta,
Mylycente, Mylysent, Mylysenta, Mylysente

Millie, Milly (English) familiar forms of
Amelia, Camille, Emily, Kamila, Melissa,
Mildred, Millicent.
Milee, Milei, Mileigh, Miley, Mili, Milie,
Millee, Millei, Milleigh, Milley, Milli, Mylee,
Mylei, Myleigh, Myli, Mylie, Myllee, Myllei,
Mylleigh, Mylley, Mylli, Myllie, Mylly, Myly

Mima (Burmese) woman.
Mimah, Mimma, Mimmah, Myma, Mymah,
Mymma, Mymmah

Mimi (French) a familiar form of Miriam.
Mimea, Mimee, Mimey, Mimie, Mimmea,
Mimmee, Mimmey, Mimmi, Mimmie, Mimmy,
Mimy, Mymea, Mymee, Mymey, Mymi,
Mymie, Mymmea, Mymmee, Mymmey,
Mymmi, Mymmie, Mymmy, Mymy

Mina (German) love. (Persian) blue sky.
(Arabic) harbor. (Japanese) south. A short
form of names ending in "mina."
Min, Minah, Myna, Mynah

Minal (Native American) fruit.
Minala, Minalah, Mynala, Mynalah

Minda (Hindi) knowledge.
Mindah, Mynda, Myndah

Mindi, Mindy (Greek) familiar forms of
Melinda.
Mindea, Mindee, Mindey, Mindie, Mindyanne,
Mindylee, Myndea, Myndee, Myndey, Myndi,
Myndie, Myndy

Mine (Japanese) peak; mountain range.
Minee, Mineko, Miney, Mini, Myne, Mynee

Minerva (Latin) wise. Mythology: the god-
dess of wisdom.
Merva, Minervah, Minivera, Mynerva,
Mynervah

Minette (French) faithful defender.
Minetta, Minitta, Minitte, Minnette, Minnita,
Mynetta, Mynette, Mynnetta, Mynnette

Minia (German) great; strong.

Minikin (Dutch) dear, darling.
Minikina, Minikinah, Minikine, Minikyna,
Minikynah, Minikyne, Mynikin, Mynikina,
Mynikinah, Mynikine

Minka (Polish) a short form of Wilhelmina.
Minkah, Mynka, Mynkah

Minkie (Australian) daylight.
Minkee, Minkey, Minki, Minky, Mynkee,
Mynkey, Mynki, Mynkie, Mynky

Minna (German) a short form of
Wilhelmina.
Minnah, Minta, Mynna, Mynnah

Minnehaha (Native American) laughing
water; waterfall.
Minehaha, Mynehaha, Mynnehaha

Minnie (American) a familiar form of Mina,
Minerva, Minna, Wilhelmina.
Mini, Minie, Minne, Minnee, Minney, Minni,
Minny, Myni, Mynie, Mynnee, Mynney,
Mynni, Mynnie, Mynny, Myny

Minore (Australian) white blossom.
Minora, Minoree, Mynora, Mynorah, Mynoree

Minowa (Native American) singer.
Minowah, Mynowa, Mynowah

Minta (Latin) mint, minty.
Minnta, Minntah, Mintah, Minty, Mynnta,
Mynntah, Mynta, Myntah

Minya (Osage) older sister.

Mio (Japanese) three times as strong.
Myo

Mío (Spanish) mine.

Miquela (Spanish) a form of Michaela.
Miquel, Miquelah, Miquella, Miquelle

Mira (Latin) wonderful. (Spanish) look, gaze.
A short form of Almira, Amira, Marabel,
Mirabel, Miranda.
Mirae, Mirra

Mirabel (Latin) beautiful.
Mirabela, Mirabele, Mirabell, Mirabella,
Mirabellah, Mirabelle, Mirable, Myrabell,
Myrabella, Myrabellah, Myrabelle

Miracle GB (Latin) wonder, marvel.
Mirica, Miricah

Mirah (Latin, Spanish) a form of Mira.
Mirrah

Mirana (Spanish) a form of Miranda.

Miranda (Latin) strange; wonderful;
admirable. Literature: the heroine of
Shakespeare's *The Tempest*. See also
Randee.
Marenda, Miran, Miranada, Mirandah,
Mirandia, Mirinda, Mirindé, Mironda, Muranda

Mirari (Spanish) miracle.

Mireia (Spanish) a form of Mireya.

Mireille (Hebrew) God spoke. (Latin) won-
derful.
Mireil, Mirel, Mirela, Mirele, Mirelle, Mirelys,
Miriell, Miriella, Mirielle, Mirilla, Mirille,
Myrella, Myrelle, Myrilla, Myrille

Mirella (German, Irish) a form of Meryl.
(Hebrew, Latin) a form of Mireille.

Miren (Hebrew) bitter.

Mirena (Hawaiian) beloved.
Mirenah, Myrena, Myrenah

Mireya (Hebrew) a form of Mireille.
Mireea, Mireyda, Miryah

Miri (Gypsy) a short form of Miriam.
Myri, Myry

Miriah (Hebrew) a form of Mireille. (Gypsy)
a form of Miriam.
Miria

Miriam (Hebrew) bitter; sea of bitterness.
Bible: the original form of Mary. See also
Macia, Mimi, Mitzi.
Mairwen, Meriame, Miram, Mirham,
Miriama, Miriame, Mirit, Mirjam, Mirriam

Míriam (Hebrew) a form of Miriam.

Mirian (Hebrew) a form of Miriam.
Miriain, Mirjana, Mirrian, Miryan

Mirna (Irish) polite. (Slavic) peaceful.
Merna, Mernah, Mirnah

Mirranda (Latin) a form of Miranda.

Mirrin (Australian) cloud.
Mirrina, Mirrine, Mirryn, Mirryna, Myrrina,
Myrrinah, Myrrine, Myrryn, Myrryna,
Myrrynah, Myrryne, Myryna, Myrynah,
Myryne

Mirta, Mirtha (Greek) crown of myrtle.

Mirya (French) a form of Mira.

Miryam (Hebrew) a form of Miriam.

Misericordia (Spanish) mercy.

Misha GB (Russian) a form of Michaela.
Mischa, Mishae, Mishela

Missy (English) a familiar form of Melissa,
Millicent.
Mise, Misey, Misi, Misie, Missee, Missey,
Missi, Missie, Mysea, Mysee, Mysey, Mysi,
Mysie, Myssea, Myssee, Myssi, Myssie, Myssy,
Mysy

Misti, Mistie (English) forms of Misty.

Misty (English) shrouded by mist.
Missty, Mistea, Mistee, Mistey, Mistin,
Mistina, Mistral, Mistylynn, Mystea, Mystee,
Mystey, Mysti, Mystie, Mysty

Mitra (Hindi) Religion: god of daylight.
(Persian) angel.
Mita

Mituna (Moquelumnan) like a fish wrapped
up in leaves.

Mitzi, Mitzy (German) forms of Mary,
Miriam.
Mieze, Mitzee, Mitzey, Mitzie, Mytzee,
Mytzey, Mytzi, Mytzie, Mytzy

Miwa (Japanese) wise eyes.
Miwah, Miwako, Mywa, Mywah, Mywako

Mixcóatl (Nahuatl) serpent of the sky.

Miya (Japanese) temple.
Miyana, Miyanna

Miyah (Japanese) a form of Miya.

Miyaoaxochitl (Nahuatl) maize tassel
flower.

Miyo (Japanese) beautiful generation.
Myo

Miyoko (Japanese) beautiful generation's
child.
Miyuko, Myyoko

Miyuki (Japanese) snow.
Miyukee, Myyukee, Myyuki

Mizquixaual (Nahuatl) mesquite face paint.

Moana (Hawaiian) ocean; fragrance.
*Moanah, Moane, Moann, Moanna, Moannah,
Moanne*

Mocha (Arabic) chocolate-flavored coffee.
Mochah, Moka, Mokah

Modesta (Italian, Spanish) a form of
Modesty.
Modestah, Modestia

Modestine (French) a form of Modesty.
*Modesteen, Modesteena, Modesteene,
Modestina, Modestyn, Modestyna, Modestyne*

Modesty (Latin) modest.
*Modesta, Modeste, Modestee, Modestey,
Modestie, Modestine, Modestus*

Moema (Tupi) sweet.

Moesha (American) a short form of
Monisha.
Moeisha, Moeysha

Mohala (Hawaiian) flowers in bloom.
Moala, Mohalah

Mohini (Sanskrit) enchantress.
*Mohinee, Mohiney, Mohinie, Mohiny, Mohynee,
Mohyney, Mohyni, Mohynie, Mohyny*

Moira (Irish) great. A form of Mary. See also
Maura.
*Moirae, Moirah, Moire, Mouira, Moya, Moyra,
Moyrah*

Molara (Basque) a form of Mary.
Molarah, Molarra, Molarrah

Moledina (Australian) creek.
*Moledin, Moledinah, Moledine, Moledyn,
Moledyna, Moledynah, Moledyne*

Moli (Tongan) orange.
*Molea, Molee, Molei, Moleigh, Moley, Molie,
Moly*

Molli, Mollie (Irish) forms of Molly.

Molly ☀ (Irish) a familiar form of Mary.
Moll, Mollea, Mollee, Mollei, Molleigh, Molley

Momoztli (Nahuatl) altar.

Mona GB (Irish) noble. (Greek) a short form
of Monica, Ramona, Rimona.
*Moina, Moinah, Monah, Mone, Monea,
Monna, Monnah, Moyna, Moynah*

Monae (American) a form of Monet.

Monegunda (German) overprotective.

Moneisha (American) a form of Monisha.

Monesa (German) protection.

Monet (French) Art: Claude Monet was a
leading French impressionist remembered
for his paintings of water lilies.
Monay, Monaye, Monee

Monica (Greek) solitary. (Latin) advisor.
*Monca, Moneeca, Moneecah, Monia, Monic,
Monicah, Monice, Monicia, Monicka, Monise,
Monn, Monnica, Monnicah, Monnicka,
Monnie, Monnyca, Monya, Monyca, Monycah,
Monycka*

Mónica (Greek) a form of Monica.

Monifa (Yoruba) I have my luck.
Monifah, Monyfa, Monyfah

Monika (German) a form of Monica.
*Moneeka, Moneekah, Moneeke, Moneik,
Moneka, Monieka, Monikah, Monike,
Monnika, Monnikah, Monnyka, Monyka,
Monykah*

Moniqua (French) a form of Monica.
Moniquea, Monniqua

Monique (French) a form of Monica.
Moniquie, Monnique, Monyque, Munique

Monisha (American) a combination of Monica + Aisha.
Monesha, Monishia

Monita (Spanish) noble.

Monserrat (Catalan) serrated mountain.

Montana GB (Spanish) mountain. Geography: a U.S. state.
Montanah, Montania, Montaniah, Montanna, Montannah, Monteen, Monteena, Monteenah, Montina, Montinah, Montyna, Montynah

Monteen (French) a form of Montana.
Monteene, Montine, Montyn, Montyne

Montgomery BG (English) rich man's mountain.
Montgomerie, Mountgomery

Monti (Spanish) a familiar form of Montana. (English) a short form of Montgomery.
Monte, Montea, Montey, Montia, Montie, Monty

Moona (English) moon. (Australian) plenty.
Moonah, Moone, Moonee, Mooney, Mooni, Moonia, Mooniah, Moonie, Moony, Moonya, Moonyah

Mora (Spanish) blueberry.
Morae, Morah, Morea, Moreah, Moria, Morita, Morite, Moryta, Morytah, Moryte

Moraima (Latin) she who is beautiful as the blueberry tree.

Moree (Australian) water.
Morey, Mori, Morie, Mory

Morela (Polish) apricot.
Morelah, Morelia, Morell, Morella, Morellah, Morelle

Morena (Irish) a form of Maureen.
Mo, Mooreen, Mooreena, Mooreenah, Mooreene, Morain, Moraina, Morainah, Moraine, Morayn, Morayna, Moraynah, Morayne, Moreen, Moreena, Moreenah, Moreene, Morein, Moreina, Moreinah, Moreine, Moren, Morenah, Morene, Morin, Morina, Morinah, Morine, Morreen, Moryn, Moryna, Morynah, Moryne

Morgan ✿ GB (Welsh) seashore. Literature: Morgan le Fay was the half-sister of King Arthur.
Morgain, Morgaina, Morgainah, Morgana, Morganah, Morgance, Morganetta, Morganette, Morganica, Morganna, Morgayn, Morgayna, Morgaynah, Morgayne, Morghen, Morghin, Morghyn, Morgin, Morgon, Morrigan

Morganda (Spanish) a form of Morgan.

Morgane, Morgann, Morganne, Morghan, Morgyn (Welsh) forms of Morgan.

Morgen GB (Welsh) a form of Morgan.

Moriah (Hebrew) God is my teacher. (French) dark skinned. Bible: the mountain on which the Temple of Solomon was built. See also Mariah.
Moria, Moriel, Morria, Morriah, Morya, Moryah

Morie (Japanese) bay.
Morea, Moree, Morey, Mori, Mory

Morina (Irish) mermaid.
Morinah, Morinna, Morinnah, Moryna, Morynah, Morynna, Morynnah

Morit (Hebrew) teacher.
Moritt, Moritta, Morittah, Morryt, Morryta, Morrytah, Morryte, Moryt, Moryta, Moryte, Morytt, Morytta, Moryttah, Morytte

Morowa (Akan) queen.
Morowah

Morrin (Irish) long-haired.
Morin, Morine, Moryn, Moryne

Morrisa (Latin) dark skinned; moor; marshland.
Morisa, Morisah, Moriset, Morisett, Morisetta, Morisette, Morissa, Morissah, Morrisah, Morrissa, Morrissah, Morysa, Morysah, Moryssa, Moryssah, Morysse

Moselle (Hebrew) drawn from the water. (French) a white wine.
Mosel, Mosela, Moselah, Mosele, Mosella, Mosellah, Mosina, Mozel, Mozela, Mozelah, Mozele, Mozella, Mozellah, Mozelle

Mosi BG (Swahili) first-born.
Mosea, Mosee, Mosey, Mosie, Mosy

Mosina (Hebrew) a form of Moselle.
Mosinah, Mosine, Mozina, Mozinah, Mozine, Mozyna, Mozynah, Mozyne

Moswen BG (Tswana) white.
Moswena, Moswenah, Moswin, Moswina, Moswinah, Moswine, Moswyn, Moswyna, Moswynah, Moswyne

Mouna (Arabic) wish, desire.
Mounah, Mounia

Moyolehuani (Nahuatl) enamored one.

Moztla (Nahuatl) tomorrow.

Mrena (Slavic) white eyes.
Mren, Mrenah

Mucamutara (Egyptian) born during the war.

Mumtaz (Arabic) distinguished.

Muna (Greek, Irish) a form of Mona. (Arabic) a form of Mouna.
Munah, Munia

Munira (Arabic) she who is the source of light.

Mura (Japanese) village.
Murah

Muriel (Arabic) myrrh. (Irish) shining sea. A form of Mary. See also Meryl.
Muire, Murial, Muriell, Muriella, Murielle, Muryel, Muryela, Muryele, Muryell, Muryella, Muryelle

Murphy BG (Irish) sea warrior.
Merffee, Merffey, Merffi, Merffie, Merffy, Murffee, Murffey, Murffi, Murffie, Murffy, Murphee, Murphey, Murphi, Murphie

Muse (Greek) inspiration. Mythology: the Muses were nine Greek goddesses of the arts and sciences.

Musetta (French) little bagpipe.
Muset, Museta, Musetah, Musete, Musettah, Musette

Mushira (Arabic) counselor.

Musidora (Greek) beautiful muse.
Musidorah, Musidore, Musydor, Musydora, Musydorah, Musydore

Musika (Tongan) music.
Musica, Musicah, Musicka, Musyca, Musycah, Musycka, Musyckah, Musyka, Musykah

Muslimah (Arabic) devout believer.

My (Burmese) a short form of Mya.

Mya (Burmese) emerald. (Italian) a form of Mia.
Meia, Meiah

Myah (Burmese, Italian) a form of Mya.

Mycah (Hebrew) a form of Micah.
Myca

Mychaela (American) a form of Michaela.
Mychael, Mychal, Mychala, Mychall, Mychela, Mychelah, Myshela, Myshelah

Myeisha (American) a form of Moesha.

Myesha (American) a form of Moesha.

Myeshia (American) a form of Moesha.

Myia (Burmese, Italian) a form of Mya.
Myiah

Myiesha (American) a form of Moesha.

Myisha (American) a form of Moesha.

Myka (Hebrew, Japanese, Russian, Native American) a form of Mika.
Mykah

Mykaela (American) a form of Michaela.
Mykael, Mykaelah, Mykyla

Mykaila (American) a form of Michaela.
Mykailah

Mykala (American) a form of Michaela.
Mykal, Mykaleen

Mykayla (American) a form of Michaela.
Mykaylah

Mykel BG (American) a form of Michael.
Mykela, Mykelah

Myla (English) merciful.
Mylah, Mylla, Myllah

Mylene (Greek) dark.
Mylaine, Mylana, Mylee, Myleen

Myra (Latin) fragrant ointment.
Myrah, Myrena, Myria, Myrra, Myrrah, Myrrha

Myranda (Latin) a form of Miranda.
Myrandah, Myrandia, Myrannda

Myriah (Hebrew, Gypsy) a form of Miriah.
Myria, Myrya, Myryah

Myriam GB (American) a form of Miriam.
Myriame, Myryam, Myryame

Myrissa (American) a form of Marisa.
Myrisa, Myrisah, Myrissah

Myrna (Irish) beloved.
*Merna, Morna, Muirna, Murna, Murnah,
Myrnah*

Myrtle (Greek) evergreen shrub.
*Mertal, Mertel, Mertell, Mertella, Mertelle,
Mertis, Mertle, Mirtal, Mirtel, Mirtil, Mirtle,
Mirtyl, Murtal, Murtel, Murtella, Murtelle,
Myrta, Myrtia, Myrtias, Myrtice, Myrtie,
Myrtilla, Myrtis*

Myune (Australian) clear water.
Miuna, Miunah, Myuna, Myunah

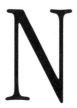

Nabila (Arabic) born to nobility.
Nabeela, Nabiha, Nabilah, Nabyla, Nabylah

Nacha (Latin) a form of Ignacia.

Nachine (Spanish) hot, fiery.
*Nachina, Nachinah, Nachyna, Nachynah,
Nachyne*

Nada GB (Arabic) a form of Nadda.
Nadah

Nadal (Catalan) a form of Natividad.

Nadda (Arabic) generous; dewy.
Naddah

Nadeen, Nadine (French, Slavic) forms of
Nadia.
*Nadean, Nadeana, Nadeanah, Nadeane,
Nadeena, Nadeenah, Nadeene, Nadena,
Nadene, Nadien, Nadin, Nadina, Nadyn,
Nadyna, Nadynah, Nadyne, Naidene, Naidine*

Nadette (French) a short form of
Bernadette.

Nadia (French, Slavic) hopeful.
*Nadea, Nadenka, Nadezhda, Nadiah, Nadie,
Nadija, Nadijah, Nadka, Nadusha*

Nadía (Egyptian) one who received the call
of God.

Nadira (Arabic) rare, precious.
Naadirah, Nadirah, Nadyra, Nadyrah

Nadiyah (French, Slavic) a form of Nadia.
Nadiya

Nadja, Nadya (French, Slavic) forms of
Nadia.
Nadjae, Nadjah, Nady, Nadyah

Nadyenka (Russian) a form of Nadia.

Naeva (French) a form of Eve.
Naeve, Nahvon

Nafisa (Arabic) a form of Nafisah.

Nafisah (Arabic) precious thing; gem.
Nafeesa

Nafuna (Luganda) born feet first.
Nafunah

Nagida (Hebrew) noble; prosperous.
Nagda, Nagdah, Nageeda, Nagyda

Nahama (Hebrew) sweetness.

Nahid (Persian) Mythology: another name
for Venus, the goddess of love and beauty.
Nahyd

Nahimana (Dakota) mystic.

Nahir (Arabic) clear; bright.

Nahuatl (Nahuatl) four waters; the Nahuatl
language.

Nahum (Hebrew) consolation.

Naiara (Spanish) reference to the Virgin
Mary.

Naida (Greek) water nymph.
Naiad, Nayad, Nyad

Naila (Arabic) successful.
Nayla, Naylah

Nailah GB (Arabic) a form of Naila.

Naima (Arabic) comfort; peace. (Indian)
belonging to one.
Na'ima, Na'imah

Nairi (Armenian) land of rivers. History: a name for ancient Armenia.
Naira, Naire, Nairee, Nairey, Nairia, Nairiah, Nairie, Nairy, Nayra

Naís (Spanish) a form of Inés.

Naiya (Greek) a form of Naida.
Naia, Naiyana, Naya

Naja, Najah (Greek) forms of Naida. (Arabic) short forms of Najam, Najila.

Najam (Arabic) star.

Najee BG (Arabic) a form of Naji (see Boys' Names).
Najae, Najée, Najei, Najiee

Najila (Arabic) brilliant eyes.
Najia, Najilah, Najja

Najla (Arabic) a short form of Najila.

Najma (Arabic) a form of Najam.

Nakayla (American) a form of Nicole.
Nakaylah

Nakea (Arabic) a form of Nakia.
Nakeea, Nakeeah

Nakeia (Arabic) a form of Nakia.

Nakeisha (American) a combination of the prefix Na + Keisha.
Nakeasha, Nakeesha, Nakeysha, Nakysha, Nakyshah, Nekeisha

Nakeita (American) a form of Nikita.
Nakeata, Nakeatah, Nakeeta, Nakeitah, Nakeitha, Nakeithia, Nakeithiah, Nakeithra, Nakeitra, Nakeitress, Nakeitta, Nakeitte, Nakeittia, Naketta, Nakette, Nakieta

Nakesha (American) a form of Nakeisha.
Nakeshea, Nakeshia

Nakeya (Arabic) a form of Nakia.
Nakeyah, Nakeyia

Nakia GB (Arabic) pure.
Nakiaya, Nakiea

Nakiah (Arabic) a form of Nakia.

Nakiesha (American) a form of Nakeisha.

Nakisha (American) a form of Nakeisha.
Nakishia, Nakishiah, Nakishya, Nakishyah

Nakita (American) a form of Nikita.
Nakitha, Nakitia, Nakitta, Nakitte, Nakkita, Nakyta, Nakytta, Nakytte, Naquita

Nakiya (Arabic) a form of Nakia.
Nakiyah

Nala (Tanzanian) queen.

Nalani (Hawaiian) calm as the heavens.
Nalanea, Nalaneah, Nalanee, Nalaney, Nalania, Nalaniah, Nalanie, Nalany, Nalanya, Nalanyah

Nalda (Spanish) strong.

Nalleli (Spanish) a form of Najla.

Ñambi (Guarani) curative herb.

Nami (Japanese) wave.
Namee, Namey, Namie, Namika, Namiko, Namy

Nan (German) a short form of Fernanda. (English) a form of Ann.
Nanice, Nanine, Nann, Nanon

Nana BG (Hawaiian) spring.
Nanah, Nanna, Nannah

Naná (Greek) she who is very young.

Nanci (English) a form of Nancy.
Nancia, Nanciah, Nancie

Nancy (English) gracious. A familiar form of Nan.
Nainsi, Nance, Nancea, Nancee, Nancey, Nancine, Nancsi, Nancya, Nancyah, Nancye, Nanice, Nanncey, Nanncy, Nanouk, Nansee, Nansey, Nansi, Nanuk

Nandalia (Australian) fire.
Nandalea, Nandaleah, Nandalee, Nandalei, Nandaleigh, Nandaley, Nandali, Nandaliah, Nandaly, Nandalya, Nandalyah

Nanette (French) a form of Nancy.
Nanet, Naneta, Nanetah, Nanete, Nanett, Nanetta, Nanettah, Nannet, Nanneta, Nannetah, Nannete, Nannett, Nannetta, Nannettah, Nannette, Nineta, Ninete, Ninetta, Ninette, Nini, Ninita, Ninnetta, Ninnette, Nynette

Nani (Greek) charming. (Hawaiian) beautiful.
Nanee, Naney, Nania, Naniah, Nanie,

Nannee, Nanney, Nanni, Nannie, Nanny,
Nany, Nanya, Nanyah

Nanon (French) a form of Ann.
Nanona, Nanonah, Nanone, Nanonia,
Nanoniah, Nanonya, Nanonyah

Nantilde (German) daring in combat.

Naolin (Spanish) Mythology: the Aztec sun
god.

Naomi (Hebrew) pleasant, beautiful. Bible:
Ruth's mother-in-law.
Naoma, Naomah, Naome, Naomee, Naomey,
Naomia, Naomiah, Neoma, Neomah,
Neomee, Neomi, Neomie, Neomy

Naomí (Hebrew) a form of Naomi.

Naomie, Naomy (Hebrew) forms of
Naomi.

Napea (Latin) from the valleys.

Nara (Greek) happy. (English) north.
(Japanese) oak.
Naara, Naarah, Narah, Narra, Narrah

Narcissa (Greek) daffodil. Mythology:
Narcissus was the youth who fell in love
with his own reflection.
Narcessa, Narcisa, Narcissah, Narcisse,
Narcissus, Narcyssa, Narkissa

Narda (Latin) fervently devoted.

Narelle (Australian) woman from the sea.
Narel, Narela, Narelah, Narele, Narell,
Narella, Narellah

Nari (Japanese) thunder.
Narea, Naree, Narey, Naria, Nariah, Narie,
Nariko, Nary, Narya, Naryah

Narissa (Greek) a form of Narcissa, Nerissa.

Narmada (Hindi) pleasure giver.
Narmadah

Naroa (Basque) tranquil, peaceful.

Nashawna (American) a combination of the
prefix Na + Shawna.
Nashan, Nashana, Nashanda, Nashaun,
Nashauna, Nashaunda, Nashawn,
Nashawnda, Nasheena, Nashounda,
Nashuana

Nashota (Native American) double; second-
born twin.

Nasrin (Muslim, Arabic) wild rose.

Nastasia (Greek) a form of Anastasia.
Nastasha, Nastashia, Nastasja, Nastassa,
Nastassia, Nastassiya, Nastazia, Nastisija,
Naztasia, Naztasiah

Nastassja (Greek) a form of Nastasia.
Nastassya, Nastasya, Nastasyah, Nastya

Nasya (Hebrew) miracle.
Nasia, Nasiah, Nasyah

Nata (Sanskrit) dancer. (Latin) swimmer.
(Native American) speaker; creator. (Polish,
Russian) a form of Natalie. See also Nadia.
Natah, Natia, Natiah, Natka, Natya, Natyah

Natacha (Russian) a form of Natasha.
Natachia, Natacia, Naticha

Natalee, Natali, Nataly (Latin) forms of
Natalie.
Natally, Natallye, Nattalee, Nattali, Nattaly

Natalí (Spanish) a form of Natalie.

Natalia (Russian) a form of Natalie. See also
Talia.
Nacia, Natala, Natalah, Natalea, Nataleah,
Nataliah, Nataliia, Natalija, Nataliya,
Nataliyah, Natalja, Natalka, Natalla,
Natallah, Natallea, Natallia, Natelea,
Nateleah, Natelia, Nateliah, Natilea,
Natileah, Natilia, Natiliah, Natlea, Natleah,
Natlia, Natliah, Nattalea, Nattaleah,
Nattaleya, Nattaleyah, Nattalia, Nattaliah,
Nattlea, Nattleah, Nattlia, Nattliah, Natylea,
Natyleah, Natylia, Natyliah

Natália (Hungarian, Portuguese) a form of
Natalie.

Natalie ☆ (Latin) born on Christmas day.
See also Nata, Natasha, Noel, Talia.
Nat, Nataleh, Natalei, Nataleigh, Nataley,
Nataliee, Natallie, Natelee, Natelei, Nateleigh,
Nateley, Nateli, Natelie, Nately, Natilee,
Natilei, Natileigh, Natili, Natilie, Natily,
Natlee, Natlei, Natleigh, Natley, Natli, Natlie,
Natly, Nattalei, Nattaleigh, Nattaley, Nattalie,
Nattilie, Nattlee, Nattlei, Nattleigh, Nattley,
Nattli, Nattlie, Nattly, Natylee, Natylei,
Natyleigh, Natyley, Natyli, Natylie, Natyly

Nataline (Latin) a form of Natalie.
Natalean, Nataleana, Nataleanah, Nataleane, Nataleena, Nataleenah, Nataleene, Natalena, Natalenah, Natalene, Nataléne, Natalina, Natalinah, Natalyn, Natalyna, Natalynah, Natalyne

Natalle (French) a form of Natalie.
Natale

Natalya (Russian) a form of Natalia.
Natalyah, Natelya, Natelyah, Natilya, Natilyah, Nattalya, Nattalyah, Nattlya, Nattlyah, Natylya, Natylyah

Natane (Arapaho) daughter.
Natana, Natanah, Natanna, Natannah, Natanne

Natania (Hebrew) gift of God.
Nataniah, Nataniela, Nataniele, Nataniell, Nataniella, Natanielle, Natanja, Natanjah, Natanya, Natanyah, Natée, Nathania, Nathaniah, Nathanya, Nathanyah, Nathenia, Natonia, Natoniah, Natonya, Natonyah, Netania, Nethania

Natara (Arabic) sacrifice.
Natarah, Nataria, Natariah, Natarya, Nataryah

Natascha (Russian) a form of Natasha.

Natasha (Russian) a form of Natalie. See also Stacey, Tasha.
Nahtasha, Nastenka, Nastia, Nastja, Natasa, Natashah, Natashea, Natashenka, Natashy, Natasza, Natausha, Natawsha, Nathasha, Nathassha, Netasha

Natashia (Russian) a form of Natasha.
Natashiea, Natashja, Natashya, Natashyah

Natasia, Natassia (Greek) forms of Nastasia.
Natasiah, Natasie

Natassja (Greek) a form of Nastasia.
Natassija, Natasya

Natesa (Hindi) cosmic dancer. Religion: another name for the Hindu god Shiva.
Natisa, Natissa

Natesha (Russian) a form of Natasha.
Nateshia

Nathalia (Latin) a form of Natalie.
Nathalea, Nathaleah, Nathaliah, Nathalya, Nathalyah

Nathália (Portuguese) a form of Natalie.

Nathalie, Nathaly (Latin) forms of Natalie.
Nathalee, Nathalei, Nathaleigh, Nathaley, Nathali, Nathaly

Nathifa (Egyptian) pure.

Natie (English) a familiar form of Natalie.
Nati, Natti, Nattie, Natty

Natisha (Russian) a form of Natasha.
Natishia

Natividad (Spanish) a form of Natividade.

Natividade (Latin) birth, nativity.

Natori (Arabic) a form of Natara.
Natoria

Natosha (Russian) a form of Natasha.
Natoshia, Natoshya, Netosha, Notosha

Nature (Latin) nature; essence; life.
Natural, Naturee, Naturey, Naturia, Naturiah, Naturie, Natury, Naturya, Naturyah

Naudia (French, Slavic) a form of Nadia.
Naudiah

Naunet (Egyptian) Mythology: goddess of the underworld.

Nava (Hebrew) beautiful; pleasant. See also Naomi.
Navah, Naveh, Navit

Navdeep BG (Sikh) new light.
Navdip

Naveen BG (Hindi) a form of Navin (see Boys' Names).

Naveena (Indian) new.

Navit (Hebrew) a form of Nava.
Navita, Navitah, Navyt, Navyta, Navytah

Nayara (Basque) swallow.

Nayeli, Nayelly, Nayely (Irish) forms of Neila.
Naeyli, Nayela, Nayelia, Nayelli, Nayla, Naylea, Naylia

Nayila (Arabic) a form of Najla.

Nazarena (Hebrew) a form of Nazareth.

Nazaret (Spanish) a form of Nazareth.

Nazareth (Hebrew) Religion: Jesus' birthplace.

Nazaria (Spanish) dedicated to God.

Neala (Irish) a form of Neila.
Nealah, Nealee, Nealia, Nealie, Nealy

Nebthet (Egyptian) a form of Nephthys.

Necahual (Nahuatl) survivor; left behind.

Necana, Necane (Spanish) sorrows.

Necha (Spanish) a form of Agnes.
Necho

Neci BG (Hungarian) fiery, intense.
Necee, Necey, Necia, Neciah, Necie, Necy

Necole (French) a form of Nicole.
Nechola, Necholah, Nechole, Necol, Necola, Necolah, Necoll, Necolle

Neda (Slavic) born on Sunday.
Nedah, Nedi, Nedia, Nedya, Nedyah

Nedda (English) prosperous guardian.
Neddah, Neddi, Neddie, Neddy

Neelam (Indian) sapphire.

Neely (Irish) a familiar form of Nelia.
Neela, Neelee, Neeley, Neeli, Neelia, Neelie, Neelya

Neema BG (Swahili) born during prosperous times.
Neemah

Neena (Spanish) a form of Nina.
Neana, Neanah, Neenah

Neera (Greek) young one.

Nefertari (Egyptian) most beautiful. History: an Egyptian queen.

Neftali, Neftalí (Hebrew) she who fights and is victorious.

Neha (Indian) rain.

Neida (Slavic) a form of Neda.

Neila (Irish) champion. See also Neala, Neely.
Neilah, Neile, Neili, Neilia, Neilie, Neilla, Neille

Neisha (Scandinavian, American) a form of Niesha.
Neishia, Neissia

Nekeisha (American) a form of Nakeisha.
Nechesa, Neikeishia, Nekeasha, Nekeashia, Nekeashiah, Nekeesha, Nekeeshia, Nekeeshiah, Nekesha, Nekeshia, Nekeysha, Nekeyshah, Nekeyshia, Nekeyshya, Nekeyshyah, Nekiesha, Nekisha, Nekysha

Nekia (Arabic) a form of Nakia.
Nekeya, Nekiya, Nekiyah, Nekya, Nekyah

Nelia (Spanish) yellow. (Latin) a familiar form of Cornelia.
Nela, Nelah, Nelea, Neleah, Neliah, Nelka, Nella, Nellah, Nellea, Nelleah, Nellia, Nelliah, Nellya, Nellyah, Nelya, Nelyah

Nelida, Nélida (Greek, Hebrew, Spanish) forms of Eleanor.

Nell (Greek) a form of Nelle. (English) a short form of Nellie.
Nel

Nelle (Greek) stone.
Nele

Nelli (Nahuatl) truth.

Nellie GB (English) a familiar form of Cornelia, Eleanor, Helen, Prunella.
Nelee, Nelei, Neleigh, Neley, Neli, Nellee, Nellei, Nelleigh, Nelley, Nelli, Nellianne, Nellice, Nellis, Nelma

Nellwyn (English) Nellie's friend.
Nellwin, Nellwina, Nellwinah, Nellwine, Nellwinn, Nellwinna, Nellwinnah, Nellwinne, Nellwyna, Nellwynah, Nellwyne, Nellwynn, Nellwynna, Nellwynnah, Nellwynne, Nelwin, Nelwina, Nelwinah, Nelwine, Nelwinn, Nelwinna, Nelwinnah, Nelwinne, Nelwyn, Nelwyna, Nelwynah, Nelwyne, Nelwynn, Nelwynna, Nelwynnah, Nelwynne

Nelly (English) a familiar form of Cornelia, Eleanor, Helen, Prunella.

Nemesia (Greek) she who administers justice.

Nena (Spanish) a form of Nina.

Nenet (Egyptian) born near the sea.
Neneta, Nenetah, Nenete, Nennet, Nenneta, Nennetah, Nennete, Nennett, Nennetta, Nennettah, Nennette

Nenetl (Nahuatl) doll.

Neola (Greek) youthful.
Neolah, Neolla

Neoma (Greek) new moon.
Neomah

Neomisia (Greek) beginning of the month.

Nephthys (Egyptian) mistress of the house.
Mythology: the goddess of the underworld.

Nerea (Spanish) mine.

Nereida (Greek) a form of Nerine.
Nerida, Neridah

Nereyda (Greek) a form of Nerine.
Nereyida, Neryda, Nerydah

Nerine (Greek) sea nymph.
Nerina, Nerinah, Nerita, Nerline, Neryn,
Neryna, Nerynah, Neryne

Nerissa (Greek) sea nymph. See also Rissa.
Nerisa, Nerrisa, Neryssa

Nerys (Welsh) lady.
Narice, Nereace, Nerease, Nereece, Nereese,
Nereice, Nereise, Nereyce, Nereyse, Nerice,
Nerise, Nerisse, Neryce, Neryse

Nesha (Greek) a form of Nessa.
Neshia

Nessa (Scandinavian) promontory. (Greek) a
short form of Agnes. See also Nessie.
Neisa, Neisah, Nesa, Nesia, Nesiah, Nessah,
Nessia, Nessiah, Nessya, Nessyah, Nesta,
Nevsa

Nessie (Greek) a familiar form of Agnes,
Nessa, Vanessa.
Nese, Nesee, Nesey, Neshie, Nesho, Nesi,
Nesie, Ness, Nessee, Nessey, Nessi, Nessy,
Nest, Nesy

Neta (Hebrew) plant, shrub. See also Nettie.
Netah, Netai, Netia, Netiah, Netta, Nettah,
Nettia, Nettiah, Nettya, Nettyah, Netya,
Netyah

Netanya (Hebrew) a form of Nathaniel (see
Boys' Names).

Netis (Native American) trustworthy.
Netisa, Netisah, Netise, Netissa, Netissah,
Netisse, Nettys, Nettysa, Nettysah, Nettyse,
Netys, Netysa, Netysah, Netyse, Netyssa,
Netyssah, Netysse

Nettie (French) a familiar form of Annette,
Antoinette, Nanette.
Netee, Netey, Neti, Netie, Nette, Nettee,
Nettey, Netti, Netty, Nety

Neva (Spanish) snow. (English) new.
Geography: a river in Russia.
Neiva, Nevah, Neve, Nevia, Neyva, Nieve,
Niva, Nivea, Nivia

Nevada GB (Spanish) snow. Geography: a
western U.S. state.
Nevadah

Neve (Hebrew) life.
Neiv, Neive, Nevee, Nevia, Neviah, Neyva,
Neyve, Nieve, Nyev, Nyeva, Nyevah, Nyeve

Neves (Portuguese) a form of Nieves.

Nevina (Irish) worshipper of the saint.
Neveen, Neveena, Neveenah, Neveene,
Nevein, Nevena, Nevenah, Nevene, Neveyan,
Nevin, Nevinah, Nevine, Nivena, Nivenah,
Nivina, Nivinah, Nivine, Nyvina, Nyvinah,
Nyvine, Nyvyn, Nyvyna, Nyvynah, Nyvyne

Neylan (Turkish) fulfilled wish.
Nealana, Nealanah, Nealanee, Nealaney,
Nealani, Nealania, Nealaniah, Nealanya,
Nealanyah, Neilana, Neilanah, Neilane,
Neilanee, Neilaney, Neilani, Neilania,
Neilaniah, Neilany, Neilanya, Neilanyah,
Nelana, Nelanah, Nelane, Nelanee, Nelaney,
Nelani, Nelania, Nelaniah, Nelanie, Nelany,
Nelanya, Nelanyah, Neyla, Neylanah,
Neylane, Neylanee, Neylaney

Neysa (Greek, Scandinavian) a form of
Nessa.
Neysah, Neysha, Neyshia

Neza (Slavic) a form of Agnes.
Nezah, Nezza, Nezzah

Ngoc (Vietnamese) jade.

Nguyen BG (Vietnamese) a form of Ngu
(see Boys' Names).

Nia (Irish) a familiar form of Neila.
Mythology: Nia Ben Aur was a legendary
Welsh woman.
Neya, Neyah, Niah, Niajia

Niabi (Osage) fawn.
Niabia, Niabiah, Niabie, Niaby, Nyabya, Nyabyah

Niam (Irish) bright.
Niama, Niamah, Nyam, Nyama, Nyamah

Niamh (Irish) a form of Niam.

Nicanora (Spanish) victorious army.

Nicasia (Greek) triumphant woman.

Nicerata (Greek) worth of victories.

Niceta (Spanish) victorious one.

Nichelle (American) a combination of Nicole + Michelle. Culture: Nichelle Nichols was the first African American woman featured in a television drama (*Star Trek*).
Nechel, Nechela, Nechelah, Nechele, Nechell, Nechella, Nechellah, Nechelle, Nichela, Nichelah, Nichele, Nichell, Nichella, Nichellah, Nishell, Nishella, Nishellah, Nishelle, Nychel, Nychela, Nychelah, Nychele, Nychell, Nychella, Nychellah, Nychelle

Nichol, Nichole, Nicholle (French) forms of Nicole.

Nicholas BG (French) victorious people.

Nicholette (French) a form of Nicole.

Nicki, Nickie (French) familiar forms of Nicole. See also Nikki.
Nicci, Nickee, Nickey, Nickeya, Nickia, Nickiya, Nyc, Nyck, Nyckee, Nyckey, Nycki, Nyckie, Nycky

Nickole (French) a form of Nicole.
Nickol

Nicky BG (French) a familiar form of Nicole.

Nicola GB (Italian) a form of Nicole.
Nacola, Nacolah, Necola, Necolah, Necolla, Necollah, Nicala, Nicalah, Nichala, Nichalah, Nichola, Nicholah, Nickala, Nickalah, Nickola, Nickolah, Nicolah, Nicolea, Nicolla, Nikkola, Nikola, Nikolia, Nycala, Nycalah, Nychala, Nychalah, Nychola, Nycholah, Nyckala, Nyckalah, Nyckola, Nyckolah, Nycola, Nycolah, Nykola, Nykolah

Nicolas BG (French) a form of Nicholas.

Nicolasa (Spanish) a form of Nicole.

Nicole ⭐ GB (French) a form of Nicholas. See also Colette, Cosette, Lacole, Nikita.
Nacole, Nica, Nicia, Nicol, Nicoli, Nicolia, Nicolie, Niquole, Nocole

Nicolette, Nicollette (French) forms of Nicole.
Necholet, Necholeta, Necholetah, Necholete, Necholett, Necholetta, Necholettah, Necholette, Necolet, Necoleta, Necoletah, Necolete, Necolett, Necoletta, Necolettah, Necolette, Nickolet, Nickoleta, Nickoletah, Nickolete, Nickolett, Nickoletta, Nickolettah, Nickolette, Nicolet, Nicoleta, Nicoletah, Nicolete, Nicolett, Nicoletta, Nicolettah, Nicollete, Nyckolet, Nyckoleta, Nyckoletah, Nyckolete, Nyckolett, Nyckoletta, Nyckolettah, Nyckolette, Nycolet, Nycoleta, Nycoletah, Nycolete, Nycolett, Nycoletta, Nycolettah, Nycolette, Nykolet, Nykoleta, Nykoletah, Nykolete, Nykolett, Nykoletta, Nykolettah, Nykolette

Nicolina (French) a form of Nicoline.

Nicoline (French) a familiar form of Nicole.
Nicholine, Nicholyn, Nicoleen, Nicolene, Nicolyn, Nicolyne, Nicolynn, Nicolynne, Nikolene, Nikoline

Nicolle (French) a form of Nicole.

Nidia (Latin) nest.
Nidi, Nidiah, Nidya

Nidía (Greek) a form of Nidia.

Niesha (American) pure. (Scandinavian) a form of Nissa.
Neesha, Nesha, Neshia, Nesia, Nessia, Neysha, Niessia

Nieves (Latin) refers to the Virgin Mary.

Nige (Latin) dark night.
Nigea, Nigela, Nigelah, Nigele, Nigell, Nigella, Nigellah, Nigelle, Nygel, Nygela, Nygelah, Nygele, Nygell, Nygella, Nygelle

Nija, Nijah (Latin) forms of Nige.
Nijae

Nika GB (Russian) belonging to God.
Nikah, Nikka, Nyka, Nykah

Nikayla (American) a form of Nicole.
Nykala, Nykalah

Nike BG (Greek) victorious. Mythology: the goddess of victory.

Nikelle (American) a form of Nicole.
Nikeille, Nikel, Nikela, Nikelie

Niki GB (Russian) a short form of Nikita.
(American) a familiar form of Nicole.
Nikee, Nikey, Nikie, Niky, Nykee, Nykey,
Nyki, Nykie, Nyky

Nikia, Nikkia (Arabic) forms of Nakia.
(Russian, American) forms of Niki, Nikki.
Nikiah, Nikkea, Nikkiah

Nikita GB (Russian) victorious people.
Nakeita, Nicheata, Nicheatah, Nicheeta,
Nicheetah, Nickeata, Nickeatah, Nickeeta,
Nickeetah, Nikeata, Nikeatah, Nikeeta,
Nikeetah, Nikeita, Nikeitah, Nikitah, Nikitia,
Nikitta, Nikitte, Niquita, Niquitah, Niquite,
Niquitta, Nykeata, Nykeatah, Nykeeta,
Nykeetah, Nykeita, Nykeitah, Nykeyta,
Nykeytah, Nykita, Nykitah, Nykytah

Nikki GB (American) a familiar form of
Nicole. See also Nicki.
Nikkee, Nikkey, Nikkie, Nikko, Nikky,
Niquee, Niquey, Niqui, Niquie, Niquy, Nyk,
Nykee, Nykey, Nyki, Nykie, Nykkee,
Nykkey, Nykki, Nykkie, Nykky, Nyky,
Nyquee, Nyquey, Nyqui, Nyquie, Nyqy

Nikkita (Russian) a form of Nikita.
Nikkitah

Nikkole, Nikole (French) forms of Nicole.
Nikkolie, Nikola, Nikolah, Nikolle

Nikolaevna (Russian) on the side of God.

Nikolette (French) a form of Nicole.
Nikkolette, Nikolet, Nikoleta, Nikoletah,
Nikolete, Nikolett, Nikoletta, Nikolettah

Nikolina (French) a form of Nicole.
Nikolena

Nila GB (Latin) Geography: the Nile River
in Africa. (Irish) a form of Neila.
Nilah, Nile, Nilea, Nileah, Nilesia, Nilla,
Nillah, Nillea, Nilleah

Nilda (Spanish) a short form of Brunhilda.

Nima BG (Hebrew) thread. (Arabic) blessing.
Neema, Nema, Nemah, Niama, Nimah,
Nimali, Nimalie, Nimaly, Nyma, Nymah

Nimia (Latin) she who is ambitious.

Nina (Spanish) girl. (Native American)
mighty. (Hebrew) a familiar form of
Hannah.
Ninacska, Ninah, Ninja, Ninna, Ninosca,
Ninoshka, Nyna, Nynah

Ninette (French) small.
Ninet, Nineta, Ninetah, Ninete, Ninett,
Ninetta, Ninettah, Nynet, Nyneta, Nynetah,
Nynete, Nynett, Nynetta, Nynettah, Nynette

Ninfa (Greek) young wife.

Ninfodora (Greek) gift of the nymphs.

Niní (French) a form of Virginia.

Niñita (Russian) victory of the community.

Ninon (French) a form of Nina.
Ninona, Ninonah, Ninone

Ninoska (Russian) a form of Nina.

Niobe (Greek) she who rejuvenates.

Nirali (Hebrew) a form of Nirel.

Niranjana (Sanskrit) night of the full moon.

Nirel (Hebrew) light of God.
Nirela, Nirelah, Nirele, Nirell, Nirella,
Nirellah, Nirelle, Nyrel, Nyrela, Nyrelah,
Nyrele, Nyrell, Nyrella, Nyrellah, Nyrelle

Nirveli (Hindi) water child.
Nirvlea, Nirvleah, Nirvlee, Nirvlei,
Nirvleigh, Nirvley, Nirvlie, Nirvly,
Nyrvlea, Nyrvleah, Nyrvlee, Nyrvlei,
Nyrvleigh, Nyrvley, Nyrvlie, Nyrvly

Nisa (Arabic) woman.
Nisah, Nysa, Nysah

Nisha (American) a form of Niesha, Nissa.
Niasha, Nishay

Nishi (Japanese) west.
Nishee, Nishey, Nishie, Nishy

Nissa (Hebrew) sign, emblem.
(Scandinavian) friendly elf; brownie. See
also Nyssa.
Nissah, Nisse, Nissi, Nissie, Nissy

Nita (Hebrew) planter. (Choctaw) bear.
(Spanish) a short form of Anita, Juanita.
Nitah, Nitai, Nitha, Nithai, Nitika, Nyta,
Nytah

Nitara (Hindi) deeply rooted.
Nitarah, Nitarra, Nitarrah, Nytara, Nytarah, Nytarra, Nytarrah

Nitasha (American) a form of Natasha.
Nitashah, Nitasia, Niteisha, Nitisha, Nitishah, Nitishia, Nitishiah, Nytasha, Nytashia, Nytashiah, Nytashya, Nytashyah

Nitsa (Greek) a form of Helen.
Nitsah, Nytsa, Nytsah

Nituna (Native American) daughter.
Nitunah, Nytuna, Nytunah

Nitza (Hebrew) flower bud.
Nitzah, Nitzana, Niza, Nizah, Nytza, Nytzah

Nixie (German) water sprite.
Nixee, Nixey, Nixi, Nixy, Nyxee, Nyxey, Nyxi, Nyxie, Nyxy

Niya, Niyah (Irish) forms of Nia.
Niyana, Niyia

Nizana (Hebrew) a form of Nitza.
Nitzana, Nitzania, Nitzanit, Nitzanita, Zana

Noah BG (Hebrew) peaceful, restful. Bible: the patriarch who built the ark to survive the Flood.

Nochtli (Nahuatl) prickly pear fruit.

Noe, Noé (Hebrew) forms of Noah.

Noel BG (Latin) Christmas. See also Natalie, Noelle.
Noël, Noele, Novelenn, Novelia, Nowel, Nowele

Noelani (Hawaiian) beautiful one from heaven. (Latin) a form of Noel.
Noelanee, Noelaney, Noelania, Noelaniah, Noelanie, Noelannee, Noelanney, Noelanni, Noelannie, Noelanny, Noelany, Noelanya, Noelanyah

Noelia (Latin) a form of Noel.

Noeline (Latin) a form of Noel.
Noelean, Noeleana, Noeleanah, Noeleane, Noeleen, Noeleena, Noeleenah, Noeleene, Noelene, Noelin, Noelina, Noelinah, Noelleen, Noellin, Noellina, Noellinah, Noelline, Noellyn, Noellyna, Noellynah, Noellyne, Noelyn, Noelynn, Noleen, Nolein, Noleina,

Noleinah, Noleine, Noleyn, Noleyna, Noleynah, Noleyne, Noweleen

Noella (French) a form of Noelle.
Noela, Noelah, Noellah, Nowela, Nowelah, Nowella, Nowellah

Noelle (French) Christmas.
Noell, Nowell, Nowelle

Noely (Latin) a form of Noel.
Noeli, Noelie, Noelly

Noemi, Noemie, Noemy (Hebrew) forms of Naomi.
Noam, Noami, Noamy, Nomee, Nomey, Nomi, Nomia, Nomiah, Nomie

Noemí (Hebrew) a form of Naomi.

Noga (Hebrew) morning light.
Nogah

Noheli, Nohely (Latin) forms of Noel.
Nohal

Nohemi (Hebrew) a form of Naomi.

Nokomis (Dakota) moon daughter.
Nokoma, Nokomas, Nokomys

Nola (Latin) small bell. (Irish) famous; noble. A short form of Fionnula.

Nolana (Irish) a form of Nola.
Noelan, Noelana, Noelanah, Noelanna, Noelannah, Noelannia, Noelanniah, Noelannya, Noelannyah, Nolanah, Nolanee, Nolaney, Nolani, Nolania, Nolaniah, Nolanie, Nolany, Nolanya, Nolanyah

Noleta (Latin) unwilling.
Noleata, Noleatah, Noleeta, Noleetah, Nolita, Nolitah, Nolyta, Nolytah

Nollie BG (English) a familiar form of Magnolia.
Nolia, Nolle, Nolley, Nolli, Nolly

Noma (Hawaiian) a form of Norma.
Nomah

Nominanda (Latin) she who will be elected.

Nona (Latin) ninth.
Nonah, Nonee, Noney, Noni, Nonia, Noniah, Nonie, Nonna, Nonnah, Nony, Nonya, Nonyah

Noor GB (Aramaic) a form of Nura.
Noora, Noorah, Noorie, Nour, Nur

Nora (Greek) light. A familiar form of
Eleanor, Honora, Leonor.
Norra

Norah (Greek) a form of Nora.
Norrah

Norberta (Scandinavian) brilliant hero.
*Norbertah, Norbirta, Norbirtah, Norburta,
Norburtah, Norbyrta, Norbyrtah*

Nordica (Scandinavian) from the north.
*Nordic, Nordicah, Nordik, Nordika, Nordikah,
Nordiqua, Nordiquah, Nordyca, Nordycah,
Nordycka, Nordyckah, Nordyka, Nordykah,
Nordyqua, Nordyquah*

Noreen (Irish) a form of Eleanor, Nora.
(Latin) a familiar form of Norma.
*Noorin, Noreena, Noreene, Noren, Norena,
Norene, Norina, Norine, Nureen*

Norell (Scandinavian) from the north.
*Narel, Narell, Narelle, Norel, Norela, Norele,
Norella, Norellah, Norelle, Norely*

Nori (Japanese) law, tradition.
*Noree, Norey, Noria, Noriah, Norico, Norie,
Noriko, Norita, Nory, Norya, Noryah*

Norleen (Irish) honest.
*Norlan, Norlana, Norlanah, Norlane, Norlean,
Norleana, Norleanah, Norleane, Norleena,
Norleenah, Norleene, Norlein, Norleina,
Norleinah, Norleine, Norleyn, Norleyna,
Norleynah, Norleyne, Norlin, Norlina,
Norlinah, Norline, Norlyn, Norlyna,
Norlynah, Norlyne*

Norma (Latin) rule, precept.
Noma, Normi, Normie

Notburga (German) protected beauty.

Nour GB (Aramaic) a short form of Nura.
Noura

Nova (Latin) new. A short form of Novella,
Novia. (Hopi) butterfly chaser. Astronomy:
a star that releases bright bursts of energy.
Novah

Novella (Latin) newcomer.
*Novel, Novela, Novelah, Novele, Novell,
Novellah, Novelle*

Novia (Spanish) sweetheart.
Noviah, Novka, Novya, Novyah, Nuvia

Noxochicoztli (Nahuatl) my necklace of
flowers.

Nu (Burmese) tender. (Vietnamese) girl.
Nue

Nuala (Irish) a short form of Fionnula.
Nualah, Nula

Nubia (Egyptian) mother of a nation.

Nuela (Spanish) a form of Amelia.

Numa, Numas (Greek) she who establishes
laws.

Numeria (Latin) she who enumerates.

Numilla (Australian) scout, lookout.
*Numil, Numila, Numilah, Numile, Numill,
Numillah, Numille, Numyl, Numyla, Numylah,
Numyle, Numyll, Numylla, Numyllah, Numylle*

Nuna (Native American) land.
Nunah

Nuncia (Latin) she who announces.

Nunciata (Latin) messenger.
Nunzia, Nunziata, Nunziatah

Nunila (Spanish) ninth daughter.

Nunilona (Latin) a form of Nunila.

Nur (Aramaic) a short form of Nura.

Nura (Aramaic) light.
Nurah

Nuria (Aramaic) the Lord's light.
Nuri, Nuriah, Nuriel, Nurin, Nurya, Nuryah

Núria (Basque) buried deep among the hills.

Nuru BG (Swahili) daylight.

Nusi (Hungarian) a form of Hannah.
Nusie, Nusy

Nuwa (Chinese) mother goddess.
Mythology: another name for Nü-gua, the
creator of mankind.

Nya, Nyah (Irish) forms of Nia.
Nyaa, Nyia

Nyasia (Greek) a form of Nyssa.

Nycole (French) a form of Nicole.
Nycol, Nycole, Nycolle

Nydia (Latin) nest.
Nyda, Nydiah, Nydya, Nydyah

Nydía (Greek) a form of Nydia.

Nyeisha (American) a form of Niesha.

Nyesha (American) a form of Niesha.
Nyeshia

Nyia (Irish) a form of Nia.

Nykia (Arabic) a form of Nakia.
Nykiah

Nyla (Latin, Irish) a form of Nila.
Nylah, Nyle, Nylea, Nyleah, Nylla, Nyllah, Nylle, Nyllea, Nylleah

Nyoko (Japanese) gem, treasure.
Nioko

Nyomi (Hebrew) a form of Naomi.
Nyoma, Nyome, Nyomee, Nyomey, Nyomia, Nyomiah, Nyomie, Nyomy, Nyomya, Nyomyah

Nyree (Maori) sea.
Niree, Nyra, Nyrie

Nyssa (Greek) beginning. See also Nissa.
Nysa, Nysah, Nyssah

Nyusha (Russian) a form of Agnes.
Nyushenka, Nyushka

Nyx (Greek) night.

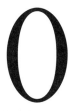

O'shea BG (Irish) a form of O'Shea.

O'Shea BG (Irish) child of Shea.

Oba BG (Yoruba) chief, ruler.
Obah

Obdulia (Latin) she who takes away sadness and pain.

Obelia (Greek) needle.
Obeliah, Obelya, Obelyah

Ocean BG (Greek) ocean.
Oceanne, Oceon

Oceana (Greek) ocean. Mythology: Oceanus was the god of the ocean.
Oceanah, Oceananna, Oceania, Oceanna, Oceaonna

Oceane (Greek) a form of Ocean.

Ocilia (Greek) a form of Othelia.

Octavia (Latin) eighth. See also Tavia.
Actavia, Octabia, Octaviah, Octaviais, Octavian, Octavice, Octavie, Octavienne, Octavio, Octavious, Octavise, Octavya, Octawia, Octivia, Oktavia, Oktavija, Otavia

Octaviana (Spanish) a form of Octavia.

Odanda (Spanish) famous land.

Odda (Scandinavian) rich.
Oda, Odah, Oddah, Oddia, Oddiah

Ode BG (Nigerian) born during travels.
Odee, Odey, Odi, Ody, Odya, Odyah

Odeda (Hebrew) strong; courageous.
Odeada, Odeadah, Odedah

Odele (Greek) melody, song.
Odel, Odell, Odelle

Odelette (French) a form of Odele.
Odelat, Odelatt, Odelatta, Odelattah, Odelatte, Odelet, Odeleta, Odeletah, Odelete, Odelett, Odeletta

Odelia (Greek) ode; melodic. (Hebrew) I will praise God. (French) wealthy. See also Odetta.
Odeelia, Odeleya, Odeliah, Odelina, Odelinah, Odelinda, Odeline, Odellah, Odelyn, Odila, Odilah, Odile, Odilia, Odille, Odyla, Odylah, Odyle, Odyll, Odylla, Odyllah, Odylle

Odella (English) wood hill.
Odela, Odelah, Odelle, Odelyn

Odera (Hebrew) plough.

Odessa (Greek) odyssey, long voyage.
Adesha, Adeshia, Adessa, Adessia, Odesa, Odesah, Odessah, Odessia, Odissa, Odissah, Odysa, Odysah, Odyssa, Odyssah

Odetta (German, French) a form of Odelia.
Oddeta, Oddetta, Odeta, Odetah, Odettah

Odette (German, French) a form of Odelia.
Oddet, Oddete, Oddett, Odet, Odete, Odett

Odina (Algonquin) mountain.
Odeana, Odeanah, Odeane, Odeen, Odeena, Odeenah, Odeene, Odinah, Odyn, Odyna, Odynah, Odyne

Ofelia (Greek) a form of Ophelia.
Ofeelia, Ofellia, Ofilia

Ofélia (Portuguese) a form of Ophelia.

Ofira (Hebrew) gold.
Ofara, Ofarra, Ofarrah, Ophira, Ophirah, Ophyra, Ophyrah

Ofra (Hebrew) a form of Aphra.
Ofrah, Ofrat, Ophra, Ophrah

Ogin (Native American) wild rose.
Ogina, Ogyn, Ogyna, Ogynah

Ohanna (Hebrew) God's gracious gift.
Ohana, Ohanah, Ohannah

Ohtli (Nahuatl) road.

Oihane (Spanish) from the forest.

Okalani (Hawaiian) heaven.
Okalana, Okalanah, Okalanea, Okalanee, Okalaney, Okalania, Okalaniah, Okalanie, Okalany, Okalanya, Okalanyah, Okiilanee, Okiilaney, Okiilani, Okiilanie, Okiilany, Okilani

Oki (Japanese) middle of the ocean.
Okie

Oksana (Latin) a form of Osanna.
Oksanna

Oksanochka (Russian) praises of God.

Ola GB (Scandinavian) ancestor. (Greek) a short form of Olesia.
Olah

Olalla (Greek) sweetly spoken.
Olallah

Olathe (Native American) beautiful.
Olanth, Olantha, Olanthah, Olanthye, Olathia

Olaya (Greek) she who speaks well.

Oldina (Australian) snow.
Oldeena, Oldeenah, Oldenia, Oldeniah, Oldinah, Oldine, Oldyn, Oldyna, Oldynah, Oldyne

Oleander (Latin) Botany: a poisonous evergreen shrub with fragrant white, rose, or purple flowers.
Oleanda, Oleandah, Oleeanda, Oleeandah, Oliannda, Olianndah, Oliannde

Olechka (Russian) a form of Helga.

Oleda (Spanish) a form of Alida. See also Leda.
Oleta, Olida, Olita

Olen BG (Russian) deer.
Olian, Olien, Olienah, Oliene, Olyan, Olyen, Olyene

Olena (Russian) a form of Helen.
Alena, Alyona, Oleena, Olenah, Olenia, Oleniah, Olenka, Olenna, Olenya, Olya, Olyena, Olyenah, Olyona

Olesia (Greek) a form of Alexandra.
Cesya, Olecia, Oleesha, Oleishia, Olesha, Olesiah, Olesya, Olesyah, Olexa, Olice, Olicia, Olisha, Olishia, Ollicia

Oletha (Scandinavian) nimble.
Oleta, Oletah, Yaletha

Olethea (Latin) truthful. See also Alethea.
Oleathea, Oleatheah, Oleathya, Oleathyah, Oleta

Olga (Scandinavian) holy. See also Helga, Olivia.
Olgah, Olgy, Olia, Olva

Olia (Russian) a form of Olga.
Olja, Ollya, Olya, Olyah

Oliana (Polynesian) oleander.
Olianah, Oliane, Oliann, Olianna, Oliannah, Olianne, Olyan, Olyana, Olyanah, Olyane, Olyann, Olyanna, Olyannah, Olyanne

Olimpe (French) a form of Olympia.
Olympe

Olimpíades (Greek) a form of Olympia.

Olina (Hawaiian) filled with happiness.
Olinah, Olyna, Olynah

Olinda (Latin) scented. (Spanish) protector of property. (Greek) a form of Yolanda.
Olindah, Olynda, Olyndah

Olisa (Ibo) God.
Olisah, Olysa, Olysah, Olyssa, Olyssah

Olive (Latin) olive tree.
Oliff, Oliffe, Oliv, Olivet, Olivette, Olliv,
Ollive, Ollyv, Ollyve, Olyv, Olyve

Oliveria (Latin) affectionate.

Olivia ☆ (Latin) a form of Olive. (English) a
form of Olga. See also Liv, Livia.
Alivia, Alyvia, Olevia, Oliva, Olivea, Oliveia,
Olivetta, Olivette, Olivi, Oliviah, Olivianne,
Olivya, Olivyah, Oliwia, Olva

Ollie **BG** (English) a familiar form of Olivia.
Olla, Olly, Ollye

Olwen (Welsh) white footprint.
Olwena, Olwenah, Olwene, Olwenn,
Olwenna, Olwennah, Olwenne, Olwin,
Olwina, Olwinah, Olwine, Olwinn, Olwinna,
Olwinnah, Olwinne, Olwyn, Olwyna,
Olwynah, Olwyne, Olwynn, Olwynna,
Olwynnah, Olwynne

Olympia (Greek) heavenly.
Olimpe, Olimpia, Olimpiah, Olimpias,
Olympiah, Olympias, Olympie, Olympya,
Olympyah

Olympie (German) a form of Olympia.
Olympy

Olyvia (Latin) a form of Olivia.
Olyviah, Olyvya, Olyvyah

Oma (Hebrew) reverent. (German) grandmother. (Arabic) highest.
Omah

Omaira (Arabic) red.
Omar, Omara, Omarah, Omari, Omaria,
Omariah, Omarra, Omarya, Omaryah

Omega (Greek) last, final, end. Linguistics:
the last letter in the Greek alphabet.
Omegah

Ona (Latin, Irish) a form of Oona. (English)
river.
Onah, Onna

Onatah (Iroquoian) daughter of the earth
and the corn spirit.
Onata

Onawa (Native American) wide awake.
Onaiwa, Onaiwah, Onaja, Onajah, Onawah,
Onowa, Onowah

Ondine (Latin) a form of Undine.
Ondene, Ondin, Ondina, Ondinah, Ondyn,
Ondyna, Ondynah, Ondyne

Ondrea (Czech) a form of Andrea.
Ohndrea, Ohndreea, Ohndreya, Ohndria,
Ondra, Ondrah, Ondraya, Ondreana,
Ondreea, Ondreya, Ondri, Ondria,
Ondrianna, Ondrie, Ondriea, Ondry, Ondrya,
Ondryah

Oneida (Native American) eagerly awaited.
Oneidah, Oneyda, Oneydah, Onida, Onidah,
Onyda, Onydah

Oneisha (American) a form of Onesha.

Onella (Hungarian) a form of Helen.
Onela, Onelah, Onellah

Onesha (American) a combination of
Ondrea + Aisha.
Oneshia, Onesia, Onessa, Onessia, Onethia,
Oniesha, Onisha

Onésima (Latin) she who is burdened.

Onfalia (Egyptian) she who does good
deeds.

Oni (Yoruba) born on holy ground.
Onee, Oney, Onie, Onnie, Ony

Onike (Tongan) onyx.
Onika, Onikah, Onikee

Onila (Latin) a form of Petronella.

Onofledis (German) she who shows her
sword.

Onora (Latin) a form of Honora.
Onorah, Onoria, Onoriah, Onorina, Onorine,
Onoryn, Onoryna, Onorynah, Ornora

Ontario **BG** (Native American) beautiful
lake. Geography: a province and a lake in
Canada.
Oniatario, Ontaryo

Onyx (Greek) onyx.
Onix

Oona (Latin, Irish) a form of Una.
Onnie, Oonagh, Oonie

Opa (Choctaw) owl. (German) grandfather.
Opah

Opal (Hindi) precious stone.
Opala, Opalah, Opale, Opalia, Opalina, Opell, Opella, Opelle

Opalina (Hindi) a form of Opal.
Opaleana, Opaleena, Opalin, Opalinah, Opaline, Opalyn, Opalyna, Opalynah, Opalyne

Opeli (Tongan) opal.
Opelea, Opeleah, Opelee, Opelei, Opeleigh, Opelia, Opeliah, Opelie, Opely, Opelya, Opelyah

Ophelia (Greek) helper. Literature: Hamlet's love interest in the Shakespearean play *Hamlet*.
Filia, Opheliah, Ophélie, Ophellia, Ophellya, Ophilia, Ophillia, Ophylla, Ophyllia, Ophylliah, Ophyllya, Ophyllyah, Phelia, Pheliah, Phelya, Phelyah

Ophelie (Greek) a form of Ophelia.
Ophellie, Ophelly, Ophely

Oportuna (Latin) opportune.

Oprah (Hebrew) a form of Orpah.
Ophra, Ophrah, Opra

Ora (Latin) prayer. (Spanish) gold. (English) seacoast. (Greek) a form of Aura.
Ohra, Orah, Orlice, Orra

Orabella (Latin) a form of Arabella.
Orabel, Orabela, Orabele, Orabell, Orabelle, Oribel, Oribela, Oribele, Oribell, Oribella, Oribelle, Orybel, Orybela, Orybele, Orybell, Orybella, Orybelle

Oraida (Arabic) eloquent.

Oralee (Hebrew) the Lord is my light. See also Yareli.
Areli, Oralea, Oraleah, Oralei, Oraleigh, Oraley, Orali, Oralie, Oralit, Oraly, Oralye, Orelee, Orelie

Oralia (French) a form of Aurelia. See also Oriana.
Oraliah, Oralis, Oralya, Oralyah, Orelia, Oreliah, Oriel, Orielda, Orielle, Oriena, Orla, Orlah, Orlena, Orlene

Oran BG (Irish) queen.

Orana (Australian) welcome.
Oranah, Oranna, Orannah

Orane (French) rising.

Orazia (Italian) keeper of time.
Orazya, Orazyah, Orzaiah, Orzaya, Orzayah

Orea (Greek) mountains.
Oreah, Oreal, Oria, Oriah

Orela (Latin) announcement from the gods; oracle.
Oreal, Orel, Orelah, Orell, Orella, Orelle

Orenda (Iroquoian) magical power.
Orendah

Oretha (Greek) a form of Aretha.
Oreta, Oretah, Oretta, Orettah, Orette

Orfelina (Italian) orphan.

Orfilia (German) female wolf.

Oriana (Latin) dawn, sunrise. (Irish) golden.
Orane, Orania, Orelda, Ori, Oria, Orian, Oriane, Orianna, Oriannah, Orieana, Oryan, Oryana, Oryanah, Oryane, Oryann, Oryanna, Oryannah, Oryanne

Oriel (Latin) fire. (French) golden; angel of destiny.
Orial, Oriale, Oriall, Orialle, Oriele, Oriell, Orielle, Oryal, Oryale, Oryall, Oryalle, Oryel, Oryell, Oryelle

Oriella (Irish) fair; white skinned.
Oriala, Orialah, Orialla, Oriallah, Oriela, Orielah, Oriellah, Oryala, Oryalah, Oryalla, Oryallah, Oryela, Oryelah, Oryella, Oryellah

Orieta (Spanish) a form of Oriana.

Orina (Russian) a form of Irene.
Orinah, Orya, Oryna, Orynah

Orinda (Hebrew) pine tree. (Irish) light skinned, white.
Orenda, Orendah, Orindah, Orynda, Oryndah

Orino (Japanese) worker's field.
Oryno

Oriole (Latin) golden; black-and-orange bird.
Auriel, Oriol, Oriola, Oriolah, Orioll, Oriolla, Oriollah, Oriolle, Oryel, Oryela, Oryelah, Oryele, Oryell, Oryella, Oryellah, Oryelle, Oryol, Oryola, Oryolah, Oryole, Oryoll, Oryolla, Oryollah, Oryolle

Orla (Irish) golden woman.
Orlagh, Orlah

Orlanda (German) famous throughout the land.
Orlandah, Orlandia, Orlantha, Orlinda

Orlena (Latin) golden.
Orlana, Orlanah, Orleana, Orleanah, Orleena, Orleenah, Orleene, Orlenah, Orlene, Orlina, Orlinah, Orline, Orlyn, Orlyna, Orlynah, Orlyne

Orlenda (Russian) eagle.
Orlendah

Orli (Hebrew) light.
Orelea, Oreleah, Orlee, Orlei, Orleigh, Orley, Orlia, Orliah, Orlie, Orly, Orlya, Orlyah

Ormanda (Latin) noble. (German) mariner.
Orma, Ormandah, Ormandia, Ormandiah, Ormandya, Ormandyah

Ornat (Irish) green.
Ornait, Ornaita, Ornaitah, Ornata, Ornatah, Ornate, Ornete, Ornetta, Ornette, Ornit, Ornita, Ornitah, Ornite, Ornitt, Ornitta, Ornittah, Ornitte, Ornyt, Ornyta, Ornytah, Ornyte, Ornytt, Ornytta, Ornyttah, Ornytte

Ornella (Latin) she who is like an ash tree.

Ornice (Hebrew) cedar tree. (Irish) pale; olive colored.
Orna, Ornah

Orofrigia (Greek, Spanish) Phrygian gold. Geography: Phrygia was an ancient region in Asia Minor.

Orosia (Greek) a form of Eurosia.

Orpah (Hebrew) runaway. See also Oprah.
Orpa, Orpha, Orphie

Orquidea (Spanish) orchid.
Orquidia

Orquídea (Italian) beautiful as a flower.

Orsa (Latin) a short form of Orseline. See also Ursa.
Orsah, Orse

Orseline (Latin) bearlike. (Greek) a form of Ursula.
Orsalin, Orsalina, Orsalinah, Orsaline, Orsalyn, Orsalyna, Orsalynah, Orsalyne,

Orsel, Orselina, Orselinah, Orselyn, Orselyna, Orselynah, Orselyne, Orsola, Orsolah

Ortensia (Italian) a form of Hortense.

Orva (French) golden; worthy. (English) brave friend.
Orvah

Orwina (Hebrew) boar friend.
Orwin, Orwinah, Orwine, Orwyn, Orwyna, Orwynah, Orwyne

Osane (Spanish) health.

Osanna (Latin) praise the Lord.
Osana, Osanah, Osannah

Osen (Japanese) one thousand.
Osena, Osenah

Oseye (Benin) merry.
Osey

Osita (Spanish) divinely strong.
Ositah, Osith, Ositha, Osithah, Osithe, Osyta, Osytah, Osyte, Osyth, Osytha, Osythah

Osma (English) divine protector.
Osmah, Ozma, Ozmah

Oswalda (English) God's power; God's crest.
Osvalda, Osvaldah, Oswaldah

Otavia (Italian) a form of Octavia.
Otaviah, Otavya, Otavyah, Ottavia, Ottaviah, Ottavya, Ottavyah

Othelia (Spanish) rich.
Othilia

Otilie (Czech) lucky heroine.
Otila, Otilah, Otka, Ottili, Ottyli, Otyla, Otylah

Otylia (Polish) rich.
Otilia, Ottylia, Ottyliah, Ottyllia, Ottylliah, Ottylya, Ottylyah, Otyliah, Otylya, Otylyah

Ovia (Latin, Danish) egg.
Ova, Ovah, Oviah, Ovya, Ovyah

Ovidia, Ovidía (German) she who takes care of the sheep.

Owena (Welsh) born to nobility; young warrior.
Owenah, Owina, Owinah, Owyna, Owynah

Oya BG (Moquelumnan) called forth.
Oia, Oiah, Oyah

Oz BG (Hebrew) strength.
Ozz

Ozara (Hebrew) treasure, wealth.
Ozarah, Ozarra, Ozarrah

Ozera (Hebrew) helpful. (Russian) lake.
Ozerah, Ozira, Ozirah, Ozyra, Ozyrah

P

Pabla (Spanish) a form of Paula.

Paca (Spanish) a short form of Pancha. See also Paka.

Paciana (Latin) peaceful woman.

Pacífica (Spanish) peaceful.

Pacomia (Greek) large woman.

Padget BG (French) a form of Page.
Padgett, Paget, Pagett

Padma (Hindi) lotus.
Padmah, Padmar

Padmani (Sri Lankan) blossom, flower.
Padmanee, Padmaney, Padmania, Padmaniah, Padmanie, Padmany

Pagan GB (Latin) from the country.
Pagen, Pagin, Pagon, Pagun, Pagyn

Page GB (French) young assistant.
Pagi

Paige ☆ GB (English) young child.

Paisley (Scottish) patterned fabric first made in Paisley, Scotland.
Paislay, Paislee, Paisleyann, Paisleyanne, Paizlei, Paizleigh, Paizley, Pasley, Pazley

Paiton (English) warrior's town.
Paitan, Paiten, Paitin, Paityn, Paityne, Paiyton, Paten, Patton, Peita, Peiten, Peitin, Peiton, Peityn, Petan

Paka (Swahili) kitten. See also Paca.
Pakah

Pakuna (Moquelumnan) deer bounding while running downhill.

Pala (Native American) water.
Palah, Palla, Pallah

Palaciada, Palaciata (Greek) mansion.

Paladia (Spanish) a form of Palas.

Palas (Greek) a form of Pallas.

Palba (Basque) blond.

Palila (Polynesian) bird.
Palilah, Palyla, Palylah

Palixena (Greek) she who returns from the foreign land.

Pallas (Greek) wise. Mythology: another name for Athena, the goddess of wisdom.
Palace, Pallass, Pallassa

Palma (Latin) palm tree.
Pallma, Pamar

Palmela (Greek) a form of Pamela.
Palmelah, Palmelia, Palmeliah, Palmelina, Palmeline, Palmelyn, Palmelyna, Palmelyne

Palmer BG (Spanish) a short form of Palmira.
Palmir

Palmera, Palmiera (Spanish) forms of palm tree.

Palmira (Spanish) a form of Palma.
Pallmirah, Pallmyra, Palmara, Palmarah, Palmaria, Palmariah, Palmarya, Palmaryah, Palmirah, Palmyra, Palmyrah

Paloma (Spanish) dove. See also Aloma.
Palloma, Palomah, Palomar, Palomara, Palomarah, Palomaria, Palomariah, Palomarya, Palomaryah, Palometa, Palomita, Paluma, Peloma

Pamela (Greek) honey.
Palmela, Pam, Pama, Pamala, Pamalah, Pamalia, Pamaliah, Pamalla, Pamalya, Pamalyah, Pamelia, Pameliah, Pamelina, Pamella, Pamelya, Pamelyah, Pami, Pamie, Pamila, Pamilla, Pamm, Pammela, Pammi, Pammie, Pammy, Pamula, Pamy

Pana (Native American) partridge.
Panah, Panna, Pannah

Panambi (Guarani) butterfly.

Pancha (Spanish) free; from France.
Paca, Panchah, Panchita

Panchali (Sanskrit) princess from Panchala, a former country in what is now India.
Panchalea, Panchaleah, Panchalee, Panchalei, Panchaleigh, Panchaley, Panchalie, Panchaly

Pancracia (Greek) all-powerful.

Pandita (Hindi) scholar.

Pandora (Greek) all-gifted. Mythology: a woman who opened a box out of curiosity and released evil into the world. See also Dora.
Pandi, Pandorah, Pandorra, Pandorrah, Pandy, Panndora, Panndorah, Panndorra, Panndorrah

Pánfila (Greek) friend of all.

Pansofia (Greek) wise, knowledgeable.
Pansofee, Pansofey, Pansoffee, Pansoffey, Pansoffi, Pansoffia, Pansofi, Pansofiah, Pansofie, Pansophee, Pansophey, Pansophi, Pansophia, Pansophiah, Pansophie, Pansophy, Pansophya, Pansophyah

Pansy (Greek) flower; fragrant. (French) thoughtful.
Pansea, Panseah, Pansee, Pansey, Pansi, Pansia, Pansiah, Pansie, Pansya, Pansyah

Panthea (Greek) all the gods.
Panfia, Panfiah, Pantheah, Pantheia, Pantheya, Panthia, Panthiah, Panthya, Panthyah

Panya (Swahili) mouse; tiny baby. (Russian) a familiar form of Stephanie.
Pania, Paniah, Panyah, Panyia

Panyin (Fante) older twin.

Paola (Italian) a form of Paula.
Paoli, Paolina, Paoline

Papan (Nahuatl) flag.

Papina (Moquelumnan) vine growing on an oak tree.
Papinah, Papyna, Papynah

Paquita (Spanish) a form of Frances.
Paqua

Paradise (Persian) the garden of Eden.

Paramita (Sanskrit) virtuous; perfect.
Paramitah, Paramyta, Paramytah

Parasha, Parashie (Russian) born on Good Friday.

Pari (Persian) fairy eagle.

Paris GB (French) Geography: the capital of France. Mythology: the Trojan prince who started the Trojan War by abducting Helen.
Parice, Paries, Parise, Parish, Pariss, Parisse, Parys, Paryse, Paryss, Parysse

Parisa (French) a form of Paris.
Parisha, Parissa, Parrisha, Parysa, Paryssa

Parker BG (English) park keeper.
Park, Parke

Parmenia (Greek) constant, faithful.

Parmenias (Spanish) a form of Parmenia.

Parnel (French) a form of Pernella.
Parnela, Parnelah, Parnele, Parnell, Parnella, Parnellah, Parnelle

Parris GB (French) a form of Paris.
Parrise, Parrish, Parrys, Parrysh

Partenia (Greek) she who is as pure as a virgin.

Parthenia (Greek) virginal.
Partheenia, Parthena, Parthene, Partheniah, Parthenie, Parthenya, Parthenyah, Parthinia, Pathina

Parvati (Sanskrit) mountain climber.
Parvatee, Parvatey, Parvatia, Parvatiah, Parvatie, Parvaty, Parvatya, Parvatyah

Parveen (Indian) star.

Parveneh (Persian) butterfly.

Pascale (French) born on Easter or Passover.
Pascala, Pascalette, Pascalina, Pascaline, Pascalle, Pascalyn, Pascalyna, Pascalyne, Paschal, Paschale, Paskel, Pasqua, Pasquah

Pascasia (Greek) Easter.

Pascua, Pascualina (Hebrew) forms of Pascale.

Pascuala (Spanish) a form of Pascale.

Pascuas (Hebrew) sacrificed for the good of the village.

Pasha BG (Greek) sea.
Palasha, Pascha, Paschah, Pasche, Pashae,
Pashe, Pashel, Pashela, Pashelah, Pashele,
Pashell, Pashelle, Pashka, Pasia, Passia

Pasifiki (Tongan) Pacific Ocean.
Pacific, Pacifica, Pacificah, Pacificka, Pacifiqua,
Pacifiquah, Pacifique, Pacifyca, Pacifycah,
Pacifyqua, Pacifyquah, Pacifyque, Pacyfica,
Pacyficah, Pacyficka, Pacyfickah, Pacyfiqua,
Pacyfiquah, Pacyfique, Pacyfyca, Pacyfycah,
Pacyfycka, Pacyfyka, Pacyfyqua, Pacyfyquah,
Pacyfyque

Passion (Latin) passion.
Pashion, Pashonne, Pasion, Passionaé,
Passionate, Passionette

Pastora (German) shepherd.

Pasua (Swahili) born by cesarean section.

Pat BG (Latin) a short form of Patricia, Patsy.
Patt

Patam (Sanskrit) city.
Patem, Patim, Patom, Pattam, Pattem, Pattim,
Pattom, Pattym, Patym

Patamon BG (Native American) raging.

Pati (Moquelumnan) fish baskets made of
willow branches.
Patee, Patey, Patie

Patia (Gypsy, Spanish) leaf. (Latin, English) a
familiar form of Patience, Patricia.
Patiah, Patya, Patyah

Patience (English) patient.
Paciencia, Patiance, Patient, Patince, Patishia

Patli (Nahuatl) medicine.

Patra (Greek, Latin) a form of Petra.
Patria, Patriah

Patrice GB (French) a form of Patricia.
Patrease, Patrece, Patreece, Patreese, Patreice,
Patriece, Patryce, Patryse, Pattrice

Patricia (Latin) noblewoman. See also
Payten, Peyton, Tricia, Trisha, Trissa.
Patresa, Patrica, Patricah, Patricea, Patriceia,
Patrichea, Patriciah, Patriciana, Patricianna,
Patricja, Patricka, Patrickia, Patrisia, Patrissa

Patrisha (Latin) a form of Patricia.
Patrishah, Patrishia

Patrizia (Italian) a form of Patricia.
Patreeza, Patriza, Patrizah, Patrizzia

Patrocinio (Spanish) sponsorship.

Patrycja (American) a form of Patricia.
Patrycia, Patrycya, Patrycyah

Patsy (Latin) a familiar form of Patricia.
Patsee, Patsey, Patsi, Patsie

Patty (English) a familiar form of Patricia.
Patte, Pattee, Pattey, Patti, Pattie, Paty

Paula (Latin) small. See also Pavla, Polly.
Paliki, Paulane, Paulann, Paulla, Pavia

Paulette (Latin) a familiar form of Paula.
Paoleta, Paulet, Pauleta, Pauletah, Paulete,
Paulett, Pauletta, Paulettah, Paulita, Paullett,
Paulletta, Paullette

Paulie (Latin) a familiar form of Paula.
Paili, Pali, Pauli, Pauly

Paulina (Slavic) a form of Paula.
Paulena, Paulenia, Paulia, Pauliah, Pauliana,
Paulianne, Paullena, Paulya, Paulyah,
Paulyna, Paulynah, Pawlina, Polena, Polina,
Polinia

Pauline (French) a form of Paula.
Paule, Pauleen, Paulene, Paulien, Paulin,
Paulyn, Paulyne, Paulynn, Pouline

Paun (Indigenous) cloud.

Pavla (Czech, Russian) a form of Paula.
Pavlina, Pavlinka

Paxton BG (Latin) peaceful town.
Paxtin, Paxtynn

Payal (Indian) anklet, foot ornament.

Payge (English) a form of Paige.
Payg

Payten (Irish) a form of Patricia.
Paydon, Paytan, Paytin, Paytn, Paytton,
Paytyn

Payton GB (Irish) a form of Patricia.

Paz GB (Spanish) peace.
Pazz

Pazi (Ponca) yellow bird.

Pazia (Hebrew) golden.
Paza, Pazice, Pazise, Pazit, Pazya, Pazyah,
Pazyce, Pazyse

Peace (English) peaceful.
Peece

Pearl (Latin) jewel.
Pearle, Pearleen, Pearlena, Pearlene, Pearlette, Pearlina, Pearline, Pearlisha, Pearlyn, Perl, Perle, Perlette, Perlie, Perline, Perlline

Peata (Maori) bringer of joy.
Peatah, Peita, Peitah, Peyta, Peytah

Pedra (Portuguese) rock.

Pedrina (Spanish) a form of Pedra.

Peggy (Greek) a familiar form of Margaret.
Peg, Pegee, Pegeen, Pegey, Pegg, Peggee, Peggey, Peggi, Peggie, Pegi, Pegie, Pegy

Peighton (Irish) a form of Patricia.

Peke (Hawaiian) a form of Bertha.

Pela (Polish) a short form of Penelope.
Pele

Pelagia (Greek) sea.
Pelage, Pelageia, Pelagiah, Pelagie, Pelagya, Pelagyah, Pelga, Pelgia, Pellagia

Pelipa (Zuni) a form of Philippa.

Pemba (Bambara) the power that controls all life.

Penda (Swahili) loved.
Pandah, Pendah, Pendana

Penelope (Greek) weaver. Mythology: the clever and loyal wife of Odysseus, a Greek hero.
Pen, Peneli, Penelia, Peneliah, Penelie, Penelopa, Penelopea, Penelopee, Penelopey, Penelopi, Penelopia, Penelopiah, Penelopie, Penelopy, Penna, Pennelope, Pennelopea, Pennelopee, Pennelopey, Pennelopi, Pennelopia, Pennelopiah, Pennelopie, Pennelopy, Pinelopi

Penélope (Greek) a form of Penelope.

Peñen (Indigenous) promise.

Peni (Carrier) mind.

Peninah (Hebrew) pearl.
Paninah, Panine, Penina, Penine, Peninit, Peninnah, Penyna, Penynah, Penyne

Pennie, Penny (Greek) familiar forms of Penelope, Peninah.
Penee, Peney, Peni, Penie, Pennee, Penney, Penni, Pennia, Penniah, Peny

Penthea (Greek) fifth-born; mourner.
Pentheah, Penthia, Penthiah, Penthya, Penthyah

Peony (Greek) flower.
Peonee, Peoney, Peoni, Peonie

Pepita (Spanish) a familiar form of Josephine.
Pepa, Pepee, Pepi, Pepie, Pepitah, Pepite, Pepitta, Pepitte, Peppy, Pepy, Pepyta, Pepytah, Pepyte, Peta

Pepper (Latin) condiment from the pepper plant.

Perah (Hebrew) flower.

Perdita (Latin) lost. Literature: a character in Shakespeare's play *The Winter's Tale*.
Perdida, Perditah, Perdy, Perdyta, Perdytah

Peregrina (Latin) pilgrim, traveler.

Perfecta (Spanish) flawless.
Perfect, Perfection

Peri (Greek) mountain dweller. (Persian) fairy or elf.
Perea, Peree, Perey, Peria, Periah, Perie, Perita, Pery

Peridot (French) yellow-green gem.
Peridota, Peridotah, Perydot, Perydota, Perydotah

Perilla (Latin) Botany: an ornamental plant with leaves often used in cooking.
Perila, Perilah, Perillah, Peryla, Perylah, Peryll, Perylla, Peryllah

Perla (Latin) a form of Pearl.
Pearla, Pearlea, Pearleah, Perlah

Perlie (Latin) a familiar form of Pearl.
Pearlee, Pearlei, Pearleigh, Pearley, Pearli, Pearlie, Pearly, Perley, Perli, Perly, Purley, Purly

Perlita (Italian) pearl.
Perleta, Perletta, Perlitta, Perlyta, Perlytta

Pernella (Greek, French) rock. (Latin) a short form of Petronella.
Parnel, Pernel, Pernela, Pernelah, Pernele, Pernell, Pernellah, Pernelle

Perpetua (Spanish) perpetual.

Perri (Greek, Latin) small rock; traveler. (French) pear tree. (Welsh) child of Harry. (English) a form of Perry.
Peree, Peri, Perie, Perre, Perree, Perriann, Perrie, Perrin, Perrine, Perya, Peryah

Perry BG (English) a familiar form of Peregrine, Peter (see Boys' Names). See also Perri.
Parry, Perey, Perrey, Perrye, Pery

Persephone (Greek) Mythology: the goddess of the underworld.
Persephanie, Persephany, Persephonie

Perseveranda (Latin) she who perseveres.

Pérsida (Latin) a form of Persis.

Persis (Latin) from Persia.
Persia, Persiah, Perssis, Persy, Persys, Persysa, Persysah

Peta (Blackfoot) golden eagle.

Petra (Greek, Latin) small rock. A short form of Petronella.
Pet, Peta, Petraann, Petrah, Petrea, Petrova, Petrovna, Peytra, Pietra

Petrina (Greek) a form of Petronella.
Perinna, Perinnah, Perrine, Petena, Peterina, Petrin, Petrinah, Petrine, Petrona, Petroni, Petronia, Petronie, Petronija, Petrony, Petryn, Petryna, Petryne

Petrisse (German) a form of Petronella.
Petrice, Petriss, Petrissa

Petronella (Greek) small rock. (Latin) of the Roman clan Petronius.
Peronel, Peronella, Peronelle, Peternella, Petrenela, Petrina, Petrisse, Petronela, Petronelle, Petronilla, Petronille

Petronila (Latin) a form of Petronella.

Petula (Latin) seeker.
Petulah

Petunia (Native American) flower.
Petuniah, Petunya, Petunyah

Peyeche (Mapuche) unforgettable woman.

Peyton BG (Irish) a form of Patricia.
Peyden, Peydon, Peyten, Peytin, Peytyn

Phaedra (Greek) bright.
Faydra, Phadra, Phadrah, Phae, Phaedrah, Phaidra, Phe, Phedra, Phedre

Phallon (Irish) a form of Fallon.
Phalaine, Phalen, Phallan, Phallie, Phalon, Phalyn

Phebe (Greek) a form of Phoebe.
Pheba, Pheby

Phelia (Greek) immortal and wise.
Felia, Feliah, Felya, Felyah, Pheliah, Phelya, Phelyah

Phemie (Scottish) a short form of Euphemia.
Phemea, Phemee, Phemey, Phemi, Phemia, Phemiah, Phemy, Phemya, Phemyah

Pheodora (Greek, Russian) a form of Feodora.
Phedora, Phedorah, Pheodorah, Pheydora, Pheydorah

Philana (Greek) lover of mankind.
Filana, Phila, Philanna, Phileen, Phileene, Philene, Philiane, Philina, Philine, Phillane, Phylana, Phylanah, Phylane, Phyllan, Phyllana, Phyllanah, Phyllane

Philantha (Greek) lover of flowers.
Philanthe, Phylantha, Phylanthe

Philberta (English) brilliant.
Filberta, Filbertah, Filberte, Philbertah, Philberte, Phylbert, Phylberta, Phylbertah, Phylberte, Phyllberta, Phyllbertah, Phyllberte

Philicia (Latin) a form of Phylicia.
Philecia, Philesha, Philica, Philicha, Philiciah, Philycia

Philippa (Greek) lover of horses. See also Filippa.
Phil, Philipa, Philipine, Philippe, Philippina, Phillie, Phillipa, Phillipe, Phillipina, Phillippine, Philly, Phylipa, Phylipah, Phyllipa, Phyllipah, Phyllypa, Phyllypah

Philomela (Greek) lover of songs.
Filomela, Filomelah, Philomelah, Phylomela, Phylomelah

Philomena (Greek) love song; loved one. Religion: a first-century saint. See also Filomena, Mena.
Philoméne, Philomina, Philomine, Phylomina, Phylomine, Phylomyna, Phylomyne

Philyra (Greek) lover of music.
Philira, Philirah, Phylyra, Phylyrah

Phoebe (Greek) shining. See also Febe.
Phaebe, Phebea, Pheebea, Pheebee, Pheibee, Pheibey, Pheobe, Pheybee, Pheybey, Phoebey

Phoenix BG (Latin) phoenix, a legendary bird.
Phenix, Pheonix, Phynix

Photina (Greek) a form of Fotina.
Photine, Photyna, Photyne

Phoung (Vietnamese) phoenix.

Phylicia (Latin) fortunate; happy. (Greek) a form of Felicia.
Phylecia, Phylesha, Phylesia, Phylica, Phyliciah, Phylisha, Phylisia, Phylissa, Phyllecia, Phyllicia, Phylliciah, Phyllisha, Phyllisia, Phyllissa, Phyllyza

Phyllida (Greek) a form of Phyllis.
Fillida, Philida, Philidah, Phillida, Phillidah, Phillyda, Phillydah, Phylida, Phylidah, Phyllidah, Phyllyda, Phyllydah, Phylyda, Phylydah

Phyllis (Greek) green bough.
Filise, Fillis, Fillys, Fyllis, Philis, Phillis, Phillisia, Philliss, Philys, Philyss, Phylis, Phylliss, Phyllys

Pia (Italian) devout.
Piah, Pya, Pyah

Pía (Latin) a form of Pia.

Piedad (Spanish) devoted; pious.
Piedada

Piedade (Latin) pity.

Piencia (Latin) a form of Pía.

Pier (French) a form of Petra.
Peret, Peretta, Perette, Pieret, Pierett, Pieretta, Pierette, Pierra, Pierre, Pierrette, Pieryn, Pieryna, Pieryne

Pier Ann (American) a combination of Pier + Ann.
Pier Anne, Pier-Ann, Pier-Anne

Pierce BG (English) a form of Petra.

Pila (Italian) a form of Pilar.

Pilar GB (Spanish) pillar, column.
Peelar, Peeler, Pilár, Pilla, Pillar, Pylar, Pyllar

Pili (Spanish) a form of Pilar.

Pililani (Hawaiian) close to heaven.
Pililanee, Pililaney, Pililanie, Pililany

Pilmayquen (Araucanian) swallow.

Pimpinela (Latin) fickle one.

Ping (Chinese) duckweed. (Vietnamese) peaceful.

Pinga (Eskimo) Mythology: the goddess of game and the hunt.
Pingah

Pink (American) the color pink.

Pinterry (Australian) star.
Pinterree, Pinterrey, Pinterri, Pinterrie

Piper (English) pipe player.
Pipper, Pyper

Pipina (Hebrew) a form of Josefina.

Pippa (English) a short form of Philippa.
Pipa, Pipah, Pippah, Pypa, Pypah, Pyppa, Pyppah

Pippi (French) rosy cheeked.
Pipee, Pipey, Pipi, Pipie, Pippee, Pippen, Pippey, Pippie, Pippin, Pippy, Pipy

Piro (Mapuche) snows.

Piscina (Italian) water.
Pischina, Pishina, Pishinah, Pychina, Pychinah, Pychyna, Pychynah, Pycina, Pycinah, Pyshina, Pyshinah, Pyshyna, Pyshynah

Pita (African) fourth daughter.
Peeta, Peetah, Pitah, Pyta, Pytah

Pitrel (Mapuche) small woman.

Piula (Catalan) a form of Paula.

Piuque (Araucanian) heart.

Pixie (English) mischievous fairy.
Pixee, Pixey, Pixi, Pixy, Pyxee, Pyxey, Pyxi, Pyxie, Pyxy

Placencia (Latin) pleasant woman.

Plácida (Latin) a form of Placida.

Placidia (Latin) serene.
Placida, Placide, Placinda, Placyda, Placydah, Placynda

Platona (Greek) broad shouldered.
Platonah, Platonia, Platoniah, Platonya, Platonyah

Pleasance (French) pleasant.
Pleasence

Plena (Latin) abundant; complete.

Pocahontas (Native American) playful.
Pocohonta

Poeta (Italian) poetry.
Poetah, Poetree, Poetrey, Poetri, Poetrie, Poetry, Poett, Poetta, Poette

Polibia (Greek) full of life.

Policarpa (Greek) fertile.

Polidora (Greek) generous woman.

Polimnia (Greek) many hymns. Mythology: Polyhymnia is one of the Muses.

Polixena (Greek) a form of Polyxena.

Polla (Arabic) poppy.
Pola, Polah, Pollah

Polly (Latin) a familiar form of Paula, Pauline.
Polea, Poleah, Polee, Polei, Poleigh, Poley, Poli, Polie, Poll, Pollea, Polleah, Pollee, Polleigh, Polley, Polli, Pollie, Poly

Pollyanna (English) a combination of Polly + Anna. Literature: an overly optimistic heroine created by Eleanor Porter.
Polian, Poliana, Polianah, Poliane, Poliann, Polianna, Poliannah, Polianne, Polliann, Pollianna, Polliannah, Pollianne, Pollyana, Pollyanah, Pollyane, Pollyann, Pollyannah, Pollyanne, Polyan, Polyana, Polyanah, Polyane, Polyann, Polyanna, Polyannah, Polyanne

Poloma (Choctaw) bow.
Polomah, Polome

Polyxena (Greek) welcoming.
Polyxeena, Polyxeenah, Polyxenah, Polyxina, Polyxinah, Polyxyna, Polyxynah, Polyzeena,

Polyzeenah, Polyzena, Polyzenah, Polyzina, Polyzinah, Polyzyna, Polyzynah

Pomona (Latin) apple. Mythology: the goddess of fruit and fruit trees.
Pomma, Pommah, Pomme, Pomonah

Pompeya (Latin) lavish.

Pompilia (Latin) fifth daughter.

Pomposa (Latin) lavish, magnificent.

Ponciana (Greek) blouse.

Poni (African) second daughter.
Ponee, Poney, Ponie, Pony

Pooja (Indian) worship.

Poonam (Indian) merit; full moon.
Punam

Poppy (Latin) poppy flower.
Popea, Popeah, Popee, Popey, Popi, Popie, Poppea, Poppee, Poppey, Poppi, Poppie

Pora, Poria (Hebrew) fruitful.
Porah, Poriah, Porya, Poryah

Porcha (Latin) a form of Portia.
Porchae, Porchai

Porche (Latin) a form of Portia.

Porchia (Latin) a form of Portia.
Porcia

Porfiria (Greek) purple.

Porscha (German) a form of Portia.
Porcsha, Porschah, Porsché, Porschea, Porschia

Porsche (German) a form of Portia.
Porcshe, Pourche

Porsha (Latin) a form of Portia.
Porshai, Porshay, Porshe, Porshea, Porshia

Porter 🅱🅶 (Latin) gatekeeper.
Port, Portie, Porty

Portia (Latin) offering. Literature: the heroine of Shakespeare's play *The Merchant of Venice*.
Porta, Portah, Portiah, Portiea, Portya, Portyah

Posy (English) flower, small bunch of flowers.
Posee, Posey, Posi, Posia, Posiah, Posie, Posya, Posyah

Potamia, Potamiena (Greek) she who lives on the river.

Potenciana (Latin) powerful.

Prairie (French) prairie.

Praxedes, Práxedes (Greek) she who has firm intentions.

Preciosa (Latin) a form of Precious.

Precious (French) precious; dear.
Pracious, Preciouse, Precisha, Prescious, Preshious, Presious

Premilla (Sanskrit) loving girl.
Premila, Premilah, Premillah, Premyla, Premylah, Premylla, Premyllah

Prepedigna (Greek) worthy.

Presencia (Spanish) presence.

Presentación (Latin) presentation.

Presley GB (English) priest's meadow.
Preslea, Preslee, Preslei, Presli, Preslie, Presly, Preslye, Pressley, Presslie, Pressly

Presta (Spanish) hurry, quick.

Pricilla (Latin) a form of Priscilla.
Pricila, Pricilia

Prima (Latin) first, beginning; first child.
Prema, Primah, Primalia, Primara, Primaria, Primariah, Primetta, Primina, Priminia, Pryma, Prymah, Prymaria, Prymariah, Prymarya, Prymaryah

Primavera (Italian, Spanish) spring.
Primaverah, Prymavera, Prymaverah

Primitiva (Latin) a form of Prima.

Primrose (English) primrose flower.
Primrosa, Primula, Prymrosa, Prymrose

Princess (English) daughter of royalty.
Princcess, Princes, Princesa, Princessa, Princetta, Princie, Princilla, Pryncess, Pryncessa, Pryncessah

Prisca (Latin) a short form of Priscilla.

Priscila (Latin) a form of Priscilla.
Priscilia

Prisciliana (English) a form of Prisca.

Priscilla (Latin) ancient.
Cilla, Piri, Precila, Precilla, Prescilla, Presilla, Pressilia, Priscela, Priscella, Priscill, Priscille, Priscillia, Priscillie, Prisella, Prisila, Prisilla, Prissila, Prissilla, Prycyla, Prycylah, Pryscylla, Prysilla, Prysillah, Prysylla, Prysyllah

Prissy (Latin) a familiar form of Priscilla.
Pris, Prisi, Priss, Prissi, Prissie

Priya (Hindi) beloved; sweet natured.
Pria, Priyah

Priyanka (Indian) dear one.
Priyasha

Procopia (Latin) declared leader.

Promise (Latin) promise, pledge.
Promis, Promisea, Promisee, Promisey, Promisi, Promisie, Promiss, Promissa, Promisse, Promissee, Promissey, Promissi, Promissie, Promissy, Promisy, Promys, Promyse

Proserpina (Greek) Mythology: the queen of the underworld.

Prospera (Latin) prosperous.
Prosperitee, Prosperitey, Prosperiti, Prosperitie, Prosperity

Próspera (Greek) a form of Prospera.

Providencia (Spanish) providence, destiny.

Pru (Latin) a short form of Prudence.
Prue

Prudence (Latin) cautious; discreet.
Prudance, Prudencia, Prudens

Prudenciana (Spanish) a form of Prudence.

Prudy (Latin) a familiar form of Prudence.
Prudee, Prudi, Prudie

Prunella (Latin) brown; little plum. See also Nellie.
Prunel, Prunela, Prunelah, Prunele, Prunell, Prunellah, Prunelle

Psyche (Greek) soul. Mythology: a beautiful mortal loved by Eros, the Greek god of love.
Psyke, Syche, Syke

Pua (Hawaiian) flower.
Puah

Puakea (Hawaiian) white flower.
Puakeah, Puakia, Puakiah, Puakya, Puakyah

Pualani (Hawaiian) heavenly flower.
Pualanee, Pualaney, Pualania, Pualaniah,
Pualanie, Pualany, Puni

Publia (Latin) from the village.

Pudenciana (Latin) a form of Prudenciana.

Puebla (Spanish) Geography: a city in
Mexico.

Puja (Indian) worship.

Pulqueria (Latin) pretty.

Purificación (Spanish) purification.

Purísima (Spanish) pure.

Purity (English) purity.
Pura, Purah, Pure, Pureza, Purisima, Puritee,
Puritey, Puriti, Puritia, Puritiah, Puritie,
Puritya

Pusina (Latin) child.

Pyralis (Greek) fire.
Piralis, Piralissa, Pyralissa

Pyrena (Greek) fiery.
Pirena, Pirenah, Pyrenah, Pyrene

Pythia (Greek) prophet.
Pithea, Pitheah, Pithia, Pithiah, Pythea,
Pytheah, Pythiah, Pythis, Pythya, Pythyah

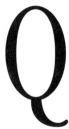

Qadesh (Egyptian) Mythology: an Egyptian
goddess.
Qadesha, Qadeshah, Quedesh, Quedesha

Qadira (Arabic) powerful.
Kadira, Kadirah, Qadirah, Qadyra

Qamra (Arabic) moon.
Kamra, Qamrah

Qiana (American) a form of Quiana.

Qitarah (Arabic) fragrant.
Qitara, Qytara, Qytarah

Quaashie BG (Ewe) born on Sunday.
Quashi, Quashie, Quashy

Quadeisha (American) a combination of
Qadira + Aisha.
Quadaishia, Quadajah, Quadasha, Quadasia,
Quadayshia, Quadaza, Quadejah, Quadesha,
Quadeshia, Quadiasha, Quaesha, Qudaisha

Quaneisha (American) a combination of
the prefix Qu + Niesha.
Quaneasa, Quanece, Quanecia, Quaneesha,
Quaneice, Quansha, Quneasha, Quynecia,
Qwanisha, Qynecia, Qynisha

Quanesha (American) a form of
Quaneisha.
Quamesha, Quaneshia, Quanesia, Quanessa,
Quanessia, Quannesha, Quanneshia,
Quannezia, Quayneshia, Quonesha,
Quynesha, Quynesia

Quanika (American) a combination of the
prefix Qu + Nika.
Quanikka, Quanikki, Quaniqua, Quanique,
Quantenique, Quanyka, Quanykka,
Quanykki, Quanyque, Quawanica,
Quawanyca, Queenika, Queenique

Quanisha (American) a form of Quaneisha.
Quaniesha, Quanishia, Quarnisha,
Quaynisha, Queenisha, Quynisha, Quynishia,
Quynsha, Qynisha, Qynysha

Quarralia (Australian) star.
Quaralia, Quaraliah, Quaralya, Quaralyah,
Quarraliah, Quarralya, Quarralyah

Quartilla (Latin) fourth.
Quantilla, Quartila, Quartilah, Quartile,
Quartillah, Quartille, Quartyla, Quartylah,
Quartyle, Quartylla, Quartyllah, Quartylle,
Quintila, Quintilah, Quintile, Quintilla,
Quintillah, Quintille, Quintyla, Quintylah,
Quintyle, Quintylla, Quintyllah, Quintylle,
Quyntila, Quyntilah, Quyntile, Quyntilla,
Quyntillah, Quyntille, Quyntyla, Quyntylah,
Quyntyle, Quyntylla, Quyntyllah, Quyntylle

Qubilah (Arabic) agreeable.
Quabila, Quabilah, Quabyla, Quabylah,
Qubila, Qubyla, Qubylah

Queen (English) queen. See also Quinn.
Quean, Queena, Queenah, Quenna

Queenie (English) a form of Queen.
*Queanee, Queaney, Queani, Queania,
Queaniah, Queanie, Queany, Queanya,
Queanyah, Queenation, Queenee, Queeneste,
Queenet, Queeneta, Queenete, Queenett,
Queenetta, Queenette, Queeney, Queeni,
Queenia, Queeniah, Queenika, Queenique,
Queeny, Queenya, Queenyah*

Queisha (American) a short form of
Quaneisha.
*Qeysha, Qeyshia, Qeyshiah, Queishah,
Queshia, Queshiah, Queshya, Queshyah,
Queysha*

Quelidonia (Greek) swallow.

Quelita (American) a combination of
Queen + Lita.
*Queleata, Queleatah, Queleeta, Queleetah,
Queleta, Queletah, Quelitah, Quelyta,
Quelytah*

Quella (English) quiet, pacify.
Quela, Quele, Quellah, Quelle

Quenby BG (Scandinavian) feminine.
*Queenbea, Queenbee, Queenbey, Queenbi,
Queenbie, Quenbye*

Quenisha (American) a combination of
Queen + Aisha.
*Queneesha, Quenesha, Quenishia,
Quennisha, Quensha, Quonisha, Quonnisha*

Quenna (English) a form of Queen.
*Queana, Queanah, Quena, Quenell,
Quenella, Quenelle, Quenessa, Quenesse,
Queneta, Quenete, Quenetta, Quenette,
Quennah*

Queralt (Celtic) high rock.

Querida (Spanish) dear; beloved.
Queridah, Queryda, Querydah

Querima, **Querina** (Arabic) the generous
one.

Quesara (Latin) youthful.

Quesare (Spanish) long-haired.

Questa (French) searcher.
Quest, Questah, Queste

Queta (Spanish) a short form of names ending in "queta" or "quetta."
Quetah, Quetta

Quetromán (Mapuche) restrained soul.

Quetzalxochitl (Nahuatl) precious flower;
queen.

Quiana, Quianna (American) combinations
of the prefix Qu + Anna.
*Quian, Quianah, Quianda, Quiane, Quiani,
Quianita, Quiann, Quiannah, Quianne,
Quionna, Quyana, Quyanah, Quyane,
Quyann, Quyanna, Quyannah, Quyanne*

Quíbele (Turkish) Mythology: another
name for Cybele, the goddess mother.

Quieta (English) quiet.
*Quietah, Quiete, Quietta, Quiettah, Quiette,
Quyeta, Quyetah, Quyete, Quyetta,
Quyettah, Quyette*

Quiliana (Spanish) substantial; productive.

Quilla (Incan) Mythology: Mama Quilla was
the goddess of the moon.
*Quila, Quilah, Quill, Quillah, Quille, Quyla,
Quylah, Quyle, Quylla, Quyllah, Quylle*

Quillen (Spanish) woman of the heights.

Quillén (Araucanian) tear.

Quimey (Mapuche) beautiful.

Quinby (Scandinavian) queen's estate.
*Quinbea, Quinbee, Quinbey, Quinbi,
Quinbie, Quynbea, Quynbee, Quynbey,
Quynbi, Quynbia, Quynbie, Quynby*

Quincey BG (Irish) a form of Quincy.
Quincee, Quinncee, Quinncey

Quincy BG (Irish) fifth.
*Quinci, Quincia, Quincie, Quinnci, Quinncia,
Quinncie, Quinncy, Quyncee, Quyncey,
Quynci, Quyncia, Quyncie, Quyncy,
Quynncee, Quynncey, Quynnci, Quynncie,
Quynncy*

Quinella (Latin) a form of Quintana.
*Quinel, Quinela, Quinelah, Quinell,
Quinellah, Quinelle, Quynel, Quynela,
Quynelah, Quynele, Quynell, Quynella,
Quynellah, Quynelle*

Quinesburga (Anglo-Saxon) royal strength.

Quinesha (American) a form of Quenisha.
Quineshia, Quinessa, Quinessia, Quinnesha, Quinneshia

Quinetta (Latin) a form of Quintana.
Quinette, Quinita, Quinnette

Quinisha (American) a form of Quenisha.
Quinisa, Quinishia, Quinnisha

Quinn BG (German, English) queen. See also Queen.
Quin, Quina, Quinah, Quinna, Quinnah, Quinne, Quiyn, Quyn, Quynn

Quinshawna (American) a combination of Quinn + Shawna.
Quinshea

Quintana (Latin) fifth. (English) queen's lawn. See also Quinella, Quinetta.
Quinta, Quintah, Quintanah, Quintane, Quintann, Quintanna, Quintannah, Quintanne, Quintara, Quintarah, Quintina, Quintona, Quintonah, Quintonice, Quynta, Quyntah, Quyntana, Quyntanah, Quyntanna, Quyntannah, Quyntanne, Quyntara, Quyntarah

Quintessa (Latin) essence. See also Tess.
Quintaysha, Quintesa, Quintesha, Quintessah, Quintesse, Quintessia, Quintice, Quinticia, Quintisha, Quintosha, Quyntessa, Quyntessah, Quyntesse

Quintilia (Latin) she who was born in the fifth month.

Quintiliana (Spanish) a form of Quintilia.

Quintina (Latin) a form of Quintana.
Quinntina, Quinntinah, Quinntine, Quintia, Quintiah, Quintila, Quintilla, Quintinah, Quintine, Quintyn, Quintyna, Quintynah, Quintyne, Quyntia, Quyntiah, Quyntila, Quyntilah, Quyntilla, Quyntillah, Quyntin, Quyntina, Quyntinah, Quyntine, Quyntyn, Quyntyna, Quyntynah, Quyntyne

Quintrell (American) a combination of Quinn + Trella.
Quintrela, Quintrella, Quintrelle

Quintruy (Mapuche) investigator.

Quintuqueo (Mapuche) she who searches for wisdom.

Quinturay (Mapuche) she who has a flower.

Quionia (Greek) she who is fertile.

Quirina (Latin) she who carries the lance.

Quirita (Latin) citizen.
Quiritah, Quirite, Quiritta, Quirittah, Quiritte, Quiryta, Quirytah, Quiryte, Quirytta, Quiryttah, Quirytte, Quyryta, Quyrytah, Quyryte, Quyrytta, Quyryttah, Quyrytte

Quisa (Egyptian) sister of twins.

Quisilinda (Scandinavian) sweet arrow.

Quiterie (Latin, French) tranquil.
Quita, Quitah, Quiteree, Quiteri, Quiteria, Quiteriah, Quitery, Quyteree, Quyteri, Quyteria, Quyteriah, Quyterie, Quytery

Qwanisha (American) a form of Quaneisha.
Qwanechia, Qwanesha, Qwanessia, Qwantasha

R

Ráa (Spanish) a form of Ria.

Raanana (Hebrew) fresh; luxuriant.
Ranana, Rananah

Rabecca (Hebrew) a form of Rebecca.
Rabbeca, Rabbecah, Rabbecca, Rabeca, Rabecka, Rabekah

Rabi BG (Arabic) breeze.
Raby

Rabia (Arabic) a form of Rabi.
Rabiah, Rabya, Rabyah

Rachael (Hebrew) a form of Rachel.
Rachaele, Rachaell

Rachal (Hebrew) a form of Rachel.
Rachall, Rachalle

Racheal (Hebrew) a form of Rachel.

Rachel ☀ GB (Hebrew) female sheep. Bible: the second wife of Jacob. See also Lahela, Rae, Rochelle.
Rachail, Rachela, Rachelann, Rahel, Raiche,

Raichel, Raichele, Raichell, Raichelle, Raishel, Raishele, Ruchel, Ruchelle

Rachele, Rachell, Rachelle (French) forms of Rachel. See also Shelley.
Rachella

Racquel (French) a form of Rachel.
Rackel, Racquele, Racquell, Racquella, Racquelle

Radegunda (German) battle counselor.

Radella (German) counselor.
Radela, Radelah, Radelia, Radeliah, Radellah, Radelle, Radiliah, Radillia, Radilliah, Radyla, Radylah, Radyllya, Radyllyah

Radeyah (Arabic) content, satisfied.
Radeeyah, Radhiya, Radhiyah, Radiah, Radiyah

Radhika (Indian) beloved. (Swahili) agreeable.

Radiante (Latin) radiant.

Radinka (Slavic) full of life; happy, glad.
Radinkah, Radynka, Radynkah

Radmilla (Slavic) worker for the people.
Radmila, Radmilah, Radmile, Radmill, Radmilla, Radmillah, Radmille, Radmyla, Radmylah, Radmyle, Radmyll, Radmylla, Radmyllah, Radmylle

Rae (English) doe. (Hebrew) a short form of Rachel.
Raeh, Raeneice, Raeneisha, Raesha, Rai, Raii, Ray, Raycene, Raye, Rayetta, Rayette, Rayma, Rey

Raeann, Raeanne (American) combinations of Rae + Ann. See also Rayan.
Raea, Raean, Raeane, Raiane, Raiann, Raianne

Raeanna (American) a combination of Rae + Anna.
Raeana, Raeanah, Raeannah, Raeona, Raiana, Raianah, Raianna, Raiannah

Raeca (Spanish) beautiful; unique.

Raechel, Raechelle (Hebrew) forms of Rachel.
Raechael, Raechal, Raechele, Raechell, Raechyl

Raeden (Japanese) Mythology: Raiden was the god of thunder and lightning.
Raeda, Raedeen

Raegan (Irish) a form of Reagan.
Raegen, Raegene, Raegine, Raegyn

Raelene (American) a combination of Rae + Lee.
Rael, Raela, Raelani, Raele, Raeleah, Raelean, Raeleana, Raeleanah, Raeleane, Raelee, Raeleen, Raeleena, Raeleenah, Raeleene, Raeleia, Raeleigh, Raeleigha, Raelein, Raelennia, Raelesha, Raelin, Raelina, Raelinah, Raeline, Raelle, Railean, Raileana, Raileanah, Raileane, Raileen, Raileena, Raileenah, Raileene, Ralean, Raleana, Raleanah, Raleane, Raleen, Raleena, Raleenah, Raleene, Ralin, Ralina, Ralinah, Raline

Raelyn, Raelynn (American) forms of Raelene.
Raelyna, Raelynah, Raelynda, Raelyne, Raelynne, Railyn, Railyna, Railynah, Railyne, Ralyn, Ralyna, Ralynah, Ralyne

Raena (German) a form of Raina.
Raeinna, Raen, Raenah, Raenee, Raeni, Raenia, Raenie, Raenna, Raeny, Raeonna, Raeyauna, Raeyn, Raeyonna

Raetruda (German) powerful advice.

Raeven (English) a form of Raven.
Raevin, Raevion, Raevon, Raevonna, Raevyn, Raevynne, Raewyn, Raewynne

Rafa (Arabic) happy; prosperous.
Rafah, Raffa, Raffah

Rafaela (Hebrew) a form of Raphaela.
Rafaelah, Rafaelia, Rafaeliah, Rafaella, Rafaellah, Raffaela, Raffaelah, Raffaella, Raffaellah, Rafia, Rafiah, Rafya, Rafyah

Rafaelle GB (French) a form of Raphaelle.
Rafael, Rafaele, Rafaell, Raffaele, Raffaell, Raffaelle

Ragan, Ragen (Irish) forms of Reagan.
Ragean, Rageane, Rageen, Ragene, Rageni, Ragenna, Raggan

Ragine (English) a form of Regina.
Ragin, Ragina, Raginee

Ragnild (Scandinavian) battle counsel.
*Ragna, Ragnah, Ragnel, Ragnela, Ragnele,
Ragnell, Ragnella, Ragnelle, Ragnhild,
Ragnilda, Ragnildah, Ragnyld, Ragnylda,
Renilda, Renilde, Renyld, Renylda, Renylde*

Raheem BG (Punjabi) compassionate God.
Raheema, Rahima

Rahel (German) a form of Rachel.
Rahela, Rahil

Ráidah (Arabic) leader.
Raeda, Raedah, Raida, Rayda, Raydah

Raimunda (Spanish) a form of Ramona.

Rain (Latin) a short form of Regina. A form
of Raina, Rane.
Raene, Reyne

Raina (German) mighty. (English) a short
form of Regina. See also Rayna.
*Raheena, Rainah, Rainai, Rainea, Rainia,
Rainiah, Rainna, Rainnah, Rainnia,
Rainniah*

Rainbow (English) rainbow.
*Raenbo, Raenbow, Rainbeau, Rainbeaux,
Rainbo, Rainebo, Rainebow, Raynbow,
Reinbow, Reynbow*

Raine GB (Latin) a short form of Regina. A
form of Raina, Rane.

Rainee, Rainy (Latin) familiar forms of
Regina.
Rainie

Rainelle (English) a combination of Raina
+ Elle.
*Rainel, Rainela, Rainelah, Rainele, Rainell,
Rainella, Raynel, Raynela, Raynell, Raynella,
Raynelle*

Rainey GB (Latin) a familiar form of
Regina.

Raingarda (German) prudent defender.

Raini GB (Latin) a familiar form of Regina.

Raisa (Russian) a form of Rose.
*Raisah, Raissa, Raissah, Raiza, Raysa,
Raysah, Rayssa, Rayssah, Rayza, Razia*

Raizel (Yiddish) a form of Rose.
*Raizela, Raizelah, Raizele, Rayzil, Rayzila,
Rayzile, Rayzill, Rayzilla, Rayzille, Rayzyl,
Rayzyla, Rayzylah, Rayzyle, Razil, Razila,*

*Razile, Razill, Razilla, Razillah, Razille,
Razyl, Razyla, Razylah, Razyle, Razyll,
Razylla, Razyllah, Razylle, Reizel, Resel*

Raja GB (Arabic) hopeful.
Raia, Rajaah, Rajae, Rajai

Rajah (Arabic) a form of Raja.

Rajani (Hindi) evening.
Rajanee, Rajaney, Rajanie, Rajany

Rajel (Hebrew) bee.

Raku (Japanese) pleasure.

Raleigh BG (Irish) a form of Riley.
Ralea, Raleiah

Raley (Irish) a form of Riley.

Rama (Hebrew) lofty, exalted. (Hindi) godlike. Religion: an incarnation of the Hindu
god Vishnu.
Ramah

Raman (Spanish) a form of Ramona.

Ramandeep GB (Sikh) covered by the light
of the Lord's love.

Ramira (Spanish) judicious.

Ramla (Swahili) fortuneteller.
Ramlah

Ramona (Spanish) mighty; wise protector.
See also Mona.
*Raemona, Raimona, Raimonah, Raimone,
Ramonda, Raymona, Raymonah, Romona,
Romonda*

Ramosa (Latin) branch.
Ramosah, Ramose

Ramsey BG (English) ram's island.
Ramsha, Ramsi, Ramsie, Ramza

Ramya (Hindi) beautiful, elegant.
Ramia, Ramiah, Ramyah

Ran (Japanese) water lily. (Scandinavian)
destroyer. Mythology: the Norse sea goddess who destroys.

Rana (Sanskrit) royal. (Arabic) gaze, look.
Rahna, Rahnah, Ranah, Ranna, Rannah

Ranait (Irish) graceful; prosperous.
*Ranaita, Ranaitah, Ranaite, Ranayt,
Ranayta, Ranaytah, Ranayte*

Randa (Arabic) tree.
Randah

Randall BG (English) protected.
Randal, Randala, Randalah, Randale,
Randalea, Randaleah, Randalee, Randalei,
Randaleigh, Randaley, Randali, Randalie,
Randaly, Randel, Randela, Randelah,
Randele, Randell, Randella, Randelle,
Randilee, Randilynn, Randlyn, Randyl

Randee, Randi, Randie (English) familiar
forms of Miranda, Randall.
Rande, Randea, Randean, Randeana,
Randeane, Randeen, Randena, Randene,
Randey, Randii, Randin, Randina, Randine,
Randyn, Randyna, Randyne

Randy BG (English) a familiar form of
Miranda, Randall.

Rane (Scandinavian) queen.
Raen, Raene

Raneisha (American) a combination of Rae
+ Aisha.

Ranesha (American) a form of Raneisha.

Rangi (Maori) sky.
Rangee, Rangia, Rangiah, Rangie, Rangy

Rani GB (Sanskrit) queen. (Hebrew) joyful.
A short form of Kerani.
Rahnee, Rahney, Rahni, Rahnie, Rahny,
Ranee, Raney, Ranice, Ranie, Ranique,
Rannee, Ranney, Ranni, Rannie, Ranny,
Rany

Rania (Sanskrit, Hebrew) a form of Rani.
Raniah

Ranielle (American) a combination of Rani
+ Elle.
Rannielle, Rannyelle, Ranyelle

Ranisha (American) a form of Raneisha.

Ranita (Hebrew) song; joyful.
Ranata, Raneata, Raneatah, Raneate,
Raneatt, Raneatta, Raneattah, Raneatte,
Raneet, Raneeta, Raneetah, Raneete, Ranit,
Ranitah, Ranite, Ranitta, Ranittah, Ranitte,
Ranyta, Ranytah, Ranyte, Ranytta, Ranyttah,
Ranytte, Ronita

Raniyah (Arabic) gazing.
Raniya

Ranya (Sanskrit, Hebrew) a form of Rani.
(Arabic) a short form of Raniyah.
Ranyah

Rapa (Hawaiian) moonbeam.
Rapah

Raphaela (Hebrew) healed by God.
Raphaelah, Raphaella, Raphaellah

Raphaelle (French) a form of Raphaela.
Raphael, Raphaele, Raphaell

Raquel, Raquelle (French) forms of Rachel.
Rakel, Rakhil, Rakhila, Raqueal, Raquela,
Raquele, Raquell, Raquella, Ricquel,
Ricquelle, Rikell, Rikelle, Rockell

Raquilda (German) a form of Radegunda.

Raquildis (German) fighting princess.

Rasha (Arabic) young gazelle.
Rahshea, Rahshia, Rahshiah, Rashae, Rashai,
Rashea, Rashi, Rashia, Rashya, Rashyah

Rashanda (American) a form of Rashawna.
Rashunda

Rashawn BG (American) a short form of
Rashawna.
Raseane, Rashane, Rashaun, Rashaune,
Rashawne, Rashon

Rashawna (American) a combination of the
prefix Ra + Shawna.
Raseana, Raseanah, Rashana, Rashanae,
Rashanah, Rashani, Rashanna, Rashanta,
Rashauna, Rashaunah, Rashaunda,
Rashaundra, Rashawnah, Rashawnna,
Rashona

Rashawnda (American) a form of
Rashawna.

Rasheda (Swahili) a form of Rashida.
Rasheada, Rasheadah, Rashedah, Rasheeda,
Rasheedah, Rasheeta, Rasheida

Rashel, Rashell, Rashelle (American)
forms of Rachel.
Raeshelle, Raishell, Raishelle, Rashele,
Rashella, Rayshel, Rayshele, Rayshell,
Rayshelle

Rashida GB (Swahili, Turkish) righteous.
Rahshea, Rahsheda, Rahsheita, Rashdah,
Rashidah, Rashidee, Rashidi, Rashidie,
Rashyda, Rashydah

Rashieka (Arabic) descended from royalty.
Rasheeka, Rasheekah, Rasheika, Rasheka,
Rashekah, Rashika, Rashikah, Rasika,
Rasike, Rasiqua, Rasiquah, Rasyqua,
Rasyquah, Rasyque

Rashonda (American) a form of Rashawna.

Rasia (Greek) rose.
Rasiah, Rasya, Rasyah

Ratana (Tai) crystal.
Ratania, Rataniah, Ratanya, Ratna, Ratnah,
Rattan, Rattana, Rattane

Rathtyen (Welsh) child of Clememyl.

Ratri (Hindi) night. Religion: the goddess of
the night.
Ratree, Ratrey, Ratria, Ratriah, Ratrie, Ratry,
Ratrya, Ratryah

Ratrudis (German) faithful counselor.

Raula (French) wolf counselor.
Raolah, Raole, Raoula, Raulla, Raullah,
Raulle

Raveen (English) a form of Raven.
Raveene, Raveenn

Raveena (English) a form of Raven.
Raveenah

Raven GB (English) blackbird.
Raivan, Raiven, Raivin, Raivyn, Ravan,
Ravana, Ravanah, Ravanna, Ravannah,
Ravena, Ravenah, Ravene, Ravenn, Ravenna,
Ravennah, Ravenne, Raveon, Revena

Ravin, Ravyn (English) forms of Raven.
Ravi, Ravina, Ravinah, Ravine, Ravinne,
Ravion, Ravyna, Ravynah, Ravyne, Ravynn

Ravon BG (English) a form of Raven.

Rawan (Gypsy) a form of Rawnie.

Rawnie (Gypsy) fine lady.
Rawna, Rawnah, Rawnee, Rawney, Rawni,
Rawnia, Rawniah, Rawnii, Rawny, Rawnya,
Rawnyah, Rhawna, Rhawnah, Rhawnee,
Rhawney, Rhawni, Rhawnie, Rhawny,
Rhawnya, Rhawnyah

Raya (Hebrew) friend.
Raia, Raiah, Raiya, Rayah

Rayan BG (American) a form of Raeann.
Ray-Ann, Rayane, Reyan, Reyann, Reyanne

Rayann, Rayanne (American) forms of
Raeann.

Rayanna (American) a form of Raeanna.
Rayana, Rayanah, Rayannah, Rayeanna,
Reyana, Reyanna

Raychel, Raychelle (Hebrew) forms of
Rachel.
Raychael, Raychela, Raychele, Raychell,
Raychil

Rayelle (American) a form of Raylyn.
Rayel, Rayele

Rayén (Araucanian, Mapuche) flower.

Raylee (American) a familiar form of
Raylyn.
Rayleigh

Rayleen, Raylene (American) forms of
Raylyn.
Raylean, Rayleana, Rayleanah, Rayleane,
Rayleena, Rayleenah, Rayleene, Raylena,
Rayline

Raylyn, Raylynn (American) combinations
of Rae + Lyn.
Raylin, Raylina, Raylinah, Raylinn, Raylona,
Raylyna, Raylynah, Raylyne, Raylynne

Raymonde (German) wise protector.
Raemond, Raemonda, Raemondah,
Raemonde, Raimond, Raimonda, Raimondah,
Raimonde, Rayma, Raymae, Raymay,
Raymie, Raymond, Raymonda, Raymondah

Rayna (Scandinavian) mighty. (Yiddish)
pure, clean. (English) king's advisor.
(French) a familiar form of Lorraine. See
also Raina.
Raynah, Raynel, Raynell, Raynella, Raynelle,
Raynette, Rayney, Rayni, Raynia, Rayniah,
Raynie, Rayny, Raynya, Raynyah

Rayne GB (Scandinavian, Yiddish, French) a
form of Rane, Rayna.
Rayn

Raynisha (American) a form of Raneisha.

Rayonna (American) a form of Raeanna.
Rayona

Rayven (English) a form of Raven.
Rayvan, Rayvana, Rayvein, Rayvenne,
Rayveona, Rayvin, Rayvon, Rayvonia

Rayya (Arabic) thirsty no longer.

Razi BG (Aramaic) secretive.
Rayzil, Rayzilee, Raz, Razia, Raziah,
Raziela, Razilea, Razileah, Razilee, Razilei,
Razileigh, Raziley, Razili, Razilia, Raziliah,
Razilie, Razilla, Razillah, Razille, Razyl,
Razyla, Razylah, Razylea, Razyleah,
Razylee, Razylei, Razyleigh, Razyley,
Razyli, Razylia, Razyliah, Razylie, Razyly

Raziya (Swahili) agreeable.
Raziyah

Rea (Greek) poppy flower.
Reah

Reagan GB (Irish) little ruler.
Raygan, Raygen, Raygene, Rayghan, Raygin,
Reagen, Reaghan, Reagin, Reagine, Reagon,
Reagyn, Reigan, Reigana, Reiganah, Reigane,
Reygan, Reygana, Reyganah, Reygane

Real (Spanish) real, true.

Reanna (German, English) a form of Raina.
(American) a form of Raeann.
Reana, Reanah, Reannah, Reeana Reiana,
Reianah, Reianna, Reiannah, Reyana,
Reyanah, Reyanna, Reyannah

Reanne (American) a form of Raeann,
Reanna.
Rean, Reane, Reann, Reannan, Reannen,
Reannon, Reian, Reiane, Reiann, Reianne,
Reyan, Reyane, Reyann, Reyanne

Reba (Hebrew) fourth-born child. A short
form of Rebecca. See also Reva, Riva.
Rabah, Reaba, Reabah, Rebah, Reeba,
Reebah, Reiba, Reibah, Reyba, Reybah,
Rheba, Rhebah, Rheiba, Rheibah, Rheyba,
Rheybah

Rebbecca, Rebeca, Rebeccah (Hebrew)
forms of Rebecca.
Rebbeca, Rebbecah, Rebecah

Rebecca ⭐ (Hebrew) tied, bound. Bible:
the wife of Isaac. See also Becca, Becky.
Rebeccea, Rebecha, Rebecqua, Rebecquah,
Rebequa, Rebequah, Rebeque

Rebecka, Rebeckah (Hebrew) forms of
Rebecca.
Rebeccka, Rebecckah, Rebeckia, Rebecky

Rebekah, Rebekka, Rebekkah (Hebrew)
forms of Rebecca.
Rebeka, Rebekha, Rebekke

Rebi (Hebrew) a familiar form of Rebecca.
Rebbie, Rebe, Rebie, Reby, Ree, Reebie

Redempta (Latin) redemption.

Reed BG (English) a form of Reid.
Raeed, Rheed

Reem (Arabic) a short form of Rima.

Reema, Reemah (Arabic) forms of Rima.
Reama, Reamah, Rema, Remah

Reena (Greek) peaceful. (English) a form of
Rina. (Hebrew) a form of Rinah.
Reen, Reenah, Reene, Reenia, Reeniah,
Reenie, Reeny, Reenya, Reenyah

Reet (Estonian) a form of Margaret.
Reat, Reata, Reatah, Reate, Reatha, Reeta,
Reetah, Reete, Reit, Reita, Reitah, Reite,
Reta, Retha, Reyt, Reyta, Reytah, Reyte

Refugio (Latin) refuge.

Regan GB (Irish) a form of Reagan.
Regana, Reganah, Regane, Regann, Reganna,
Regannah, Regen, Regin

Reganne (Irish) a form of Reagan.

Regenfrida (German) peaceful advice.

Reggie BG (English) a familiar form of
Regina.
Reggi, Reggy, Regi, Regia, Regiah, Regie

Reghan (Irish) a form of Reagan.

Regina (Latin) queen. (English) king's advi-
sor. Geography: the capital of
Saskatchewan. See also Gina.
Raegina, Rega, Regeana, Regeanah, Regeena,
Regeenah, Regena, Regennia, Regiena,
Reginah, Reginia, Regis, Regyna, Regynah,
Reygina, Reyginah, Reygyna, Reygynah

Regine (Latin) a form of Regina.
Regeane, Regeene, Regin, Regyne, Reygin,
Reygine, Reygyn, Reygyne

Regla (Spanish) rule.

Régula (Latin) small king.

Rei GB (Japanese) polite, well behaved.

Reia, Reya, Reyes (Spanish) forms of
Reina.

Reid BG (English) redhead.
Read, Reide, Reyd, Reyde, Ried

Reiko (Japanese) grateful.
Reyko

Reilly BG (Irish) a form of Riley.
Reilee, Reileigh, Reiley, Reili, Reilley, Reily

Reina (Spanish) a short form of Regina. See
also Reyna.
*Rein, Reinah, Reine, Reinie, Reinna, Reiny,
Reiona, Renia*

Rekha (Hindi) thin line.
Reka, Rekah, Rekia, Rekiah, Rekiya, Rekiyah

Relinda (German) kind-hearted princess.

Remedios (Spanish) remedy.

Remei (Catalan) a form of Remedios.

Remi BG (French) from Rheims, France.
*Raymi, Reims, Remee, Remey, Remia,
Remiah, Remie, Remmee, Remmi, Remmia,
Remmiah, Remmie*

Remigia (Latin) rower.

Remington BG (English) raven estate.
Remmington

Remy BG (French) a form of Remi.
Remmey, Remmy

Ren (Japanese) arranger; water lily; lotus.

Rena (Hebrew) song; joy. A familiar form of
Irene, Regina, Renata, Sabrina, Serena.
Renah

Renae (French) a form of Renée.
*Renai, Renaia, Renaiah, Renay, Renaya,
Renaye, Rennae, Rennay, Rennaya, Rennaye,
Wrenae, Wrenai, Wrenay, Wrennae, Wrennai,
Wrennay*

Renata (French) a form of Renée.
*Ranata, Reinet, Reineta, Reinete, Reinett,
Reinetta, Reinette, Renada, Renatah, Renate,
Renatta, Reneata, Reneatah, Rennie,
Renyatta, Rinada, Rinata*

Rene BG (Greek) a short form of Irene,
Renée.
Reen, Reene, Renne

Renea (French) a form of Renée.
Reneah, Rennea, Renneah

Renee GB (French) a form of Renée.

Renée (French) born again.
Reenee, Reeney, Reneigh, Rennee, Rinee

Reneisha (American) a form of Raneisha.

Renelle (French) a form of Renée.
Renell

Renesha (American) a form of Raneisha.

Renisha (American) a form of Raneisha.

Renita (French) a form of Renata.
*Reneeta, Reneetae, Reneetah, Reneita,
Reneitah, Renetta, Renitah, Renitta,
Renittah, Renitte, Renitza, Renyta, Renytah,
Renyte*

Rennie (English) a familiar form of Renata.
*Reenie, Reney, Reni, Renie, Renney, Renni,
Renny, Reny*

Reparada (Latin) renewed.

Reseda (Spanish) fragrant mignonette blos-
som.
*Reseada, Reseadah, Resedah, Reseeda,
Reseedah, Resida, Residah, Resyda, Resydah,
Seda, Sedah*

Reshawna (American) a combination of the
prefix Re + Shawna.
*Resaunna, Reschauna, Reschaunah,
Reschaune, Reschawna, Reschawnah,
Reschawne, Rescheana, Rescheanah,
Rescheane, Reseana, Reseanah, Reshana,
Reshauna, Reshaunah, Reshaunda,
Reshawnah, Reshawnda, Reshawnna,
Reshonda, Reshonn, Reshonta*

Resi (German) a familiar form of Theresa.
*Resee, Resey, Resia, Resie, Ressa, Resse,
Ressee, Ressi, Ressie, Ressy, Resy, Reza,
Rezee, Rezey, Rezi, Rezie, Rezka, Rezy,
Rezzee, Rezzey, Rezzi, Rezzie, Rezzy*

Restituta (Latin) restitution.

Reta (African) shaken.
*Reata, Reatah, Reate, Reatee, Reatey, Reati,
Reatie, Reatta, Reattah, Reaty, Reita, Reitah,
Reitta, Reittah, Retah, Retee, Retey, Retta,
Rettah, Reyta, Reytah, Reytta, Reyttah,*

Rheata, Rheatah, Rheta, Rhetah, Rhetta, Rhettah

Retha (Greek) a short form of Aretha.
Reatha, Reitha, Rethah, Rethia, Rethiah, Rethya, Rethyah, Reti, Retie, Rety, Ritha

Reubena (Hebrew) behold a child.
Reubina, Reubinah, Reuvena, Reuvenah, Rubena

Reva (Latin) revived. (Hebrew) rain; one-fourth. A form of Reba, Riva.
Reava, Reavah, Ree, Reeva, Reevah, Revah, Revia, Reviah, Revida, Revidah, Revya, Revyah, Revyda, Revydah

Reveca, Reveka (Slavic) forms of Rebecca, Rebekah.
Reve, Revecca, Reveccah, Revecka, Reveckah, Revekah, Revekka

Revocata (Latin) call again.

Rewuri (Australian) spring.
Rewuree, Rewurey, Rewurie, Rewury

Rexanne (American) queen.
Rexan, Rexana, Rexanah, Rexane, Rexann, Rexanna, Rexannah, Rexanne

Reyhan BG (Turkish) sweet-smelling flower.
Reihan, Reihana, Reihanah, Reihane, Reyhana, Reyhanah, Reyhane

Reyna (Greek) peaceful. (English) a form of Reina.
Reyn, Reynah, Reyne, Reynee, Reyni, Reynie, Reynna, Reyny

Reynalda (German) king's advisor.
Reinald, Reinalda, Reinaldah, Reinalde, Reynaldah, Reynalde

Réz BG (Latin, Hungarian) copper-colored hair.
Res, Rezz

Reza BG (Czech) a form of Theresa.
Rezah, Rezi, Rezie, Rezka, Rezza, Rezzah

Rhea (Greek) brook, stream. Mythology: the mother of Zeus.
Rheá, Rhéa, Rheah, Rhealyn, Rhia

Rheanna (Greek) a form of Rhea.
Rheana, Rheanah, Rheannah, Rheeanna, Rheeannah

Rheannon (Welsh) a form of Rhiannon.
Rheanan, Rheannan, Rheannin, Rheanon

Rhedyn (Welsh) fern.
Readan, Readen, Readin, Readon, Readyn, Reedan, Reeden, Reedin, Reedon, Reedyn, Rheadan, Rheaden, Rheadin, Rheadon, Rheadyn, Rhedan, Rhedin, Rhedon, Rheedan, Rheeden, Rheedin, Rheedon, Rheedyn

Rhian (Welsh) a short form of Rhiannon.
Rheane, Rheann, Rheanne, Rheean, Rheeane, Rheeann, Rheeanne, Rhiane, Rhiann, Rhianne

Rhiana, Rhianna (Greek) forms of Rheanna. (Welsh) forms of Rhian. (Arabic) forms of Rihana.
Rhianah, Rhiannah, Rhiauna

Rhiannon (Welsh) witch; nymph; goddess.
Rhianen, Rhiannan, Rhiannen, Rhianon, Rhianwen, Rhianyn, Rhinnon, Rhyanan, Riannon, Rianon, Ryanan, Ryanen, Ryanin, Ryanyn

Rhoda (Greek) from Rhodes, Greece.
Rhodah, Rhodeia, Rhodia, Rhodiah, Rhodya, Rhodyah, Roda, Rodina

Rhodelia (Greek) rosy.
Rhodeliah, Rhodelya, Rhodelyah, Rodelia, Rodeliah, Rodelya, Rodelyah

Rhody (Greek) rose.
Rhode, Rhodea, Rhodee, Rhodey, Rhodi, Rhodie, Rhody, Rodi, Rodie

Rhona (Scottish) powerful, mighty. (English) king's advisor.
Rhonae, Rhonnie

Rhonda (Welsh) grand.
Rhondah, Rhondene, Rhondia, Rhondiah, Rhondiesha, Rhondya, Rhondyah, Ronelle, Ronnette

Rhonwyn (Irish) a form of Bronwyn.
Rhonwena, Rhonwenah, Rhonwin, Rhonwina, Rhonwinah, Rhonwine, Rhonwinn, Rhonwinna, Rhonwinnah, Rhonwinne, Rhonwyna, Rhonwynah, Rhonwyne, Rhonwynn, Rhonwynna, Rhonwynnah, Rhonwynne, Ronwen, Ronwena, Ronwenah, Ronwene, Ronwin, Ronwina, Ronwinah, Ronwine, Ronwyn, Ronwyna, Ronwynah, Ronwyne, Ronwynn, Ronwynna, Ronwynnah, Ronwynne

Rhyan BG (Welsh) a form of Rhian.
Rhyane, Rhyann, Rhyanne

Rhyanna (Greek) a form of Rheanna.
Rhyana, Rhyanah, Rhyannah

Ria (Spanish) river.
Rhia, Rhiah, Rhya, Rhyah, Riah, Rya, Ryah

Ría (Spanish) a form of Ria.

Rian GB (Welsh) a form of Rhian.
Riann, Riayn, Rioann, Rioanne

Riana, Rianna (Irish) short forms of Briana.
(Arabic) forms of Rihana.
Rianah, Riannah

Riane, Rianne (Welsh) forms of Rhian.

Rica (Spanish) a short form of Erica,
Frederica, Ricarda. See also Enrica,
Sandrica, Terica, Ulrica.
*Rhica, Rhicah, Rhicca, Rhiccah, Rhyca,
Rhycah, Ricah, Ricca, Riccah, Ricka, Rickah,
Rieca, Riecka, Rieka, Riqua, Riquah, Ryca,
Rycah, Rycca, Ryccah, Rycka, Ryckah,
Ryqua, Ryquah*

Ricadonna (Italian) a combination of
Ricarda + Donna.
*Ricadona, Ricadonah, Ricadonnah, Riccadona,
Riccadonah, Riccadonna, Riccadonnah,
Rickadona, Rickadonah, Rickadonna,
Rickadonnah, Rikadona, Rikadonah,
Rikadonna, Rikadonnah, Rycadona,
Rycadonah, Rycadonna, Rycadonnah,
Ryckadona, Ryckadonah, Ryckadonna,
Ryckadonnah, Rykadona, Rykadonah,
Rykadonna, Rykadonnah*

Ricarda (Spanish) rich and powerful ruler.
*Riccarda, Riccardah, Richanda, Richarda,
Richardah, Richardena, Richardina, Richena,
Richenza, Richi, Rickarda, Rickardah,
Rikarda, Rikardah, Ritcarda, Ritcharda,
Rycadra, Rycardah, Rycharda, Rychardah,
Ryckarda, Ryckardah, Rykarda, Rykardah*

Ricci (American) a familiar form of Erica,
Frederica, Ricarda. See also Ricki, Riki.
*Riccy, Rici, Ricquie, Rique, Ryckee, Ryckey,
Rycki, Ryckie, Rykee, Rykey, Ryki, Rykie,
Ryky*

Richa (Spanish) a form of Rica.

Richael (Irish) saint.
*Ricael, Rickael, Rikael, Rycael, Ryckael,
Rykael*

Richelle (German, French) a form of
Ricarda.
*Richel, Richela, Richelah, Richele, Richell,
Richella, Richellah, Richia, Rishel, Rishela,
Rishelah, Rishele, Rishell, Rishella, Rishellah,
Rishelle, Rychel, Rychela, Rychelah, Rychele,
Rychell, Rychella, Rychellah, Rychelle,
Ryshel, Ryshela, Ryshelah, Ryshele, Ryshell,
Ryshella, Ryshellah, Ryshelle*

Rickelle (American) a form of Raquel.
Rickel, Rickela, Rickell

Ricki GB (American) a familiar form of
Erica, Frederica, Ricarda. See also Ricci,
Riki.
Rickee, Rickey, Rickilee, Ricky

Rickia (American) a form of Ricki.
Rickina, Rickita, Rikia, Rikita, Rikkia

Rickie BG (American) a familiar form of
Erica, Frederica, Ricarda.

Rickma (Hebrew) woven.
*Rickmah, Ricma, Ricmah, Ryckma, Ryckmah,
Rycma, Rycmah, Rykma, Rykmah*

Ricquel (American) a form of Raquel.
Rickquel, Rickquell, Ricquelle, Rikell, Rikelle

Rictruda (German) powerful strength.

Rida BG (Arabic) favored by God.
Ridah, Ryda, Rydah

Rigel (Spanish) foot. Astronomy: one of the
stars in the constellation Orion.

Rigoberta (German) brilliant advisor.

Rihana (Arabic) sweet basil. See also
Rhiana, Riana.

Rika (Swedish) ruler.
*Rhika, Rhikah, Rhikka, Rhikkah, Rikah,
Rikka, Rikkah, Ryka, Rykah, Rykka,
Rykkah*

Riki GB (American) a familiar form of Erica,
Frederica, Ricarda. See also Ricci, Ricki.
*Rikee, Rikey, Rikie, Rikka, Rikke, Rikkee,
Rikkey, Rikkie, Rikky, Riko, Riky*

Rikki GB (American) a familiar form of
Erica, Frederica, Ricarda.

Rilee, Rileigh (Irish) forms of Riley.

Riley ⭐ BG (Irish) valiant. See also Rylee.
Rielee, Rieley, Rielle, Rielly, Riely, Rilea, Rileah, Rilei, Rili, Rilie, Rily

Rilla (German) small brook.
Rhila, Rhilah, Rhilla, Rhillah, Rhyla, Rhylah, Rhylla, Rhyllah, Rila, Rilah, Rillah, Ryla, Rylah, Rylla, Ryllah

Rim (Arabic) a short form of Rima.

Rima (Arabic) white antelope.
Rheama, Rheamah, Rheema, Rheemah, Rheyma, Rheymah, Rhima, Rhimah, Rhime, Rhyma, Rhymah, Rhymia, Rimah, Ryma, Rymah

Rimona (Hebrew) pomegranate. See also Mona.
Reamona, Reamonah, Reamone, Reemona, Reemonah, Reemone, Remona, Remonah, Remone, Rheimona, Rheimonah, Rheimone, Rheymona, Rheymonah, Rheymone, Rhimona, Rhimonah, Rhimone, Rhymona, Rhymonah, Rhymone, Rimonah, Rimone, Rymona, Rymonah, Rymone

Rin (Japanese) park. Geography: a Japanese village.
Rini, Ryn, Rynn, Ryny

Rina (English) a short form of names ending in "rina." (Hebrew) a form of Rena, Rinah.
Rheena, Rheenah, Rinea, Riney, Rini, Rinie, Rinn, Rinna, Rinnah, Rinne, Rinnee, Rinney, Rinni, Rinnie, Rinny, Riny, Ryna, Ryne, Rynea, Rynee, Ryney, Ryni, Rynie, Ryny

Rinah (Hebrew) joyful.
Rynah

Rio BG (Spanish) river. Geography: Rio de Janeiro is a seaport in Brazil.
Ryo

Río (Spanish) a form of Rio.

Riona (Irish) saint.
Reaona, Reaonah, Reeona, Reeonah, Reona, Reonah, Rheaona, Rheaonah, Rheeona, Rheeonah, Rheiona, Rheionah, Rheona, Rheonah, Rheyona, Rheyonah, Rhiona, Rhionah, Rhyona, Rhyonah, Rionah, Ryona, Ryonah

Risa (Latin) laughter.
Reasa, Reasah, Reesa, Reesah, Reisa, Reisah, Resa, Resah, Risah, Rysa, Rysah

Risha (Hindi) Vrishabha is another name for the zodiac sign Taurus.
Rishah, Rishay, Rysha, Ryshah

Rishona (Hebrew) first.
Rishina, Rishon, Rishonah, Ryshona, Ryshonah

Rissa (Greek) a short form of Nerissa.
Rissah, Ryssa, Ryssah

Rita (Sanskrit) brave; honest. (Greek) a short form of Margarita.
Reda, Reeta, Reetah, Reetta, Reettah, Reida, Rheeta, Rheetah, Riet, Ritah, Ritamae, Ritamarie, Ritta, Rittah, Ryta, Rytah, Rytta, Ryttah

Ritsa (Greek) a familiar form of Alexandra.
Ritsah, Ritsi, Ritsie, Ritsy, Rytsa, Rytsah

Riva (French) river bank. (Hebrew) a short form of Rebecca. See also Reba, Reva.
Rivah, Rivalee, Rivi, Rivvy, Ryva, Ryvah

Rivalea (American) a combination of Riva + Lea.
Rivaleah, Rivalee, Rivalei, Rivaleigh, Rivaley, Rivali, Rivalia, Rivaliah, Rivaly, Rivalya, Rivalyah, Riverlea, Riverleah, Ryvalea, Ryvaleah, Ryvalee, Ryvalei, Ryvaleigh, Ryvali, Ryvalia, Ryvaliah, Ryvalie, Ryvaly, Ryvalya, Ryvalyah

River BG (Latin, French) stream, water.
Rivana, Rivanah, Rivane, Rivanna, Rivannah, Rivanne, Rivers, Riviane, Ryvana, Ryvanah, Ryvane, Ryvanna, Ryvannah, Ryvanne, Ryver

Rivka (Hebrew) a short form of Rebecca.
Rivca, Rivcah, Rivkah, Ryvka, Ryvkah

Riza (Greek) a form of Theresa.
Riesa, Riesah, Rizah, Rizus, Rizza, Rizzah, Ryza, Ryzah, Ryzza, Ryzzah

Roanna (American) a form of Rosana.
Ranna, Rhoanna, Rhoannah, Roan, Roana, Roanae, Roanah, Roanda, Roane, Roann, Roannae, Roannah, Roanne

Robbi (English) a familiar form of Roberta.
Robby, Robbye, Robey, Robi, Robia, Roby

Robbie BG (English) a familiar form of Roberta.

Robert BG (English) famous brilliance.

Roberta (English) a form of Robert. See also Bobbette, Bobbi, Robin.
Roba, Robertah, Robertena, Robertha, Robertina, Robette, Robettia, Robettiah, Roburta, Roburtah, Ruperta, Ryberta, Rybertah

Robin GB (English) robin. A form of Roberta.
Rebin, Rebina, Rebinah, Rebine, Rebyn, Rebyna, Rebynah, Rebyne, Robann, Robban, Robbana, Robbanah, Robbane, Robben, Robbena, Robbenah, Robbene, Robbin, Robbina, Robbinah, Robbine, Robbon, Robeen, Roben, Robena, Robenah, Robenia, Robeniah, Robian, Robina, Robinah, Robine, Robinia, Robiniah, Robinn, Robon

Robinette (English) a familiar form of Robin.
Robernetta, Robinatta, Robinet, Robinett, Robinetta, Robinita, Robinta, Robynett, Robynetta, Robynette

Robustiana (Latin) well-built woman.

Robyn GB (English) a form of Robin.
Robbyn, Robbyna, Robbynah, Robbyne, Robbynn, Robyna, Robyne, Robynne

Robynn (English) a form of Robin.

Rochel (Hebrew, French) a form of Rochelle.

Rochelle (French) large stone. (Hebrew) a form of Rachel. See also Shelley.
Reshelle, Roch, Rocheal, Rochealle, Rochele, Rochell, Rochella, Rochette, Rockelle, Rohcell, Rohcelle, Roshel, Roshele, Roshell, Roshelle

Rochely (Latin) a form of Rochelle.

Rocio (Spanish) dewdrops.
Rocío, Rocyo

Roderica (German) famous ruler.
Rodericka, Roderik, Roderika, Roderocah, Roderyc, Roderyca, Roderycah, Roderyck, Roderycka, Roderyka, Rodreicka, Rodricka, Rodrika

Roderiga, Rodriga (Spanish) forms of Roderica.

Rodia (Greek) rose.

Rodnae (English) island clearing.
Rodna, Rodnah, Rodnai, Rodnay, Rodneta, Rodnete, Rodnett, Rodnetta, Rodnette, Rodnicka

Rodneisha (American) a combination of Rodnae + Aisha.
Rodesha, Rodisha, Rodishah, Rodnecia, Rodneycia, Rodneysha

Rodnesha (American) a form of Rodneisha.
Rodneshia

Rodnisha (American) a form of Rodneisha.

Rogaciana (Latin) forgiving woman.

Rogelia (Teutonic) beautiful one.

Rohana (Hindi) sandalwood. (American) a combination of Rose + Hannah.
Rochana, Rochanah, Rohan, Rohanah, Rohane, Rohanna, Rohannah, Rohanne, Rohena, Rohenah

Rohini (Hindi) woman.
Rohine, Rohiney, Rohinie, Rohiny, Rohynee, Rohyney, Rohyni, Rohynie, Rohyny

Roisin (Irish) a short form of Roisina.
Roisine, Roisyn, Roisyne, Roysyn, Roysyne

Roisina (Irish) rose.
Roisinah, Roisyna, Roisynah, Roysyna, Roysynah

Roja (Spanish) red.

Rolanda (German) famous throughout the land.
Ralna, Rolandah, Rolande, Rolandia, Rolandiah, Rolando, Rolandya, Rolandyah, Rolaunda, Roleesha, Rolinda, Rollande

Roldana (Spanish) a form of Rolanda.

Rolene (German) a form of Rolanda.
Rolaine, Rolena, Rolleen, Rollene

Rolonda (German) a form of Rolanda.

Roma (Latin) from Rome.
Romah, Romai, Rome, Romeise, Romeka, Romesha, Rometta, Romini, Romma, Romola

Romaine (French) from Rome.
Romain, Romaina, Romainah, Romana,
Romanah, Romanda, Romanel, Romanela,
Romanele, Romanella, Romanelle, Romania,
Romanique, Romany, Romayna, Romaynah,
Romayne, Romina, Rominah, Romine,
Romona, Romonia, Romyn, Romyna,
Romynah, Romyne

Romelda (German) Roman fighter.
Romeld, Romeldah, Romelde, Romilda,
Romildah, Romilde, Romildia, Romildiah,
Romylda, Romyldah, Romylde

Romelia (Hebrew) God's beloved one.

Romero (Spanish) romero plant.

Romia (Hebrew) praised.
Romiah, Romya, Romyah

Romola (Latin) a form of Roma.
Romel, Romela, Romelah, Romele, Romell,
Romella, Romellah, Romelle, Romellia,
Romelliah, Romila, Romilah, Romile,
Romilla, Romillah, Romille, Romillia,
Romolah, Romole, Romolla, Romollah,
Romolle, Romyla, Romylah, Romyle,
Romylla, Romyllah, Romylle

Romualda (German) glorious governess.

Rómula (Spanish) possessor of great
strength.

Romy GB (French) a familiar form of
Romaine. (English) a familiar form of
Rosemary.
Romee, Romey, Romi, Romie

Rona, Ronna (Scandinavian) short forms of
Ronalda.
Ronah, Ronalee, Ronnae, Ronnah, Ronnay,
Ronne, Ronsy

Ronaele (Greek) the name Eleanor spelled
backwards.

Ronalda (Scottish) powerful, mighty.
(English) king's advisor.
Rhonalda, Rhonaldah, Rhonaldia,
Rhonaldiah, Ronaldah, Ronaldia, Ronaldiah,
Ronaldya, Ronaldyah

Ronda (Welsh) a form of Rhonda.
Rondah, Rondai, Rondesia, Rondi, Rondie,
Ronelle, Ronnette

Rondelle (French) short poem.
Rhondelle, Rondel, Ronndelle

Roneisha (American) a combination of
Rhonda + Aisha.
Roneasha, Ronecia, Roneeka, Roneesha,
Roneice, Ronese, Ronessa, Ronesse, Roneysha,
Roniesha, Ronneisha, Ronnesa, Ronniesha,
Ronnysha, Ronysha

Ronelle (Welsh) a form of Rhonda, Ronda.
Ranell, Ranelle, Ronel, Ronela, Ronelah,
Ronele, Ronell, Ronella, Ronielle, Ronnel,
Ronnela, Ronnele, Ronnell, Ronnella,
Ronnelle

Ronesha (American) a form of Roneisha.
Ronnesha

Roneshia (American) a form of Roneisha.
Ronesia, Ronessia, Ronneshia

Roni GB (American) a familiar form of
Veronica and names beginning with
"Ron."
Rone, Ronea, Ronee, Roney, Ronia, Roniah,
Ronie, Ronnee, Ronney, Rony, Ronya,
Ronyah, Ronye

Ronica, Ronika, Ronique (Latin) short
forms of Veronica.
Ronicah, Ronikah, Roniqua, Ronnica,
Ronnicah, Ronnika, Ronnikah

Ronisha, Ronnisha (American) forms of
Roneisha.
Ronice, Ronichia, Ronicia, Ronise, Ronnisa,
Ronnise, Ronnishia

Ronli (Hebrew) joyful.
Ronlea, Ronleah, Ronlee, Ronlei, Ronleigh,
Ronley, Ronlia, Ronliah, Ronlie, Ronly,
Ronnlea, Ronnleah, Ronnlee, Ronnlei,
Ronnleigh, Ronnley, Ronnlia, Ronnliah,
Ronnlie, Ronnly

Ronnette (Welsh) a familiar form of
Rhonda, Ronda.
Ronet, Roneta, Ronetah, Ronete, Ronett,
Ronetta, Ronettah, Ronette, Ronit, Ronita,
Ronnetta, Ronnit, Ronny

Ronni (American) a familiar form of
Veronica and names beginning with
"Ron."

Ronnie, Ronny BG (American) familiar
forms of Veronica and names beginning
with "Ron."

Roquelia (German) war cry.

Roquelina (Latin) a form of Rochelle.

Rori (Irish) famous brilliance; famous ruler.
*Roarea, Roaree, Roarey, Roari, Roarie, Roary,
Rorea, Roree, Roria, Roriah, Rorie, Rorya,
Roryah*

Rory BG (Irish) famous brilliance; famous
ruler.

Ros (English) a short form of Rosalind,
Rosalyn. See also Roz.

Rosa (Italian, Spanish) a form of Rose.
History: Rosa Parks inspired the American
Civil Rights movement by refusing to give
up her bus seat to a white man in
Montgomery, Alabama. See also Charo,
Roza.
Rosae, Rosah

Rosa de Lima (Spanish) Rose from Lima,
the capital of Peru.

Rosabel (French) beautiful rose.
*Rosabela, Rosabelah, Rosabele, Rosabelia,
Rosabell, Rosabella, Rosabellah, Rosabelle,
Rosabellia, Rosabelliah, Rosebel, Rosebela,
Rosebelah, Rosebele, Rosebell, Rosebella,
Rosebellah, Rosebelle, Rosebellia, Rosebelliah,
Rozabel, Rozabela, Rozabelah, Rozabele,
Rozabell, Rozabella, Rozabellah, Rozabelle,
Rozebel, Rozebela, Rozebelah, Rozebele,
Rozebell, Rozebella, Rozebellah, Rozebelle*

Rosalba (Latin) white rose.
Rosalbah, Roselba

Rosalee, Rosalie (English) forms of
Rosalind.
*Rosalea, Rosaleen, Rosalei, Rosaleigh,
Rosalene, Rosali, Rosalle, Rosaly, Rosealee,
Rosealie, Roselee, Roselei, Roseleigh, Roseley,
Roseli, Roselie, Rosely, Rosilee, Rosli,
Rozalee, Rozalei, Rozaleigh, Rozaley,
Rozali, Rozalie, Rozaly, Rozele, Rozlee,
Rozlei, Rozleigh, Rozley, Rozli, Rozlie,
Rozly*

Rosalia (English) a form of Rosalind.
*Rosaleah, Rosaliah, Rosalla, Rosallah,
Roselea, Roseleah, Roselia, Roseliah, Rozalea,
Rozaleah, Rozália, Rozaliah, Rozlea,
Rozleah, Rozlia, Rozliah*

Rosalía (Spanish) a form of Rosalia.

Rosalín, Roselín (Spanish) forms of
Rosalyn.

Rosalina (Spanish) a form of Rosalind.
*Rosaleana, Rosaleanah, Rosaleena,
Rosaleenah, Rosaleina, Rosaleinah, Rosalinah,
Rosalyna, Rosalynah, Rozalaina, Rozalainah,
Rozalana, Rozalanah, Rozalina, Rozalinah*

Rosalind (Spanish) fair rose.
*Rosalinde, Rosalynd, Rosalynde, Roselind,
Rozalind, Rozalinde, Rozelynd, Rozelynde,
Rozland*

Rosalinda (Spanish) a form of Rosalind.
*Rosalindah, Rosalynda, Rosalyndah,
Roslynda, Roslyndah, Rozalinda,
Rozalindah, Rozelynda, Rozelyndah*

Rosalva (Latin) a form of Rosalba.

Rosalyn (Spanish) a form of Rosalind.
*Rosalean, Rosaleane, Rosaleen, Rosaleene,
Rosalein, Rosaleine, Rosalin, Rosaline,
Rosalyne, Rosalynn, Rosalynne, Rosilyn,
Rozalain, Rozalaine, Rozalan, Rozalane,
Rozalin, Rozaline, Rozalyn*

Rosamaria (English) a form of Rose Marie.
Rosamarie

Rosamaría (Spanish) a form of Rosamaria.

Rosamond (German) famous guardian.
*Rosamonda, Rosamondah, Rosamonde,
Rosiemond, Rozamond, Rozamonda,
Rozmond, Rozmonda, Rozmondah*

Rosamund (Spanish) a form of Rosamond.
*Rosamunda, Rosamundah, Rosamunde,
Rosemund, Rosemunda, Rosemundah,
Rosiemund, Rosiemunda, Rozmund,
Rozmunda, Rozmundah*

Rosana, Rosanna, Roseanna (English)
combinations of Rose + Anna.
*Rosanah, Rosania, Rosaniah, Rosannae,
Rosannah, Rosannia, Rosanniah, Roseana,
Roseanah, Roseania, Roseaniah, Roseannah,
Roseannia, Roseanniah, Rosehanah,*

Rosehannah, Rosiana, Rosianah, Rosianna, Rosiannah, Rossana, Rossanna, Rosyana, Rosyanah, Rosyanna, Rosyannah, Rozana, Rozanah, Rozanna, Rozannah, Rozannia, Rozanniah, Rozannya, Rozeana, Rozeanah, Rozeanna, Rozeannah, Rozzanna, Rozzannah, Rozzannia, Rozzanniah, Rozzanya, Rozzanyah

Rosangelica (American) a combination of Rose + Angelica.
Rosangelika, Roseangelica, Roseangelika

Rosanne, Roseann, Roseanne (English) combinations of Rose + Ann.
Rosan, Rosane, Rosann, Rose Ann, Rose Anne, Rosean, Roseane, Rosian, Rosiane, Rosiann, Rosianne Rossann, Rossanne, Rosyan, Rosyane, Rosyann, Rosyanne, Rozan, Rozane, Rozann, Rozanne, Rozannie, Rozanny, Rozean, Rozeane, Rozeann, Rozeanne, Rozzann, Rozzanne

Rosario GB (Filipino, Spanish) rosary.
Rosaria, Rosariah, Rosarie, Rosary, Rosarya, Rosaryah, Rozaria, Rozariah, Rozarya, Rozaryah, Rozaryo

Rosaura (Filipino, Spanish) a form of Rosario.
Rosarah

Rose (Latin) rose. See also Chalina, Raisa, Raizel, Roza.
Rada, Rasia, Rasine, Rois, Róise, Rosea, Roses, Rosina, Rosse, Roze, Rozelle

Rose Marie, Rosemarie (English) combinations of Rose + Marie.
Rosemarea, Rosemaree, Rosemari, Rosemaria, Rosemariah, Rozmari, Rozmaria, Rozmariah, Rozmarie

Roselani (Hawaiian) heavenly rose.
Roselana, Roselanah, Roselanea, Roselanee, Roselaney, Roselania, Roselaniah, Roselanie, Roselany, Roselanya, Roslanea, Roslanee, Roslaney, Roslani, Roslania, Roslaniah, Roslanie, Roslany, Roslanya, Roslanyah

Roseline, Roselyn (Spanish) forms of Rosalind.
Roselean, Roseleana, Roseleanah, Roseleane, Roseleen, Roseleena, Roseleenah, Roseleene, Roselein, Roseleina, Roseleinah, Roseleine, Roselene, Roselin, Roselina, Roselinah, Roselyna, Roselynah, Roselyne, Roselynn,

Roselynne, Rozelain, Rozelaina, Rozelainah, Rozelaine, Rozelan, Rozelana, Rozelanah, Rozelane, Rozelin, Rozelina, Rozelinah, Rozeline, Rozelyn, Rozelyna, Rozelynah, Rozelyne

Rosella (Latin) a form of Rose.
Rosela, Roselah, Rosellah, Rozela, Rozelah, Rozella, Rozellah, Rozellia, Rozelliah

Rosemary (English) a combination of Rose + Mary.
Rosemarey, Rosemarya, Rosemaryah, Rozmary, Rozmarya, Rozmaryah

Rosemonde (French) a form of Rosamond.
Rosemonda, Rosemondah, Rozmonde, Rozmunde

Rosenda (German) excellent lady.

Roser (Catalan) a form of Rosario.

Rosetta (Italian) a form of Rose.
Roset, Roseta, Rosetah, Rosete, Rosett, Rosettah, Rosette, Rozet, Rozeta, Rozetah, Rozete, Rozett, Rozetta, Rozettah, Rozette

Roshan BG (Sanskrit) shining light.
Roshaina, Roshainah, Roshaine, Roshana, Roshanah, Roshane, Roshani, Roshania, Roshaniah, Roshanie, Roshany, Roshanya, Roshanyah

Roshawna (American) a combination of Rose + Shawna.
Roseana, Roseanah, Roseane, Roshanda, Roshann, Roshanna, Roshanta, Roshaun, Roshauna, Roshaunah, Roshaunda, Roshawn, Roshawnah, Roshawnda, Roshawnna, Rosheen, Rosheena, Rosheene, Roshona, Roshowna

Roshni (Indian) brighteners.

Roshonda (American) a form of Roshawna.

Roshunda (American) a form of Roshawna.

Rosicler (French) a combination of Rosa + Clara.

Rosie, Rosy (English) familiar forms of Rosalind, Rosana, Rose.
Rosea, Roseah, Rosee, Rosey, Rosi, Rosia, Rosiah, Rosse, Rosya, Rosyah, Rosye, Rozsi, Rozy

Rosilda (German) horse-riding warrior.

Rosina (English) a familiar form of Rose.
Roseena, Roseenah, Roseene, Rosena, Rosenah, Rosene, Rosinah, Rosine, Rosyna, Rosynah, Rosyne, Roxina, Roxinah, Roxine, Roxyna, Roxynah, Roxyne, Rozeana, Rozeanah, Rozeane, Rozeena, Rozeenah, Rozeene, Rozena, Rozenah, Rozene, Rozina, Rozinah, Rozine, Rozyna, Rozynah, Rozyne

Rosinda, Rosuinda (Teutonic) famous warrior.

Rosio (Spanish) a form of Rosie.

Rosita (Spanish) a familiar form of Rose.
Roseat, Roseata, Roseatah, Roseate, Roseet, Roseeta, Roseetah, Roseete, Rosit, Rositah, Rosite, Rositt, Rositta, Rosittah, Rositte, Rosyt, Rosyta, Rosytah, Rosyte, Rozit, Rozita, Rozitah, Rozite, Rozyt, Rozyta, Rozytah, Rozyte, Rozytt, Rozytta, Rozyttah, Rozytte

Roslyn (Scottish) a form of Rossalyn.
Roslain, Roslan, Roslana, Roslanah, Roslane, Roslin, Roslina, Roslinah, Rosline, Roslinia, Rosliniah, Roslyne, Roslynn, Rosslyn, Rosslynn, Rozlain, Rozlayn, Rozlayna, Rozlin, Rozlina, Rozlinah, Rozline, Rozlyn, Rozlyna, Rozlynah, Rozlyne, Rozlynn, Rozlynna, Rozlynnah, Rozlynne

Rosmarí (Spanish) a form of Rosamaría.

Rosmira (German) a form of Rosilda.

Rosó (Catalan) a form of Rosario.

Rosoínda (Latin) a form of Rosa.

Rossalyn (Scottish) cape; promontory.
Rosalin, Rosaline, Rosalyne, Rossalin, Rossaline, Rossalyne, Rosselyn, Rosylin, Roszaliyn

Rósula (Latin) a form of Rosa.

Rosura (Latin) golden rose.

Roswinda (Germanic) a form of Rosinda.

Rotrauda (Germanic) celebrated counselor.

Rowan 🅱🅶 (English) tree with red berries. (Welsh) a form of Rowena.
Rhoan, Rhoane, Rhoann, Rhoanne, Rhoen, Rhoin, Rhoina, Rhoinah, Rhoine, Rhoinn, Rhoinna, Rhoinnah, Rhoinne, Rowana, Rowanah, Rowane, Rowon, Rowona, Rowonah, Rowone

Rowena (Welsh) fair-haired. (English) famous friend. Literature: Ivanhoe's love interest in Sir Walter Scott's novel *Ivanhoe*.
Ranna, Row, Rowe, Roweana, Roweanah, Roweena, Roweenah, Rowein, Roweina, Rowen, Rowenah, Rowene, Rowin, Rowina, Rowinah, Rowine, Rowyn, Rowyna, Rowynah, Rowyne, Rowynn, Rowynna, Rowynnah, Rowynne

Roxana, Roxanna (Persian) forms of Roxann.
Rexana, Rexanah, Rexanna, Rexannah, Rocsana, Roxanah, Roxannah, Roxannia, Roxanniah, Roxannie, Roxanny

Roxane (Persian) a form of Roxann.

Roxann, Roxanne (Persian) sunrise. Literature: Roxanne is the heroine of Edmond Rostand's play *Cyrano de Bergerac*.
Rocxann, Roxan, Roxianne

Roxie, Roxy (Persian) familiar forms of Roxann.
Roxi

Roya (English) a short form of Royanna.

Royale (English) royal.
Roial, Roiala, Roiale, Roiell, Roielle, Royal, Royala, Royalene, Royalle, Royel, Royela, Royele, Royell, Royella, Royelle, Roylee, Roylene, Ryal, Ryale

Royanna (English) queenly, royal.
Roiana, Roianah, Roiane, Roianna, Roiannah, Roianne, Royana, Royanah, Royane, Royannah, Royanne

Roz (English) a short form of Rosalind, Rosalyn. See also Ros.
Rozz, Rozzey, Rozzi, Rozzie, Rozzy

Roza (Slavic) a form of Rosa.
Rozah, Rozalia, Rozea, Rozeah, Rozelli, Rozia, Rozsa, Rozsi, Rozyte, Rozza, Rozzie

Rozelle (Latin) a form of Rose.
Rosel, Rosele, Rosell, Roselle, Rozel, Rozele, Rozell

Rozene (Native American) rose blossom.
Rozeana, Rozeanah, Rozeane, Rozeena, Rozeenah, Rozeene, Rozena, Rozenah,

Rozin, Rozina, Rozinah, Rozine, Rozyn,
Rozyna, Rozynah, Rozyne, Ruzena,
Ruzenah, Ruzene

Ruana (Spanish) poncho.
Ruan, Ruanah, Ruane, Ruann, Ruanna,
Ruannah, Ruanne, Ruon

Ruba (French) a form of Ruby.

Rubena (Hebrew) a form of Reubena.
Rubenah, Rubenia, Rubeniah, Rubina,
Rubinah, Rubine, Rubinia, Rubyn, Rubyna,
Rubynah

Rubi (French) a form of Ruby.
Rubbie, Rubia, Rubiah, Rubiann, Rubie

Rubí (Latin) a form of Ruby.

Ruby GB (French) precious stone.
Rubby, Rube, Rubea, Rubee, Rubetta,
Rubette, Rubey, Rubyann, Rubye

Ruchi (Hindi) one who wishes to please.
Ruchee, Ruchey, Ruchie, Ruchy

Rudecinda (Spanish) a form of Rosenda.

Rudee (German) a short form of Rudolfa.
Rudea, Rudeline, Rudey, Rudi, Rudia,
Rudiah, Rudie, Rudina, Rudy, Rudya,
Rudyah

Rudelle (American) a combination of
Rudee + Elle.
Rudel, Rudela, Rudele, Rudell, Rudella,
Rudellah

Rudolfa (German) famous wolf.
Rudolfea, Rudolfee, Rudolfia, Rudolfiah,
Rudolphee, Rudolphey, Rudolphia,
Rudolphiah

Rudra (Hindi) Religion: another name for
the Hindu god Shiva.
Rudrah

Rue (German) famous. (French) street.
(English) regretful; strong-scented herbs.
Roo, Ru, Ruey

Ruel (English) path.
Rual, Ruela, Ruelah, Ruele, Ruell, Ruella,
Ruellah, Ruelle

Rufa (Latin) a form of Ruffina.

Ruffina (Italian) redhead.
Rufeana, Rufeanah, Rufeane, Rufeena,

Rufeenah, Rufeene, Rufeine, Rufina, Rufinah,
Rufinia, Rufiniah, Rufynia, Rufyniah,
Rufynya, Rufynyah, Ruphina, Ruphinah,
Ruphinia, Ruphiniah, Ruphyna, Ruphynia,
Ruphyniah, Ruphynya, Ruphynyah

Rui (Japanese) affectionate.

Rukan (Arabic) steady; confident.
Rukana, Rukanah, Rukane, Rukann,
Rukanna, Rukannah, Rukanne

Rula (Latin, English) ruler.
Rulah, Rular, Rule, Ruler, Rulla, Rullah,
Rulor

Rumer (English) gypsy.
Rouma, Roumah, Roumar, Ruma, Rumah,
Rumar, Rumor

Runa (Norwegian) secret; flowing.
Runah, Rune, Runna, Runnah, Runne

Ruperta (Spanish) a form of Roberta.

Rupinder (Sanskrit) beautiful.

Ruri (Japanese) emerald.
Ruriko

Rusalka (Czech) wood nymph. (Russian)
mermaid.
Rusalkah

Russhell (French) redhead; fox colored.
Rushel, Rushela, Rushelah, Rushele, Rushell,
Rushella, Rushellah, Rushelle, Russellynn,
Russhel, Russhela, Russhelah, Russhele,
Russhella, Russhellah, Russhelle

Rusti (English) redhead.
Russet, Ruste, Rustee, Rustey, Rustie, Rusty

Rústica (Latin) country dweller, rustic.

Rut (Hebrew) a form of Ruth.

Rute (Portuguese) a form of Ruth.

Ruth (Hebrew) friendship. Bible: daughter-
in-law of Naomi.
Rooth, Routh, Rueth, Rute, Rutha,
Ruthalma, Ruthe, Ruthella, Ruthetta,
Ruthina, Ruthine, Ruthven

Ruthann (American) a combination of
Ruth + Ann.
Ruthan, Ruthanna, Ruthannah, Ruthanne

Ruthie (Hebrew) a familiar form of Ruth.
Ruthey, Ruthi, Ruthy

Rutilda (German) strong because of her fame.

Rutilia (German) she who shines brightly.

Ruza (Czech) rose.
Ruz, Ruze, Ruzena, Ruzenah, Ruzenka, Ruzha, Ruzsa

Ryan BG (Irish) little ruler.
Raiann, Raianne, Rye, Ryen, Ryenne

Ryane, Ryanne (Irish) forms of Ryan.

Ryann GB (Irish) little ruler.

Ryanna (Irish) a form of Ryan.
Ryana, Ryanah, Ryannah

Ryba (Czech) fish.
Riba, Ribah, Rybah

Rylee GB (Irish) valiant. See also Riley.
Ryelee, Ryeley, Ryelie, Rylea, Ryleah, Rylei, Ryli, Rylina, Rylly, Ryly, Rylyn

Ryleigh (Irish) a form of Rylee.
Rylleigh, Ryllie

Ryley BG (Irish) a form of Rylee.

Rylie GB (Irish) a form of Rylee.

Ryo BG (Japanese) dragon.
Ryoko

S

Saarah (Arabic) princess.
Saara, Saarra, Saarrah

Saba (Arabic) morning. (Greek) a form of Sheba.
Sabaah, Sabah, Sabba, Sabbah

Sabana (Latin) a form of Savannah.

Sabelia (Spanish) a form of Sabina.

Sabi (Arabic) young girl.

Sabina (Latin) a form of Sabine. See also Bina.
Sabena, Sabenah, Sabiny, Saby, Sabyna, Savina, Sebina, Sebinah, Sebyna, Sebynah

Sabine (Latin) History: the Sabine were a tribe in ancient Italy.
Sabeen, Sabene, Sabienne, Sabin, Sabyne, Sebine, Sebyn, Sebyne

Sabiniana (Latin) a form of Sabina.

Sabiya (Arabic) morning; eastern wind.
Sabaya, Sabayah, Sabea, Sabia, Sabiah, Sabiyah, Sabya, Sabyah

Sable (English) sable; sleek.
Sabel, Sabela, Sabelah, Sabele, Sabella, Sabelle

Sabra (Hebrew) thorny cactus fruit. (Arabic) resting. History: a name for native-born Israelis, who were said to be hard on the outside and soft and sweet on the inside.
Sabara, Sabarah, Sabarra, Sabarrah, Sabera, Sabira, Sabrah, Sabre, Sebra

Sabreen (English) a short form of Sabreena.
Sabreane, Sabreene, Sabrene

Sabreena (English) a form of Sabrina.
Sabreana, Sabreanah, Sabreenah

Sabrena (English) a form of Sabrina.

Sabria (Hebrew, Arabic) a form of Sabra.
Sabrea, Sabreah, Sabree, Sabreea, Sabri, Sabriah, Sabriya

Sabrina GB (Latin) boundary line. (English) princess. (Hebrew) a familiar form of Sabra. See also Bree, Brina, Rena, Xabrina, Zabrina.
Sabrinah, Sabrinas, Sabrinia, Sabriniah, Sabrinna, Sebree, Subrina

Sabrine (Latin, Hebrew) a short form of Sabrina.
Sabrin

Sabryna (English) a form of Sabrina.
Sabrynah, Sabryne, Sabrynna

Sacha BG (Russian) a form of Sasha.
Sachah, Sache, Sachia

Sachi (Japanese) blessed; lucky.
Saatchi, Sachie, Sachiko

Sacnite (Mayan) white flower.

Sacramento (Latin) consecrated. Geography: the capital of California.

Sada (Japanese) chaste. (English) a form of Sadie.
Sadá, Sadah, Sadako, Sadda, Saddah

Sadaf (Indian) pearl. (Iranian) seashell.

Sade (Hebrew) a form of Chadee, Sarah, Shardae.
Sáde, Sadea, Saedea, Shadae, Shadai, Shaday

Sadé (Hebrew) a form of Sade.

Sadee (Hebrew) a form of Sade, Sadie.

Sadella (American) a combination of Sade + Ella.
Sadel, Sadela, Sadelah, Sadele, Sadell, Sadellah, Sadelle, Sydel, Sydell, Sydella, Sydelle

Sadhana (Hindi) devoted.
Sadhanah, Sadhanna, Sadhannah

Sadi (Hebrew) a form of Sadie. (Arabic) a short form of Sadiya.

Sadia (Arabic) a form of Sadiya.
Sadiah

Sadie (Hebrew) a familiar form of Sarah. See also Sada.
Saddie, Sadey, Sadiey, Sady, Sadye, Saedee, Saedi, Saedie, Saedy, Saide, Saidea, Saidee, Saidey, Saidi, Saidia, Saidie, Saidy, Seidy

Sadira (Persian) lotus tree. (Arabic) star.
Sadirah, Sadire, Sadra, Sadrah, Sadyra, Sadyrah, Sadyre

Sadiya (Arabic) lucky, fortunate.
Sadiyah, Sadiyyah, Sadya, Sadyah

Sadzi (Carrier) sunny disposition.
Sadzee, Sadzey, Sadzia, Sadziah, Sadzie, Sadzya, Sadzyah

Safa (Arabic) pure.
Safah, Saffa, Saffah

Saffi (Danish) wise.
Safee, Safey, Saffee, Saffey, Saffie, Saffy, Safi, Safie, Safy

Saffron (English) Botany: a plant with purple or white flowers whose orange stigmas are used as a spice.
Saffrona, Saffronah, Saffrone, Safron, Safrona, Safronah, Safrone, Safronna, Safronnah, Safronne

Safia (Arabic) a form of Safiya.
Safiah

Safiya (Arabic) pure; serene; best friend.
Safeia, Safeya, Safiyah

Safo (Greek) she who sees with clarity.

Sagara (Hindi) ocean.
Sagarah

Sage BG (English) wise. Botany: an herb used as a seasoning.
Saeg, Saege, Sagia, Sayg, Sayge

Sagrario (Spanish) tabernacle.

Sahar, Saher (Arabic) short forms of Sahara.
Saheer

Sahara (Arabic) desert; wilderness.
Saharah, Sahari, Saharra, Saharrah, Sahira

Sahra (Hebrew) a form of Sarah.
Sahrah

Sai (Japanese) talented.
Saiko, Say

Saida (Arabic) happy; fortunate. (Hebrew) a form of Sarah.
Saeda, Saedah, Said, Saidah, Saide, Saidea, Sayda, Saydah

Saída (Arabic) a form of Saida.

Saige GB (English) a form of Sage.
Saig

Saira (Hebrew) a form of Sara.
Sairah, Sairi

Sakaë (Japanese) prosperous.
Sakai, Sakaie, Sakay

Sakari (Hindi) sweet.
Sakara, Sakarah, Sakaree, Sakari, Sakaria, Sakariah, Sakarie, Sakary, Sakarya, Sakaryah, Sakkara, Sakkarah

Saki (Japanese) cloak; rice wine.
Sakee, Sakia, Sakiah, Sakie, Saky, Sakya, Sakyah

Sakina (Indian) friend. (Muslim) tranquility, calmness.
Sakinah

Sakti (Hindi) energy, power.
Saktea, Saktee, Saktey, Saktia, Saktiah,
Saktie, Sakty, Saktya, Saktyah

Sakuna (Native American) bird.
Sakunah

Sakura (Japanese) cherry blossom; wealthy;
prosperous.
Sakurah

Sala (Hindi) sala tree. Religion: the sacred
tree under which Buddha died.
Salah, Salla, Sallah

Salaberga, Solaberga (German) she who
defends the sacrifice.

Salali (Cherokee) squirrel.
Salalea, Salaleah, Salalee, Salalei, Salaleigh,
Salalia, Salaliah, Salalie, Salaly, Salalya,
Salalyah

Salama (Arabic) peaceful. See also Zulima.
Salamah

Salbatora (Spanish) a form of Salvadora.

Saleena (French) a form of Salina.
Saleen, Saleenah, Saleene, Salleen, Salleena,
Salleenah, Salleene

Salem 🇬🇧 (Arabic) a form of Salím (see
Boys' Names).
Saleem

Salena (French) a form of Salina.
Salana, Salanah, Salane, Salean, Saleana,
Saleanah, Saleane, Salen, Salenah, Salene,
Salenna, Sallene

Salette (English) a form of Sally.
Salet, Saleta, Saletah, Salete, Salett, Saletta,
Salettah, Sallet, Salletta, Sallettah, Sallette

Salima (Arabic) safe and sound; healthy.
Saleema, Salema, Salim, Salimah, Salyma,
Salymah

Salina (French) solemn, dignified. See also
Xalina, Zalina.
Salin, Salinah, Salinda, Saline, Salinee, Sallin,
Sallina, Sallinah, Salline, Sallyn, Sallyna,
Sallynah, Sallyne, Sallynee, Salyn, Salyna,
Salynah, Salyne

Salinas (Spanish) salt mine.

Salliann (English) a combination of Sally +
Ann.
Saleann, Saleanna, Saleannah, Saleanne,
Saleean, Saleeana, Saleeanah, Saleeane,
Saleeann, Saleeanna, Saleeannah, Saleeanne,
Salian, Saliana, Salianah, Saliane, Saliann,
Salianna, Saliannah, Salianne, Salleeann,
Salleeanna, Salleeannah, Salleeanne, Sallian,
Salliana, Sallianah, Salliane, Sallianna,
Salliannah, Sallianne, Sally-Ann, Sally-Anne,
Sallyann, Sallyanna, Sallyannah, Sallyanne

Sallie (English) a form of Sally.
Sali, Salia, Saliah, Salie, Saliee, Salli, Sallia,
Salliah

Sally (English) princess. History: Sally Ride,
an American astronaut, became the first
U.S. woman in space.
Sailee, Saileigh, Sailey, Saili, Sailia, Sailie,
Saily, Sal, Salaid, Salea, Saleah, Salee, Salei,
Saleigh, Salette, Saley, Sallea, Salleah, Sallee,
Sallei, Salleigh, Salley, Sallya, Sallyah, Sallye,
Saly, Salya, Salyah, Salye

Salma (Arabic) a form of Salima.

Salome (Hebrew) peaceful. History: Salome
Alexandra was a ruler of ancient Judea.
Bible: the niece of King Herod.
Salaome, Saloma, Salomah, Salomé, Salomea,
Salomee, Salomei, Salomey, Salomi, Salomia,
Salomiah, Salomya, Salomyah

Salud (Spanish) a form of Salustiana.

Salustiana (Latin) healthy.

Salvadora (Spanish) savior.
Salvadorah

Salvatora (Italian) a form of Salvadora.

Salvia (Spanish) healthy; saved. (Latin) a
form of Sage.
Sallvia, Sallviah, Salviah, Salviana, Salvianah,
Salviane, Salvianna, Salviannah, Salvianne,
Salvina, Salvinah, Salvine, Salvyna, Salvynah,
Salvyne

Samah (Hebrew, Arabic) a form of Sami.
Sama

Samala (Hebrew) asked of God.
Samalah, Samale, Sammala, Sammalah

Samanatha (Aramaic, Hebrew) a form of Samantha.
Samanath

Samanfa (Hebrew) a form of Samantha.
Samanffa, Samenffa, Sammanfa, Sammanffa, Semenfa, Semenfah, Semenffah

Samanta (Hebrew) a form of Samantha.
Samantah, Smanta

Samantha ★ GB (Aramaic) listener. (Hebrew) told by God. See also Xamantha, Zamantha.
Samana, Samanitha, Samanithia, Samanth, Samanthe, Samanthi, Samanthia, Samanthiah, Semantha, Sementha, Simantha, Smantha

Samara (Latin) elm-tree seed.
Saimara, Samaira, Samar, Samarie, Samarra, Samary, Samera, Sammar, Sammara, Samora

Samarah (Latin) a form of Samara.

Samaria (Latin) a form of Samara.
Samari, Samariah, Samarrea, Sameria

Samatha (Hebrew) a form of Samantha.
Sammatha

Sameera (Hindi) a form of Samira.

Sameh (Hebrew) listener. (Arabic) forgiving.
Samaiya, Samaya

Sami BG (Arabic) praised. (Hebrew) a short form of Samantha, Samuela. See also Xami, Zami.
Samea, Samee, Samey, Samie, Samy, Samye

Samia (Arabic) exalted.
Samiha, Sammia, Sammiah, Sammya, Sammyah, Samya, Samyah

Samiah (Arabic) a form of Samia.

Samina (Hindi) happiness. (English) a form of Sami.
Saminah, Samyna, Samynah

Samira (Arabic) entertaining.
Samir, Samirah, Samire, Samiria, Samirra, Samyra, Samyrah, Samyre

Samiya (Arabic) a form of Samia.

Sammantha (Aramaic, Hebrew) a form of Samantha.
Sammanth, Sammanthia, Sammanthiah, Sammanthya, Sammanthyah

Sammi (Hebrew) a familiar form of Samantha, Samuel, Samuela. (Arabic) a form of Sami.
Samm, Samma, Sammah, Sammee, Sammey, Sammijo, Sammyjo

Sammie BG (Hebrew) a familiar form of Samantha, Samuel, Samuela. (Arabic) a form of Sami.

Sammy BG (Hebrew) a familiar form of Samantha, Samuel, Samuela. (Arabic) a form of Sami.

Samone (Hebrew) a form of Simone.
Samoan, Samoane, Samon, Samona, Samoné, Samonia

Samuel BG (Hebrew) heard God; asked of God. Bible: a famous Old Testament prophet and judge.

Samuela (Hebrew) a form of Samuel. See also Xamuela, Zamuela.
Samelia, Sammila, Sammile

Samuelle (Hebrew) a form of Samuel.
Samella, Samiella, Samielle, Samilla, Samille, Samuella

Sana (Arabic) mountaintop; splendid; brilliant.
Sanaa, Sanáa, Sanaah, Sanah, Sane

Sancia (Spanish) holy, sacred.
Sanceska, Sancha, Sancharia, Sanche, Sancheska, Sanchia, Sanchiah, Sanchie, Sanchya, Sanchyah, Sanciah, Sancie, Sanctia, Sancya, Sancyah, Santsia, Sanzia, Sanziah, Sanzya, Sanzyah

Sandeep BG (Punjabi) enlightened.
Sandip

Sandi (Greek) a familiar form of Sandra. See also Xandi, Zandi.
Sandea, Sandee, Sandia, Sandiah, Sandie, Sandiey, Sandine, Sanndie

Sandía (Spanish) watermelon.

Sandra (Greek) defender of mankind. A short form of Cassandra. History: Sandra Day O'Connor was the first woman appointed to the U.S. Supreme Court. See also Xandra, Zandra.
Sahndra, Sandira, Sandrea, Sandria, Sandrica, Sanndra

Sandrea (Greek) a form of Sandra.
Sandreah, Sandreea, Sandreia, Sandreiah, Sandrell, Sandrella, Sandrellah, Sandrelle, Sandria, Sandriah, Sanndria

Sandrica (Greek) a form of Sandra. See also Rica.
Sandricah, Sandricka, Sandrickah, Sandrika, Sandrikah, Sandryca, Sandrycah, Sandrycka, Sandryckah, Sandryka, Sandrykah

Sandrine (Greek) a form of Alexandra. See also Xandrine, Zandrine.
Sandreana, Sandreanah, Sandreane, Sandreen, Sandreena, Sandreenah, Sandreene, Sandrene, Sandrenna, Sandrennah, Sandrenne, Sandrianna, Sandrina, Sandrinah, Sandryna, Sandrynah, Sandryne

Sandy GB (Greek) a familiar form of Cassandra, Sandra.
Sandey, Sandya, Sandye

Sanne (Hebrew, Dutch) lily.
Sanea, Saneh, Sanna, Sanneen, Sanneena

Santana GB (Spanish) saint.
Santa, Santah, Santania, Santaniah, Santaniata, Santena, Santenah, Santenna, Shantana, Shantanna

Santanna (Spanish) a form of Santana.
Santanne

Santina (Spanish) little saint. See also Xantina, Zantina.
Santin, Santinah, Santine, Santinia, Santyn, Santyna, Santynah, Santyne

Sanura (Swahili) kitten.
Sanora, Sanurah

Sanuye (Moquelumnan) red clouds at sunset.

Sanya (Sanskrit) born on Saturday.
Saneiya, Sania, Sanyah, Sanyia

Sanyu BG (Luganda) happiness.

Sapata (Native American) dancing bear.
Sapatah

Saphire (Greek) a form of Sapphire.
Saphir, Saphyre

Sapphira (Hebrew) a form of Sapphire.
Saffira, Saffirah, Safira, Safirah, Safyra, Safyrah, Sapheria, Saphira, Saphirah, Saphyra, Sapir, Sapira, Sapphirah, Sapphyra, Sapphyrah, Sapyr, Sapyra, Sapyrah, Sephira

Sapphire (Greek) blue gemstone.
Saffir, Saffire, Safir, Safire, Safyr, Sapphir, Sapphyr, Sapphyre

Saqui (Mapuche) chosen one; kind soul.

Sara ☆ (Hebrew) a form of Sarah.
Saralee

Sara Eve, Sarah Eve (American) combinations of Sarah + Eve.
Sara-Eve, Sarah-Eve

Sara Jane, Sarah Jane (American) combinations of Sarah + Jane.
Sara-Jane, Sarah-Jane

Sara Maude, Sarah Maud, Sarah Maude (American) combinations of Sarah + Maud.
Sara Maud, Sara-Maud, Sara-Maude, Sarah-Maud, Sarah-Maude

Sarafina (Hebrew) a form of Serafina.

Sarah ☆ GB (Hebrew) princess. Bible: the wife of Abraham and mother of Isaac. See also Sadie, Saida, Sally, Saree, Sharai, Xara, Zara, Zarita.
Sarae, Saraha, Sorcha

Sarah Ann, Sarah Anne (American) combinations of Sarah + Ann.
Sara Ann, Sara Anne, Sara-Ann, Sara-Anne, Sarah-Ann, Sarah-Anne, Sarahann, Sarahanne, Sarann

Sarah Jeanne (American) a combination of Sarah + Jeanne.
Sara Jeanne, Sara-Jeanne, Sarah-Jeanne, Sarahjeanne, Sarajeanne

Sarah Marie (American) a combination of Sarah + Marie.
Sara Marie, Sara-Marie, Sarah-Marie, Sarahmarie, Saramarie

Sarahi (Hebrew) a form of Sarah.

Sarai, Saray (Hebrew) forms of Sarah.
Saraya

Saralyn (American) a combination of Sarah + Lynn.
Saralena, Saraly, Saralynn

Saree (Arabic) noble. (Hebrew) a familiar form of Sarah.
Sarry, Sary, Sarye

Sarena (Hebrew) a form of Sarina.
Saren, Sarenah, Sarene, Sarenna

Sarha (Hebrew) a form of Sarah.

Sari (Hebrew, Arabic) a form of Saree.
Sarie, Sarri, Sarrie

Saria, Sariah (Hebrew) forms of Sarah.
Sahria, Sahriah, Sahrya, Sahryah, Sarea, Sareah, Sarria, Sarriah, Sarya, Saryah, Sayria, Sayriah, Sayrya, Sayryah

Sarika (Hebrew) a familiar form of Sarah. See also Xarika, Zarika.
Sareaka, Sareakah, Sareeka, Sareekah, Sareka, Sarekah, Sarica, Saricah, Saricka, Sarickah, Sarikah, Sarka, Saryca, Sarycah, Sarycka, Saryckah, Saryka, Sarykah

Sarila (Turkish) waterfall.
Sarilah, Sarill, Sarilla, Sarillah, Sarille, Saryl, Saryla, Sarylah, Saryle, Saryll, Sarylla, Saryllah, Sarylle

Sarina (Hebrew) a familiar form of Sarah. See also Xarina, Zarina.
Sarana, Saranah, Sarane, Saranna, Sarannah, Saranne, Sareana, Sareanah, Sareane, Sareen, Sareena, Sareenah, Sareene, Sarin, Sarinah, Sarine, Sarinna, Sarinne, Saryna, Sarynah, Saryne, Sarynna, Sarynnah, Sarynne

Sarita (Hebrew) a familiar form of Sarah.
Sareata, Sareatah, Sareate, Sareatta, Sareattah, Sareatte, Sareeta, Sareetah, Sareete, Saret, Sareta, Saretah, Sarete, Sarett, Saretta, Sarettah, Sarette, Sarit, Saritah, Sarite, Saritia, Saritt, Saritta, Sarittah, Saritte, Saryt, Saryta, Sarytah, Saryte, Sarytt, Sarytta, Saryttah, Sarytte

Sarolta (Hungarian) a form of Sarah.
Saroltah

Sarotte (French) a form of Sarah.
Sarot, Sarota, Sarotah, Sarote, Sarott, Sarotta, Sarottah

Sarra, Sarrah (Hebrew) forms of Sara.

Sasa (Japanese) assistant. (Hungarian) a form of Sarah, Sasha.
Sasah

Sasha GB (Russian) defender of mankind. See also Zasha.
Sahsha, Sascha, Saschae, Sashae, Sashah, Sashai, Sashana, Sashay, Sashea, Sashel, Sashenka, Sashey, Sashi, Sashia, Sashiah, Sashira, Sashsha, Sashya, Sashyah, Sasjara, Sauscha, Sausha, Shasha, Shashi, Shashia

Saskia, Sasquia (Teutonic) one who carries a knife.

Sass (Irish) Saxon.
Sas, Sasi, Sasie, Sassi, Sassie, Sassoon, Sassy, Sasy

Sata (Spanish) princess.

Satara (American) a combination of Sarah + Tara.
Satarah, Sataria, Satariah, Satarra, Satarrah, Satarya, Sataryah, Sateria, Sateriah, Saterra, Saterrah, Saterria, Saterriah, Saterya, Sateryah

Satin (French) smooth, shiny.
Satean, Sateana, Sateane, Sateen, Sateena, Sateene, Satina, Satinah, Satinder, Satine, Satyn, Satyna, Satynah, Satyne

Satinka (Native American) sacred dancer.
Satinkah

Sato (Japanese) sugar.
Satu

Saturia (Latin) she who has it all.

Saturniana (Latin) healthy.

Saturnina (Spanish) gift of Saturn.

Saula (Greek) desired woman.

Saundra (English) a form of Sandra, Sondra.
Saundee, Saundi, Saundie, Saundrea, Saundree, Saundrey, Saundri, Saundria, Saundriah, Saundrie, Saundry, Saundrya, Saundryah

Saura (Hindi) sun worshiper.
Saurah

Savana, Savanah, Savanna (Spanish) forms of Savannah.

Savannah ☀ (Spanish) treeless plain. See also Zavannah.
Sahvana, Sahvanna, Sahvannah, Savan, Savanha, Savania, Savann, Savannha, Savannia, Savanniah, Savauna, Savona, Savonna, Savonnah, Savonne, Sevan, Sevana, Sevanah, Sevanh, Sevann, Sevanna, Sevannah, Svannah

Saveria (Teutonic) from the new house.

Savhanna (Spanish) a form of Savannah.
Savhana, Savhanah

Savina (Latin) a form of Sabina.
Savean, Saveana, Saveanah, Saveane, Saveen, Saveena, Saveenah, Saveene, Savinah, Savine, Savyna, Savynah, Savyne

Sawa (Japanese) swamp. (Moquelumnan) stone.
Sawah

Sawyer 🅱🅶 (English) wood worker.
Sawyar, Sawyor

Sayde, Saydee (Hebrew) forms of Sadie.
Saydea, Saydi, Saydia, Saydie, Saydy, Saydye

Sayén (Mapuche) sweet woman.

Sayo (Japanese) born at night.
Saio, Sao

Sayra (Hebrew) a form of Sarah.
Sayrah, Sayre, Sayri

Scarlet (English) a form of Scarlett.
Scarleta, Scarlete

Scarlett (English) bright red. Literature: Scarlett O'Hara is the heroine of Margaret Mitchell's novel *Gone with the Wind*.
Scarletta, Scarlette, Scarlit, Scarlitt, Scarlotte, Scarlyt, Scarlyta, Scarlyte, Skarlette

Schyler 🅶🅱 (Dutch) sheltering.
Schiler, Schuyla, Schuyler, Schuylia, Schylar

Scotti (Scottish) from Scotland.
Scota, Scotea, Scoteah, Scotee, Scotey, Scoti, Scotia, Scotiah, Scottea, Scotteah, Scottee, Scottey, Scottia, Scottiah, Scottie, Scotty, Scoty, Scotya, Scotyah

Scout (French) scout. Literature: Scout is a protagonist in Harper Lee's *To Kill a Mockingbird*.

Seaira, Seairra (Irish, Spanish) forms of Sierra.

Sealtiel (Hebrew) my desire is God.

Sean 🅱🅶 (Hebrew, Irish) God is gracious.
Seaghan, Seain, Seaine, Seán, Séan, Seane, Seann, Seayn, Seayne, Shaan, Shon, Siôn

Seana, Seanna (Irish) forms of Jane, Sean. See also Shauna, Shawna.
Seaana, Seanah, Seannae, Seannah, Seannalisa, Seanté

Searra (Irish, Spanish) a form of Sierra.
Seara, Searria

Sebastiane (Greek) venerable. (Latin) revered. (French) a form of Sebastian (see Boys' Names).
Sebastene, Sebastia, Sebastiana, Sebastianah, Sebastiann, Sebastianna, Sebastiannah, Sebastianne, Sebastien, Sebastienne, Sebastyana, Sebastyann, Sebastyanna, Sebastyanne, Sevastyana

Seble (Ethiopian) autumn.

Sebrina (English) a form of Sabrina.
Sebrena, Sebrenna, Sebria, Sebriana, Sebrinah

Secilia (Latin) a form of Cecilia.
Saselia, Saseliah, Sasilia, Sasiliah, Secylia, Secyliah, Secylya, Secylyah, Sesilia, Sesiliah, Sesilya, Sesilyah, Sesylia, Sesyliah, Sesylya, Sesylyah, Sileas, Siselea, Siseleah

Secret (Latin) secret.

Secunda (Latin) second.
Seconda, Secondah, Secondea, Secondee, Secondia, Secondiah, Secondya, Secondyah

Secundila (Latin) a form of Secundina.

Secundina (Latin) second daughter.

Seda (Armenian) forest voices.
Sedah

Sedna (Eskimo) well-fed. Mythology: the goddess of sea animals.
Sednah

Sedofa (Latin) silk.

Sedona (French) a form of Sidonie.

Seelia (English) a form of Sheila.

Seema (Greek) sprout. (Afghan) sky; profile.
Seama, Seamah, Seemah, Sima, Simah, Syma, Symah

Sefa (Swiss) a familiar form of Josefina.
Sefah, Seffa, Seffah

Séfora (Hebrew) like a small bird.

Segene (German) victorious.

Segismunda (German) victorious protector.

Segunda (Spanish) a form of Secundina.

Seina (Basque) innocent.

Seirra (Irish) a form of Sierra.
Seiara, Seiarra, Seira, Seirria

Sejal (Indian) river water.

Seki (Japanese) wonderful.
Seka, Sekah, Sekee, Sekey, Sekia, Sekiah, Sekie, Seky, Sekya, Sekyah

Sela, Selah (English) short forms of Selena.
Seeley, Sella, Sellah

Selam (Ethiopian) peaceful.
Selama, Selamah

Selda (German) a short form of Griselda. (Yiddish) a form of Zelda.
Seldah, Selde, Sellda, Selldah

Selena (Greek) a form of Selene. See also Celena, Zelena.
Saleena, Selana, Seleana, Seleanah, Seleena, Seleenah, Selen, Selenah, Séléné, Selenia, Selenna, Syleena, Sylena

Selene (Greek) moon. Mythology: Selene was the goddess of the moon.
Selean, Seleane, Seleen, Seleene, Seleni, Selenie, Seleny

Seleste (Latin) a form of Celeste.

Selestina (Latin) a form of Celestina.
Selesteana, Selesteanah, Selesteane, Selesteena, Selesteenah, Selesteene, Selestin, Selestina, Selestinah, Selestine, Selestyna, Selestynah, Selestyne

Selia (Latin) a short form of Cecilia.
Seel, Seelia, Seil, Seila, Selea, Seleah, Selee, Selei, Seleigh, Seley, Seli, Seliah, Selie, Sellia, Selliah, Sellya, Sellyah, Sely, Silia

Selima (Hebrew) peaceful.
Selema, Selemah, Selimah, Selyma, Selymah

Selin (Greek) a short form of Selina.
Selyn, Selyne, Selynne, Sillyn, Sylin, Sylyn, Sylyne

Selina (Greek) a form of Celina, Selena.
Selinah, Selinda, Seline, Selinia, Seliniah, Selinka, Sellina, Selyna, Selynah, Silina, Silinah, Siline, Sillina, Sillinah, Silline, Sillyna, Sillynah, Sillyne, Sylina, Sylinah, Syline, Sylyna, Sylynah

Selma (German) divine protector. (Irish) fair, just. (Scandinavian) divinely protected. (Arabic) secure. See also Zelma.
Sellma, Sellmah, Selmah

Selva (Latin) a form of Silvana.

Sema (Turkish) heaven; divine omen.
Semah

Semaj BG (Turkish) a form of Sema.

Semele (Latin) once.

Seminaris, Semíramis (Assyrian) she who lives harmoniously with the doves.

Sempronia (Spanish) a form of Semproniana.

Semproniana (Latin) eternal.

Sena (Greek) a short form of Selena. (Spanish) a short form of Senalda.
Senda

Senalda (Spanish) sign.

Seneca (Iroquoian) a tribal name.
Senaka, Seneka, Senequa, Senequae, Senequai, Seneque

Senia (Greek) a form of Xenia.
Seniah, Senya, Senyah

Senona (Spanish) lively.

Senorina (Latin) aged.

Sephora (English) a form of Séfora.

September (Latin) born in the ninth month.

Septima (Latin) seventh.
Septime, Septym, Septyma, Septyme, Sevann, Sevanna, Sevanne, Sevena, Sevenah

Sequoia (Cherokee) giant redwood tree.
Seqoiyia, Seqouyia, Seqoya, Sequoi, Sequoiah, Sequora, Sikoya

Sequoya, Sequoyah (Cherokee) forms of Sequoia.

Sera, Serah (American) forms of Sarah.
Serra

Serafia (Spanish) a form of Seraphina.

Serafín (Hebrew) a form of Seraphina.

Serafina (Hebrew) burning; ardent. Bible: seraphim are an order of angels.
Seafina, Seaphina, Serafeena, Seraphe, Serapheena, Seraphina, Seraphita, Seraphyna, Seraphynah, Seraphyne, Serapia, Serephyna, Serephynah, Serofina

Seraphyne (French) a form of Serafina.
Serafeen, Serafeene, Serafin, Serafine, Serapheen, Serapheene, Seraphin, Seraphine, Serephyn

Serén (Welsh) star.

Serena (Latin) peaceful. See also Rena, Xerena, Zerena.
Sareana, Sareanah, Sareena, Sareenah, Saryna, Seraina, Serana, Sereana, Sereanah, Sereina, Serenah, Serenea, Serenia, Serenna, Serreana, Serrena, Serrenna

Serene (French) a form of Serena.
Serean, Sereane, Sereen, Seren

Serenela (Spanish) a form of Seren.

Serenity (Latin) peaceful.
Serenidy, Serenitee, Serenitey, Sereniti, Serenitie, Serenitiy, Serinity, Serrennity

Sergia (Greek) attendant.

Serica (Greek) silky smooth.
Sericah, Sericka, Serickah, Serika, Serikah, Seryca, Serycah, Serycka, Seryckah, Seryka, Serykah

Serilda (Greek) armed warrior woman.
Sarilda, Sarildah, Serildah, Serylda, Seryldah

Serina (Latin) a form of Serena.
Sereena, Serin, Serinah, Serine, Serreena, Serrin, Serrina, Seryn, Seryna, Serynah, Seryne

Serita (Hebrew) a form of Sarita.
Seritah, Serite, Seritt, Seritta, Serittah, Seritte, Seryt, Seryta, Serytah, Seryte, Serytt, Serytta, Seryttah, Serytte

Serotina (Latin) dusk.

Servanda, Sevanda (Latin) she who must be saved and protected.

Servia (Latin) daughter of those who serve the Lord.

Severa (Spanish) severe.

Severina (Italian, Portuguese, Croatian, German, Ancient Roman) severe.

Sevilla (Spanish) from Seville, Spain.
Sevil, Sevila, Sevilah, Sevile, Sevill, Sevillah, Seville, Sevyl, Sevyla, Sevylah, Sevyle, Sevyll, Sevylla, Sevyllah, Sevylle

Sexburgis (German) shelter of the victorious one.

Shaba (Spanish) rose.
Shabah, Shabana, Shabanah, Shabina, Shabinah, Shabine, Shabyna, Shabynah, Shabyne

Shada (Native American) pelican.
Shadah, Shadee, Shadi, Shadie, Shaida, Shaidah, Shayda, Shaydah

Shaday (American) a form of Sade.
Shadae, Shadai, Shadaia, Shadaya, Shadayna, Shadei, Shadeziah, Shaiday

Shade BG (English) shade.
Shaed, Shaede, Shaid, Shaide, Shayd, Shayde

Shadia (Native American) a form of Shada.
Shadea, Shadeana, Shadiah, Shadiya

Shadow BG (English) shadow.

Shadrika (American) a combination of the prefix Sha + Rika.
Shadreeka, Shadreka, Shadrica, Shadricah, Shadricka, Shadrieka, Shadrikah, Shadriqua, Shadriquah, Shadrique, Shadryca, Shadrycah, Shadrycka, Shadryckah, Shadryka, Shadrykah, Shadryqua, Shadryquah, Shadryque

Shae GB (Irish) a form of Shea.
Shaenel, Shaeya

Shae-Lynn, Shaelyn, Shaelynn (Irish)
forms of Shea. See also Shailyn.
Shael, Shaelaine, Shaelan, Shaelanie,
Shaelanna, Shaelean, Shaeleana, Shaeleanah,
Shaeleane, Shaeleen, Shaeleena, Shaeleenah,
Shaeleene, Shaelena, Shaelenah, Shaelene,
Shaelin, Shaelina, Shaelinah, Shaeline,
Shaelyna, Shaelynah, Shaelyne, Shaelynne

Shaela (Irish) a form of Sheila.
Shaeyla

Shaelee (Irish) a form of Shea.
Shaelea, Shaeleah, Shaelei, Shaeleigh, Shaeley,
Shaeli, Shaelia, Shaeliah, Shaelie, Shaely

Shaena (Irish) a form of Shaina.
Shaeina, Shaeine, Shaenah

Shafira (Swahili) distinguished.
Shaffira, Shafirah, Shafyra, Shafyrah

Shahar (Arabic) moonlit.
Shahara, Shaharah, Shaharia, Shahariah,
Shaharya, Shaharyah

Shahina (Arabic) falcon.
Shahean, Shaheana, Shaheanah, Shaheane,
Shaheen, Shaheena, Shaheenah, Shaheene,
Shahi, Shahin, Shahinah, Shahine, Shahyna,
Shahynah, Shahyne

Shahira (Arabic) famous.
Shahirah, Shahyra, Shahyrah

Shahla (Afghan) beautiful eyes.
Shahlah

Shai BG (Irish) a form of Shea.
Shaia, Shaiah

Shaianne (Cheyenne) a form of Cheyenne.
Shaeen, Shaeine, Shaian, Shaiana, Shaiandra,
Shaiane, Shaiann, Shaianna

Shaila (Latin) a form of Sheila.
Shailah, Shailla

Shailee (Irish) a form of Shea.
Shailea, Shaileah, Shailei, Shaileigh, Shailey,
Shaili, Shailia, Shailiah, Shailie, Shaily

Shailyn, Shailynn (Irish) forms of Shea. See
also Shae-Lynn.
Shailean, Shaileana, Shaileanah, Shaileen,
Shaileena, Shaileenah, Shaileene, Shailin,
Shailina, Shailinah, Shailine, Shailyna,
Shailynah, Shailyne

Shaina (Yiddish) beautiful.
Schaina, Schainah, Schayna, Schaynah,
Shainah, Shainna, Shajna, Shayndel, Sheina,
Sheinah, Sheindel, Sheyna, Sheynah

Shajuana (American) a combination of the
prefix Sha + Juanita. See also Shawana.
Shajana, Shajanah, Shajuan, Shajuanda,
Shajuanita, Shajuanna, Shajuanne, Shajuanza

Shaka BG (Hindi) a form of Shakti. A short
form of names beginning with "Shak." See
also Chaka.
Shakah, Shakha

Shakala (Arabic) a form of Shakila.

Shakara, Shakarah (American) combina-
tions of the prefix Sha + Kara.
Shacara, Shacarah, Shaccara, Shaccarah,
Shakarya, Shakaryah, Shakkara, Shikara,
Shykara, Shykarah

Shakari (American) a form of Shakara.
Shacari, Shacaria, Shakaria, Shakariah

Shakayla (Arabic) a form of Shakila.
Shakaela, Shakail, Shakaila

Shakeena (American) a combination of the
prefix Sha + Keena.
Shakean, Shakeana, Shakeanah, Shakeane,
Shakeen, Shakeena, Shakeenah, Shakeene,
Shakein, Shakeina, Shakeinah, Shakeine,
Shakeyn, Shakeyna, Shakeynah, Shakeyne,
Shakin, Shakina, Shakinah, Shakine, Shakyn,
Shakyna, Shakynah, Shakyne

Shakeita (American) a combination of the
prefix Sha + Keita. See also Shaqueita.
Shakeata, Shakeatah, Shakeatia, Shakeatiah,
Shakeeta, Shakeetah, Shakeetia, Shakeetiah,
Shakeitah, Shakeitha, Shakeithia, Shaketa,
Shaketah, Shaketha, Shakethia, Shaketia,
Shaketiah, Shakeyta, Shakeytah, Shakyta,
Shakytah, Shakytia, Shakytiah, Sheketa,
Sheketah, Sheketia, Shekita, Shekitah,
Shikita, Shikitha, Shikyta, Shikytah, Shykita,
Shykitah, Shykitia, Shykyta, Shykytah,
Shykytia, Shykytiah, Shykytya, Shykytyah

Shakela (Arabic) a form of Shakila.
Shakelah

Shakera, Shakerra (Arabic) forms of
Shakira.
Shakerah

Shakeria, Shakerria (Arabic) forms of Shakira.
Chakeria, Shakeriah, Shakeriay, Shakerri, Shakerya, Shakeryia

Shakeya (American) a form of Shakia.

Shakia (American) a combination of the prefix Sha + Kia.
Shakeeia, Shakeeiah, Shakeeya, Shakeeyah, Shakeia, Shakeiah, Shakiah, Shakiya, Shakiyah, Shakya, Shakyah, Shekeia, Shekia, Shekiah, Shekya, Shekyah, Shikia

Shakiera (Arabic) a form of Shakira.
Shakierra

Shakila (Arabic) pretty.
Chakila, Shakeala, Shakealah, Shakeela, Shakeelah, Shakeena, Shakilah, Shakyla, Shakylah, Shekela, Shekila, Shekilla, Shikeela, Shikila

Shakima (African) beautiful one.

Shakira (Arabic) thankful.
Shaakira, Shacora, Shaka, Shakeera, Shakeerah, Shakeeria, Shakeira, Shakeirra, Shakeyra, Shakir, Shakirah, Shakirat, Shakirea, Shakora, Shakuria, Shekiera, Shekira, Shikira, Shikirah, Shikyra, Shikyrah, Shykira, Shykirah, Shykyra, Shykyrah

Shakirra (Arabic) a form of Shakira.

Shakita (American) a form of Shakeita.
Shakitah, Shakitra

Shakti (Hindi) energy, power. Religion: a form of the Hindu goddess Devi.
Sakti, Shaktea, Shaktee, Shaktey, Shaktia, Shaktiah, Shaktie, Shakty

Shakyra (Arabic) a form of Shakira.
Shakyrah, Shakyria

Shalana (American) a combination of the prefix Sha + Lana.
Shalaana, Shalain, Shalaina, Shalainah, Shalaine, Shalanah, Shalane, Shalann, Shalanna, Shalannah, Shalanne, Shalaun, Shalauna, Shalaunah, Shallan, Shallana, Shallanah, Shelan, Shelana, Shelanah, Shelanda, Shelane, Shelayna, Shelaynah, Shelayne, Sholaina, Sholainah, Sholaine, Sholana, Sholanah, Sholane, Sholayna, Sholaynah, Sholayne

Shalanda (American) a form of Shalana.
Shaland

Shalayna (American) a form of Shalana.
Shalayn, Shalaynah, Shalayne, Shalaynna

Shaleah (American) a combination of the prefix Sha + Leah.
Shalea, Shalei, Shaleigh, Shaley, Shali, Shalia, Shaliah, Shalie, Shaly

Shalee (American) a form of Shaleah.
Shaleea

Shaleen, Shalene (American) short forms of Shalena.
Shalean, Shaleane, Shaleene, Shalen, Shalenne, Shaline

Shaleisha (American) a combination of the prefix Sha + Aisha.
Shalesha, Shaleshah, Shalesia, Shalesiah, Shalicia, Shaliciah, Shalisha, Shalishah, Shalysha, Shalyshah

Shalena (American) a combination of the prefix Sha + Lena. See also Chalina.
Shaleana, Shaleanah, Shaleena, Shaleenah, Shálena, Shalenah, Shalené, Shalenna, Shalennah, Shalina, Shalinah, Shalinda, Shalinna, Shalyna, Shalynah, Shelena, Shelenah

Shalini (American) a form of Shalena.

Shalisa (American) a combination of the prefix Sha + Lisa.
Shalesa, Shalesah, Shalese, Shalessa, Shalice, Shalicia, Shaliece, Shalisah, Shalise, Shalisha, Shalishea, Shalisia, Shalisiah, Shalissa, Shalissah, Shalisse, Shalyce, Shalys, Shalysa, Shalysah, Shalyse, Shalyss, Shalyssa, Shalyssah, Shalysse

Shalita (American) a combination of the prefix Sha + Lita.
Shaleata, Shaleatah, Shaleeta, Shaleetah, Shaleta, Shaletah, Shaletta, Shalettah, Shalida, Shalidah, Shalitta, Shalittah, Shalyta, Shalytah, Shalytta, Shalyttah

Shalon (American) a short form of Shalona.
Shalone, Shalonne

Shalona (American) a combination of the prefix Sha + Lona.
Shalonah, Shálonna, Shalonnah

Shalonda (American) a combination of the prefix Sha + Ondine.
Shalondah, Shalonde, Shalondina, Shalondine, Shalondra, Shalondria, Shalondyna, Shalondyne

Shalyn, Shalynn, Shalynne (American) combinations of the prefix Sha + Lynn.
Shalin, Shalina, Shalinda, Shaline, Shalyna, Shalynda, Shalyne, Shalynna

Shamara (Arabic) ready for battle.
Shamar, Shamarah, Shamare, Shamarra, Shammara, Shamora, Shamorah, Shamori, Shamoria, Shamoriah, Shamorra, Shamorrah, Shamorria, Shamorriah, Shamorya, Shamoryah

Shamari BG (Arabic) a form of Shamara.
Shamaree, Shamarri

Shamaria (Arabic) a form of Shamara.
Shamarea, Shamariah, Shamarria, Shamarya, Shamaryah

Shameka (American) a combination of the prefix Sha + Meka.
Shameca, Shamecca, Shamecha, Shamecia, Shameika, Shameke, Shamekia, Shamekya, Shamekyah

Shamia (American) a combination of the prefix Sha + Mia.
Shamea, Shamiah, Shamyia, Shamyiah, Shamyne

Shamika (American) a combination of the prefix Sha + Mika.
Shameaka, Shameakah, Shameeca, Shameeka, Shamica, Shamicah, Shamicia, Shamicka, Shamickah, Shamieka, Shamikah, Shamikia, Shamyca, Shamycah, Shamycka, Shamyckah, Shamyka, Shamykah

Shamira (Hebrew) precious stone.
Shamir, Shamirah, Shamiran, Shamiria

Shamiya (American) a form of Shamia.
Shamiyah

Shamyra (Hebrew) a form of Shamira.
Shamyrah, Shamyria, Shamyriah, Shamyrya, Shamyryah

Shana (Hebrew) God is gracious. (Irish) a form of Jane.
Shaana, Shaanah, Shan, Shanah

Shanae, Shanea (Irish) forms of Shana.
Shanay

Shanaya (American) a form of Shania.
Shaneah

Shanda (American) a form of Chanda, Shana.
Shandae, Shandah, Shannda

Shandi (English) a familiar form of Shana.
Shandea, Shandee, Shandei, Shandeigh, Shandey, Shandice, Shandie

Shandra (American) a form of Shanda. See also Chandra.
Shandrah

Shandria (American) a form of Shandra.
Shandrea, Shandri, Shandriah, Shandrice, Shandrie, Shandry, Shandrya, Shandryah

Shandrika (American) a form of Shandria.
Shandreka

Shane BG (Irish) a form of Shana.
Schain, Schaine, Schayn, Schayne, Shaen, Shaene, Shain, Shaine, Shayn

Shanece (American) a form of Shanice.

Shanee (Irish) a familiar form of Shane. (Swahili) a form of Shany. See also Shanie.
Shanée

Shaneice (American) a form of Shanice.
Shanneice

Shaneika (American) a form of Shanika.
Shaneikah

Shaneisha (American) a combination of the prefix Sha + Aisha.
Shanesha, Shaneshia, Shanessa, Shaneysha, Shaneyshah, Shanisha, Shanishia, Shanishiah, Shanissa, Shanysha, Shanyshah

Shaneka (American) a form of Shanika.
Shaneaca, Shaneacah, Shaneacka, Shaneackah, Shaneaka, Shaneakah, Shaneca, Shanecka, Shaneeca, Shaneecah, Shaneecka, Shaneeckah, Shaneeka, Shaneekah, Shanekah, Shanekia, Shanekiah, Shaneyka, Shonneka

Shanel, Shanell, Shanelle, Shannel
(American) forms of Chanel.
Schanel, Schanela, Schanelah, Schanele,
Schanell, Schanelle, Shanela, Shanelah,
Shanele, Shanella, Shanelly, Shannela,
Shannelah, Shannele, Shannell, Shannella,
Shannellah, Shannelle, Shinelle, Shonel,
Shonela, Shonelah, Shonele, Shonell, Shonella,
Shonelle, Shynelle

Shanequa (American) a form of Shanika.
Shaneaqua, Shaneaquah, Shaneaque,
Shaneequa, Shaneequah, Shaneeque,
Shaneiqua, Shaneiquah, Shaneique,
Shanequah, Shaneque

Shanese (American) a form of Shanice.
Shanesse

Shaneta (American) a combination of the
prefix Sha + Neta.
Seanette, Shaneata, Shaneatah, Shaneate,
Shaneeta, Shaneetah, Shanetah, Shanetha,
Shanethia, Shanethis, Shanetta, Shanette,
Shineta, Shonetta

Shani GB (Swahili) a form of Shany.
Shaenee, Shaeni, Shaenie, Shainee, Shaini,
Shainie

Shania, Shaniah, Shaniya (American)
forms of Shana.
Shaenea, Shaenia, Shaeniah, Shaenya,
Shaenyah, Shainia, Shainiah, Shainya,
Shainyah, Shanasia, Shannea, Shannia,
Shanya, Shanyah, Shenia

Shanice (American) a form of Janice. See
also Chanice.
Shaneace, Shanease, Shaneece, Shaneese,
Shaneise, Shanicea, Shannice, Sheneice,
Shenyce

Shanida (American) a combination of the
prefix Sha + Ida.
Shaneeda, Shaneedah, Shannida, Shannidah,
Shanyda, Shanydah

Shanie (Irish) a form of Shane. (Swahili) a
form of Shany. See also Shanee.
Shanni, Shannie

Shaniece (American) a form of Shanice.

Shanika (American) a combination of the
prefix Sha + Nika.
Shanica, Shanicah, Shanicca, Shanicka,

Shanickah, Shanieka, Shanikah, Shanike,
Shanikia, Shanikka, Shanikqua, Shanikwa,
Shanyca, Shanycah, Shanycka, Shanyckah,
Shanyka, Shanykah, Shineeca, Shonnika

Shaniqua, Shanique (American) forms of
Shanika.
Shaniqa, Shaniquah, Shaniquia, Shaniquwa,
Shaniqwa, Shanyqua, Shanyquah, Shanyque,
Shinequa, Shiniqua

Shanise (American) a form of Shanice.
Shanisa, Shanisah, Shanisha, Shanisia,
Shaniss, Shanissa, Shanissah, Shanisse,
Shanysa, Shanysah, Shanyse, Shanyssa,
Shanyssah, Shineese

Shanita (American) a combination of the
prefix Sha + Nita.
Shanitah, Shanitha, Shanitra, Shanitt,
Shanitta, Shanittah, Shanitte, Shanyt,
Shanyta, Shanytah, Shanyte, Shanytt,
Shanytta, Shanyttah, Shanytte, Shinita

Shanley GB (Irish) hero's child.
Shanlea, Shanleah, Shanlee, Shanlei,
Shanleigh, Shanli, Shanlie, Shanly

Shanna, Shannah (Irish) forms of Shana,
Shannon.
Shannea

Shannen, Shanon (Irish) forms of
Shannon.
Shanen, Shanena, Shanene

Shannon GB (Irish) small and wise.
Shanadoah, Shanan, Shann, Shannan,
Shanneen, Shannie, Shannin, Shannyn,
Shanyn, Sheannon

Shanny (Swahili) a form of Shany.

Shanta (French) a form of Chantal.
Shantah

Shantae GB (French) a form of Chantal.
Shantai, Shantay, Shantaya, Shantaye, Shantée

Shantal (American) a form of Shantel.
Shantale, Shantall, Shontal

Shantana (American) a form of Santana.
Shantaina, Shantainah, Shantan, Shantanae,
Shantanah, Shantanell, Shantania,
Shantaniah, Shantanickia, Shantanika,
Shantanna, Shantanne, Shantanya,
Shantanyah, Shantayna, Shantaynah,

Shantena, Shantenah, Shantenna, Shentana, Shentanna

Shantara (American) a combination of the prefix Sha + Tara.
Shantarah, Shantaria, Shantariah, Shantarra, Shantarrah, Shantarria, Shantarriah, Shantarya, Shantaryah, Shantera, Shanterra, Shantira, Shantyra, Shantyrah, Shontara, Shuntara

Shante (French) a form of Chantal.
Shantea, Shantee, Shanteia

Shanté (French) a form of Chantal.

Shanteca (American) a combination of the prefix Sha + Teca.
Shantecca, Shantecka, Shanteka, Shantika, Shantikia, Shantikiah, Shantyca, Shantycka, Shantyckah, Shantyka, Shantykah

Shantel, Shantell, Shantelle (American) song. See also Shauntel.
Seantelle, Shanntell, Shanteal, Shanteil, Shantela, Shantelah, Shantele, Shantella, Shantellah, Shantyl, Shantyle, Shentel, Shentelle, Shontal, Shontalla, Shontalle

Shanteria, Shanterria (American) forms of Shantara.
Shanterica, Shanterrie, Shantieria, Shantirea, Shonteria

Shantesa (American) a combination of the prefix Sha + Tess.
Shantesah, Shantese, Shantessa, Shantessah, Shantesse, Shantice, Shantise, Shantisha, Shontecia, Shontessia

Shanti (American) a short form of Shantia.
Shantey, Shantie, Shanty

Shantia (American) a combination of the prefix Sha + Tia.
Shanteia, Shanteya, Shantiah, Shantida, Shantya, Shantyah, Shaunteya, Shauntia, Shauntya, Shauntyah

Shantille (American) a form of Chantilly.
Shanteil, Shantil, Shantilea, Shantileah, Shantilee, Shantiley, Shantili, Shantilie, Shantillea, Shantilleah, Shantillee, Shantillei, Shantilleigh, Shantilli, Shantillie, Shantilly, Shantyl, Shantyle, Shantylea, Shantyleah, Shantylee, Shantylei, Shantyleigh, Shantyley, Shantylli, Shantyllie, Shantylly, Shantyly

Shantina (American) a combination of the prefix Sha + Tina.
Shanteana, Shanteanah, Shanteena, Shanteenah, Shanteina, Shanteinah, Shanteyna, Shanteynah, Shantinah, Shantine, Shantyna, Shantynah, Shontina

Shantora (American) a combination of the prefix Sha + Tory.
Shantorah, Shantoree, Shantorey, Shantori, Shantorie, Shantory, Shantoya

Shantoria (American) a form of Shantora.
Shantorya, Shanttoria

Shantrell (American) a form of Shantel.

Shantrice (American) a combination of the prefix Sha + Trice. See also Chantrice.
Shanteace, Shantease, Shantrece, Shantrecia, Shantreece, Shantreese, Shantrese, Shantress, Shantrezia, Shantricia, Shantriece, Shantriese, Shantris, Shantrisa, Shantrisah, Shantrise, Shantrissa, Shantrisse, Shantryce, Shantryse, Shontrice

Shany (Swahili) marvelous, wonderful. See also Shani.
Shaeney, Shaeny, Shaenye, Shainey, Shainy, Shaney, Shannai, Shanya

Shanyce (American) a form of Shanice.
Shannyce

Shappa (Native American) red thunder.
Shapa, Shapah, Shappah

Shaquan BG (American) a short form of Shaquanda.

Shaquana, Shaquanna (American) forms of Shaquanda.
Shaquanah, Shaquannah

Shaquanda (American) a combination of the prefix Sha + Wanda.
Shaquand, Shaquandah, Shaquandra, Shaquandrah, Shaquandria, Shaquanera, Shaquani, Shaquania, Shaquanne, Shaquanta, Shaquantae, Shaquantay, Shaquante, Shaquantia, Shaquona, Shaquonda, Shaquondah, Shaquondra, Shaquondria

Shaquandey (American) a form of Shaquanda.

Shaqueita (American) a form of Shakeita.

Shaquetta (American) a form of Shakeita.
Shaqueta, Shaquetah, Shaquettah, Shaquette

Shaquia (American) a short form of
Shakila.

Shaquila, Shaquilla (American) forms of
Shakila.
*Shaquilah, Shaquillah, Shaquillia, Shequela,
Shequele, Shequila, Shquiyla*

Shaquille 🅱🅶 (American) a form of Shakila.
Shaquail, Shaquil, Shaquile, Shaquill

Shaquira (American) a form of Shakira.
*Shaquirah, Shaquire, Shaquirra, Shaqura,
Shaqurah, Shaquri*

Shaquita, Shaquitta (American) forms of
Shakeita.
*Shaquitah, Shequida, Shequidah, Shequita,
Shequitah, Shequittia, Shequitya, Shequityah,
Shequytya*

Shara (Hebrew) a short form of Sharon.
*Shaara, Sharah, Sharal, Sharala, Sharalee,
Sharlyn, Sharlynn, Sharra, Sharrah*

Sharai (Hebrew) princess. See also Sharon.
*Sharae, Sharaé, Sharah, Sharaiah, Sharay,
Sharaya, Sharayah, Sharrai, Sharray*

Sharan (Hindi) protector.
Sharaine, Sharanda, Sharanjeet

Sharda (Punjabi, Yoruba, Arabic) a form of
Shardae.

Shardae, Sharday (Punjabi) charity. (Yoruba)
honored by royalty. (Arabic) runaway. Forms
of Chardae.
*Shadae, Shar-Dae, Shar-Day, Shardah,
Shardai, Sharde, Shardea, Shardee, Shardée,
Shardei, Shardeia, Shardey, Shardi, Shardy*

Sharee (English) a form of Shari.
Share, Sharea, Shareah, Sharree

Sharen (English) a form of Sharon.
Sharene, Sharenn, Sharren, Sharrene, Sharrona

Shari (French) beloved, dearest. (Hungarian) a
form of Sarah. See also Sharita, Sheree,
Sherry.
Sharie, Sharri, Sharrie, Sharry, Shary

Shariah (French, Hungarian) a form of Shari.
*Sharia, Sharria, Sharriah, Sharrya, Sharryah,
Sharya, Sharyah*

Shariann, Sharianne (English) combina-
tions of Shari + Ann.
*Sharian, Shariana, Sharianah, Sharianna,
Shariannah*

Sharice (French) a form of Cherice.
*Shareace, Sharease, Shareese, Sharese, Sharesse,
Shariece, Sharis, Sharise, Sharish, Shariss,
Sharisse, Sharyce, Sharyse, Shereece*

Sharik (African) child of God.
*Sharica, Sharicka, Sharicke, Sharika, Sharike,
Shariqua, Sharique, Sharyk, Sharyka, Sharyque*

Sharina (English) a form of Sharon.
*Shareana, Shareena, Sharena, Sharenah,
Sharenna, Sharennah, Sharrena, Sharrina*

Sharissa (American) a form of Sharice.
*Sharesa, Sharessia, Sharisa, Sharisha,
Shereeza, Shericia, Sherisa, Sherissa*

Sharita (French) a familiar form of Shari.
(American) a form of Charity. See also
Sherita.
Shareeta, Sharrita

Sharla (French) a short form of Sharlene,
Sharlotte.
Sharlah

Sharleen (French) a form of Sharlene.
Sharlee, Sharleena, Sharleenah, Sharleene

Sharlene (French) little and strong.
*Scharlane, Scharlene, Shar, Sharlaina,
Sharlaine, Sharlane, Sharlanna, Sharlean,
Sharleana, Sharleanah, Sharleane, Sharlein,
Sharleina, Sharleine, Sharlena, Sharleyn,
Sharleyna, Sharleyne, Sharlin, Sharlina,
Sharlinah, Sharline, Sharlyn, Sharlyna,
Sharlynah, Sharlyne, Sharlynn, Sharlynne,
Sherlean, Sherleen, Sherlene, Sherline*

Sharlotte (American) a form of Charlotte.
*Sharlet, Sharleta, Sharletah, Sharlete, Sharlett,
Sharletta, Sharlettah, Sharlette, Sharlot,
Sharlota, Sharlotah, Sharlote, Sharlott,
Sharlotta, Sharlottah*

Sharma (American) a short form of
Sharmaine.
Sharmae, Sharmah, Sharme

Sharmaine (American) a form of
Charmaine.
*Sharmain, Sharmaina, Sharman, Sharmane,
Sharmanta, Sharmayn, Sharmayna,*

Sharmayne, Sharmeen, Sharmeena, Sharmena,
Sharmene, Sharmese, Sharmin, Sharmina,
Sharmine, Sharmon, Sharmona, Sharmone,
Sharmyn, Sharmyna, Sharmyne

Sharna (Hebrew) a form of Sharon.
Sharnae, Sharnah, Sharnai, Sharnay, Sharne,
Sharnea, Sharnee, Sharneta, Sharnete,
Sharnett, Sharnetta, Sharnette, Sharney,
Sharnie

Sharnell (American) a form of Sharon.
Sharnelle

Sharnice (American) a form of Sharon.
Sharnease, Sharneesa, Sharneese, Sharnesa,
Sharnese, Sharnisa, Sharnise, Sharnissa,
Sharnisse, Sharnyc, Sharnyce, Sharnys,
Sharnysa, Sharnysah, Sharnyse

Sharolyn (American) a combination of
Sharon + Lynn.
Sharolean, Sharoleana, Sharoleanah,
Sharoleane, Sharoleen, Sharoleena,
Sharoleenah, Sharoleene, Sharolin, Sharolina,
Sharolinah, Sharoline, Sharolyna, Sharolynah,
Sharolyne, Sharolynn, Sharolynna,
Sharolynnah, Sharolynne

Sharon (Hebrew) desert plain. A form of
Sharai.
Shaaron, Sharan, Sharean, Shareane, Shareen,
Shareene, Sharin, Sharine, Sharone, Sharran,
Sharrane, Sharrin, Sharrinae, Sharrine,
Sharryn, Sharryne, Sharyn, Sharyon, Sheren,
Sheron, Sherryn

Sharonda (Hebrew) a form of Sharon.
Sharronda, Sheronda, Sherrhonda

Sharron GB (English) a form of Sharon.

Sharrona (Hebrew) a form of Sharon.
Sharona, Sharonah, Sharone, Sharonia,
Sharonna, Sharony, Sharrana, Sharronne,
Sharryna, Shirona

Shatara (Hindi) umbrella. (Arabic) good;
industrious. (American) a combination of
Sharon + Tara.
Shatarah, Shatarea, Shatari, Shataria,
Shatariah, Shatarra, Shatarrah, Shataura,
Shateira, Shatherian, Shatierra, Shatiria,
Shatyra, Shatyrah, Sheatara

Shateria (American) a form of Shatara.
Shateriah, Shaterri, Shaterria

Shaterra (American) a form of Shatara.
Shatera, Shaterah

Shatoria (American) a combination of the
prefix Sha + Tory.
Shatora, Shatorah, Shatorea, Shatori, Shatoriah,
Shatorri, Shatorria, Shatory, Shatorya, Shatoryah

Shatoya (American) a form of Shatoria.

Shaun BG (Irish) a form of Sean. See also
Shawn.
Schaun, Schaune, Shaughan, Shaughn, Shaugn,
Shaunahan, Shaune, Shaunn, Shaunne

Shauna (Hebrew, Irish) a form of Shana,
Shaun. See also Seana, Shawna, Shona.
Schauna, Schaunah, Schaunee, Shaunah,
Shaunee, Shauneen, Shaunelle, Shaunette,
Shauni, Shaunie, Shaunika, Shaunisha,
Shaunnea, Shaunua, Sheann, Sheaon,
Sheaunna

Shaunda (Irish) a form of Shauna. See also
Shanda, Shawnda, Shonda.
Shaundal, Shaundala, Shaundra, Shaundrea,
Shaundree, Shaundria, Shaundrice

Shaunice (Irish) a form of Shauna.
Shaunicy

Shaunna (Hebrew, Irish) a form of Shauna.

Shaunta (Irish) a form of Shauna. See also
Shawnta, Shonta.
Schaunta, Schauntah, Schaunte, Schauntea,
Schauntee, Schunta, Shauntah, Shaunte,
Shauntea, Shauntee, Shauntée, Shaunteena,
Shauntia, Shauntier, Shauntrel, Shauntrell,
Shauntrella, Sheanta

Shauntae (Irish) a form of Shaunta.
Schauntae, Schauntay, Shauntay, Shauntei

Shauntel (American) song. See also Shantel.
Shauntela, Shauntele, Shauntell, Shauntella,
Shauntelle, Shauntrel, Shauntrell, Shauntrella,
Shauntrelle

Shaunya (Hebrew, Irish) a form of Shauna.

Shavon GB (American) a combination of
the prefix Sha + Yvonne. See also Siobhan.
Schavon, Schevon, Shavan, Shavaun, Shavone,
Shavonia, Shavonn, Shavonni, Shavonnia,
Shavonnie, Shavontae, Shavonte, Shavonté,
Shavoun, Sheavon, Shivaun, Shivawn, Shivon,
Shivonne, Shyvon, Shyvonne

Shavonda (American) a form of Shavon.
Shavondra

Shavonna (American) a form of Shavon.
Shavana, Shavanna, Shavona, Shavonah

Shavonne (American) a combination of the prefix Sha + Yvonne.

Shawana, Shawanna (American) combinations of the prefix Sha + Wanda. See also Shajuana, Shawna.
Shawan, Shawanah, Shawanda, Shawannah, Shawanta, Shawante, Shiwani

Shawn BG (Irish) a form of Sean. See also Shaun.
Schawn, Schawne, Shawen, Shawne, Shawnee, Shawnn, Shawon

Shawna (Hebrew, Irish) a form of Shana, Shawn. See also Seana, Shauna, Shona.
Sawna, Schawna, Schawnah, Shaw, Shawnae, Shawnah, Shawnai, Shawnell, Shawnette, Shawnra, Sheona

Shawnda (Irish) a form of Shawna. See also Shanda, Shaunda, Shonda.
Shawndan, Shawndra, Shawndrea, Shawndree, Shawndreel, Shawndrell, Shawndria

Shawndelle (Irish) a form of Shawna.
Schaundel, Schaundela, Schaundele, Schaundell, Schaundella, Schaundelle, Schawndel, Schawndela, Schawndele, Schawndell, Schawndelle, Seandel, Seandela, Seandele, Seandell, Seandella, Seandelle, Shaundel, Shaundela, Shaundele, Shaundell, Shaundella, Shaundelle, Shawndal, Shawndala, Shawndel, Shawndela, Shawndele, Shawndella

Shawnee (Irish) a form of Shawna.
Schawne, Schawnea, Schawnee, Shawne, Shawneea, Shawneen, Shawneena, Shawney, Shawni, Shawnie

Shawnika (American) a combination of Shawna + Nika.
Shawnaka, Shawneika, Shawnequa, Shawnicka

Shawnna (Hebrew, Irish) a form of Shawna.

Shawnta GB (Irish) a form of Shawna. See also Shaunta, Shonta.
Shawntae, Shawntah, Shawntay, Shawnte, Shawnté, Shawntee, Shawnteria, Shawntia,

Shawntina, Shawntish, Shawntrese, Shawntriece

Shawntel (American) song. See also Shantel, Shauntel.
Shawntela, Shawntelah, Shawntele, Shawntell, Shawntella, Shawntellah, Shawntelle, Shawntil, Shawntile, Shawntill, Shawntille

Shay BG (Irish) a form of Shea.
Shayda, Shayha, Shayia, Shey, Sheye

Shaya (Irish) a form of Shay.
Shayah

Shayann, Shayanne (Irish) combinations of Shay + Ann.
Shay Ann, Shay Anne, Shay-Ann, Shay-Anne

Shaye GB (Irish) a form of Shea.

Shayla, Shaylah (Irish) forms of Shay.
Shaylagh, Shaylain, Shaylan, Shaylea, Shayleah, Shaylla, Sheyla

Shaylee, Shayli, Shaylie (Irish) forms of Shea.
Shaylei, Shayleigh, Shayley, Shaylia, Shayliah, Shayly

Shayleen, Shaylene (Irish) forms of Shea.
Shaylean, Shayleana, Shayleanah, Shayleane, Shayleena, Shayleenah, Shayleene

Shaylen, Shaylin, Shaylyn, Shaylynn (Irish) forms of Shealyn.
Shaylina, Shaylinah, Shayline, Shaylinn, Shaylyna, Shaylynah, Shaylyne, Shaylynne

Shayna (Hebrew) beautiful.
Shaynae, Shaynah, Shaynee, Shayney, Shayni, Shaynia, Shaynie, Shaynna, Shaynne, Shayny

Shayne BG (Hebrew) a form of Shayna. (Irish) a form of Shane.

Shea GB (Irish) fairy palace.
Shearra

Shealyn (Irish) a form of Shea. See also Shaylen.
Shealy, Sheylyn

Sheba (Hebrew) a short form of Bathsheba. Geography: an ancient country of south Arabia.
Sheaba, Sheabah, Shebah, Sheeba, Sheebah, Sheiba, Sheibah, Sheyba, Sheybah

Sheena (Hebrew) God is gracious. (Irish) a form of Jane.
Sheana, Sheanah, Sheanna, Sheenagh, Sheenah, Sheenan, Sheeneal, Sheenna, Sheina, Sheinah, Sheyna, Sheynah, Shiona

Sheila (Latin) blind. (Irish) a form of Cecelia. See also Cheyla, Zelizi.
Sheela, Sheelagh, Sheelah, Sheilagh, Sheilah, Sheileen, Sheiletta, Sheilia, Sheilla, Sheillah, Sheillia, Sheilliah, Sheillynn, Sheilya, Shela, Shelagh, Shelah, Shiela, Shielah

Shelbe, Shelbee, Shelbey, Shelbi, Shelbie, Shellbie, Shellby (English) forms of Shelby.
Shelbbie, Shellbee, Shellbi

Shelby **GB** (English) ledge estate.
Chelby, Schelby, Shel, Shelbea, Shelbye, Shellbea, Shellbey

Sheldon **BG** (English) farm on the ledge.
Sheldina, Sheldine, Sheldrina, Sheldyn, Shelton

Shelee (English) a form of Shelley.
Shelea, Sheleah, Shelee, Sheleen, Shelei, Sheleigh, Shelena, Sheley, Sheli, Shelia, Shelie, Shelina, Shelinda, Shelita, Shely

Shelia (Latin, Irish) a form of Sheila.
Sheliah

Shelisa (American) a combination of Shelley + Lisa.
Sheleza, Shelica, Shelicia, Shelise, Shelisse, Sheliza

Shelley **GB** (English) meadow on the ledge. (French) a familiar form of Michelle. See also Chelley, Rochelle.
Shell, Shella, Shellaine, Shellana, Shellany, Shellea, Shelleah, Shellee, Shellei, Shelleigh, Shellene, Shelli, Shellian, Shelliann, Shellina

Shellie, Shelly (English) meadow on the ledge. (French) familiar forms of Michelle.

Shelsea (American) a form of Chelsea.
Shellsea, Shellsey, Shelsey, Shelsie, Shelsy

Shena (Irish) a form of Sheena.
Shenada, Shenah, Shenda, Shene, Sheneda, Shenee, Sheneena, Shenina, Shenita, Shenna, Shennah, Shenoa

Shenae (Irish) a form of Sheena.
Shenay, Shenea, Shennae

Shenandoa (Algonquin) beautiful star.
Shenandoah

Shenell, Shenelle (American) forms of Shanel.
Shenel, Shenela, Shenelah, Shenele, Shenella, Shenellah, Shenelly

Shenice, Shenise (American) forms of Shanice.
Shenece, Sheniece

Shenika, Sheniqua (American) forms of Shanika, Shena.
Sheenika, Shenequa, Shenica

Shera (Aramaic) light.
Sheara, Shearah, Sheera, Sheerah, Sherae, Sherah, Sheralla, Sheralle, Sheray, Sheraya

Sheralee (American) a combination of Shera + Lee.
Sheralea, Sheraleah, Sheraley

Sheree (French) beloved, dearest.
Scherea, Scheree, Scherey, Scherie, Sheerea, Sheeree, Shere, Sherea, Shereé, Sherey, Sherrea, Sherree, Sherrey

Shereen (French) a form of Sheree.
Shereena

Sherell, Sherelle, Sherrell (French) forms of Cherelle, Sheryl.
Sherel, Sherela, Sherelah, Sherele, Sherella, Sheriel, Sherrel, Sherrelle, Shirelle

Sheri, Sherie, Sherri, Sherrie (French) forms of Sherry.
Sheria, Sheriah, Sherria, Sherriah

Sherian, Sheriann (American) combinations of Sheri + Ann.
Sherianne, Sherrina

Sherica (Punjabi, Arabic) a form of Sherika.
Shericah, Sherrica

Sherice (French) a form of Cherice.
Scherise, Sherece, Shereece, Sherees, Shereese, Sherese, Shericia, Sherise, Sherisse, Sherrish, Sherryse, Sheryce

Sheridan GB (Irish) wild.
Cherida, Cheriden, Sherida, Sheridane,
Sherideen, Sheriden, Sheridian, Sheridin,
Sheridon, Sheridyn, Sherridan, Sherridana,
Sherridane, Sherridanne, Sherridon, Sherrydan,
Sherrydana, Sherrydane, Sherrydin,
Sherrydon, Sherrydyn, Sherydan, Sherydana,
Sherydane

Sherika (Punjabi) relative. (Arabic) easterner.
Shereka, Sherekah, Shericka, Sherikah,
Sheriqua, Sheriquah, Sherricka, Sherrika,
Sheryca, Sherycah, Sherycka, Sheryckah,
Sheryka, Sheryqua, Sheryquah

Sherilyn (American) a form of Sherylyn.
Sharilyn, Sherilin, Sherilina, Sherilinah,
Sheriline, Sherilyna, Sherilynah, Sherilyne,
Sherilynn, Sherilynna, Sherilynnah, Sherilynne

Sherissa (French) a form of Sherry, Sheryl.
Shereesa, Shereese, Shereeza, Shereeze,
Sheresa, Shericia, Sherisa, Sherisah, Sherise,
Sheriss, Sherissah, Sherisse, Sheriza, Sherizah,
Sherize, Sherizza, Sherizzah, Sherizze,
Sherrish, Sherys, Sherysa, Sherysah, Sheryse,
Sheryss, Sheryssa, Sheryssah, Sherysse

Sherita (French) a form of Sherry, Sheryl.
See also Sharita.
Shereata, Shereatah, Shereeta, Shereetah,
Shereta, Sheretta, Sherette, Sheritah, Sherrita,
Sheryta, Sherytah

Sherleen (French, English) a form of
Sheryl, Shirley.
Sherileen, Sherlene, Sherlin, Sherlina, Sherline,
Sherlyn, Sherlyne, Sherlynne

Sherley (English) a form of Shirley.
Sherlee, Sherli, Sherlie

Shermaine (American) a form of
Sharmaine.

Sherron (Hebrew) a form of Sharon.
Sheron, Sherona, Sheronna, Sherronna,
Sherronne

Sherry (French) beloved, dearest. A familiar
form of Sheryl. See also Sheree.
Scheri, Scherie, Schery, Sheerey, Sheeri,
Sheerie, Sheery, Sherey, Sherissa, Sherrey,
Shery, Sherye, Sheryy

Sheryl (French) beloved. A familiar form of
Shirley. See also Sherry.
Sharel, Sharil, Sharyl, Sharyll, Sheral, Sheriel,
Sheril, Sherile, Sherill, Sherille, Sherily,
Sherral, Sherril, Sherrill, Sherryl, Sheryle,
Sheryll, Sherylle, Sherylly

Sherylyn (American) a combination of
Sheryl + Lynn. See also Cherilyn.
Sharolin, Sharolyn, Sharyl-Lynn, Sheralin,
Sheralina, Sheraline, Sheralyn, Sheralyna,
Sheralyne, Sheralynn, Sheralynne, Sherralyn,
Sherralynn, Sherrilyn, Sherrilynn, Sherrilynne,
Sherrylyn, Sherylanne, Sherylin, Sherylina,
Sherylinah, Sheryline, Sherylyna, Sherylynah,
Sherylyne

Shevonne (American) a combination of the
prefix She + Yvonne.
Shevaun, Shevon, Shevonda, Shevone

Sheyanne, Sheyenne (Cheyenne) forms of
Cheyenne. See also Shyan.
Shayhan, Sheyan, Sheyane, Sheyann,
Sheyanna, Sheyannah, Sheyen, Sheyene

Shi (Japanese) a short form of Shika.
She

Shian, Shiane, Shiann, Shianne
(Cheyenne) forms of Cheyenne.
Shiante, Shiany, Shieann, Shieanne, Shiene,
Shienn, Shienne

Shiana, Shianna (Cheyenne) forms of
Cheyenne.
Shianah, Shianda, Shiannah, Shieana, Shiena,
Shienna

Shifra (Hebrew) beautiful.
Schifra, Shifrah, Shyfra, Shyfrah

Shika (Japanese) gentle deer.
Shikah

Shikha (Japanese) a form of Shika.

Shilah (Latin, Irish) a form of Sheila.
Shila, Shilea

Shilo BG (Hebrew) a form of Shiloh.

Shiloh GB (Hebrew) God's gift. Bible: a
sanctuary for the Israelites where the Ark
of the Covenant was kept.

Shilpa (Indian) well proportioned.
Shilpta

Shina (Japanese) virtuous, good; wealthy. (Chinese) a form of China.
Shinae, Shinay, Shine, Shinna

Shino (Japanese) bamboo stalk.

Shinobu (Japanese) to support.

Shiquita (American) a form of Chiquita.
Shiquata, Shiquitta

Shira (Hebrew) song.
Shirah, Shiray, Shire, Shiree, Shiri, Shirit

Shirin (Persian) charming, sweet.

Shirlene (English) a form of Shirley.
Shirleen, Shirlena, Shirlina, Shirline, Shirlyn, Shirlynn

Shirley (English) bright meadow. See also Sheryl.
Shir, Shirl, Shirlee, Shirlie, Shirlly, Shirly, Shurlee, Shurley

Shivani (Hindi) life and death.
Shiva, Shivana, Shivanie, Shivanna

Shizu (Japanese) silent.
Shizue, Shizuka, Shizuko, Shizuyo

Shona (Irish) a form of Jane. A form of Shana, Shauna, Shawna.
Shiona, Shonagh, Shonah, Shonalee, Shone, Shonee, Shonette, Shoni, Shonie

Shonda (Irish) a form of Shona. See also Shanda, Shaunda, Shawnda.
Shondalette, Shondalyn, Shondel, Shondelle, Shondi, Shondia, Shondie, Shondra, Shondreka, Shounda

Shonna (Irish) a form of Shona.
Shonnah

Shonta (Irish) a form of Shona. See also Shaunta, Shawnta.
Shontá, Shontai, Shontalea, Shontasia, Shontedra, Shonteral, Shontol, Shontoy, Shontrail

Shontae (Irish) a form of Shonta.
Shontay, Shontaya, Shonté, Shountáe

Shontavia (Irish) a form of Shonta.
Shontaviea

Shonte (Irish) a form of Shonta.
Shontee, Shonti

Shontel, Shontell (American) forms of Shantel.
Shontela, Shontelah, Shontele, Shontella, Shontellah, Shontelle

Shontia (American) a form of Shantia.

Shoshana (Hebrew) a form of Susan.
Shosha, Shoshan, Shoshanah, Shoshane, Shoshanha, Shoshann, Shoshanna, Shoshannah, Shoshauna, Shoshaunah, Shoshawna, Shoshona, Shoshone, Shoshonee, Shoshoney, Shoshoni, Shoushan, Shushana, Sosha, Soshana

Shreya (Indian) better.

Shu (Chinese) kind, gentle.

Shug (American) a short form of Sugar.

Shula (Arabic) flaming, bright.
Shulah

Shulamith (Hebrew) peaceful. See also Sula.
Shulamit, Sulamith

Shunta (Irish) a form of Shonta.
Shuntae, Shunté, Shuntel, Shuntell, Shuntelle, Shuntia

Shura (Russian) a form of Alexandra.
Schura, Shurah, Shuree, Shureen, Shurelle, Shuritta, Shurka, Shurlana

Shy, Shye (Cheyenne) short forms of Shyan.

Shyan, Shyann, Shyanne, Shyenne (Cheyenne) forms of Cheyenne. See also Sheyanne.
Shyane, Shyene, Shynee

Shyanna (Cheyenne) a form of Cheyenne.
Shyana, Shyanah, Shyandra, Shyannah, Shyenna

Shyla (English) a form of Sheila.
Shya, Shyah, Shylah, Shylan, Shylana, Shylane, Shylayah, Shyle, Shyleah, Shylee, Shyley, Shyli, Shylia, Shylie, Shylyn

Shylo (Hebrew) a form of Shilo.
Shyloe, Shyloh, Shylon

Shyra (Hebrew) a form of Shira.
Shyrae, Shyrah, Shyrai, Shyrie, Shyro

Sianna (Irish) a form of Seana.
Sian, Siana, Sianae, Sianai, Sianey, Siannah, Sianne, Sianni, Sianny, Siany, Sina, Sion, Syon

Siara, Siarra (Irish) forms of Sierra.
Siarah, Siarrah

Sibeta (Moquelumnan) finding a fish under a rock.

Sibila, Sibilia, Sibilina (Greek) forms of Sybil.

Sibley (English) sibling; friendly. (Greek) a form of Sybil.
Sybley

Sidnee, Sidnie (French) forms of Sydney.
Sidne, Sidnei, Sidneya, Sidni, Sidny, Sidnye

Sidney 🇬🇧 (French) a form of Sydney.

Sidonia (Hebrew) enticing.
Sydania, Syndonia

Sidonie (French) from Saint-Denis, France. See also Sydney.
Sidaine, Sidanni, Sidelle, Sidoine, Sidona, Sidonae, Sidonia, Sidony

Sidra (Latin) star child.
Sidrah, Sidras

Siena, Sienna (American) forms of Ciana.
Seini

Siera, Sierrah (Irish) forms of Sierra.
Sierah

Sierra ☀ 🇬🇧 (Irish) black. (Spanish) saw toothed. Geography: any rugged range of mountains that, when viewed from a distance, has a jagged profile. See also Ciara.
Seera, Sieara, Siearra, Sieria, Sierre, Sierrea, Sierriah

Sigfreda (German) victorious peace. See also Freda.
Sigfreida, Sigfrida, Sigfrieda, Sigfryda

Siglinda (Germanic) protective victory.

Sigmunda (German) victorious protector.
Sigmonda

Signe (Latin) sign, signal. (Scandinavian) a short form of Sigourney.
Sig, Signa, Signy, Singna, Singne

Sigolena (Scandinavian) gentle victory.

Sigourney (English) victorious conquerer.
Sigournee, Sigourny

Sigrada (German) famous because of the victory.

Sigrid (Scandinavian) victorious counselor.
Siegrid, Siegrida, Sigritt

Sihu (Native American) flower; bush.

Siko (African) crying baby.

Silenia (Latin) belongs to the earthly gods.

Silvana (Latin) a form of Sylvana.
Silvaine, Silvanna, Silviane

Silver (English) a precious metal.

Silveria, Silvina (Spanish) forms of Selva.

Silvia (Latin) a form of Sylvia.
Silivia, Silva, Silvya

Simcha 🅱🇬 (Hebrew) joyful.

Simona (Hebrew, French) a form of Simone.
Simmona, Simonetta, Simonia, Simonina

Simone (Hebrew) she heard. (French) a form of Simon (see Boys' Names). See also Ximena, Zimena.
Siminie, Simmi, Simmie, Simmone, Simoane, Simonette, Simonne, Somone

Simran 🇬🇧 (Sikh) absorbed in God.
Simren, Simrin, Simrun

Sina 🅱🇬 (Irish) a form of Seana.
Seena, Sinai, Sinaia, Sinan, Sinay

Sinclair 🇬🇧 (French) a form of Sinclaire.

Sinclaire (French) prayer.

Sinclética (Greek) she who is invited.

Sindy (American) a form of Cindy.
Sinda, Sindal, Sindea, Sindeah, Sindee, Sindey, Sindi, Sindia, Sindie, Sinnedy, Synda, Syndal, Syndea, Syndeah, Syndee, Syndey, Syndi, Syndia, Syndie, Syndy

Sinead (Irish) a form of Jane.
Seonaid, Sine, Sinéad

Sinforiana (Greek) a form of Sinforosa.

Sinforosa (Latin) full of misfortunes.

Sinovia, Sinya (Russian) foreign.

Sintiques, Síntiques (Greek) fortunate.

Siobhan (Irish) a form of Joan. See also Shavon.
Shibahn, Shibani, Shibhan, Shioban, Shobana, Shobha, Shobhana, Siobahn, Siobhana, Siobhann, Siobhon, Siovaun, Siovhan

Sión (Latin) a form of Asunción.

Sira (Latin) she who comes from Syria.

Sirena (Greek) enchanter. Mythology: Sirens were sea nymphs whose singing enchanted sailors and made them crash their ships into nearby rocks. See also Cyrena, Xirena, Zirina.
Sireena, Siren, Sirenah, Sirene, Sirine

Siri (Scandinavian) a short form of Sigrid.
Siree, Sirey, Siry

Sisika (Native American) songbird.

Sissy (American) a familiar form of Cecelia.
Sisi, Sisie, Sissey, Sissi, Sissie

Sita (Hindi) a form of Shakti.
Sitah, Sitha

Sitara (Sanskrit) morning star.
Sitarah, Sithara

Siti (Swahili) respected woman.

Sky BG (Arabic, Dutch) a form of Skye.
Skky

Skye GB (Arabic) water giver. (Dutch) a short form of Skyler. Geography: an island in the Inner Hebrides, Scotland.
Ski, Skie, Skii

Skyla (Dutch) a form of Skyler.
Skya, Skylah

Skylar BG (Dutch) a form of Skyler.
Skyllar, Skyylar

Skyler BG (Dutch) sheltering.
Skila, Skilah, Skyela, Skyelar, Skyeler, Skyelur, Skylair, Skylee, Skylena, Skyli, Skylia, Skylie, Skylin, Skylor, Skylyn, Skylynn, Skylyr, Skyra

Skyy (Arabic, Dutch) a form of Skye.

Sloan BG (Irish) a form of Sloane.

Sloane (Irish) warrior.
Sloanne

Socorro (Spanish) helper.

Sofia ⭐ (Greek) a form of Sophia. See also Zofia, Zsofia.
Sofeea, Sofeeia, Soficita, Sofija, Sofiya, Sofka, Sofya

Sofía (Greek) a form of Sofia.

Sofie (Greek) a form of Sofia.
Soffi, Sofi

Sol (Latin) sun.

Solada (Tai) listener.

Solana (Spanish) sunshine.
Solande, Solanna, Soleil, Solena, Soley, Solina, Solinda

Solange (French) dignified.

Soledad (Spanish) solitary.
Sole, Soleda

Soledada (Spanish) a form of Soledad.

Solenne (French) solemn, dignified.
Solaine, Solene, Soléne, Solenna, Solina, Soline, Solonez, Souline, Soulle

Solita (Latin) alone.
Soleata, Soleatah, Soleeta, Soleetah, Soleete, Soleighta, Soleita, Soleitah, Solitah, Solite, Solitta, Solittah, Solitte, Solyta, Solytah, Solytta, Solyttah, Solytte

Solomon BG (Hebrew) peaceful.

Soma (Hindi) lunar.

Somer (English, Arabic) a form of Sommer.

Sommer (English) summer; summoner. (Arabic) black. See also Summer.
Somara, Sommar, Sommara, Sommers

Somoche (Mapuche) distinguished woman.

Sondra (Greek) defender of mankind.
Sondre, Sonndra, Sonndre

Sonia (Russian, Slavic) a form of Sonya.
Sonica, Sonida, Sonita, Sonna, Sonni, Sonnia, Sonnie, Sonny

Sonja (Scandinavian) a form of Sonya.
Sonjae, Sonjia

Sonora (Spanish) pleasant sounding.

Sonsoles (Spanish) they are suns.

Sonya (Greek) wise. (Russian, Slavic) a form of Sophia.
Sonnya, Sonyae, Sunya

Sook (Korean) pure.

Sopatra (Greek) father's savior.

Sopheary (Cambodian) beautiful girl.

Sophia ☆ (Greek) wise. See also Sofia, Sonya, Zofia.

Sophie (Greek) a familiar form of Sophia. See also Zocha.
Sophey, Sophi, Sophy

Sophronia (Greek) wise; sensible.
Soffrona, Sofronia

Sora (Native American) chirping songbird.

Soraya (Persian) princess.
Suraya

Sorne (Basque) a form of Concepción.

Sorrel GB (French) reddish brown. Botany: a plant whose leaves are used as salad greens.

Sorya (Spanish) she who is eloquent.

Soso (Native American) tree squirrel dining on pine nuts; chubby-cheeked baby.

Sotera (Greek) savior.

Soterraña (Spanish) burier; burial site.

Souzan (Persian) burning fire.
Sousan, Souzanne

Spencer, Spenser BG (English) dispenser of provisions.

Speranza (Italian) a form of Esperanza.
Speranca

Spica (Latin) ear of wheat. Astronomy: a star in the constellation Virgo.

Spring (English) springtime.
Spryng

Stacee, Staci, Stacie (Greek) forms of Stacey.

Stacey GB (Greek) resurrection. (Irish) a short form of Anastasia, Eustacia, Natasha.
Stacci, Stace, Staceyan, Staceyann, Staicy, Stasey, Stayce, Staycee, Stayci, Steacy

Stacia, Stasia (English) short forms of Anastasia.
Staysha

Stacy GB (Greek) resurrection. (Irish) a short form of Anastasia, Eustacia, Natasha.

Star (English) star.
Staria, Starisha, Starleen, Starlet, Starlette, Starley, Starlight, Starre, Starri, Starria, Starrika, Starrsha, Starsha, Starshanna, Startish

Starla (English) a form of Star.
Starrla

Starleen (English) a form of Star.
Starleena, Starlena, Starlene

Starley (English) a familiar form of Star.
Starle, Starlee, Starly

Starling BG (English) bird.

Starlyn (English) a form of Star.
Starlin, Starlynn, Starrlen

Starr GB (English) star.

Stasha (Greek, Russian) a form of Stasya.
Stashia

Stasya (Greek) a familiar form of Anastasia. (Russian) a form of Stacey.
Stasa, Stasja, Staska

Stefani, Stefanie, Stefany, Steffani, Steffanie, Steffany (Greek) forms of Stephanie.
Stafani, Stafanie, Staffany, Stefane, Stefanee, Stefaney, Stefanié, Stefanni, Stefannie, Stefanny, Stefenie, Steffane, Steffanee, Steffaney, Stefini, Stefinie, Stefoni

Stefania (Greek) a form of Stephanie.
Stefanija, Stefanya

Stefanía (Greek) a form of Stephanie.

Steffi (Greek) a familiar form of Stefani, Stephanie.
Stefa, Stefcia, Steffee, Steffie, Steffy, Stefi, Stefka, Stefy, Stepha, Stephi, Stephie, Stephy

Stella (Latin) star. (French) a familiar form of Estelle.
Steile, Stellina

Stella Maris (Hispanic) star of the sea.

Stepania (Russian) a form of Stephanie.
Stepa, Stepahny, Stepanida, Stepanie,
Stepanyda, Stepfanie

Stephaine (Greek) a form of Stephanie.

Stephani, Stephannie, Stephany (Greek)
forms of Stephanie.
Stephanni, Stephanye

Stephania (Greek) a form of Stephanie.
Stephanida

Stephanie ⭐ **GB** (Greek) crowned. See also
Estefani, Estephanie, Panya, Stevi, Zephania.
Stamatios, Stephaija, Stephana, Stephanas,
Stephane, Stephanee, Stephaney, Stéphanie,
Stephanine, Stephann, Stephianie, Stephinie,
Stesha, Steshka, Stevanee

Stephene (Greek) a form of Stephanie.

Stephenie (Greek) a form of Stephanie.
Stephena, Stephenee, Stepheney, Stepheni,
Stephenny, Stepheny

Stephine (Greek) a form of Stephanie.
Stephina, Stephyne

Stephney (Greek) a form of Stephanie.
Stephne, Stephni, Stephnie, Stephny

Sterling **BG** (English) valuable; silver penny.

Stevi (Greek) a familiar form of Stephanie.
Steva, Stevana, Stevanee, Stevee, Stevena,
Stevey, Stevy, Stevye

Stevie **GB** (Greek) a familiar form of
Stephanie.

Stina (German) a short form of Christina.
Steena, Stena, Stine, Stinna

Stockard (English) stockyard.

Storm **BG** (English) storm.
Storme, Stormm

Stormi, Stormie (English) forms of Stormy.
Stormii

Stormy **GB** (English) impetuous by nature.
Stormee, Stormey

Su (Chinese) revive, resurrect.

Suchin (Tai) beautiful thought.

Sue (Hebrew) a short form of Susan,
Susana.

Sueann (American) a combination of Sue +
Ann.
Suann, Suanne, Sueanne

Sueanna (American) a combination of Sue
+ Anna.
Suanna, Suannah

Suela (Spanish) consolation.
Suelita

Sugar (American) sweet as sugar.

Sugi (Japanese) cedar tree.

Suke (Hawaiian) a form of Susan.

Sukey (Hawaiian) a familiar form of Susan.
Suka, Sukee, Suky

Sukhdeep (Sikh) light of peace and bliss.
Sukhdip

Suki (Japanese) loved one. (Moquelumnan)
eagle-eyed.
Sukie

Sula (Icelandic) large sea bird. (Greek,
Hebrew) a short form of Shulamith,
Ursula.

Sulamita (Hebrew) peaceful woman.

Suleika (Arabic) most beautiful woman.

Suletu (Moquelumnan) soaring bird.

Sulia (Latin) a form of Julia.
Suliana

Sullivan **BG** (Irish) black eyed.
Sullavan, Sullevan, Sully, Syllyvan

Sulpicia (Latin) Literature: a woman poet
from ancient Rome.

Sulwen (Welsh) bright as the sun.

Suma (English) born in the summertime.

Sumalee (Tai) beautiful flower.

Sumati (Hindi) unity.

Sumaya (American) a combination of Sue
+ Maya.
Sumayah, Sumayya, Sumayyah

Sumer (English) a form of Summer.

Sumi (Japanese) elegant, refined.
Sumiko

Summer (English) summertime. See also Sommer.
Summar, Summerann, Summerbreeze, Summerhaze, Summerine, Summerlee, Summerlin, Summerlyn, Summerlynn, Summers, Summyr, Sumrah, Sumyr

Sun (Korean) obedient.
Suncance, Sundee, Sundeep, Sundi, Sundip, Sundrenea, Sunta, Sunya

Sun-Hi (Korean) good; joyful.

Sunday (Latin) born on the first day of the week.

Sunee (Tai) good.

Suni (Zuni) native; member of our tribe.
Sunita, Sunitha, Suniti, Sunne, Sunnilei

Suniva (Latin) radiant; enlightened.

Sunki (Hopi) swift.
Sunkia

Sunny BG (English) bright, cheerful.
Sunni, Sunnie

Sunshine (English) sunshine.
Sunshyn, Sunshyne

Surata (Pakistani) blessed joy.

Suri (Todas) pointy nose.
Suree, Surena, Surenia

Surya BG (Sanskrit) Mythology: a sun god.
Suria, Suriya, Surra

Susammi (French) a combination of Susan + Aimee.
Suzami, Suzamie, Suzamy

Susan (Hebrew) lily. See also Shoshana, Sukey, Zsa Zsa, Zusa.
Sawsan, Siusan, Sosan, Sosana, Suesan, Sueva, Suisan, Susen, Suson

Susana, Susanna, Susannah (Hebrew) forms of Susan. See also Xuxa, Zanna, Zsuzsanna.
Sonel, Sosana, Suesanna, Susanah, Susane, Susanka

Susanita (Spanish) a familiar form of Susana.

Susanne (Hebrew) a form of Susan.
Susann

Suse (Hawaiian) a form of Susan.

Susette (French) a familiar form of Susan, Susana.
Susetta

Susie (American) a familiar form of Susan, Susana.
Susey, Susi, Sussi, Sussy, Susy

Susima (Greek) elected.

Suyapa (Spanish) Geography: a village in Honduras.

Suzan (English) a form of Susan.

Suzana, Suzanna, Suzannah (Hebrew) forms of Susan.
Suzenna, Suzzanna

Suzanne (English) a form of Susan.
Suszanne, Suzane, Suzann, Suzzane, Suzzann, Suzzanne

Suzette (French) a form of Susan.
Suzetta, Suzzette

Suzie (American) a familiar form of Susan, Susana.
Suze, Suzi, Suzy, Suzzie

Suzu (Japanese) little bell.
Suzue, Suzuko

Suzuki (Japanese) bell tree.

Svetlana (Russian) bright light.
Sveta, Svetochka

SyÀ (Chinese) summer.

Sybella (English) a form of Sybil.
Sebila, Sibbella, Sibella, Sibilla, Sibylla, Sybila, Sybilla

Sybil (Greek) prophet. Mythology: sibyls were oracles who relayed the messages of the gods. See also Cybele, Sibley.
Sib, Sibbel, Sibbie, Sibbill, Sibby, Sibeal, Sibel, Sibell, Sibelle, Sibyl, Sibylle, Sibylline, Sybel, Sybelle, Sybille, Syble

Sydne, Sydnee, Sydnei, Sydni, Sydnie (French) forms of Sydney.

Sydney ☀ GB (French) from Saint-Denis, France. See also Sidnee, Sidonie.
Cidney, Cydney, Sy, Syd, Sydel, Sydelle, Sydna, Sydnea, Sydny, Sydnye, Syndona, Syndonah

Syerra (Irish, Spanish) a form of Sierra.
Syera

Sying BG (Chinese) star.

Sylvana (Latin) forest.
Sylva, Sylvaine, Sylvanah, Sylvania, Sylvanna, Sylvina, Sylvinnia, Sylvonah, Sylvonia, Sylvonna

Sylvia (Latin) forest. Literature: Sylvia Plath was a well-known American poet. See also Silvia, Xylia.
Sylvette

Sylviann, Sylvianne (American) combinations of Sylvia + Ann.
Sylvian

Sylvie (Latin) a familiar form of Sylvia.
Silvi, Silvie, Silvy, Sylvi

Sylwia (Latin) a form of Sylvia.

Symantha (American) a form of Samantha.

Symone (Hebrew) a form of Simone.
Symmeon, Symmone, Symona, Symoné, Symonne

Symphony (Greek) symphony, harmonious sound.
Symfoni, Symphanée, Symphanie, Symphany, Symphoni, Symphonie

Synthia (Greek) a form of Cynthia.
Sinthea, Sinthia, Sinthiah, Sinthya, Sinthyah, Synthea, Synthiah, Synthya, Synthyah

Syreeta (Hindi) good traditions. (Arabic) companion.
Syretta, Syrrita

Syrena (Greek) a form of Sirena.
Syreana, Syreanah, Syreane, Syreen, Syreena, Syreenah, Syreene, Syren, Syrenah, Syrenia, Syreniah, Syrenna, Syrenya, Syrenyah, Syrin, Syrina, Syrinah, Syrine, Syryn, Syryna, Syrynah, Syryne

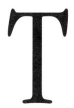

T'keyah (American) a form of Takia.

Tabatha, Tabbatha (Greek, Aramaic) forms of Tabitha.
Tabathe, Tabathia

Tabbitha (Greek, Aramaic) a form of Tabitha.

Tabby (English) a familiar form of Tabitha.
Tabbee, Tabbey, Tabbi, Tabbie

Tabea (Swahili) a form of Tabia.

Tabetha (Greek, Aramaic) a form of Tabitha.
Tabbetha

Tabia (Swahili) talented.
Tabya, Tabyah

Tabina (Arabic) follower of Muhammad.
Tabinah, Tabyna, Tabynah

Tabitha (Greek, Aramaic) gazelle.
Tabiatha, Tabita, Tabithia, Tabotha, Tabtha

Tabora (Arabic) plays a small drum.

Tabytha (Greek, Aramaic) a form of Tabitha.
Tabbytha

Tacey (English) a familiar form of Tacita.
Tace, Tacea, Tacee, Taci, Tacy, Tacye, Taicea, Taicee, Taicey, Taici, Taicie, Taicy, Taycea, Taycee, Taycey, Tayci, Taycie, Taycy

Taci (Zuni) washtub. (English) a form of Tacey.
Tacia, Taciana, Tacie

Tacita (Latin) silent.
Taceta, Tacetah, Tasita, Tasitah, Taycita, Taycitah, Taycyta, Taycytah

Tácita (Latin) a form of Tacita.

Taddea (Greek) a form of Thaddea.
Taddeah, Tadea, Tadeah, Tadia, Tadiah, Tadya, Tadyah

Tadita (Omaha) runner.
Tadeta, Tadetah, Taditah, Tadra, Tadyta,
Tadytah

Taelar, Taeler, Taelor (English) forms of
Taylor.
Taellor, Taelore, Taelyr

Taesha (Latin) a form of Tisha. (American) a
combination of the prefix Ta + Aisha.
Tadasha, Taeshayla, Taeshia, Taheisha, Tahisha,
Taiesha, Tayesha

Taffline (Welsh) beloved.
Taflina, Taflinah, Tafline, Taflyn, Taflyna,
Taflynah, Taflyne

Taffy GB (Welsh) a familiar form of Taffline.
Taafe, Taffea, Taffee, Taffey, Taffi, Taffia, Taffie,
Taffine, Taffye, Tafia, Tafisa, Tafoya, Tafy

Tafne (Egyptian) Mythology: the goddess of
light.
Taffnee, Taffney, Taffni, Taffnie, Taffny, Tafna,
Tafnah, Tafnee

Tahira (Arabic) virginal, pure.
Taheera, Taheerah, Tahera, Tahere, Taheria,
Taherri, Tahiara, Tahirah, Tahireh, Tahyra,
Tahyrah

Tahiti (Polynesian) rising sun. Geography: an
island in the southern Pacific Ocean.
Tahitea, Tahitee, Tahitey, Tahitia, Tahitie, Tahity

Tahlia (Greek, Hebrew) a form of Talia.
Tahleah, Tahleia

Tai BG (Vietnamese) weather; prosperous;
talented.

Taija (Hindi) a form of Taja.
Taiajára

Tailer, Tailor (English) forms of Taylor.
Tailar, Tailara, Taillor, Tailora, Tailore, Tailyr

Taima GB (Native American) clash of thun-
der.
Taimah, Taimi, Taimia, Taimy, Tayma, Taymah,
Taymi, Taymie, Taymmi, Taymmie, Taymmy,
Taymy

Taimani (Tongan) diamonds.
Taimanee, Taimaney, Taimania, Taimaniah,
Taimanie, Taimany, Taimanya, Taimanyah

Taipa (Moquelumnan) flying quail.
Taipah, Taypa, Taypah

Taira (Aramaic, Irish, Arabic) a form of Tara.
Tairra

Tais (Greek) bound.
Taisa, Taisah, Tays, Taysa, Taysah

Taisha (American) a form of Taesha.
Taishae

Taite (English) cheerful.
Tait, Taita, Taitah, Tayt, Tayta, Tayte, Tayten

Taja (Hindi) crown.
Tahai, Tajae, Teja, Tejah, Tejal

Tajah (Hindi) a form of Taja.

Taka (Japanese) honored.
Takah

Takala (Hopi) corn tassel.

Takara (Japanese) treasure.
Takarah, Takaria, Takariah, Takarra, Takarrah,
Takarya, Takaryah, Takra

Takayla (American) a combination of the
prefix Ta + Kayla.
Takayler, Takeyli

Takeia (Arabic) a form of Takia.
Takeiah, Takeiya, Takeiyah

Takeisha (American) a combination of the
prefix Ta + Keisha.
Takecia, Tekeesha, Tekeisha, Tekeshi, Tekeysia,
Tekisha, Tikesha, Tikisha, Tokesia

Takenya (Hebrew) animal horn.
(Moquelumnan) falcon. (American) a com-
bination of the prefix Ta + Kenya.
Takenia, Takeniah, Takenja, Takenjah,
Takenyah

Takeria (American) a form of Takira.
Takeara, Takearah, Takera, Takeri, Takerian,
Takerra, Takerria, Takierria, Takoria, Taquera,
Taquerah, Tekeria, Tekeriah

Takesha (American) a form of Takeisha.
Takeshia, Takesia

Takeya (Arabic) a form of Takia.
Takeyah

Taki (Japanese) waterfall.
Takee, Takey, Takie, Taky, Tiki

Takia (Arabic) worshiper.
Takhiya, Takiah, Takija, Takijah, Takkia,
Takkiah, Takkya, Takkyah, Takya, Takyah,

Takyia, Taqiya, Taqiyah, Taqiyya, Taquaia, Taquaya, Taquiia, Taquiiah, Tikia

Takila (American) a form of Tequila.
Takeila, Takela, Takelia, Takella, Takeyla, Takiela, Takilah, Takilla, Takilya, Takyla, Takylia, Tatakyla, Tehilla, Tekeila, Tekela, Tekelia, Tekilaa, Tekilia, Tekilla, Tekilyah, Tekla

Takira (American) a combination of the prefix Ta + Kira.
Takeera, Takeira, Takeirah, Takera, Takiara, Takiera, Takierah, Takierra, Takirah, Takiria, Takiriah, Takirra, Takora, Takyra, Takyrah, Takyrra, Taquira, Taquirah, Tekyra, Tekyria, Tekyriah, Tekyrya, Tikara, Tikarah, Tikira, Tikirah, Tikiria, Tikiriah, Tikirya, Tikiryah

Takisha (American) a form of Takeisha.
Takishea, Takishia

Takiya, Takiyah (Arabic) forms of Takia.

Tala (Native American) stalking wolf.
Talah

Talasi (Hopi) corn tassel.
Talasea, Talasee, Talasia, Talasiah, Talasy, Talasya, Talasyah

Talaya (American) a form of Talia.
Talayah, Talayia

Talea, Taleah (American) forms of Talia.
Taleana, Taleea, Taleéi, Taleia, Taleiya, Tylea, Tyleah

Taleebin (Australian) young.
Taleabin, Taleabina, Taleabine, Taleabyn, Taleabyna, Taleabyne, Taleebina, Taleebine, Taleebyn, Taleebyna, Taleebyne

Taleisha (American) a combination of Talia + Aisha.
Taileisha, Taleasha, Taleashia, Taleashiah, Taleashya, Taleesha, Taleeshia, Taleeshiah, Taleeshya, Taleise, Taleysha, Taleyshia, Taleyshiah, Taleyshya, Taleyshyah, Talicia, Taliesha, Talysha, Tilisha, Tyleasha, Tyleisha, Tylicia, Tylisha, Tylishia

Talena (American) a combination of the prefix Ta + Lena.
Talayna, Taleana, Taleanah, Taleane, Taleena, Taleenah, Taleene, Talenah, Talene, Talihna, Tallenia, Talná, Tilena, Tilene, Tylena

Talesha (American) a form of Taleisha.
Taleesha, Talesa, Talese, Taleshia, Talesia, Tallese, Tallesia, Tylesha, Tyleshia, Tylesia

Talia (Greek) blooming. (Hebrew) dew from heaven. (Latin, French) birthday. A short form of Natalie. See also Thalia.
Taleya, Taleyah, Taliatha, Taliea, Talieya, Tallia, Tylia

Talía (Greek) a form of Talia.

Taliah (Greek, Hebrew, Latin, French) a form of Talia.
Talliah

Talina (American) a combination of Talia + Lina.
Talin, Talinah, Talinda, Taline, Tallyn, Talyn, Talyna, Talynah, Talyne, Talynn, Tylina, Tyline

Talisa, Talissa (English) forms of Tallis.
Talisah, Talisia, Talisiah, Talissah, Tallisa, Tallisah, Tallysa, Tallysah, Talysa, Talysah, Talysha, Talysia, Talysiah, Talyssa, Talyssah

Talisha (American) a form of Taleisha. (English) a form of Talisa.
Talishia

Talitha (Arabic) young girl.
Taleetha, Taletha, Talethia, Taliatha, Talita, Talith, Talithah, Talithe, Talithia, Talyth, Talytha, Talythe, Telita, Tiletha

Taliyah (Greek) a form of Talia.
Taliya, Talliyah

Talley (French) a familiar form of Talia.
Talee, Talei, Taleigh, Taley, Tali, Talie, Talle, Tallee, Tallei, Talleigh, Talli, Tallie, Tally, Taly, Talye, Tylee

Tallis BG (French, English) forest.
Taleace, Talease, Taleece, Taleese, Taleice, Taleise, Taleyce, Taleyse, Talice, Taliece, Taliese, Talise, Taliss, Talisse, Talliss, Tallisse, Tallys, Tallyse, Talyce, Talys, Talyse, Talyss, Talysse

Tallulah (Choctaw) leaping water.
Tallou, Tallula, Talula

Talma (Native American) thunder.
Talmah

Talman BG (Hebrew) to injure, oppress.

Talon BG (French, English) claw, nail.
Taelon, Taelyn, Talen, Tallin, Tallon, Talyn

Talor GB (Hebrew) dew.
Talora, Talorah, Talore, Talorey, Talori, Taloria, Taloriah, Talorie, Talory, Talorya, Taloryah, Talorye

Talya (Greek) a form of Talia.
Tallya, Talyah, Talyia

Tam BG (Vietnamese) heart.

Tama (Japanese) jewel.
Tamaa, Tamah, Tamaiah, Tamala, Tema

Tamaira (American) a form of Tamara.
Tamairah

Tamaka (Japanese) bracelet.
Tamakah, Tamaki, Tamakia, Tamakiah, Tamako, Tamaky, Tamakya, Tamakyah, Timaka

Tamanna (Hindi) desire.
Tamana, Tamanah, Tamannah

Tamar GB (Russian) History: a twelfth-century Georgian queen. (Hebrew) a short form of Tamara.
Tamer, Tamor, Tamour

Tamara (Hebrew) palm tree. See also Tammy.
Tamará, Tamarae, Tamaree, Tamarin, Tamarla, Tamarria, Tamarrian, Tamarsha, Tamary, Tamarya, Tamaryah, Tamma, Tammara, Tamora, Tamoya, Tamura, Temara, Temarian, Thamara, Tomara, Tymara

Tamarah, Tamarra (Hebrew) forms of Tamara.
Tamarrah

Tamaria (Hebrew) a form of Tamara.
Tamari, Tamariah, Tamarie

Tamassa (Hebrew) a form of Thomasina.
Tamas, Tamasa, Tamasah, Tamasin, Tamasine, Thamasa

Tamaya (Quechua) in the center.

Tameisha (American) a form of Tamesha.

Tameka (Aramaic) twin.
Tameca, Tamecah, Tamecka, Tameckah, Tameeca, Tameecah, Tameeka, Tameekah, Tamekah, Tamiecka, Tamieka, Temeka, Tomeka, Trameika, Tymeka, Tymmeeka, Tymmeka

Tamekia (Aramaic) a form of Tameka.
Tamecia, Tomekia

Tamela (American) a form of Tamila.
Tamelia

Tamera (Hebrew) a form of Tamara.
Tamer, Tamerai, Tameran, Tameria, Tamerra, Tammera, Thamer, Timera

Tamesha (American) a combination of the prefix Ta + Mesha.
Tameesha, Tameshah, Tamnesha, Tamysha, Tamyshah, Temisha, Tomesha, Tomiese, Tomise, Tomisha, Tramesha, Tramisha, Tymesha

Tameshia (American) a form of Tamesha.
Tameeshia, Tameeshiah, Tameeshya, Tameshkia, Tameshya, Tamishia, Tamishiah, Tamyshia, Tamyshiah, Tamyshya, Tamyshyah

Tami, Tammi, Tammie (English) forms of Tammy.
Tamie

Tamia (Hebrew, English) a form of Tammy.
Tameia, Tamiah

Tamika (Japanese) a form of Tamiko.
Tameika, Tamica, Tamicah, Tamicka, Tamickah, Tamieka, Tamikah, Tamikia, Tamikka, Tammika, Tamyca, Tamycah, Tamycka, Tamyckah, Tamyka, Tamykah, Timika, Timikia, Tomika, Tomyka, Tymika, Tymmicka

Tamiko (Japanese) child of the people.
Tameeko, Tameko, Tamike, Tamiqua, Tamiyo, Tammiko, Tamyko

Tamila (American) a combination of the prefix Ta + Mila.
Tamala, Tamilah, Tamilla, Tamillah, Tamille, Tamillia, Tamilya, Tamyla, Tamylah, Tamylla, Tamyllah

Tamira (Hebrew) a form of Tamara.
Tamir, Tamirae, Tamirah, Tamiria, Tamirra

Tamisha (American) a form of Tamesha.
Tamishah

Tamiya (Hebrew, English) a form of Tammy.

Tammy GB (English) twin. (Hebrew) a familiar form of Tamara.
Tamee, Tamey, Tamijo, Tamilyn, Tamlyn, Tammee, Tammey, Tamy, Tamya

Tamra (Hebrew) a short form of Tamara.
Tammra, Tammrah, Tamrah

Tamrika (American) a combination of Tammy + Erika.
Tamricka, Tamrickah, Tamrikah, Tamriqua, Tamriquah, Tamrique, Tamryca, Tamrycah, Tamrycka, Tamryckah, Tamryka, Tamrykah, Tamryqua, Tamryquah, Tamryque

Tamsin (English) a short form of Thomasina.
Tamsen, Tamsina, Tamsinah, Tamsine, Tamsyn, Tamsyna, Tamsynah, Tamsyne, Tamzen, Tamzin, Tamzina, Tamzinah, Tamzine, Tamzyn, Tamzyna, Tamzynah, Tamzyne

Tamyra (Hebrew) a form of Tamara.
Tamyria, Tamyrra

Tana, Tanna (Slavic) short forms of Tanya.
Taina, Tanae, Tanaeah, Tanah, Tanalia, Tanara, Tanavia, Tanaz, Tannah

Tanaya (Russian, Slavic) a form of Tanya.

Tandra (English) a form of Tandy.
Tandrea, Tandria

Tandy (English) team.
Tanda, Tandalaya, Tandea, Tandee, Tandey, Tandi, Tandia, Tandiah, Tandie, Tandis, Tandya, Tandyah, Tandye

Tanea (Russian, Slavic) a form of Tanya.
Taneah, Taneé, Taneeia, Taneia

Tanechka, Tanichka (Russian) forms of Tania.

Taneesha (American) a form of Tanesha.
Taneeshah

Taneisha (American) a form of Tanesha.
Tahniesha

Tanesha (American) a combination of the prefix Ta + Nesha.
Taineshia, Tanasha, Tanashah, Tanashia, Tanaysia, Taneasha, Taneshea, Taneshia, Taneshya, Tanesia, Tanesian, Tanessa, Tanessia, Tannesha, Tanneshia, Tanniecia, Tanniesha, Tantashea

Taneya (Russian, Slavic) a form of Tanya.
Taneeya, Taneeyah

Tangela (American) a combination of the prefix Ta + Angela.
Tangel, Tangelah, Tangele, Tangell, Tangella, Tangellah, Tangelle, Tanjel, Tanjela, Tanjelah, Tanjele, Tanjell, Tanjella, Tanjelle

Tangi, Tangie (American) short forms of Tangia.
Tanji, Tanjie, Tanjy

Tangia (American) a form of Tangela.
Tangiah, Tangya, Tangyah

Tani **GB** (Japanese) valley. (Slavic) stand of glory. A familiar form of Tania.
Tahnee, Tahney, Tahni, Tahnie, Tahny, Tanee, Taney, Tanie, Tany

Tania (Russian, Slavic) fairy queen.
Tahnia, Tahniah, Taneea, Taniah, Tanija, Tannia, Tanniah, Tarnia

Taniel **GB** (American) a combination of Tania + Danielle.
Taniela, Tanielah, Taniele, Taniell, Taniella, Taniellah, Tanielle, Tanyel, Tanyela, Tanyelah, Tanyele, Tanyell, Tanyella, Tanyellah, Tanyelle

Taniesha (American) a form of Tanesha.

Tanika, Taniqua (American) forms of Tania.
Taneek, Tanikka, Tanikqua, Tanique, Tannica, Tannika, Tianeka, Tianika

Tanis **GB** (Slavic) a form of Tania, Tanya.
Tanas, Tanese, Taniese, Tanise, Tanisia, Tanisse, Tannese, Tanniece, Tanniese, Tannise, Tannisse, Tannus, Tannyce, Tannys, Tanys, Tiannis, Tonise, Tranice, Tranise, Tynice, Tyniece, Tyniese, Tynise

Tanisha (American) a combination of the prefix Ta + Nisha.
Tahniscia, Tahnisha, Tanasha, Tanashea, Tanicha, Tanish, Tanishah, Tanishia, Tanitia, Tannicia, Tannisha, Tanysha, Tanyshah

Tanissa (American) a combination of the prefix Tania + Nissa.
Tanesa, Tanisa, Tanisah, Tanissah, Tannesa, Tannisa, Tannisah, Tannissa, Tannissah, Tannysa, Tannysah, Tannyssa, Tannyssah, Tennessa, Tranissa

Tanita (American) a combination of the prefix Ta + Nita.
Taneeta, Taneetah, Taneta, Tanetta, Tanitah, Tanitra, Tanitta, Tanyta, Tanytah, Tanyte, Teneta, Tenetta, Tenita, Tenitta, Tyneta, Tynetta, Tynette, Tynita, Tynitra, Tynitta

Tanith (Phoenician) Mythology: Tanit is the goddess of love.
Tanitha, Tanithah, Tanithe, Tanyth, Tanytha, Tanythah, Tanythe

Taniya (Russian, Slavic) a form of Tania, Tanya.

Tanja (American) a short form of Tangela.
Tanjia

Tanner BG (English) leather worker, tanner.
Tannor

Tannis GB (Slavic) a form of Tania, Tanya.

Tansy (Greek) immortal. (Latin) tenacious, persistent.
Tancy, Tansea, Tansee, Tansey, Tanshay, Tansi, Tansia, Tansiah, Tansie, Tansya, Tansyah, Tansye, Tanzey

Tanya (Russian, Slavic) fairy queen. See also Tania.
Tahnya, Tahnyah, Taniya, Tanniya, Tannya, Tannyah, Tanoya, Tany, Tanyah, Tanyia, Taunya, Thanya

Tao (Chinese, Vietnamese) peach.

Tara (Aramaic) throw; carry. (Irish) rocky hill. (Arabic) a measurement.
Taraea, Taráh, Tarai, Taralee, Tarali, Tarasa, Tarasha, Taraya, Tarha, Tayra, Tehra

Tarah, Tarra, Tarrah (Irish) forms of Tara.

Taralyn (American) a form of Teralyn.

Taran BG (Persian) a short form of Taraneh. (Irish) a form of Tara.

Taraneh (Persian) melody.
Tarana, Taranah, Tarane

Tararia (Spanish) a form of Teresa.

Tarati (Maori) God's gift.
Taratea, Taratee, Taratey, Taratia, Taratiah, Taratie, Taraty, Taratya, Taratyah

Tarbula (Arabic) square, block.

Tarcisia (Greek) valiant.

Taree GB (Japanese) arching branch.
Tarea, Tarey, Tareya, Tari

Tareixa (Galician) wild animal.

Tari (Irish) a familiar form of Tara.
Taria, Tariah, Tarie, Tarila, Tarilyn, Tarita, Tary, Tarya, Tayah

Tarian (Welsh) coat of arms.

Tarika (Hindi) star.
Tarikah, Taryka, Tarykah

Tarin, Tarryn (Irish) forms of Tara.
Tareen, Tareena, Taren, Tarene, Tarina, Tarinah, Tarine, Taron, Tarren, Tarrena, Tarrin, Tarrina, Tarrinah, Tarrine, Tarron, Tarryna, Tarrynah, Tarryne, Taryna, Tarynah, Taryne, Tarynn, Tarynna, Tarynnah, Tarynne

Tarissa (American) a combination of Tara + Rissa.
Taris, Tarisa, Tarise, Tarisha

Tarne (Scandinavian) lake in the mountains. (Australian) salty water.
Tarnea, Tarnee, Tarney, Tarni, Tarnia, Tarnie, Tarny, Tarnya, Tarnyah

Tarsicia (Latin) she who was born in Tarso, the Turkish city where St. Paul was born.

Társila (Greek) valiant.

Tarsilia (Greek) basket weaver.

Taryn GB (Irish) a form of Tara.

Tasarla (Gypsy) dawn.
Tasarlea, Tasarleah, Tasarlee, Tasarleigh, Tasarley, Tasarli, Tasarlia, Tasarliah, Tasarlie, Tasarly, Tasarlya, Tasarlyah, Tasarlye

Taseem (Indian) salute of praise.

Tasha (Greek) born on Christmas day. (Russian) a short form of Natasha. See also Tashi, Tosha.
Tacha, Tachiana, Tahsha, Tasenka, Tashe, Tasheka, Taska, Taysha, Thasha, Tiaisha, Tysha

Tashana (American) a combination of the prefix Ta + Shana.
Tashan, Tashanah, Tashanda, Tashaney, Tashani, Tashania, Tashaniah, Tashanie, Tashanika, Tashanna, Tashany, Tashanya, Tashanyah, Tashina, Tishana, Tishani, Tishanna, Tishanne, Toshanna, Toshanti, Tyshana

Tashara (American) a combination of the prefix Ta + Shara.
Tashar, Tasharah, Tasharia, Tasharna, Tasharra, Tashera, Tasherey, Tasheri, Tasherra, Tashira, Tashirah

Tashauna (American) a form of Tashawna.
Tashaugna, Tashaugnah, Tashaunah, Tashauni, Tashaunia, Tashauniah, Tashaunie, Tashaunna, Tashaunya, Tashaunyah, Toshauna

Tashawna (American) a combination of the prefix Ta + Shawna.
Taseana, Taseanah, Taseania, Taseanya, Tashawanna, Tashawn, Tashawnah, Tashawnda, Tashawnia, Tashawniah, Tashawnna, Tashawnnia, Tashawnya, Tashawnyah, Tashonda, Tashondra, Tiashauna, Tishawn, Tishunda, Tishunta, Toshawna, Tyshauna, Tyshawna

Tashay (Greek, Russian) a form of Tasha.
Tashae

Tasheena (American) a combination of the prefix Ta + Sheena.
Tasheana, Tasheeana, Tasheeni, Tasheona, Tashina, Tisheena, Tosheena, Tysheana, Tysheena, Tyshyna

Tashelle (American) a combination of the prefix Ta + Shelley.
Tachell, Tashel, Tashela, Tashelah, Tashele, Tashelia, Tasheliah, Tashelie, Tashell, Tashella, Tashellah, Tashellea, Tashelleah, Tashellee, Tashelleigh, Tashelley, Tashelli, Tashellia, Tashelliah, Tashellie, Tashelly, Tashellya, Tashellyah, Techell, Techelle, Teshell, Teshelle, Tochell, Tochelle, Toshelle, Tychell, Tychelle, Tyshell, Tyshelle

Tashena (American) a form of Tasheena.
Tashenna, Tashennia

Tashi (Hausa) a bird in flight. (Slavic) a form of Tasha.
Tashe, Tashea, Tashee, Tashey, Tashie, Tashika, Tashima, Tashy

Tashia (Slavic, Hausa) a form of Tashi.
Tashiah, Tashiya, Tashya, Tashyah

Tashiana (American) a form of Tashana.
Tashianna

Tasia (Slavic) a familiar form of Tasha.
Tachia, Tasiah, Tasija, Tasiya, Tassia, Tassiah, Tassiana, Tasya, Tasyah

Tasmin (English) a short form of Thomasina.
Tasma, Tasmyn, Tasmyna, Tasmynah, Tasmyne, Tasmynn, Tasmynna, Tasmynnah, Tasmynne, Tazmin, Tazmina, Tazminah, Tazmine, Tazmyn, Tazmyna, Tazmynah, Tazmyne

Tassie (English) a familiar form of Tasmin.
Tasee, Tasey, Tasi, Tasie, Tassee, Tassey, Tassi, Tassy, Tazee, Tazey, Tazi, Tazie, Tazy, Tazzee, Tazzey, Tazzi, Tazzie, Tazzy

Tassos (Greek) a form of Theresa.
Tasos

Tata (Russian) a familiar form of Tatiana.
Tatah, Tatia, Tatiah, Tatya, Tatyah

Tate BG (English) a short form of Tatum. A form of Taite, Tata.

Tatiana (Slavic) fairy queen. See also Tania, Tanya, Tiana.
Taitiann, Taitianna, Tatania, Tataniah, Tatanya, Tatanyah, Tateana, Tateanna, Tateonna, Tateyana, Tati, Tatia, Tatianah, Tatiania, Tatianiah, Tatiayana, Tatie, Tatihana, Tationna, Tatiyona, Tatiyonna, Tiatiana

Tatianna (Slavic) a form of Tatiana.
Tatiann, Tatiannah

Tatiyana (Slavic) a form of Tatiana.
Tatiyanna

Tatjana (Slavic) a form of Tatiana.

Tatum GB (English) cheerful.
Taitam, Taitem, Taitim, Taitom, Taitum, Taitym, Tatam, Tatem, Tatim, Tatom, Tatumn, Taytam, Taytem, Taytim, Taytom, Taytum, Taytym

Tatyana, Tatyanna (Slavic) forms of Tatiana.
Tatyanah, Tatyani, Tatyannah, Tatyanne, Tatyona, Tatyonna

Taura (Latin) bull. Astrology: Taurus is a sign of the zodiac.
Taurae, Taurah, Tauria, Tauriah, Taurina, Taurya, Tauryah

Tauri (English) a form of Tory.
Taure, Taurie, Taury

Tavia (Latin) a short form of Octavia. See also Tawia.
Taiva, Tauvia, Tava, Tavah, Taviah, Tavita, Tavya, Tavyah

Tavie (Scottish) twin.
Tavee, Tavey, Tavi

Tawana, Tawanna (American) combinations of the prefix Ta + Wanda.
Taiwana, Taiwanna, Taquana, Taquanna, Tawan, Tawanda, Tawandah, Tawannah, Tawannda, Tawanndah, Tawanne, Tequana, Tequanna, Tequawna, Tewanna, Tewauna, Tiquana, Tiwanna, Tiwena, Towanda, Towanna, Tywania, Tywanna

Tawia (African) born after twins. (Polish) a form of Tavia.
Tawiah, Tawya, Tawyah

Tawnee, Tawney, Tawni, Tawnie (English) forms of Tawny.
Tawnnie

Tawny (Gypsy) little one. (English) brownish yellow, tan.
Tahnee, Tany, Tauna, Tauné, Tauni, Taunisha, Tawnesha, Tawnye, Tawnyell, Tiawna, Tiawni

Tawnya (American) a combination of Tawny + Tonya.
Taunia, Tawna, Tawnea, Tawnia, Tawniah, Tawnyah

Taya (English) a short form of Taylor.
Taia, Taiah, Tayah, Tayiah, Tayna, Tayra, Taysha, Taysia, Tayva, Tayvonne, Tiaya, Tiya, Tiyah, Tye

Tayana (English) a form of Taya.

Tayanita (Cherokee) beaver.
Taianita, Taianitah, Tayanitah, Tayanyta, Tayanytah

Taye (English) a short form of Taylor.
Tay

Tayla (English) a short form of Taylor.
Taila, Tailah, Tailea, Taileah, Tailee, Tailei, Taileigh, Tailey, Taili, Tailia, Tailiah, Tailie, Taylah, Taylea, Tayleah, Taylee, Taylei, Tayleigh, Tayley, Tayli, Taylia, Tayliah, Taylie, Tayly

Taylar, Taylore, Taylour, Taylre (English) forms of Taylor.
Taylara, Taylare, Tayllar, Tayller, Tayllore

Tayler GB (English) a form of Taylor.

Taylor ☀ GB (English) tailor.
Taiylor, Talar, Tayllor, Tayloir, Taylora, Taylorann, Taylorr, Taylur

Tazu (Japanese) stork; longevity.
Taz, Tazi, Tazoo

Tea (Spanish) a short form of Dorothy.

Teagan GB (Welsh) beautiful, attractive.
Taegan, Taegen, Taegin, Taegon, Taegun, Taegyn, Teage, Teagen, Teaghan, Teaghanne, Teaghen, Teaghin, Teaghon, Teaghun, Teaghyn, Teagin, Teagon, Teague, Teagun, Teagyn, Teegan, Teegen, Teeghan, Teegin, Teegon, Teegun, Teegyn, Teigan, Teigen, Teigin, Teigon, Teigun, Teigyn, Tejan, Teygan, Teygen, Teygin, Teygon, Teygun, Teygyn, Tiegan, Tigan, Tigen, Tigin, Tigon, Tigun, Tigyn, Tijan, Tijana, Tygan, Tygen, Tygin, Tygon, Tygun, Tygyn

Teah (Greek, Spanish) a form of Tia.
Téa

Teaira, Teairra (Latin) forms of Tiara.
Teair, Teairre, Teairria

Teal (English) river duck; blue green.
Teale, Teel, Teele, Teil

Teala (English) a form of Teal.
Tealah, Tealia, Tealisha, Teyla, Teylah

Teana, Teanna (American) combinations of the prefix Te + Anna. Forms of Tiana.
Tean, Teanah, Teane, Teann, Teannah, Teanne, Teaunna, Teiana, Teianah, Teiane, Teiann, Teianna, Teiannah, Teianne, Teuana

Teara, Tearra (Latin) forms of Tiara.
Tearah, Téare, Teareya, Teari, Tearia, Teariea, Tearria

Teasha (Latin, American) a form of Taesha.
Teashia, Teashiah, Teashya, Teashyah

Teca (Hungarian) a form of Theresa.
Tecah, Techa, Tecka, Teckah, Teka, Tekah, Tica, Ticah, Tika, Tikah, Tyca, Tycah, Tyka, Tykah

Tecla (Greek) God's fame.
Tekla, Theckla

Tecusa (Latin) covered, hidden.

Teda (Greek) a form of Teodora.

Teddi, Tedi (Greek) familiar forms of Theodora.
Tedde, Teddea, Teddee, Teddey, Teddia, Teddiah, Teddie, Teddy, Tediah, Tedie, Tedy

Tedra (Greek) a short form of Theodora.
Teddra, Teddrah, Teddreya, Tedera, Tedrah, Teedra, Teidra

Tedya (Russian) a form of Teodora.

Teela (English) a form of Teala.

Teena (Spanish, American) a form of Tina.
Teenah, Teenia, Teeniah, Teenya, Teenyah

Teesha (Latin) a form of Tisha.
Teeshia, Teeshiah

Tegan GB (Welsh) a form of Teagan.
Tega, Tegana, Tegane, Tegen, Teggan, Teghan, Tegin, Tegyn

Tehya (Hindi) a form of Taja.

Teia (Greek, Spanish) a form of Tia.
Teiah

Teicuih (Nahuatl) younger sister.

Teila (English) a form of Teala.

Teira, Teirra (Latin) forms of Tiara.

Teisha (Latin, American) a form of Taesha.

Tejana (Spanish) Texan.

Tekia (Arabic) a form of Takia.
Tekeiya, Tekeiyah, Tekeyia, Tekiah, Tekiya, Tekiyah

Teleri (Welsh) child of Paul.

Telisha (American) a form of Taleisha.
Teleesha, Teleisia, Telesa, Telesha, Teleshia, Telesia, Telicia, Telisa, Telishia, Telisia, Telissa, Telisse, Tellisa, Tellisha, Telsa, Telysa

Telmao (Greek) loving with her fellow people.

Temira (Hebrew) tall.
Temora, Timora

Temis (Greek) she who establishes order and justice.

Tempany (Australian) a form of Tempest.
Tempanee, Tempaney, Tempani, Tempania, Tempaniah, Tempanie, Tempanya, Tempanyah

Tempest GB (French) stormy.
Tempesta, Tempestah, Tempeste, Tempist, Tempistt, Tempress, Tempteste

Tempestt (French) a form of Tempest.
Tempestta, Tempestte

Tenesha (American) a form of Tenisha.
Tenecia, Teneesha, Teneisha, Teneshia, Tenesia, Tenessa, Teneusa

Tenestina (Greek) bandage.

Tenille, Tennille (American) combinations of the prefix Te + Nellie.
Teneal, Teneall, Tenealla, Tenealle, Teneil, Teneille, Teniel, Teniele, Tenielle, Tenil, Tenila, Tenilah, Tenile, Tenill, Tenilla, Tenillah, Tenneal, Tenneill, Tenneille, Tennia, Tennie, Tennielle, Tennil, Tennila, Tennilah, Tennile, Tennill, Tennilla, Tennillah, Tennyl, Tennyla, Tennylah, Tennyle, Tennyll, Tennylla, Tennyllah, Tennylle, Tenyl, Tenyla, Tenylah, Tenyle, Tenyll, Tenylla, Tenyllah, Tenylle, Tineal, Tiniel, Tonielle, Tonille

Tenise (Slavic) a form of Tanis.
Tenice, Tenyse

Tenisha (American) a combination of the prefix Te + Nisha.
Teniesha, Tenishia, Tenishka

Teo (Greek) a short form of Teodora.

Teoctistes (Greek) created by God.

Teodelina, Teodolinda (German) she who loves her village.

Teodequilda (German) warrior of her village.

Teodomira (Spanish) important woman in the village.

Teodora (Czech) a form of Theodora.
Teadora, Teodory

Teodota (Greek) a form of Teodora.

Teofania, Teofanía (Greek) forms of Theophania.

Teófila (Greek) a form of Theophilia.

Teolinda (German) a short form of Teodelinda.

Teona, Teonna (Greek) forms of Tiana.
Teon, Teoni, Teonia, Teonie, Teonney, Teonnia, Teonnie

Teopista, Teopistes (Greek) dignity of God.

Teorítgida (Greek) converted to God.

Teotista (Greek) drunk with the love of God.

Teoxihuitl (Nahuatl) turquoise; precious and divine.

Tepin (Nahuatl) little one.

Tequila (Spanish) a kind of liquor. See also Takila.
Taquela, Taquella, Taquila, Taquilla, Tequilia, Tiquila, Tiquilia

Tequilla (Spanish) a form of Tequila.

Tera, Terah, Terra, Terrah (Latin) earth. (Japanese) swift arrow. (American) forms of Tara.
Terai, Terrae

Teralyn (American) a combination of Teri + Lynn.
Teralin, Teralina, Teralinah, Teraline, Teralyna, Teralynah, Teralyne, Teralynn, Terralin, Terralina, Terralinah, Terraline, Terralyn, Terralyna, Terralynah, Terralyne

Terceira, Tercera, Terciera (Spanish) born third.

Teresa (Greek) a form of Theresa. See also Tressa.
Taresa, Taressa, Tarissa, Terasa, Tercza, Tereasa, Tereasah, Tereatha, Tereesa, Tereesah, Teresah, Teresea, Teresha, Teresia, Teresina, Tereson, Teretha, Tereza, Terezia, Terezie, Terezijya, Terezon, Terezsa, Terisa, Terisah, Terisha, Teriza, Terrasa, Terreasa, Terreasah, Terresa, Terresha, Terresia, Terrisa, Terrisah, Terrysa, Terrysah, Teruska, Teté, Tyresa, Tyresia

Terese (Greek) a form of Teresa.
Tarese, Taress, Taris, Tarise, Terease, Tereece, Terees, Tereese, Teress, Terez, Teris, Terise, Terreas, Terrease, Terrise, Terrys, Terryse

Teresina (Italian) a form of Teresa.
Terezinha, Terrosina, Theresina

Teresinha (Portuguese) a form of Teresa.

Teresita (Spanish) a form of Teresa.

Teressa (Greek) a form of Teresa.
Terressa

Teri, Terri, Terrie (Greek) familiar forms of Theresa.
Tere, Teree, Tereey, Terie, Terree, Terrey, Terrye, Tery

Teria, Terria (Irish) forms of Tera. (Greek) forms of Teri.
Teriah, Terriah, Terrya, Terryah

Terica, Terrica, Terricka (American) combinations of Teri + Erica. See also Rica.
Tericka, Tyrica, Tyricka, Tyronica

Terika, Terrika (American) forms of Terica.
Tereka, Terreka, Tyrika, Tyrikka

Terpsícore (Greek) she who enjoys dancing.

Terrelle BG (German) thunder ruler.
Tarrell, Teral, Terall, Terel, Terela, Terele, Terell, Terella, Teriel, Terral, Terrall, Terrel, Terrell, Terrella, Terriel, Terriell, Terrielle, Terrill, Terryelle, Terryl, Terryll, Terrylle, Teryl, Tyrell, Tyrelle

Terrene (Latin) smooth.
Tareena, Tarena, Teran, Teranee, Terean, Tereana, Tereane, Tereen, Tereena, Tereene, Terena, Terencia, Terene, Terenia, Terentia, Terentya, Terentyah, Terran, Terrean, Terreana, Terreane, Terreen, Terreena, Terreene, Terren, Terrena, Terron, Terrosina, Terun, Tyreen, Tyrene

Terriana, Terrianna (American) combinations of Teri + Anna.
Teriana, Terianna, Terriauna, Terrina, Terriyana, Terriyanna, Terryana, Terryauna, Tyrina

Terriann (American) a combination of Teri + Ann.
Terian, Teriann, Terianne, Teriyan, Terrian, Terrianne, Terryann

Terrin BG (Latin) a form of Terrene.
Terin, Terina, Terine, Terrina, Terrine, Terryna, Terryne, Teryna, Terynn

Terriona (American) a form of Terriana.
Terrionna

Terrwyn (Welsh) valiant.

Terry BG (Greek) a familiar form of Theresa.

Terry-Lynn (American) a combination of Teri + Lynn.
Terelyn, Terelynn, Terri-Lynn, Terrilynn, Terrylynn

Terryn, Teryn (Latin) forms of Terrene.

Tersea (Greek) a form of Teresa.
Tersa, Terza

Tertia (Latin) third.
Tercia, Tercina, Tercine, Terecena, Tersia, Tertiah, Tertya, Tertyah, Terza

Tesa (Greek) a form of Tessa.
Tesah

Tesha (Latin, American) a form of Taesha, Tisha.

Tesia, Tessia (Greek) forms of Tessa.

Tesira (Greek) founder.

Tesla (American) a unit of magnetic flux density, named after its creator, Nikola Tesla, a Croatian-born physicist.

Tess (Greek) a short form of Quintessa, Theresa.
Tes, Tese

Tessa (Greek) reaper.
Tessah, Tezia

Tessie (Greek) a familiar form of Theresa.
Tesi, Tessey, Tessi, Tessy, Tezi

Tessla (American) a form of Tesla.

Tetis (Greek) nurse for the new mother.

Tetsu (Japanese) strong as iron.
Tetsoo

Tetty (English) a familiar form of Elizabeth.

Teuicui (Nahuatl) younger sister.

Tevy (Cambodian) angel.
Teva, Tevee, Tevey, Tevi, Tevie

Teya (English) a form of Taya. (Greek, Spanish) a form of Tia.

Teyacapan (Nahuatl) first born.

Teyana, Teyanna (American) forms of Teana.
Teyan, Teyanah, Teyane, Teyann, Teyannah, Teyanne, Teyuna

Teylor (English) a form of Taylor.
Teighlor, Teylar

Teyona (American) a form of Teana.

Thaddea (Greek) courageous. (Latin) praiser.
Taddea, Thada, Thadda, Thadia, Thadiah, Thadie, Thadina, Thadya, Thadyah, Thadyna, Thadyne

Thais (Greek) a form of Tais.
Thays

Thaís (Greek) bond.

Thalassa (Greek) sea, ocean.
Thalassah

Thalia (Greek) a form of Talia. Mythology: the Muse of comedy.
Thaleia, Thaliah, Thalie, Thalya, Thalyah

Thamara (Hebrew) a form of Tamara.
Thama, Thamar, Thamarah, Thamare, Thamaria, Thamariah, Thamarra, Thamarya, Thamaryah

Thana (Arabic) happy occasion.
Thaina, Thainah, Thayna, Thaynah

Thandie BG (Zulu) beloved.
Thandee, Thandey, Thandi, Thandy

Thanh BG (Vietnamese) bright blue. (Punjabi) good place.

Thania (Arabic) a form of Thana.
Thanie

Thao (Vietnamese) respectful of parents.

Thea (Greek) goddess. A short form of Althea.
Theah, Theia, Theiah, Theo, Theya, Theyah

Theadora (Greek) a form of Theodora.

Thelma (Greek) willful.
Telma, Telmah, Thelmai, Thelmalina

Thema (African) queen.
Themah

Theodora (Greek) gift of God. See also Dora, Dorothy, Feodora.
Taedra, Tedra, Teodora, Theda, Thedorsha, Thedrica, Theo, Theodore, Theodoria, Theodorian, Theodosia, Theodra

Theodosia (Greek) a form of Theodora.
Teodosia, Teodosiah, Teodosya, Teodosyah, Thedosia, Thedosiah, Thedosya, Thedosyah, Theodosiah, Theodosya, Theodosyah

Theone (Greek) gift of God.
Theona, Theonah, Theondra, Theonee, Theoni, Theonie

Theophania (Greek) God's appearance. See also Epiphany, Tiffany.
Theophaniah, Theophanie, Theophano, Theophanya, Theophanyah

Theophila (Greek) loved by God.
Teofila, Theofilia, Theofilie, Theophyla, Theophylah, Theophylla, Theophyllah

Theresa (Greek) reaper. See also Resi, Reza, Riza, Tassos, Teca, Tracey, Zilya.
Thereasa, Theresah, Theresia, Theresie, Theresita, Theressa, Thereza, Therisa, Therisah, Therissie, Therrisa, Therrisah, Therrysa, Therrysah, Thersea, Therysa, Therysah

Therese (Greek) a form of Theresa.
Thérése, Theresse, Therise, Therra, Therressa, Therris, Therrise, Therrys, Therryse, Theryse

Thérèse (French) a form of Teresa.

Theta (Greek) Linguistics: a letter in the Greek alphabet.

Thetis (Greek) disposed. Mythology: the mother of Achilles.
Thetisa, Thetisah, Thetise, Thetiss, Thetissa, Thetisse, Thetys, Thetysa, Thetyse, Thetyss, Thetyssa, Thetysse

Thi (Vietnamese) poem.
Thia, Thy, Thya

Thirza (Hebrew) pleasant. See also Tirza.
Thersa, Therza, Thirsa, Thirzah, Thursa, Thurza, Thyrza, Thyrzah, Tirshka

Thomasina (Hebrew) twin. See also Tamassa, Tasmin.
Thamasin, Thamasina, Thamasine, Thomasa, Thomasah, Thomasia, Thomasin, Thomasinah, Thomasine, Thomason, Thomassine, Thomassyn, Thomassyna, Thomassynah, Thomassyne, Thomasyn, Thomasyna, Thomasynah, Thomasyne, Thomazine, Thomencia, Thomethia, Thomisha, Thomsina, Toma, Tomasa, Tomasin, Tomasina, Tomasinah, Tomasine, Tomasyn, Tomasyna, Tomasynah, Tomasyne, Tomina, Tommina

Thora (Scandinavian) thunder.
Thorah, Thorri

Thordis (Scandinavian) Thor's spirit.
Thordia, Thordisa, Thordisah, Thordise, Thordiss, Thordissa, Thordissah, Thordisse, Thordys, Thordysa, Thordysah, Thordyse, Thordyss, Thordyssa, Thordyssah, Thordysse

Thrina (Greek) a form of Trina.
Thrinah, Thrine, Thryn, Thryna, Thrynah, Thryne

Thu (Vietnamese) autumn; poem.

Thuy (Vietnamese) gentle.

Tia (Greek) princess. (Spanish) aunt.
Teea, Teeah, Teeya, Ti, Tiah, Tialeigh, Tiamarie, Tianda, Tiandria, Tiante, Tiia, Tiye, Tya, Tyah, Tyja

Tía (Spanish, Greek) a form of Tia.

Tiaira (Latin) a form of Tiara.

Tiana, Tianna (Greek) princess. (Latin) short forms of Tatiana. See also Tyana.
Tiahna, Tian, Tianah, Tiane, Tiann, Tiannah, Tianne, Tiannee, Tianni, Tiaon, Tiena

Tiani (Greek, Latin) a form of Tiana.
Tianea, Tianee

Tiara (Latin) crowned.
Teearia, Tiarah, Tiarea, Tiareah, Tiari, Tiaria, Tyara, Tyarah

Tiare (Latin) a form of Tiara.

Tiarra (Latin) a form of Tiara.
Tiairra, Tiarrah, Tyarra

Tiauna (Greek) a form of Tiana.
Tiaunah, Tiaunia, Tiaunna

Tiberia (Latin) Geography: the Tiber River in Italy.
Tib, Tibbie, Tibby, Tiberiah, Tyberia, Tyberiah, Tyberya, Tyberyah

Tiburcia (Spanish) born in the place of pleasures.

Tichina (American) a combination of the prefix Ti + China.
Tichian, Tichin, Tichinia

Ticiana (Latin) valiant defender.

Tida (Tai) daughter.
Tidah, Tyda, Tydah

Tieara (Latin) a form of Tiara.

Tiera, Tierra (Latin) forms of Tiara.
Tiéra, Tierah, Tierre, Tierrea, Tierria

Tierney GB (Irish) noble.
Tieranae, Tierani, Tieranie, Tieranni, Tierany, Tiernan, Tiernee, Tierni, Tiernie, Tierny, Tyernee, Tyerney, Tyerni, Tyernie, Tyerny

Tiesha (Latin) a form of Tisha.
Tieshia, Tieshiah

Tifani, Tiffaney, Tiffani, Tiffanie (Latin)
forms of Tiffany.

Tifara (Hebrew) happy.
*Tifarah, Tifarra, Tifarrah, Tyfara, Tyfarah,
Tyfarra, Tyfarrah*

Tiff (Latin) a short form of Tiffany.

Tiffany (Latin) trinity. (Greek) a short form
of Theophania. See also Tyfany.
*Taffanay, Taffany, Teffani, Tephanie, Tifanee,
Tifaney, Tifanie, Tifany, Tiffanee, Tiffanny,
Tiffayne, Tiffeney, Tiffeni, Tiffenie, Tiffennie,
Tiffiani, Tiffianie, Tiffiany, Tiffynie, Triffany*

Tiffini (Latin) a form of Tiffany.
Tiffine, Tiffiney, Tiffinie, Tiffiny

Tiffney (Latin) a form of Tiffany.
Tiffnay, Tiffni, Tiffny, Tifni

Tiffy (Latin) a familiar form of Tiffany.
Tiffey, Tiffi, Tiffie

Tigris (Irish) tiger. Geography: a river in
southwest Asia that flows from Turkey,
through Iraq, to the Euphrates River.
Tiger, Tigress, Tyger, Tygris, Tygriss, Tygrys, Tygryss

Tijuana (Spanish) Geography: a border town
in Mexico.
*Tajuana, Tajuanah, Tajuanna, Thejuana,
Thejuanah, Tiajuana, Tiajuanah, Tiajuanna,
Tiawanna, Tyawanna*

Tikvah (Hebrew) hope.
Tikva

Tilda (German) a short form of Matilda.
*Tildah, Tilde, Tildea, Tildeah, Tildee, Tildey,
Tildi, Tildie, Tildy, Tylda, Tyldah, Tyldee,
Tyldey, Tyldi, Tyldie, Tyldy*

Tillie (German) a familiar form of Matilda.
*Tilia, Tillea, Tilleah, Tillee, Tillei, Tilleigh,
Tilley, Tilli, Tillia, Tilly, Tillye, Tily, Tylee,
Tylei, Tyleigh, Tyley, Tyli, Tylie, Tyllea, Tyllee,
Tyllei, Tylleigh, Tylley, Tylli, Tyllie, Tylly, Tyly*

Timara (Hebrew) a form of Tamara.

Timber (English) wood.

Timeka (Aramaic) a form of Tameka.
Timeeka

Timesha (American) a form of Tamesha.
Timisha

Timi (English) a familiar form of Timothea.
*Timee, Timey, Timie, Timmee, Timmey, Timmi,
Timmie, Timmy, Timy, Tymee, Tymey, Tymi,
Tymie, Tymmee, Tymmey, Tymmi, Tymmie,
Tymmy, Tymy*

Timia (English) a form of Timi.
Timea, Timmea, Tymea, Tymmea

Timotea (Greek) a form of Timothea.

Timothea (English) honoring God.
*Timathea, Timithea, Timythea, Tymathea,
Tymithea, Tymythea*

Tina (Spanish, American) a short form of
Augustine, Martina, Christina, Valentina.
*Teina, Tena, Tenae, Tenah, Tiena, Tienah,
Tienna, Tiennah, Tinah, Tinai, Tine, Tinea,
Tinia, Tiniah, Tinna, Tinnia*

Tinble (English) sound bells make.
Tynbal, Tynble

Tíndara (Greek) she who is willing to love.

Tinesha (American) a combination of the
prefix Ti + Niesha.
*Timnesha, Tinecia, Tineisha, Tinesa, Tineshia,
Tinessa, Tiniesha, Tinieshia, Tinsia*

Tinisha (American) a form of Tenisha.
Tinishia, Tinishya

Tiona, Tionna (American) forms of Tiana.
*Tionda, Tiondra, Tiondre, Tioné, Tionette,
Tioni, Tionia, Tionie, Tionja, Tionnah, Tionne,
Tionya*

Tiphanie (Latin) a form of Tiffany.
*Tiphane, Tiphanee, Tiphaney, Tiphani,
Tiphania, Tiphany*

Tiponya (Native American) great horned
owl.
*Tiponia, Tiponiah, Tiponyah, Typonia,
Typoniah, Typonya, Typonyah*

Tipper (Irish) water pourer. (Native
American) a short form of Tiponya.

Tippi (Greek) a familiar form of Xanthippe.

Tira (Hindi) arrow.
Tirah, Tirea, Tirena

Tirranna (Australian) stream of water.
Tirran, Tirrann, Tirrannah, Tirranne, Tyran, Tyrana, Tyranah, Tyrane, Tyrann, Tyranna, Tyrannah, Tyranne, Tyrran, Tyrrana, Tyrranah, Tyrrane, Tyrrann, Tyrranna, Tyrrannah, Tyrranne

Tirtha (Hindi) ford.

Tirza (Hebrew) pleasant. See also Thirza.
Tierza, Tirsa, Tirzha, Tyrza, Tyrzah

Tirzah (Hebrew) a form of Tirza.

Tisa (Swahili) ninth-born.
Tisah, Tysa, Tyssa

Tish (Latin) a short form of Tisha.

Tisha ⚏ (Latin) joy. A short form of Leticia.
Teisha, Tish, Tishah, Tishal, Tishia, Tishiah, Tysha, Tyshah, Tyshia, Tyshiah

Tita (Greek) giant. (Spanish) a short form of names ending in "tita." A form of Titus (see Boys' Names).

Titania (Greek) giant. Mythology: the Titans were a race of giants.
Teata, Titaniah, Titanna, Titanya, Titanyah, Tiziana, Tytan, Tytania, Tytaniah, Tytanya, Tytanyah

Titiana (Greek) a form of Titania.
Titianay, Titiania, Titianna, Titiayana, Titionia, Titiyana, Titiyanna, Tityana

Tivona (Hebrew) nature lover.
Tibona, Tivonah, Tivone, Tivoni, Tivonie, Tivony, Tyvona, Tyvonah, Tyvone

Tiwa (Zuni) onion.
Tiwah, Tywa, Tywah

Tiyana, Tiyanna (English) forms of Tayana. (Greek) forms of Tiana.
Tiyan, Tiyani, Tiyania, Tiyonna

Tj ⚏ (American) a form of TJ.

TJ ⚏ (American) a combination of the initials T. + J.

Tkeyah (American) a form of Takia.

Tlachinolli (Nahuatl) fire.

Tlaco (Nahuatl) a short form of Tlacoehua.

Tlacoehua (Nahuatl) middle one.

Tlacotl (Nahuatl) osier twig.

Tlahutli (Nahuatl) sir.

Tlalli (Nahuatl) earth.

Tlanextli (Nahuatl) radiance; majesty.

Tlazohtzin (Nahuatl) one who is loved.

Tlexictli (Nahuatl) fire navel.

Tobi ⚏ (Hebrew) God is good.
Toba, Tobe, Tobea, Tobee, Tobey, Tobia, Tobiah, Tobie, Tobit, Toby, Tobya, Tobyah, Tobyas, Tobye, Tove, Tovi, Tybi, Tybie, Tyby

Tocarra (American) a combination of the prefix To + Cara.
Tocara, Tocarah, Tocarrah, Toccara

Toinette (French) a short form of Antoinette.
Toinet, Toineta, Toinete, Toinett, Toinetta, Tonetta, Tonette, Toniette, Toynet, Toyneta, Toynete, Toynett, Toynetta, Toynette, Tuanetta, Tuanette, Twanette

Toki (Japanese) hopeful.
Tokee, Tokey, Toko, Tokoya, Tokyo

Tokoni ⚏ (Tongan) helpful.
Tokonee, Tokoney, Tokonia, Tokoniah, Tokony, Tokonya, Tokonyah

Tola (Polish) a form of Toinette.
Tolah, Tolla, Tollah, Tolsia

Toltecatl, Toltecatli (Nahuatl) artist.

Tomi ⚏ (Japanese) rich.
Tomea, Tomee, Tomey, Tomie, Tomiju, Tomy

Tomiko (Japanese) wealthy.

Tommi (Hebrew) a short form of Thomasina.
Tomme, Tommea, Tommee, Tommey, Tommia, Tommy

Tommie ⚏ (Hebrew) a short form of Thomasina.

Tomo (Japanese) intelligent.
Tomoko

Tonalnan (Nahuatl) mother of light.

Tonatzin (Nahuatl) goddess of the earth.

Toneisha (American) a combination of the prefix To + Niesha.
Toneisheia, Tonesia, Toniece, Toniesha, Tonneshia

Tonesha (American) a form of Toneisha.

Toni GB (Greek) flourishing. (Latin) praise-worthy.
Tonee, Toney, Tonneli, Tonni, Tony, Tonye

Tonia (Latin, Slavic) a form of Toni, Tonya.
Tonea, Toneea, Toniah, Toniea, Tonja, Tonje, Tonna, Tonnia, Tonniah, Tonnja

Tonie (Greek, Latin) a form of Toni.
Toniee, Tonnie

Tonisha (American) a form of Toneisha.
Tonisa, Tonise, Tonisia, Tonnisha

Tonneli (Swiss) a form of Toni.
Tonelea, Toneleah, Tonelee, Tonelei, Toneleigh, Toneley, Toneli, Tonelia, Toneliah, Tonelie, Tonely, Tonnelea, Tonneleah, Tonnelee, Tonnelei, Tonneleigh, Tonneley, Tonnelie, Tonnely

Tonya (Slavic) fairy queen.
Tonnya, Tonnyah, Tonyah, Tonyea, Tonyetta, Tonyia

Topaz (Latin) golden yellow gem.
Topaza, Topazah, Topazia, Topaziah, Topazz, Topazza, Topazzah, Topazzia, Topazziah

Topsy (English) on top. Literature: a slave in Harriet Beecher Stowe's novel *Uncle Tom's Cabin.*
Toppsy, Topsea, Topsee, Topsey, Topsi, Topsia, Topsie

Tora (Japanese) tiger.
Torah, Torra, Torrah

Torcuata (Latin) adorned.

Toree, Torie, Torri (English) forms of Tori, Tory.
Tore, Torre, Torree

Toreth (Welsh) abundant.

Torey BG (English) a form of Tori, Tory.

Tori GB (Japanese) bird. (English) a form of Tory.
Torei, Torrita

Toria (English) a form of Tori, Tory.
Torea, Toriah, Torreya, Torria, Torya, Toryah

Toriana (English) a form of Tori.
Torian, Torianah, Toriane, Toriann, Torianna, Toriannah, Torianne, Toriauna, Torin, Torina, Torine, Torinne, Torion, Torionna, Torionne,

Toriyanna, Torrina, Toryan, Toryana, Toryanah, Toryane, Toryann, Toryanna, Toryannah, Toryanne

Toribia (Latin) a form of Tránsito.

Torilyn (English) a combination of Tori + Lynn.
Torilynn, Torrilyn, Torrilynn

Torlan (Welsh) comes from the river.

Torrey BG (English) a form of Tori, Tory.

Torrie GB (English) a form of Tori, Tory.

Tory BG (English) victorious. (Latin) a short form of Victoria.
Tauri, Torry, Torrye, Torye

Tosca, Toscana (Latin) native of Tuscany, a region in Italy.

Tosha (Punjabi) armaments. (Polish) a familiar form of Antonia. (Russian) a form of Tasha.
Toshea, Toshia, Toshiea, Toshke, Tosia, Toska

Toshi (Japanese) mirror image.
Toshee, Toshey, Toshie, Toshiko, Toshikyo, Toshy

Toski (Hopi) squashed bug.
Toskee, Toskey, Toskie, Tosky

Totsi (Hopi) moccasins.
Totsee, Totsey, Totsia, Totsie, Totsy, Totsya

Tottie (English) a familiar form of Charlotte.
Tota, Totee, Totey, Toti, Totie, Tottee, Tottey, Totti, Totty, Toty

Tova (Hebrew) a form of Tovah.

Tovah (Hebrew) good.
Tovia

Toya (Spanish) a form of Tory.
Toia, Toiah, Toyah, Toyanika, Toyanna, Toyea, Toylea, Toyleah, Toylenn, Toylin, Toylyn

Tracey GB (Latin) warrior. (Greek) a familiar form of Theresa.
Trace, Tracea, Tracee, Tracell, Traice, Traicee, Traicey, Traicy, Traisea, Traisee, Traisey, Traisy, Trasea, Trasee, Trasey, Trasy, Traycea, Traycee, Traycy, Traycya, Traysea, Traysee, Traysey, Traysy, Treacy, Treesy

Traci, Tracie (Latin) forms of Tracey.
Tracia, Traciah, Tracilee, Tracilyn, Tracilynn,
Tracina, Traeci, Traici, Traicie, Traisi, Traisie,
Trasi, Trasia, Trasie, Trayci, Traycia, Traycie,
Traysi, Traysie

Tracy GB (Latin) warrior. (Greek) a familiar
form of Theresa.

Tralena (Latin) a combination of Tracey +
Lena.
Traleen, Tralene, Tralin, Tralinda, Tralyn,
Tralynn, Tralynne

Tranesha (American) a combination of the
prefix Tra + Niesha.
Traneice, Traneis, Traneise, Traneisha, Tranese,
Traneshia, Tranice, Traniece, Traniesha, Tranisha,
Tranishia

Trang (Vietnamese) intelligent, knowledgeable; beautiful.

Tranquila, Tranquilla (Spanish) forms of
Tranquilina.

Tranquilina (Latin) tranquil.

Tránsito (Latin) she who moves on to
another life.

Trashawn BG (American) a combination of
the prefix Tra + Shawn.
Trashan, Trashana, Trashauna, Trashon,
Trayshauna

Trava (Czech) spring grasses.
Travah

Traviata (Italian) straying.
Traviatah, Travyata, Travyatah

Treasure (Latin) treasure, wealth; valuable.
Treasa, Treasur, Treasura, Treasurah, Treasuré,
Treasury

Trella (Spanish) a familiar form of Estelle.

Tresha (Greek) a form of Theresa.
Trescha, Trescia, Treshana, Treshia

Tressa (Greek) a short form of Theresa. See
also Teresa.
Treaser, Tresa, Tresca, Trese, Treska, Tressia,
Tressie, Trez, Treza, Trisa

Treva (Irish, Welsh) a short form of Trevina.

Trevina (Irish) prudent. (Welsh) homestead.
Trevanna, Treveana, Treveanah, Treveane,

Treveena, Treveenah, Treveene, Trevena,
Trevenia, Treveon, Trevia, Treviana, Trevien,
Trevin, Trevinah, Trevine, Trevyn, Trevyna,
Trevynah, Trevyne

Trevona (Irish) a form of Trevina.
Trevion, Trevon, Trevonah, Trevone, Trevonia,
Trevonna, Trevonne, Trevonye

Triana (Latin) third. (Greek) a form of Trina.
Tria, Trianah, Triane, Triann, Trianna,
Triannah, Trianne, Tryan, Tryana, Tryanah,
Tryane, Tryann, Tryanna, Tryannah, Tryanne

Trice (Greek) a short form of Theresa.
Treece

Tricia (Latin) a form of Trisha.
Trica, Tricha, Trichelle, Tricina, Trickia

Trifena (Greek) delicate.
Trifenah, Trifene, Trifenna, Trifennah, Tryfena,
Tryfenah, Tryfenna, Tryfennah, Tryphena,
Tryphenah

Trifina, Trifonia (Greek) fun.

Trifosa (Greek) she who delights in God.

Trilby (English) soft hat.
Tribi, Trilbea, Trilbee, Trilbey, Trilbi, Trilbie,
Trillby, Trylbea, Trylbee, Trylbeey, Trylbi, Trylbie,
Trylby

Trina (Greek) pure.
Thrina, Treana, Treanah, Treena, Treenah,
Treina, Trenna, Trinah, Trind, Trinda, Trine,
Trinette, Trinia, Triniah, Trinica, Trinice,
Triniece, Trinika, Trinique, Trinisa, Tryna,
Trynah, Trynya, Trynyah

Trindade, Trinidad (Latin) forms of Trinity.

Trini GB (Greek) a form of Trina.
Treanee, Treaney, Treani, Treanie, Treany,
Treenee, Treeney, Treeni, Treenie, Trinia, Trinie,
Triny

Trinity ⭐ GB (Latin) triad. Religion: the
Father, the Son, and the Holy Spirit.
Trinita, Trinite, Trinitee, Trinitey, Triniti,
Trinitie, Trinnette, Trinty, Trynitee, Tryniti,
Trynitie, Trynity

Tripaileo (Mapuche) passionate woman.

Trish (Latin) a short form of Beatrice, Trisha.
Trishell, Trishelle

Trisha (Latin) noblewoman. (Hindi) thirsty.
See also Tricia.
*Treasha, Trishann, Trishanna, Trishanne,
Trishara, Trishia, Trishna, Trissha, Trysha,
Tryshah*

Trissa (Latin) a familiar form of Patricia.
*Trisa, Trisanne, Trisia, Trisina, Trissi, Trissie,
Trissy, Tryssa*

Trista (Latin) a short form of Tristan.
*Tristah, Tristal, Tristess, Tristia, Trysta, Trystah,
Trystia*

Tristabelle (English) a combination of
Tristan + Belle.
*Tristabel, Tristabela, Tristabelah, Tristabele,
Tristabell, Tristabella, Tristabellah, Trystabel,
Trystabela, Trystabelah, Trystabele, Trystabell,
Trystabella, Trystabellah, Trystabelle*

Tristan BG (Latin) bold.
*Tristana, Tristanah, Tristane, Tristann,
Tristanni, Tristany*

Tristen BG (Latin) a form of Tristan.
Tristene, Tristine, Tristinye, Tristn, Tristony

Tristian BG (Irish) a short form of
Tristianna.
*Tristiane, Tristiann, Tristianne, Trystiane,
Trystiann, Trystianne, Trystyane, Trystyann,
Trystyanne*

Tristianna (Irish) a combination of Tristan +
Anna.
*Tristiana, Tristianah, Tristiannah, Tristina,
Trystian, Trystiana, Trystianah, Trystianna,
Trystiannah, Trystyan, Trystyana, Trystyanah,
Trystyanna, Trystyannah*

Tristin BG (Latin) a form of Tristan.

Triston BG (Latin) a form of Tristan.

Tristyn BG (Latin) a form of Tristan.

Trixie (American) a familiar form of
Beatrice.
*Tris, Trissie, Trissina, Trix, Trixe, Trixee, Trixey,
Trixi, Trixy, Tryxee, Tryxey, Tryxi, Tryxie,
Tryxy*

Troy BG (Irish) foot soldier. (French) curly
haired. (English) water.
Troi, Troye, Troyton

Troya (Irish) a form of Troy.
Troia, Troiah, Troiana, Troianah, Troiane,

*Troiann, Troianna, Troianne, Troiya, Troyan,
Troyana, Troyanah, Troyane, Troyann, Troyanna,
Troyanne*

Trudel (Dutch) a form of Trudy.
*Trudela, Trudelah, Trudele, Trudell, Trudella,
Trudellah, Trudelle*

Trudy (German) a familiar form of
Gertrude.
*Truda, Trudah, Trude, Trudee, Trudessa, Trudey,
Trudi, Trudia, Trudiah, Trudie, Trudya*

Trycia (Latin) a form of Trisha.

Tryna (Greek) a form of Trina.
Tryane, Tryanna, Trynee

Tryne (Dutch) pure.
Trine

Trynel (Bavarian) a form of Katherine.
*Treinel, Treinela, Treinele, Treinell, Treinella,
Treinelle, Trynela, Trynelah, Trynele, Trynell,
Trynella, Trynellah, Trynelle*

Trystan BG (Latin) a form of Tristan.
Trystane, Trystann, Trystanne, Trysten, Trystin

Trystyn (Latin) a form of Tristan.

Tsigana (Hungarian) a form of Zigana.
Tsigane, Tzigana, Tzigane

Tu BG (Chinese) jade.

Tuesday (English) born on the third day of
the week.
*Tuesdae, Tuesdai, Tuesdea, Tuesdee, Tuesdey,
Tusdai*

Tuhina (Hindi) snow.
Tuhinah, Tuhyna, Tuhynah

Tula (Teutonic) a form of Gertrudes.

Tulip (French) tulip flower.
Tullip, Tullop, Tullyp, Tulyp

Tullia (Irish) peaceful, quiet.
Tulia, Tulliah, Tullya, Tullyah, Tulya, Tulyah

Tully BG (Irish) at peace with God.
*Tulea, Tuleah, Tulee, Tulei, Tuleigh, Tuley, Tuli,
Tulie, Tullea, Tulleah, Tullee, Tullei, Tulleigh,
Tulley, Tulli, Tullie, Tuly*

Tulsi (Hindi) basil, a sacred Hindu herb.
Tulsia, Tulsiah, Tulsy, Tulsya, Tulsyah

Tura (Catalan) ox.

Turquoise (French) blue-green semi-precious stone.
Turkois, Turkoise, Turkoys, Turkoyse, Turquois

Tusa (Zuni) prairie dog.
Tusah

Tusnelda (German) she who fights giants.

Tuyen GB (Vietnamese) angel.

Tuyet (Vietnamese) snow.

Twyla (English) woven of double thread.
Twila, Twilla

Ty BG (English) a short form of Tyler.
Ti, Tie, Tye

Tyana, Tyanna (Greek) forms of Tiana.
(American) combinations of Ty + Anna.
Tyanah, Tyannah, Tyannia

Tyann (Greek, American) a short form of
Tyana.
Tyan, Tyane, Tyanne

Tyasia (American) a form of Tyesha.
Tyasiah

Tyeesha (American) a form of Tyesha.

Tyeisha (American) a form of Tyesha.
Tyeishia

Tyesha (American) a combination of Ty +
Aisha.
*Tyasha, Tyashia, Tyeyshia, Tyieshia, Tyisha,
Tyishea, Tyishia, Tyishya, Tyshia, Tyshya*

Tyeshia (American) a form of Tyesha.

Tyfany (American) a short form of Tiffany.
*Tyfani, Tyfanny, Tyffanee, Tyffaney, Tyffani,
Tyffanie, Tyffanni, Tyffany, Tyffini, Typhanie,
Typhany*

Tyiesha (American) a form of Tyesha.
Tyieshia

Tykeisha (American) a form of Takeisha.
*Tykeesha, Tykeisa, Tykeishia, Tykesha,
Tykeshia, Tykeysha, Tykeza, Tykisha*

Tykera (American) a form of Takira.
*Tykeira, Tykeirah, Tykiera, Tykierra, Tykira,
Tykirah, Tykirra, Tykyra, Tykyrah*

Tykeria (American) a form of Tykera.
Tykereiah, Tykeriah, Tykerria, Tykiria

Tykia (American) a form of Takia.
Tykeia, Tykeiah, Tykiah, Tykya, Tykyah

Tylar BG (English) a form of Tyler.

Tyler BG (English) tailor.
Tyller

Tylor BG (English) a form of Tyler.

Tyna (Czech) a short form of Kristina.
Tynae, Tynea, Tynia

Tyne (English) river.
Tine, Tyna, Tynelle, Tynessa, Tynetta

Tyneisha (American) a form of Tynesha.
Tyneicia, Tyneisia

Tynesha (American) a combination of Ty +
Niesha.
Tynaise, Tynece, Tynesa, Tynessia, Tyniesha

Tyneshia (American) a form of Tynesha.

Tynisha (American) a form of Tynesha.
Tynisa, Tynise, Tynishi

Tyonna (American) a form of Tiana.
Tyona

Tyra (Scandinavian) battler. Mythology: Tyr
was the god of war. A form of Thora.
(Hindi) a form of Tira.
Thyra, Tyraa, Tyran, Tyria

Tyrah (Scandinavian, Hindi) a form of Tyra.

Tyree BG (Scandinavian, Hindi) a form of
Tyra.

Tyshanna (American) a combination of Ty
+ Shawna.
*Tyshana, Tyshanae, Tyshane, Tyshaun,
Tyshaunda, Tyshawn, Tyshawna, Tyshawnah,
Tyshawnda, Tyshawnna, Tysheann, Tysheanna,
Tyshonia, Tyshonna, Tyshonya*

Tytiana, Tytianna (Greek) forms of Titania.
*Tytana, Tytanna, Tyteana, Tyteanna, Tytianni,
Tytionna, Tytiyana, Tytiyanna, Tytyana,
Tytyauna*

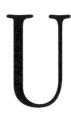

U (Korean) gentle.

Ualani (Hawaiian) rain from heaven.
Ualana, Ualanah, Ualanea, Ualanee, Ualaney, Ualania, Ualanie, Ualany

Ubaldina (Teutonic) audacious; intelligent.

Udalrica (Scandinavian) rich country.

Udele (English) prosperous.
Uda, Udah, Udella, Udelle, Yudelle

Ugolina (German) bright mind; bright spirit.
Hugolina, Hugolinah, Hugoline, Hugolyna, Hugolynah, Hygolyne, Ugolin, Ugolinah, Ugoline, Ugolyna, Ugolynah, Ugolyne

Ujana (Breton) noble; exellent. (African) youth.
Jana, Janah, Ujanah, Uyana, Uyanah

Ula (Irish) sea jewel. (Scandinavian) wealthy. (Spanish) a short form of Eulalia.
Eula, Oola, Uli, Ulia

Ulalia (Greek) sweet; soft-spoken.
Ulaliah, Ulalya, Ulalyah

Ulani (Polynesian) cheerful.
Ulana, Ulanah, Ulane, Ulanee, Ulaney, Ulania, Ulanie, Ulany, Ulanya, Ulanyah

Ulima (Arabic) astute; wise.
Uleama, Uleamah, Uleema, Uleemah, Ulemah, Ulimah, Ullima, Ulyma, Ulymah

Ulla (German, Swedish) willful. (Latin) a short form of Ursula.
Ula, Ulah, Ullah, Ulli

Ulrica (German) wolf ruler; ruler of all. See also Rica.
Ulka, Ullrica, Ullricka, Ullrika, Ulricah, Ulricka, Ulrickah, Ulrika, Ulrikah, Ulrike, Ulrique, Ulryca, Ulrycah, Ulrycka, Ulryckah, Ulryka, Ulrykah, Ulryqua

Ultima (Latin) last, endmost, farthest.
Ultimah, Ultyma, Ultymah

Ululani (Hawaiian) heavenly inspiration.
Ululanee, Ululaney, Ululania, Ululanie, Ululany, Ululanya

Ulva (German) wolf.
Ulvah

Uma (Hindi) mother. Religion: another name for the Hindu goddess Devi.
Umah

Umay (Turkish) hopeful.
Umai

Umbelina (Latin) she who gives protective shade.

Umeko (Japanese) plum-blossom child; patient.
Ume, Umeyo

Umiko (Japanese) child of the sea.

Una (Latin) one; united. (Hopi) good memory. (Irish) a form of Agnes. See also Oona.
Unagh, Unah, Unna, Uny

Undine (Latin) little wave. Mythology: the undines were water spirits. See also Ondine.
Undeen, Undene, Undina, Undinah, Undyn, Undyna, Undynah, Undyne

Unice (English) a form of Eunice.

Unika GB (American) a form of Unique.
Unica, Unicka, Unik, Unikue

Uniqua (Latin) a form of Unique.
Unikqua

Unique GB (Latin) only one.
Uniqia, Uniquia

Unity GB (English) unity.
Uinita, Unita, Unite, Unitea, Unitee, Unitey, Unyta, Unytea, Unytee, Unytey, Unyti, Unytie, Unyty

Unn (Norwegian) she who is loved.

Unna (German) woman.
Unnah

Unnea (Scandinavian) linden tree.
Unea, Uneah, Unneah

Urania (Greek) heavenly. Mythology: the Muse of astronomy.
Uraina, Urainah, Urainia, Urainiah, Uranie, Uraniya, Uranya, Uranyah

Urbana (Latin) city dweller.
Urabannah, Urbanah, Urbanna

Uri BG (Hebrew) my light.
Uree, Urie, Ury

Uriana (Greek) heaven; the unknown.
*Urianna, Uriannah, Urianne, Uryan, Uryana,
Uryanah, Uryane, Uryann, Uryanna, Uryanne*

Uriel (Hebrew) light of God.

Urika (Omaha) useful to everyone.
*Ureka, Urica, Uricah, Uricka, Urickah,
Urikah, Uriqua, Uryca, Urycah, Uryka,
Urykah, Uryqua*

Urit (Hebrew) bright.
Urice, Urita, Uritah, Uryt, Uryta, Urytah

Urith (German) worthy.
Uritha, Urithah, Urithe, Uryth, Urythah

Urola (Russian) a form of Ursula.

Urraca (German) magpie.

Ursa (Greek) a short form of Ursula. (Latin)
a form of Orsa.
Ursah, Ursea, Ursey, Ursi, Ursie, Ursy

Ursicina (Latin) bear meat.

Ursina (Latin) a form of Ursula.

Ursula (Greek) little bear. See also Sula,
Ulla, Vorsila.
*Irsaline, Ursala, Ursel, Ursela, Ursella, Ursely,
Ursilla, Ursillane, Ursola, Ursule, Ursulina,
Ursuline, Ursulyna, Ursylyn, Urszula,
Urszuli, Urzsulah, Urzula, Urzulah*

Usha (Hindi) sunrise.
Ushah

Ushi (Chinese) ox. Astrology: a sign of the
Chinese zodiac.
Ushee, Ushie, Ushy

Usoa (Spanish) dove.

Uta (German) rich. (Japanese) poem.
Utah, Utako

Utano (Japanese) field of songs.
Utan, Utana, Utanah

Utina (Native American) woman of my
country.
*Utahna, Uteana, Uteanah, Uteena, Uteenah,
Utinah, Utona, Utonna, Utyna, Utynah*

Uxía (Greek) born from a good family.

Uxue (Basque) dove.

Uzza (Arabic) strong.
Uza, Uzah, Uzzah

Uzzia (Hebrew) God is my strength.
*Uzia, Uziah, Uzya, Uzyah, Uzziah, Uzzya,
Uzzyah*

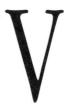

Vachya (Hindi) talking.
Vachia, Vachiah, Vachyah

Vail BG (English) valley.
*Vaile, Vale, Valee, Valey, Vali, Valie, Valy, Vayl,
Vayle*

Vailea (Polynesian) talking water.
*Vaileah, Vailee, Vailei, Vaileigh, Vailey, Vaili,
Vailie, Vaily, Vailya, Vaylea, Vayleah, Vaylee,
Vaylei, Vayleigh, Vayley, Vayli, Vaylie, Vayly*

Val BG (Latin) a short form of Valentina,
Valerie.
Vall, Valle

Vala (German) singled out.
Valah, Valla, Vallah

Valarie (Latin) a form of Valerie.
*Valarae, Valaree, Valarey, Valari, Valaria,
Vallarie, Vallary*

Valborga (Swedish) mighty mountain.
Valborg, Valborgah

Valburga (German) she who defends on the
battlefield.

Valda (German) famous ruler.
Valdah, Valida, Velda

Valdrada (German) she who gives advice.

Valencia (Spanish) strong. Geography: a
region in eastern Spain.
*Valanca, Valancia, Valecia, Valence, Valenciah,
Valencya, Valencyah, Valenica, Valenzia*

Valene (Latin) a short form of Valentina.
*Valaina, Valainah, Valaine, Valean, Valeana,
Valeanah, Valeane, Valeda, Valeen, Valeena,*

Valeenah, Valeene, Valen, Valena, Valenah, Valeney, Valien, Valina, Valine, Vallan, Vallana, Vallanah, Vallane, Vallen, Vallena, Vallenah, Vallene, Vallina, Vallinah, Valline, Vallyna, Vallynah, Vallyne, Valyn, Valynn

Valentia (Italian) a form of Valentina.
Valentiah, Valentya, Valentyah

Valentina (Latin) strong. History: Valentina Tereshkova, a Soviet cosmonaut, was the first woman in space. See also Tina, Valene, Valli.
Valantina, Valenteana, Valenteane, Valenteen, Valenteena, Valenteene, Valentena, Valentia, Valentijn, Valentin, Valentine, Valentyn, Valentyna, Valentyne, Valtina

Valera (Russian) a form of Valerie. See also Lera.

Valeria (Latin) a form of Valerie.
Valaria, Valariah, Valeriah, Valeriana, Valeriane, Veleria

Valéria (Hungarian, Portuguese) a form of Valerie.

Valerie (Latin) strong.
Vairy, Valaree, Vale, Valeree, Valeri, Valeria, Valérie, Valerye, Valka, Valleree, Valleri, Vallerie, Vallirie, Valry, Valya, Velerie, Waleria

Valery (Latin) a form of Valerie.
Valerye, Vallery

Valeska (Slavic) glorious ruler.
Valesca, Valese, Valeshia, Valeshka, Valeskah, Valezka, Valisha

Valkiria (German) Mythology: the Valkyries were Norse handmaidens who carried warriors' souls to Valhalla.

Valli (Latin) a familiar form of Valentina, Valerie. Botany: a plant native to India.
Valee, Valei, Valeigh, Valey, Vali, Valie, Vallee, Vallei, Valleigh, Vallie, Vally, Valy

Vallia (Spanish) strong protector.
Valea, Valeah, Valia, Valiah, Vallea, Valleah, Valliah, Vallya, Vallyah, Valya, Valyah

Valma (Finnish) loyal defender.
Valmah, Valmai

Valonia (Latin) shadow valley.
Valione, Valioney, Valioni, Valionia, Valioniah, Valionie, Valiony, Valionya, Valionyah, Vallon,

Vallonia, Valloniah, Vallonya, Vallonyah, Valona, Valoniah, Valonya, Valonyah, Valyona, Valyonah, Valyonia, Valyoniah, Valyony, Valyonya, Valyonyah

Valora (Latin) a form of Valerie.
Valorah, Valore, Valoria, Valoriah, Valorya, Valoryah, Velora

Valorie (Latin) a form of Valerie.
Vallori, Vallory, Valoree, Valorey, Valori, Valory, Valorye

Valtruda (German) strong dynasty.

Van **BG** (Greek) a short form of Vanessa.

Vanda **GB** (German) a form of Wanda.
Vandah, Vandana, Vandella, Vandetta, Vandi, Vannda

Vandani (Hindi) worthy, honorable.
Vandanee, Vandaney, Vandanie, Vandany

Vanesa, Vannesa, Vannessa (Greek) forms of Vanessa.
Vanesha, Vaneshah, Vaneshia, Vanesia, Vanisa, Vannesha, Vannesse, Vannessee

Vanessa ☆ (Greek) butterfly. Literature: a name invented by Jonathan Swift as a nickname for Esther Vanhomrigh. See also Nessie.
Vanassa, Vanesse, Vanessee, Vanessia, Vanessica, Vanetta, Vaneza, Vaniece, Vaniessa, Vanika, Vaniss, Vanissa, Vanisse, Vanissee, Vanneza, Vannysa, Vannysah, Vannyssa, Vanysa, Vanysah Vanyssa, Vanyssah, Varnessa

Vanetta (English) a form of Vanessa.
Vaneta, Vanetah, Vanete, Vanett, Vanettah, Vanette, Vanita, Vanitah, Vanneta, Vannetta, Vannita, Venetta

Vani (Hindi) voice. (Italian) a form of Ann.
Vanee, Vaney, Vanie, Vannee, Vanney, Vanni, Vannie, Vanny, Vany

Vania (Russian) a familiar form of Anna.
Vanea, Vaneah, Vaniah, Vanija, Vanijah, Vanina, Vaniya, Vanja, Vanka, Vannea, Vanneah, Vannia, Vanniah, Vannya, Vannyah, Vanyah

Vanity (English) vain.
Vanitee, Vanitey, Vaniti, Vanitie, Vanittee, Vanittey, Vanitti, Vanittie, Vanitty, Vanyti, Vanytie, Vanyty

Vanna (Cambodian) golden. (Greek) a short form of Vanessa.
Vana, Vanae, Vanah, Vanelly, Vannah, Vannalee, Vannaleigh, Vannie, Vanny

Vanora (Welsh) white wave.
Vannora, Vanorah, Vanorea, Vanoree, Vanorey, Vanori, Vanoria, Vanoriah, Vanorie, Vanory, Vanorya, Vanoryah

Vantrice (American) a combination of the prefix Van + Trice.
Vantrece, Vantricia, Vantriciah, Vantricya, Vantricyah, Vantrisa, Vantrise, Vantrisia, Vantrisiah, Vantrissa, Vantrisya, Vantrisyah, Vantrysia, Vantrysiah, Vantrysya, Vantrysyah

Vanya BG (Russian) a familiar form of Anna.

Vara (Scandinavian) careful.
Varah, Varia, Variah

Varana (Hindi) river.
Varanah, Varanna, Varannah

Varda (Hebrew) rose.
Vardia, Vardiah, Vardice, Vardina, Vardis, Vardissa, Vardisse, Vardit, Vardita, Vardyce, Vardys, Vardysa, Vardyse, Vardyta, Vardytah

Vardina (Hebrew) a form of Varda.
Vardin, Vardinah, Vardine, Vardinia, Vardiniah, Vardyn, Vardyna, Vardynah, Vardyne

Varina (English) thorn.
Varinah, Varyna, Varynah, Varyne

Varinia (Roman, Spanish) versatile.

Varvara (Slavic) a form of Barbara.
Varenka, Varinka, Varya, Varyusha, Vava, Vavka

Vashti (Persian) lovely. Bible: the wife of Ahasuerus, king of Persia.
Vashtee, Vashtie, Vashty

Vasilisa, Vasillisa (Russian) royal.

Vassy (Persian) beautiful.
Vasi, Vasie, Vassee, Vassey, Vassi, Vassie, Vasy

Vasya (Russian) royal.

Veanna (American) a combination of the prefix Ve + Anna.
Veannah, Veeana, Veeanah, Veeann, Veeanna, Veeannah, Veeanne, Veena, Veenah, Veenaya, Veeona

Veda (Sanskrit) sacred lore; knowledge. Religion: the Vedas are the sacred writings of Hinduism.
Vedad, Vedah, Veida, Veleda

Vedette (Italian) sentry; scout. (French) movie star.
Vedet, Vedeta, Vedetah, Vedete, Vedett, Vedetta, Vedettah

Vedis (German) spirit from the forest.
Vediss, Vedissa, Vedisse, Vedys, Vedyss, Vedyssa, Vedysse

Vega (Arabic) falling star.
Vegah

Velda (German) a form of Valda.
Veldah

Velia (Latin) concealed.

Velika (Slavic) great, wondrous.
Velikah, Velyka, Velykah

Velinda (American) a combination of the prefix Ve + Linda.
Velindah, Velynda, Velyndah

Velma (German) a familiar form of Vilhelmina.
Valma, Valmah, Vellma, Vellmah, Vilma, Vilmah, Vilna, Vylma, Vylmah

Velvet (English) velvety.
Velveta, Velvetah, Velvete, Velvett, Velvetta, Velvettah, Velvette, Velvit, Velvyt

Venancia (Latin) hunter.

Venecia (Italian) from Venice, Italy.
Vanecia, Vaneciah, Vanetia, Veneece, Veneise, Venesha, Venesher, Venicia, Veniece, Veniesa, Venise, Venisha, Venishia, Vennice, Vennise, Venyce, Vonizia, Vonizya, Vonysia, Vonysiah, Vonysya, Vonysyah

Veneranda (Latin) worthy of veneration.

Venessa (Latin) a form of Vanessa.
Veneese, Venesa, Venese, Veneshia, Venesia, Venessah, Venesse, Venessia, Venisa, Venissa, Vennesa, Vennessa, Vennisa

Venetia (Italian) a form of Venecia.
Veneta, Venetiah, Venetta, Venette, Venetya, Venetyah, Venita, Venitia, Vinetia, Vinetiah, Vinita, Vinitah, Vonita, Vonitia, Vynita, Vynitah, Vynyta, Vynytah

Venezia (Italian) a form of Venecia.
Veniza, Venize

Venice (Italian) from Venice, Italy.

Venidle (German) flag of the warrior.

Ventana (Spanish) window.

Ventura (Spanish) good fortune.

Venus (Latin) love. Mythology: the goddess of love and beauty.
Venis, Venusa, Venusina, Venussa, Venys, Vinny, Vynys

Venustiana (Latin) a form of Venus.

Vera (Latin) true. (Slavic) faith. A short form of Elvera, Veronica. See also Verena, Wera.
Vara, Veera, Veira, Verah, Verasha, Vere, Verka, Verla, Verra, Verrah, Viera, Vira, Vjera, Vyra, Vyrah

Veradis (Latin) truthful.
Veradissa, Veradisse, Veradys, Veradysa, Veradyss, Veradyssa

Verbena (Latin) sacred plants.
Verbeen, Verbeena, Verbeene, Verben, Verbene, Verbin, Verbina, Verbine, Verbyn, Verbyna, Verbyne

Verda (Latin) young, fresh.
Verdah, Verdea, Verdee, Verdey, Verdi, Verdie, Verdy, Virida

Verdad (Spanish) truthful.
Verdada

Verdianna (American) a combination of Verda + Anna.
Verdian, Verdiana, Verdiane, Verdiann, Verdianne, Verdyan, Verdyana, Verdyane, Verdyann, Verdyanna, Verdyanne, Virdian, Virdiana, Virdiane, Virdiann, Virdianna, Virdianne, Vyrdian, Vyrdiana, Vyrdiane, Vyrdiann, Vyrdianna, Vyrdianne, Vyrdyan, Vyrdyana, Vyrdyane, Vyrdyann, Vyrdyanna, Vyrdyanne

Veredigna (Latin) she who has earned great honors for her dignity.

Verena (Latin) truthful. A familiar form of Vera, Verna.
Varyn, Varyna, Varyne, Verean, Vereana, Vereane, Vereen, Vereena, Vereene, Verenah, Verene, Verin, Verina, Verine, Verinka,

Veroshka, Verunka, Verusya, Veryn, Veryna, Veryne, Virna

Verenice (Latin) a form of Veronica.
Verenis, Verenise, Vereniz

Veridiana (Latin) truthful.

Verity (Latin) truthful.
Verita, Veritah, Veritea, Veritee, Veritey, Veriti, Veritie, Veryta, Verytah, Verytea, Verytee, Verytey, Veryti, Verytie, Veryty

Verlene (Latin) a combination of Veronica + Lena.
Verleen, Verlena, Verlin, Verlina, Verlinda, Verline, Verlyn

Verna (Latin) springtime. (French) a familiar form of Laverne. See also Verena, Wera.
Verasha, Verla, Vernah, Verne, Verneta, Vernetia, Vernetta, Vernette, Vernia, Vernita, Viera, Virida, Virna, Virnah, Virnell, Vyrna, Vyrnah

Vernice (Latin) a form of Bernice, Verna.
Vernese, Vernesha, Verneshia, Vernessa, Vernica, Vernicca, Verniccah, Verniece, Vernika, Vernique, Vernis, Vernise, Vernyca, Vernycah, Vernycca, Vernyccah, Vyrnessa, Vyrnessah, Vyrnesse

Vernisha (Latin) a form of Vernice.
Vernisheia, Vernissia

Veronic (Latin) a short form of Veronica.

Veronica (Latin) true image. See also Ronica, Roni, Weronika.
Varonica, Varonicca, Varoniccah, Verhonica, Verinica, Verohnica, Veron, Verona, Verone, Véronic, Veronice, Veronne, Veronnica, Veruszhka, Vironica, Vironicah, Vironicca, Vironiccah, Vironiqua, Vron, Vronica, Vronicah, Vyronica, Vyronicah, Vyronicca, Vyroniccah

Verónica (Spanish) a form of Veronica.

Verônica (Portuguese) a form of Veronica.

Veronika (Latin) a form of Veronica.
Varonika, Veronick, Véronick, Veronicka, Veronik, Veronike, Veronka, Veronkia, Veruka, Vironika, Vronika, Vyronika, Vyronikah

Veronique, Véronique (French) forms of Veronica.
Veranique, Veroniqua, Vironique, Vroniqua, Vronique, Vyroniqua, Vyronique

Vespasiana (Latin) wasp.

Vespera (Latin) evening star.
Vesperah

Vesta (Latin) keeper of the house.
Mythology: the goddess of the home.
Vessy, Vest, Vestah, Vestea, Vestee, Vesteria,
Vestey

Veta (Slavic) a familiar form of Elizabeth.
Vetah

Vevila (Irish) melodious voice.
Vevilla, Vevillia, Vevilliah, Vevyla, Vevylah,
Vevyle, Vevylla, Vevyllah, Vevylle

Vevina (Irish) pleasant, sweet.
Vevinah, Vevine, Vevyna, Vevynah, Vevyne

Vi (Latin, French) a short form of Viola,
Violet.

Vianca (Spanish) a form of Bianca.
Vianeca, Vianica, Vianka, Vyaneca, Vyanica,
Vyanka

Vianey, Vianney (American) familiar forms
of Vianna.
Viany

Vianna (American) a combination of Vi +
Anna.
Viana, Vianah, Viann, Viannah, Vianne, Vyan,
Vyana, Vyanah, Vyane, Vyanna, Vyannah,
Vyanne

Vica (Hungarian) a form of Eve.
Vicah, Vyca, Vycah

Vicka, Vika (Latin) familiar forms of
Victoria.
Vickah, Vikah, Vikka, Vikkah, Vikkia, Vycka,
Vyckah, Vyka, Vykah, Vykka, Vykkah

Vicki, Vickie, Vicky (Latin) familiar forms of
Victoria. See also Vikki.
Vic, Viccey, Vicci, Viccy, Vicke, Vickee, Vickey,
Vickia, Vickiana, Vickilyn, Vickkee, Vickkey,
Vickki, Vickkie, Vickky, Vycke, Vyckee, Vyckey,
Vycki, Vyckie, Vycky, Vykki, Vykkie, Vykky,
Vyky

Victoria ☀ (Latin) victorious. See also Tory,
Wicktoria, Wisia.
Victoriya, Victorria, Victorriah, Victorya,
Vitoria, Vyctoria, Vyctoriah

Victorine (Latin) a form of Victoria.
Victoreana, Victoreane, Victoreene, Victoriana,
Victorianna, Victorina, Victorinah, Victoryn,

Victoryna, Victoryne, Viktorina, Viktorine,
Vyctorina, Vyctorine, Vyctoryn, Vyctoryna,
Vyctorynah, Vyctoryne, Vyktorin, Vyktorina,
Vyktorinah, Vyktorine, Vyktoryn, Vyktoryna,
Vyktorynah, Vyktoryne

Victory (Latin) victory.
Victoire, Victorie, Victorine, Vitorie

Vida (Sanskrit) a form of Veda. (Hebrew) a
short form of Davida.
Veeda, Vidah, Vidamarie, Vyda, Vydah

Vidal BG (Latin) life.
Vital, Vydal, Vytal

Vidalina (Spanish) a form of Vidal.

Vidonia (Portuguese) branch of a vine.
Vedonia, Vidoniah, Vidonya, Vidonyah,
Vydonia, Vydoniah, Vydonya, Vydonyah

Vienna (Latin) Geography: the capital of
Austria.
Vena, Venah, Venia, Venna, Vennah, Vennia,
Vienetta, Vienette, Vienne

Vigilia (Latin) wakeful, watching.
Vigiliah, Vijilia, Vijiliah, Vygilia, Vygiliah,
Vygylia, Vyjilia

Vignette (French) small vine.
Vignet, Vigneta, Vignete, Vignett, Vignetta,
Vygnet, Vygneta, Vygnete, Vygnett, Vygnetta,
Vygnette

Vikki (Latin) a familiar form of Victoria. See
also Vicki.
Vika, Viki, Vikie, Vikkee, Vikkey, Vikkie,
Vikky, Viky

Viktoria (Latin) a form of Victoria.
Viktoriah, Viktorie, Viktorija, Viktorya,
Viktoryah

Vila (Latin) from a house in the country.
Vilah, Villa, Villah, Vyla, Vylah, Vylla, Vyllah

Vilana (Latin) inhabitant of a small village.

Vilhelmina (German) a form of Wilhelmina.
Vilhalmine, Vilhelmine, Vylhelmina,
Vylhelmine

Villette (French) small town.
Vietta, Vilet, Vileta, Viletah, Vilete, Vilett,
Viletta, Vilette, Villet, Villeta, Villetah, Villete,
Villett, Villetta, Villettah, Vylet, Vyleta,
Vyletah, Vylete, Vylett, Vyletta, Vylettah,

Vylette, Vyllet, Vylleta, Vylletah, Vyllete,
Vyllette

Vilma (German) a short form of Vilhelmina.
Vilmah, Vylma, Vylmah

Vina (Hindi) Religion: a musical instrument
played by the Hindu goddess of wisdom.
(Spanish) vineyard. (Hebrew) a short form
of Davina. (English) a short form of Alvina.
See also Lavina.
Veena, Veenah, Viña, Vinesha, Vinessa, Viniece,
Vinique, Vinisha, Viñita, Vinna, Vinnah,
Vinora, Vyna, Vynah, Vynna, Vynnah

Vincent BG (Latin) victor, conqueror.

Vincentia (Latin) a form of Vincent.
Vicenta, Vincensa, Vincensah, Vincensia,
Vincensiah, Vincenta, Vincentah, Vincentena,
Vincentina, Vincentine, Vincenza, Vincenzah,
Vincenzia, Vincenziah, Vincy, Vinnie,
Vyncenzia, Vyncenziah, Vyncenzya,
Vyncenzyah

Vinia (Latin) wine.
Viniah, Vynia, Vyniah, Vynya, Vynyah

Viñita (Spanish) a form of Vina.
Viñeet, Viñeeta, Viñeete, Viñetta, Viñette,
Viñitha, Viñta, Viñti, Viñtia, Vyñetta, Vyñette,
Vyñita, Vyñyta, Vyñytta, Vyñytte

Viola (Latin) violet; stringed instrument in
the violin family. Literature: the heroine of
Shakespeare's play *Twelfth Night*.
Violah, Violaina, Violaine, Violainee, Violainey,
Violaini, Violainia, Violanta, Violante, Viole,
Violeine, Vyoila, Vyoilah, Vyola, Vyolah,
Vyolani, Vyolania, Vyolanie, Vyolany,
Vyolanya

Violet (French) Botany: a plant with pur-
plish blue flowers.
Violete, Violett, Violette, Vyolet, Vyolete,
Vyolett, Vyolette

Violeta, Violetta (French) forms of Violet.
Violatta, Violetah, Vyoleta, Vyoletah, Vyoletta

Virgilia (Latin) rod bearer, staff bearer.
Virgilea, Virgileah, Virgilee, Virgileigh, Virgili,
Virgilie, Virgillia, Virgily, Virgilya, Virjil,
Virjilea, Virjileah, Virjilee, Virjileigh, Virjiley,
Virjili, Virjilie, Virjily, Vylgiliah, Vyrgilia,
Vyrgylya, Vyrgylyah

Virginia (Latin) pure, virginal. Literature:
Virginia Woolf was a well-known British
writer. See also Gina, Ginger, Ginny, Jinny.
Verginia, Verginya, Virge, Virgeen, Virgeena,
Virgeenah, Virgeenia, Virgeeniah, Virgen,
Virgene, Virgenia, Virgenya, Virgie, Virgine,
Virginio, Virginnia, Virgy, Virjeana, Virjinea,
Virjineah, Virjinia, Virjiniah, Vyrginia,
Vyrginiah, Vyrgynia, Vyrgyniah, Vyrgynya,
Vyrgynyah

Virginie (French) a form of Virginia.
Virgeenee, Virginië, Virjinee

Viridiana (Latin) a form of Viridis.

Viridis (Latin) green.
Virdis, Virida, Viridia, Viridiss, Viridissa,
Viridys, Viridyss, Viridyssa, Vyridis, Vyridiss,
Vyridissa, Vyridys, Vyridyss, Vyridyssa

Virtudes (Latin) blessed spirit.

Virtue (Latin) virtuous.
Vertue, Virtu, Vyrtu, Vyrtue

Virxinia (Latin) pure.

Visia (Latin) strength, vigor.

Visitación (Latin) refers to the Virgin Mary
visiting Saint Elizabeth.

Vita (Latin) life.
Veeta, Vitah, Vitaliana, Vitalina, Vitel, Vitella,
Vitia, Vitka, Vitke, Vitta, Vyta, Vytah, Vytta,
Vyttah

Vitalia (Latin) a form of Vita.

Vitoria, Vittoria (Spanish, Italian) forms of
Victoria.
Vitoriah, Vittoriah, Vittorya, Vittoryah,
Vytoria, Vytoriah, Vyttoria, Vyttoriah

Vitória (Portuguese) a form of Victoria.

Viv (Latin) a short form of Vivian.
Vive, Vyv

Viva (Latin) a short form of Aviva, Vivian.
Vica, Vivah, Vivan, Vivva, Vyva, Vyvah

Vivalda (Latin) alive; brave in battle.

Viveca (Scandinavian) a form of Vivian.
Vivecah, Vivecca, Vivecka, Viveka, Vivica,
Vivieca, Vyveca

Vivian (Latin) full of life.
Vevay, Vevey, Viv, Viva, Viveca, Vivi, Vivia, Viviann, Vivina, Vivion, Vivyan, Vivyann, Vivyanne, Vyvian, Vyvyan, Vyvyann, Vyvyanne

Viviana, Vivianna (Latin) forms of Vivian.
Viviannah, Vivyana, Vyvyana, Vyvyanna

Viviane, Vivianne, Vivien (Latin) forms of Vivian.
Vivee, Vivie, Vivienne

Voleta (Greek) veiled.
Volet, Voletah, Volett, Voletta, Volette, Volita, Volitt, Volitta, Volitte, Volyta, Volyta, Volyte, Volytt, Volytta, Volyttah, Volytte

Volupia (Greek) voluptuous woman.

Vondra (Czech) loving woman.
Vonda, Vondrah, Vondrea

Voneisha (American) a combination of Yvonne + Aisha.
Voneishia, Vonesha, Voneshia

Vonna (French) a form of Yvonne.
Vona, Vonah, Vonia, Voniah, Vonnah, Vonnia, Vonnya, Vonya

Vonny (French) a familiar form of Yvonne.
Vonney, Vonni, Vonnie, Vony

Vontricia (American) a combination of Yvonne + Tricia.
Vontrece, Vontrese, Vontrice, Vontriece, Vontrisha, Vontrishia, Vontrycia, Vontryciah, Vontrycya, Vontrycyah

Vorsila (Greek) a form of Ursula.
Vorsilla, Vorsula, Vorsulah, Vorsulla, Vorsyla

Vulpine (English) like a fox.
Vulpina, Vulpinah, Vulpyna, Vulpynah, Vulpyne

Vy (Latin, French) a form of Vi.
Vye

Vyoma (Hindi) sky.
Vioma, Viomah, Vyomah

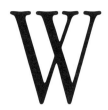

Wadd (Arabic) beloved.
Wad

Wahalla (Scandinavian) immortal.
Valhalla, Walhalla

Waheeda (Arabic) one and only.

Wainani (Hawaiian) beautiful water.
Wainanee, Wainanie, Wainany

Wakana (Japanese) plant.
Wakanah

Wakanda (Dakota) magical power.
Wakandah, Wakenda

Wakeisha (American) a combination of the prefix Wa + Keisha.
Wakeishah, Wakeishia, Wakesha, Wakeshia, Wakesia, Wakesiah, Wakeysha, Wakeyshah, Wakeyshia, Wakeyshiah, Wakeyshya, Wakeyshyah

Walad (Arabic) newborn.
Waladah, Walida, Walidah, Walyda, Walydah

Walda (German) powerful; famous.
Waldah, Waldina, Waldine, Waldyna, Waldyne, Walida, Wallda, Walldah, Welda, Weldah, Wellda, Welldah

Waleria (Polish) a form of Valerie.
Wala, Waleriah, Walerya, Waleryah, Walleria, Walleriah, Wallerya, Walleryah

Walker BG (English) cloth; walker.
Wallker

Wallis GB (English) from Wales.
Walice, Walise, Wallie, Wallisa, Wallise, Walliss, Wally, Wallys, Wallysa, Wallyse

Wanda (German) wanderer. See also Wendy.
Vanda, Wahnda, Wandah, Wandely, Wandie, Wandis, Wandja, Wandzia, Wannda, Wanndah, Wonda, Wondah, Wonnda, Wonndah

Wandie (German) a familiar form of Wanda.
Wandea, Wandee, Wandey, Wandi, Wandy

Waneta (Native American) charger. See also Juanita.
Waneata, Waneatah, Waneeta, Waneetah, Waneita, Waneitah, Wanetah, Wanete, Wanita, Wanitah, Wanite, Wanneata, Wanneatah, Wanneeta, Wanneetah, Wanneita, Wanneitah, Wanneta, Wannetah, Wannete, Waunita, Wonita, Wonnita, Wonnitah, Wonyta, Wonytah, Wonyte, Wynita

Wanetta (English) pale face.
Wanette, Wannetta, Wannette, Wonnitta, Wonnitte, Wonytta, Wonyttah, Wonytte

Wanika (Hawaiian) a form of Juanita.
Waneeka, Wanicka, Wanikah, Wanyka, Wanykah

Warda (German) guardian.
Wardah, Wardeh, Wardena, Wardenia, Wardia, Wardine

Washi (Japanese) eagle.
Washee, Washie, Washy

Wasila (English) healthy.
Wasilah, Wasilla, Wasillah, Wasyla, Wasylah, Wasylla, Wasyllah

Wattan (Japanese) homeland.
Watan

Wauna (Moquelumnan) snow geese honking.
Waunah, Waunakee

Wava (Slavic) a form of Barbara.
Wavah, Wavia, Waviah, Wavya, Wavyah

Waverly GB (English) quaking aspen-tree meadow.
Waverley, Waverli, Wavierlee

Wayca (Aboriginal) sauce.

Wayna (Quechua) young.

Waynesha (American) a combination of Waynette + Niesha.
Wayneesha, Wayneisha, Waynie, Waynisha

Waynette (English) wagon maker.
Wainet, Waineta, Wainetah, Wainete, Wainetta, Wainettah, Wainette, Waynel, Waynelle, Waynet, Wayneta, Waynete, Waynetta, Waynlyn

Wednesday (Latin, English) born on the fourth day of the week.

Weeko (Dakota) pretty girl.
Weiko, Weyko

Wehilani (Hawaiian) heavenly adornment.

Wenda (Welsh) a form of Wendy.
Wendah, Wendaine, Wendayne

Wendelle (English) wanderer.
Wendalina, Wendalinah, Wendaline, Wendall, Wendalla, Wendallah, Wendalle, Wendalyn, Wendalyna, Wendalynah, Wendalyne, Wendelin, Wendelina, Wendelinah, Wendeline, Wendella, Wendelline, Wendelly, Wendelyn, Wendelyna, Wendelynah, Wendelyne

Wendi (Welsh) a form of Wendy.
Wendia, Wendie

Wendy (Welsh) white; light skinned. A familiar form of Gwendolyn, Wanda.
Wende, Wendea, Wendee, Wendey, Wendya, Wendye, Wuendy

Wera (Polish) a form of Vera. See also Verna.
Werah, Wiera, Wiercia, Wierka

Wereburga (Germanic) protector of the army.

Weronika (Polish) a form of Veronica.
Weronica, Weronicah, Weronicka, Weronickah, Weronikah, Weronike, Weronikra, Weroniqua, Weronique, Weronyca, Weronycah, Weronycka, Weronyckah, Weronyka, Weronykah, Weronyqua, Weronyque

Wesisa (Musoga) foolish.
Wesisah, Wesysa, Wesysah

Weslee (English) a form of Wesley.

Wesley BG (English) western meadow.
Wesla, Weslah, Weslea, Wesleah, Weslei, Wesleigh, Weslene, Wesli, Weslia, Weslie, Wesly, Weslya, Weslyah, Weslyn

Whaley (English) whale meadow.
Whalea, Whaleah, Whalee, Whalei, Whaleigh, Whali, Whalia, Whaliah, Whalie, Whaly, Whalya

Whisper (English, German) whisper.

Whitley GB (English) white field.
Whitely, Whitlea, Whitleah, Whitlee, Whitlei, Whitleigh, Whitli, Whitlia, Whitlie, Whitly, Whitlya, Whittley, Whytlea, Whytleah, Whytlee, Whytlei, Whytleigh, Whytley, Whytli, Whytlia, Whytlie, Whytly, Whytlya

Whitnee, Whitni, Whitnie, Whittney
(English) forms of Whitney.
Whittnee, Whittni, Whittnie

Whitney GB (English) white island.
*Whitani, Whiteney, Whitne, Whitné, Whitnei,
Whitneigh, Whitny, Whitnye, Whittaney,
Whittanie, Whittany, Whitteny, Whittnay,
Whytne, Whytnee, Whytney, Whytni, Whytnie,
Whytny, Witney*

Whoopi (English) happy; excited.
Whoopee, Whoopey, Whoopie, Whoopy

Wicktoria (Polish) a form of Victoria.
*Wicktoriah, Wicktorja, Wiktoria, Wiktoriah,
Wiktorja, Wycktoria, Wycktoriah, Wycktorja,
Wyktoria, Wyktoriah, Wyktorja*

Wila (Hawaiian) loyal, faithful.
Wilah, Wyla, Wylah

Wilda (German) untamed. (English) willow.
Wildah, Willda, Wylda, Wyldah, Wylder

Wileen (English) a short form of
Wilhelmina.
*Wilean, Wileana, Wileane, Wileena, Wileenah,
Wileene, Wilene, Wilin, Wilina, Wilinah,
Wiline, Willeen, Willene, Wilyn, Wilyna,
Wilynah, Wilyne, Wylean, Wyleana,
Wyleanah, Wyleane, Wyleen, Wyleena,
Wyleenah, Wyleene, Wylin, Wylina, Wylinah,
Wyline, Wylyn, Wylyna, Wylynah, Wylyne*

Wilhelmina (German) a form of Wilhelm
(see Boys' Names). See also Billie,
Guillerma, Helma, Minka, Minna, Minnie.
*Vilhelmina, Wilhelmine, Willamina,
Willaminah, Willamine, Willemina,
Willeminah, Willemine, Williamina,
Williamine, Willmina, Willmine, Wimina,
Wimine, Wylhelmin, Wylhelmina,
Wylhelminah, Wylhelmine, Wylhelmyn,
Wylhelmyna, Wylhelmynah, Wylhelmyne,
Wyllhelmin, Wyllhelmina, Wyllhelminah,
Wyllhelmine, Wyllhelmyn, Wyllhelmyna,
Wyllhelmynah, Wyllhelmyne*

Wilikinia (Hawaiian) a form of Virginia.
Wilikiniah

Willa (German) a short form of Wilhelmina,
William.
Wylla, Wyllah

Willabelle (American) a combination of
Willa + Belle.
*Wilabel, Wilabela, Wilabele, Willabel,
Willabela, Willabele, Willabell, Willabella,
Williabelle, Wylabel, Wylabela, Wylabele,
Wylabell, Wylabella, Wylabelle, Wyllabel,
Wyllabela, Wyllabele, Wyllabell, Wyllabella,
Wyllabelle*

Willette (English) a familiar form of
Wilhelmina, Willa, William.
Wiletta, Wilette, Willetta, Williette

William BG (English) determined guardian.

Willie BG (English) a familiar form of
Wilhelmina, William.
*Wilea, Wileah, Wilee, Wilei, Wileigh, Wiley,
Wili, Wilie, Willea, Willeah, Willee, Willei,
Willeigh, Willi, Willina, Willisha, Willishia,
Willy*

Willow (English) willow tree.
Willo, Willough, Wyllo, Wyllow, Wylo, Wylow

Wilma (German) a short form of
Wilhelmina.
*Williemae, Wilmah, Wilmanie, Wilmayra,
Wilmetta, Wilmette, Wilmina, Wilmyne,
Wylma, Wylmah*

Wilona (English) desired.
*Willona, Willone, Wilonah, Wilone, Wylona,
Wylonah, Wylone*

Win BG (German) a short form of Winifred.
See also Edwina, Wynne.
Winn, Winne

Winda (Swahili) hunter.

Windy (English) windy.
*Windea, Windee, Windey, Windi, Windie,
Wyndea, Wyndee, Wyndey, Wyndi, Wyndie,
Wyndy*

Winefrida, Winifreda (Germanic) forms of
Winifred.

Winema (Moquelumnan) woman chief.
Winemah, Wynema, Wynemah

Wing GB (Chinese) glory.
Wing-Chiu, Wing-Kit

Winifred (German) peaceful friend. (Welsh)
a form of Guinevere. See also Freddi, Una,
Winnie.
Winafred, Winefred, Winefrid, Winefride,

Winfreda, Winfrieda, Winiefrida, Winifrid,
Winifryd, Winifryda, Winnafred, Winnafreda,
Winnefred, Winniefred, Winnifred, Winnifreda,
Winnifrid, Winnifrida, Wynafred, Wynafreda,
Wynafrid, Wynafrida, Wynefred, Wynefreda,
Wynefryd, Wynifred, Wynnifred

Winna (African) friend.
Wina, Winnah, Wyna, Wynah, Wynna,
Wynnah

Winnie (English) a familiar form of Edwina,
Gwyneth, Winifred, Winona, Wynne. History:
Winnie Mandela kept the anti-aparteid
movement alive in South Africa while her
then-husband, Nelson Mandela, was impris-
oned. Literature: the lovable bear in A. A.
Milne's children's story Winnie-the-Pooh.
Winee, Winey, Wini, Winie, Winnee, Winney,
Winni, Winny, Winy, Wynee, Wyney, Wyni,
Wynie, Wynnee, Wynney, Wynni, Wynnie,
Wynny, Wyny

Winola (German) charming friend.
Winolah, Wynola, Wynolah

Winona (Lakota) oldest daughter.
Wanona, Wanonah, Wenona, Wenonah,
Winonah

Winter GB (English) winter.
Wintr

Wira (Polish) a form of Elvira.
Wirah, Wiria, Wirke, Wyra, Wyrah

Wisia (Polish) a form of Victoria.
Wicia, Wiciah, Wikta, Wisiah, Wysia, Wysiah,
Wysya, Wysyah

Wren BG (English) wren, songbird.
Wrena, Wrenah, Wrene, Wrenee, Wrenie,
Wrenn, Wrenna, Wrennah, Wrenny

Wulfilde (Germanic) one who fights with
the wolves.

Wyanet (Native American) legendary
beauty.
Wianet, Wianeta, Wianete, Wianett, Wianetta,
Wianette, Wianita, Wyaneta, Wyanete,
Wyanett, Wyanetta, Wyanette, Wyanita,
Wynette

Wynne (Welsh) white, light skinned. A short
form of Blodwyn, Guinevere, Gwyneth.
See also Win.
Wyn, Wyne, Wynn

Wynonna (Lakota) a form of Winona.
Wynnona, Wynona, Wynonah

Wynter (English) a form of Winter.
Wynteria

Wyoming (Native American) Geography: a
western U.S. state.
Wy, Wye, Wyoh, Wyomia, Wyomya

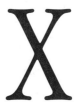

Xabrina (Latin) a form of Sabrina.
Xabrinah, Xabrine, Xabryna, Xabrynah,
Xabryne

Xalbadora, Xalvadora (Spanish) forms of
Salvadora.

Xalina (French) a form of Salina.
Xalean, Xaleana, Xaleanah, Xaleane, Xaleen,
Xaleena, Xaleenah, Xaleene, Xalena, Xalenah,
Xalinah, Xaline, Xalyna, Xalynah, Xalyne

Xamantha (Hebrew) a form of Samantha.
Xamanfa, Xamanfah, Xamanffa, Xamanffah,
Xamanthah, Xamanthia, Xamanthiah,
Xammantha, Xammanthia, Xammanthya

Xami (Hebrew) a form of Sami.
Xama, Xamah, Xamee, Xamey, Xamia,
Xamiah, Xamie, Xamm, Xamma, Xammah,
Xammi, Xammia, Xammiah, Xammie,
Xammy, Xammya, Xammyah, Xamy, Xamya,
Xamyah

Xamuela (Hebrew) a form of Samuela.
Xamuelah, Xamuele, Xamuell, Xamuella,
Xamuellah, Xamuelle

Xana (Greek) a form of Xanthe.
Xanna, Xanne

Xandi (Greek) a form of Sandi.
Xandea, Xandee, Xandey, Xandia, Xandiah,
Xandie, Xandy

Xandra (Greek) a form of Sandra. (Spanish)
a short form of Alexandra.
Xander, Xandrah

Xandria (Greek, Spanish) a form of Xandra.
*Xandrea, Xandreah, Xandreia, Xandreiah,
Xandriah, Xandrya, Xandryah*

Xàndria (Catalan) a form of Alexandria.

Xandrine (Greek) a form of Sandrine.
*Xandrean, Xandreana, Xandreanah,
Xandreane, Xandreen, Xandreena,
Xandreenah, Xandreene, Xandrina,
Xandrinah, Xandryna, Xandrynah*

Xanthe (Greek) yellow, blond. See also
Zanthe.
Xantha, Xanthia, Xanthiah

Xanthippe (Greek) a form of Xanthe.
History: Socrates's wife.
Xantippie, Zanthippe, Zantippie

Xantina (Spanish) a form of Santina.
*Xantinah, Xantine, Xantyna, Xantynah,
Xantyne*

Xara (Hebrew) a form of Sarah.
*Xarah, Xari, Xaria, Xariah, Xarie, Xarra,
Xarrah, Xarri, Xarria, Xarriah, Xarrie, Xarry,
Xary, Xarya, Xaryah*

Xarika (Hebrew) a form of Sarika.
*Xareaka, Xareakah, Xareeka, Xareekah,
Xareka, Xarekah, Xarikah, Xarka, Xarkah*

Xarina (Hebrew) a form of Sarina.
*Xareana, Xareanah, Xareane, Xareena,
Xareenah, Xareene, Xarena, Xarenah, Xarene,
Xarinah, Xarine, Xarinna, Xarinnah, Xarinne,
Xaryna, Xarynah, Xaryne, Xarynna, Xarynnah*

Xavier 🅑🅖 (Arabic) bright. (Basque) owner
of the new house.
*Xabier, Xaiver, Xavaeir, Xaver, Xavery, Xavian,
Xaviar, Xaviero, Xavior, Xavon, Xavyer,
Xizavier, Xxavier, Xzavier*

Xaviera (Basque, Arabic) a form of Xavier.
See also Javiera, Zaviera.
*Xavia, Xavierah, Xaviére, Xavyera, Xavyerah,
Xavyere, Xiveria*

Xela (Quiché) my mountain home.
Xelah, Xella, Xellah, Zela, Zelah, Zella, Zellah

Xema (Latin) precious.

Xena (Greek) a form of Xenia.
*Xeena, Xenah, Xene, Xina, Xinah, Xyna,
Xynah*

Xenia (Greek) hospitable. See also Senia,
Zena, Zina.
*Xeenia, Xeeniah, Xenea, Xeniah, Xenya,
Xenyah, Xinia*

Xenobia (Greek) a form of Cenobia.

Xenosa (Greek) stanger.
Xenosah, Zenosa, Zenosah

Xerena (Latin) a form of Serena.
Xeren, Xerenah, Xerene

Xesca (Catalan) a form of Francesca.

Xevera, Xeveria (Spanish) forms of Xavier.

Xiang (Chinese) fragrant. See also Ziang.
Xeang, Xeeang, Xyang

Xihuitl (Nahuatl) year; comet.

Xilda (Celtic) tribute.

Xiloxoch (Nahuatl) calliandra flower.

Xima (Catalan) a form of Joaquina.

Ximena (Spanish) a form of Simone.
*Ximenah, Ximona, Ximonah, Ximone,
Xymena, Xymenah, Xymona, Xymonah*

Xiomara (Teutonic) glorious forest.
Xiomaris, Xiomayra

Xipil (Nahuatl) noble of the fire.

Xirena (Greek) a form of Sirena.
*Xireena, Xireenah, Xirenah, Xirene, Xirina,
Xirinah, Xyren, Xyrena, Xyrenah, Xyrene,
Xyrina, Xyrinah, Xyrine, Xyryna, Xyrynah*

Xita (Catalan) a form of Conchita.

Xitlali (Nahuatl) a form of Citlali.

Xiu Mei (Chinese) beautiful plum.

Xiuhcoatl (Nahuatl) fire serpent.

Xiuhtonal (Nahuatl) precious light.

Xoana (Hebrew) God is compassionate and
merciful.

Xochicotzin (Nahuatl) little necklace of
flowers.

Xochilt (Aztec) a form of Xochitl.

Xochiquetzal (Nahuatl) most beautiful
flower.

Xochitl (Aztec) place of many flowers.
Xochil, Xochilth, Xochiti

Xochiyotl (Nahuatl) heart of a gentle flower.

Xoco (Nahuatl) youngest sister.

Xocotzin (Nahuatl) youngest daughter.

Xocoyotl (Nahuatl) youngest child.

Xosefa (Hebrew) seated by God.

Xuan (Vietnamese) spring.
Xuana, Zuan

Xuxa (Portuguese) a familiar form of Susanna.
Xuxah

Xyleena (Greek) forest dweller. See also
Zylina.
Xilean, Xileana, Xileanah, Xileane, Xileen,
Xileena, Xileenah, Xileene, Xilin, Xilina, Xilinah,
Xiline, Xilyn, Xilyna, Xilynah, Xilyne, Xylean,
Xyleana, Xyleanah, Xyleane, Xyleen, Xyleenah,
Xyleene, Xylin, Xylina, Xylinah, Xyline, Xylona,
Xylyn, Xylyna, Xylynah, Xylyne

Xylia (Greek) a form of Sylvia.
Xilia, Xiliah, Xylya, Xylyah

Xylona (Greek) a form of Xyleena.
Xilon, Xilona, Xilonah, Xilone, Xilonia,
Xiloniah, Xylon, Xylonah, Xylone, Xylonia,
Xyloniah, Xylonya, Xylonyah

Xylophia (Greek) forest lover.
Xilophia, Xilophiah, Xylophiah, Xylophila,
Xylophilah, Zilophia, Zylophia

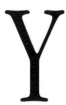

Yachne (Hebrew) hospitable.
Yachnee

Yadira (Hebrew) friend.
Yadirah, Yadirha, Yadyra

Yadra (Spanish) mother.

Yael GB (Hebrew) strength of God. See also
Jael.
Yaela, Yaele, Yaeli, Yaell, Yaella, Yaelle, Yeala

Yaffa (Hebrew) beautiful. See also Jaffa.
Yafeal, Yaffah, Yaffit, Yafit

Yahaira (Hebrew) a form of Yakira.
Yahara, Yahayra, Yahira

Yaíza (Guanche) rainbow.

Yajaira (Hebrew) a form of Yakira.
Yajara, Yajayra, Yajhaira

Yakira (Hebrew) precious; dear.
Yakirah, Yakyra, Yakyrah

Yalanda (Greek) a form of Yolanda.
Yalandah, Yalando, Yalonda, Ylana, Ylanda

Yalena (Greek, Russian) a form of Helen.
See also Lena, Yelena.
Yalana, Yalanah, Yalane, Yaleana, Yaleanah,
Yaleane, Yaleena, Yaleenah, Yaleene, Yalina,
Yalinah, Yaline, Yalyna, Yalynah, Yalyne

Yaletha (American) a form of Oletha.
Yelitsa

Yamary (American) a combination of the
prefix Ya + Mary.
Yamairee, Yamairey, Yamairi, Yamairie, Yamairy,
Yamaree, Yamarey, Yamari, Yamaria, Yamarie,
Yamaris, Yamarya, Yamaryah, Yamayra

Yamelia (American) a form of Amelia.
Yameily, Yameliah, Yamelya, Yamelyah, Yamelys,
Yamilya, Yamilyah

Yamila (Arabic) a form of Jamila.
Yamela, Yamely, Yamil, Yamile, Yamiley, Yamill,
Yamilla, Yamille, Yamyl, Yamyla, Yamyle,
Yamyll, Yamylla, Yamylle

Yamilet (Arabic) a form of Jamila.

Yamileta (Germanic) a form of Yamilet.

Yaminah (Arabic) right, proper.
Yamina, Yamini, Yamyna, Yamynah, Yemina,
Yeminah, Yemini

Yaminta (Native American) mint, minty.
Yamintah, Yamynta, Yamyntah, Yiminta

Yamka (Hopi) blossom.

Yamuna (Hindi) sacred river.
Yamunah

Yana BG (Slavic) a form of Jana.
Yanae, Yanah, Yanay, Yanaye, Yanesi, Yaney, Yania, Yaniah, Yanina, Yanis, Yanisha, Yanitza, Yanna, Yannah, Yannia, Yanniah, Yannica, Yannina, Yannya, Yannyah, Yannyna

Yanaba (Navajo) brave.
Yanabah

Yanamaría (Slavic) bitter grace.

Yaneli, Yanely (American) combinations of the prefix Ya + Nellie.
Yanela, Yanelis, Yaneliz, Yanelle, Yanelli, Yanelys

Yanet (American) a form of Janet.
Yanete, Yanette, Yannet, Yannette

Yaneta (Russian) a form of Jeannette.

Yaneth (American) a form of Janet.
Yanethe, Yanneth

Yáng (Chinese) sun.

Yani (Australian) peaceful. (Hebrew) a short form of Yannis.
Yanee, Yaney, Yanie, Yannee, Yanney, Yanni, Yannie, Yanny, Yany

Yannis (Hebrew) gift of God.
Yanis, Yannys, Yanys

Yaotl (Nahuatl) war; warrior.

Yara (Iranian) courage.

Yareli, Yarely (American) forms of Oralee.
Yaresly

Yarina (Slavic) a form of Irene.
Yarinah, Yarine, Yaryna, Yarynah, Yaryne

Yaritza (American) a combination of Yana + Ritsa.
Yaritsa, Yaritsah

Yarkona (Hebrew) green.
Yarkonah

Yarmilla (Slavic) market trader. See also Jarmilla.
Yarmila, Yarmilah, Yarmillah, Yarmille, Yarmyla, Yarmylah, Yarmylla, Yarmyllah, Yarmylle

Yasemin (Persian) a form of Yasmin.
Yasemeen

Yashira (Afghan) humble; takes it easy. (Arabic) wealthy.

Yasmeen, Yasmen (Persian) forms of Yasmin.
Yasmeene, Yasmene, Yasmenne, Yassmeen, Yassmen

Yasmin, Yasmine (Persian) jasmine flower.
Yashmine, Yasiman, Yasimine, Yasma, Yasmain, Yasmaine, Yasmeni, Yasmon, Yasmyn, Yasmyne, Yesmean, Yesmeen, Yesmin, Yesmine, Yesmyn

Yasmín, Yazmín (Persian) forms of Yasmin.

Yasmina (Persian) a form of Yasmin.
Yasmeena, Yasmeenah, Yasminah, Yasminda, Yasmyna, Yasmynah, Yesmina

Yasu (Japanese) resting, calm.
Yasuko, Yasuyo, Yazoo

Yasú (Japanese) calm.

Yayauhqui (Nahuatl) black smoking mirror.

Yayoi (Japanese) spring.

Yazmin, Yazmine (Persian) forms of Yasmin.
Yazmeen, Yazmen, Yazmene, Yazmina, Yazminah, Yazmyn, Yazmyna, Yazmynah, Yazmyne, Yazzmien, Yazzmine, Yazzmyn, Yazzmyne

Yecenia (Arabic) a form of Yesenia.

Yedida (Hebrew) dear friend.
Yedidah, Yedyda, Yedydah

Yegane (Persian) incomparable beauty.

Yehudit (Hebrew) a form of Judith.
Yuta

Yei (Japanese) flourishing.

Yeira (Hebrew) light.
Yeirah, Yeyra, Yeyrah

Yekaterina (Russian) a form of Katherine.

Yelena (Russian) a form of Helen, Jelena. See also Lena, Yalena.
Yelain, Yelaina, Yelainah, Yelaine, Yelana, Yelanah, Yelane, Yeleana, Yeleanah, Yeleane, Yeleena, Yeleenah, Yeleene, Yelen, Yelenah, Yelenna, Yelenne, Yelina, Yelinah, Yeline, Yellaina, Yellaine, Yellayna, Yellaynah, Yellena, Yellenah, Yellene, Yelyna, Yelynah, Yelyne, Yileana, Yileanah, Yileane, Yileena, Yileenah, Yileene, Yilina, Yilinah, Yiline, Yilyna, Yilynah, Yilyne, Ylena, Ylenia, Ylenna

Yelisabeta (Russian) a form of Elizabeth.
Yelizaveta

Yemena (Arabic) from Yemen.
Yemina, Yeminah, Yemyna, Yemynah

Yen (Chinese) yearning; desirous.
Yeni, Yenih, Yenny

Yenay (Chinese) she who loves.

Yenene (Native American) shaman.
Yenena, Yenenah, Yenina, Yeninah, Yenyna, Yenynah, Yenyne

Yenifer (Welsh) a form of Jennifer.
Yenefer, Yennifer

Yeo (Korean) mild.
Yee

Yepa (Native American) snow girl.
Yepah, Yeppa, Yeppah

Yeruti (Guarani) turtledove.

Yesenia (Arabic) flower.
Yasenya, Yeseniah, Yesenya, Yesenyah, Yesinia, Yesnia

Yesica, Yessica (Hebrew) forms of Jessica.
Yesicah, Yesicka, Yesickah, Yesika, Yesikah, Yesiko, Yessicah, Yessicka, Yessickah, Yessika, Yessikah, Yesyka

Yésica (Hebrew) a form of Jessica.

Yesim (Turkish) jade.

Yessenia (Arabic) a form of Yesenia.
Yessena, Yessenah, Yesseniah, Yessenya, Yessenyah, Yissenia

Yetta (English) a short form of Henrietta.
Yeta, Yette, Yitta, Yitty

Yeva (Ukrainian) a form of Eve.
Yevah

Yevgenia (Russian) a form of Eugenia.
Yevgena, Yevgeniah, Yevgenya, Yevgenyah, Yevgina, Yevginah, Yevgyna

Yexalén (Indigenous) star.

Yiesha (Arabic, Swahili) a form of Aisha.
Yiasha, Yieshah

Yildiz (Turkish) star.

Yín (Chinese) silver.

Ynés, Ynéz (Spanish) forms of Ines, Inez.

Ynez (Spanish) a form of Agnes. See also Ines.
Ynes, Ynesita

Yoana, Yoanna (Hebrew) forms of Joana.

Yocasta (Greek) a form of Yolanda.

Yocceline (Latin) a form of Jocelyn.

Yocelin, Yocelyn (Latin) forms of Jocelyn.
Yoceline, Yocelyne, Yuceli

Yoconda (Italian) happy and jovial.

Yohana (Hebrew) a form of Joana.
Yohanka, Yohanna, Yohannah

Yoi (Japanese) born in the evening.

Yoki (Hopi) bluebird.
Yokee, Yokie, Yoky

Yoko (Japanese) good girl.
Yo

Yolanda (Greek) violet flower. See also Iolanthe, Jolanda, Olinda.
Yolaine, Yolana, Yoland, Yolande, Yolane, Yolanna, Yolantha, Yolanthe, Yolette, Yorlanda, Youlanda, Yulanda, Yulonda

Yole (Greek) a form of Yolanda.

Yolencia (Greek) a form of Yolie.

Yolie (Greek) a familiar form of Yolanda.
Yola, Yolah, Yolee, Yoley, Yoli, Yoly

Yolihuani (Nahuatl) source of life.

Yolonda (Greek) a form of Yolanda.

Yolotli (Nahuatl) heart.

Yoloxochitl, Yoloxóhitl (Nahuatl) flower of the heart.

Yoltzin (Nahuatl) small heart.

Yoluta (Native American) summer flower.
Yolutah

Yolyamanitzin (Nahuatl) just; tender and considerate person.

Yomara (American) a combination of Yolanda + Tamara.
Yomaira, Yomarie, Yomira

Yomaris (Spanish) I am the sun.

Yon (Burmese) rabbit. (Korean) lotus blossom.
Yona, Yonna

Yone (Greek) a form of Yolanda.

Yoné (Japanese) wealth; rice.

Yonie (Hebrew) a familiar form of Yonina.
Yonee, Yoney, Yoni, Yony

Yonina (Hebrew) a form of Jonina.
Yona, Yonah, Yoneena, Yoneene, Yoninah, Yonine, Yonyna, Yonynah

Yonita (Hebrew) a form of Jonita.
Yonat, Yonati, Yonit, Yonitah, Yonyta, Yonytah

Yoomee (Coos) star.
Yoome

Yordana (Basque) descendant. See also Jordana.
Yordanah, Yordanna, Yordannah

Yori (Japanese) reliable.
Yoriko, Yoriyo

Yoselin, Yoseline, Yoselyn (Latin) forms of Jocelyn.
Yosselin, Yosseline, Yosselyn

Yosepha (Hebrew) a form of Josephine.
Yosefa, Yosifa, Yosyfa, Yuseffa

Yoshi (Japanese) good; respectful.
Yoshee, Yoshey, Yoshie, Yoshiko, Yoshiyo, Yoshy

Yovela (Hebrew) joyful heart; rejoicer.
Yovelah, Yovella, Yovelle

Yoyotli (Nahuatl) bell of the tree.

Yris (Greek) a form of Iris.

Ysabel (Spanish) a form of Isabel.
Ysabela, Ysabelah, Ysabele, Ysabell, Ysabella, Ysabellah, Ysabelle, Ysbel, Ysbella, Ysibel, Ysibela, Ysibelah, Ysibele, Ysibell, Ysibella, Ysibellah, Ysibelle, Ysobel, Ysobela, Ysobele, Ysobell, Ysobella, Ysobelle, Ysybel, Ysybela, Ysybelah, Ysybele, Ysybell, Ysybella, Ysybellah, Ysybelle

Ysann, Ysanne (American) combinations of Ysabel + Ann.
Ysande, Ysanna, Ysannah

Ysbail (Welsh) to trip.

Ysbaíl (Welsh) spoiled.

Yseult (German) ice rule. (Irish) fair; light skinned. (Welsh) a form of Isolde.
Yseulte, Ysolde, Ysolt

Yu BG (Chinese) universe.
Yue

Yuana (Spanish) a form of Juana.
Yuan, Yuanah, Yuanna, Yuannah

Yudelle (English) a form of Udele.
Yudela, Yudelah, Yudele, Yudelia, Yudeliah, Yudell, Yudella, Yudellah, Yudelya, Yudelyah

Yudita (Russian) a form of Judith.
Yudit, Yuditah, Yudith, Yuditt, Yuditta, Yudyta, Yudytah, Yudytta, Yudyttah

Yuki BG (Japanese) snow.
Yukee, Yukey, Yukie, Yukiko, Yukiyo, Yuky

Yulene (Basque) a form of Julia.
Yulean, Yuleana, Yuleanah, Yuleane, Yuleen, Yuleena, Yuleenah, Yuleene, Yulena, Yulenah

Yulia (Russian) a form of Julia.
Yula, Yulah, Yulenka, Yulinka, Yulka, Yulya, Yulyah

Yuliana (Spanish) a form of Juliana.
Yulenia, Yuliani

Yuliya (Russian) a form of Julia.

Yuri GB (Japanese) lily.
Yuree, Yuriko, Yuriyo, Yury

Yvanna (Slavic) a form of Ivana.
Yvan, Yvana, Yvanah, Yvania, Yvaniah, Yvannah, Yvannia, Yvannya, Yvannyah

Yvette (French) a familiar form of Yvonne. See also Evette, Ivette.
Yavette, Yevett, Yevetta, Yevette, Yvet, Yveta, Yvett, Yvetta

Yvonne (French) young archer. (Scandinavian) yew wood; bow wood. See also Evonne, Ivonne, Vonna, Vonny, Yvette.
Yavanda, Yavanna, Yavanne, Yavonda, Yavonna, Yavonne, Yveline, Yvon, Yvone, Yvonna, Yvonnah, Yvonnia, Yvonnie, Yvonny

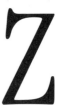

Zaba (Hebrew) she who offers a sacrifice to God.

Zabrina (American) a form of Sabrina.
Zabreana, Zabreanah, Zabreane, Zabreena, Zabreenah, Zabreenia, Zabreeniah, Zabrinah, Zabrine, Zabrinia, Zabriniah, Zabrinna,

Zabrinnah, Zabrinnia, Zabrinniah, Zabryna, Zabrynah, Zabryne, Zabrynia, Zabryniah, Zabrynya, Zabrynyah

Zacharie BG (Hebrew) God remembered.
Zacara, Zacarah, Zacaree, Zacari, Zacaria, Zacariah, Zaccaree, Zaccari, Zacceaus, Zacchaea, Zachoia, Zackaria, Zackeisha, Zackeria, Zakaria, Zakariah, Zakelina, Zakeshia, Zakira, Zechari, Zecharie

Zachary BG (Hebrew) a form of Zacharie.
Zacarey, Zaccarey, Zackery, Zakary, Zakarya, Zakaryah, Zechary

Zada (Arabic) fortunate, prosperous.
Zayda, Zayeda

Zafina (Arabic) victorious.
Zafinah, Zafyna, Zafynah

Zafirah (Arabic) successful; victorious.
Zafira, Zafire, Zafyra, Zafyrah, Zafyre

Zahar (Hebrew) daybreak; dawn.
Zaher, Zahir, Zahyr

Zahara (Swahili) a form of Zahra.
Zaharra, Zahera, Zaherah, Zahira, Zahirah, Zahyra, Zahyrah, Zeeherah

Zahavah (Hebrew) golden.
Zachava, Zachavah, Zahavya, Zahavyah, Zechava, Zechavah, Zehava, Zehavah, Zehavi, Zehavia, Zehaviah, Zehavit, Zeheva, Zehuva

Zahra (Swahili) flower. (Arabic) white.
Sahra, Zahraa, Zahrah, Zahreh, Zahria, Zahriah

Zaida (Arabic) a form of Zada.

Zaída (Arabic) a form of Zada.

Zaidee (Arabic) rich.
Zaidea, Zaidey, Zaidi, Zaidie, Zaidy, Zaydea, Zaydee, Zaydi, Zaydie, Zaydy

Zaina (Spanish, English) a form of Zanna.
Zainah, Zainna

Zainab (Iranian) child of Ali.

Zainabu (Swahili) beautiful.

Zaira (Hebrew) a form of Zara.
Zairah, Zairea, Zirrea

Zaire BG (Hebrew) a short form of Zara.
Zair

Zakelina (Russian) a form of Zacharie.
Zacelina, Zacelinah, Zaceline, Zacelyn, Zacelyna, Zacelynah, Zacelyne, Zackelin, Zackelina, Zackelinah, Zackeline, Zackelyn, Zackelyna, Zackelynah, Zackelyne, Zakeleana, Zakeleanah, Zakeleane, Zakeleen, Zakeleena, Zakeleene, Zakelin, Zakelinah, Zakeline, Zakelyn, Zakelyna, Zakelynah, Zakelyne

Zakia GB (Swahili) smart. (Arabic) chaste.
Zakea, Zakeia, Zakiah

Zakira (Hebrew) a form of Zacharie.
Zaakira, Zakiera, Zakierra, Zakir, Zakirah, Zakiria, Zakiriya, Zykarah, Zykera, Zykeria, Zykerria, Zykira, Zykuria

Zakiya (Arabic) a form of Zakia.
Zakaya, Zakeya, Zakeyia, Zakiyaa, Zakiyah, Zakiyya, Zakiyyah, Zakkiyya, Zakkiyyah, Zakkyyah, Zakya, Zakyah, Zakyya, Zakyyah

Zali (Polish) a form of Sara.
Zalea, Zaleah, Zalee, Zalei, Zaleigh, Zaley, Zalia, Zaliah, Zalie, Zaly, Zalya, Zalyah

Zalika (Swahili) born to royalty.
Salika, Zalik, Zalikah, Zalyka, Zalykah, Zuleika

Zalina (French) a form of Salina.
Zalean, Zaleana, Zaleanah, Zaleane, Zaleen, Zaleena, Zaleenah, Zaleene, Zalena, Zalenah, Zalene, Zalinah, Zaline, Zalyna, Zalynah, Zalyne

Zaltana (Native American) high mountain.
Zaltanah

Zamantha (Hebrew) a form of Samantha.
Zamanthia, Zamanthiah, Zammantha, Zammanthah, Zammanthia, Zammanthiah, Zammanthya, Zammanthyah

Zami (Hebrew) a form of Sami.
Zama, Zamah, Zamee, Zamey, Zamia, Zamiah, Zamie, Zamm, Zamma, Zammah, Zammi, Zammia, Zammiah, Zammie, Zammy, Zammya, Zammyah, Zamy, Zamya, Zamyah

Zamuela (Hebrew) a form of Samuela.
Zamuelah, Zamuele, Zamuell, Zamuella, Zamuellah, Zamuelle

Zana (Spanish, English) a form of Zanna.

Zandi (Greek) a form of Sandi.
Zandea, Zandee, Zandey, Zandia, Zandiah,
Zandie, Zandy

Zandra (Greek) a form of Sandra.
Zahndra, Zandrah, Zandrie, Zandry,
Zanndra, Zondra

Zandria (Greek) a form of Zandra.
Zandrea, Zandreah, Zandriah, Zandrya,
Zandryah

Zandrine (Greek) a form of Sandrine.
Zandreen, Zandreena, Zandreenah, Zandreene,
Zandreina, Zandreinah, Zandreine, Zandrina,
Zandrinah, Zandryn, Zandryna, Zandrynah,
Zandryne

Zaneta (Spanish) a form of Jane.
Saneta, Sanete, Sanetta, Zaneata, Zaneatah,
Zaneeta, Zaneetah, Zanetah, Zanete, Zanett,
Zanetta, Zanettah, Zanette, Zanita, Zanitah,
Zanitra, Zanyta, Zanytah

Zanna (Spanish) a form of Jane. (English) a
short form of Susanna.
Zanae, Zanah, Zanella, Zanette, Zannah,
Zannette, Zannia, Zannie, Zannya, Zannyah

Zanthe (Greek) a form of Xanthe.
Zanth, Zantha, Zanthia, Zanthiah

Zantina (Spanish) a form of Santina.
Zantinah, Zantine, Zantyna, Zantynah,
Zantyne

Zara, Zarah (Hebrew) forms of Sarah, Zora.
Zareh, Zarra, Zarrah

Zari (Hebrew) a form of Zara.
Zaree, Zareen, Zarie, Zarri, Zarrie, Zarry, Zary

Zaria (Hebrew) a form of Zara.
Zarea, Zareea, Zareena, Zareya, Zariah,
Zariya, Zarria, Zarriah, Zarya, Zaryah

Zarifa (Arabic) successful.
Zarifah, Zaryfa, Zaryfah

Zarika (Hebrew) a form of Sarika.
Zareaka, Zareakah, Zareeka, Zareekah,
Zareka, Zarekah, Zarikah, Zarka, Zarkah

Zarina (Hebrew) a form of Sarina.
Zareana, Zareanah, Zareane, Zareena,
Zareenah, Zareene, Zarena, Zarenah, Zarene,
Zarinah, Zarine, Zarinna, Zarinnah, Zarinne,
Zaryna, Zarynah, Zaryne, Zarynna,
Zarynnah

Zarita (Spanish) a form of Sarah.
Zareata, Zareatah, Zareate, Zareeta, Zareetah,
Zareete, Zaritah, Zarite, Zaritta, Zarittah,
Zaritte, Zaryt, Zaryta, Zarytah, Zaryte

Zasha (Russian) a form of Sasha.
Zascha, Zashenka, Zashka, Zasho

Zavannah (Spanish) a form of Savannah.
Zavana, Zavanah, Zavanna, Zevana,
Zevanah, Zevanna, Zevannah

Zaviera (Spanish) a form of Xaviera.
Zavera, Zaverah, Zavierah, Zaviere, Zavira,
Zavirah, Zavyera, Zavyerah

Zavrina (English) a form of Sabrina.

Zawati (Swahili) gift.
Zawatia, Zawatiah, Zawaty, Zawatya,
Zawatyah

Zayit BG (Hebrew) olive.
Zayita

Zayna (Arabic) a form of Zaynah.

Zaynab (Iranian) a form of Zainab.

Zaynah (Arabic) beautiful.
Zayn

Zayra (Hebrew) a form of Zara.

Zaza (Hebrew) golden.
Zazah, Zazu

Zea (Latin) grain. See also Zia.
Sea, Zeah

Zebina (Greek) hunter's dart.

Zecharia BG (Hebrew) a form of Zachariah
(see Boys' Names).

Zedislava (German) glory, honor.

Zefiryn (Polish) a form of Zephyr.
Zafirin, Zafirina, Zafirinah, Zefiryna,
Zefirynah, Zefyrin, Zefyrina, Zefyrinah,
Zefyryn, Zefyryna, Zefyrynah

Zeina (Greek, Ethiopian, Persian) a form of
Zena.
Zein

Zeinab (Somali) good.

Zelda (Yiddish) gray haired. (German) a
short form of Griselda. See also Selda.
Zeldah, Zelde, Zella, Zellda

Zelena (Greek) a form of Selena.
Zeleana, Zeleanah, Zeleena, Zeleenah,
Zelenah, Zelina, Zelinah, Zelyna, Zelynah

Zelene (English) sunshine.
Zelean, Zeleane, Zeleen, Zeleene, Zelen,
Zeline, Zelyn, Zelyne

Zelia (Spanish) sunshine.
Zele, Zeliah, Zelie, Zélie, Zelya, Zelyah

Zelizi (Basque) a form of Sheila.
Zelizia, Zeliziah, Zelzya, Zelzyah

Zelma (German) a form of Selma.
Zalmah

Zelmira (Arabic) brilliant one.

Zeltzin (Nahuatl) delicate.

Zemirah (Hebrew) song of joy.
Senira, Senyra, Zemir, Zemira, Zemyr,
Zemyra, Zemyrah, Zimira, Zimirah, Zymira,
Zymirah, Zymyra, Zymyrah

Zena (Ethiopian) news. (Persian) woman.
(Greek) a form of Xenia. See also Zina.
Zanae, Zanah, Zeena, Zeenat, Zeenet,
Zenah, Zenana, Zenna, Zennah

Zenadia (Greek) she who is dedicated to
God.

Zenaida (Greek) white-winged dove.
Zenaidah, Zenayda, Zenochka

Zenaide (Greek) a form of Zenaida.
Zenaïde, Zenayde

Zenda GB (Persian) sacred; feminine.
Senda, Zendah

Zenia (Greek, Ethiopian, Persian) a form of
Zena.
Zeenia, Zeenya, Zenea, Zeniah, Zennia,
Zenya, Zenyah

Zenobia (Greek) sign, symbol. History: a
queen who ruled the city of Palmyra in
ancient Syria.
Senobe, Senobia, Senovia, Zeba, Zeeba,
Zenobiah, Zenobie, Zenobya, Zenobyah,
Zenovia

Zeonchka (Russian) comes from Zeus.

Zephania (Greek) a form of Stephanie.
Zepania, Zephanas, Zephaniah, Zephanya,
Zephanyah

Zephanie (Greek) a form of Stephanie.
Zephanee, Zephaney, Zephani, Zephany

Zephrine (English) breeze.
Sephrine, Zephrean, Zephreana, Zephreanah,
Zephreane, Zephreen, Zephreena, Zephreenah,
Zephreene, Zephrin, Zephrina, Zephrinah,
Zephryn, Zephryna, Zephrynah, Zephryne,
Zephyrine

Zephyr BG (Greek) west wind.
Zephra, Zephria, Zephyer

Zera (Hebrew) seeds.
Zerah, Zeriah

Zerdali (Turkish) wild apricot.
Zerdalia, Zerdaly, Zerdalya

Zerena (Latin) a form of Serena.
Zerenah, Zirena, Zirenah, Zyrena, Zyrenah

Zerlina (Latin, Spanish) beautiful dawn.
Music: a character in Mozart's opera *Don
Giovanni*.
Serlina, Serlyna, Serlyne, Zerla, Zerlean,
Zerleana, Zerleanah, Zerleane, Zerlee,
Zerleen, Zerleena, Zerleenah, Zerleene,
Zerlinah, Zerlinda, Zerline, Zerlyn, Zerlyna,
Zerlynah, Zerlyne

Zerrin (Turkish) golden.
Zerran, Zerren, Zerron, Zerryn

Zeta (English) rose. Linguistics: a letter in
the Greek alphabet.
Zetana

Zetta (Portuguese) rose.

Zhana (Slavic) a form of Jane.
Zhanae, Zhanay, Zhanaya, Zhanea, Zhanee,
Zhaney, Zhani, Zhaniah, Zhanna

Zhane (Slavic) a form of Jane.

Zhané (Slavic) a form of Jane.

Zhen (Chinese) chaste.
Zen, Zenn, Zhena

Zi (Chinese) beautiful; with grace.

Zia GB (Latin) grain. (Arabic) light. See also
Zea.
Sia, Ziah, Zya, Zyah

Ziang (Chinese) a form of Xiang.
Zeang, Zeeang, Zyang

Zidanelia (Greek) she who is God's judge.

Zigana (Hungarian) gypsy girl. See also
Tsigana.
Ziganah, Zigane, Zygana, Zyganah

Zihna (Hopi) one who spins tops.
Zihnah, Zyhna, Zyhnah

Zilia (Greek) a form of Sylvia.
Ziliah, Zylia, Zyliah, Zylina, Zylyna

Zilla (Hebrew) shadow.
*Sila, Zila, Zilah, Zillah, Zyla, Zylah, Zylla,
Zyllah*

Zilpah (Hebrew) dignified. Bible: Jacob's wife.
Silpah, Zilpha, Zylpa, Zylpah, Zylpha

Zilya (Russian) a form of Theresa.
Zilyah, Zylya, Zylyah

Zimena (Spanish) a form of Simone.
*Zimenah, Zimene, Zimona, Zimonah,
Zimone, Zymena, Zymenah, Zymona,
Zymonah*

Zimra 🅱🅶 (Hebrew) song of praise.
*Zamira, Zamora, Zamyra, Zemira, Zemora,
Zemyra, Zimria, Zimrria, Zymria, Zymriah,
Zymrya, Zymryah*

Zina (African) secret spirit. (English) hospitable. (Greek) a form of Zena.
Zeena, Zinah, Zine, Zyhna, Zyna, Zynah

Zinerva (Italian) fair, light-haired.
Zinervah, Zynerva, Zynervah

Zinnia (Latin) Botany: a plant with beauti-
ful, colorful flowers.
*Zeenia, Zinia, Ziniah, Zinniah, Zinny,
Zinnya, Zinya, Zynia, Zyniah, Zynyah*

Zipporah (Hebrew) bird. Bible: Moses' wife.
*Cipora, Sipora, Sippora, Zipora, Ziporah,
Zipporia, Ziproh, Zypora, Zyporah, Zyppora,
Zypporah*

Zirina (Greek) a form of Sirena.
*Zireena, Zireenah, Zirinah, Ziryna, Zirynah,
Zyreena, Zyreenah, Zyrina, Zyrinah, Zyryna,
Zyrynah*

Zita (Spanish) rose. (Arabic) mistress. A short
form of names ending in "sita" or "zita."
Zeeta, Zitah, Zyta, Zytah, Zytka

Ziva (Hebrew) bright; radiant.
*Zeeva, Ziv, Zivanka, Zivi, Zivit, Zyva,
Zyvah*

Zizi (Hungarian) a familiar form of
Elizabeth.
Zsi Zsi, ZyZy

Zoa (Greek) a form of Zoe.

Zobeida (Arabic) pleasant as cream.

Zocha (Polish) a form of Sophie.
Zochah

Zoe ☀ 🅶🅱 (Greek) life.
*Zoé, Zoë, Zoee, Zoelie, Zoeline, Zoelle, Zowe,
Zowey, Zowie*

Zoey (Greek) a form of Zoe.
Zooey

Zofia (Slavic) a form of Sophia. See also
Sofia.
*Zofee, Zofey, Zofi, Zofiah, Zofie, Zofka, Zofy,
Zophee, Zophey, Zophi, Zophia, Zophiah,
Zophie, Zophya, Zophyah*

Zohar 🅱🅶 (Hebrew) shining, brilliant.
Zohara, Zoharah, Zohera, Zoheret

Zohra (Hebrew) blossom.
Zohrah

Zohreh (Persian) happy.
Zahreh, Zohrah

Zoie (Greek) a form of Zoe.
Zoi, Zoye

Zoila (Italian) a form of Zola.

Zola 🅶🅱 (Italian) piece of earth.
Zoela, Zolah

Zona (Latin) belt, sash.
Zonah, Zonia

Zondra (Greek) a form of Zandra.
*Zohndra, Zohndria, Zohndriah, Zohndrya,
Zohndryah, Zondrah, Zondria, Zondriah,
Zondrya, Zondryah*

Zora (Slavic) aurora; dawn. See also Zara.
*Sora, Zorah, Zorane, Zorna, Zorra, Zorrah,
Zory, Zorya*

Zoraida (Arabic) she who is eloquent.

Zorina (Slavic) golden.
*Sorina, Zorana, Zoranah, Zorean, Zoreana,
Zoreanah, Zoreane, Zoreen, Zoreena,
Zoreenah, Zoreene, Zori, Zorie, Zorin,
Zorinah, Zorine, Zoryna, Zorynah, Zoryne*

Zósima (Greek) vital, vigorous.

Zoya (Slavic) a form of Zoe.
Zoia, Zoiah, Zoy, Zoyah, Zoyara, Zoyechka, Zoyenka, Zoyya, Zoyyah

Zsa Zsa (Hungarian) a familiar form of Susan.
Zhazha

Zsofia (Hungarian) a form of Sofia.
Zsofi, Zsofiah, Zsofie, Zsofika, Zsofy, Zsophee, Zsophey, Zsophi, Zsophia, Zsophiah, Zsophie, Zsophy

Zsuzsanna (Hungarian) a form of Susanna.
Zsuska, Zsuzsa, Zsuzsi, Zsuzsika, Zsuzska

Zubaida (Arabic) excellent.

Zubaidah (Arabic) excellent.

Zudora (Sanskrit) laborer.
Zudorah

Zulecia, Zuleica, Zuleyca (Arabic) plump, chubby.

Zuleika (Arabic) brilliant.
Zeleeka, Zul, Zulay, Zulekha, Zuleyka

Zuleima (Arabic) a form of Zulima.

Zulema (Arabic) a form of Zulima.
Zulemah

Zuleyma (Arabic) a form of Zulima.
Zuleymah

Zulima (Arabic) a form of Salama.
Zalama, Zalamah, Zulimah, Zulyma, Zulymah

Zulma (Arabic) healthy and vigorous woman.

Zulmara (Spanish) a form of Zulma.

Zuly (Arabic) a short form of Zulma.

Zurafa (Arabic) lovely.
Ziraf, Zirafa, Zuruf, Zurufa

Zuri (Basque) white; light skinned. (Swahili) beautiful.
Zuree, Zurey, Zuria, Zuriah, Zurie, Zurisha, Zury, Zurya, Zuryah

Zurina, Zurine (Basque) white.

Zurisaday (Arabic) over the earth.

Zusa (Czech, Polish) a form of Susan.
Zusah, Zuza, Zuzah, Zuzana, Zuzanka, Zuzia, Zuzka, Zuzu

Zuwena (Swahili) good.
Zwena

Zyanya (Zapotec) always.

Zylina (Greek) a form of Xyleena.
Zilin, Zilina, Zilinah, Ziline, Zilyna, Zilynah, Zylin, Zylinah, Zyline, Zylyn, Zylyna, Zylynah

Zytka (Polish) rose.

Boys

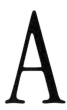

'Aziz (Arabic) strong.
Azizz

Aabha (Indian) light.

Aabharan (Indian) jewel.

Aabheer, Aabher, Abheer (Indian) cowherd.

Aacharya, Acharya (Indian) teacher.

Aadarsh (Indian) one who has principles.

Aadesh (Indian) command; message.

Aadhishankar (Indian) another name for Sri Shankaracharya, founder of Adwaitha philosophy.

Aadhunik (Indian) modern; new.

Aadi (Indian) first; most important.

Aadinath (Indian) God, supreme ruler of the universe, the first god.

Aaditey (Indian) son of Aditi.

Aafreen (Indian) encouragement.

Aagney (Indian) son of the fire god.

Aahlaad (Indian) delight.

Aahlaadith (Indian) joyous person.

Aahwaanith (Indian) one who has been invited; wanted.

Aakaash, Aakash, Akaash, Akash (Indian) the sky; vast like the sky.

Aakanksh (Indian) desire.

Aakar (Indian) form, shape.

Aakash (Hindi) a form of Akash.

Aalam (Indian) ruler, king.

Aalap (Indian) musical prelude.

Aalok (Indian) cry of victory.

Aamir (Hebrew, Punjabi, Arabic) a form of Amir.
Aamer

Aamod (Indian) pleasant.

Aandaleeb (Indian) bulbul bird.

Aaran (Hebrew) a form of Aaron. (Scottish) a form of Arran.

Aaron ☀ 🅱🅶 (Hebrew) enlightened. (Arabic) messenger. Bible: the brother of Moses and the first high priest. See also Ron.
Aahron, Aaren, Aareon, Aarin, Aaronn, Aeron, Arek, Arren, Arrin, Arryn

Aarón (Hebrew) a form of Aaron.

Aaronjames (American) a combination of Aaron + James.
Aaron James, Aaron-James

Aarron, Aaryn (Hebrew, Arabic) forms of Aaron.
Aarronn, Aarynn

Aashish (Indian) blessings.

Abaco (Hebrew) abacus.

Aban (Persian) Mythology: a figure associated with water and the arts.

Abasi (Swahili) stern.
Abasee, Abasey, Abasie, Abasy

Abban (Latin) white.
Abben, Abbin, Abbine, Abbon

Abbas (Arabic) lion.

Abbey 🅶🅱 (Hebrew) a familiar form of Abe.
Abbee, Abbi, Abbie, Abby, Abee, Abey, Abi, Aby

Abbón (Hebrew) a form of Abbott.

Abbott (Hebrew) father; abbot.
Ab, Abad, Abba, Abbah, Abbán, Abbé, Abboid, Abbot, Abot, Abott

Abbud (Arabic) devoted.

Abd-El-Kader (Arabic) servant of the powerful.

Abda (Hebrew) servant of God.

Abdalongo (Hebrew) servant of Elon.

Abdecalas (Hebrew) server of a dog.

Abdénago (Hebrew) Abdenago is the Babylonian name for Azarilts, one of the three companions of the prophet Daniel.

Abderico (Hebrew) rich and powerful servant.

Abdi (African) my servant.

Abdías (Hebrew) God's servant.

Abdiel (Hebrew) I serve God.

Abdikarim (Somali) slave of God.

Abdirahman (Arabic) a form of Abdulrahman.
Abdirehman

Abdiraxman (Somali) servant of divine grace.

Abdón (Hebrew) servant of God; the very helpful man.

Abdul (Arabic) servant.
Abdal, Abdeel, Abdel, Abdoul, Abdual, Abdull, Abul

Abdulaziz (Arabic) servant of the Mighty.
Abdelazim, Abdelaziz, Abdulazaz, Abdulazeez

Abdullah (Arabic) servant of Allah.
Abdala, Abdalah, Abdalla, Abdallah, Abdela, Abduala, Abdualla, Abduallah, Abdula, Abdulah, Abdulahi, Abdulha, Abdulla

Abdullahi (Arabic) a form of Adullah.

Abdulmalik (Arabic) servant of the Master.

Abdulrahman (Arabic) servant of the Merciful.
Abdelrahim, Abdelrahman, Abdolrahem, Abdularahman, Abdurrahman, Abdurram

Abe (Hebrew) a short form of Abel, Abraham. (German) a short form of Abelard.
Ab, Abb, Abbe

Abebe (Amharic) one who has flourished, thrived.

Abel (Hebrew) breath. (Assyrian) meadow. (German) a short form of Abelard. Bible: Adam and Eve's second son.
Abele, Abell, Able, Adal, Avel

Abelard (German) noble; resolute.
Abalard, Abelarde, Abelhard, Abilard

Abelardo (Spanish) a form of Abelard.

Abercio (Greek) first son.

Abernethy (Scottish) river's beginning.
Abernathie, Abernethi

Abi (Turkish) older brother.
Abbi, Abee

Abiah (Hebrew) God is my father.
Abia, Abiel, Abija, Abijah, Aviya, Aviyah, Avyya, Avyyah

Abibo (Hebrew) beloved.

Abibón (Hebrew) a form of Abibo.

Abidan (Hebrew) father of judgment.
Abiden, Abidin, Abidon, Abydan, Abyden, Abydin, Abydon, Abydyn

Abie (Hebrew) a familiar form of Abraham.
Abbie

Abiel (Hebrew) a form of Abiah.

Abihú (Hebrew) he is my father.

Abilio (Latin) expert; able.

Abimael (Hebrew) my father is God.

Abir (Hebrew) strong.
Abyr

Abiram (Hebrew) my father is great.

Abisha (Hebrew) gift of God.
Abijah, Abishai, Abishal, Abysha, Abyshah

Ableberto (Germanic) brilliant strength.

Abner (Hebrew) father of light. Bible: the commander of Saul's army.
Ab, Avner, Ebner

Abo (Hebrew) father.

Abraam (Hebrew) a form of Abraham.

Abrafo (Ghanaian) warrior.

Abraham (Hebrew) father of many nations. Bible: the first Hebrew patriarch. See also Avram, Bram, Ibrahim.
Abarran, Aberham, Abey, Abhiram, Abie, Abrahaim, Abrahame, Abrahamo, Abraheem, Abrahem, Abrahim, Abrahm, Abrao, Arram, Avram

Abrahan (Spanish) a form of Abraham.
Abrahán, Abrahin, Abrahon, Abrán

Abram (Hebrew) a short form of Abraham. See also Bram.
Abrama, Abramo, Abrams, Avram

Abrúnculo (Latin) shattered; devastated.

Absalom (Hebrew) father of peace. Bible: the rebellious third son of King David. See also Avshalom, Axel.
Absalaam, Absalon, Abselon, Absolam, Absolom, Absolum

Absalón (Hebrew) a form of Absalom.

Abubakar (Egyptian) noble.

Abudemio (Latin) one who speaks in a sweet, refined way.

Abundancio (Latin) rich, affluent.

Abundio (Latin) he who has a lot of property.

Acab (Hebrew) uncle.

Acacio (Greek) honorable.

Acañir (Mapuche) freed fox.

Acapana (Quechua) lightning; swirl of wind, small hurricane.

Acar (Turkish) bright.

Acario (Greek) without grace.

Ácatl (Nahuatl) giant reed.

Acayo (Greek) out of step; ill-timed.

Accas (Hebrew) winding.

Ace (Latin) unity.
Acer, Acey, Acie

Acel (French) nobility.

Acesto (Greek) one who can fix; useful.

Achachic (Aymara) ancestor; grandfather.

Achcauhtli (Nahuatl) leader.

Achic (Quechua) luminous, resplendent.

Achilles (Greek) Mythology: a hero of the Trojan War. Literature: the hero of Homer's epic poem *Iliad*.
Achil, Achill, Achille, Achillea, Achilleus, Achillios, Achyl, Achyll, Achylle, Achylleus, Akilles

Acilino (Spanish) sharp.

Acindino (Greek) out of danger, safe.

Acisclo (Latin) a pick used to work on rocks.

Ackerley (English) meadow of oak trees.
Accerlee, Accerleigh, Accerley, Ackerlea, Ackerlee, Ackerleigh, Ackerli, Ackerlie, Ackersley, Ackley, Akerlea, Akerlee, Akerleigh, Akerley, Akerli, Akerlie, Akerly

Ackley (English) a form of Ackerley.
Acklea, Acklee, Ackleigh, Ackli, Acklie, Ackly, Aklea, Aklee, Akleigh, Akley, Akli, Aklie, Akly

Aconcauac (Quechua) stone sentinel.

Acton (English) oak-tree settlement.
Actan, Acten, Actin, Actun, Actyn

Acucio (Latin) sharp; shrewd.

Acursio (Latin) he who heads toward God.

Adabaldo (German) noble and bold.

Adacio (Latin) determined; active.

Adael (Hebrew) eternity of God.

Adahy (Cherokee) in the woods.
Adahi

Adair GB (Scottish) oak-tree ford.
Adaire, Adare, Adayr, Adayre, Addair, Addaire, Addar, Addare, Addayr, Addyre

Adalbaro (Greek) the combatant of nobility.

Adalbergo (German) village.

Adalberón (Spanish) a form of Adalbergo.

Adalberto (Italian, Spanish, Portuguese) a form of Alberto.

Adalgiso, Adalvino (Greek) the lance of nobility.

Adalhardo (Scandinavian) noble and strong.

Adalrico (Greek) noble chief of his lineage.

Adam ☼ (Phoenician) man; mankind. (Hebrew) earth; man of the red earth. Bible: the first man created by God. See also Adamson, Addison, Damek, Keddy, Macadam.
Ad, Adama, Adamec, Adamo, Adão, Adas, Adem, Adham, Adhamh, Adim, Adné, Adok, Adom, Adomas, Adym, Edam, Edem, Edim, Edym

Adám (Hebrew) a form of Adam.

Adamec (Czech) a form of Adam.
Adamek, Adamik, Adamka, Adamko, Adamok

Adamnán (Hebrew) a form of Adan.

Adamson (Hebrew) son of Adam.
Adams, Adamsson, Addams, Addamson

Adan (Irish) a form of Aidan.
Adian, Adun

Adar GB (Syrian) ruler; prince. (Hebrew) noble; exalted.
Addar, Addare

Adarius (American) a combination of Adam + Darius.
Adareus, Adarias, Adarrius, Adarro, Adarruis, Adaruis, Adauris

Adaucto (Latin) increase.

Adauto (Roman) increased.

Addam (Phoenician, Hebrew) a form of Adam.

Addison BG (English) son of Adam.
Addis, Addisen, Addisun, Addoson, Addyson

Addo (Ghanaian) king of the path.

Addy GB (Hebrew) a familiar form of Adam, Adlai. (German) a familiar form of Adelard.
Addey, Addi, Addie, Ade, Adi

Ade (Yoruba) royal.

Adeel (Arabic) a form of Adil.
Adeele

Adel (German) a short form of Adelard.
Adal, Addel, Adél, Adell

Adelard (German) noble; courageous.
Adalar, Adalard, Adalarde, Adelar, Adelarde, Adelhard

Adelardo (Greek) the daring prince.

Adelelmo, Adelmo (German) noble protector.

Adelfo (Greek) male friend.

Adelgario (German) noble lance.

Adelino (Greek) the daring prince.

Adelio (Spanish) father of the noble prince.

Adelmaro (Greek) distinguished because of his lineage.

Adelric (German) noble ruler.
Adalric, Adelrich, Adelrick, Adelrik, Adelryc, Adelryck, Adelryk

Ademar, Ademaro, Adhemar, Adimar (German) he whose battles have made him distinguished; celebrated and famous combatant.

Aden (Arabic) Geography: a region in southern Yemen. (Irish) a form of Aidan.

Aderito (German) strong and powerful.

Adham (Arabic) black.

Adhelmar (Greek) ennobled by his battles.

Adiel (Hebrew) he was adorned by God.

Adif (Hebrew) the preferred one.

Adil (Arabic) just; wise.
Adill, Adyl, Adyll

Adilón (Spanish) noble.

Adin (Hebrew) pleasant.
Addin, Addyn, Adyn

Adín (Hebrew) a form of Adin.

Adino (Hebrew) adorned.

Adiosdado (Latin) given by God.

Adir (Hebrew) majestic; noble.
Adeer

Adirán (Latin) from the Adriatic Sea.

Adisa (Ghanaian) one who teaches us.

Adison BG (English) a form of Addison.
Adisson, Adyson

Aditya (Hindi) sun.

Adiv (Hebrew) pleasant; gentle.
Adeev, Adev

Adjatay (Cameroon) prince.

Adjutor (Latin) one who helps.

Adlai (Hebrew) my ornament.
Ad, Addlai, Addlay, Adlay

Adler (German) eagle.
Ad, Addlar, Addler, Adlar

Adli (Turkish) just; wise.
Adlea, Adlee, Adleigh, Adley, Adlie, Adly

Admiel (Hebrew) land of God.

Admon (Hebrew) peony.

Adnan (Arabic) pleasant.
Adnaan, Adnane

Adney (English) noble's island.
Adnee, Adni, Adnie, Adny

Ado (Hebrew) beauty.

Adofo (Ghanaian) one who loves us.

Adolf (German) noble wolf. History: Adolf
Hitler's German army was defeated in
World War II. See also Dolf.
Ad, Addof, Addoff, Adof

Adolfo (Spanish) a form of Adolf.
*Addofo, Adolffo, Adolpho, Andolffo, Andolfo,
Andolpho*

Adolph (German) a form of Adolf.
Adolphe

Adolphus (French) a form of Adolf.
Adolfius, Adolfus, Adolphius, Adulphus

Adom (Akan) help from God.

Adon (Hebrew) Lord. (Greek) a short form
of Adonis.

Adón (Hebrew) a form of Adon.

Adonai (Hebrew) my Lord.

Adonías (Hebrew) God is my Lord.

Adonis (Greek) highly attractive.
Mythology: the attractive youth loved by
Aphrodite.
Adonise, Adonnis, Adonys, Adonyse

Adri (Indo-Pakistani) rock.
Adree, Adrey, Adrie, Adry

Adrian ☀ 🅱🅶 (Greek) rich. (Latin) dark.
(Swedish) a short form of Hadrian.
*Adarian, Ade, Adorjan, Adrain, Adreian,
Adreyan, Adriaan, Adriane, Adriann,
Adrianne, Adrianus, Adriean, Adrin, Adrion,
Adrionn, Adrionne, Adron, Adryan, Adryn,
Adryon*

Adrián (Latin) a form of Adrian.

Adriano (Italian) a form of Adrian.
Adrianno

Adriel (Hebrew) member of God's flock.
Adrial, Adriall, Adriell, Adryel, Adryell

Adrien 🅱🅶 (French) a form of Adrian.
Adriene, Adrienne, Adryen

Adrik (Russian) a form of Adrian.
Adric

Adrodato (Germanic) daring father.

Adulfo (Germanic) of noble heritage.

Adwin (Ghanaian) creative.
Adwyn

Adyuto, Adyutor (Latin) one who helps.

Aeneas (Greek) praised. (Scottish) a form of
Angus. Literature: the Trojan hero of Vergil's
epic poem *Aeneid*. See also Eneas.
Oneas

Afework (Ethiopian) one who speaks of
pleasing things.

Afonso (German) prepared for combat.

Afram (African) Geography: a river in
Ghana, Africa.

África (Greek) left to the sun.

Afrodisio (Greek) amorous.

Afton 🅶🅱 (English) from Afton, England.
Affton, Aftan, Aften, Aftin, Aftyn

Aftonio (Greek) one who does not have
jealousy.

Agabio (Greek) of much life, vigor.

Ágabos (Greek) magnificent.

Agacio (Greek) good.

Agamemnon (Greek) resolute. Mythology:
the king of Mycenae who led the Greeks
in the Trojan War.

Agamenón (Greek) a form of Agamemnon.

Ágape (Latin) love.

Agapito (Hebrew) the beloved one.

Agar (Hebrew) he who escaped.

Agatángel (Greek) good angel.

Agatodoro (Greek) worthy of admiration.

Agatón (Greek) the victor.

Agatónico (Greek) good victory.

Agatopo (Greek) nice scenery.

Agatópode, Agatópodis (Greek) good feet.

Agberto (German) famous for the sword.

Agenor (Greek) the strong man.

Agento (Latin) efficient; active.

Ageo (Hebrew) having a festive character, makes people happy.

Agerico (Latin) powerful sword.

Agesislao (Greek) leader of villages.

Agila (Teutonic) he who possesses combat support.

Agilberto (German) famous sword from combat.

Agileo (German) spade of a fighter.

Agilulfo (German) spear of the warrior.

Agliberto (German) a form of Agilberto.

Agnelo (Latin) reference to the lamb of God.

Agni (Hindi) Religion: the Hindu fire god.

Agoardo (German) strong sword.

Agobardo (German) strong spear.

Agofredo (German) spear that brings peace.

Agomar (German) distinguished sword.

Agostino (Italian) a form of Augustine.
Agostine, Agosto, Agoston, Agostyne

Agresto (Latin) rugged, rustic.

Agrícola (Latin) farmer.

Agrippa (Latin) born feet first. History: the commander of the Roman fleet that defeated Mark Antony and Cleopatra at Actium.
Agripa, Agripah, Agrippah, Agrypa, Agrypah, Agryppa, Agryppah

Agu (Ibo) leopard.

Aguinaldo (Germanic) one who rules by the sword.

Agur (Hebrew) accumulation.

Agús (Spanish) a form of Agustín.

Agustin (Latin) a form of Augustine.
Aguistin, Agustein, Agusteyne, Agustis, Agusto, Agustus, Agustyn

Agustín (Latin) a form of Agustin.

Agustine (Latin) a form of Augustine.
Agusteen, Agustyne

Ahab (Hebrew) father's brother. Literature: the captain of the Pequod in Herman Melville's novel *Moby-Dick*.

Ahanu (Native American) laughter.

Aharon (Hebrew, Arabic) a form of Aaron.
Ahren

Ahdik (Native American) caribou; reindeer.
Ahdic, Ahdick, Ahdyc, Ahdyck, Ahdyk

Ahearn (Scottish) lord of the horses. (English) heron.
Ahearne, Aherin, Ahern, Aherne, Aheron, Aheryn, Hearn, Hearne

Ahir (Turkish) last.

Ahkeem (Hebrew) a form of Akeem.
Ahkiem, Ahkieme, Ahkyem, Ahkyeme

Ahmad (Arabic) most highly praised. See also Muhammad.
Achmad, Ahamad, Ahamada, Ahmaad, Ahmaud, Amad, Amahd

Ahmed (Swahili) praiseworthy.
Achmed, Ahamed, Amed

Ahsan (Arabic) charitable.

Ahuatzi (Nahuatl) small oak.

Ahuiliztli (Nahuatl) joy.

Ahuv (Hebrew) loved.

Ahuviá (Hebrew) loved by God.

Aicardo (German) strong sword.

Aidan ☆ BG (Irish) fiery.
Aidun, Aydan, Aydin

Aidano (Teutonic) he who distinguishes himself.

Aiden ☆ BG (Irish) a form of Aidan.
Aidon, Aidwin, Aidwyn, Aidyn

Aiken (English) made of oak.
Aicken, Aikin, Ayken, Aykin

Aimario (German) strong lineage.

Aimery (French) a form of Emery.
Aime, Aimeree, Aimerey, Aimeri, Aimeric,
Aimerie, Ameree, Amerey, Ameri, Americ,
Amerie, Aymeree, Aymerey, Aymeri, Aymeric,
Aymerie, Aymery

Aimon (French) house. (Irish) a form of
Eamon.

Aindrea (Irish) a form of Andrew.
Aindreas, Ayndrea, Ayndreas

Aingeru (Basque) angel.

Ainsley GB (Scottish) my own meadow.
Ainslea, Ainslee, Ainslei, Ainsleigh, Ainsli,
Ainslie, Ainsly, Ansley, Aynslea, Aynslee,
Aynsley, Aynsli, Aynslie, Aynsly

Aitalas (Greek) eternally young.

Aitor (Basque) father.

Aizik (Russian) a form of Isaac.
Ayzik

Aj (Punjabi, American) a form of Ajay.

Ajab (Hebrew) uncle.

Ajala (Yoruba) potter.
Ajalah

Aján (Hebrew) problem.

Ajay (Punjabi) victorious; undefeatable.
(American) a combination of the initials A.
+ J.
Aja, Ajae, Ajai, Ajaye, Ajaz, Ajé, Ajee, Ajit

Ajidan (Hebrew) my brother judges.

Ajiel (Hebrew) my brother is God.

Ajiezer (Hebrew) my brother is help.

Ajimán (Hebrew) my brother is manna.

Ajiram (Hebrew) my brother exalted.

Ajishar (Hebrew) my brother sings.

Ajit (Sanskrit) unconquerable.
Ajeet, Ajith

Ajitov (Hebrew) my brother is good.

Ajshalom (Hebrew) brother of peace.

Akar (Turkish) flowing stream.
Akara, Akare

Akash (Hindi) sky.
Akasha

Akbar (Arabic) great.
Akbara, Akbare

Akecheta (Sioux) warrior.
Akechetah

Akeem (Hebrew) a short form of Joachim.
Ackeem, Akeam, Akee, Akiem, Arkeem

Akemi (Japanese) dawn.
Akemee, Akemie, Akemy

Akhil (Arabic) a form of Akil.
Ahkeel

Akia (African) first born.

Akiiki (Egyptian) friendly.

Akil (Arabic) intelligent. (Greek) a form of
Achilles.
Akeel, Akeil, Akeyla, Akiel, Akila, Akilah,
Akile, Akyl, Akyle

Akili BG (Greek) a form of Achilles. (Arabic)
a form of Akil.

Akim (Hebrew) a short form of Joachim.
Achim, Achym, Ackim, Ackime, Ackym,
Ackyme, Akima, Akym

Akins (Yoruba) brave.
Akin, Akyn, Akyns, Atkins, Atkyns

Akinsanya (Nigerian) courage for the
rematch.

Akintunde (Nigerian) courageous return.

Akinyemi (Nigerian) destined to be a warrior.

Akio (Japanese) bright.
Akiyo, Akyo

Akira GB (Japanese) intelligent.
Akihito, Akirah, Akyra, Akyrah

Akiva (Hebrew) a form of Jacob.
Akiba

Akmal (Arabic) perfect.
Ackmal

Akram (Arabic) most generous.

Aksel (Norwegian) father of peace.
Aksell

Akshat (Sanskrit) unable to be injured.

Akshay (American) a form of Akash.
Akshaj, Akshaya

Akule (Native American) he looks up.
Akul

Al (Irish) a short form of Alan, Albert, Alexander.

Alaa GB (Arabic) a short form of Aladdin.
Ala

Alacrino (Latin) alive; outgoing.

Aladdin (Arabic) height of faith. Literature: the hero of a story in the *Arabian Nights*.
Alaaddin, Aladan, Aladdan, Aladden, Aladdyn, Aladean, Aladen, Aladin, Aladino, Aladyn

Alain (French) a form of Alan.
Alaen, Alaine, Alainn, Alayn, Alein, Aleine, Aleyn, Aleyne, Allain, Allayn, Allayne

Alaire (French) joyful.
Alair, Alayr, Alayre

Alam (Arabic) universe.
Alame

Alan (Irish) handsome; peaceful.
Ailan, Ailin, Alaan, Aland, Alande, Alando, Alane, Alani, Alann, Alano, Alanson, Alao, Alon, Alun, Alune, Alyn, Alyne

Alán (Celtic) a form of Alan.

Alante, Allante, Allanté (Spanish) forms of Alan.

Alardo (Greek) the courageous prince.

Alaric (German) ruler of all. See also Ulrich.
Alarich, Alarick, Alarico, Alarik, Alaryc, Alaryck, Alaryk, Aleric, Allaric, Allarick, Alric, Alrick, Alrik

Alastair (Scottish) a form of Alexander.
Alaisdair, Alaistair, Alaister, Alasdair, Alasteir, Alaster, Alastor, Aleister, Alester, Allaistar, Allastair, Allaster, Allastir, Allysdair, Alystair

Alba (Latin) town on the white hill.

Alban (Latin) from Alba, Italy.
Albain, Albany, Albean, Albein, Alby, Auban, Auben

Albano (Germanic) a form of Alban.

Alberic (German) smart; wise ruler.
Alberich, Alberick, Alberyc, Alberyck, Alberyk

Alberico (German) a form of Alberic.

Albern (German) noble; courageous.
Alberne, Alburn, Alburne

Alberón (German) noble bear.

Albert (German, French) noble and bright. See also Elbert, Ulbrecht.
Adelbert, Ailbert, Albertik, Albertus, Albrecht, Albret, Albyrt, Albyrte, Alvertos, Aubert

Alberte (German) a form of Albert.

Alberto (Italian) a form of Albert.
Albertino, Berto

Albie, Alby (German, French) familiar forms of Albert.
Albee, Albey, Albi

Albin (Latin) a form of Alvin.
Alben, Albeno, Albinek, Albino, Albins, Albinson, Albun, Alby, Albyn, Auben

Albion (Latin) white cliffs. Geography: a reference to the white cliffs in Dover, England.
Albon, Albyon, Allbion, Allbyon

Albón (German, Spanish) brave ruler.

Albuino (German) powerful; noble home.

Alcandor (Greek) manly; strong.

Alceo (Greek) man of great strength and vigor.

Alcibiades (Greek) generous and violent.

Alcibíades (Greek) strong and valiant man.

Alcides (Greek) strong and vigorous.

Alcott (English) old cottage.
Alcot, Alkot, Alkott, Allcot, Allcott, Allkot, Allkott

Alcuino (Teutonic) friend of sacred places, friend of the temple.

Aldair (German, English) a form of Alder.
Aldahir, Aldayr

Aldano (Celtic) noble; full of experience, experienced man.

Aldeberto (German) famous leader.

Aldebrando (German) governs with the sword.

Aldelmo (German) old helmet.

Aldemar (German) famous for nobility.

Alden 🅱🅶 (English) old; wise protector.
Aldan, Aldean, Aldin, Aldon, Aldyn

Alder (German, English) alder tree.
Aldar, Aldare, Aldyr

Alderidge (English) alder ridge.
Alderige, Aldridge, Aldrige, Aldrydge, Aldryge, Alldridge

Aldetrudis (Germanic) strong leader.

Aldino (Celtic) noble, full of experience.

Aldis (English) old house. (German) a form of Aldous.
Aldise, Aldiss, Aldys

Aldo (Italian) old; elder. (German) a short form of Aldous.
Alda

Aldobrando (Germanic) ancient sword.

Aldous (German) a form of Alden.
Aldis, Aldon, Aldos, Aldus, Elden

Aldred (English) old; wise counselor.
Alldred, Eldred

Aldrich (English) wise counselor. See also Uldric.
Aldric, Aldrick, Aldritch, Aldryc, Aldryck, Aldryk, Alldric, Alldrich, Alldrick, Eldridge

Aldwin (English) old friend.
Aldwan, Aldwen, Aldwon, Aldwyn, Eldwin, Eldwyn

Alec, Aleck, Alek (Greek) short forms of Alexander.
Aleik, Alekko, Aleko, Elek, Ellec, Elleck

Aleczander (Greek) a form of Alexander.
Alecander, Aleckxander, Alecsandar, Alecsander, Alecxander

Alefrido (Germanic) total peace.

Aleixo (Greek) defender.

Alejandrino (Spanish) a form of Alexander.

Alejandro ☆ (Spanish) a form of Alexander.
Alejandra, Aléjo, Alexjandro

Alejándro (Spanish) a form of Alejandro.

Alejo (Greek) he who protects and defends.

Aleksandar, Aleksander, Aleksandr (Greek) forms of Alexander.
Aleksandor, Aleksandras, Aleksandur

Aleksei (Russian) a short form of Alexander.
Aleks, Aleksey, Aleksi, Aleksis, Aleksy

Alekzander (Greek) a form of Alexander.
Alekxander, Alekxzander

Alem (Arabic) wise.
Alym

Alen, Allan, Allen (Irish) forms of Alan.
Allane, Allayne, Allene, Alley, Alleyn, Alleyne, Allie, Allin, Alline, Allon, Allyn, Allyne

Aleo (German) governor.

Aleric (German) a form of Alaric.
Alerick, Alerik, Alleric, Allerick, Alleryc, Alleryck, Alleryk

Aleron (Latin) winged.
Aleronn

Alerón (French) a form of Aleron.

Alesio (Italian) a form of Alejo.

Alessandro (Italian) a form of Alexander.
Alessand, Alessander, Alessandre, Allessandro

Alex ☆ 🅱🅶 (Greek) a short form of Alexander.
Alax, Alexx, Alixx, Allax, Allex, Allix, Allixx, Allyx, Allyxx, Alyx, Elek

Alexandar, Alexandr (Greek) forms of Alexander.

Alexander ☆ 🅱🅶 (Greek) defender of mankind. History: Alexander the Great was the conqueror of the civilized world. See also Alastair, Alistair, Iskander, Jando, Leks, Lex, Lexus, Macallister, Oleksandr, Olés, Sander, Sándor, Sandro, Sandy, Sasha, Xan, Xander, Zander, Zindel.
Alekos, Alexandor, Alexxander

Alexandra 🅶🅱 (Greek) a form of Alexander.

Alexandre BG (French) a form of Alexander.

Alexandro (Greek) a form of Alexander.
Alexandru

Alexandros (Greek) a form of Alexander.
Alexandras

Alexei (Russian) a form of Aleksei. (Greek) a short form of Alexander.
Alexey

Alexi GB (Greek) a short form of Alexander.
Alexe, Alexee, Alexie, Alexio, Alezio

Alexis GB (Greek) a short form of Alexander.
Alexes, Alexey, Alexios, Alexius, Alexiz, Alexsis, Alexsus, Alexus, Alexys

Alexsander (Greek) a form of Alexander.

Alexy (Greek) a short form of Alexander.

Alexzander (Greek) a form of Alexander.
Alexkzandr, Alexzandr, Alexzandyr

Aleydis (Teutonic) born into a noble family.

Alfa (African) leader.

Alferio (Greek) saint who suffered a great disease and promised to become a monk if cured.

Alfie BG (English) a familiar form of Alfred.
Alfy

Alfio (Greek) he who has a white complexion.

Alfonso, Alfonzo (Italian, Spanish) forms of Alphonse.
Affonso, Alfons, Alfonse, Alfonsus, Alfonza, Alfonzus

Alford (English) old river ford.
Allford

Alfred (English) elf counselor; wise counselor. See also Fred.
Ailfrid, Ailfryd, Alf, Alfeo, Alfredus, Alfrid, Alfried, Alfryd, Alured, Elfrid

Alfredo (Italian, Spanish) a form of Alfred.
Alfrido

Alger (German) noble spearman. (English) a short form of Algernon. See also Elger.
Aelfar, Algar, Algor, Allgar

Algerico (German) a form of Algerio.

Algerio (German) noble governor prepared for combat.

Algernon (English) bearded, wearing a moustache.
Aelgernon, Algenon, Algin, Algon

Algie (English) a familiar form of Algernon.
Algee, Algia, Algy

Algis (German) spear.
Algiss

Algiso (Greek) the lance of nobility.

Algrenon (French) beard.

Ali BG (Arabic) greatest. (Swahili) exalted.
Aly

Alí (Arabic) a form of Ali.

Alic (Greek) a short form of Alexander.
Alick, Aliek, Alik, Aliko, Alyc, Alyck, Alyk, Alyko, Ellic, Ellick

Alicio (Greek) truth.

Alijah (Hebrew) a form of Elijah.

Alim (Arabic) scholar. A form of Alem.
Alym

Alîm (Arabic) wise.

Alinando (German) daring ruler.

Alipio (Greek) he who suffering does not affect.

Alisander (Greek) a form of Alexander.
Alisandre, Alisaunder, Alissander, Alissandre, Alsandair, Alsandare, Alsander

Alistair (English) a form of Alexander.
Alisdair, Alistaire, Alistar, Allistair, Allistar, Alstair, Alystair, Alystayr, Alystyre

Alix GB (Greek) a short form of Alixander.

Alixander (Greek) a form of Alexander.
Alixandre, Alixandru, Alixsander, Alixxander, Alixxzander, Alixzander, Alyxxander, Alyxxsander, Alyxxzander, Alyxzander

Aliz (Hebrew) happy.

Alladin (Arabic) nobility of faith.

Allambee (Australian) quiet place.
Alambee, Alambey, Alambi, Alambie, Alamby, Allambey, Allambi, Allambie, Allamby

Allard (English) noble, brave.
Alard, Ellard

Allison GB (English) Alice's son.
Allisan, Allisen, Allisun, Allisyn, Allysan,
Allysen, Allysin, Allyson, Allysun, Allysyn

Allister (English) a form of Alistair.
Alister, Allistir

Almagor (Hebrew) indestructible.

Almano (German) famous for nobility.

Almanzor (Arabic) triumphant.

Almaquio (Greek) foreign combatant.

Almárico (German) rich family; powerful.

Almeric (German) powerful ruler.
Almauric, Amaurick, Amaurik, Amauryc,
Amauryck, Amauryk, Americk, Amerik,
Ameryc, Ameryck, Ameryk

Almodis (Germanic) totally spirited.

Almon (Hebrew) widower.
Alman, Almen, Almin, Almyn

Aloín (French) noble friend.

Alois (German) a short form of Aloysius.
Alaois, Aloys

Aloisio (Spanish) a form of Louis.

Alok (Sanskrit) victorious cry.

Alon (Hebrew) oak.
Allon, Alonn

Alón (Hebrew) a form of Alon.

Alonso, Alonzo (Spanish) forms of Alphonse.
Alano, Alanzo, Allonzo, Alonz, Alonze

Alonza BG (Spanish) a form of Alphonse.
Allonza

Aloyoshenka, Aloysha (Russian) defender of humanity.

Aloysius (German) a form of Louis.
Aloisius

Alpha (African) leader.

Alphonse (German) noble and eager.
Alf, Alfons, Alphons, Alphonsa, Alphonsus,
Alphonza, Alphonzus

Alphonso (Italian) a form of Alphonse.
Alphanso, Alphonzo, Fonso

Alpin (Irish) attractive.
Alpine, Alpyn, Alpyne

Alpiniano (Swiss) belongs to the Alps mountains.

Alquimio (Greek) strong.

Alredo (German) advice from the governor.

Alroy (Spanish) king.
Alroi

Alston (English) noble's settlement.
Allston, Alstan, Alsten, Alstin, Alstun, Alstyn

Altair BG (Greek) star. (Arabic) flying eagle.
Altayr, Altayre

Alterio (Greek) like a starry night.

Altman (German) old man.
Altmann, Altmen, Atman

Alton (English) old town.
Alten

Alucio (Latin) he is lucid and illustrious.

Aluín (French) noble friend.

Alula (Latin) winged, swift.

Alva BG (Hebrew) sublime.
Alvah

Alvan (German) a form of Alvin.
Alvand, Alvun

Alvar (English) army of elves.
Alvara

Àlvar, Álvaro (Spanish) forms of Alvaro.

Alvaro (Spanish) just; wise.

Alvern (Latin) spring.
Alverne, Elvern

Alvero (Germanic) completely prudent.

Alví (German) friend.

Alvin (Latin) white; light skinned. (German) friend to all; noble friend; friend of elves. See also Albin, Elvin.
Aloin, Aluin, Alvan, Alven, Alvie, Alvon, Alvy,
Alvyn, Alwin, Elwin

Alvino (Spanish) a form of Alvin.
Aluino

Alvis (Scandinavian) all-knowing.

Alwin (German) a form of Alvin.
Ailwyn, Alwan, Alwen, Alwon, Alwun,
Alwyn, Alwynn, Aylwin

Amable (Latin) one who loves; nice.

Amadeo (Italian) a form of Amadeus.

Amadeus (Latin) loves God. Music:
Wolfgang Amadeus Mozart was a famous
eighteenth-century Austrian composer.
Amad, Amadeaus, Amadée, Amadei, Amadis,
Amadou, Amando, Amedeo, Amodaos

Amado (Spanish) a form of Amadeus.
Amadio

Amador (Spanish) a form of Amadeus.

Amal GB (Hebrew) worker. (Arabic) hopeful.
Amahl

Amalio (Greek) a man who is carefree.

Aman BG (Arabic) a short form of Amani.

Amancio (Latin) he who loves God.

Amanda GB (Latin) lovable.

Amandeep BG (Punjabi) light of peace.
Amandip, Amanjit, Amanjot

Amando (French) a form of Amadeus.
Amand, Amandio, Amaniel, Amato

Amani GB (Arabic) believer. (Yoruba)
strength; builder.
Amanee

Amanpreet BG (Punjabi) a form of
Amandeep.

Amar (Punjabi) immortal. (Arabic) builder.
Amare, Amario, Amaris, Amarjit, Amaro,
Amarpreet

Amaranto (Greek) he who does not slow
down.

Amari BG (Punjabi, Arabic) a form of Amar.
Amaree, Amarri

Amaru (Quechua) sacred serpent.

Amaruquispe (Quechua) free, like the
Amaru.

Amarutopac (Quechua) glorious, majestic
Amaru.

Amaruyupanqui (Quechua) he who honors
Amaru.

Amato (French) loved.
Amat, Amatto

Amauri, Amaury (French) name of a count.

Amazu (Nigerian) no one knows
everything.

Ambar GB (Sanskrit) sky.

Amber GB (French) amber. (Sanskrit) a form
of Ambar.

Amberto (German) brilliant work.

Ambico (Latin) one who is ambitious.

Ambroise (French) a form of Ambrose.
Ambrois

Ambrose (Greek) immortal.
Ambie, Ambrogio, Ambroisius, Ambros,
Ambrosi, Ambrosio, Ambrosios, Ambrosius,
Ambrossye, Ambrosye, Ambrotos, Ambroz,
Ambrus, Amby

Ameen (Hebrew, Arabic, Hindi) a form of
Amin.

Ameer (Hebrew) a form of Amir.
Ameir, Amere

Amelio (Teutonic) very hard worker, energetic.

Amenhotep (Egyptian) name of a count.

Amenophis (Egyptian) name of the
pharaoh.

Amenra (Egyptian) personification of the
universe's power.

Amer (Hebrew) a form of Amir.

Américo (Germanic) the prince in action.

Amerigo (Teutonic) industrious. History:
Amerigo Vespucci was the Italian explorer
for whom America is named.
Americo, Americus, Amerygo

Ames (French) friend.
Amess

Amfiloquio (Greek) distinguished sword.

Amfión (Greek) argumentative.

Ami (Hebrew) the builder.

Amiano (Hebrew) a form of Amon.

Amicus (English, Latin) beloved friend.
Amic, Amick, Amicko, Amico, Amik, Amiko,
Amyc, Amyck, Amycko, Amyk, Amyko

Amiel (Hebrew) God of my people.
Amiell, Ammiel, Amyel, Amyell

Amiezer (Hebrew) my community is
helped.

Amijai (Hebrew) my community is alive.

Amílcar (Punic) he who governs the city.

Amin (Hebrew, Arabic) trustworthy; honest.
(Hindi) faithful.
Amen, Ammen, Ammin, Ammyn, Amyn,
Amynn

Amín (Arabic) a form of Amin.

Amine (Hebrew, Arabic, Hindi) a form of
Amin.

Amintor (Greek) the protector.

Amior (Hebrew) my community is light.

Amir (Hebrew) proclaimed. (Punjabi)
wealthy; king's minister. (Arabic) prince.
Amire, Amiri, Amyr

Amiram (Hebrew) my community is lifted
high.

Amish (Sanskrit) honest.

Amishalom (Hebrew) my community is
peace.

Amishar (Hebrew) my community sings.

Amistad (Spanish) friendship.

Amit (Punjabi) unfriendly. (Arabic) highly
praised.
Amita, Amitan

Amitai (Hebrew) my truth.

Ammar (Punjabi, Arabic) a form of Amar.
Ammer

Ammâr (Arabic) builder.

Ammon (Egyptian) hidden. Mythology: the
ancient god associated with reproduction.
Amman

Amnas (Greek, Latin) young lamb.

Amnicado (Latin) one who lives close to
the river.

Amol (Hindi) priceless, valuable.
Amul

Amoldo (Spanish) power of an eagle.

Amon (Hebrew) trustworthy; faithful.
Amun

Amón (Hebrew) a form of Amon.

Amory (German) a form of Emory.
Ameree, Amerey, Ameri, Amerie, Amery,
Ammeree, Ammerey, Ammeri, Ammerie,
Ammery, Ammoree, Ammorey, Ammori,
Ammorie, Ammory, Amor, Amoree, Amorey,
Amori, Amorie

Amos (Hebrew) burdened, troubled. Bible:
an Old Testament prophet.
Amose, Amous

Amós (Hebrew) a form of Amos.

Amoxtli (Nahuatl) book.

Amparo (Latin) to prepare oneself.

Ampelio (Greek) he who makes wine from
his own grapes.

Ampelos (Greek) a satyr and good friend of
Dionysus.

Ampliato (Latin) illustrious.

Ampodio (Greek) well-behaved.

Amram (Hebrew) mighty nation.
Amarien, Amran, Amren, Amryn

Amrit BG (Sanskrit) nectar. (Punjabi, Arabic)
a form of Amit.
Amreet, Amryt

Amritpal (Sikh) protector of the Lord's nectar.

Amsi (Egyptian) embodiment of the power
of the universe.

Amsu (Egyptian) embodiment of reproduction.

Amuillan (Mapuche) he who warmly serves
others.

An BG (Chinese, Vietnamese) peaceful.
Ana

Anacario (Greek) not without grace.

Anacleto (Greek) he who was called upon.

Anaías (Hebrew) the Lord answers.

Anan, Anán (Hebrew) cloudy.

Anand (Hindi) blissful.
Ananda, Anant, Ananth

Ananías (Hebrew) he who has the grace of God.

Anantas (Hindi) infinite.

Anas (Greek) a short form of Anastasius.

Anastario, Anastasón (Greek) forms of Anastasios.

Anastasios (Greek) a form of Anastasius.
Anastasio

Anastasius (Greek) resurrection.
Anastacio, Anastacios, Anastagio, Anastas, Anastase, Anastasi, Anastatius, Anastice, Anastisis, Anaztáz, Athanasius

Anasvindo (German) strength of God.

Anatalón (Greek) one who grows and flourishes.

Anatole (Greek) east.
Anatol, Anatoley, Anatoli, Anatolie, Anatolijus, Anatolio, Anatolis, Anatoliy, Anatoly, Anitoly, Antoly

Anatolii (Russian) what comes from the east.

Anayantzin (Basque) small.

Anbesa, Anbessa (Spanish) governor of Spain.

Anca (Quechua) black eagle.

Ancasmayu (Quechua) blue like the river.

Ancaspoma, Ancaspuma (Quechua) bluish puma.

Ancavil (Mapuche) identical mythological being.

Ancavilo (Mapuche) snake's body.

Anchali (Taos) painter.
Anchalee, Anchaley, Anchalie, Anchaly

Ancil (French) of nobility.

Ancuguiyca (Quechua) having sacred resistance.

Anders (Swedish) a form of Andrew.
Andar, Ander

Anderson (Swedish) son of Andrew.
Andersen

Andomarro (German) notable God.

Andoni (Greek) a form of Anthony.
Andonny

Andonios (Greek) a form of Anthony.
Andonis

Andoquino (Greek) without comparison.

Andor (Hungarian) a form of Andrew, Anthony.

Andra GB (French) a form of Andrew.

Andrae (French) a form of Andrew.

András (Hungarian) a form of Andrew.
Andraes, Andri, Andris, Andrius, Andriy, Aundras, Aundreas

Andre, André (French) forms of Andrew.
Andrecito, Andree, Andrie, Aundré

Andrea GB (Greek) a form of Andrew.
Andrean, Andreani

Andreas (Greek) a form of Andrew.
Andries

Andrei, Andrey (Bulgarian, Romanian, Russian) forms of Andrew.
Andreian, Andrej, Andreyan, Andrie, Aundrei

Andreo (Greek) manly.

Andres, Andrez (Spanish) forms of Andrew.
Andras, Andrés

Andrew ⭐ (Greek) strong; manly; courageous. Bible: one of the Twelve Apostles. See also Bandi, Drew, Endre, Evangelos, Kendrew, Ondro.
Aindrea, Andery, Andonios, Andrews, Anker, Anndra, Antal, Audrew

Andrian (Greek) a form of Andrew.

Androcles (Greek) man covered with glory.

Andrónico (German) victorious man.

Andros (Polish) sea. Mythology: the god of the sea.
Andris, Andrius, Andrus

Andru, Andrue (Greek) forms of Andrew.
Andrus

Andrzej (Polish) a form of Andrew.

Andy (Greek) a short form of Andrew.
Ande, Andee, Andey, Andi, Andie, Andino, Andis, Andje

Anecto (Greek) tolerable.

Anesio (Greek) a form of Anisio.

Aneurin (Welsh) honorable; gold. See also Nye.
Aneirin

Anfernee (Greek) a form of Anthony.
Anferney, Anfernie, Anferny, Anfonee, Anfoney, Anfoni, Anfonie, Anfony, Anfranee, Anfrene, Anfrenee, Anpherne

Anfión (Greek) Mythology: Amphion is the son of Antiope and Jupiter.

Anfos (Catalan) a form of Alfonso.

Angel ☀ 🇧🇬 (Greek) angel. (Latin) messenger. See also Gotzon.
Ange, Angell, Angie, Angy, Anjel, Anjell

Ángel (Greek) a form of Angel.

Angelino (Latin) messenger.

Angelo (Italian) a form of Angel.
Angeleo, Angelito, Angello, Angelos, Angelous, Angiolo, Anglo, Anjello, Anjelo

Ángelo (Spanish) a form of Angelo.

Angilberto (Teutonic) a combination of Ángel and Alberto.

Angulo (German) lance.

Angus (Scottish) exceptional; outstanding. Mythology: Angus Og was the Celtic god of youth, love, and beauty. See also Ennis, Gus.
Aonghas

Anh 🇬🇧 (Vietnamese) peace; safety.

Aniano (Greek) he who is sad and upset.

Anías (Hebrew) God answers.

Anibal (Phoenician) a form of Hannibal.

Aníbal (Punic) a form of Anibal.

Anicet, Aniceto (Greek) invincible man of great strength.

Anil (Hindi) wind god.
Aneal, Aneel, Anel, Aniel, Aniello, Anielo, Anyl, Anyll

Aniol (Catalan) a form of Aniano.

Anîs (Arabic) intimate friend.

Anish (Greek) a form of Annas.

Anisio (Greek) reliable.

Anka 🇬🇧 (Turkish) phoenix.

Anker (Danish) a form of Andrew.
Ankor, Ankur

Annan (Scottish) brook. (Swahili) fourth-born son.
Annen, Annin, Annon, Annun, Annyn

Annas (Greek) gift from God.
Anis, Anna, Annais

Anno (German) a familiar form of Johann.
Ano

Anoki (Native American) actor.
Anokee, Anokey, Anokie, Anoky

Anón (Latin) yearly.

Anoop (Sikh) beauty.

Anpu (Egyptian) God of death.

Ansaldo (German) he who represents God.

Ansano (Latin) ear.

Ansbaldo (Germanic) peaceful God.

Ansberto (German) brilliant God.

Ansejiso (German) lance.

Ansel (French) follower of a nobleman.
Ancell, Ansa, Anselino, Ansell, Ansellus, Anselyno, Ansyl

Anselm (German) divine protector. See also Elmo.
Anse, Anselme, Anselmi

Anselmo (Italian) a form of Anselm.

Anserico (German) rich in God.

Ansfrido (German) peaceful God.

Ansis (Latvian) a form of Janis.

Ansley **GB** (Scottish) a form of Ainsley.
Anslea, Anslee, Ansleigh, Ansli, Anslie, Ansly, Ansy

Anson (German) divine. (English) Anne's son.
Ansan, Ansen, Ansin, Ansun, Ansyn

Ansovino (German) friend of God.

Anta (Quechua) copper-like

Antal (Hungarian) a form of Anthony.
Antek, Anti, Antos

Antares (Greek) giant, red star. Astronomy: the brightest star in the constellation Scorpio.
Antar, Antario, Antarious, Antarius, Antarr, Antarus

Antauaya (Quechua) copper-colored meadow.

Antavas (Lithuanian) a form of Anthony.
Antaeus

Antavious (Lithuanian) a form of Antavas.
Antavius

Antay (Quechua) copper-colored.

Ante (Lithuanian) a short form of Antavas.
Antae, Anteo

Antelmo (Germanic) protector of the homeland.

Antem (Germanic) giant who wears a helmet.

Antenor (Greek) he who is a fighter.

Anteros (Greek) god of mutual love.

Anthany (Latin, Greek) a form of Anthony.
Antanas, Antanee, Antanie, Antenee, Anthan, Antheny, Anthine, Anthney

Anthoney, Anthonie (Latin, Greek) forms of Anthony.
Anthone, Anthonee, Anthoni, Anthonia

Anthony ☆ **BG** (Latin) praiseworthy. (Greek) flourishing. See also Tony.
Anathony, Anothony, Anthawn, Anthey, Anthian, Anthino, Anthonio, Anthonu, Anthonysha, Anthoy, Anthyoine, Anthyonny

Antico (Latin) old; venerable.

Antidio (Greek) one who radiates God in his actions.

Antígono (Greek) he who stands out amongst all of his fellow men.

Antilaf (Mapuche) happy day.

Antimo (Greek) flourishing.

Antininan (Quechua) copper-colored, like fire.

Antinko (Russian) invaluable.

Antinógenes (Greek) a saint.

Antioco (Greek) he who commands the chariot in the fight against the enemy.

Antíoco (Greek) firm; liberator.

Antione (French) a form of Anthony.
Antion, Antionio, Antionne, Antiono

Antipan (Mapuche) sunny branch of a clear brown color.

Antipas (Greek) he is the enemy of all, in opposition to everyone.

Antivil (Mapuche) sunny snake.

Antjuan (Spanish) a form of Anthony.
Antajuan, Anthjuan, Antuan, Antuane

Antoan (Vietnamese) safe, secure.

Antoine (French) a form of Anthony.
Anntoin, Anthoine, Antoiné, Antoinne, Atoine

Antolín (Greek) flourishing, beautiful like a flower.

Anton (Slavic) a form of Anthony.
Anthon, Antonn, Antons, Antos

Antón (Spanish) a form of Antonio.

Antone (Slavic) a form of Anthony.
Antonne

Antoni (Latin) a form of Anthony.
Antini

Antonia **GB** (Greek, Latin) a form of Anthony.

Antonino (Italian) a form of Anthony.

Antonio ☆ (Italian) a form of Anthony. See also Tino, Tonio.
Anthonio, Antinio, Antoinio, Antoino, Antonello, Antoneo, Antonin, Antonín, Antonnio, Antonyia, Antonyio

Antonios (Italian) a form of Anthony.

Antonius (Italian) a form of Anthony.

Antony (Latin) a form of Anthony.
Antin, Antius, Antonee, Antoney, Antonie, Antonin, Antonyia, Antonyio

Antonyo (Italian) a form of Antonio.

Antosha (Russian) invaluable.

Antoshika (Catalan) a form of Antonio.

Antti (Finnish) manly.
Anthey, Anthi, Anthie, Anthy, Anti, Antty, Anty

Antu (Indigenous) salt.

Antwain, Antwane (Arabic) forms of Antwan.
Antwaina, Antwaine, Antwainn, Antwaion, Antwanne

Antwan, Antwaun, Antwoine, Antwon, Antwone (Arabic) forms of Anthony.
Antaw, Antawan, Antawn, Anthawn, Antowan, Antowaun, Antowine, Antown, Antowne, Antowyn, Antuwan, Antuwon, Antwann, Antwarn, Antwen, Antwian, Antwine, Antwion, Antwione, Antwoan, Antwonn, Antwonne, Antwoun, Antwuan, Antwun, Antwyné, Antwyon, Antwyone, Antyon, Antyonne, Antywon

Anubis (Egyptian) god of death.

Anum (Egyptian) fifth birth.

Anwar (Arabic) luminous.
Anouar, Anour, Anwi

Anxo (Greek) messenger.

Anyaypoma, Anyaypuma (Quechua) he who roars and becomes angry like the puma.

Aparicio (Latin) he who refers to the appearances of the Virgin in different stages.

Apeles (Greek) he who is in a sacred place.

Apelio (Greek) of clear skin.

Aperio (Greek) wild pig.

Apfiano (Greek) a form of Apfias.

Apfías (Greek) youthful term for father.

Apiatan (Kiowa) wooden lance.

Apo, Apu (Quechua) chief; he who moves forward.

Apodemio (Greek) one who travels far from his country.

Apolinar (Greek) a form of Apollo.
Apolinario

Apólito (Latin) dedicated to the god Apollo.

Apollo (Greek) manly. Mythology: the god of prophecy, healing, music, poetry, and light. See also Polo.
Apollos, Apolo, Apolonio, Appollo, Appolo, Appolonio

Apolodoro (Greek) the skill of Apollo.

Aprión (Greek) convincing.

Apro (Greek) a form of Aperio.

Apronio (Greek) a form of Aperio.

Apucachi (Quechua) salty.

Apucatequil, Apucatiquil (Quechua) God of lightning.

Apumaita (Quechua) where are you, master?

Apurimac (Quechua) eloquent master.

Apuyurac (Quechua) white chief.

Aquías (Hebrew) brother of God.

Aquila GB (Latin, Spanish) eagle.
Acquilla, Aquil, Aquilas, Aquileo, Aquiles, Aquilino, Aquill, Aquilla, Aquille, Aquillino, Aquyl, Aquyla, Aquyll, Aquylla

Ara BG (Syrian) a form of Aram.
Arra

Arador (Latin) farmer; laborer.

Arafat (Arabic) mountain of recognition.

Araldo (Spanish) a form of Harold.
Aralodo, Aralt, Aroldo, Arry

Aram (Syrian) high, exalted.
Aramia, Arem, Arim, Arram, Arum, Arym

Aramis (French) Literature: one of the title characters in Alexandre Dumas's novel *The Three Musketeers*.
Airamis, Aramith, Aramys

Aran (Tai) forest. (Danish) a form of Aren. (Hebrew, Scottish) a form of Arran.
Arane

Arapey (Indigenous) aquatic plant that forms floating islands.

Arbel (Hebrew) divine night.

Arbogastro (French) inheriting guest.

Arcadio (Spanish) a form of Archibald.

Arcángel (Greek) the prince of all angels.

Archard (French) powerful.

Archenbaud (French) courageous.

Archer (English) bowman.
Archar, Archor

Archibald (German) bold. See also Arkady.
Arch, Archaimbaud, Archambault, Archibaldes, Archibaldo, Archibold, Archybald, Archybalde, Archybaldes, Archybauld, Archybaulde

Archie (German, English) a familiar form of Archer, Archibald.
Arche, Archee, Archey, Archi, Archy

Arconcio (Greek) one who governs.

Ardal (Irish) a form of Arnold.
Ardale, Ardall

Ardalión (Greek) Ardalion was a martyr who professed Christ while performing on stage.

Ardell (Latin) eager; industrious.
Ardel

Arden GB (Latin) ardent; fiery.
Ard, Ardan, Ardene, Ardent, Ardian, Ardie, Ardin, Ardint, Ardn, Arduino, Ardyn, Ardynt

Ardley (English) ardent meadow.
Ardlea, Ardlee, Ardleigh, Ardli, Ardlie, Ardly

Ardon (Hebrew) bronzed.
Ardun

Arecio (Latin) the god of war.

Arelí (Hebrew) lion of God.

Aren (Danish) eagle; ruler. (Hebrew, Arabic) a form of Aaron.
Aaren

Aretas (Arabic) metal forger.

Aretino (Greek, Italian) victorious.
Aretin, Aretine, Artyn, Artyno

Argar (Greek) shining; gleaming.

Argénides (Greek) white.

Argenis (Greek) he who has a great whiteness.

Argentino, Argento (Latin) shines like silver.

Argimiro (Greek) careful, vigilant.

Argimundo (German) defending army.

Argus (Danish) watchful, vigilant.
Agos, Arguss

Argyle (Irish) from Ireland.
Argile, Argiles, Argyles

Ari BG (Hebrew) a short form of Ariel. (Greek) a short form of Aristotle.
Aree, Arey, Arieh, Arih, Arij, Ario, Arri, Ary, Arye

Aria GB (Greek, Hebrew) a form of Ari.
Arias

Arian BG (Greek) a form of Arion.
Ariana, Ariane, Ariann, Arianne, Arrian

Ariano (Greek) a form of Arian.

Aric, Arick, Arik (Scandinavian) forms of Eric. (German) forms of Richard.
Aaric, Aarick, Aarik, Arec, Areck, Arich, Ariek, Arrek, Arric, Arrick, Arrik, Aryc, Aryck, Aryk

Arie BG (Greek, Hebrew) a form of Ari. (Greek, Latin) a form of Aries.

Ariel GB (Hebrew) lion of God. Bible: another name for Jerusalem. Literature: the name of a sprite in the Shakespearean play *The Tempest*.
Airal, Airel, Arel, Areli, Ariele, Ariell, Arielle, Ariya, Ariyel, Arrial, Arriel, Aryel, Aryell, Aryl, Aryll, Arylle

Aries GB (Latin) ram. Astrology: the first sign of the zodiac.
Arees, Ares, Ariez, Aryes

Arif (Arabic) knowledgeable.
Areef, Aryf

Arin BG (Hebrew, Arabic) a form of Aaron. (Danish) a form of Aren.

Arion (Greek) enchanted. (Hebrew) melodious.
Arien, Ario, Arione, Aryon

Aristarco (Greek) the best of the princes.

Aristeo (Greek) the outstanding one, the most significant one.

Aristides (Greek) son of the best.
Aris, Aristede, Aristedes, Aristeed, Aristide, Aristides, Aristidis, Arystides, Arystydes

Arístides (Greek) a form of Aristides.

Aristión (Greek) selective person.

Aristóbulo (Greek) the greatest and best counselor, he who gives very good advice.

Aristofanes (Greek) the best, the optimum.

Aristónico (Greek) perfect victory.

Aristóteles (Greek) the best; the most optimistic.

Aristotle (Greek) best; wise. History: a third-century B.C. philosopher who tutored Alexander the Great.
Aris, Aristito, Aristo, Aristokles, Aristotal, Aristotel, Aristotelis, Aristotol, Aristott, Aristotyl, Arystotle

Arjun (Hindi) white; milk colored.
Arjen, Arjin, Arju, Arjuna, Arjune

Arkady (Russian) a form of Archibald.
Arkadee, Arkadey, Arkadi, Arkadie, Arkadij, Arkadiy

Arkin (Norwegian) son of the eternal king.
Aricin, Arkeen, Arkyn

Arledge (English) lake with the hares.
Arlege, Arlidge, Arlledge, Arllege

Arlen (Irish) pledge.
Arlan, Arland, Arlend, Arlin, Arlinn, Arlon, Arlyn, Arlynn

Arley (English) a short form of Harley.
Arleigh, Arlie, Arly

Arlo (Spanish) barberry. (English) fortified hill. A form of Harlow. (German) a form of Charles.
Arlow

Armaan (Persian) a form of Arman.

Arman (Persian) desire, goal.
Armahn, Armaine, Armann

Armand (Latin, German) a form of Herman. See also Mandek.
Armad, Armanda, Armands, Armanno, Armaude, Armenta

Armando (Spanish) a form of Armand.
Armondo

Armani 🅱🅶 (Hungarian) sly. (Hebrew) a form of Armon.
Armanee, Armaney, Armanie, Armany, Armoni, Armonie, Armonio, Armonni, Armony

Armelio (Greek) union.

Armen, Armin (Hebrew) forms of Armon.
Armino

Armengol (German) ready for combat.

Armentario (Greek) herder of livestock.

Armentaro (Latin) winner.

Armogastes (German) guest of the eagle.

Armon (Hebrew) high fortress, stronghold.
Armonn, Armons, Armyn

Armond (Latin, German) a form of Armand.

Armstrong (English) strong arm. History: astronaut Neil Armstrong was the commander of Apollo 11 and the first person to walk on the moon.
Armstron, Armstronge

Arnaldo (Spanish) a form of Arnold.

Arnau (Catalan) a form of Arnaldo.

Arnaud (French) a form of Arnold.
Arnaude, Arnauld, Arnault, Arnoll

Arne (German) a form of Arnold.
Arna, Arnay, Arnel, Arnele, Arnell, Arnelle

Arnette 🅱🅶 (English) little eagle.
Arnat, Arnatt, Arnet, Arnett, Arnetta, Arnot, Arnott

Arniano (Latin) lamb.

Arnie (German) a familiar form of Arnold.
Arnee, Arney, Arni, Arnny, Arny

Arno (German) a short form of Arnold. (Czech) a short form of Ernest.
Arnou, Arnoux

Arnold (German) eagle ruler.
Ardal, Arnald, Arndt, Arne, Arnhold, Arnol, Arnoldas, Arnolde, Arnoll, Arnolt, Arnot, Arnott, Arnoud, Arnyld

Arnoldo (Spanish) a form of Arnold.

Arnon (Hebrew) rushing river.
Arnan, Arnen, Arnin, Arnyn

Arnulfo (German) a form of Arnold.

Aron, Arron (Hebrew) forms of Aaron. (Danish) forms of Aren.
Aronek, Aronne, Aronos, Arrion

Aroon (Tai) dawn.
Aroone

Arquelao (Greek) governor of his village.

Arquimedes (Greek) he who has profound thoughts.

Arquímedes (Greek) deep thinker.

Arquipo (Greek) horse-breaker.

Arran (Scottish) island dweller. Geography: an island off the west coast of Scotland. (Hebrew) a form of Aaron.
Aeran, Ahran, Aranne

Arrigo (Italian) a form of Harry.
Alrigo, Arrighetto

Arrio (Spanish) warlike.
Ario, Arrow, Arryo, Aryo

Arsalan (Pakistani) lion of the mountain.

Arsenio (Greek) masculine; virile. History: Saint Arsenius was a teacher in the Roman Empire.
Arsen, Arsène, Arseneo, Arsenius, Arseny, Arsenyo, Arsinio, Arsinyo, Arsynio, Arsynyo

Arsha (Persian) venerable.
Arshah

Art (English) a short form of Arthur.
Arte

Artemio (Spanish) a form of Artemus.

Artemón (Greek) consecrated by the goddess Artemis.

Artemus (Greek) gift of Artemis. Mythology: Artemis was the goddess of the hunt and the moon.
Artemas, Artemis, Artimas, Artimis, Artimus

Arthur (Irish) noble; lofty hill. (Scottish) bear. (English) rock. (Icelandic) follower of Thor. See also Turi.
Artair, Artek, Arth, Arther, Arthor, Arthyr, Artor, Artus, Aurthar, Aurther, Aurthur

Artie (English) a familiar form of Arthur.
Artee, Artian, Arty, Atty

Artis BG (English) a form of Artie.

Artur (Italian) a form of Arthur.

Arturo (Italian) a form of Arthur.
Arthuro

Artzi (Hebrew) my land.

Arun (Cambodian, Hindi) sun.
Aruns

Arundel (English) eagle valley.

Arve (Norwegian) heir, inheritor.
Arv

Arvel (Welsh) wept over.
Arval, Arvell, Arvelle, Arvil, Arvol, Arvyl

Arvid (Hebrew) wanderer. (Norwegian) eagle tree. See also Ravid.
Arv, Arvad, Arve, Arvie, Arvyd, Arvydas

Arvin (German) friend of the people; friend of the army.
Arv, Arvan, Arven, Arvie, Arvon, Arvy, Arvyn, Arwan, Arwen, Arwin, Arwon, Arwyn

Arvind (Hebrew, Norwegian) a form of Arvid. (German) a form of Arvin.
Arvinder

Arya (Hebrew) a form of Aria.

Aryan (Greek) a form of Arion.

Aryeh (Hebrew) lion.
Arye

Aryn GB (Hebrew, Arabic) a form of Aaron. (Danish) a form of Aren.

Asa BG (Hebrew) physician, healer. (Yoruba) falcon.
Asaa, Asah, Ase

Asad (Arabic) a form of Asád. (Turkish) a form of Azad.

Asád (Arabic) lion.
Asaad, Asid, Assad

Asadel (Arabic) prosperous.
Asadour, Asadul, Asadyl, Asael

Asaf (Hebrew) the one chosen by God.

Asafo (Spanish) Yahweh has chosen.

Asaiá (Hebrew) God did it.

Asante (African) thank you.

Ascensión (Spanish) alludes to the ascension of Jesus Christ to heaven.

Ascot (English) eastern cottage; style of necktie. Geography: a village near London and the site of the Royal Ascot horseraces.
Ascott

Asdrúbal (Punic) he who is protected by God.

Asedio (Latin) stable.

Asgard (Scandinavian) court of the gods.

Ash (Hebrew) ash tree.

Ashanti GB (Swahili) from a tribe in West Africa.
Ashan, Ashani, Ashante, Ashantee, Ashaunte

Ashburn (English) from the ash-tree stream.
Ashbern, Ashberne, Ashbirn, Ashbirne, Ashborn, Ashborne, Ashbourn, Ashbourne, Ashburne, Ashbyrn, Ashbyrne

Ashby (Scandinavian) ash-tree farm. (Hebrew) a form of Ash.
Ashbee, Ashbey, Ashbi, Ashbie

Asher (Hebrew) happy; blessed.
Ashar, Ashir, Ashor, Ashyr

Ashford (English) ash-tree ford.
Ashforde

Ashley GB (English) ash-tree meadow.
Asheley, Ashelie, Ashely, Ashlan, Ashlea, Ashlee, Ashleigh, Ashlen, Ashli, Ashlie, Ashlin, Ashling, Ashlinn, Ashlone, Ashly, Ashlyn, Ashlynn, Aslan

Ashon (Swahili) seventh-born son.

Ashraf (Arabic) most honorable.

Ashten GB (English) a form of Ashton.

Ashtin GB (English) a form of Ashton.

Ashton ☆ BG (English) ash-tree settlement.
Ashtan, Ashtian, Ashtion, Ashtonn, Ashtown, Ashtun, Ashtyn

Ashur (Swahili) Mythology: the principal Assyrian deity.

Ashwani (Hindi) first. Religion: the first of the twenty-seven galaxies revolving around the moon.
Ashwan

Ashwin (Hindi) star.
Ashwan, Ashwen, Ashwon, Ashwyn

Asiel (Hebrew) created by God.
Asyel

Asif (Arabic) forgiveness.

Asker (Turkish) soldier.

Aspacio, Aspasio (Greek) welcome.

Aspen GB (English) aspen tree.

Asprén, Asprenio (Latin) hard; rough.

Aster (Greek) a form of Asterio.

Asterio (Greek) mythical figure that was thrown into the sea because of his escape from Zeus.

Astío (Latin) one who belongs.

Astley (Greek) starry field.
Asterlea, Asterlee, Asterleigh, Asterley, Asterli, Asterlie, Asterly, Astlea, Astlee, Astleigh, Astli, Astlie, Astly

Asto, Astu (Quechua) bird of the Andes.

Astolfo (Greek) he who helps with his lance.

Aston (English) eastern town.
Astan, Asten, Astin, Astown, Astyn

Astuguaraca (Quechua) he who hunts Astus with a sling.

Aswad (Arabic) dark skinned, black.
Aswald

Aswaldo (Germanic) lance of the leader.

Ata (Fante) twin.
Atah

Atahualpa (Quechua) bird of fortune.

Atalas, Ataleno, Atalo (Greek) young; energetic.

Atanasio, Atansasio (Greek) immortal.

Atau (Quechua) fortunate.

Atauaipa (Quechua) bird of fortune.

Atauanca (Quechua) fortunate eagle.

Atauchi (Quechua) he who makes us good fortunes.

Ataulfo (Germanic) noble warrior.

Âtef (Arabic) nice.

Atek (Polish) a form of Tanek.

Atenodoro (Greek) gift of wisdom.

Atenógenes (Greek) descendent of Atenas.

Athan (Greek) immortal.
Athen, Athens, Athin, Athon, Athons, Athyn, Athyns

Atherton (English) town by a spring.
Atharton, Atherton, Athorton

Athol (Scottish) from Ireland.
Affol, Athal, Athel, Athil, Atholton, Athyl

Ático (Greek) top floor; loft.

Atid (Tai) sun.
Atyd

Atif (Arabic) caring.
Ateef, Atef, Atyf

Atkins (English) from the home of the relatives.
Akin, Akins, Akyn, Akyns, Atkin, Atkyn, Atkyns

Atl (Nahuatl) water.

Atlas (Greek) lifted; carried. Mythology: Atlas was forced by Zeus to carry the heavens on his shoulders as a punishment for his share of the war of the Titans.

Atley (English) meadow.
Atlea, Atlee, Atleigh, Atli, Atlie, Atly, Attlea, Attlee, Attleigh, Attley, Attli, Attlie, Attly

Atoc, Atuc (Quechua) sly as a fox.

Atocuaman (Quechua) he who possesses the strength of a falcon and the shrewdness of a fox.

Atón (Egyptian) sundial.

Atonatihu (Nahuatl) sun of water.

Atsu (Egyptian) twins.

Atticus (Latin) from Attica, a region outside Athens.

Attila (Gothic) little father. History: the Hun leader who invaded the Roman Empire.
Atalik, Atila, Atilio, Atilla, Atiya, Attal, Attilah, Attilio, Attyla, Attylah

Atu (Ghanaian) born on Sunday.

Atur (Hebrew) crowned.

Atwater (English) at the water's edge.
Attwater

Atwell (English) at the well.
Attwel, Atwel

Atwood (English) at the forest.
Attwood

Atworth (English) at the farmstead.
Attworth

Atzel (Hebrew) noble, generous.

Auberon (German) a form of Oberon.
Auberron, Aubrey

Aubrey GB (German) noble; bearlike. (French) a familiar form of Auberon. See also Avery.
Aubary, Aube, Aubery, Aubie, Aubré, Aubree, Aubreii, Aubri, Aubrie, Aubry, Aubury

Auburn GB (Latin) reddish brown.
Abern, Aberne, Abirn, Abirne, Aburn, Aburne, Abyrn, Abyrne, Aubern, Auberne, Aubin, Aubirn, Aubirne, Aubun, Auburne, Aubyrn, Aubyrne

Audacto (Latin) bold.

Audas (Latin) valiant, bold.

Auden (English) old friend.
Audan, Audin, Audyn

Audie (German) noble; strong. (English) a familiar form of Edward.
Audee, Audey, Audi, Audiel, Audley, Audy

Audífaz (Latin) hatred and acts.

Audomaro (Greek) famous because of his riches.

Audon (French) old; rich.
Audelon

Audrey GB (English) noble strength.
Audra, Audre, Audrea, Audri, Audrius, Audry

Audric (English) wise ruler.
Audrick, Audrik, Audryc, Audryck, Audryk

Audun (Scandinavian) deserted, desolate.

Augie (Latin) a familiar form of August.
Auggie, Augy

Augurio (Latin) name of priests specializing in understanding divine will through the flight and sounds of birds.

August BG (Latin) a short form of Augustine, Augustus.
Augie, Auguste, Augusto

Augustin (Latin) a form of Augustine.

Augustine BG (Latin) majestic. Religion: Saint Augustine was the first archbishop of Canterbury. See also Austin, Gus, Tino.
Augusteen, Augustein, Augusteyn, Augusteyne, Augustinas, Augustino, Augusto, Augustyn, Augustyne

Augustus (Latin) majestic; venerable. History: an honorary title given to the first Roman emperor, Octavius Caesar.
Agustas, Agustus, Agustys, Auguste

Aukai (Hawaiian) seafarer.
Aukay

Aundre (Greek) a form of Andre.
Aundrae, Aundray, Aundrea, Aundrey, Aundry

Auqui (Quechua) master, prince.

Auquipuma (Quechua) prince who is as strong as a puma.

Auquitupac (Quechua) glorious prince.

Auquiyupanqui (Quechua) he who honors his masters.

Aurek (Polish) golden haired.
Aurec

Aurelia (Latin) gold.

Aureliano (Latin) a form of Aurelius.

Aurelio (Latin) a short form of Aurelius.
Aurel, Aurele, Aureli, Aurellio

Aurelius (Latin) golden. History: Marcus Aurelius was a second-century A.D. philosopher and emperor of Rome.
Arelian, Areliano, Aurèle, Aurelien, Aurélien, Aurelyus, Aurey, Auriel, Aury

Auremundo (Germanic) old army.

Áureo (Latin) golden.

Aurick (German) protecting ruler.
Auric, Aurik, Auryc, Auryck, Auryk

Auriville (French) one who comes from the city of gold.

Auspicio (Latin) protector.

Austen BG (Latin) a short form of Augustine.
Austan, Austun, Austyne

Austin ☀ BG (Latin) a short form of Augustine.
Astin, Austine, Oistin, Ostin

Austín (Latin) a form of Austin.

Auston (Latin) a short form of Augustine.

Austyn BG (Latin) a short form of Augustine.

Autónomo (Greek) one who values himself.

Auxano (Greek) one who grows.

Auxencio (Greek) a form of Auxano.

Auxibio (Greek) powerful; alive.

Auxilio (Latin) he who saves, who brings help.

Avdel (Hebrew) servant of God.

Avel (Greek) breath.
Avell

Avelino (Latin) he who was born in Avella, Italy.

Avenall, Aveneil, Avenelle (French) lives close to the oat field.

Avent (French) born during Advent.
Advent, Aventin, Aventino, Aventyno

Averill (French) born in April.
Ave, Averal, Averall, Averel, Averell, Averiel, Averil, Averyl, Averyll, Avrel, Avrell, Avrill, Avryll

Avertano (Latin) one who moves away.

Avery BG (English) a form of Aubrey.
Avary, Aveary, Avere, Averee, Averey, Averi, Averie, Avrey, Avry

Avi (Hebrew) God is my father.
Avian, Avidan, Avidor, Avie, Aviel, Avion, Avy

Aviezri (Hebrew) my father is my help.

Avimael (Hebrew) my father is of divine origin.

Avimelej (Hebrew) my father is king.

Avinatán (Hebrew) my father provided for me.

Aviramv (Hebrew) my father is lifted up.

Aviraz (Hebrew) father of the secret.

Avishajar (Hebrew) father of the morning.

Avitio, Avito (Latin) from grandfather.

Avitzedek (Hebrew) father of justice.

Aviv (Hebrew) youth; springtime.
Avyv

Avner (Hebrew) a form of Abner.
Avneet, Avniel

Avraham (Hebrew) a form of Abraham.

Avram (Hebrew) a form of Abraham, Abram.
Arram, Avraam, Avrahom, Avrohom, Avrom, Avrum

Avshalom (Hebrew) father of peace. See also Absalom.
Avsalom

Awan (Native American) somebody.
Awen, Awin, Awon, Awun, Awyn

Awar (Lebanese) the brightest.

Axel (Latin) axe. (German) small oak tree; source of life. (Scandinavian) a form of Absalom.
Aksel, Ax, Axe, Axell, Axil, Axill, Axle, Axyl, Axyle

Axl (Latin, German, Scandinavian) a form of Axel.

Ayar (Quechua) wild quinoa.

Ayden (Irish) a form of Aidan. (Turkish) a form of Aydin.
Aydean, Aydon, Aydyn

Aydin (Turkish) intelligent.
Aydan, Aydon, Aydyn

Ayers (English) heir to a fortune.

Ayinde (Yoruba) we gave praise and he came.

Aylmer (English) a form of Elmer.
Aillmer, Ailmer, Allmer, Ayllmer

Aylwin (English) noble friends.
Ailwan, Ailwen, Ailwin, Ailwyn, Alwan, Alwen, Aylwan, Aylwen, Aylwon, Aylwyn

Ayman, Aymon (French) forms of Raymond.
Aiman, Aimen, Aimin, Aimon, Aimyn, Aymen, Aymin, Aymyn

Aymán (Lebanese) skillful.

Aymil (Greek) a form of Emil.
Aimil, Aimyl, Aymyl

Ayo (Yoruba) happiness.

Ayraldo (Germanic) noble, honorable.

Ayub (Arabic) penitent.

Ayyûb (Arabic) a form of Job.

Azad (Turkish) free.
Azzad

Azadanes (Hebrew) strong.

Azades (Hebrew) a form of Azadanes.

Azael (Hebrew) made from God.

Azahar (Arabic) alludes to the flower of the orange tree.

Azái (Hebrew) strong.

Azanías (Hebrew) God hears him.

Azare (Hebrew) God helped.

Azarias, Azarías (Hebrew) the Lord sustains me.

Azariel (Hebrew) he who has control over the waters.

Azas (Hebrew) strong.

Azazael (Hebrew) name of an evil spirit.

Azazel (Hebrew) cancerous spirit.

Azeca (Hebrew) strong

Azeem (Arabic) a form of Azim.
Aseem, Azzeem

Azekel (Angolan) praise from God.

Azhar (Arabic) luminous.

Azi (Nigerian) youth.
Azee, Azie, Azy

Azikiwe (African) full of vigor.

Azim (Arabic) defender.
Asim, Azeem, Azym

Azîm (Arabic) a form of Azim.

Azizi (Swahili) precious.

Azriel (Hebrew) God is my aid.

Azul (Arabic) the color of the sky without clouds.

Azuriah (Hebrew) aided by God.
Azaria, Azariah, Azuria, Azuruah, Azurya

Azzâm (Arabic) resolved, decided.

B

Baal (Chaldean) he who dominates a territory.

Babatunde (Nigerian) father has returned.

Bábilas (Hebrew) mouth of God.

Babu (African) grandfather.

Baco (Greek) he who creates disturbances.

Badal (Indian) cloud; rain.

Baden (German) bather.
Badan, Bade, Badin, Badon, Badyn, Baedan, Baede, Baeden, Baedin, Baedon, Baedyn, Bayden, Baydon

Badilón (Spanish) bold, courageous.

Badri, Badrinath (Indian) other names for the Hindu god Vishnu.

Badrick (English) axe ruler.
Badric, Badrik, Badryc, Badryck, Badryk

Badriprasad, Bhadriprasad (Indian) Bhadri's gift.

Badru (Swahili) born from a full moon.

Badu (Ghanaian) tenth born.

Baez (Welsh) boar.

Bahir (Arabic) brilliant, dazzling.
Bahur

Bahram (Persian) ancient king.
Bairam

Bahubali (Indian) son of the first Tirthankar, a type of Jain god.

Bahuleya (Indian) another name for the Hindu god Kartikeya.

Bail (English) a form of Vail.
Bale, Balle, Bayl, Bayle

Bailey GB (French) bailiff, steward.
Bailea, Bailee, Baileigh, Baili, Bailie, Bailio, Baillea, Baillee, Bailleigh, Bailley, Bailli, Baillie, Bailly, Baily, Bailye, Baley

Bain (Irish) a short form of Bainbridge.
Baine, Bayn, Bayne, Baynn

Bainbridge (Irish) fair bridge.
Baenbridge, Baenebridge, Bainebridge, Baynbridge, Baynebridge

Baird (Irish) traveling minstrel, bard; poet.
Bairde, Bard, Bayrd, Bayrde

Bajrang (Indian) another name for the Hindu monkey god Hanuman.

Bakari BG (Swahili) noble promise.
Bacari, Baccari, Bakarie, Bakary

Baker (English) baker. See also Baxter.
Bakir, Bakker, Bakory, Bakr

Bal (Sanskrit) child born with lots of hair.

Balaaditya (Indian) young sun.

Balachandra (Indian) young moon.

Balagopal, Balagovind, Balakrishna, Balgopal (Indian) the Hindu god Krishna as a baby.

Balaji (Indian) another name for the Hindu god Vishnu.

Balamani (Indian) young jewel.

Balamohan (Indian) one who is attractive; the Hindu god Krishna as a youth.

Balaraj, Balbir, Baldev, Balvinder, Balvindra, Balwant (Indian) strong.

Balaram (Indian) brother of the Hindu god Krishna.

Balasi (Basque) flat footed.

Balbino (Latin) he who mumbles.

Balbo (Latin) stammerer.
Bailby, Balbi, Balbie, Balby, Ballbo

Baldemar (German) bold; famous.
Baldemer, Baldmar, Baldmare, Baumar, Baumer

Balder (Scandinavian) bald. Mythology: the Norse god of light, summer, purity, and innocence.
Baldier, Baldur, Baudier, Baulder

Balderico (German) a form of Baldemar.

Baldomero (German) a form of Baldemar.

Baldomiano (German) governor.

Baldovín (Spanish) a form of Balduino.

Baldric (German) brave ruler.
Baldrick, Baldrik, Baldryc, Baldryck, Baldryk, Baudric

Balduino (Germanic) the valiant friend.

Baldwin (German) bold friend.
Bald, Baldewin, Baldewyn, Baldovino, Balduin, Baldwinn, Baldwyn, Baldwynn, Balldwin, Baudoin, Baudoiun, Bealdwine

Balfour (Scottish) pastureland.
Balfor, Balfore

Balin (Hindi) mighty soldier.
Bali, Baline, Balyn, Balyne, Baylen, Baylin, Baylon, Valin

Ballard (German) brave; strong.
Balard, Balerd, Ballerd

Balraj (Hindi) strongest.

Balsemio (Latin) balm.

Baltazar (Greek) a form of Balthasar.
Baltasar

Balthasar (Greek) God save the king. Bible: one of the three wise men who bore gifts for the infant Jesus.
Badassare, Baldassare, Balthasaar, Balthazar, Balthazzar, Baltsaros, Belshazar, Belshazzar, Boldizsár

Banan (Irish) white.
Banen, Banin, Banon, Banun, Banyn

Banbihari (Indian) another name for the Hindu god Krishna.

Bancroft (English) bean field.
Ban, Bancrofft, Bank, Bankroft, Banky

Bandarido (Latin) flag.

Bandhu (Indian) friend.

Bandhul (Indian) pleasing.

Bandi BG (Hungarian) a form of Andrew.
Bandee, Bandey, Bandie, Bandy

Bandit (German) outlaw, robber.
Badyt, Banditt, Bandytt

Bane (Hawaiian) a form of Bartholomew.
Baen, Baene, Ban

Banner (Scottish, English) flag bearer.
Banna, Bannar, Bannor, Banny

Banning (Irish) small and fair.
Baning, Bannie, Banny

Bao GB (Chinese) treasure.

Baptist (Greek) baptised.
Baptista, Baptiste, Baptysta, Battista

Baradine (Australian) small kangaroo.
Baradin, Baradyn, Baradyne

Barak (Hebrew) lightning bolt. Bible: the valiant warrior who helped Deborah.
Barrack, Barrak, Baruch

Baram (Hebrew) son of the people.
Barem, Barim, Barom, Barym

Baran (Russian) ram.
Baren, Barran, Barren

Barasa (Kikuyu) meeting place.
Barasah

Barbaciano (Latin) full of hair.

Barclay (Scottish, English) birch-tree
meadow.
*Bar, Barcklae, Barcklaey, Barcklai, Barcklaie,
Barclae, Barclaey, Barclai, Barclaie, Barcley,
Barkclay, Barklay, Barklea, Barklee, Barkleigh,
Barkley, Barkli, Barklie, Barkly, Barrclay,
Berkeley*

Bard (Irish) a form of Baird.
Bar, Barde, Bardia, Bardiya, Barr

Barden (English) barley valley.
*Bairdan, Bairden, Bairdin, Bairdon, Bairdyn,
Bardan, Bardon, Bardyn, Bayrdan, Bayrden,
Bayrdin, Bayrdon, Bayrdyn*

Bardolf (German) bright wolf.
*Bardo, Bardolfe, Bardolph, Bardolphe, Bardou,
Bardoul, Bardulf, Bardulph*

Bardrick (Teutonic) axe ruler.
Bardric, Bardrik, Bardryck, Bardryk

Bareh (Lebanese) able.

Baris (Turkish) peaceful.
Barris, Barrys, Barys

Barker (English) lumberjack; advertiser at a
carnival.
Barkker

Barlaán (Hebrew) son of the community.

Barlow (English) bare hillside.
Barloe, Barlowe, Barrlow, Barrlowe

Barnabas (Greek, Hebrew, Aramaic, Latin)
son of the missionary. Bible: Christian
apostle and companion of Paul on his first
missionary journey.
*Bane, Barna, Barnaba, Barnabe, Barnabus,
Barnaby, Barnebas, Barnebus, Barney,
Barnibas, Barnibus, Barnybas, Barnybus,
Burnabas*

Barnabás (Hebrew) a form of Barnabas.

Barnabe (French) a form of Barnabas.
Barnabé

Barnaby (English) a form of Barnabas.
*Barnabee, Barnabey, Barnabi, Barnabie,
Bernabé, Bernabee, Bernabey, Bernabi,
Bernabie, Bernaby, Birnabee, Birnabey,
Birnabi, Birnabie, Birnaby, Burnabee,
Burnabey, Burnabi, Burnabie, Burnaby,
Byrnabee, Byrnabey, Byrnabi, Byrnabie,
Byrnaby*

Barnard (French) a form of Bernard.
Barn, Barnard, Barnhard, Barnhardo, Barnhart

Barnes (English) bear; son of Barnett.

Barnett (English) nobleman; leader.
*Barn, Barnet, Barnete, Barnette, Barney,
Baronet, Baronett*

Barney (English) a familiar form of
Barnabas, Barnett.
Barnee, Barni, Barnie, Barny

Barnum (German) barn; storage place.
(English) baron's home.
Barnham

Baron (German, English) nobleman, baron.
Baaron, Barin, Barion, Baronie, Baryn, Beron

Baroncio (Latin) clumsy.

Barret (German) a form of Barrett.
Barrat, Barrhet, Barrit, Berrit

Barrett BG (German) strong as a bear.
*Bar, Baret, Barett, Barit, Baritt, Barretta,
Barrette, Barrhett, Barritt, Baryt, Barytt,
Berrett*

Barric (English) grain farm.
*Barrick, Barrik, Baryc, Baryck, Baryk, Beric,
Berric, Berrick, Berrik, Beryc, Beryck, Beryk*

Barrington (English) fenced town.
Geography: a town in England.
Barington

Barron (German, English) a form of Baron.
Barrin, Barrion, Barryn, Berron

Barry (Welsh) son of Harry. (Irish) spear,
marksman. (French) gate, fence.
*Baree, Barey, Bari, Barie, Barree, Barrey, Barri,
Barrie, Bary*

Barsabás, Bársabas (Hebrew) son of the
time away.

Bart (Hebrew) a short form of
Bartholomew, Barton.
Barrt, Barte, Bartel, Bartie, Barty

Bartel (German) a form of Bartholomew.
Barthel, Barthol, Bartholdy

Bartelemy (French) a form of Barthelemy.

Barthelemy (French) a form of Bartholomew.
Barholomee, Barthelemi, Barthélemy, Barthélmy, Bartholome, Bartholomy, Bartolome, Bartolomé

Bartholomew (Hebrew) son of Talmaí. Bible: one of the Twelve Apostles. See also Jerney, Parlan, Parthalán.
Balta, Bartek, Barteleus, Bartelmes, Barteo, Barth, Barthelemy, Bartho, Bartholo, Bartholomaus, Bartholomeo, Bartholomeus, Bartholomieu, Bartholomu, Bartimous, Bartolomeo, Bartolomeô, Bartolommeo, Bartome, Bartz

Bartlet (English) a form of Bartholomew.
Bartlett

Bartley (English) barley meadow.
Bartlea, Bartlee, Bartleigh, Bartli, Bartlie, Bartly

Barto (Spanish) a form of Bartholomew.
Bardo, Bardol, Bartol, Bartoli, Bartolo, Bartos

Barton (English) barley town; Bart's town.
Barrton, Bartan, Barten, Bartin, Bartyn

Bartram (English) a form of Bertram.
Barthram

Baruc, Baruj (Hebrew) he who is blessed by God.

Baruch (Hebrew) blessed.
Boruch

Baruti (Egyptian) teacher.

Basam (Arabic) smiling.
Basem, Basim, Bassam, Bassem, Bassim

Basiano (Latin) short and stout.

Basil (Greek, Latin) royal, kingly. Religion: a saint and founder of monasteries. Botany: an herb often used in cooking. See also Vasilis, Wasili.
Bas, Basal, Base, Baseal, Basel, Basile, Basilius, Basino, Basle, Bassel, Bazek, Bazel, Bazil, Bazyli

Basile (French) a form of Basil.

Basílides (Greek) son of the king.

Basilio (Greek, Latin) a form of Basil.
Basilios

Basir (Turkish) intelligent, discerning.
Bashar, Basheer, Bashir, Bashiyr, Basyr, Bechir, Bhasheer

Basistha (Indian) an ancient Indian sage.

Bassett (English) little person.
Baset, Basett, Basit, Basset, Bassit

Bastet (Egyptian) cat.

Bastien (German) a short form of Sebastian.
Baste, Bastiaan, Bastian, Bastiane, Bastion, Bastyan, Bastyane

Basudha (Indian) earth.

Bat (English) a short form of Bartholomew.
Bato

Batildis (Germanic) intrepid revolutionary.

Baudilio (Teutonic) he who is brave and valiant.

Baul (Gypsy) snail.

Bauterio (Germanic) heroic army.

Bautista (Greek) he who baptizes.

Bavol (Gypsy) wind; air.
Baval, Bavel, Bavil, Bavyl, Beval, Bevel, Bevil, Bevol, Bevyl

Baxter (English) a form of Baker.
Bax, Baxie, Baxty, Baxy

Bay (Vietnamese) seventh son. (French) chestnut brown color; evergreen tree. (English) howler.
Bae, Bai, Baye

Bayard (English) reddish brown hair.
Baeyard, Baiardo, Baiyard, Bay, Bayardo, Bayerd, Bayrd

Baylee GB (French) a form of Bailey.
Baylea, Bayleigh, Bayli, Baylie, Bayly, Beylea, Beylee, Beyleigh, Beyley, Beyli, Beylie, Beyly

Bayley GB (French) a form of Bailey.

Bayron (German, English) a form of Baron.

Beacan (Irish) small.
Beacán, Beacen, Becan, Becen, Becin, Becon, Becyn

Beacher (English) beech trees.
Beach, Beachy, Beech, Beecher, Beechy

Beagan (Irish) small.
Beagen, Beagin, Beegan

Beale (French) a form of Beau.
Beal, Beall, Bealle, Beals, Beil, Beill, Beille, Beyl, Beyll, Beylle

Beaman (English) beekeeper.
Beamann, Beamen, Beeman, Beemen, Beman

Beamer (English) trumpet player.
Beemer

Beasley (English) field of peas.
Beaslea, Beaslee, Beasleigh, Beasli, Beaslie, Beasly, Peaslee, Peasley

Beato (Latin) happy; blessed.

Beattie (Latin) blessed; happy; bringer of joy.
Beatie, Beatti, Beatty, Beaty, Beeti, Beetie, Beety

Beau (French) handsome.
Beale, Beaux, Bo

Beaufort (French) beautiful fort.
Bofort

Beaumont (French) beautiful mountain.
Bomont

Beauregard (French) handsome; beautiful; well regarded.
Beaureguard, Boregard, Boreguard

Beaver (English) beaver.
Beav, Beavo, Beever, Beve, Bevo

Bebe BG (Spanish) baby.

Beck (English, Scandinavian) brook.
Beckett

Beda (Teutonic) he who orders and provides for.

Bede (English) prayer. Religion: the patron saint of lectors.

Bedir (Turkish) full moon.
Bedire, Bedyr, Bedyre

Bee BG (American) the letter B.

Beethoven (German) Music: Ludwig van Beethoven was a German musical genius.

Beinvenido (Spanish) welcome.

Bejay (American) a combination of Beau + Jay.
Beajae, Beajai, Beajay, Beejae, Beejai, Beejay, Beejaye

Bekele (Ethiopian) he has grown.

Bela BG (Czech) white. (Hungarian) bright.
Béla, Belah, Belay

Belal (Czech, Hungarian) a form of Bela.
Belaal, Belall, Bellal

Belarmino (Germanic) having beautiful armor.

Belden (French, English) pretty valley.
Baliden, Balidin, Balidon, Balidyn, Beldan, Beldin, Beldon, Beldyn, Belidan, Belldan, Bellden, Belldin, Belldon, Belldyn

Belen GB (Greek) arrow.

Belén (Hebrew) house of bread.

Beli (Welsh) white.
Belee, Beley, Belie, Bely

Belino (Latin) man of war.

Belisario (Greek) he who shoots arrows skillfully.

Bell (French) handsome. (English) bell ringer.
Bel

Bellamy (French) beautiful friend.
Belami, Belamie, Belamy, Bellamey, Bellamie

Bello (African) helper or promoter of Islam.
Belo

Belmiro (Portuguese) good-looking; attractive.
Belmirow, Belmyro, Belmyrow

Beltane (French) classic name.

Belveder (Italian) beautiful.
Belvedear, Belvedere, Belvidere, Belvydear, Belvydere

Bem (Tiv) peace.
Behm

Bemabé (Spanish) son of comfort.

Bembé (Spanish) prophet.

Ben (Hebrew) a short form of Benjamin.
Behn, Benio, Benn

Ben Zion (Hebrew) son of Zion.
Benzi

Ben-ami (Hebrew) son of my people.
Baram, Barami

Benaiá (Hebrew) God has built.

Benedict (Latin) blessed. See also
Venedictos, Venya.
*Benci, Bendict, Bendix, Bendrick, Benedictas,
Benedictus, Benediktas, Benedit, Benedyct*

Benedicto (Spanish) a form of Benedict.

Benedikt (German, Slavic) a form of
Benedict.
*Bendek, Bendic, Bendick, Bendik, Benedek,
Benedic, Benedick, Benedik, Benedix, Benedyc,
Benedyck, Benedyk*

Benedito (Latin) a form of Benedict.

Benevento (Latin) welcome.

Bengt (Scandinavian) a form of Benedict.
Beng, Benke, Bent

Beniam (Ethiopian) a form of Benjamin.
Beneyam, Beniamin, Beniamino

Benicio (Latin) riding friend.

Benigno (Latin) the prodigal son; he who
does good deeds.

Benildo (Teutonic) fights against bears.

Benincasa (Arabic) child of Qasim.

Benito (Italian) a form of Benedict. History:
Benito Mussolini led Italy during World
War II.
*Banyto, Bendetto, Bendino, Benedetto, Benedo,
Benino, Bennito, Benno, Beno, Beto, Betto*

Benjamen (Hebrew) a form of Benjamin.
*Banjamen, Benejamen, Bengamen, Benjermen,
Benjjmen, Bennjamen*

Benjamin ✰ (Hebrew) son of my right
hand. See also Peniamina, Veniamin.
*Banjamin, Banjamyn, Behnjamin, Bejamin,
Benejaminas, Bengamin, Bengamon,
Bengamyn, Beniam, Beniamino, Benja,
Benjahmin, Benjaim, Benjam, Benjamain,
Benjamine, Benjaminn, Benjamino, Benjamon,
Benjamyn, Benjamynn, Benjemin,
Benjermain, Benjermin, Benkamin,*

*Bennjamin, Bennjamon, Bennjamyn,
Benyamin, Benyamino, Binyamin, Mincho*

Benjamín (Hebrew) a form of Benjamin.

Benjiman (Hebrew) a form of Benjamin.
*Banjaman, Bemjiman, Bengaman, Benjaman,
Benjimen, Benjimin, Benjimon, Benjmain,
Bennjaman*

Benjiro (Japanese) enjoys peace.

Benjy (Hebrew) a familiar form of
Benjamin.
*Bengee, Bengey, Bengi, Bengie, Bengy, Benjee,
Benjey, Benji, Benjie, Bennjee, Bennjey,
Bennji, Bennjie, Bennjy*

Bennett BG (Latin) little blessed one.
*Benet, Benett, Benette, Benit, Benitt, Bennet,
Bennete, Bennette, Benyt, Benytt*

Bennie, Benny (Hebrew) familiar forms of
Benjamin.
*Bene, Benee, Beney, Beni, Benie, Benne,
Bennee, Benney, Benni, Beny*

Beno (Hebrew) son. (Mwera) band member.
Benno

Benoit (French) a form of Benedict.
Benoitt, Benott, Benoyt, Benoytt

Benoni (Hebrew) son of my sorrow. Bible:
Ben-oni was the son of Jacob and Rachel.
Ben-Oni, Benonee, Benoney, Benonie, Benony

Benson (Hebrew) son of Ben. A short form
of Ben Zion.
*Bennsan, Bennsen, Bennsin, Bennson,
Bennsyn, Bensan, Bensen, Bensin, Benssen,
Bensson, Bensyn*

Bentivolio (Latin) I love you; I desire you.

Bentley (English) moor; coarse grass
meadow.
*Bent, Bentlea, Bentlee, Bentleigh, Bentli,
Bentlie, Bently, Lee*

Bento (Latin) well-named.

Benton (English) Ben's town; town on the
moors.
Bent

Benxamín (Hebrew) a form of Benjamin.

Benzi (Hebrew) a familiar form of Ben Zion.
Benzee, Benzey, Benzie, Benzy

Beppe (Italian) a form of Joseph.
Bepe, Beppy

Ber (English) boundary. (Yiddish) bear.

Beraco (Celtic) bear.

Berardo (Germanic) a form of Bernard.

Bercario (German) prince of the army.

Beredei (Russian) a form of Hubert.
Berdry, Berdy, Beredej, Beredy

Beregiso (Germanic) blade of the bear.

Berengario (Germanic) blade of the warrior.

Berenger (French) courageous as a bear.
Berengir, Berynger

Berenguer (Teutonic) a form of Berenger.

Berg (German) mountain.
Berdj, Berge, Bergh, Berje

Bergen (German, Scandinavian) hill dweller.
Bergan, Bergin, Bergon, Bergyn, Birgin

Berger (French) shepherd.

Bergren (Scandinavian) mountain stream.
Berggren, Bergrin

Berhanu (Ethiopian) your light.

Berk (Turkish) solid; rugged.
Berc, Berck, Berke

Berkeley (English) a form of Barclay.
Berkelea, Berkelee, Berkeleigh, Berkeli, Berkelie, Berkely, Berkie, Berklea, Berklee, Berkleigh, Berkli, Berklie, Berkly, Berky, Burkley

Berkley BG (English) a form of Barclay.

Berl (German) a form of Burl.
Bearl, Bearle, Berle, Berlea, Berlee, Berli, Berlie, Birl, Birle

Berlyn (German) boundary line. See also Burl.
Berlin, Burlin, Burlyn

Bermo (Greek) from Thesalia, a region in Greece.

Bermudo (German) valiant bear; warrior.

Bern (German) a short form of Bernard.
Berne

Bernabe (French) a form of Barnabas.

Bernal (German) strong as a bear.
Bernald, Bernall, Bernalle, Bernhald, Bernhold, Bernold, Burnal

Bernaldino (German) strong bear.

Bernard (German) brave as a bear. See also Bjorn.
Barnard, Bear, Bearnard, Benek, Ber, Berend, Bern, Bernad, Bernadas, Bernal, Bernardel, Bernardin, Bernardus, Bernardyn, Bernarr, Bernat, Bernek, Bernel, Bernerd, Berngards, Bernhard, Bernhards, Bernhardt, Bernhart, Burnard

Bernardino (Spanish) a form of Bernard.
Barnardino

Bernardo (Spanish) a form of Bernard.
Barnardo, Barnhardo, Benardo, Bernaldo, Bernhardo, Berno, Burnardo, Nardo

Bernbe (Spanish) a form of Barnaby.

Bernd (German) a form of Bernardo.

Bernie (German) a familiar form of Bernard.
Bernee, Berney, Berni, Berny, Birnee, Birney, Birni, Birnie, Birny

Bernón (German, Spanish) bear.

Bernstein (German) amber stone.
Bernsteen, Bernsteyn, Bernsteyne

Berry BG (English) berry; grape.
Berri, Berrie

Bersh (Gypsy) one year.
Besh

Bert (German, English) bright, shining. A short form of Berthold, Berton, Bertram, Bertrand, Egbert, Filbert.
Bertus, Birt, Byrt

Bertadio (German) a form of Burton.

Bertario (Germanic) brilliant army.

Berthold (German) bright; illustrious; brilliant ruler.
Berthoud, Bertoide, Bertold, Bertoldi, Bertolt, Burthold, Burtholde

Bertie (English) a familiar form of Bert, Egbert.
Berty, Birt, Birtie, Birty

Bertil (Scandinavian) bright; hero.
Bertyl, Birtil, Birtyl, Burtil, Burtyl, Byrtil, Byrtyl

Bertín (Spanish) distinguished friend.
Bertyn, Burtin, Burtyn

Bertino (German) brilliant; famous.

Berto (Spanish) a short form of Alberto.
Burto

Bertoldi (Italian) a form of Berthold.
Bertolde, Bertuccio

Bertoldo (Germanic) the splendid boss.

Berton (English) bright settlement; fortified town.
Bertan, Berten, Burtan, Burten

Bertram (German) bright; illustrious.
(English) bright raven. See also Bartram.
Beltran, Beltrán, Beltrano, Bertrae, Bertraim, Bertramus, Bertraum, Bertrem, Bertron

Bertrán (Spanish) a form of Bertram.

Bertrand (German) bright shield.
Bertran, Bertrando, Bertranno, Burtrand

Bertualdo (German) community; illustrious leader.

Bertuino (German) brilliant.

Bertulfo (Teutonic) the warrior who shines.

Berwick (English) barley farm.
Berwic, Berwik, Berwyc, Berwyck, Berwyk

Berwyn BG (Welsh) white head.
Berwin, Berwynn, Berwynne

Besa (Greek) man of the valley.

Besarión (Greek) the walker.

Besín (Greek) relative of Bessa.

Betel, Betue (Hebrew) house of God.

Betsabé (Hebrew) oath of God.

Beval (English) like the wind.
Bevel, Bevil, Bevyl

Bevan (Welsh) son of Evan.
Beavan, Beaven, Beavin, Bev, Beve, Beven, Bevin, Bevo, Bevon, Bevyn

Beverly GB (English) beaver meadow.
Beverlea, Beverlee, Beverleigh, Beverley, Beverli, Beverlie

Bevis (French) from Beauvais, France; bull.
Beauvais, Beavis, Beavys, Beuves, Bevys

Bhagwandas (Hindi) servant of God.

Bibiano (Spanish) small man.

Bickford (English) axe-man's ford.
Bickforde, Bikford, Bycford, Byckford, Bykford

Bieito, Bieto (Latin) well-named.

Bienvenido (Filipino) welcome.

Bijan (Persian) ancient hero.
Bihjan, Bijann, Bijhan, Bijhon, Bijon, Byjan

Bilal (Arabic) chosen.
Bila, Bilaal, Bilale, Bile, Bilel, Billaal, Billal

Bill (German) a short form of William.
Bil, Billee, Billijo, Billye, Byll, Will

Billie GB (German) a familiar form of Bill, William.
Bilea, Bilee, Bileigh, Biley, Bili, Bilie, Bille, Billea, Billee, Billey, Billi, Bily, Willie

Billy BG (German) a familiar form of Bill, William.

Binah (Hebrew) understanding; wise.
Bina, Byna, Bynah

Bing (German) kettle-shaped hollow.
Byng

Binh (Vietnamese) peaceful.
Bin

Binkentios (Greek) a form of Vincent.

Binky (English) a familiar form of Bancroft, Vincent.
Bink, Binki, Binkie

Birch (English) white; shining; birch tree.
Berch, Berche, Birche, Birk, Burch, Byrch, Byrche

Birger (Norwegian) rescued.
Berger

Birin (Australian) cliff.
Biryn, Byrin, Byryn

Birino (Latin) reddish.

Birkey (English) island with birch trees.
*Berkee, Berkey, Berki, Berkie, Berky, Birk,
Birkee, Birki, Birkie, Birky*

Birkitt (English) birch-tree coast.
*Berket, Berkett, Berkette, Birk, Birket, Birkett,
Birkit, Burket, Burkett, Burkette, Burkitt,
Byrket, Byrkett*

Birley (English) meadow with the cow barn.
*Berlea, Berlee, Berleigh, Berley, Berli, Berlie,
Berly, Birlea, Birlee, Birleigh, Birlie, Birly*

Birney (English) island with a brook.
*Birne, Birnee, Birni, Birnie, Birny, Burnee,
Burney, Burni, Burnie, Burny*

Birtle (English) hill with birds.

Bishop (Greek) overseer. (English) bishop.
Bish, Bishup

Bjorn (Scandinavian) a form of Bernard.
Bjarne, Bjorne

Blackburn (Scottish) black brook.
Blackbern, Blackberne, Blackburne

Blade (English) knife, sword.
*Bladen, Bladon, Bladyn, Blae, Blaed, Blaid,
Blaide, Blayd, Blayde*

Bladimir (Russian) a form of Vladimir.
Bladimer

Bladimiro (Slavic) prince of peace.

Blain (Irish, English) a form of Blaine.

Blaine ⓑⓖ (Irish) thin, lean. (English) river
source.
Blayne

Blair ⓑⓖ (Irish) plain, field. (Welsh) place.
Blaire, Blare, Blayr, Blayre

Blaise ⓑⓖ (French) a form of Blaze.
*Ballas, Balyse, Blais, Blaisot, Blase, Blasi,
Blasien, Blasius*

Blaize (French) a form of Blaze.

Blake ☀★ ⓑⓖ (English) attractive; dark.
Blaec, Blaek, Blaik, Blaike, Blakeman, Blakey

Blakely ⓑⓖ (English) dark meadow.
Blakelea, Blakelee, Blakeleigh, Blakeley,

*Blakeli, Blakelie, Blakelin, Blakelyn, Blakeny,
Blakley, Blakney*

Blanco (Spanish) light skinned; white;
blond.
Blanko

Blandino (Latin) he who is flattered.

Blane (Irish) a form of Blaine.
Blaney, Blanne

Blas (French) a form of Blaze.
Blass, Blaz

Blasco (Latin) of a pale color.

Blayke (English) a form of Blake.
Blayk

Blayne ⓑⓖ (Irish) a form of Blaine.
Blayn, Blayney

Blayze (French) a form of Blaze.
Blayse, Blayz, Blayze, Blayzz

Blaze (Latin) stammerer. (English) flame; trail
mark made on a tree.
Balázs, Biaggio, Biagio, Blazen, Blazer

Bliss ⓖⓑ (English) blissful; joyful.
Blis, Blys, Blyss

Blondel (French) blond.
Blondell, Blundel, Blundell, Blundelle

Bly (Native American) high.
Bli, Bligh

Blythe ⓖⓑ (English) carefree; merry, joyful.
Blith, Blithe, Blyth

Bo ⓑⓖ (English) a form of Beau, Beauregard.
(German) a form of Bogart.
Boe

Boaz (Hebrew) swift; strong.
Boas, Booz, Bos, Boz

Bob (English) a short form of Robert.
Bobb, Rob

Bobbie ⓖⓑ (English) a familiar form of Bob,
Robert.
*Bobbee, Bobbey, Bobbi, Bobbye, Bobee, Bobey,
Bobi, Bobie, Boby*

Bobby (English) a familiar form of Bob,
Robert.

Bobek (Czech) a form of Bob, Robert.

Bobo (Ghanaian) born on a Tuesday.

Boden (Scandinavian) sheltered. (French) messenger, herald.
Bodene, Bodin, Bodine, Bodyn, Bodyne, Boe

Bodhi (American) a form of Bodie.

Bodie (Scandinavian) a familiar form of Boden.
Boddie, Bode, Bodee, Bodey, Bodi, Boedee, Boedi, Boedy

Bodil BG (Norwegian) mighty ruler.
Bodyl

Bodua (Akan) animal's tail.
Boduah

Boecio (Greek) he who helps; the defender, who goes into battle ready.

Bogart (German) strong as a bow. (Irish, Welsh) bog, marshland.
Bogar, Bogey, Bogie, Bogy

Bohdan (Ukrainian) a form of Donald.
Bogdan, Bogdashka, Bogden, Bogdin, Bogdon, Bogdyn, Bohden, Bohdon

Boleslao (Slavic) the most glorious of the glorious.

Bolívar (Basque) mill of the shore.

Bolodenka (Russian) calm.

Bolton (English) from the manor farm.
Boltan, Bolten, Boltin, Boltyn

Bomani (Egyptian) warrior.

Bonaro (Italian, Spanish) friend.
Bona, Bonar, Bonnar

Bonaventure (Italian) good luck.
Bonaventura

Bond (English) tiller of the soil.
Bondie, Bondon, Bonds, Bondy

Bonfilio, Bonfilo (Latin) good son.

Boni (Latin) man of decency.

Boniface (Latin) do-gooder.
Bonifacio, Bonifacius, Bonifacy

Bonifaci (French) a form of Boniface.

Bonito (Latin) worthy.

Bono, Bonoso (Latin) man of decency.

Booker (English) bookmaker; book lover; Bible lover.
Bookie, Bookker, Books, Booky

Boone (Latin, French) good. History: Daniel Boone was an American pioneer.
Bon, Bone, Bonne, Boon, Boonie, Boony

Booth (English) hut. (Scandinavian) temporary dwelling.
Boot, Boote, Boothe, Bothe

Borak (Arabic) lightning. Mythology: the horse that carried Muhammad to seventh heaven.
Borac, Borack

Borden (French) cottage. (English) valley of the boar; boar's den.
Bord, Bordan, Bordie, Bordin, Bordon, Bordy, Bordyn

Boreas (Greek) the north wind.

Borg (Scandinavian) castle.
Borge

Boris (Slavic) battler, warrior. Religion: the patron saint of Moscow, princes, and Russia.
Boriss, Borja, Borris, Borya, Boryenka, Borys

Borís (Russian) a form of Boris.

Borka (Russian) fighter.

Boseda (Tiv) born on Saturday.
Bosedah

Bosley (English) grove of trees.
Boslea, Boslee, Bosleigh, Bosli, Boslie, Bosly

Boswell (English) boar enclosure by the stream.
Boswel, Bozwel, Bozwell

Botan (Japanese) blossom, bud.
Boten, Botin, Boton, Botyn

Boulus (Arabic) a form of Pablo.

Bourey (Cambodian) country.
Bouree

Bourne (Latin, French) boundary. (English) brook, stream.
Born, Borne, Bourn

Boutros (Arabic) a form of Peter.
Boutro

Bowen (Welsh) son of Owen.
Bow, Bowan, Bowe, Bowie, Bowin, Bowon, Bowyn, Bowynn

Bowie (Irish) yellow haired. History: James Bowie was an American-born Mexican colonist who died during the defense of the Alamo.
Bow, Bowee, Bowey, Bowi, Bowy

Boy (French) a short form of Boyce.

Boyce (French) woods, forest.
Boice, Boise, Boycey, Boycie, Boyse

Boyd (Scottish) yellow haired.
Boid, Boydan, Boyde, Boyden, Boydin, Boydon, Boydyn

Brad (English) a short form of Bradford, Bradley.
Bradd, Brade

Bradburn (English) broad stream.
Bradbern, Bradberne, Bradborn, Bradborne, Bradbourn, Bradbourne, Braddbourn, Braddbourne

Braden (English) broad valley.
Bradan, Bradden, Bradeon, Bradin, Bradine, Bradun, Bredan, Bredon

Bradey (Irish, English) a form of Brady.

Bradford (English) broad river crossing.
Braddford, Bradforde, Ford

Bradlee, Bradly (English) forms of Bradley.
Braddlea, Braddlee, Braddleigh, Braddli, Braddlie, Braddly, Bradlea, Bradleigh, Bradlie

Bradley 🅱🅶 (English) broad meadow.
Braddley, Bradlay, Bradlyn, Bradney

Bradon (English) broad hill.

Bradshaw (English) broad forest.
Braddshaw

Brady 🅱🅶 (Irish) spirited. (English) broad island.
Bradi, Bradie, Bradye, Braedee, Braedey, Braedi, Braedie, Braedy, Braidy

Bradyn (English) a form of Braden.
Bradynne, Braidyn, Braydyn, Breidyn

Braedan, Braedyn (English) forms of Braden.
Braedin

Braeden 🅱🅶 (English) a form of Braden.

Braedon (English) a form of Bradon.
Breadon

Bragi (Scandinavian) poet. Mythology: the god of poetry, eloquence, and song.
Brage

Braham (Hindi) creator.
Braheem, Braheim, Brahiem, Brahima, Brahm

Braiden (English) a form of Braden.
Braidan, Braidin

Braidon (English) a form of Bradon.

Brainard (English) bold raven; prince.
Brainerd, Braynard

Bram (Scottish) bramble, brushwood. (Hebrew) a short form of Abraham, Abram.
Bramdon, Brame, Bramm

Bramwell (English) bramble spring.
Brammel, Brammell, Bramwel, Bramwele, Bramwyll

Branch (Latin) paw; claw; tree branch.

Brand (English) firebrand; sword. A short form of Brandon.
Brandall, Brande, Brandel, Brandell, Brander, Brandley, Brann

Brandan (English) a form of Brandon.

Brandán (Celtic) a form of Brandan.

Brandeis (Czech) dweller on a burned clearing.
Brandis

Branden 🅱🅶 (English) beacon valley.
Brandden, Brandene, Breandan

Brandin (English) a form of Branden.
Brandine

Brando (English) a form of Brand.
Brandol

Brandon ☀ 🅱🅶 (English) beacon hill.
Bran, Branddon, Brandone, Brandonn, Brandyn, Branndan, Branndon, Breandon, Brendon

Brandt (English) a form of Brant.

Brandy GB (Dutch) brandy. (English) a familiar form of Brand.
Branddy, Brandey, Brandi, Brandie

Brandyn (English) a form of Branden, Brandon.
Brandynn

Brannen, Brannon (Irish) forms of Brandon.
Branen, Brannan, Brannin, Branon

Bransen (English) a form of Branson.

Branson (English) son of Brandon, Brant. A form of Bronson.
Bransan, Bransin, Bransyn, Brantson

Brant (English) proud.
Brannt, Brante, Branton

Brantley, Brantly (English) forms of Brant.
Brantlee, Brantleigh, Brantlie, Brentlee, Brentley, Brently

Branton (English) Brant's town.

Brasil (Irish) brave; strong in conflict.
Brasill, Brasyl, Brasyll, Brazil, Brazill, Brazyl, Brazyll, Brazylle

Braulio (Italian) a form of Brawley.
Brauli, Brauliuo

Brawley (English) meadow on the hillside.
Brawlea, Brawlee, Brawleigh, Brawli, Brawlie, Brawly

Braxton BG (English) Brock's town.
Brax, Braxdon, Braxston, Braxtan, Braxten, Braxtin, Braxtyn, Braxxton

Brayan (Irish, Scottish) a form of Brian.
Brayn, Brayon

Brayden (English) a form of Braden.
Braydan, Braydin, Braydn, Breydan, Breyden

Braydon (English) a form of Bradon.
Braydoon, Breydon

Braylon (American) a combination of Braydon + Lynn.

Brayton (English) a form of Brighton. (Scottish) a form of Bret.
Braten, Braton

Breck BG (Irish) freckled.
Brec, Breckan, Brecken, Breckie, Breckin, Breckke, Breckyn, Breik, Brek, Brexton

Brede (Scandinavian) iceberg, glacier.
Bred

Brencis (Latvian) a form of Lawrence.
Brence, Brencys

Brendan (Irish) little raven. (English) sword.
Breandan, Breendan, Bren, Brenden, Brendis, Brendon, Brenn, Brenndan, Bryn

Brenden, Brendin (Irish) forms of Brendan.
Bren, Brendene, Brendine, Brennden, Brenndin

Brendon (English) a form of Brandon. (Irish, English) a form of Brendan.
Brenndon

Brendyn (Irish, English) a form of Brendan.
Brenndyn, Brenyan

Brenen, Brennen, Brennon (English, Irish) forms of Brendan.
Bren, Brenan, Brenin, Brenn, Brenna, Brennann, Brennin, Brennun, Brennyn, Brenon

Brennan BG (English, Irish) a form of Brendan.

Brenner (English, Irish) a form of Brendan.
Brennor

Brent (English) a short form of Brenton.
Brendt, Brente, Brentson, Brentt

Brenten (English) a form of Brenton.
Brentten

Brentley (English) a form of Brantley.
Brentlee, Brently

Brenton (English) steep hill.
Brentan, Brentin, Brentton, Brentun, Brentyn

Breogán (Spanish) indicative of family or origin.

Breon, Breyon (Irish, Scottish) forms of Brian.
Breyan

Bret BG (Scottish) from Great Britain. See also Britton.
Bhrett, Bretley, Bretlin, Brette

Breton, Bretton (Scottish) forms of Bret.
Bretan, Breten, Bretin, Brettan, Bretten, Brettun, Brettyn, Bretyn

Brett BG (Scottish) from Great Britain.

Brewster (English) brewer.
Brew, Brewer, Brewstar, Brewstarr, Brewstir,
Brewstor, Bruwster

Brian ☀ (Irish, Scottish) strong; virtuous;
honorable. History: Brian Boru was an
eleventh-century Irish king and national
hero. See also Palaina.
Braiano, Briana, Briann, Brianna, Brianne,
Briano, Briant, Briante, Briaun, Briayan, Brin,
Briny

Briar BG (French) heather.
Brier, Brierly

Briccio, Bricio (Celtic) strength.

Brice BG (Welsh) alert; ambitious. (English)
son of Rice.
Bricen, Briceton, Brise, Brisen, Bryce

Brick (English) bridge.
Bric, Bricker, Bricklen, Brickman, Brik, Bryc,
Bryck, Bryk

Bridgely (English) meadow near a bridge.
Bridgelea, Bridgelee, Bridgelei, Bridgeleigh,
Bridgeley, Bridgeli, Bridgelie

Bridger (English) bridge builder.
Bridd, Bridgar, Bridge, Bridgir, Bridgor

Brien (Irish, Scottish) a form of Brian.
Brience, Brient

Brigham (English) covered bridge. (French)
troops, brigade.
Brig, Brigg, Briggs, Bringham

Brighton BG (English) bright town.
Breighton, Bright, Brightin, Bryton

Brigliadoro (French) classic name.

Brinley (English) tawny.
Brinlea, Brinlee, Brinlei, Brinleigh, Brinli,
Brinlie, Brinly, Brynlea, Brynlee, Brynlei,
Brynleigh, Brynley, Brynli, Brynlie, Brynly

Brion (Irish, Scottish) a form of Brian.
Brieon, Brione, Brionn, Brionne

Brishan (Gypsy) born during a rain.
Brishen, Brishin, Brishon, Bryshan, Bryshen,
Bryshin, Bryshon, Bryshyn

Brit (Scottish) a form of Bret. See also
Britton.
Brityce

Britanic (Catalan) a form of Bruno.

Briton BG (Scottish) a form of Britton.
Britain, Briten, Britian, Brittain, Brittian

Britt BG (Scottish) a form of Bret.

Brittan BG (Scottish) a form of Britton.

Britten BG (Scottish) a form of Britton.

Britton BG (Scottish) from Great Britain.
See also Bret, Brit.
Britin, Brittin, Brittun, Brittyn

Britvaldo (Germanic) leader of the British.

Broc (English) a form of Brock.

Brocardo (Breton) armed warrior.

Brock (English) badger.
Brocke, Brockett, Brockie, Brockley, Brocky,
Brok, Broque

Brockton (English) a form of Brock.

Brod (English) a short form of Broderick.
Brode

Broden (Irish) a form of Brody. (English) a
form of Brod.

Broderick (Welsh) son of the famous ruler.
(English) broad ridge. See also Roderick.
Brodaric, Brodarick, Brodarik, Brodderick,
Brodderrick, Broderic, Broderik, Broderrick,
Broderyc, Broderyck, Broderyk, Brodrick

Brodie BG (Irish) a form of Brody.
Broddie, Brodee, Brodi, Broedi

Brodrick (Welsh, English) a form of
Broderick.
Broddrick, Brodric, Brodryck

Brody (Irish) ditch; canal builder.
Broddy, Brodey, Broedy

Brogan BG (Irish) a heavy work shoe.
Brogen, Broghan, Broghen

Bromley (English) brushwood meadow.
Bromlea, Bromlee, Bromleigh, Bromli, Bromlie,
Bromly

Bron (Afrikaans) source.
Brone

Bronislaw (Polish) weapon of glory.
Bronislav, Bronyslav, Bronyslaw

Bronson (English) son of Brown.
Bransin, Bron, Bronnie, Bronnson, Bronny, Bronsan, Bronsen, Bronsin, Bronsonn, Bronsson, Bronsun, Bronsyn, Brunson

Brook GB (English) brook, stream.
Brooc, Brooker, Brookin, Brooklyn

Brooke GB (English) a form of Brook.

Brooks BG (English) son of Brook.
Brookes, Broox

Brown (English) brown; bear.
Browne

Bru (Catalan) a form of Bruno.

Bruce (French) brushwood thicket; woods.
Brooce, Broose, Brucey, Brucy, Brue, Bruis, Bruse

Brunelle (French) black hair.

Bruno (German, Italian) brown haired; brown skinned.
Brunon, Bruns

Brutus (Latin) coarse, stupid. History: a Roman general who conspired to assassinate Julius Caesar.
Brootus, Brutas, Brutis, Brutiss, Brutos, Brutoss, Brutuss

Bryan ☆ (Irish) a form of Brian.
Brayan, Bryann, Bryen

Bryant (Irish) a form of Bryan.
Bryent

Bryar, Bryer (French) forms of Briar.
Bryor

Bryce BG (Welsh) a form of Brice.
Brycen, Bryceton, Bryse, Bryston

Bryden, Brydon (English) forms of Braden.
Brydan

Bryn GB (Welsh) mountain. (German, English) a form of Bryon.
Brin, Brinn, Bryne, Brynn, Brynne

Brynmor (Welsh) big mountain.
Brinmor, Brinmore, Brynmore

Bryon (German) cottage. (English) bear.
Bryeon, Bryone

Brys (French) comes from Brys.

Brysen (Welsh) a form of Bryson.

Bryson (Welsh) son of Brice.
Brysan, Brysun, Brysyn

Bryton (English) a form of Brighton.
Brayten, Breyton, Bryeton, Brytan, Bryten, Brytin, Brytten, Brytton

Bubba (German) a boy.
Babba, Babe, Bebba

Buck (German, English) male deer.
Buc, Buckie, Buckley, Buckner, Bucko, Bucky, Buk

Buckley (English) deer meadow.
Bucklea, Bucklee, Buckleigh, Buckli, Bucklie, Buckly, Buclea, Buclee, Bucleigh, Bucley, Bucli, Buclie, Bucly, Buklee, Bukleigh, Bukley, Bukli, Buklie, Bukly

Buckminster (English) preacher.

Bucolo (Greek) voyeur.

Bud (English) herald, messenger.
Budd

Buddy (American) a familiar form of Bud.
Budde, Buddee, Buddey, Buddi, Buddie, Budi, Budie, Budy

Buell (German) hill dweller. (English) bull.
Buel

Buenaventura (Latin) he who predicts happiness.

Buford (English) ford near the castle.
Burford

Buinton, Buintón (Spanish) born fifth.

Bundy (English) free.
Bundee, Bundey, Bundi, Bundie

Bunyan (Australian) home of pigeons.
Bunyen, Bunyin, Bunyon, Bunyyn

Burbank (English) from the castle on a slope.
Berbanc, Berbanck, Berbank, Burbanc, Burbanck

Burcardo (Germanic) daring protector; the defender of the fortress.

Burcet (French) comes from the stronghold.

Burdan (English) birch valley.
Berdan, Berden, Berdin, Berdon, Berdyn, Birdan, Birden, Birdon, Birdyn, Burden, Burdin, Burdon, Burdun, Burdyn

Burdett (French) small shield.
Berdet, Berdett, Berdette, Burdet, Burdette

Burford (English) birch ford.
Berford, Berforde, Birford, Birforde, Burforde, Byrford, Byrforde

Burgess (English) town dweller; shopkeeper.
Bergess, Birgess, Burg, Burges, Burgh, Burgiss, Burr, Byrgess

Burian (Ukrainian) lives near weeds.
Berian, Beriane, Beryan, Beryane, Birian, Biriane, Biryan, Biryane, Buriane, Byrian, Byriane, Byryan, Byryane

Burke (German, French) fortress, castle.
Birk, Birke, Bourke, Burk, Byrk, Byrke

Burl (English) cup bearer; wine servant; knot in a tree. (German) a short form of Berlyn.
Berl, Burle, Byrl, Byrle

Burleigh (English) meadow with knotted tree trunks.
Berleigh, Berley, Birlea, Birlee, Birleigh, Birley, Birli, Birlie, Birly, Burlea, Burlee, Burley, Burli, Burlie, Burly, Byrlee, Byrleigh

Burne (English) brook.
Beirne, Burn, Byrne

Burnell (French) small; brown haired.
Bernel, Bernell, Bernelle, Birnel, Birnell, Birnelle, Burnel, Burnele, Burnelle, Byrnel, Byrnell, Byrnelle

Burnett (English) burned nettle.
Bernet, Bernett, Birnet, Birnett, Burnet

Burney (English) island with a brook. A familiar form of Rayburn.
Burnee, Burni, Burnie, Burny, Byrnee, Byrney, Byrni, Byrnie, Byrny

Burr (Swedish) youth. (English) prickly plant.
Bur

Burrell (French) purple skin.

Burril (Australian) wallaby.
Bural, Burel, Buril, Burol, Burral, Burrel, Burril, Burrol, Burryl, Buryl

Burris (English) town dweller.
Buris, Buriss, Buryss, Byris

Burt (English) a form of Bert. A short form of Burton.
Burrt, Burtt, Burty

Burton (English) fortified town.
Bertan, Berten, Bertin, Bertyn, Birtan, Birten, Birtin, Birton, Birtyn, Burtan, Burten, Burtin, Burtyn, Byrtan, Byrten, Byrtin, Byrton, Byrtyn

Busby (Scottish) village in the thicket; tall military hat made of fur.
Busbee, Busbey, Busbi, Busbie, Buzbi, Buzbie, Buzby, Buzz

Buster (American) hitter, puncher.
Bustar

Butch (American) a short form of Butcher.

Butcher (English) butcher.
Butch

Butrus (Arabic) a form of Peter.

Buz (Hebrew) rebelliousness; disdain.

Buzz (Scottish) a short form of Busby.
Buzzy

Bwana (Swahili) gentleman.

Byford (English) by the ford.
Biford, Biforde, Byforde

Byram (English) cattle yard.
Biram

Byran (French, English) a form of Byron.
Biran, Byrann

Byrd (English) birdlike.
Bird, Birdie, Byrdie

Byrne (English) a form of Burne.
Byrn, Byrnes

Byron (French) cottage. (English) barn.
Beyren, Beyron, Biren, Birin, Biron, Buiron, Byren, Byrom, Byrone

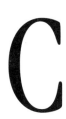

Cable (French, English) rope maker.
Cabell

Cachayauri (Quechua) hard as a shard of copper.

Cadao (Vietnamese) folksong.

Cadby (English) warrior's settlement.
Cadbee, Cadbey, Cadbi, Cadbie

Caddock (Welsh) eager for war.
Cadock, Cadok

Cade (Welsh) a short form of Cadell.
Cady, Caid, Cayd

Cadell (Welsh) battler.
Cadel, Caidel, Caidell, Caydel, Cedell

Caden (American) a form of Kadin.
Cadan, Caddon, Cadian, Cadien, Cadin, Cadon, Cadyn, Caeden, Caedon

Cadman (Irish) warrior.
Cadmen, Caedman, Caidman, Caydman

Cadmar (Irish) brave warrior.
Cadmer, Cadmir, Caedmar, Caidmar, Caydmar

Cadmus (Greek) from the east. Mythology: a Phoenician prince who founded Thebes and introduced writing to the Greeks.

Caelan (Scottish) a form of Nicholas.
Cael, Caelen, Caelin, Caellin, Caelon, Caelyn, Cailan, Cailean, Cailen, Cailin, Caillan, Cailon, Cailun, Cailyn, Callin, Caylen, Cayley, Caylin, Caylon, Caylyn

Caesar (Latin) long-haired. History: a title for Roman emperors. See also Kaiser, Kesar, Sarito.
Caesarae, Caesare, Caesario, Caesarius, Caeser, Caezar, Casar, Casare, Caseare, Czar, Saecer, Saeser, Seasar

Caesear (Latin) a form of Caesar.

Cagnoaldo (German) illustrious.

Cahil (Turkish) young, naive. See also Kahil.
Cahill

Cai BG (Welsh) a form of Gaius.
Cae, Caio, Caius, Caw, Cay

Caiden (American) a form of Kadin.
Caid

Caifas (Assyrian) man of little energy.

Cain (Hebrew) spear; gatherer. Bible: Adam and Eve's oldest son. See also Kabil, Kane, Kayne.
Caen, Caene, Cayn, Cayne

Caín (Hebrew) a form of Cain.

Cainán (Hebrew) blacksmith.

Caine (Hebrew) a form of Cain.
Cainaen, Cainan, Cainen, Caineth

Cairn (Welsh) landmark made of a mound of stones.
Cairne, Carn, Carne, Cayrn, Cayrne, Cayrnes

Cairo (Arabic) Geography: the capital of Egypt.
Cayro, Kairo

Caitan (Latin) a form of Caín.

Caitán (Galician) a form of Cayetano.

Caiya (Quechua) close, nearby.

Cal (Latin) a short form of Calvert, Calvin.

Calan (Scottish) a form of Caelan. (Australian) a form of Callan.
Caleon, Calon, Calyn

Calánico (Greek) blend of to yell and victory.

Caldeolo (Latin) hot.

Calder (Welsh, English) brook, stream.

Caldwell (English) cold well.
Caldwel, Kaldwel, Kaldwell

Cale (Hebrew) a short form of Caleb.
Cael, Caell, Cail, Caill, Calle, Cayl, Cayll

Caleb ⭐ (Hebrew) dog; faithful. (Arabic) bold, brave. Bible: one of the twelve spies sent by Moses. See also Kaleb, Kayleb.
Caelab, Caeleb, Cailab, Calab, Calabe, Callob, Calob, Calyb, Caylab, Cayleb, Caylebb, Caylob

Calen, Calin (Scottish) forms of Caelan.
Calean

Calepodio (Greek) he who has beautiful feet.

Caley GB (Irish) a familiar form of Calan, Caleb.
Calea, Calee, Caleigh, Cali, Calie, Callea, Callee, Calleigh, Calley, Calli, Callie, Cally, Caly

Calfumil (Mapuche) glazed ceramic tile, brilliant blue.

Calhoun (Irish) narrow woods. (Scottish) warrior.
Calhoon, Colhoun, Colhoune, Colquhoun, Kalhoon, Kalhoun

Calib (Hebrew, Arabic) a form of Caleb.
Calieb, Caylib

Calícrates (Greek) excellent government.

Calígula (Latin) he who wears sandals.

Calimaco, Calímaco (Greek) excellent fighter.

Calimerino (Greek) a form of Calimero.

Calimerio (Greek) he who ushers in a beautiful day.

Calimero (Greek) beautiful body.

Calinico, Calínico (Greek) he who secures a beautiful victory.

Calistenes (Greek) beautiful and strong.

Calisto, Calixto (Greek) the best and the most beautiful.

Calistrato, Calístrato (Greek) he who commands a great army.

Calistro (Galician) a form of Calisto.

Calixtrato (Greek) a form of Calisto.

Callahan (Irish) descendant of Ceallachen.
Calaghan, Calahan, Callaghan, Kallaghan, Kallahan

Callan GB (Australian) sparrow hawk. (Scottish) a form of Caelan.
Callin, Callon, Callyn

Callen (Scottish) a form of Caelan. (Australian, Scottish) a form of Callan.

Callis (Latin) chalice, goblet.
Calliss, Callys, Calyss, Kallis, Kalliss, Kallys, Kallyss

Callum (Irish) dove.
Callam, Callem, Callim, Callym, Kallum

Calminio (Latin) calmed.

Calócero (Greek) well traveled.

Calogero (Greek) the wise one.

Calros (German) free man.

Calum (Irish) a form of Callum.
Calam, Calem, Calim, Calym, Colum, Kalum

Calvert (English) calf herder.
Calbert, Calburt, Calvirt, Kalbert, Kalvert

Calvin (Latin) bald. See also Kalvin, Vinny.
Calv, Calvan, Calven, Calvien, Calvino, Calvon, Calvun, Calvyn

Calvucura (Mapuche) blue stone.

Cam BG (Gypsy) beloved. (Scottish) a short form of Cameron. (Latin, French, Scottish) a short form of Campbell.
Camm, Cammie, Cammy, Camy, Kam

Camara (West African) teacher.

Camaron (Scottish) a form of Cameron.
Camar, Camaran, Camaren, Camari

Camden BG (Scottish) winding valley.
Camdan, Camdin, Camdon, Camdyn, Kamden

Cameren (Scottish) a form of Cameron.

Cameron ☀ BG (Scottish) crooked nose. See also Kameron.
Cameran, Camerin, Cameroun, Camerron, Camerson, Camerun, Cameryn, Camiren, Camiron, Cammeron

Camille GB (French) young ceremonial attendant.
Camile

Camilo (Latin) child born to freedom; noble.
Camiel, Camillo, Camillus, Camilow, Kamilo

Campbell BG (Latin, French) beautiful field. (Scottish) crooked mouth.
Cambel, Cambell, Camp, Campy, Kampbell

Camren, Camrin, Camron (Scottish) short forms of Cameron.
Cammrin, Cammron, Camran, Camreon, Camrynn

Camryn **GB** (Scottish) a short form of Cameron.

Canaan (French) a form of Cannon. History: an ancient region between the Jordan River and the Mediterranean.
Canan, Cannan, Caynan

Cancio (Latin) founder of the city of Anzio.

Candide (Latin) pure; sincere.
Candid, Candida, Kandide

Candido (Latin) a form of Candide.
Candonino

Cándido (Latin) a form of Candido.

Canión (Latin) dog.

Cannon (French) church official; large gun. See also Kannon.
Cannen, Cannin, Canning, Cannyn

Canon (French) a form of Cannon.
Canen, Canin, Canyn

Cantidio (Latin) song.

Canute (Latin) white haired. (Scandinavian) knot. History: a Danish king who became king of England after 1016. See also Knute.
Cnut, Cnute

Canuto (Latin) a form of Canute.

Canyon (Latin) canyon.
Cannyon, Cañon, Canyan, Canyen, Canyin, Kanyon

Capac, Capah (Quechua) rich in kindness.

Capacuari (Quechua) kind-hearted master and untamable like the Vicuna.

Capaquiupanqui (Quechua) he who honors his master.

Capitón (Latin) big head.

Cappi (Gypsy) good fortune.
Cappee, Cappey, Cappie, Cappy, Kappi

Caprasio (Latin) regarding the goat.

Caquia (Quechua) thunder.

Car (Irish) a short form of Carney.
Kar

Caralampio (Greek) to shine with happiness.

Caralipo (Greek) saddened heart.

Carden (French) wool comber. (Irish) from the black fortress.
Cardan, Cardin, Cardon, Cardyn

Carey **BG** (Greek) pure. (Welsh) castle; rocky island. See also Karey.
Care, Caree, Cari, Carre, Carree, Carrey, Carrie, Cary

Carilao (Greek) grace of the community.

Carim (Arabic) generous.

Carino (Greek) smiley; friendly.

Carión (Greek) beautiful; graceful.

Carísimo (Latin) loved; appreciated.

Caritón (Greek) person that loves.

Carl (German, English) a short form of Carlton. A form of Charles. See also Carroll, Kale, Kalle, Karl, Karlen, Karol.
Carle, Carles, Carless, Carlis, Carll, Carlson

Carleton (English) a form of Carlton.
Karleton

Carlin **BG** (Irish) little champion.
Carlan, Carlen, Carley, Carlie, Carling, Carlino, Carlon, Carly

Carlisle (English) Carl's island.
Karlisle

Carlito (Spanish) a familiar form of Carlos.
Carlitos

Carlo (Italian) a form of Carl, Charles.
Carolo, Charlo, Karlo

Carlomagno (Spanish) Charles the great.

Carlomán (Germanic) one who lives.

Carlos ☆ (Spanish) a form of Carl, Charles.
Carlus, Carolos, Charlos, Karlos

Carlton (English) Carl's town.
Carllton, Carlston, Carltonn, Carltton, Karlton

Carlyle **BG** (English) a form of Carlisle.
Carlysle, Karlyle

Carmel GB (Hebrew) vineyard, garden. See also Carmine.
Carmeli, Carmiel, Karmel

Carmelo (Hebrew) a form of Carmel.
Carmello

Carmen GB (Latin, Italian) a form of Carmine.
Carman, Carmon, Carmyn

Carmichael (Scottish) follower of Michael.
Karmichael

Carmine BG (Latin) song; crimson. (Italian) a form of Carmel.
Carmain, Carmaine, Carmyne, Karmine

Carnelius (Greek, Latin) a form of Cornelius.
Carnealius, Carneilius, Carnellius, Carnilious

Carnell (English) defender of the castle. (French) a form of Cornell.
Carnel, Karnel, Karnell

Carney (Irish) victorious. (Scottish) fighter. See also Kearney.
Car, Carnee, Carnie, Carny, Karney

Carolas (French) strong.

Carpo (Greek) valuable fruit.

Carpóforo (Greek) he who carries nuts and dried fruit.

Carponio (Greek) a form of Carpo.

Carr (Scandinavian) marsh. See also Kerr.
Karr

Carrick (Irish) rock.
Carooq, Carric, Carricko, Carrik, Karric, Karrick

Carrington BG (Welsh) rocky town.

Carroll (Irish) champion. (German) a form of Carl.
Carel, Carell, Cariel, Cariell, Carol, Carole, Carollan, Carolo, Carols, Carolus, Carrol, Caryl

Carsen (English) a form of Carson.

Carson BG (English) son of Carr.
Carrson, Carsan, Carsin, Carsino, Karson

Carsten (Greek) a form of Karsten.
Carston

Carter ☀ BG (English) cart driver.
Cart, Cartar, Cartor, Kartar, Karter, Kartor

Carterio (Greek) solid, sensible.

Cartland (English) cart builder's island.
Cartlan, Kartlan, Kartland

Cartwright (English) cart builder.
Cartright

Caruamayu (Quechua) yellow river.

Carvell (French, English) village on the marsh.
Carvel, Carvelle, Carvellius, Karvel, Karvell, Karvelle

Carver (English) wood-carver; sculptor.
Carvar, Carvir, Carvor, Karvar, Karver, Karvir, Karvor

Cary BG (Welsh) a form of Carey. (German, Irish) a form of Carroll.
Carray, Carry

Casandro (Greek) the hero's brother.

Case (Irish) a short form of Casey. (English) a short form of Casimir.

Caseareo (Italian) a form of Caesar.

Casey BG (Irish) brave.
Casee, Casi, Casie, Cassee, Cassey, Cassi, Cassie, Casy, Casye, Cayse, Caysey, Cazzee, Cazzey, Cazzi, Cazzie, Cazzy

Cash (Latin) vain. (Slavic) a short form of Casimir.
Cashe

Cashlin (Irish) little castle.
Cashlind, Cashlyn, Cashlynd, Kashlin, Kashlyn

Casiano (Latin) he who is equipped with a helmet.

Casildo (Arabic) the youth that carries the lance.

Casimir (Slavic) peacemaker.
Cachi, Cas, Cashemere, Cashi, Cashmeire, Cashmere, Casimere, Casimire, Casimiro, Castimer, Cazimier, Cazimir, Kasimir, Kazio

Casiodoro (Greek) gift from a friend.

Casper (Persian) treasurer. (German) imperial. See also Gaspar, Jasper, Kasper.
Caspar, Caspir

Cass **BG** (Irish, Persian) a short form of Casper, Cassidy.

Cassidy **GB** (Irish) clever; curly haired. See also Kazio.
Casidy, Cassady, Cassidee, Cassidey, Cassidi, Cassidie, Kassidy

Cassie **GB** (Irish) a familiar form of Cassidy.
Casi, Casie, Casio, Cassey, Cassi, Cassy, Casy, Cazi, Cazie, Cazy

Cassius (Latin, French) box; protective cover.
Casius, Cassia, Cassio, Cazzie, Cazzius, Kasius, Kassio, Kassius, Kazzius

Casta (Spanish) pure.

Castle (Latin) castle.
Cassle, Castal, Castel

Casto (Greek) pure, clean; honest.

Castor (Greek) beaver. Astrology: one of the twins in the constellation Gemini. Mythology: one of the patron saints of mariners.
Castar, Caster, Castir, Caston, Kastar, Kaster, Kastor, Kastyr

Cástor (Greek) a form of Castor.

Castrense (Latin) castle.

Cataldo (Greek) outstanding in war.

Catari (Aymara) serpent.

Catequil, Catiquil (Quechua) ray of light.

Cater (English) caterer.

Cathal (Irish) strong; wise.
Cathel, Cathol, Kathal, Kathel, Kathol

Catherine **GB** (Greek) pure. (English) a form of Katherine (see Girls' Names).

Cathmor (Irish) great fighter.
Cathmoor, Cathmoore, Cathmore, Kathmoor, Kathmoore, Kathmor, Kathmore

Catlin **GB** (Irish) a form of Caitlin (see Girls' Names).

Cato (Latin) knowledgeable, wise.
Caton, Catón, Kato

Catricura (Mapuche) cut stone.

Catuilla (Quechua) ray of light.

Catulino, Catulo (Latin) little dog.

Cauac (Quechua) sentinel, he who guards.

Cauachi (Quechua) he who makes us attentive, vigilant.

Cauana (Quechua) he who is in a place where all can be seen.

Cautaro (Araucanian) daring and enterprising.

Cavan (Irish) handsome. See also Kavan, Kevin.
Caven, Cavon, Cawoun

Cavell (French) small and active.
Cavel, Kavel, Kavell

Cavin (Irish) a form of Cavan.

Cawley (Scottish) ancient. (English) cow meadow.
Cawlea, Cawleah, Cawlee, Cawleigh, Cawli, Cawlie, Cawly, Kawlee, Kawleigh, Kawley, Kawli, Kawlie, Kawly

Cayden (American) a form of Caden.
Cayde, Caydin

Cayetano (Latin) he who is from Gaeta, an ancient Italian city in the Lazio region.

Caylan (Scottish) a form of Caelan.
Caylans, Caylen, Caylon

Cayo (Latin) happy and fun.

Cayua (Quechua) he who follows.

Cazzie (American) a familiar form of Cassius.
Caz, Cazz, Cazzy

Ceadas (Anglo-Saxon) battle.

Ceasar (Latin) a form of Caesar.
Ceaser

Ceasario (Italian) a form of Caesar.

Cecil (Latin) blind.
Cacelius, Cece, Cecile, Cecilius, Cecill, Cecilus, Cecyl, Siseal

Cecilio (Latin) a form of Cecil.
Celio, Cesilio

Cedar BG (Latin) a kind of evergreen conifer.

Cederic (English) a form of Cedric.
Cederick, Cederrick, Cedirick

Cedric (English) battle chieftain. See also Kedric, Rick.
Cad, Caddaric, Ced, Cedrec, Cédric, Cedryche, Sedric

Cedrick, Cedrik (English) forms of Cedric.
Ceddrick

Cedro (Spanish) strong gift.

Ceejay (American) a combination of the initials C. + J.
C.J., Cejay

Cefas (Hebrew) rock.

Ceferino (Greek) he who caresses like the wind.

Celedonio, Celonio (Latin) he who is like the swallow.

Celerino (Latin) fast.

Celestine GB (Latin) celestial, heavenly.
Celestyn, Selestin, Selestine, Selestyn

Celestino (Latin) a form of Celestine.
Selestino

Celso (Italian, Spanish, Portuguese) tall.

Cemal (Arabic) attractive.

Cencio (Italian) a form of Vicente.

Cenerico (German) bold; rich and powerful.

Cenobio (Latin) he who rejects the strangers.

Censurio (Latin) critic.

Cephas (Latin) small rock. Bible: the term used by Jesus to describe Peter.
Cepheus, Cephus

Cepos (Egyptian) pharaoh.

Cerano (Greek) thunder.

Cerdic (Welsh) beloved.
Caradoc, Caradog, Ceredig, Ceretic

Cerek (Polish) lordly. (Greek) a form of Cyril.
Cerik

Cerni (Catalan) a form of Saturno.

Cesar (Spanish) a form of Caesar.
Casar, César, Cesare, Cesareo, Cesario, Cesaro, Ceseare, Ceser, Cesit, Cesor, Cessar

Cesáreo (Latin) relating to Caesar.

Cesarión (Latin) Caesar's follower.

Cesidio (Latin) blue.

Ceslao (Greek) one who is with the community.

Cestmir (Czech) fortress.

Cezar (Slavic) a form of Caesar.
Cézar, Cezary, Cezek, Chezrae, Sezar

Chace (French) a form of Chase.
Chaice

Chad (English) warrior. A short form of Chadwick. Geography: a country in north-central Africa.
Ceadd, Chaad, Chaddi, Chaddie, Chaddy, Chade, Chadleigh, Chadler, Chadley, Chadlin, Chadlyn, Chadmen, Chado, Chadron, Chady

Chadd (English) a form of Chad.

Chadrick (German) mighty warrior.
Chaddrick, Chaderic, Chaderick, Chaderik, Chadrack, Chadric, Chadrik, Chadryc, Chadryck, Chadryk

Chadwick (English) warrior's town.
Chaddwick, Chadvic, Chadwic, Chadwik, Chadwyc, Chadwyck, Chadwyk

Chafulumisa (Egyptian) quickly.

Chago (Spanish) a form of Jacob.
Chango, Chanti

Chaicu (Aymara) he who has great strength to fling stones.

Chaim (Hebrew) life. See also Hyman.
Chai, Chaimek, Chaym, Chayme, Haim, Khaim

Chaise (French) a form of Chase.
Chais, Chaisen, Chaison

Chaitanya (Indian) consciousness.

Chakir (Arabic) the chosen one.

Chakor (Indian) a bird enamored of the moon.

Chakrapani (Indian) another name for the Hindu god Vishnu.

Chakshu (Indian) eye.

Chal (Gypsy) boy; son.
Chalie, Chalin

Chale (Spanish) strong and youthful.

Chalmers (Scottish) son of the lord.
Chalmer, Chalmr, Chamar, Chamarr

Chalten (Tehuelche) bluish.

Cham (Vietnamese) hard worker.
Chams

Chaman, Chamanlal (Indian) garden.

Chambi (Aymara) he who brings good news.

Chambigüiyca, Champigüiyca (Aymara) beam of sunlight.

Champak (Indian) flower.

Champi (Aymara) he who brings good news.

Chan BG (Sanskrit) shining. (English) a form of Chauncey. (Spanish) a form of Juan.
Chann, Chano, Chayo

Chanan (Hebrew) cloud.
Chanen, Chanin, Channan, Channen, Channin, Channon, Channyn, Chanon, Chanyn

Chance BG (English) a short form of Chancellor, Chauncey.
Chanc, Chants, Chaynce

Chancellor (English) record keeper.
Chancellar, Chancellen, Chancelleor, Chanceller, Chansellor

Chancelor (English) a form of Chancellor.
Chancelar, Chancelen, Chanceleor, Chanceler, Chanselor, Chanslor

Chancey BG (English) a familiar form of Chancellor, Chauncey.
Chancee, Chancie, Chancy

Chanchal (Indian) restless.

Chandak, Chandra, Chandrabhan, Chandrakanta, Chandrakishore, Chandrakumar, Chandran, Chandranath (Indian) moon.

Chander (Hindi) moon.
Chand, Chandan, Chandany, Chandara, Chandon

Chandler BG (English) candle maker.
Chandelar, Chandlan, Chandlar, Chandlier, Chandlor, Chandlyr

Chandrachur (Indian) another name for the Hindu god Shiva.

Chandrahas (Indian) bow of the Hindu god Shiva.

Chandrak (Indian) peacock feather.

Chandramohan (Indian) attractive like the moon.

Chandraraj (Indian) moonbeam.

Chandrashekhar (Indian) one who holds moon in his hair knot; another name for the Hindu god Shiva.

Chandresh (Indian) lord of the moon.

Chane (Swahili) dependable.
Chaen, Chaene, Chain, Chaine, Chayn, Chayne, Cheyn

Chaney BG (French) oak.
Chaynee, Cheaney, Cheney

Chankrisna (Cambodian) sweet smelling tree.

Chanler (French) a form of Chandler.

Channing BG (English) wise. (French) canon; church official.
Chane, Chanin, Chaning, Chann, Channin, Channyn, Chanyn

Chanse (English) a form of Chance.
Chans, Chansey, Chansy

Chante BG (French) singer.
Chant, Chantha, Chanthar, Chantra, Chantry, Shantae

Chanten (Galician) colored blue.

Chantz (English) a form of Chance.
Chanz, Chanze

Chapal (Indian) quick.

Chapin (French) scholar.

Chapman (English) merchant.
Chap, Chapmann, Chapmen, Chapmin, Chapmyn, Chappie, Chappy

Chappel, Chappell (French) one who comes from the chapel.

Charan (Indian) feet.

Charanjeet, Charanjit (Indian) one who has won over the lord.

Charanjiv (Hindi) long lived.

Charif (Lebanese) honest.

Charles ⚝ (German) farmer. (English) strong and manly. See also Carl, Searlas, Tearlach, Xarles.
Arlo, Chareles, Charels, Charl, Charle, Charlen, Charlese, Charlot, Charlz, Charlzell

Charleston (English) a form of Carlton.
Charlesten

Charley BG (German, English) a familiar form of Charles.
Charle, Charlea, Charlee, Charleigh, Charli

Charlie BG (German, English) a familiar form of Charles.

Charlton (English) a form of Carlton.
Charleton, Charlotin

Charly BG (German, English) a familiar form of Charles.

Charro (Spanish) cowboy.
Charo

Chas (English) a familiar form of Charles.

Chase ⚝ BG (French) hunter.
Chass, Chasse, Chastan, Chasten, Chastin, Chastinn, Chaston, Chasyn, Chayse

Chasen, Chason (French) forms of Chase.

Chaska (Sioux) first-born son.
Chaskah

Chatha (African) ending.

Chatham (English) warrior's home.
Chathem, Chathim, Chathom, Chathym

Chatuluka (Egyptian) to divert.

Chaturbhuj (Indian) strong; broad-shouldered.

Chauar (Quechua) fiber, rope.

Chauki (Lebanese) my wishes, desires.

Chauncey (English) chancellor; church official.
Chaunce, Chauncee, Chauncei, Chaunci, Chauncie, Chaunecy, Chaunesy, Chaunszi

Chauncy (English) a form of Chauncey.

Chaupi (Quechua) he who is in the middle of everything.

Chavez (Hispanic) a surname used as a first name.
Chavaz, Chaves, Chaveze, Chavies, Chavius, Chevez, Cheveze, Cheviez, Chevious, Chevis, Chivez

Chávez (Spanish) a form of Chavez.

Chavis (Hispanic) a form of Chavez.
Chivass

Chayanne (Cheyenne) a form of Cheyenne.
Chayann, Shayan

Chayce, Chayse (French) forms of Chase.
Chaysea, Chaysen, Chayson, Chaysten

Chayton (Lakota) falcon.
Chaiton

Chaz, Chazz (English) familiar forms of Charles.
Chasz, Chaze, Chazwick, Chazy, Chez

Che, Ché (Spanish) familiar forms of Jose. History: Ernesto "Che" Guevara was a revolutionary who fought at Fidel Castro's side in Cuba.
Chay

Checha (Spanish) a familiar form of Jacob.

Cheche (Spanish) a familiar form of Joseph.

Chee (Chinese, Nigerian) a form of Chi.

Cheikh (African) to learn.

Chen (Chinese) great, tremendous.

Chenche (Spanish) conquer.

Chencho (Spanish) a familiar form of Lawrence.

Cheney (French) from the oak forest.
Chenee, Cheni, Chenie, Cheny

Chenzira (Egyptian) born on a trip.

Chepe (Spanish) a familiar form of Joseph.
Cepito

Cherokee GB (Cherokee) people of a different speech.
Cherokey, Cheroki, Cherokie, Cheroky, Cherrakee

Chesmu (Native American) gritty.
Chesmue

Chester (English) a short form of Rochester.
Ches, Cheslav

Cheston (English) a form of Chester.

Chet (English) a short form of Chester.
Chett, Chette

Chetan (Indian) consciousness; life.

Chetana (Indian) consciousness.

Cheung (Chinese) good luck.

Chevalier (French) horseman, knight.
Chev, Chevalyer

Chevy (French) a familiar form of Chevalier. Geography: Chevy Chase is a town in Maryland. Culture: a short form of Chevrolet, an American automobile company.
Chev, Chevee, Chevey, Chevi, Chevie, Chevvy, Chewy

Cheyenne GB (Cheyenne) a tribal name.
Cheienne, Cheyeenne, Cheyene, Chyenne

Cheyne (French) a form of Chaney.
Cheyney

Chhandak (Indian) charioteer of Buddha.

Chi BG (Chinese) younger generation. (Nigerian) personal guardian angel.

Chicahua (Nahuatl) strong.

Chican (Quechua) unique.

Chicho (Spanish) a form of Chico.

Chick (English) a familiar form of Charles.
Chic, Chickie, Chicky

Chico (Spanish) boy.

Chidambar (Indian) one whose heart is as big as the sky.

Chidananda (Indian) the Hindu god Shiva.

Chik (Gypsy) earth.
Chic, Chyc, Chyk

Chike (Ibo) God's power.

Chiko (Japanese) arrow; pledge.
Chyko

Chilo (Spanish) a familiar form of Francisco.
Chylo

Chilton (English) farm by the spring.
Chil, Chill, Chillton, Chilt, Chiltown, Chylt, Chylton

Chim (Vietnamese) bird.
Chym

Chimalli (Nahuatl) shield.

Chincolef (Mapuche) swift squad; rapid.

Chinmay, Chinmayananda (Indian) blissful.

Chintamani (Indian) philosopher's stone.

Chinua (Ibo) God's blessing.
Chino, Chinou, Chinuah, Chynua, Chynuah

Chioke (Ibo) gift of God.
Chyoke

Chip (English) a familiar form of Charles.
Chipman, Chipp, Chyp, Chypp

Chipahua (Nahuatl) clean.

Chipper (English) a form of Chip.

Chippia (Australian) duck.
Chipia, Chipiah, Chippiah, Chippya, Chipya, Chipyah, Chypia, Chypiah, Chyppia, Chyppiah, Chyppya, Chyppyah, Chypya, Chypyah

Chirag (Indian) lamp.

Chiram (Hebrew) exalted; noble.
Chyram

Chiranjeev, Chirantan, Chirayu (Indian) immortal.

Chisisi (Egyptian) secret.

Chitrabhanu (Indian) fire.

Chitraksh (Indian) beautiful-eyed.

Chitral (Indian) variegated.

Chitrarath (Indian) the sun.

Chitrasen (Indian) a king of the Gandharvas, Hindu spirits of the air, forests, and mountains.

Chitta (Indian) mind.

Chittaranjan (Indian) joy of the inner mind.

Chittaswarup (Indian) the supreme spirit.

Chittesh (Indian) lord of the soul.

Choque, Chuqui (Quechua) lance.

Chorche (Aragonese) a form of George.

Chris BG (Greek) a short form of Christian, Christopher. See also Kris.
Chriss, Christ, Chrys, Chryss, Cris, Criss, Crist

Christain BG (Greek) a form of Christian.
Christai, Christane, Christaun, Christein

Christan BG (Greek) a form of Christian.
Christensen

Christapher (Greek) a form of Christopher.

Christen, Christin GB (Greek) forms of Christian.

Christian ☀ BG (Greek) follower of Christ; anointed. See also Cristian, Jaan, Kerstan, Khristian, Kit, Krister, Kristian, Krystian.
Chretien, Christa, Christé, Christiaan, Christiana, Christiane, Christiann, Christianna, Christianno, Christiano, Christianos, Christino, Christion, Christon, Christyan, Christyon, Chritian, Chrystian, Crystek

Christien (Greek) a form of Christian.
Christienne, Christinne, Chrystien

Christofer, Christoffer (Greek) forms of Christopher.
Christafer, Christaffer, Christaffur, Christafur, Christeffor, Christefor, Christerfer, Christifer, Christofher, Christoforo, Christofper, Chrystofer

Christoff (Russian) a form of Christopher.
Chrisof, Chrisstof, Chrisstoff, Christif, Christof, Cristofe

Christoper (Greek) a form of Christopher.
Christopehr

Christoph (French) a form of Christopher.
Chrisstoph, Chrisstophe

Christophe BG (French) a form of Christopher.

Christopher ☀ BG (Greek) Christ-bearer. Religion: the patron saint of travelers. See also Cristopher, Kester, Kit, Kristopher, Risto, Stoffel, Tobal, Topher.
Chrisopherson, Christepher, Christerpher, Christhoper, Christipher, Christobal, Christoher, Christopherr, Christophor, Christophr, Christophre, Christophyer, Christophyr, Christorpher, Christovao, Christpher, Christphere, Christphor, Christpor, Christrpher, Chrystopher

Christophoros (Greek) a form of Christopher.
Christoforos, Christophor, Christophorus, Christphor

Christos (Greek) a form of Christopher. See also Khristos.
Cristos

Chrysander (Greek) golden.
Chrisander, Chrisandor, Chrisandre, Chrysandor, Chrysandre

Chucho (Hebrew) a familiar form of Jesus.

Chuck (American) a familiar form of Charles.
Chuckee, Chuckey, Chucki, Chuckie, Chucky, Chuk, Chuki, Chukie, Chuky

Chucri (Lebanese) my grace.

Chudamani (Indian) jewel adorned by the gods.

Chui (Swahili) leopard.

Chul (Korean) firm.

Chuma (Ibo) having many beads, wealthy. (Swahili) iron.

Chuminga (Spanish) a familiar form of Dominic.
Chumin, Chumingah

Chumo (Spanish) a familiar form of Thomas.

Chun BG (Chinese) spring.

Chung (Chinese) intelligent.
Chungo, Chuong

Chuquigüaman (Quechua) dancing falcon; golden falcon.

Chuquigüiyca (Quechua) sacred dance.

Chuquilla (Quechua) ray of light, golden light.

Churchill (English) church on the hill. History: Sir Winston Churchill served as British prime minister and won a Nobel Prize for literature.
Churchil, Churchyl, Churchyll

Chuscu (Quechua) fourth son.

Chuya (Quechua) clear as water, pure.

Cian BG (Irish) ancient.
Céin, Cianán, Cyan, Kian

Ciaran (Irish) black; little.

Cibardo (German) strong offering.

Cibrán, Cibrao (Latin) inhabitant of Chipre.

Cicero (Latin) chickpea. History: a famous Roman orator, philosopher, and statesman.
Cicerón, Cicerone, Ciceroni, Cyro

Cid (Spanish) lord. History: title for Rodrigo Díaz de Vivar, an eleventh-century Spanish soldier and national hero.
Cidd, Cyd, Cydd

Cidro (Spanish) strong gift.

Cilistro (Galician) a form of Celestino.

Cindeo (Greek) one who escapes danger.

Cipactli (Nahuatl) crocodile.

Cipactonal (Nahuatl) production of the day.

Ciqala (Dakota) little.

Cireneo, Cirineo (Greek) native from Cyrene.

Ciriaco, Ciríaco (Greek) Lord.

Cirilo, Cirrillo (Italian) forms of Cyril.
Cirilio Cirillo, Cyrilo, Cyryllo, Cyrylo

Ciro (Italian) a form of Cyril. (Persian) a form of Cyrus. (Latin) a form of Cicero.

Cisco (Spanish) a short form of Francisco.
Cisca, Cysco

Citino (Latin) quick to act.

Citlali (Nahuatl) star.

Clancey (Irish) a form of Clancy.

Clancy BG (Irish) redheaded fighter.
Clance, Clancee, Clanci, Clancie, Claney, Clanse, Clansee, Clansey, Clansi, Clansie, Clansy

Clare GB (Latin) a short form of Clarence.
Clair, Clarey, Clary

Clarence (Latin) clear; victorious.
Clarance, Clare, Clarin, Clarince, Claronce, Clarrance, Clarrence, Clarynce, Clearence

Clarencio (Latin) a form of Clarence.

Clark (French) cleric; scholar.
Clarke, Clerc, Clerk

Claro (Latin) he who is clean and transparent.

Clateo (Greek) honored.

Claude BG (Latin, French) lame.
Claud, Claudan, Claudanus, Claudel, Claudell, Claudey, Claudi, Claudian, Claudianus, Claudie, Claudien, Claudin, Claudis, Claudy

Claudino (Italian) a form of Claudio.

Claudio (Italian) a form of Claude.

Claudius (German, Dutch) a form of Claude.
Claudios, Klaudius

Claus (German) a short form of Nicholas. See also Klaus.
Claas, Claes, Clause

Clay (English) clay pit. A short form of Clayborne, Clayton.
Clae, Clai, Klay

Clayborne (English) brook near the clay pit.
Claeborn, Claeborne, Claebourn, Claebourne, Claeburn, Claeburne, Claibern, Claiborn, Claiborne, Claibrone, Claiburn, Claiburne, Claybon, Clayborn, Claybourn, Claybourne, Clayburn, Clayburne, Clebourn

Clayton (English) town built on clay.
Claeton, Claiton, Clayten, Cleighton, Cleyton, Clyton, Klayton

Cleandro (Greek) glorious man.

Cleary (Irish) learned.
Clearey, Cleari, Clearie

Cleavon (English) cliff.
Clavin, Clavion, Clavon, Clavone, Clayvon, Claywon, Cleavan, Cleaven, Cleavin, Cleavon, Cleavyn, Clevan, Cleven, Clevin, Clévon, Clevonn, Clevyn, Clyvon

Clem (Latin) a short form of Clement.
Cleme, Clemmy, Clim

Clemence GB (French) a form of Clement.
Clemens

Clemencio (Italian) a form of Clemence.

Clement (Latin) merciful. Bible: a coworker of Paul. See also Klement, Menz.
Clément, Clementius, Clemmons

Clemente (Italian, Spanish) a form of Clement.
Clemento, Clemenza

Cleo BG (Greek) a form of Clio (see Girls' Names).

Cleóbulo (Greek) glorious counselor.

Cleofas (Greek) he is the glory of his father.

Cleómaco (Greek) he who fights gloriously.

Cleómenes (Greek) glorious courage.

Cleon (Greek) famous.
Kleon

Cleónico (Greek) a form of Cleon.

Cleto (Greek) he was chosen to fight.

Cletus (Greek) illustrious. History: a Roman pope and martyr.
Cleatus, Cledis, Cleotis, Clete, Cletis, Cleytus

Cleve (English) a short form of Cleveland. A form of Clive.
Cleave, Cleeve, Clevey, Clevie

Cleveland (English) land of cliffs.
Cleaveland, Cleavland, Clevelend, Clevelynn

Clicerio (Greek) sweet.

Cliff (English) a short form of Clifford, Clifton.
Clif, Cliffe, Clift, Clyf, Clyfe, Clyff, Clyffe, Clyph, Kliff

Clifford (English) cliff at the river crossing.
Cliford, Clyfford, Clyford, Klifford

Clifton (English) cliff town.
Cliffton, Clift, Cliften, Clyffton, Clyfton

Climaco, Clímaco (Greek) he who climbs the ladder.

Clímene (Greek) famous, celebrated.

Clint (English) a short form of Clinton.
Clynt, Klint

Clinton (English) hill town.
Clenten, Clindon, Clintan, Clinten, Clintin, Clintion, Clintton, Clyndon, Clynten, Clyntin, Clynton, Clynttan, Klinton

Clio (Greek) one who celebrates.

Clitarco (Greek) wing of the army.

Clive (English) a form of Cliff.
Cleiv, Cleive, Cliv, Clivans, Clivens, Clyv, Clyve, Klyve

Clodio (German) glorious.

Clodoaldo (Teutonic) illustrious captain.

Clodomiro (Germanic) he of illustrious fame.

Clodoveo (Spanish) famous warrior.

Clodulfo (Germanic) glory.

Clorindo (Greek) he who is like the grass.

Clotario (Gothic) a form of Lotario.

Clove (Spanish) a nail.

Clovis (German) famous soldier. See also Louis.
Clovys

Cluny (Irish) meadow.
Clunee, Cluney, Cluni, Clunie

Clyde (Welsh) warm. (Scottish) Geography: a river in Scotland.
Clide, Cly, Clyd, Clywd, Klyde

Coady (English) a form of Cody.

Coatl (Nahuatl) snake.

Cobi, Coby (Hebrew) familiar forms of Jacob.
Cob, Cobby, Cobe, Cobee, Cobey, Cobia, Cobie

Coburn (English) meeting of streams.
Cobern, Coberne, Cobirn, Cobirne, Cobourn, Cobourne, Coburne, Cobyrn, Cobyrne

Cochise (Apache) hardwood. History: a famous Chiricahua Apache leader.
Cochyse

Coco GB (French) a familiar form of Jacques.
Coko, Koko

Codey (English) a form of Cody.
Coadi, Coday, Code, Codea, Codee

Codi BG (English) a form of Cody.

Codie BG (English) a form of Cody.

Cody ☆ BG (English) cushion. History: William "Buffalo Bill" Cody was an American frontier scout who toured America and Europe with his Wild West show. See also Kodey.
Coddy, Codell, Codiak, Coedy

Coffie (Ewe) born on Friday.
Cofi, Cofie

Coique, Cuiycui (Quechua) silver.

Coiquiyoc (Quechua) he who is rich with silver.

Cola (Italian) a familiar form of Nicholas, Nicola.
Colah, Colas, Kola

Colar (French) a form of Nicholas.

Colbert (English) famous seafarer.
Calbert, Calburt, Colburt, Colvert, Culbert, Culvert

Colbey (English) a form of Colby.

Colby BG (English) dark; dark haired.
Colbee, Colbi, Colbie, Colbin, Colebee, Coleby, Collby

Cole ☆ (Latin) cabbage farmer. (English) a short form of Colbert, Coleman. (Greek) a short form of Nicholas.
Coal, Coale, Col, Colet, Colie, Kole

Coleman (Latin) cabbage farmer. (English) coal miner.
Colemann, Colm, Koleman

Colen, Colyn (Greek, Irish) forms of Colin.

Coley (Greek, Latin, English) a familiar form of Cole. (English) a form of Colley.

Colin ☆ (Irish) young cub. (Greek) a short form of Nicholas.
Cailean, Colan, Coleon, Colinn, Kolin

Colla, Culla (Quechua) eminent, excellent.

Collacapac, Collatupac, Cullacapac, Cullatupac (Quechua) eminent and kind-hearted lord.

Collana, Cullana (Quechua) the best.

Collen (Scottish) a form of Collin.

Colley (English) black haired; swarthy.
Colea, Colee, Coleigh, Coley, Coli, Colie, Collea, Collee, Colleigh, Colli, Collie, Collis, Colly, Coly

Collier (English) miner.
Colier, Collayer, Collie, Collyer, Colyer

Collin (Scottish) a form of Colin, Collins.
Collan, Collian, Collon, Collyn

Collins (Greek) son of Colin. (Irish) holly.
Colins, Collis, Collyns, Colyns

Colman (Latin, English) a form of Coleman.
Colmann

Colombino (Latin) dove.

Colon (Latin) he has the beauty of a dove.

Colón (Spanish) a form of Colon.

Colson (Greek, English) son of Nicholas.
Colsan, Colsen, Colsin, Colsyn, Coulson

Colt (English) young horse; frisky. A short form of Colbert, Colter, Colton.
Colte, Kolt

Coltan, Colten, Coltin, Coltyn (English) forms of Colton.
Coltinn, Colttan, Coltyne

Colter (English) herd of colts.
Kolter

Colton (English) coal town.
Coltn, Coltrane, Coltton, Coltun, Kolton

Columba BG (Latin) dove.
Coim, Colum, Columb, Columbah, Columbas, Columbia, Columbias, Columbus

Columbo (Latin) a form of Columba.

Colwyn (Welsh) Geography: a river in Wales.
Colwin, Colwinn, Colwyne, Colwynn, Colwynne

Coman (Arabic) noble. (Irish) bent.
Cómán, Comin, Comyn

Coñalef (Mapuche) rapid; agile.

Conall (Irish) high, mighty.
Conal, Conel, Conell, Conelle, Connal, Connall, Connolly

Conan (Irish) praised; exalted. (Scottish) wise.
Conant, Conary, Connen, Connon, Conon, Konan

Conary (Irish) a form of Conan.
Conaire

Concordio (Latin) harmony; union.

Condel (Celtic) intrepid.

Congal (Celtic) tall.

Coni (Quechua) warm.

Coniraya, Cuñiraya (Quechua) heat from the sun.

Conlan (Irish) hero.
Conlen, Conlin, Conlon, Conlyn

Conley (Irish) a form of Conlan.

Connar (Irish) a form of Connor.
Connary, Conneer, Connery, Konner

Connell (Irish) a form of Conall.
Connel, Connelle, Connelly

Conner BG (Irish) a form of Connor.

Connie GB (English, Irish) a familiar form of Conan, Conrad, Constantine, Conway.
Con, Conn, Conney, Conny

Connor ☀ BG (Scottish) wise. (Irish) a form of Conan.
Connoer, Connory, Connyr, Konner, Konnor

Cono (Mapuche) ringdove.

Conón (Greek) dust.

Conor (Irish) a form of Connor.
Conar, Coner, Conour, Konner

Conrad (German) brave counselor.
Coenraad, Conrade, Konrad

Conrado (Spanish) a form of Conrad.
Corrado, Currado

Conroy (Irish) wise.
Conroi, Conry, Roy

Constable (Latin) established

Constancio (Latin) the perseverant one.

Constant (Latin) a short form of Constantine.
Constante

Constantine (Latin) firm, constant. History: Constantine the Great was the Roman emperor who adopted the Christian faith. See also Dinos, Konstantin, Stancio.
Considine, Constadine, Constandine, Constandios, Constanstine, Constant, Constantin, Constantinos, Constantinus, Constantios, Costa, Costandinos, Costantinos

Constantino (Latin) a form of Constantine.

Consuelo (Spanish) consolation.

Contardo (Teutonic) he who is daring and valiant.

Conun-Huenu (Mapuche) entrance to the sky; elevated hill.

Conway (Irish) hound of the plain.
Conwai, Conwy

Cook (English) cook.
Cooke, Cooki, Cookie, Cooky

Cooper BG (English) barrel maker. See also Keifer.
Coop, Couper, Kooper, Kuepper

Copres (Greek) gentile from Atenas.

Corban, Corben (Latin) forms of Corbin.

Corbett (Latin) raven.
Corbbitt, Corbet, Corbette, Corbit, Corbitt, Korbet, Korbett

Corbin BG (Latin) raven.
Corbon, Corbyn, Korbin

Corbiniano (Latin) raven, crow.

Corby (Latin) a familiar form of Corbett, Corbin.
Corbey, Corbie

Corcoran (Irish) ruddy.

Cord (French) a short form of Cordell, Cordero.

Cordarius (Spanish) a form of Cordero.
Cordarious, Cordarrius, Cordarus

Cordaro (Spanish) a form of Cordero.
Coradaro, Cordairo, Cordara, Cordarel, Cordarell, Cordarelle, Cordareo, Cordarin, Cordario, Cordarion, Cordarrel, Cordarrell, Cordarris, Cordarro, Cordarrol, Cordarryl, Cordaryal, Corddarro, Corrdarl

Cordel (French) a form of Cordell.
Cordele

Cordell (French) rope maker.
Cordae, Cordale, Corday, Cordeal, Cordeil, Cordelle, Cordie, Cordy, Kordell

Cordero (Spanish) little lamb.
Cordaro, Cordeal, Cordeara, Cordearo, Cordeiro, Cordelro, Corder, Cordera, Corderall, Corderias, Corderious, Corderral, Corderro, Corderryn, Corderun, Corderus, Cordiaro, Cordierre, Cordy, Corrderio, Corrderyo

Córdulo (Latin) heart.

Corentino (Latin) he who helps.

Corey BG (Irish) hollow. See also Korey, Kory.
Core, Corea, Coree, Corian, Corio, Cory

Cori GB (Irish) a form of Corey.

Corie GB (Irish) a form of Corey.

Coriguaman (Quechua) golden falcon.

Corin BG (Irish) a form of Corrin.
Coren, Corion, Coryn, Korin, Koryn

Coriñaui, Curiñaui (Quechua) he who has eyes that are the color gold.

Coripoma (Quechua) golden puma.

Corliss BG (English) cheerful; goodhearted.

Cormac (Irish) raven's son. History: a third-century king of Ireland who was a great lawmaker.
Cormack, Cormick

Cornelius (Greek) cornel tree. (Latin) horn colored. See also Kornel, Kornelius, Nelek.
Carnelius, Conny, Cornealous, Corneili, Corneilius, Corneille, Corneilus, Cornelias, Corneliaus, Cornelious, Cornelis, Corneliu,

Cornellious, Cornellis, Cornellius, Cornellus, Cornelous, Corneluis, Cornelus, Corney, Cornie, Cornielius, Corniellus, Corny, Cournelius, Cournelyous, Nelius, Nellie

Cornell (French) a form of Cornelius.
Cornall, Corneil, Cornel, Cornelio, Corney, Cornie, Corny, Nellie

Cornwallis (English) from Cornwall.
Cornwalis

Corona (Latin) crown.

Corpus (Latin) body.

Corradeo (Italian) bold.

Corrado (Italian) a form of Conrad.
Carrado

Corrigan (Irish) spearman.
Carrigan, Carrigen, Corigan, Corogan, Corrigon, Corrigun, Corrogun, Korrigan

Corrin GB (Irish) spear carrier.
Corren, Corrion, Corryn, Korrin, Korryn

Corry (Latin) a form of Corey.
Corree, Correy, Corria, Corrie, Corrye

Cort (German) bold. (Scandinavian) short. (English) a short form of Courtney.
Corte, Cortie, Corty, Court, Kort

Cortez (Spanish) conqueror. History: Hernando Cortés was a Spanish conquistador who conquered Aztec Mexico.
Cartez, Cortes, Cortis, Cortize, Courtes, Courtez, Curtez, Kortez

Cortland (English) a form of Courtland.

Cortney GB (English) a form of Courtney.
Cortnay, Cortne, Kortney

Corwin (English) heart's companion; heart's delight.
Corwinn, Corwyn, Corwyne, Corwynn, Corwynne, Korwin, Korwyn, Korwynn

Cory BG (Latin) a form of Corey. (French) a familiar form of Cornell. (Greek) a short form of Corydon.
Corye

Corydon (Greek) helmet, crest.
Coridan, Coriden, Coridon, Coridyn, Corradino, Coryden, Corydin, Corydyn, Coryell, Korydon

Cosgrove (Irish) victor, champion.

Cósima (Greek) gifted; adorned.

Cosimus (Italian) a form of Cosme.

Cosino (Greek) name of a Greek family.

Cosme (Greek) a form of Cosmo.
Cosmé

Cosmo (Greek) orderly; harmonious; universe.
Cos, Cosimo, Cosma, Cosmas, Cosmos,
Cozmo, Kosmo

Cosnoaldo (German) daring ruler.

Costa (Greek) a short form of Constantine.
Costah, Costas, Costes

Cótido (Latin) every day.

Coty (French) slope, hillside.
Cote, Cotee, Cotey, Coti, Cotie, Cottee,
Cottey, Cotti, Cottie, Cotty, Cotye

Coulter (English) a form of Colter.

Courtland (English) court's land.
Court, Courtlan, Courtlana, Courtlandt,
Courtlin, Courtlind, Courtlon, Courtlyn,
Kourtland

Courtney 🅶🅱 (English) court.
Court, Courten, Courtenay, Courteney,
Courtnay, Courtnee

Cowan (Irish) hillside hollow.
Coe, Coven, Covin, Cowen, Cowey, Cowie,
Cowin, Cowyn

Coy (English) woods.
Coi, Coye, Coyie, Coyt

Coyahue (Mapuche) meeting place for
speaking and debating.

Coyle (Irish) leader in battle.
Coil, Coile

Coyne (French) modest.
Coine, Coyan, Coyn

Coyotl (Nahuatl) coyote.

Craddock (Welsh) love.
Caradoc, Caradog, Craddoc, Craddoch, Cradoc,
Cradoch, Cradock

Craig (Irish, Scottish) crag; steep rock.
Craeg, Craege, Craegg, Crag, Craige, Craigen,

Craigery, Craigg, Craigh, Craigon, Crayg,
Crayge, Craygg, Creag, Creage, Creg, Cregan,
Cregg, Creig, Creigh, Creyg, Creyge, Creygg,
Criag, Crieg, Criege, Criegg, Kraig

Cramer (English) full.
Crammer, Kramer, Krammer

Crandall (English) crane's valley.
Cran, Crandal, Crandel, Crandell, Crendal

Crane (English) crane.
Crain, Craine, Crayn, Crayne

Cranston (English) crane's town.
Crainston, Craynston

Cratón (Greek) he who rules.

Crawford (English) ford where crows fly.
Craw, Crow, Crowford, Ford

Creed (Latin) belief.
Creeden, Creedin, Creedon, Creedyn

Creighton (English) town near the rocks.
(Welsh) a form of Crichton.
Craighton, Cray, Crayton, Creigh, Creight,
Creighto, Creightown, Crichtyn

Crepin (French) a form of Crispin.
Crepyn

Crescencio (Latin) he who constantly
increases his virtue.

Crescente (Latin) growing.

Cretien (French) Christian.

Crevan (Irish) fox.
Creven, Crevin, Crevon, Crevyn

Crichton (Welsh) from the town on the hill.
Crighton, Cryghton

Cripín, Cripo (Latin) forms of Crispin.

Crisantemo (Latin) the plant of the golden
flowers.

Crisanto (Greek) golden flower.

Crisiant (Welsh) crystal.
Crisient, Crisyant, Crysiant, Crysyant,
Krisiant

Crisipo (Greek) golden horse.

Crisoforo (Greek) he who wears gold.

Crisóforo (Greek) he who gives advice that
has value.

Crisógono (Greek) of golden roots; creator of richness.

Crisol (Latin) cross; light.

Crisologo (Greek) he who says words that are like gold.

Crisólogo (Greek) a form of Crisologo.

Crisostomo, Crisóstomo (Greek) mouth of gold.

Crisóteles (Greek) one who has golden aims.

Crispin (Latin) curly haired.
Crepin, Cris, Crispian, Crispien, Crispino, Crispo, Crispyn, Cryspyn, Krispin

Crispín (Latin) a form of Crispin.

Cristian BG (Greek) a form of Christian.
Crétien, Cristean, Cristhian, Cristiano, Cristien, Cristino, Cristle, Criston, Cristos, Cristy, Cristyan, Crystek, Crystian

Cristián (Latin) Christian, he who follows Christ.

Cristo (Greek) a form of Cristopher.

Cristobal (Greek) a form of Christopher.
Cristóbal, Cristoval, Cristovao

Cristódulo (Greek) slave of Christ.

Cristofer (Greek) a form of Christopher.

Cristoforo (Italian) a form of Christopher.
Christoforo, Christophoro, Cristofor

Cristopher (Greek) a form of Christopher.
Cristaph, Cristhofer, Cristifer, Cristoph, Cristophe, Crystapher, Crysteffer, Crysteffor, Crystifer

Cristovo (Greek) Christ's servant.

Crofton (Irish) town with cottages.
Krofton

Cromacio (Greek) colored; adorned.

Cromwell (English) crooked spring, winding spring.
Cromvel, Cromvill, Cromwyl, Cromwyll

Crónidas (Greek) time.

Crosby (Scandinavian) shrine of the cross.
Crosbee, Crosbey, Crosbi, Crosbie, Cross

Crosley (English) meadow of the cross.
Croslea, Croslee, Crosleigh, Crosli, Croslie, Crosly, Cross

Crowther (English) fiddler.

Cruz (Portuguese, Spanish) cross.
Cruze, Cruzz, Kruz

Crystek (Polish) a form of Christian.

Crystian (Polish) a form of Christian.

Cuadrado (Latin) complete; square.

Cuadrato (Latin) square; medium height.

Cuahutémoc (Nahuatl) eagle that falls.

Cualli (Nahuatl) good.

Cuartio, Cuarto (Spanish) born fourth.

Cuasimodo (Latin) he who is childlike.

Cuauhtemoc (Nahuatl) descending eagle.

Cuba (Spanish) tub. Geography: the largest island country in the Caribbean.

Cuetlachtli (Nahuatl) wolf.

Cuetzpalli (Nahuatl) lizard

Cuirpuma (Quechua) golden puma.

Cuixtli (Nahuatl) kite.

Cullan (Irish) a form of Cullen.

Cullen (Irish) handsome.
Culen, Cull, Cullin, Culyn

Culley (Irish) woods.
Culea, Culee, Culey, Culi, Culie, Cullea, Cullee, Culleigh, Culli, Cullie, Cully, Culy

Culmacio (Latin) elevated; important.

Culver (English) dove.
Colvar, Colver, Cull, Culvar

Cuminao (Mapuche) crimson glow.

Cumya (Quechua) thunder.

Cunac (Quechua) counselor.

Cuñi (Quechua) warm.

Cunibaldo (Greek) of noble birth.

Cuniberto (Teutonic) he who stands apart from the other noble gentlemen.

Cunningham (Irish) village of the milk pail.

Cuntur (Quechua) condor.

Cunturcanqui, Cunturchaua (Quechua) he who has all the virtues of a condor.

Cunturi (Aymara) representative of the gods.

Cunturpoma, Cunturpuma (Quechua) powerful as the puma and the condor.

Cunturuari (Quechua) untamable and savage like the vicuna and the condor.

Cunturumi (Quechua) strong as the stone and the condor.

Curamil (Mapuche) brilliant stone of gold and silver.

Curi (Quechua) golden.

Curiguaman (Quechua) golden falcon.

Curileo (Mapuche) black river.

Curiman (Mapuche) black condor.

Curipan (Mapuche) stinging nettle.

Curran 🅱🅶 (Irish) hero.
Curan, Curon, Curr, Curren, Currin, Curron

Currito (Spanish) a form of Curtis.
Curcio

Curro (Spanish) a form of Curtis.

Curry (Irish) a familiar form of Curran.
Currey, Curri, Currie

Curt (Latin) a short form of Courtney, Curtis. See also Kurt.
Court

Curtis (Latin) enclosure. (French) courteous. See also Kurtis.
Courtis, Courtys, Curio, Currito, Curtice, Curtus, Curtys

Curtiss (Latin, French) a form of Curtis.
Curtyss

Cusi (Quechua) prosperous man.

Cusiguaman (Quechua) happy falcon.

Cusiguaypa (Quechua) happy rooster.

Cusiñaui (Quechua) smiling, with happy eyes.

Cusipoma, Cusipuma (Quechua) happy puma.

Cusirimachi (Quechua) he who fills us with happy words.

Cusiyupanqui (Quechua) honored and fortunate.

Custodio (Latin) guardian spirit.

Cutberto (German) famous for knowledge.

Cuthbert (English) brilliant.
Cuthberte, Cuthburt

Cutler (English) knife maker.
Cut, Cutlir, Cutlor, Cuttie, Cutty, Kutler

Cutmano (Anglo-Saxon) the man who is famous.

Cutter (English) tailor.

Cuycusi (Quechua) he who moves happily.

Cuyquiyuc (Quechua) he who is rich with silver.

Cuyuc (Quechua) he who is restless.

Cuyuchi (Quechua) he who makes us move.

Cy (Persian) a short form of Cyrus.
Ci

Cyle (Irish) a form of Kyle.

Cynan (Welsh) chief.
Cinan, Cinen, Cinin, Cinon, Cinyn, Cynin, Cynon, Cynyn

Cyprian (Latin) from the island of Cyprus.
Ciprian, Cipriano, Ciprien, Cyprianus, Cyprien, Cyprryan

Cyrano (Greek) from Cyrene, an ancient city in North Africa. Literature: Cyrano de Bergerac is a play by Edmond Rostand about a great guardsman and poet whose large nose prevented him from pursuing the woman he loved.
Cirano

Cyril (Greek) lordly. See also Kiril.
Cerek, Cerel, Ceril, Ciril, Cirill, Cirille, Cirrillo, Cyra, Cyrel, Cyrell, Cyrelle, Cyrill, Cyrille, Cyrillus, Cyryl, Syrell, Syril

Cyrus (Persian) sun. Historial: Cyrus the Great was a king in ancient Persia. See also Kir.
Cyress, Cyris, Cyriss, Cyruss, Syris, Syrus

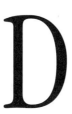

D Andre (American) a form of Deandre.

D'andre (American) a form of Dandre,
Deandre.
D'Andre, D'andré, D'andrea

D'angelo (American) a form of Dangelo,
Deangelo.
D'Angleo

D'ante (American) a form of Dante.
D'Ante, D'anté

D'anthony (American) a form of
Deanthony.
D'Anthony

D'arcy (American, French) a form of Darcy.
D'Aray, D'Arcy

D'juan, Djuan (American) forms of Dajuan,
Dejuan.
D'Juan

D'marco (American) a form of Damarco,
Demarco.
D'Marco

D'marcus (American) a form of Damarcus,
Demarcus.
D'Marcus

D'quan (American) a form of Daquan,
Dequan.
D'Quan

D'vonte (American) a form of Davonte,
Devonte.
D'Vonte, D'vonté

Da Quan, Da'quan (American) forms of
Daquan.

Da'shawn (American) a form of Dashawn.
Da'shaun, Da'shon

Da'ûd (Arabic) a form of David.

Da'von (American) a form of Davon.

Dabeet (Indian) warrior.

Dabi (Basque) a form of David.
Dabee, Dabey, Dabie, Daby

Dabir (Arabic) tutor.
Dabar, Daber, Dabor, Dabyr

Dacey GB (Latin) from Dacia, an area now
in Romania. (Irish) southerner.
*Dace, Dacee, Dache, Daci, Dacian, Dacias,
Dacie, Dacio, Dacy, Daice, Daicey, Daici,
Daicie, Daicy, Dayce, Daycee, Daycey, Dayci,
Daycie, Daycy*

Dacoda (Dakota) a form of Dakota.
Dacodah

Dacota, Dacotah (Dakota) forms of
Dakota.
Dac, Dack, Dackota, DaCota

Dada (Yoruba) curly haired.
Dadah, Dadi

Dadas (Greek) torch.

Dadio (Greek) a form of Dada.

Daegan (Irish) black haired.
*Daegen, Daegin, Daegon, Daegyn, Daigan,
Daigen, Daigin, Daigon, Daigyn, Daygan,
Daygen, Daygin, Daygon, Daygyn*

Daegel (English) from Daegel, England.
Daigel, Daygel

Daelen (English) a form of Dale.
*Daelan, Daelen, Daelin, Daelon, Daelyn,
Daelyne*

Daemon (Greek) a form of Damian.
(Greek, Latin) a form of Damon.
*Daemen, Daemeon, Daemien, Daemin,
Daemion, Daemiyn, Daemond, Daemyen*

Daequan (American) a form of Daquan.
*Daekwaun, Daekwon, Daequane, Daequon,
Daequone, Daeqwan*

Daeshawn (American) a combination of the
prefix Da + Shawn.
*Daesean, Daeshaun, Daeshon, Daeshun,
Daisean, Daishaun, Daishawn, Daishon,
Daishoun*

Daevon (American) a form of Davon.
*Daevion, Daevohn, Daevonne, Daevonte,
Daevontey*

Dafydd (Welsh) a form of David.
Dafid, Dafidd, Dafyd

Dag (Scandinavian) day; bright.
Daeg, Dagen, Dagny, Deegan

Dagan (Hebrew) corn; grain.
Dagen, Dageon, Dagin, Dagon, Dagyn

Dagoberto (Germanic) he who shines like the sun.

Dagwood (English) shining forest.

Dai ⚬🄱 (Japanese) big.
Dae, Dai, Daie, Daye

Daimian (Greek) a form of Damian.
Daemean, Daemian, Daiman, Daimean, Daimen, Daimien, Daimin, Daimiyn, Daimyan

Daimon (Greek, Latin) a form of Damon.
Daimeon, Daimeyon, Daimion, Daimone

Dain (Scandinavian) a form of Dana. (English) a form of Dane.
Daine

Daiquan (American) a form of Daquan.
Daiqone, Daiqua, Daiquane, Daiquawn, Daiquon, Daiqwan, Daiqwon

Daivon (American) a form of Davon.
Daivain, Daivion, Daivonn, Daivonte, Daiwan

Dajon (American) a form of Dajuan.
Dajean, Dajiawn, Dajin, Dajion, Dajn, Dajohn, Dajonae

Dajuan (American) a combination of the prefix Da + Juan.
Da Jon, Da-Juan, Daejon, Daejuan, Dajwan, Dajwoun, Dakuan, Dakwan, Dawaun, Dawawn, Dawon, Dawoyan, Dijuan, Diuan, Dwaun

Dakarai (Shona) happy.
Dakairi, Dakar, Dakara, Dakaraia

Dakari (Shona) a form of Dakarai.
Dakarri

Dakoda 🄱🄶 (Dakota) a form of Dakota.
Dakodah, Dakodas

Dakota 🄱🄶 (Dakota) friend; partner; tribal name.
Dak, Dakcota, Dakkota, Dakoata, Dakotha, Dakotta, Dekota

Dakotah 🄱🄶 (Dakota) a form of Dakota.
Dakottah

Daksh (Hindi) efficient.
Dakshi

Dalal (Sanskrit) broker.

Dalan, Dalen, Dalon, Dalyn (English) forms of Dale.
Dailan, Dailen, Dalaan, Dalain, Dalane, Daleon, Dalian, Dalibor, Dalione

Dalbert (English) bright, shining. See also Delbert.
Dalbirt, Dalburt, Dalbyrt

Dale 🄱🄶 (English) dale, valley.
Dael, Dail, Daile, Dal, Daley, Dalibor, Daly, Dayl, Dayle

Daley (Irish) assembly. (English) a familiar form of Dale.
Daily, Daly, Dawley

Dalin (English) a form of Dallin.

Dallan, Dallen (English) forms of Dalan, Dallin.

Dallas 🄱🄶 (Scottish) valley of the water; resting place. Geography: a town in Scotland; a city in Texas.
Dal, Dalieass, Dall, Dalles, Dallus, Dallys, Dalys, Dellis

Dallin, Dallyn (English) pride's people.
Daelin, Dailin, Dalyn

Dallis 🄱🄶 (Scottish) a form of Dallas.

Dallon (English) a form of Dallan, Dalston.

Dalmacio (Latin) from Dalmatia.

Dalman (Australian) bountiful place.
Dallman, Dallmen, Dallmin, Dallmon, Dallmyn, Dalmen, Dalmin, Dalmon, Dalmyn

Dalmazio (Italian) a form of Dalmacio.

Dalmiro (Germanic) the illustrious one.

Dalphin (French) dolphin.
Dalphine, Dalphyn, Dalphyne, Delphin, Delphine, Delphyn, Delphyne, Dolphine, Dolphyn

Dalston (English) Daegel's place.
Dalis, Dallston

Dalton BG (English) town in the valley.
Dal, Dalaton, Dalltan, Dallten, Dalltin,
Dallton, Dalltyn, Dalt, Daltan, Dalten,
Daltin, Daltyn, Delton

Dalvin (English) a form of Delvin.
Dalven, Dalvon, Dalvyn

Dalziel (Scottish) small field.
Dalzil, Dalzyel, Dalzyl

Damain (Greek) a form of Damian.
Damaian, Damaine, Damaion

Daman, Damen, Damin (Greek, Latin)
forms of Damon.

Damani (Greek) a form of Damian.
Damanni

Damar (American) a short form of
Damarcus, Damario.
Damare, Damari, Damarre, Damauri

Damarco (American) a form of Damarcus.
(Italian) a form of Demarco.
Damarkco, Damarko, Damarrco

Damarcus (American) a combination of the
prefix Da + Marcus. A form of Demarcus.
Damacus, Damarcius, Damarcue, Damarques,
Damarquez, Damarquis

Damario (Greek) gentle. (American) a com-
bination of the prefix Da + Mario.
Damarea, Damareus, Damaria, Damarie,
Damarino, Damarion, Damarrea, Damarrion,
Damaryo

Damarius (Greek, American) a form of
Damario.
Damarious, Damaris, Damarrious, Damarrius,
Dameris, Damerius

Damarkus (American) a form of Damarcus.
Damarick, Damark, Damarkis

Damaso, Dámaso (Greek) skillful horse-
breaker.

Damein (Greek) a form of Damian.

Dameion, Dameon (Greek) forms of
Damian.
Dameone

Damek (Slavic) a form of Adam.
Damick, Damicke, Damik, Damyk

Dametri (Greek) a form of Dametrius,
Demetrius.
Damitré, Damitri, Damitrie

Dametrius (Greek) a form of Demetrius.
Dametries, Dametrious, Damitric, Damitrious,
Damitrius

Damian (Greek) tamer; soother.
Damaiaon, Damaien, Damaun, Damayon,
Dame, Damean, Damián, Damiane,
Damiann, Damiano, Damianos, Damiyan,
Damján, Damyan, Damyen, Damyin,
Damyyn, Daymian, Dema, Demyan

Damien, Damion (Greek) forms of
Damian. Religion: Father Damien minis-
tered to the leper colony on the Hawaiian
island Molokai.
Daemien, Damie, Damienne, Damieon,
Damiion, Damine, Damionne, Damiyon,
Dammion, Damyen, Damyon

Damocles, Damócles (Greek) gives glory
to his village.

Damodar (Indian) another name for the
Hindu god Ganapati.

Damon (Greek) constant, loyal. (Latin) spirit,
demon.
Damoni, Damonn, Damonni, Damyn

Damond (Greek, Latin) a form of Damon.

Damone (Greek, Latin) a form of Damon.

Damonta (Greek, Latin) a form of Damon.
Damontis

Damonte (Greek, Latin) a form of Damon.
Damontae, Damontez

Dan (Vietnamese) yes. (Hebrew) a short
form of Daniel.
Dahn, Danh, Dann, Danne

Dana GB (Scandinavian) from Denmark.
Daina, Danah, Dayna

Dandin (Hindi) holy man.
Dandan, Danden, Dandon, Dandyn

Dandre (French) a combination of the pre-
fix De + Andre.
Dandrae, Dandras, Dandray, Dandrea,
Dondrea

Dandré (French) a form of Dandre.

Dane (English) from Denmark. See also Halden.
Daen, Daene, Danie, Dhane

Danek (Polish) a form of Daniel.

Danforth (English) a form of Daniel.

Dang (Italian) a short form of Deangelo.

Dangelo (Italian) a form of Deangelo.

Daniachew (Ethiopian) you will be judged.

Danial (Hebrew) a form of Daniel.
Danal, Daneal, Danieal, Daniyal, Dannal, Dannial

Danick, Danik, Dannick (Slavic) familiar forms of Daniel.
Danek, Danieko, Danika, Danyck

Daniel ☀ 🅱🅶 (Hebrew) God is my judge. Bible: a Hebrew prophet. See also Danno, Kanaiela, Taniel.
Dacso, Dainel, Dan'l, Daneel, Daneil, Danel, Daniël, Dániel, Danielius, Daniell, Daniels, Danielson, Danukas, Dasco, Deniel, Doneal, Doniel, Donois, Nelo

Daniele 🅶🅱 (Hebrew) a form of Daniel.
Danile, Danniele

Danielle 🅶🅱 (Hebrew) a form of Daniel.

Danilo (Slavic) a form of Daniel.
Danielo, Danil, Danila, Danilka, Danylo

Danior (Gypsy) born with teeth.
Danyor

Danish (English) from Denmark.

Danladi (Hausa) born on Sunday.
Danladee, Danladey, Danladie, Danlady

Dannie, Danny, Dany (Hebrew) familiar forms of Daniel.
Danee, Daney, Dani, Danie, Dannee, Danney, Danni, Dannye

Danniel (Hebrew) a form of Daniel.
Dannel, Dannil

Danno (Japanese) gathering in the meadow. (Hebrew) a familiar form of Daniel.
Dano

Dannon (American) a form of Danno.
Daenan, Daenen, Dainon, Danaan, Danen, Dannan, Dannen, Dannin, Dannyn, Danon, Danyn

Dano (Czech) a form of Daniel.
Danko

Danso (Ghanaian) trustworthy; reliable.

Dantae (Latin) a form of Dante.

Dante, Danté (Latin) lasting, enduring.
Danatay, Danaté, Dant, Dantay, Dantee, Dauntay, Dauntaye, Daunté, Dauntrae

Dantel (Latin) a form of Dante.

Danton (American) a form of Deanthony.

Dantrell (American) a combination of Dante + Darell.
Dantrel, Dantrey, Dantril, Dantyrell

Danyel 🅶🅱 (Hebrew) a form of Daniel.
Daniyel, Danya, Danyal, Danyale, Danyele, Danyell, Danyiel, Danyil, Danyill, Danyl, Danyle, Danylets, Danyll, Danylo, Donyell

Danzel (Cornish) a form of Denzell.
Danzell

Daoud (Arabic) a form of Daniel, David.
Daudi, Daudy, Dauod, Dawud

Daquan (American) a combination of the prefix Da + Quan.
Daquandre, Daquandrey, Daquann, Daquantae, Daquante, Daquaun, Daquawn, Daquin, Daquwon, Daqwain, Daqwan, Daqwann, Daqwone

Daquane (American) a form of Daquan.
Daquain, Daquaine, Daqwane

Daquarius (American) a form of Daquan.

Daquon (American) a form of Daquan.
Daqon, Daquone, Daqwon

Dar (Hebrew) pearl.
Darr

Dara 🅶🅱 (Cambodian) stars.
Darah

Daran, Darin, Darrin, Darron, Darryn (Irish, English) forms of Darren.
Daaron, Daeron, Dairon, Darann, Darawn, Darone, Daronn, Darran, Darroun, Darynn, Dayran, Dayrin, Dayron, Dearin, Dearon, Deran, Dharin, Dharon, Diron

Darby GB (Irish) free. (English) deer park.
*Dar, Darb, Darbe, Darbee, Darbey, Darbi,
Darbie, Derbe, Derbee, Derbey, Derbi, Derbie,
Derby*

Darcy GB (Irish) dark. (French) from Arcy,
France.
*Dar, Daray, Darce, Darcee, Darcel, Darcey,
Darci, Darcie, Darcio, Darse, Darsee, Darsey,
Darsi, Darsie, Darsy*

Dardo (Greek) astute and skillful.

Dareh (Persian) wealthy.
Dare

Darek, Darick, Darik, Darrick (German)
forms of Derek.
*Darec, Dareck, Daric, Darico, Darieck, Dariek,
Darrec, Darrek, Darric, Darrik, Darryc,
Darryck, Darryk, Daryk*

Darell, Darrel (English) forms of Darrell.
*Daral, Darall, Daralle, Dareal, Darel, Darelle,
Darol*

Daren (Hausa) born at night. (Irish, English)
a form of Darren.
Daran, Dare, Dayren, Dheren

Dareon (Irish, English) a form of Darren.
Daryeon, Daryon

Darian BG (Irish, English) a form of Darren.
*Dairean, Dairion, Darrione, Darriun,
Darriyun, Daryan, Derrion*

Dariel BG (French) a form of Darrell.

Darien BG (Irish, English) a form of Darren.

Dario (Spanish) affluent.
Daryo

Darío (Spanish) a form of Dario.

Darion BG (Irish, English) a form of Darren.

Darious, Darrious, Darrius (Greek) forms
of Darius.
*Darreus, Darrias, Darriuss, Darryus, Derrious,
Derrius*

Daris, Darris (Greek) short forms of
Darius.
Darrus, Derris

Darius (Greek) wealthy.
Dairus, Darieus, Darioush, Dariuse, Dariush,

*Dariuss, Dariusz, Darrias, Darrios, Darrus,
Darus, Daryos, Daryus*

Darkon (English) dark.
Darkan, Darken, Darkin, Darkun, Darkyn

Darnel (English) a form of Darnell.
Darnele

Darnell (English) hidden place.
*Dar, Darn, Darnall, Darneal, Darneil,
Darnyell, Darnyll*

Darnelle BG (English) a form of Darnell.

Daron BG (Irish, English) a form of Darren.

Darpan (Indian) mirror.

Darrell (French) darling, beloved; grove of
oak trees.
Dare, Darral, Darrall, Darril, Darrill, Darrol

Darren (Irish) great. (English) small; rocky
hill.
Dare, Darran, Darrience, Darun, Dearron

Darrian BG (Irish, English) a form of
Darren.

Darrien BG (Irish, English) a form of
Darren.

Darrion BG (Irish, English) a form of
Darren.

Darryl, Daryle (French) forms of Darrell.
*Dahrll, Daril, Darl, Darly, Daroyl, Darryle,
Darryll, Daryell, Daryll, Darylle, Derryl*

Darshan (Sanskrit) philosophy; seeing
clearly.
*Darshaun, Darshen, Darshin, Darshon,
Darshyn*

Darton (English) deer town.
*Dartan, Dartel, Darten, Dartin, Dartrel,
Dartyn*

Darvell (English) eagle town.
*Darvel, Darvele, Darvelle, Darvil, Darvile,
Darvill, Darville, Darvyl, Darvyle, Darvyll*

Darvin (English) a form of Darwin.
Darvan, Darven, Darvon, Darvyn

Darwin (English) dear friend. History:
Charles Darwin was the British naturalist
who established the theory of evolution.
Darwen, Darwyn

Darwishi (Egyptian) saint.

Daryl BG (French) a form of Darrell.

Daryn BG (Irish, English) a form of Darren.

Dasan (Pomo) leader of the bird clan.
Dasen, Dasin, Dason, Dassan, Dasyn

Dasean, Dashaun, Dashon (American) forms of Dashawn, Deshawn.

Dasharath (Indian) father of the Hindu god Rama.

Dasharathi (Indian) another name for the Hindu god Rama.

Dashawn BG (American) a combination of the prefix Da + Shawn.
Dashan, Dashane, Dashante, Dashaunte, Dashean, Dashonnie, Dashonte, Dashuan, Dashun, Dashwan

Dasio (Latin) baron.

Dat (Vietnamese) accomplished.

Dativo (Latin) term from Roman law, applied to educators.

Dato (Latin) a form of Donato.

Dauid (Swahili) a form of David.
Dawud

Daulton (English) a form of Dalton.

Daunte (Spanish) a form of Dante.

Davante, Davanté (American) forms of Davonte.
Davanta, Davantay, Davinte

Davaris (American) a combination of Dave + Darius.
Davario, Davarious, Davarius, Davarrius, Davarus

Davaughn (American) a combination of the prefix Da + Vaughn.

Dave (Hebrew) a short form of David, Davis.

Daven (Hebrew) a form of David. (Scandinavian) a form of Davin.

Daveon (American) a form of Davin.
Deaveon

Davet (French) loved.

Davey, Davy (Hebrew) familiar forms of David.
Davee, Davi, Davie

Davian, Davion (American) forms of Davin.
Davione, Davionne, Daviyon, Davyon

David ☀ BG (Hebrew) beloved. Bible: the second king of Israel. See also Dov, Havika, Kawika, Taaveti, Taffy, Taved, Tevel.
Dabi, Daevid, Daevyd, Dafydd, Dai, Daived, Daivid, Daivyd, Dauid, Dav, Daved, Daveed, Davidd, Davidde, Davide, Davidek, Davido, Davood, Davoud, Davyd, Davydas, Davydd, Davyde, Dayvid, Deved, Devid, Devidd, Devidde, Devod, Devodd, Devyd, Devydd, Devydde, Dodya

David Alexander (American) a combination of David + Alexander.
David-Alexander, Davidalexander

Davidia (Hebrew) a form of David.

Davidson (Welsh) a form of Davis.
Davison, Davyson

Davin (Scandinavian) brilliant Finn.
Daevin, Davan, Davyn, Deavan, Deaven

Davis (Welsh) son of David.
Davies, Davys

Davon BG (American) a form of Davin.
Davone, Davonn, Davonne, Deavon, Deavone

Davonta (American) a form of Davonte.
Davontah

Davontae, Davontay, Davonté (American) forms of Davonte.
Davontai, Davontaye

Davonte (American) a combination of Davon + the suffix Te.
Davonnte, Davontea, Davontee, Davonti

Dawan (American) a form of Dajuan, Davin.
Dawann, Dawante, Dawaun, Dawin, Dawine, Dawon, Dawone, Dawoon, Dawyne, Dawyun

Dawid (Polish) a form of David.
Dawed, Dawud

Dawit (Ethiopian) a form of David.
Dawyt

Dawson (English) son of David.
Dawsan, Dawsen, Dawsin, Dawsyn, Dayson

Dawûd (Arabic) a form of David.

Dax (French, English) water.

Day (English) a form of Daniel.

Daylan BG (American) a form of Dalan, Dillon.
Daelon, Dailon, Daylun, Daylyn

Daylen, Daylon (American) forms of Dalan, Dillon.

Daylin BG (American) a form of Dalan, Dillon.

Daymian (Greek) a form of Damian.
Daymayne, Daymeon, Daymiane, Daymien, Dayminn, Daymion, Daymn

Daymon (Greek, Latin) a form of Damon.
Dayman, Daymen, Daymin

Daymond (Greek, Latin) a form of Damon.

Dayne (Scandinavian) a form of Dane.
Dayn

Dayquan (American) a form of Daquan.
Dayquain, Dayquawane, Dayquin, Dayqwan

Dayshawn (American) a form of Dashawn.
Daysean, Daysen, Dayshaun, Dayshon, Dayson

Dayton BG (English) day town; bright, sunny town.
Daeton, Daiton, Daythan, Daython, Daytonn, Deyton

Daytona BG (English) a form of Dayton.
Daytonah

Dayvon (American) a form of Davin.
Dayven, Dayveon, Dayvin, Dayvion, Dayvonn

De (Chinese) virtuous.

De Andre, Deandré, Déandre (American) forms of Deandre.
De André, De Andrea, De Aundre, Déandrea

De Marcus, Démarcus (American) forms of Demarcus.

De Vante, Devanté, Dévante (American) forms of Devante.
De Vantae, De Vanté, Dévanté

Deacon (Greek) one who serves.
Deakin, Deicon, Deke, Deycon

Dean (French) leader. (English) valley. See also Dino.
Deane, Deen, Deene, Dene, Deyn, Deyne, Dyn, Dyne

Deandra GB (French) a form of Deandre.
Deaundera, Deaundra

Deandre (French) a combination of the prefix De + Andre.
Deandrae, Deandres, Deandrey, Deeandre, Deiandre, Deyandre, Dondre

Deandrea GB (French) a form of Deandre.

Deangelo (Italian) a combination of the prefix De + Angelo.
Danglo, De Angelo, Deaengelo, Deangelio, Deangello, Deangilio, Deangleo, Deanglo, Deangulo, Di'angelo, Diangello, Diangelo, Dyangello, Dyangelo

Déangelo (American) a form of Deangelo.

Deante, Deanté (Latin) forms of Dante, Deonte.
De Anté, Deanta, Deantai, Deantay, Deanteé, Deaunta

Deanthony (Italian) a combination of the prefix De + Anthony.
Dianthony

Déanthony (American) a form of Deanthony.

Dearborn (English) deer brook.
Dearborne, Dearbourn, Dearbourne, Dearburne, Deaurburn, Deerborn, Deerborne, Deerbourn, Deerbourne

Deaundre (French) a form of Deandre.
Deaundray, Deaundrey, Deaundry

Deaven (Hindi, Irish) a form of Deven.

Debashis (Indian) benediction of God.

Decarlos (Spanish) a combination of the prefix De + Carlos.
Dacarlo, Dacarlos, Decarlo, Di'carlos, Dicarlo

Decha (Tai) strong.
Dechah

Decimus (Latin) tenth.
Decymus

Decio (Latin) tenth.

Declan (Irish) man of prayer. Religion: Saint Declan was a fifth-century Irish bishop.
Daclan, Deklan, Diclan, Dyclan

Decoroso (Latin) he is practical.

Dédalo (Greek) industrious and skillful artisan.

Dedric (German) a form of Dedrick.
Dederic, Dedryc, Detric

Dedrick (German) ruler of the people. See also Derek, Theodoric.
Deadric, Deadrick, Deadrik, Deddrick, Dederick, Dederik, Dedrek, Dedreko, Dedrix, Dedrrick, Dedryck, Dedryk, Deedrick, Detrik, Diedrich

Deems (English) judge's child.
Deam, Deim, Deym, Deyms

Deenabandhu (Indian) friend of the poor.

Deep (Indian) lamp.

Deepak (Hindi) a form of Dipak.

Deepan (Indian) lighting up.

Deepankar, Deepesh (Indian) lord of light.

Deependu, Deeptendu (Indian) bright moon.

Deepit (Indian) lighted.

Deeptanshu (Indian) sun.

Deeptiman, Deeptimoy (Indian) lustrous.

Deicola, Deícola (Latin) he who cultivates a relationship with God.

Deion (Greek) a form of Deon, Dion.
Deione, Deionta, Deionte

Deiondre (American) a form of Deandre.
Deiondray, Deiondré

Deionte (American) a form of Deontae.
Deiontae, Deionté

Dejon 🅱🅶 (American) a form of Dejuan.

Déjon (American) a form of Dejuan.

Dejuan (American) a combination of the prefix De + Juan.
D'Won, Dejan, Dejuane, Dejun, Dijuan

Dekel (Hebrew, Arabic) palm tree, date tree.
Dekal, Dekil, Dekyl

Dekota (Dakota) a form of Dakota.
Decoda, Dekoda, Dekodda, Dekotes

Del (English) a short form of Delbert, Delvin, Delwin.

Delaiá (Hebrew) God has liberated me.

Delaney 🇬🇧 (Irish) descendant of the challenger.
Delaine, Delainey, Delaini, Delainie, Delainy, Delan, Delane, Delanny, Delany

Delano (French) nut tree. (Irish) dark.
Delanio, Delayno, Dellano

Delbert (English) bright as day. See also Dalbert.
Bert, Delbirt, Delburt, Delbyrt, Dilbert

Delfín (Greek) the playful one with a graceful and beautiful form.

Delfino (Latin) dolphin.
Delfin, Delfine, Delfyn, Delfyne, Delfyno, Delphino, Delphyno

Déli (Chinese) virtuous.

Dell (English) small valley. A short form of Udell.

Delling (Scandinavian) scintillating.

Delmar 🅱🅶 (Latin) sea.
Dalmar, Dalmer, Delmare, Delmario, Delmarr, Delmer, Delmor, Delmore

Delmon (French) mountain.
Delman, Delmen, Delmin, Delmyn

Delon (American) a form of Dillon.
Deloin, Delone, Deloni, Delonne

Delroy (French) belonging to the king. See also Elroy, Leroy.
Dalroi, Dalroy, Delray, Delree, Delroi

Delshawn (American) a combination of Del + Shawn.
Delsean, Delshon, Delsin, Delson

Delsin (Native American) he is so.
Delsan, Delsen, Delson, Delsyn

Delton (English) a form of Dalton.
Deltan, Delten, Deltin, Deltyn

Delvin (English) proud friend; friend from the valley.
Dalvyn, Delavan, Delvian, Delvyn

Delvon (English) a form of Delvin.

Delvonte (American) a form of Delvon.

Delwin (English) a form of Delvin.
Dalwin, Dalwyn, Dellwin, Dellwyn, Delwyn, Delwynn

Deman (Dutch) man.
Demann

Demarco (Italian) a combination of the prefix De + Marco.
Demarcco, Demarceo, Demarcio, Demarquo

Demarcus (American) a combination of the prefix De + Marcus.
Demarces, Demarcis, Demarcius, Demarcos, Demarcuse, Demarqus

Demarea (Italian) a form of Demario.
Demaree, Demareo, Demaria, Demariea

Demario (Italian) a combination of the prefix De + Mario.
Demari, Demariez, Demaris, Demarreio, Demarrio, Demaryo, Demerio, Demerrio

Demarion (Italian) a form of Demario.

Demarious (Italian) a form of Demario.
Demariuz

Demarius (American) a combination of the prefix De + Marius.

Demarko (Italian) a form of Demarco.
Demarkco, Demarkeo, Demarkes, Demarkis, Demarkos

Demarkus (Italian, American) a form of Demarco, Demarcus.

Demarquis (American) a combination of the prefix De + Marquis.
Demarques, Demarquez, Demarqui

Dembe (Luganda) peaceful.
Damba

Demetre, Demetri (Greek) short forms of Demetrius.
Demeter, Demetrea, Demetriel, Domotor

Demetric, Demetrick (Greek) forms of Demetrius.
Demeatric, Demetrics, Demetrik

Demetrice (Greek) a form of Demetrius.
Demeatrice

Demetrio (Greek) a form of Demetrius.

Demetrios (Greek) a form of Demetrius.

Demetrious (Greek) a form of Demetrius.

Demetris (Greek) a short form of Demetrius.
Demeatris, Demetres, Demetress, Demetricus, Demitrez, Demitries, Demitris

Demetrius (Greek) lover of the earth. Mythology: a follower of Demeter, the goddess of the harvest. See also Dimitri, Mimis, Mitsos.
Demeitrius, Demeterious, Demetreus, Demetrias, Demetriu, Demetrium, Demetrois, Demetrus, Demetryus, Demtrius, Demtrus, Dmetrius, Dymek, Dymetrias, Dymetrius, Dymetriys, Dymetryas, Dymetryus

Demetruis (Greek) a form of Demetrius.

Demian (Greek) he who emerged from the village.

Demián (Spanish) a form of Damian.

Demichael (American) a combination of the prefix De + Michael.
Dumichael

Demissie (Ethiopian) destructor.

Demitri (Greek) a short form of Demetrius.
Demitre, Demitrie

Demitrius (Greek) a form of Demetrius.
Demitirus, Demitrias, Demitriu, Demitrus

Demócrito (Greek) arbiter of the village.

Demófilo (Greek) friend of the community.

Demon (Greek) demon.

Demond (Irish) a short form of Desmond.
Demonde, Demonds, Demone, Dumonde

Demondre (American) a form of Demond.

Demont (French) mountain.
Démont, Demontaz, Demontez

Demonta (American) a form of Demont.

Demontae, Demonte, Demonté (American) forms of Demont.
Demontay

Demontre (American) a form of Demont.

Demorris (American) a combination of the prefix De + Morris.
Demoris, DeMorris, Demorus

Demos (Greek) people.
Demas, Demous

Demóstenes (Greek) the strength of the village.

Demothi (Native American) talks while walking.
Demoth

Dempsey (Irish) proud.
Demp, Demps, Dempsi, Dempsie, Dempsy

Dempster (English) one who judges.
Dempstar, Demster

Denham (English) village in the valley.
Denhem

Denholm (Scottish) Geography: a town in Scotland.

Denis 🅱🅶 (Greek) a form of Dennis.
Denas, Denes, Dénes, Denies, Denise, Denys, Dinis, Diniss, Dynis, Dyniss, Dynys, Dynyss

Denís (Greek) a form of Denis.

Deniz, Dennys (Greek) forms of Dennis.

Denley (English) meadow; valley.
Denlea, Denlee, Denli, Denlie, Denly

Denman (English) man from the valley.
Denmen

Dennis (Greek) Mythology: a follower of Dionysus, the god of wine. See also Dion, Nicho.
Dannis, Dannys, Dennas, Dennes, Dennet, Dennez, Denya

Dennison (English) son of Dennis. See also Dyson, Tennyson.
Denison, Denisson, Dennyson, Denyson

Denny (Greek) a familiar form of Dennis.
Den, Deni, Denie, Denney, Denni, Dennie, Deny

Denton (English) happy home.
Dent, Denten, Dentin, Dentown

Denver 🅱🅶 (English) green valley. Geography: the capital of Colorado.
Denvor

Denzel, Denzil (Cornish) forms of Denzell.
Dennzil, Dennzyl, Denzial, Denziel, Denzill, Denzille, Denzyel, Denzyl, Denzyll, Denzylle

Denzell (Cornish) Geography: a location in Cornwall, England.
Dennzel, Denzal, Denzale, Denzall, Denzalle, Denzelle, Denzle, Denzsel

Deocaro (Latin) loved by God.

Deodato (Latin) he who serves God.

Deon 🅱🅶 (Greek) a form of Dennis. See also Dion.
Deone, Deonn, Deonno

Deondra 🅶🅱 (French) a form of Deandre.

Deondre, Deondré (French) forms of Deandre.
Deondrae, Deondray, Deondrea, Deondree, Deondrei, Deondrey

Deonta, Deontá (American) forms of Deontae.

Deontae (American) a combination of the prefix De + Dontae.
Deontai, Deontea, Deonteya, Deonteye, Deontia

Deontay, Deonte, Deonté, Déonte (American) forms of Deontae.
Deontaye, Deontée, Deontie

Deontrae, Deontray, Deontre (American) forms of Deontae.
Deontrais, Deontrea, Deontrey, Deontrez, Deontreze, Deontrus

Dequan (American) a combination of the prefix De + Quan.
Dequain, Dequane, Dequann, Dequaun, Dequawn, Dequian, Dequin, Dequine, Dequinn, Dequion, Dequoin, Dequon, Dequwan, Dequwon, Dequwone

Déquan (American) a form of Dequan.

Dequante (American) a form of Dequan.
Dequantez, Dequantis

Dequavius (American) a form of Dequan.

Dereck, Deric, Derick, Derik, Derreck, Derrek, Derric, Derrick, Derrik, Deryck, Deryk (German) forms of Derek.
Derec, Derekk, Dericka, Derico, Deriek, Derikk, Derique, Derrec, Derreck, Derric, Derryc, Derryck, Derryk, Deryc, Deryke, Detrek, Dyrryc, Dyrryck, Dyrryk, Dyryc, Dyryck

Derek (German) a short form of Theodoric. See also Dedrick, Dirk.
Derak, Derecke, Derele, Derk, Derke, Deryek

Derian BG (Irish, English) a form of Darren.

Derion, Derrian, Derrion (Irish, English) forms of Darren.
Dereon, Derreon, Derrien, Deryan, Deryon

Derius, Derrius (Greek) forms of Darius.
Deriues, Derrious, Derryus, Deryus

Dermot (Irish) free from envy. (English) free. (Hebrew) a short form of Jeremiah. See also Kermit.
Der, Dermod, Dermont, Dermott, Diarmid, Diarmuid

Deron (Hebrew) bird; freedom. (American) a combination of the prefix De + Ron.
Dereon, Deronn, Deronne, Derrin, Derronn, Derronne, Derryn, Deryn, Diron, Dyron

Deror (Hebrew) lover of freedom.
Derori, Derorie

Derrell (French) a form of Darrell.
Derel, Derele, Derell, Derelle, Derrel, Dérrell, Derriel, Derril, Derrill

Derren (Irish, English) a form of Darren.
Deren, Derran, Derraun, Derrin, Derryn, Deryn

Derron (Irish, English) a form of Darren. (Hebrew, American) a form of Deron.

Derry BG (Irish) redhead. Geography: a city in Northern Ireland.
Darrie, Darry, Deri, Derie, Derri, Derrie, Derrye, Dery

Derryl (French) a form of Darryl.
Deryl, Deryle, Deryll, Derylle

Derward (English) deer keeper.
Derwood, Dirward, Durward, Dyrward

Derwin (English) a form of Darwin.
Dervin, Dervon, Dervyn, Dervyne, Derwen, Derwyn, Derwyne, Derwynn, Durwin, Durwyn, Durwyne

Deseado (Spanish) a form of Desiderio.

Desean (American) a combination of the prefix De + Sean.
D'Sean, Dusean, Dysean

Désean (American) a form of Desean.

Deshane (American) a combination of the prefix De + Shane.
Deshan, Deshayne

Deshaun (American) a combination of the prefix De + Shaun.
D'shaun, D'Shaun, Deshan, Deshane, Deshann, Deshaon, Deshaune, Dushaun, Dyshaun

Déshaun (American) a form of Deshaun.

Deshawn BG (American) a combination of the prefix De + Shawn.
D'shawn, D'Shawn, Deshauwn, Deshawan, Deshawon, Dyshawn

Déshawn (American) a form of Deshawn.

Deshea (American) a combination of the prefix De + Shea.
Deshay

Déshì (Chinese) virtuous.

Deshon (American) a form of Deshawn.
Deshondre, Deshone, Deshonn, Deshonte, Dyshon, Dyshone, Dyshyn, Dyshyne

Deshun (American) a form of Deshon.
Deshunn

Desi BG (Latin) desiring. (Irish) a short form of Desmond.
Dezi

Desiderato (Spanish) a form of Desiderio.

Desiderio (Spanish) desired.
Desideryo

Desierto (Latin) wild.

Desire (French) wish.

Desmon (Irish) a form of Desmond.
Desimon, Desman, Desmane, Desmen, Desmine, Desmyn

Desmond (Irish) from south Munster.
Des, Desmand, Desmound, Desmund

Desta (Ethiopian) happiness.

Destin BG (French) destiny, fate.
Destan, Desten, Destine, Deston, Destun, Destyn

Destry (American) a form of Destin.
Destrey, Destrie

Detrick (German) a form of Dedrick.
Detrek, Detric, Detrich, Detrik, Detrix

Deuce (Latin) two; devil.

Deusdedit (Latin) God has given to him.

Dev Kumar (Indian) son of gods.

Devabrata (Indian) another name for Bhisma, a hero of the Indian epic poem *Mahabharata*.

Devadas (Indian) follower of God.

Devajyoti (Indian) brightness of the lord.

Devak (Indian) divine.

Devan BG (Irish) a form of Devin.
Deavan, Deavyn, Devaan, Devain, Devane, Devann, Devean, Devun, Devyin, Devynn, Devynne, Diwan

Devanta (American) a form of Devante.

Devante (American) a combination of Devan + the suffix Te.
Devantae, Devantay, Devantée, Devantez, Devanty, Devaunte, Deventae, Deventay, Devente, Divante

Devaughn (American) a form of Devin.
Devaugh, Devaughntae, Devaughnte

Devaun (American) a form of Devaughn.

Devayne (American) a form of Dewayne.
Devain, Devaine, Devane, Devayn, Devein, Deveion

Devdutta (Indian) king.

Deven (Hindi) for God. (Irish) a form of Devin.
Deiven, Devein, Devenn, Devven, Diven, Dyven

Devendra (Indian) another name for the Hindu god Indra.

Deveon (American) a form of Devon.
Deveone

Deverell (English) riverbank.

Devesh, Deveshwar (Indian) other names for the Hindu god Shiva.

Devin ☀ BG (Irish) poet.
Deavin, Deivin, Dev, Devinn, Devvin, Devy, Dyvon

Devine (Latin) divine. (Irish) ox.
Devyne, Dewine

Devion (American) a form of Devon.

Devlin (Irish) brave, fierce.
Dev, Devlan, Devland, Devlen, Devlon

Devlyn (Irish) a form of Devlin.

Devon BG (American) a form of Davon. (Irish) a form of Devin.
Deavon, Deivon, Devoen, Devohn, Devonae, Devoni, Devonio, Devonn, Devontaine, Devun, Devvon, Devvonne, Dewon, Dewone, Divon, Diwon

Dévon, Devonne (American) forms of Davon. (Irish) forms of Devin.

Devone (Irish, American) a form of Devon.
Deivone, Deivonne

Devonta (American) a combination of Devon + the suffix Ta.
Deveonta, Devonnta, Devonntae, Devontai, Devontay, Devontaye

Devontá, Dévonta (American) forms of Devonta.

Devontae, Devontay, Devonté (American) forms of Devonte.

Devonte (American) a combination of Devon + the suffix Te.
Deveonte, Devionte, Devontea, Devontee, Devonti, Devontia, Devontre

Devoto (Latin) dedicated.

Devyn BG (Irish) a form of Devin.

Dewan (American) a form of Dejuan, Dewayne.
Dewaun, Dewaune, Dewon

Dewayne (American) a combination of the prefix De + Wayne. (Irish) a form of Dwayne.
Deuwayne, Devayne, Dewain, Dewaine, Dewane, Dewayen, Dewean, Dewune

Dewei (Chinese) highly virtuous.

Dewey (Welsh) prized.
Dew, Dewi, Dewie, Dewy

DeWitt (Flemish) blond.
Dewit, Dewitt, Dewyt, Dewytt, Wit

Dexter (Latin) dexterous, adroit. (English) fabric dyer.
Daxter, Decca, Deck, Decka, Dekka, Dex, Dextar, Dextor, Dextrel, Dextron, Dextur

Deyonte (American) a form of Deontae.

Dezmon (Irish) a form of Desmond.
Dezman, Dezmen, Dezmin

Dezmond (Irish) a form of Desmond.
Dezmand, Dezmund

Día (West African) champion.

Diadelfo (Greek) brother of Zeus.

Diamante, Diamonte (Spanish) forms of Diamond.
Diamanta, Diamont, Diamonta, Dimonta, Dimontae, Dimonte

Diamond GB (English) brilliant gem; bright guardian.
Diaman, Diamend, Diamenn, Diamund, Dimond, Dymond

Diandre (French) a form of Deandre.

Diante, Dianté (American) forms of Deontae.
Diantae, Diantey

Dick (German) a short form of Frederick, Richard.
Dic, Dicken, Dickens, Dickie, Dickon, Dicky, Dik

Dickran (Armenian) History: an ancient Armenian king.
Dicran, Dikran

Dickson (English) son of Dick.
Dickenson, Dickerson, Dikerson, Diksan

Dictino (Greek) goddess of the ocean.

Dídac (Catalan) a form of Diego.

Diderot (Spanish) a form of Desiderio.

Didi (Hebrew) a familiar form of Jedidiah, Yedidya.

Didier (French) desired, longed for.

Didimo, Dídimo (Greek) twin brother.

Diedrich (German) a form of Dedrick, Dietrich.
Didrich, Didrick, Didrik, Didyer, Diederick

Diego ✰ (Spanish) a form of Jacob, James.
Diaz

Dietbald (German) a form of Theobald.
Dietbalt, Dietbolt

Dieter (German) army of the people.
Deiter, Deyter

Dietrich (German) a form of Dedrick.
Deitrich, Deitrick, Deke, Didric, Didrick, Diedrich, Diedrick, Diedrik, Dierck, Dieter, Dieterich, Dieterick, Dietric, Dietrick, Dietz, Ditrik

Digby (Irish) ditch town; dike town.
Digbe, Digbee, Digbey, Digbi, Digbie

Digno (Latin) worthy of the best.

Diji (Nigerian) farmer.

Dijon (French) Geography: a city in France. (American) a form of Dejon.

Dilan, Dillen, Dillyn (Irish) forms of Dillon.
Dilun, Dilyan

Dillan BG (Irish) a form of Dillon.

Dillian BG (Irish) a form of Dillon.

Dillion (Irish) a form of Dillon.

Dillon (Irish) loyal, faithful. See also Dylan.
Dil, Dill, Dillie, Dilly, Dillyn, Dilon, Dilyn, Dilynn

Dilwyn (Welsh) shady place.
Dillwin, Dillwyn, Dilwin

Dima (Russian) a familiar form of Vladimir.
Dimah, Dimka, Dyma, Dymah

Dimano (Latin) to lose.

Dimas (Greek) loyal comrade.

Dimitri (Russian) a short form of Demetrius.
Dimetra, Dimetri, Dimetric, Dimetrie, Dimitr, Dimitric, Dimitrie, Dimitrij, Dimitrik, Dimitris, Dimitry, Dimmy, Dymetree, Dymetrey, Dymetri, Dymetrie, Dymitr, Dymitry

Dimitrios (Greek) a form of Demetrius.
Dhimitrios, Dimos, Dmitrios

Dimitrius (Greek) a form of Demetrius.
Dimetrius, Dimetrus, Dimitricus, Dmitrius

Dingbang (Chinese) protector of the country.

Dinh (Vietnamese) calm, peaceful.
Din, Dyn, Dynh

Dinís (Greek) devoted to Dionysus.

Dino (German) little sword. (Italian) a form of Dean.
Deano, Dyno

Dinos (Greek) a familiar form of Constantine, Konstantin.
Dynos

Dinsmore (Irish) fortified hill.
Dinmoar, Dinmoor, Dinmoore, Dinmor, Dinmore, Dinnie, Dinny, Dinse, Dinsmoor, Dinsmoore, Dynmoar, Dynmoor, Dynmoore, Dynmor, Dynmore

Dioclecio (Greek) a form of Diocles.

Diocles (Greek) glory of God.

Diogenes (Greek) honest. History: an ancient philosopher who searched with a lantern in daylight for an honest man.
Diogenese

Diógenes (Greek) a form of Diogenes.

Diogo (Galician) a form of Diego.

Diomedes (Greek) thoughts of God.

Diómedes (Greek) he who trusts in God's protection.

Dion (Greek) a short form of Dennis, Dionysus.
Dio, Dionigi, Dionis, Dionn, Dyon, Dyone

Dión (Greek) a form of Dion.

Diondre (French) a form of Deandre.
Diondra, Diondrae, Diondrey

Dione (American) a form of Dion.

Dionicio (Spanish) a form of Dionysus.

Dionne GB (American) a form of Dion.

Dionta (American) a form of Deontae.

Diontae, Diontay, Dionte, Dionté (American) forms of Deontae.
Diontaye, Diontea

Dionysus (Greek) celebration. Mythology: the god of wine.
Dionesios, Dionisio, Dionisios, Dionusios, Dionysios, Dionysius, Dyonisios, Dyonisus

Dioscórides (Greek) relative of Dioscoro.

Dioscoro, Dióscoro (Latin) he who is of the Lord.

Dipak (Hindi) little lamp. Religion: another name for the Hindu god Kama.

Diquan (American) a combination of the prefix Di + Quan.
Diqawan, Diqawn, Diquane

Dirk (German) a short form of Derek, Theodoric.
Derc, Derk, Dirc, Dirck, Dirke, Durc, Durk, Dyrc, Dyrck, Dyrk, Dyrrc, Dyrrck, Dyrrk

Disibodo (German) bold wise one.

Dixon (English) son of Dick.
Dix, Dixan, Dixen, Dixin, Dixyn, Dyxan, Dyxen, Dyxin, Dyxon, Dyxyn

Dmitri, Dmitry (Russian) forms of Dimitri.
Dmetriy, Dmitiri, Dmitrik, Dmitriy

Doane (English) low, rolling hills.
Doan

Dob (English) a familiar form of Robert.
Dobie

Dobry (Polish) good.
Dobri, Dobrie

Doherty (Irish) harmful.
Docherty, Dougherty, Douherty

Dolan (Irish) dark haired.
Dolin, Dollan, Dolyn

Dolf, Dolph (German) short forms of Adolf, Adolph, Rudolf, Rudolph.
Dolfe, Dolff, Dolffe, Dolfi, Dolphe, Dolphus, Dulph, Dulphe

Dom (Latin) a short form of Dominic.
Dome, Domm, Domó

Domanic (Latin) a form of Dominic.
Domanick

Doménech (Catalan) a form of Domingo.

Domenic, Domenick (Latin) forms of Dominic.
Domenik, Domenyc, Domenyck, Domenyk

Domenico (Italian) a form of Dominic.
Demenico, Domicio, Dominico, Dominiko, Menico

Dominador (Latin) to want to be loved.

Domingo (Spanish) born on Sunday. See also Mingo.
Demingo, Domingos, Domyngo

Dominic ⚝ (Latin) belonging to the Lord. See also Chuminga.
Deco, Dom, Domeka, Domini, Dominie, Dominitric, Dominy, Domminic, Domnenique, Domokos, Nick

Dominick, Dominik (Latin) forms of Dominic.
Domiku, Domineck, Dominicke, Dominiek, Dominnick, Dominyck, Dominyk, Domminick, Dommonick, Domnick, Donek, Dumin

Dominique **GB** (French) a form of Dominic.
Domeniq, Domeniqu, Domenique, Domenque, Dominiqu, Dominiqueia, Domnenique, Domnique, Domoniqu, Domonique, Domunique

Dominque **BG** (French) a form of Dominic.

Domokos (Hungarian) a form of Dominic.
Dedo, Dome, Domek, Domok, Domonkos

Domonic, Domonick (Latin) forms of Dominic.
Domonik

Don (Scottish) a short form of Donald. See also Kona.
Donn

Donahue (Irish) dark warrior.
Donahu, Donahugh, Donehue, Donohoe, Donohu, Donohue, Donohugh

Donal (Irish) a form of Donald.
Dónal, Donall, Donil

Donald (Scottish) world leader; proud ruler. See also Bohdan, Tauno.
Donalt, Donát, Donaugh, Doneld, Donild, Donyld

Donaldo (Spanish) a form of Donald.

Donardo (Celtic) a form of Donald.

Donatien (French) gift.
Donathan, Donathon, Donatyen

Donato (Italian) gift.
Dodek, Donatello, Donati, Donatien, Donatus, Doneto

Donavan, Donavin, Donavon (Irish) forms of Donovan.
Donaven, Donavyn

Dondre, Dondré (American) forms of Deandre.
Dondra, Dondrae, Dondray, Dondrea

Donell (Irish) a form of Donnell.
Doneal, Donel, Donele, Donelle, Doniel, Donielle, Donyl

Dong (Vietnamese) easterner.
Duong

Donivan (Irish) a form of Donovan.
Donnivan

Donkor (Akan) humble.

Donnell (Irish) brave; dark.
Donnel, Donnele, Donnelle, Donniel, Donnyl

Donnelly (Irish) a form of Donnell.
Donelly, Donlee, Donley

Donnie, Donny (Irish) familiar forms of Donald.
Donee, Doney, Doni, Donie, Donnee, Donney, Donni, Dony

Donovan (Irish) dark warrior.
Dohnovan, Donevan, Donevin, Donevon, Donnovan, Donnoven, Donoven, Donovin, Donvan, Donyvon

Donovon (Irish) a form of Donovan.

Donta (American) a form of Dante.

Dontae, Dontay, Donte, Donté (Latin) forms of Dante.
Dontai, Dontao, Dontate, Dontaye, Dontea, Dontee

Dontarious, Dontarius (American) forms of Dontae.

Dontavious, Dontavius (American) forms of Dontae.

Dontavis (American) a form of Dontae.

Dontez (American) a form of Dontae.

Dontray, Dontre (American) forms of Dontrell.

Dontrell (American) a form of Dantrell.
Dontral, Dontrall, Dontreal, Dontrel, Dontrelle, Dontriel, Dontriell

Donyell (Irish) a form of Donnell.
Donyel

Donzell (Cornish) a form of Denzell.
Donzeil, Donzel, Donzelle, Donzello

Dooley (Irish) dark hero.
Doolea, Doolee, Dooleigh, Dooli, Doolie, Dooly

Dor (Hebrew) generation.

Doran (Greek, Hebrew) gift. (Irish) stranger; exile.
Dore, Doren, Dorin, Doron, Dorran, Dorren, Dorrin, Dorron, Dorryn, Doryn

Dorcas (Hebrew) gazelle.

Dorian 🅱🄶 (Greek) from Doris, Greece. See also Isidore.
Dore, Dorey, Dorie, Dorján, Dorrion, Dorryen, Dorryn, Dory

Dorien, Dorion, Dorrian (Greek) forms of Dorian.
Dorrien

Doroteo (Greek) gift of God.

Dorrell (Scottish) king's doorkeeper. See also Durell.
Dorrel, Dorrelle

Dosio (Latin) rich.

Dositeo (Greek) God's possession.

Dotan (Hebrew) law.
Dothan

Doug (Scottish) a short form of Dougal, Douglas.
Douge, Dougee, Dougey, Dougi, Dougie, Dougy, Dug, Dugee, Dugey, Dugi, Dugie, Dugy

Dougal (Scottish) dark stranger. See also Doyle.
Doogal, Doogall, Dougall, Dugal, Dugald, Dugall, Dughall

Douglas (Scottish) dark river, dark stream. See also Koukalaka.
Dougles, Dugaid, Dughlas

Douglass (Scottish) a form of Douglas.
Duglass

Dov (Yiddish) bear. (Hebrew) a familiar form of David.
Dove, Dovi, Dovidas, Dowid

Dovev (Hebrew) whisper.

Dovid (Hebrew, Yiddish) a form of Dov.

Dow (Irish) dark haired.

Doyle (Irish) a form of Dougal.
Doial, Doiale, Doiall, Doil, Doile, Doy, Doyal, Doyel, Doyele, Doyell, Doyelle

Drago (Italian) a form of Drake.

Drake (English) dragon; owner of the inn with the dragon trademark.
Draek, Draik, Draike, Drayk, Drayke

Draper (English) fabric maker.
Draeper, Draiper, Dray, Drayper, Draypr

Draven (American) a combination of the letter D + Raven.
Dravian, Dravin, Dravion, Dravon, Dravone, Dravyn, Drayven

Dre (American) a short form of Andre, Deandre.
Drae, Dray, Dré

Dreng (Norwegian) hired hand; brave.

Drequan (American) a combination of Drew + Quan.

Dréquan (American) a form of Drequan.

Dreshawn (American) a combination of Drew + Shawn.
Dreshaun, Dreshon, Dreshown

Drevon (American) a form of Draven.
Drevan, Drevaun, Dreven, Drevin, Drevion, Drevone

Drew 🅱🄶 (Welsh) wise. (English) a short form of Andrew.
Drewe

Drey (American) a form of Dre.

Driscoll (Irish) interpreter.
Driscol, Driscole, Dryscol, Dryscoll, Dryscolle

Dru (English) a form of Drew.
Druan, Drud, Drugi, Drui

Drue BG (English) a form of Drew.

Drummond (Scottish) druid's mountain.
Drummund, Drumond, Drumund

Drury (French) loving. Geography: Drury Lane is a street in London's theater district.
Druree, Drurey, Druri, Drurie

Dryden (English) dry valley.
Dridan, Driden, Dridin, Dridyn, Dry, Drydan, Drydin, Drydon, Drydyn

Duane (Irish) a form of Dwayne.
Deune, Duain, Duaine, Duana

Duardo (Spanish) prosperous guardian.

Duardos (Galician) a form of Eduardo.

Duarte (Portuguese) rich guard. See also Edward.
Duart

Dubham (Irish) black.
Dubhem, Dubhim, Dubhom, Dubhym

Dubric (English) dark ruler.
Dubrick, Dubrik, Dubryc, Dubryck, Dubryk

Duc (Vietnamese) moral.
Duoc

Duce (Latin) leader, commander.

Dudd (English) a short form of Dudley.
Dud, Dudde, Duddy

Dudley (English) common field.
Dudlea, Dudlee, Dudleigh, Dudli, Dudlie, Dudly

Duer (Scottish) heroic.

Duff (Scottish) dark.
Duf, Duffey, Duffie, Duffy

Dugan (Irish) dark.
Doogan, Doogen, Dougan, Dougen, Douggan, Douggen, Dugen, Duggan

Duilio (Latin) ready to fight.

Dujuan (American) a form of Dajuan, Dejuan.
Dujuane

Duke (French) leader; duke.
Duk, Dukey, Dukie, Duky

Dukker (Gypsy) fortuneteller.
Duker

Dulani (Nguni) cutting.
Dulanee, Dulaney, Dulanie, Dulany

Dulcidio (Latin) sweet.

Dumaka (Ibo) helping hand.

Duman (Turkish) misty, smoky.
Dumen, Dumin, Dumon, Dumyn

Duncan (Scottish) brown warrior. Literature: King Duncan was Macbeth's victim in Shakespeare's play *Macbeth*.
Doncan, Dunc, Dunkan

Dunham (Scottish) brown.
Dunhem

Dunixi (Basque) a form of Dionysus.

Dunley (English) hilly meadow.
Dunlea, Dunlee, Dunleigh, Dunli, Dunlie, Dunly

Dunlop (Scottish) muddy hill.
Dunlope

Dunmore (Scottish) fortress on the hill.
Dunmoar, Dunmoor, Dunmoore, Dunmor

Dunn (Scottish) a short form of Duncan.
Dun, Dune, Dunne

Dunstan (English) brownstone fortress.
Dun, Dunsten, Dunstin, Dunston, Dunstyn

Dunstano (English) a form of Dunstan.

Dunton (English) hill town.
Duntan, Dunten, Duntin, Duntyn

Dur (Hebrew) stacked up. (English) a short form of Durwin.

Duran (Latin) a form of Durant.

Durand (Latin) a form of Durant.

Durando (Latin) a form of Durand.

Durant (Latin) enduring.
Durance, Durand, Durante, Durontae, Durrant

Durell (Scottish, English) king's doorkeeper. See also Dorrell.
Durel, Durelle, Durial

Durko (Czech) a form of George.

Duron (Hebrew, American) a form of Deron.
Durron

Durrell (Scottish, English) a form of Durell.
Durreil, Durrelle

Durriken (Gypsy) fortuneteller.

Durril (Gypsy) gooseberry.
Duril, Durryl, Durryll, Duryl

Durward (English) gatekeeper.
Derward, Durwood, Ward

Durwin (English) a form of Darwin.

Dusan (Czech) lively, spirited. (Slavic) a form of Daniel.
Dusen, Dusin, Duson, Dusyn

Dushawn (American) a combination of the prefix Du + Shawn.
Dusean, Dushan, Dushane, Dushaun, Dushon, Dushun

Dustan, Dusten, Duston, Dustyn (German, English) forms of Dustin.

Dustin BG (German) valiant fighter. (English) brown rock quarry.
Dust, Dustain, Dustine, Dustion, Dustynn

Dusty BG (English) a familiar form of Dustin.
Dustee, Dustey, Dusti, Dustie

Dutch (Dutch) from the Netherlands; from Germany.

Duval (French) a combination of the prefix Du + Val.
Duvall, Duveuil, Duvyl

Duy (Vietnamese) a form of Duc.

Dwan (American) a form of Dajuan. (Irish) a form of Dwayne.

Dwaun (American) a form of Dajuan.
Dwaunn, Dwawn, Dwon, Dwuann

Dwayne (Irish) dark. See also Dewayne.
Dawayne, Dawyne, Duwain, Duwan, Duwane, Duwayn, Duwayne, Dwain, Dwaine, Dwane, Dwayn, Dwyane, Dywan, Dywane, Dywayne, Dywone

Dwight (English) a form of DeWitt.
Dwhite, Dwite, Dwyte

Dyami (Native American) soaring eagle.
Dyani

Dyer (English) fabric dyer.

Dyke (English) dike; ditch.
Dike

Dylan ☀ BG (Welsh) sea. See also Dillon.
Dylane, Dylann, Dylen, Dylian, Dyllen, Dyllian, Dyllyn, Dylyn

Dylin, Dyllan, Dyllon, Dylon (Welsh) forms of Dylan.
Dyllin, Dyllion

Dyonis (Greek) a form of Dionicio.

Dyre (Norwegian) dear heart.
Dire

Dyson (English) a short form of Dennison.
Dysen, Dysonn

Dzigbode (Ghanaian) patience.

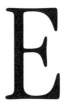

Ea (Irish) a form of Hugh.
Eah

Eabrizio (Italian) artisan.

Eabroni (Italian) blacksmith.

Eachan (Irish) horseman.
Eachen, Eachin, Eachon, Eachyn

Eadberto (Teutonic) outstanding for his riches.

Eagan (Irish) very mighty.

Eamon, Eamonn (Irish) forms of Edmond, Edmund.
Aimon, Eaman, Eamen, Eamin, Eamman, Eammen, Eammin, Eammon, Eammun, Eammyn, Eamun, Eamyn, Eiman, Eimen, Eimin, Eimon, Eimyn, Eyman, Eymen, Eymin, Eymon, Eymyn

Ean (English) a form of Ian.
Eaen, Eann, Eayon, Eon, Eonn, Eyan, Eyen, Eyon, Eyyn

Earl (Irish) pledge. (English) nobleman.
Airle, Earld, Earle, Earli, Earlie, Earlson, Early, Eorl, Erl, Erle

Earnest (English) a form of Ernest.
Earn, Earneste, Earnesto, Earnie, Eirnest, Eranest, Eyrnest

Easton (English) eastern town.
Eason, Eastan, Easten, Eastin, Eastton, Eastyn

Eaton (English) estate on the river.
Eatton, Eton, Eyton

Eb (Hebrew) a short form of Ebenezer.
Ebb, Ebbie, Ebby

Eben (Hebrew) rock.
Eban, Ebenn, Ebin, Ebyn

Ebenezer (Hebrew) foundation stone. Literature: Ebenezer Scrooge is a miserly character in Charles Dickens's *A Christmas Carol*.
Ebbaneza, Ebeneezer, Ebeneser, Ebenezar, Evanezer, Eveneser, Ibenezer

Eber (German) a short form of Eberhard.
Ebere

Eberhard (German) courageous as a boar. See also Everett.
Eberardo, Eberhardt, Evard, Everard, Everhardt, Everhart

Ebner (English) a form of Abner.
Ebnar, Ebnir, Ebnor, Ebnyr

Ebo (Fante) born on Tuesday.

Ebon (Hebrew) a form of Eben.

Ecio (Latin) possessor of great strength.

Eco (Greek) sound, resonance.

Ed (English) a short form of Edgar, Edsel, Edward.
Edd

Edan (Scottish) fire.
Eadan, Eadon, Edain, Edon, Edun

Edbert (English) wealthy; bright.
Ediberto

Edberto (Germanic) he whose blade makes him shine.

Edco (Greek) he who blows with force.

Eddie (English) a familiar form of Edgar, Edsel, Edward.
Eddee, Eddi, Eddye, Edi, Edie, Edy

Eddy BG (English) a familiar form of Edgar, Edsel, Edward.

Edel (German) noble.
Adel, Edell, Edelmar, Edelweiss

Edelberto (German) a form of Edelbert.

Edelio (Greek) person who always remains young.

Edelmiro (Germanic) celebrated for the nobility that he represents.

Eden GB (Hebrew) delightful. Bible: the garden that was first home to Adam and Eve.
Eaden, Eadin, Eadyn, Edenson, Edyn, Eiden

Eder (Hebrew) flock.
Edar, Ederick, Edir, Edor, Edyr

Edgar (English) successful spearman. See also Garek, Gerik, Medgar.
Edek, Edgars, Edger, Edgir, Edgor

Edgard (English) a form of Edgar.

Edgardo (Spanish) a form of Edgar.

Edgerrin (American) a form of Edgar.

Edik (Slavic) a familiar form of Edward.
Edic, Edick

Edilio (Greek) he who is like a statue.

Edin (Hebrew) a form of Eden.

Edipo (Greek) he who has swollen feet.

Edison (English) son of Edward.
Eddisen, Eddison, Eddisyn, Eddyson, Edisen, Edysen, Edyson

Edmond (English) a form of Edmund.
Edmen, Edmon, Edmonde, Edmondson, Edmynd, Esmond

Edmund (English) prosperous protector.
Eadmund, Edman, Edmand, Edmaund, Edmun, Edmunds

Edmundo (Spanish) a form of Edmund.
Edmando, Edmondo, Mundo

Edo (Czech) a form of Edward.

Edoardo (Italian) a form of Edward.

Edorta (Basque) a form of Edward.

Edouard (French) a form of Edward.
Édoard, Édouard

Edric (English) prosperous ruler.
*Eddric, Eddrick, Eddrik, Eddryc, Eddryck,
Eddryk, Ederic, Ederick, Ederik, Ederyc,
Ederyck, Ederyk, Edrek, Edrice, Edrick,
Edrico, Edrik, Edryc, Edryck, Edryk*

Edsel (English) rich man's house.
Edsell

Edson (English) a short form of Edison.
Eddson, Edsen

Eduard (Spanish) a form of Edward.

Eduardo (Spanish) a form of Edward.

Edur (Basque) snow.
Edure

Edvar (Czech) a form of Eduardo.

Edward (English) prosperous guardian. See also
Audie, Duarte, Ekewaka, Ned, Ted, Teddy.
*Edik, Edko, Edo, Edorta, Edus, Edvard,
Edvardo, Edwards, Edwy, Edzio, Etzio, Ewart*

Edwardo (Italian) a form of Edward.

Edwin (English) prosperous friend. See also
Ned, Ted.
*Eadwin, Eadwinn, Edlin, Eduino, Edwan,
Edwen, Edwinn, Edwon, Edwyn, Edwynn*

Effiom (African) crocodile.

Efrain (Hebrew) fruitful.
*Efraine, Efran, Efrane, Efrayin, Efrayn,
Efrayne, Efrian, Efrin, Efryn, Eifraine*

Efraín (Hebrew) a form of Efrain.

Efrat (Hebrew) honored.

Efreín, Efrén (Spanish) forms of Efraín.

Efrem (Hebrew) a short form of Ephraim.
Efe, Efraim, Efrayim, Efrim, Efrum

Efren (Hebrew) a form of Efrain, Ephraim.

Egan (Irish) ardent, fiery.
Egann, Egen, Egin, Egyn

Egbert (English) bright sword. See also Bert,
Bertie.
Egbirt, Egburt, Egbyrt

Egecatl (Nahuatl) wind serpent.

Egerton (English) Edgar's town.
Edgarton, Edgartown, Edgerton, Egeton

Egidio (Greek) he who carries the goatskin
sword in battle.

Egil (Norwegian) awe inspiring.
Egyl, Eigil, Eygel

Eginhard (German) power of the sword.
*Eginhardt, Egynhard, Egynhardt, Einhard,
Einhardt, Enno*

Egisto (Greek) raised on goat's milk.

Egon (German) formidable.
Egun

Egor (Russian) a form of George. See also
Igor, Yegor.

Ehren (German) honorable.
Eren

Eian, Eion (Irish) forms of Ean, Ian.
Ein, Eine, Einn

Eikki (Finnish) ever powerful.
Eiki

Einar (Scandinavian) individualist.
Ejnar, Inar

Eitan (Hebrew) a form of Ethan.
Eita, Eithan, Eiton

Ejau (Ateso) we have received.

Ekalavya (Indian) renowned for his devotion to his guru.

Ekambar (Indian) sky.

Ekanath (Indian) king.

Ekewaka (Hawaiian) a form of Edward.

Ekon (Nigerian) strong.

Ekram (Indian) honor.

Eladio (Greek) he who came from Greece.

Elam (Hebrew) highlands.
Elame

Elan (Hebrew) tree. (Native American)
friendly.
Elann

Elbert (English) a form of Albert.
Elberto, Elbirt, Elburt, Elbyrt

Elbio (Celtic) he who comes from the mountain.

Elchanan (Hebrew) a form of John.
Elchan, Elchonon, Elhanan, Elhannan

Elden (English) a form of Alden, Aldous.
Eldan, Eldin, Eldun, Eldyn

Elder (English) dweller near the elder trees.
Eldar, Eldir, Eldor, Eldyr

Eldon (English) holy hill. A form of Elton.

Eldred (English) a form of Aldred.
Eldrid, Eldryd

Eldridge (English) a form of Aldrich.
El, Elderydg, Elderydge, Eldredge, Eldrege, Eldrige, Elric, Elrick, Elrik

Eldwin (English) a form of Aldwin.
Eldwen, Eldwinn, Eldwyn, Eldwynn

Eleazar (Hebrew) God has helped. See also Lazarus.
Elasar, Elasaro, Elazar, Elazaro, Eleasar, Eléazar

Eleazaro (Hebrew) a form of Eleazar.

Elek (Hungarian) a form of Alec, Alex.
Elec, Eleck, Elic, Elick, Elik, Elyc, Elyck, Elyk

Elenio (Greek) he who shines like the sun.

Eleodoro (Greek) he who comes from the sun.

Eleuia (Nahuatl) wish.

Eleuterio (Greek) he who enjoys liberty for being honest.

Elfego (Germanic) spirit of the air.

Elger (German) a form of Alger.
Elfar, Elgir, Elgor, Elgyr, Ellgar, Ellger

Elgin (English) noble; white.
Elgan, Elgen, Elgon, Elgyn

Eli **BG** (Hebrew) uplifted. A short form of Elijah, Elisha. Bible: the high priest who trained the prophet Samuel. See also Elliot.
Elay, Elier, Ellie

Elia **GB** (Zuni) a short form of Elijah.
Eliah, Eliya, Elya, Elyah

Eliahu (Hebrew) a form of Elijah.

Elian (English) a form of Elijah. See also Trevelyan.
Elien, Elion, Elyan, Elyen, Elyin, Elyn, Elyon

Elián (Greek) sunshine.

Elias (Greek) a form of Elijah.
Elia, Eliasz, Elice, Eliyas, Ellias, Ellice, Ellis, Elyas, Elyes

Elías (Greek) a form of Elias.

Eliazar (Hebrew) a form of Eleazar.
Eliasar, Eliaser, Eliazer, Elizar, Elizardo

Elido (Greek) native of Elida.

Elie (Hebrew) a form of Eli.

Eliecer (Hebrew) God is his constant aid.

Eliezer (Hebrew) a form of Eleazar.
Elieser

Elifelet (Hebrew) God is my liberation.

Eligio (Latin) he who has been elected by God.

Elihu (Hebrew) a short form of Eliyahu.
Elih, Eliu, Ellihu

Elihú (Hebrew) a form of Elihu.

Elijah ⭐ **BG** (Hebrew) a form of Eliyahu. Bible: a Hebrew prophet. See also Eli, Elisha, Elliot, Ilias, Ilya.
El, Elija, Elijiah, Elijio, Elijuah, Elijuo, Eliya, Eliyah, Ellija, Ellijah, Ellyjah

Elijha (Hebrew) a form of Elijah.
Elisjsha

Elika (Hawaiian) a form of Eric.
Elyka

Elimu (African) knowledge.

Elio (Zuni) a form of Elia. (English) a form of Elliot.

Eliot (English) a form of Elliot.
Eliott, Eliud, Eliut, Elyot, Elyott

Elisandro (Greek) liberator of men.

Eliseo (Hebrew) a form of Elisha.
Elisee, Elisée, Elisei, Elisiah, Elisio

Elisha BG (Hebrew) God is my salvation. Bible: a Hebrew prophet, successor to Elijah. See also Eli, Elijah.
Elijsha, Elish, Elishah, Elisher, Elishia, Elishua, Elysha, Lisha

Eliyahu (Hebrew) the Lord is my God.
Elihu, Eliyahou

Elizabeth GB (Hebrew) consecrated to God.

Elkan (Hebrew) God is jealous.
Elkana, Elkanah, Elkin, Elkins, Elkyn, Elkyns

Elki (Moquelumnan) hanging over the top.
Elkie, Elky

Ellard (German) sacred; brave.
Allard, Elard, Ellerd

Ellery BG (English) from a surname derived from the name Hilary.
Elari, Elarie, Elery, Ellari, Ellarie, Ellary, Ellerey, Elleri, Ellerie

Elliot, Elliott (English) forms of Eli, Elijah.
Elliotte, Ellyot, Ellyott

Ellis BG (English) a form of Elias.
Elis, Ellys, Elys

Ellison GB (English) son of Ellis.
Elison, Ellson, Ellyson, Elson, Elyson

Ellsworth (English) nobleman's estate.
Ellswerth, Elsworth

Elman (German) like an elm tree.
Elmen

Elmer (English) noble; famous.
Aylmer, Elemér, Ellmer, Elmar, Elmir, Ulmer

Elmo (Greek) lovable, friendly. (Italian) guardian. (Latin) a familiar form of Anselm. (English) a form of Elmer.

Elmore (English) moor where the elm trees grow.
Ellmoar, Ellmoor, Ellmoore, Ellmor, Ellmore, Elmoar, Elmoor, Elmoore

Eloi (Hebrew) a form of Eli.

Elon (Spanish) a short form of Elonzo.

Elonzo (Spanish) a form of Alonso.
Elonso

Eloy (Latin) chosen. (Hebrew) a form of Eli.
Eloi

Elpidio (Greek) he who has hopes.

Elrad (Hebrew) God rules.
Ellrad, Elradd, Rad, Radd

Elroy (French) a form of Delroy, Leroy.
Elroi, Elroye

Elsdon (English) nobleman's hill.
Elsden, Elsdin, Elsdyn

Elston (English) noble's town.
Ellston

Elsu (Native American) swooping, soaring falcon.

Elsworth (English) noble's estate.
Ellsworth

Elton (English) old town.
Alton, Ellton, Eltan, Elten, Elthon, Eltin, Eltonia, Eltyn

Eluney (Mapuche) gift.

Elvern (Latin) a form of Alvern.
Elver, Elverne, Elvirn, Elvirne

Elvin (English) a form of Alvin.
El, Elvyn, Elwen, Elwin, Elwyn, Elwynn

Elvio (Spanish) light skinned; blond.
Elvyo

Elvío (Spanish) a form of Elvio.

Elvis (Scandinavian) wise.
El, Elviss, Elviz, Elvys, Elvyss

Elvy (English) elfin warrior.
Elvi, Elvie

Elwell (English) old well.
Elwel

Elwood (English) old forest. See also Wood, Woody.
Ellwood

Ely (Hebrew) a form of Eli. Geography: a region of England with extensive drained bogs.
Elya, Elyie

Elzeario (Hebrew) God has helped.

Eman BG (Czech) a form of Emmanuel.
Emaney, Emani

Emanuel (Hebrew) a form of Emmanuel.
Emaniel, Emannual, Emannuel, Emanual, Emanueal, Emanuele, Emanuell, Emanuelle

Emerenciano (Latin) deserving.

Emerson (German, English) son of Emery.
Emmerson, Emreson

Emery BG (German) industrious leader.
Aimery, Emari, Emarri, Emeree, Emeri, Emerich, Emerie, Emerio, Emmeree, Emmeri, Emmerich, Emmerie, Emmery, Emrick, Imrich, Inre

Emesto (Spanish) serious.

Emeterio (Greek) he who deserves affection.

Emigdio (Greek) he who has brown skin.

Emil (Latin) flatterer. (German) industrious. See also Milko, Milo.
Aymil, Emiel, Emilek, Emill, Emils, Emilyan, Emyl, Emyll

Emila (Greek) a form of Emilio.

Emile BG (French) a form of Emil.
Emiel, Emille, Emylle

Émile (French) a form of Emil.

Emiliano (Italian) a form of Emil.
Emilian, Emilion

Emilien (Latin) friendly; industrious.

Emilio (Italian, Spanish) a form of Emil.
Emielio, Emileo, Emilios, Emillio, Emilo

Emillen (Latin) a form of Emilien.

Emily GB (Latin, German) a form of Emil.

Emir (Arabic) chief, commander.

Emlyn (Welsh) waterfall.
Emelen, Emlen, Emlin

Emmanuel (Hebrew) God is with us. See also Immanuel, Maco, Mango, Manuel.
Emek, Emmahnuel, Emmanel, Emmaneuol, Emmanle, Emmanual, Emmanueal, Emmanuele, Emmanuell, Emmanuelle, Emmanuil

Emmet, Emmitt (German, English) forms of Emmett.
Emmit, Emmyt, Emmytt, Emyt, Emytt

Emmett (German) industrious; strong. (English) ant. History: Robert Emmett was an Irish patriot.
Em, Emet, Emett, Emitt, Emmette, Emmot, Emmott, Emmy

Emory BG (German) a form of Emery.
Emmo, Emmori, Emmorie, Emmory, Emorye

Emre (Turkish) brother.
Emra, Emrah, Emreson

Emrick (German) a form of Emery.
Emeric, Emerick, Emric, Emrik, Emrique, Emryc, Emryck, Emryk

Emry (Welsh) honorable.
Emree, Emrey, Emri, Emrie

Enan (Welsh) hammer.
Enen, Enin, Enon, Enyn

Enapay (Sioux) brave appearance; he appears.
Enapai

Endre (Hungarian) a form of Andrew.
Ender, Endres

Enea (Italian) ninth born.

Eneas (Greek) a form of Aeneas.
Eneias, Enné

Engelbert (German) bright as an angel. See also Ingelbert.
Bert, Engelburt, Englebert, Englebirt, Engleburt, Englebyrt

Engelberto (Germanic) a form of Engelbert.

Enio (Spanish) the second divinity of war.

Enli (Dene) that dog over there.
Enly

Enmanuel (Hebrew) a form of Emmanuel.

Ennis (Greek) mine. (Scottish) a form of Angus.
Eni, Enis, Enni, Ennys, Enys

Enoc (Hebrew) a form of Enoch.

Enoch (Hebrew) dedicated, consecrated. Bible: the father of Methuselah.
Enock, Enok

Enol (Asturian) referring to Lake Enol.

Enos (Hebrew) man.
Enosh

Enric, Enrick (Romanian) forms of Henry.
Enrica, Enrik, Enryc, Enryck, Enryk

Enrico (Italian) a form of Henry.
Enzio, Rico

Enright (Irish) son of the attacker.
Enrit, Enrite, Enryght, Enryte

Enrikos (Greek) a form of Henry.

Enrique, Enrrique (Spanish) forms of Henry. See also Quiqui.
Enrigué, Enriq, Enriqué, Enriquez

Enver (Turkish) bright; handsome.

Enyeto (Native American) walks like a bear.
Enieto

Enzi (Swahili) powerful.
Enzie, Enzy

Enzo (Italian) a form of Enrico.

Eoin (Welsh) a form of Evan.

Ephraim (Hebrew) fruitful. Bible: the second son of Joseph.
Ephraen, Ephrain, Ephram, Ephrem, Ephriam

Epicuro (Greek) he who helps.

Epifanio (Greek) he who gives off brilliance.

Epimaco (Greek) easy to attack.

Epulef (Mapuche) two quick trips.

Eraclio (Greek) a form of Hercules.

Erán (Hebrew) vigilant.

Erasmo (Greek) a form of Erasmus.

Erasmus (Greek) lovable.
Érasme, Rasmus

Erasto (East African) man of peace.

Erastus (Greek) beloved.
Éraste, Erastious, Ras, Rastus

Erato (Greek) kind, pleasant.

Erbert (German) a short form of Herbert.
Ebert, Erberto, Erbirt, Erbirto, Erburt, Erburto, Erbyrt, Erbyrto

Ercole (Italian) splendid gift.
Ercoal, Ercol

Erek, Erik (Scandinavian) forms of Eric.
Erike, Errik

Erhard (German) strong; resolute.
Erhardt, Erhart

Eri (Teutonic) vigilant.

Eriberto (Italian) a form of Herbert.
Erberto, Heriberto

Eric ☀ (Scandinavian) ruler of all. (English) brave ruler. (German) a short form of Frederick. History: Eric the Red was a Norwegian explorer who founded Greenland's first colony.
Aric, Ehric, Éric, Erica, Ericc, Erico, Erric, Rick

Erich (Czech, German) a form of Eric.
Ehrich

Erick, Errick (English) forms of Eric.
Eryck

Erickson (English) son of Eric.
Erickzon, Erics, Ericson, Ericsson, Eriks, Erikson, Erikzzon, Eriqson

Erikur (Icelandic) a form of Erek, Eric.

Erin GB (Irish) peaceful. History: an ancient name for Ireland.
Eran, Eren, Erine, Erinn, Erino, Errin, Eryn, Erynn

Eriq (American) a form of Eric.

Erland (English) nobleman's land.
Earlan, Earland, Erlan, Erlen, Erlend

Erling (English) nobleman's son.

Ermanno (Italian) a form of Herman.
Erman, Erminio

Ermano (Spanish) a form of Herman.
Ermin, Ermine, Ermon

Ermelindo (Teutonic) offers sacrifices to God.

Ermenegildo (German) strong warrior.

Ermengaldo (Germanic) dwelling of strength.

Ermengol (Catalan) a form of Armengol.

Ermino (Spanish) a form of Erminoldo.

Erminoldo (Germanic) government of strength.

Ernest (English) earnest, sincere. See also Arno.
Erneste, Ernestino, Ernestus, Ernist, Ernyst

Ernesto (Spanish) a form of Ernest.
Ernester, Ernestino, Neto

Ernie (English) a familiar form of Ernest.
Earnee, Earni, Earnie, Earny, Ernee, Erney, Erni, Erny

Erno (Hungarian) a form of Ernest.
Ernö

Ernst (German) a form of Ernest.
Erns

Erol (Turkish) strong, courageous.
Eroll

Eron, Erron (Irish) forms of Erin.
Erran, Erren, Errion

Erón (Spanish) a form of Aaron.

Eros (Greek) love, desire. Mythology: Eros was the god of love.

Errando (Basque) bold.

Errol (Latin) wanderer. (English) a form of Earl.
Erol, Erold, Erral, Errel, Erril, Erroll, Erryl, Erryll, Eryl, Eryll

Erroman (Basque) from Rome.
Eroman

Erskine (Scottish) high cliff. (English) from Ireland.
Ersin, Erskin, Erskyn, Erskyne, Kinny

Ervin, Erwin (English) sea friend. Forms of Irving, Irwin.
Earvan, Earven, Earvin, Earvon, Earvyn, Erv, Ervan, Erven, Ervon, Ervyn, Erwan, Erwinek, Erwinn, Erwyn, Erwynn

Ervine (English) a form of Irving.
Erv, Ervince, Erving, Ervins, Ervyne, Ervyng

Ervino (Germanic) he who is consistent with honors.

Eryk (Scandinavian) a form of Eric.
Eryc

Esau (Hebrew) rough; hairy. Bible: Jacob's twin brother.
Esaw

Esaú, Esav (Hebrew) forms of Esau.

Esben (Scandinavian) god.

Esbern (Danish) holy bear.
Esberne, Esbirn, Esbirne, Esburn, Esburne, Esbyrn, Esbyrne

Escipion, Escipión (Latin) man who uses a cane.

Escolástico (Latin) the man who teaches all that he knows.

Escubillón (Latin) one who is in the main seat.

Esculapio (Greek) the doctor.

Esdras, Esdrás (Hebrew) forms of Ezra.

Esequiel (Hebrew) a form of Ezekiel.

Eshkol (Hebrew) grape clusters.

Eshwar (Indian) another name for the Hindu god Shiva.

Esidore (Greek) a form of Isidore.
Easidor, Esidor, Ezador, Ezadore, Ezidor, Ezidore

Eskil (Norwegian) god vessel.
Eskyl

Esleban (Hebrew) bearer of children.

Esmond (English) rich protector.

Esopo (Greek) he who brings good luck.

Espartaco (Greek) he who plants.

Espen (Danish) bear of the gods.
Espan, Espin, Espon, Espyn

Espiridión (Greek) breadbasket.

Essâm (Arabic) shelter.

Essien (African) sixth-born son.
Esien

Estanislao (Slavic) the glory of his village.

Estanislau (Slavic) glory.

Este (Italian) east.
Estes

Esteban, Estéban (Spanish) forms of Stephen.
Estabon, Esteben, Estefan, Estefano, Estefen, Estephan, Estephen

Estebe (Basque) a form of Stephen.

Estéfan, Estévan, Estévon (Spanish) forms of Estevan.

Estevan, Esteven (Spanish) forms of Stephen.
Estevon, Estiven, Estyvan, Estyven, Estyvin, Estyvon, Estyvyn

Estevao (Spanish) a form of Stephen.
Estevez

Esteve (Catalan) a form of Estevan.

Estevo (Greek) a form of Estevan.

Estraton (Greek) man of the army.

Estuardo (Spanish) a form of Edward.
Estvardo

Etalpalli (Nahuatl) wing.

Etel (Germanic) noble.

Etelberto (Spanish) a form of Adalberto.

Eterio (Greek) as clean and pure as heaven.

Ethan ☀ (Hebrew) strong; firm.
Eathan, Eathen, Eathin, Eathon, Eathyn, Eeathen, Efan, Efen, Effan, Effen, Effin, Effon, Effyn, Efin, Efon, Efyn, Eithan, Eithen, Eithin, Eithon, Eithyn, Etan, Ethaen, Ethe, Ethian, Ethin, Ethon, Ethyn, Eythan, Eythen, Eythin, Eython, Eythyn

Ethán (Hebrew) a form of Ethan.

Ethen (Hebrew) a form of Ethan.

Etienne 🅱🅶 (French) a form of Stephen.
Etian, Etien, Étienn, Ettien

Étienne (French) a form of Stephen.

Ettore (Italian) steadfast.
Etor, Etore

Etu (Native American) sunny.
Eetu

Eubulo (Greek) good counselor.

Eucario (Greek) gracious, generous.

Eucarpo (Greek) he who bears good fruit.

Euclid (Greek) intelligent. History: the founder of Euclidean geometry.
Euclyd

Euclides (Greek) a form of Euclid.

Eudaldo (German) famous leader.

Eudoro (Greek) beautiful gift.

Eudoxio (Greek) he who is famous.

Eufemio (Greek) he who has a good reputation.

Eufrasio (Greek) he who uses words well.

Eufronio (Greek) having a good mind.

Eugen (German) a form of Eugene.

Eugene (Greek) born to nobility. See also Ewan, Gene, Gino, Iukini, Jenö, Yevgenyi, Zenda.
Eoghan, Eugeen, Eugeene, Eugen, Eugéne, Eugeni, Eugenius, Eujean, Eujeane, Eujeen, Eujein, Eujeyn

Eugène (French) a form of Eugenio.

Eugenio (Spanish) a form of Eugene.
Eugenios

Euladio (Greek) one who is pious.

Eulalio (Greek) good speaker.

Eulises (Latin) a form of Ulysses.

Eulogio (Greek) he who speaks well.

Eumenio (Greek) opportune, favorable.

Euniciano (Spanish) happy victory.

Euno (Greek) intellect.

Eupilo (Greek) warmly welcomed.

Euprepio (Greek) decent; comfortable.

Eupsiquio (Greek) having a good soul.

Euquerio (Greek) sure handed.

Eurico (Germanic) the prince to whom all pay homage.

Eusebio (Greek) with good feelings.

Eusiquio (Greek) a form of Eupsiquio.

Eustace (Greek) productive. (Latin) stable, calm. See also Stacey.
Eustacee, Eustache, Eustachio, Eustachius,

Eustachy, Eustashe, Eustasius, Eustatius, Eustazio, Eustis, Eustiss

Eustacio (Greek) healthy and strong.

Eustaquio (Greek) he who has many heads of wheat.

Eustasio (Greek) healthy and strong.

Eustoquio (Greek) good marksman.

Eustorgio (Greek) well loved.

Eustrato (Greek) good soldier.

Eutiquio (Greek) fortunate.

Eutrapio (Greek) changing, transforming.

Euxenio (Greek) born into nobility.

Evan ⭐ BG (Irish) young warrior. (English) a form of John. See also Bevan, Owen.
Eavan, Ev, Evaine, Evann, Even, Evun, Ewen

Evander (Greek) benevolent ruler; preacher.
Evandar

Evando (Greek) considered a good man.

Evangelino (Greek) he who brings glad tidings.

Evangelos (Greek) a form of Andrew.
Evagelos, Evaggelos, Evangelo

Evans (Irish, English) a form of Evan.
Evens

Evarado (Spanish) hardy, brave.

Evaristo (Greek) the excellent one.

Evelio (Hebrew) he who gives life.

Evelyn GB (English) hazelnut.
Evelin

Evencio (Latin) successful.

Ever (English) boar. A short form of Everett, Everley, Everton. (German) a short form of Everardo.

Everardo (German) strong as a boar. A form of Eberhard.
Everado, Everard, Everhard, Everhardt, Everhart

Everett BG (English) a form of Eberhard.
Ev, Evered, Everet, Everhet, Everhett, Everit, Everitt, Everrett, Evert, Everyt, Everyte, Everytt, Evrett, Evryt, Evryte, Evrytt, Evrytte

Everette (English) a form of Eberhard.

Everley (English) boar meadow.
Everlea, Everlee, Everleigh, Everli, Everlie, Everly

Everton (English) boar town.

Evgenii (Russian) a form of Evgeny.

Evgeny (Russian) a form of Eugene. See also Zhek.
Evgeni, Evgenij, Evgenyi

Evin, Evon, Evyn (Irish) forms of Evan.
Evian, Evinn, Evins

Evodio (Greek) he who follows a good road.

Ewald (German) always powerful. (English) powerful lawman.

Ewan (Scottish) a form of Eugene, Evan. See also Keon.
Euan, Euann, Euen, Ewen, Ewhen, Ewin, Ewon, Ewyn

Ewert (English) ewe herder, shepherd.
Ewart, Ewirt

Ewing (English) friend of the law.
Ewin, Ewyng, Ewynn

Exavier (Basque) a form of Xavier.
Exaviar, Exavior, Ezavier

Exequiel (Hebrew) God is my strength.

Expedito (Latin) unencumbered.

Expósito (Latin) abandoned.

Exuperancio (Latin) he who is outstanding.

Exuperio (Latin) he who exceeds expectations.

Eyén (Araucanian) God.

Eynstein (Norse) stone island.
Einstein, Einsteyn, Eynsteyn

Eyota BG (Native American) great.
Eiota, Eyotah

Ezekiel (Hebrew) strength of God. Bible: a Hebrew prophet. See also Haskel, Zeke.
Ezakeil, Ezéchiel, Ezeck, Ezeckiel, Ezeeckel, Ezekeial, Ezekeil, Ezekeyial, Ezekial, Ezekielle, Ezell, Eziakah, Eziechiele

Ezequias (Hebrew) Yahweh is my strength.

Ezequías (Hebrew) has divine power.

Ezequiel (Hebrew) a form of Ezekiel.
Eziequel

Ezer (Hebrew) a form of Ezra.
Ezera, Ezerah

Ezio (Latin) he who has a nose like an eagle.

Ezra (Hebrew) helper; strong. Bible: a Jewish priest who led the Jews back to Jerusalem.
Esra, Esrah, Ezer, Ezrah, Ezri, Ezry

Eztli (Nahuatl) blood.

Ezven (Czech) a form of Eugene.
Esven, Esvin, Ezavin, Ezavine

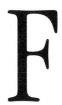

Faas (Scandinavian) wise counselor.
Fas

Faber (German) a form of Fabian.
Fabar, Fabir, Fabor, Fabyr

Fabian (Latin) bean grower.
Fabain, Fabayan, Fabe, Fabean, Fabein, Fabek, Fabeon, Faber, Fabert, Fabi, Fabijan, Fabin, Fabion, Fabius, Fabiyan, Fabiyus, Fabyan, Fabyen, Fabyous, Faybian, Faybien

Fabián (Spanish) a form of Fabian.

Fabiano (Italian) a form of Fabian.
Fabianno

Fabien (Latin) a form of Fabian.

Fabio (Latin) a form of Fabian. (Italian) a short form of Fabiano.
Fabbio

Fabrice (Italian) a form of Fabrizio.
Fabricio

Fabrizio (Italian) craftsman.
Fabrizius

Fabron (French) little blacksmith; apprentice.
Fabra, Fabre, Fabriano, Fabroni, Fabryn

Facundo (Latin) he who makes convincing arguments.

Fâdel (Arabic) generous.

Fadey (Ukrainian) a form of Thaddeus.
Faday, Faddei, Faddey, Faddi, Faddie, Faddy, Fade, Fadeyka, Fadie, Fady

Fadi (Arabic) redeemer.
Fadee, Fadhi

Fadil (Arabic) generous.
Fadal, Fadeel, Fadel, Fayl

Fadrique (Spanish) a form of Federico.

Fagan (Irish) little fiery one.
Faegan, Faegen, Faegin, Faegon, Faegyn, Fagen, Fagin, Fagon, Fagyn, Faigan, Faigen, Faigin, Faigon, Faigyn, Faygan, Faygen, Faygin, Faygon, Faygyn

Fahd (Arabic) lynx.
Fahaad, Fahad

Fai (Chinese) beginning.

Fairfax (English) blond.
Fair, Fax, Fayrfax

Faisal (Arabic) decisive.
Faisel, Faisil, Faisl, Faiyaz, Faiz, Faizal, Faize, Faizel, Faizi, Fasel, Fasil, Faysal, Fayzal, Fayzel

Fakhir (Arabic) excellent.
Fahkry, Fakher

Fakih (Arabic) thinker; reader of the Koran.

Falak (Indian) sky.

Falco (Latin) falconer.
Falcko, Falckon, Falcon, Falconn, Falk, Falke, Falken, Faulco

Falguni (Indian) born in the Hindu month of Falgun.

Falito (Italian) a familiar form of Rafael, Raphael.

Falkner (English) trainer of falcons. See also Falco.
Falconer, Falconner, Falconnor, Faulconer, Faulconner, Faulconnor, Faulkner

Fane (English) joyful, glad.
Fain, Faine, Faines, Fanes, Faniel, Fayn, Fayne

Fanibhusan (Indian) another name for the Hindu god Shiva.

Fanindra, Fanish (Indian) other names for the Hindu serpent god Shesh.

Fanishwar (Indian) lord of serpents.

Fantino (Latin) innocent.

Fanuco (Spanish) free.

Fanuel (Hebrew) vision of God.

Faraji (Swahili) consolation.
Farajy

Faraón (Egyptian) pharaoh.

Faraz (Arabic) a form of Faris.
Farhaz, Fariez

Farhad, Farhat (Indian) happiness.

Farid (Arabic) unique.
Farad, Fared, Farod, Faryd

Faris (Arabic) horseman. (Irish) a form of Ferris.
Fares, Faress, Farice, Fariss, Fariz, Farris, Farrish, Farrys, Farys

Fâris (Arabic) a form of Faris.

Farlane (English) far lane.
Farlaen, Farlaene, Farlain, Farlaine, Farlayn, Farlayne

Farley (English) bull meadow; sheep meadow. See also Lee.
Fairlay, Fairlea, Fairlee, Fairleigh, Fairley, Fairlie, Far, Farlay, Farlea, Farlee, Farleigh, Farli, Farlie, Farly, Farrleigh, Farrley

Farnell (English) fern-covered hill.
Farnal, Farnall, Farnalle, Farnel, Farnelle, Fernal, Fernald, Fernall, Fernalle, Furnal, Furnald, Furnall, Furnalle, Furnel, Furnell, Furnelle, Fyrnel, Fyrnele, Fyrnell, Fyrnelle

Farnham (English) field of ferns.
Farnam, Farnem, Farnhem, Farnum, Fernham

Farnley (English) fern meadow.
Farnlea, Farnlee, Farnleigh, Farnli, Farnlie, Farnly, Fernlea, Fernlee, Fernleigh, Fernley, Fernli, Fernlie, Fernly

Faroh (Latin) a form of Pharaoh.
Faro, Farro, Farrow

Farokh, Farukh (Indian) power of discrimination.

Farold (English) mighty traveler.

Faron (English) a form of Faren (see Girls' Names).

Farón (Spanish) pharaoh.

Farquhar (Scottish) dear.
Fark, Farq, Farquar, Farquarson, Farque, Farquharson, Farquy, Farqy

Farr (English) traveler.
Faer, Far, Farran, Farren, Farrin, Farrington, Farron, Farrun, Farryn

Farrar (English) blacksmith.
Farar, Farer, Farrer

Farrell (Irish) heroic; courageous.
Faral, Farel, Faril, Farol, Farral, Farrel, Farrill, Farryl, Farryll, Faryl, Ferol, Ferrel, Ferrell, Ferril, Ferryl

Farrow (English) piglet.
Farow

Farruco (Spanish) a form of Francis, Francisco.
Farruca, Farrucah, Farruka, Farruko, Faruca, Farucah, Faruco, Frascuelo

Faruq (Arabic) honest.
Farook, Farooq, Faroque, Farouk, Faruqh

Faste (Norwegian) firm.

Fateh (Indian) victory.

Fath (Arabic) victor.

Fatik (Indian) crystal.

Fatin (Arabic) clever.
Fatine, Fatyn, Fatyne

Fâtin (Arabic) a form of Fatin.

Fauac (Quechua) he who flies.

Fauacuaipa (Quechua) rooster in flight.

Faust (Latin) lucky, fortunate. History: the sixteenth-century German necromancer who inspired many legends.
Fauste, Faustis, Faustise, Faustos, Faustus, Faustyce, Faustys

Faustino (Italian) a form of Faust.
Faustin, Faustine, Faustyn

Fausto (Italian) a form of Faust.

Favian (Latin) understanding.
Favain, Favien, Favio, Favion, Favyen, Favyon

Fawwâz, Fawzî (Arabic) successful.

Faxon BG (German) long-haired.
Faxan, Faxen, Faxin, Faxyn

Fazio (Italian) good worker.
Fazyo

Febe, Febo (Latin) he who shines.

Federico (Italian, Spanish) a form of Frederick.
Federic, Federigo, Federoquito

Fedro (Greek) the splendid man.

Fedyenka (Russian) gift of God.

Feivel (Yiddish) God aids.
Feyvel

Feliciano (Italian) a form of Felix.
Felicio

Feliks (Russian) a form of Felix.

Felipe (Spanish) a form of Philip.
Feeleep, Felep, Felip, Felo

Felippo (Italian) a form of Philip.
Felipino, Lipp, Lippo, Pip, Pippo

Felisardo (Latin) valiant and skillful man.

Felix (Latin) fortunate; happy. See also Phelix, Pitin.
Fee, Felic, Félice, Felike, Feliks, Félix, Felizio, Felo, Filix, Filyx, Fylix, Fylyx

Felíx (Latin) a form of Felix.

Felix Antoine (Latin, French) a combination of Felix + Antoine.
Felix-Antoine

Felix Olivier (Latin, French) a combination of Felix +Olivier.
Felix-Olivier

Felton (English) field town.
Feltan, Felten, Feltin, Feltun, Feltyn

Fenton (English) marshland farm.
Fen, Fennie, Fenny, Fentan, Fenten, Fentin, Fentun, Fentyn, Fintan, Finton

Fenuku (Egyptian) born late.

Fenyang (Egyptian) conqueror.

Feo (Spanish) ugly.

Feodor (Slavic) a form of Theodore.
Dorek, Feador, Feaodor, Feaodore, Fedar, Fedinka, Fedor, Fedore, Fedya, Feedor,

Feeodor, Feeodore, Fidor, Fidore, Fiodor, Fiodore

Feoras (Greek) smooth rock.
Feora

Ferd (German) horse.
Ferda, Ferde, Ferdi, Ferdie, Ferdy

Ferdinand (German) daring, adventurous. See also Hernando.
Ferdinan, Ferdinánd, Ferdinandus, Ferdynand, Ferynand

Ferdinando (Italian) a form of Ferdinand.
Feranado, Ferdnando, Ferdynando, Ferrando, Nando

Ferenc (Hungarian) a form of Francis.
Feri, Ferke, Ferko

Fergus (Irish) strong; manly.
Fearghas, Fearghus, Feargus, Ferghas, Ferghus, Fergie, Ferguson, Fergusson, Firgus, Firgusen, Firguson, Furgus, Furgusen, Furguson, Fyrgus, Fyrgusen, Fyrgusun

Fermin (French, Spanish) firm, strong. See also Firman.
Ferman, Firmin, Furmin, Furmyn, Fyrmen, Fyrmin, Fyrmyn

Fermín (Spanish) a form of Fermin.

Fernán (Spanish) a form of Fernando.

Fernando (Spanish) a form of Ferdinand.
Ferando, Ferdo, Fernand, Fernandez, Fernendo, Ferynando

Feroz (Persian) fortunate.
Firoz, Fyroz

Ferran (Arabic) baker.
Farran, Feran, Feren, Ferin, Feron, Ferren, Ferrin, Ferron, Ferryn, Feryn

Ferrand (French) iron-gray hair.
Farand, Farrand, Farrando, Farrant, Ferand, Ferrant

Ferrell (Irish) a form of Farrell.
Ferel, Ferell, Ferrel, Ferrill, Ferryl

Ferreolo (Latin) referring to iron.

Ferris (Irish) a form of Peter.
Feris, Ferrice, Ferrise, Ferriss, Ferryce, Ferryse, Ferryss

Festus (Latin) happy.
Festys

Feta-plom (Mapuche) high and large plain.

Fhakîr (Arabic) proud; excellent.

Fiacro (Latin) the soldier.

Fico (Spanish) a familiar form of Frederick.
Ficko, Fiko, Fycko, Fyco, Fyko

Fidel (Latin) faithful. History: Fidel Castro was the Cuban revolutionary who overthrew a dictatorship in 1959 and established a communist regime in Cuba.
Fidele, Fidèle, Fidelio, Fidelis, Fidell, Fido, Fydal, Fydel, Fydil, Fydyl

Fidencio (Latin) trusting; fearless.

Fidias (Greek) unhurried, calm.

Field (English) a short form of Fielding.
Fields

Fielding (English) field; field worker.
Field

Fife (Scottish) from Fife, Scotland.
Fif, Fyf, Fyfe

Fifi GB (Fante) born on Friday.

Fil (Polish) a form of Phil.
Filipek

Filadelfo, Filademo (Greek) man who loves his brothers.

Filbert (English) brilliant. See also Bert, Philbert.
Filberte, Filberti, Filberto, Filbirt, Filburt, Filibert, Filibirt, Filiburt, Fillbert, Fillbirt, Fylbert, Fylbirt, Fylburt, Fylibert, Fylibirt, Fyliburt, Fyllbert, Fyllbirt, Fyllbyrt

Filberte (French) a form of Filbert.
Filbirte, Filburte, Filiberte, Filibirte, Filiburte, Fillberte, Fillbirte, Fylberte, Fylbirte, Fylburte, Fyliberte, Fylibirte, Fyliburte, Fyllberte, Fyllbirte, Fyllbyrte

Fileas (Greek) he who loves deeply.

Filebert (Catalan) a form of Filiberto.

Filelio (Latin) he who is trustworthy.

Filemón (Greek) horse lover.

Filiberto (Spanish) a form of Filbert.

Filip (Greek) a form of Philip.
Filippo

Fillipp (Russian) a form of Philip.
Filipe, Filipek, Filips, Fill, Fillip

Filmore (English) famous.
Fillmore, Filmer, Fyllmer, Fyllmore, Fylmer, Fylmore, Philmore

Filón (Greek) philosophical friend.

Filya (Russian) a form of Philip.
Filyah, Fylya, Fylyah

Findlay (Irish) a form of Finlay.
Findlea, Findlee, Findleigh, Findley, Fyndlay, Fyndlea, Fyndlee, Fyndleigh, Fyndley, Fynndlay, Fynndlea, Fynndlee, Fynndleigh, Fynndley

Fineas (Irish) a form of Phineas.
Finneas, Fyneas

Finian (Irish) light skinned; white. See also Phinean.
Finan, Fineen, Finien, Finnen, Finnian, Finyan, Fionan, Fionn, Fynia, Fynyan

Finlay (Irish) blond-haired soldier.
Findlay, Finlea, Finlee, Finleigh, Finley, Finnlea, Finnlee, Finnleigh, Finnley, Fynlay, Fynlea, Fynlee, Fynleigh, Fynley, Fynnlay, Fynnlea, Fynnlee, Fynnleigh, Fynnley

Finn (German) from Finland. (Irish) blond haired; light skinned. A short form of Finlay. (Norwegian) from the Lapland. See also Fynn.
Fin, Finnie, Finnis, Finny

Finnegan (Irish) light skinned; white.
Finegan, Fineghan, Finneghan, Fynegan, Fyneghan, Fynnegan, Fynneghan

Fintan (Irish) from Finn's town.
Finten, Fintin, Finton, Fintyn, Fyntan, Fynten, Fyntin, Fynton, Fyntyn

Fiorello (Italian) little flower.
Fiore, Fiorelleigh, Fiorelley, Fiorelli, Fiorellie, Fiorelly, Fyorellee, Fyorelleigh, Fyorelley, Fyorelli, Fyorellie, Fyorello, Fyorelly

Firas (Arabic) persistent.
Fira, Fyra, Fyras

Firdaus (Indian) paradise.

Firman (French) firm; strong. See also Fermin.
Firmyn, Furman, Fyrman

Firmino (Latin) firm, sure.

Firmo (Latin) morally and physically firm.

Firth (English) woodland.
Fyrth

Fischel (Yiddish) a form of Philip.
Fyschel

Fischer (English) a form of Fisher.

Fisher (English) fisherman.

Fiske (English) fisherman.
Fisk, Fysk, Fyske

Fitch (English) weasel, ermine.
Fitche, Fytch

Fito (Spanish) a form of Adolfo.

Fitz (English) son.
Filz, Fits, Fyts, Fytz

Fitzgerald (English) son of Gerald.
Fitsgerald, Fitzgeraldo, Fytsgerald, Fytsgeraldo, Fytzgerald, Fytzgeraldo

Fitzhugh (English) son of Hugh.
Fitshu, Fitshue, Fitshugh, Fitzhu, Fitzhue, Fytshu, Fytzhue, Fytzhugh

Fitzpatrick (English) son of Patrick.
Fitspatric, Fitspatrik, Fitzpatric, Fitzpatrik, Fytspatric, Fytspatrick, Fytspatrik, Fytzpatric, Fytzpatrick, Fytzpatrik

Fitzroy (Irish) son of Roy.
Fitsroi, Fitsroy, Fitzroi, Fytsroi, Fytsroy, Fytzroi, Fytzroy

Fiz (Latin) happy; fertile.

Flaminio (Spanish) Religion: Marcantonio Flaminio coauthored one of the most important texts of the Italian Reformation.

Flann (Irish) redhead.
Flainn, Flan, Flanan, Flanin, Flannan, Flannen, Flannery, Flannin, Flannon, Flanon, Flanyn

Flavian (Latin) blond, yellow haired.
Flavel, Flavelle, Flavien, Flavyan, Flawian, Flawiusz, Flawyan

Flaviano (Latin) a form of Flavian.

Flavio (Italian) a form of Flavian.
Flabio, Flavias, Flavious, Flavius, Flavyo

Fleming (English) from Denmark; from Flanders.
Flemming, Flemmyng, Flemyng

Fletcher (English) arrow featherer, arrow maker.
Flecher, Fletch

Flint (English) stream; flint stone.
Flinte, Flynt, Flynte

Flip (Spanish) a short form of Felipe. (American) a short form of Philip.
Flipp, Flyp, Flypp

Floreal (Latin) alludes to the eighth month of the French Revolution.

Florencio (Italian) a form of Florent.
Florenci, Florenzo, Florinio, Florino, Floryno

Florent (French) flowering.
Florentin, Florentine, Florentyn, Florentyne, Florentz, Florynt, Florynte

Florente (Latin) a form of Florent.

Florentino (Italian) a form of Florent.
Florentyno

Florian 🅱🅶 (Latin) flowering, blooming.
Florien, Florion, Florrian, Flory, Floryan, Floryant, Floryante

Florián (Latin) a form of Florian.

Floriano (Spanish) a form of Florian.

Floriberto (Germanic) brilliant master.

Florio (Spanish) a form of Florián.

Floro (Spanish) flower.

Florus (French) flowers.

Flósculo (Latin) wildflower.

Floyd (English) a form of Lloyd.
Floid, Floyde

Flurry (English) flourishing, blooming.
Fluri, Flurie, Flurri, Flurrie, Flury

Flynn (Irish) son of the red-haired man.
Flin, Flinn, Flyn

Focas (Greek) habitant of Focida.

Focio (Latin) illuminated, shining.

Fodjour (Ghanaian) fourth born.

Folco (Catalan) man who belongs to the community.

Folke (German) a form of Volker.
Folker

Foluke BG (Yoruba) given to God.

Foma (Bulgarian, Russian) a form of Thomas.
Fomah, Fomka

Fonso (German, Italian) a short form of Alphonso.
Fonzo

Fontaine (French) fountain.
Fontain, Fontayn, Fontayne, Fountain, Fountaine, Fountayn, Fountayne

Fonzie (German) a familiar form of Alphonse.
Fons, Fonsee, Fonsey, Fonsi, Fonsie, Fonsy, Fonz, Fonzee, Fonzey, Fonzi, Fonzy

Forbes (Irish) prosperous.
Forbe, Forbs

Ford (English) a short form of names ending in "ford."
Forde

Fordel (Gypsy) forgiving.
Fordal, Fordele, Fordell, Fordelle, Fordil, Fordile

Fordon (German) destroyer.
Fordan, Forden, Fordin, Fordyn

Forest (French) a form of Forrest.
Forestt, Foryst

Forester (English) forest guardian.
Forrestar, Forrester, Forrie, Forry, Foss

Formerio (Latin) beauty.

Forrest BG (French) forest; woodsman.
Forreste, Forrestt, Forrie

Fortino (Italian) fortunate, lucky.
Fortin, Fortine, Fortyn, Fortyne

Fortune (French) fortunate, lucky.
Fortun, Fortunato, Fortuné, Fortunio

Foster (Latin) a short form of Forester.
Forster

Fouad (Lebanese) heart.

Fowler (English) trapper of wildfowl.

Fraco (Spanish) weak.

Fran GB (Latin) a short form of Francis.
Franh

Francesco (Italian) a form of Francis.

Franchot (French) a form of Francis.

Francis BG (Latin) free; from France. Religion: Saint Francis of Assisi was the founder of the Franciscan order. See also Farruco, Ferenc.
France, Frances, Franciskus, Francys, Frannie, Franny, Franscis, Fransis, Franus, Frecis

Francisco (Portuguese, Spanish) a form of Francis. See also Chilo, Cisco, Farruco, Paco, Pancho.
Fransysco, Frasco

Franco (Latin) a short form of Francis.
Franko

Francois, François (French) forms of Francis.
Francoise

Frank (English) a short form of Francis, Franklin. See also Palani, Pancho.
Franc, Franck, Franek, Frang, Franio, Franke, Franko

Frankie BG (English) a familiar form of Frank.
Francky, Franke, Frankey, Franki, Franqui

Franklin (English) free landowner.
Francklen, Francklin, Francklyn, Francylen, Frankin, Franklen, Franklinn, Franquelin

Franklyn (English) a form of Franklin.
Franklynn

Franky (English) a familiar form of Frank.

Frans (Swedish) a form of Francis.
Frants

Fransisco (Portuguese, Spanish) a form of Francis.

Frantisek (Czech) a form of Francis.
Franta, Frantik, Frantyc, Frantyck, Frantyk

Frantz, Franz (German) forms of Francis.
Fransz, Franzen, Franzie, Franzin, Franzl, Franzy

Fraser (French) strawberry. (English) curly haired.
Frasier

Fraterno (Latin) relating to the brother.

Frayne (French) dweller at the ash tree. (English) stranger.
Frain, Fraine, Frayn, Frean, Freane, Freen, Freene, Frein, Freine, Freyn, Freyne

Frazer, Frazier (French, English) forms of Fraser.
Fraizer, Fraze, Frazyer

Fred (German) a short form of Alfred, Frederick, Manfred.
Fredd, Fredson

Freddie 🅱🄶 (German) a familiar form of Frederick.
Fredde, Freddi, Fredie

Freddrick, Fredrick (German) forms of Frederick.
Feidrik, Fredric, Fredrich, Fredricka, Fredricks, Fredrik

Freddy, Fredi, Fredy (German) familiar forms of Frederick.

Frederic, Frederik (German) forms of Frederick.
Frédéric, Frederich, Frédérik, Frederric, Frederrik

Frederick (German) peaceful ruler. See also Dick, Eric, Fico, Peleke, Rick.
Fredderick, Fredek, Fréderick, Frédérick, Frederrick, Fredwick, Fredwyck

Frederico (Spanish) a form of Frederick.
Frederigo, Fredrico

Frederique 🄶🄱 (French) a form of Frederick.

Fredo (Spanish) a form of Fred.
Freddo

Freeborn (English) child of freedom.
Freborn, Free

Freeman (English) free.
Free, Freedman, Freemin, Freemon, Friedman, Friedmann

Fremont (German) free; noble protector.
Fremonte

Frenchc (Catalan) a form of Francisco.

Fresco (Spanish) fresh.

Frewin (English) free; noble friend.
Freewan, Freewen, Frewan, Frewen, Frewon, Frewyn

Frey (English) lord. (Scandinavian) Mythology: the Norse god who dispenses peace and prosperity.
Frai, Fray, Frei

Frick (English) bold.
Fric, Frik, Friq, Frique, Fryc, Fryck, Fryk, Fryq

Fridmund (German) peaceful guardian.
Frimond, Frymond, Frymund

Fridolf (English) peaceful wolf.
Freydolf, Freydolph, Freydolphe, Freydulf, Freydulph, Freydulphe, Fridolph, Fridolphe, Fridulf, Frydolph, Frydolphe, Frydulf

Fridolino (Teutonic) he who loves peace.

Friedrich (German) a form of Frederick.
Frideric, Friderik, Fridrich, Fridrick, Friedel, Friederick, Friedrick, Friedrike, Friedryk, Fryderic, Fryderick, Fryderyk, Frydric, Frydrich, Frydrick, Frydrik

Frisco (Spanish) a short form of Francisco.

Fritz (German) a familiar form of Frederick.
Fritson, Fritts, Fritzchen, Fritzl

Froberto (Spanish) a form of Roberto.

Frode (Norwegian) wise.
Frod

Froilan, Froilán (Teutonic) rich and beloved young master.

Fronton (Latin) he who thinks.

Fructuoso (Latin) he who bears much fruit.

Frumencio (Latin) he who provides wheat.

Frutos (Latin) fertile.

Fu'ad (Arabic) heart.

Fuad (Lebanese) heart.

Fulberto (Germanic) he who shines.

Fulbright (German) very bright.
Fulbert, Fulbirt, Fulburt, Fulbyrt

Fulco (Spanish) village.

Fulgencio (Latin) he who shines and stands out.

Fuller (English) cloth thickener.
Fuler

Fulton (English) field near town.
Faulton, Folton

Fulvio (Latin) he who has reddish hair.

Funsani (Egyptian) request.

Funsoni (Nguni) requested.
Funsony

Fyfe (Scottish) a form of Fife.
Fyffe

Fynn (Ghanaian) Geography: another name for the Offin River in Ghana. See also Finn.
Fyn

Fyodor (Russian) a form of Theodore.
Fydor, Fydore, Fyodore

G

Gabby (American) a familiar form of Gabriel.
Gabbi, Gabbie, Gabi, Gabie, Gaby

Gabe (Hebrew) a short form of Gabriel.
Gab

Gabela (Swiss) a form of Gabriel.
Gabel, Gabelah, Gabell

Gabino (American) a form of Gabriel.
Gabin, Gabrino

Gábor (Hungarian) God is my strength.
Gabbo, Gabko, Gabo

Gabrial (Hebrew) a form of Gabriel.
Gaberial, Gabrail, Gabreal, Gabriael, Gabrieal

Gabriel ⭐ BG (Hebrew) devoted to God. Bible: the angel of the Annunciation.
Gabis, Gabrael, Gabraiel, Gabreil, Gabrel, Gabrell, Gabriël, Gabrielius, Gabrile, Gabris, Gebereal, Ghabriel, Riel

Gabriele GB (Hebrew) a form of Gabriel.

Gabriell GB (Hebrew) a form of Gabriel.

Gabrielle GB (Hebrew) a form of Gabriel.

Gabrielli (Italian) a form of Gabriel.
Gabriello

Gabrio (Spanish) a form of Gabriel.

Gabryel (Hebrew) a form of Gabriel.
Gabryalle, Gabryele, Gabryell, Gabryelle, Gabys

Gadi (Arabic) God is my fortune.
Gad, Gaddy, Gadie, Gadiel, Gady

Gael (Irish) Gaelic-speaking Celt. (Greek) a form of Gale.

Gaetan (Italian) from Gaeta, a region in southern Italy.
Gaetano, Gaetono

Gagan (Sikh) sky.

Gagandeep BG (Sikh) sky's light.

Gage BG (French) pledge.
Gager, Gayg, Gayge

Gahiji (Egyptian) hunter.

Gaige (French) a form of Gage.
Gaig

Gair (Irish) small.
Gaer, Gayr, Gearr, Geir, Geirr

Gaius (Latin) rejoicer. See also Cai.

Gajanand, Ganapati (Indian) other names for the Hindu god Ganesh.

Gaje (French) a form of Gage.

Gajendra (Indian) king of elephants.

Gálatas (Greek) white as milk.

Galbraith (Irish) Scotsman in Ireland.
Galbrait, Galbrayth, Galbreath

Gale (Greek) a short form of Galen.
Gail, Gaile, Gayl, Gayle

Galeaso (Latin) he who is protected by the helmet.

Galen BG (Greek) healer; calm. (Irish) little and lively.
Gaelan, Gaelen, Gaelin, Gaelyn, Gailen, Galan, Galin, Galon, Galyn

Galeno (Spanish) illuminated child. (Greek, Irish) a form of Galen.

Galileo (Hebrew) he who comes from Galilee.

Gallagher (Irish) eager helper.

Galloway (Irish) Scotsman in Ireland.
Gallowai, Gallwai, Gallway, Galwai, Galway

Galo (Latin) native of Galilee.

Galt (Norwegian) high ground.

Galton (English) owner of a rented estate.
Gallton, Galtan, Galten, Galtin, Galtyn

Galvin (Irish) sparrow.
Gal, Gall, Gallven, Gallvin, Galvan, Galven, Galvon, Galvyn

Gamal (Arabic) camel. See also Jamal.
Gamall, Gamel, Gamil

Gamaliel (Hebrew) God is your reward.

Gamble (Scandinavian) old.
Gambal, Gambel, Gambil, Gambol, Gambyl

Gamelberto (Germanic) distinguished because of his age.

Gamlyn (Scandinavian) small elder.
Gamlin

Gan (Chinese) daring, adventurous. (Vietnamese) near.

Gandharva (Indian) celestial musician.

Gandhik (Indian) fragrant.

Gandolfo (Germanic) valiant warrior.

Ganesh (Indian) Hindu god with an elephant's head, son of the god Shiva and goddess Parvati.

Gangesh, Gaurinath (Indian) other names for the Hindu god Shiva.

Gangeya (Indian) of the Ganges River.

Gangol (Indian) precious.

Ganimedes (Spanish) the most beautiful of the mortals.

Gannon (Irish) light skinned, white.
Ganan, Ganen, Ganin, Gannan, Gannen, Gannie, Ganny, Gannyn, Ganon, Ganyn

Ganya BG (Zulu) clever.
Gania, Ganiah, Ganyah

Gar (English) a short form of Gareth, Garnett, Garrett, Garvin.
Garr

Garai (Egyptian) stable.

Garcia (Spanish) mighty with a spear.
Garcias, Garcya, Garcyah, Garcyas, Garsias, Garsya, Garsyah, Garsyas

García (Spanish) a form of Garcia.

Garcilaso (Spanish) a form of Garcia.

Gardner (English) gardener.
Gard, Gardener, Gardie, Gardiner, Gardnar, Gardnor, Gardnyr, Gardy

Garek (Polish) a form of Edgar.
Garak, Garok

Garen, Garin, Garren, Garrin (English) forms of Garry.
Garan, Garon, Garran, Garron, Garryn, Garyn, Gerren, Gerron, Gerryn

Garet, Garett, Garret (Irish) forms of Garrett.
Garhett, Garit, Garitt, Garrit, Garryt, Garyt, Garytt, Gerret, Gerrot

Gareth (Welsh) gentle. (Irish) a form of Garrett.
Garef, Gareff, Garif, Gariff, Garith, Garreth, Garrith, Garyf, Garyff, Garyth

Garfield (English) field of spears; battlefield.
Garfyeld

Garibaldo (Germanic) he who is bold with a lance.

Garion (English) a form of Garry.
Garrion, Garyon

Garland BG (French) wreath of flowers; prize. (English) land of spears; battleground.
Garlan, Garlande, Garlen, Garllan, Garlund, Garlyn

Garman (English) spearman.
Garmann, Garmen, Garrman

Garner (French) army guard, sentry.
Garnar, Garnier, Garnit, Garnor, Garnyr

Garnet BG (Latin, English) a form of Garnett.

Garnett (Latin) pomegranate seed; garnet stone. (English) armed with a spear.
Garnie

Garnock (Welsh) dweller by the alder river.
Garnoc, Garnok

Garoa (Basque) dew.

Garrad (English) a form of Garrett, Gerard. See also Jared.
Gared, Garrard, Garred, Garrid, Garrod, Garrode, Garryd

Garrett (Irish) brave spearman. See also Jarrett.
Garrette, Garritt, Garrytt, Gerrett, Gerritt, Gerrott

Garrick (English) oak spear.
Gaerick, Garic, Garick, Garik, Garreck, Garrek, Garric, Garrik, Garryc, Garryck, Garryk, Garyc, Garyck, Garyk, Gerreck, Gerrick

Garrison (English) Garry's son. (French) troops stationed at a fort; garrison.
Garison, Garisson, Garris, Garryson, Garyson

Garroway (English) spear fighter.
Garraway

Garry (English) a form of Gary.
Garree, Garrey, Garri, Garrie

Garson (English) son of Gar.

Garth (Scandinavian) garden, gardener. (Welsh) a short form of Gareth.
Garthe

Garvey (Irish) rough peace. (French) a form of Gervaise.
Garbhán, Garrvey, Garrvie, Garv, Garvan, Garvi, Garvie, Garvy, Gervee

Garvin (English) comrade in battle.
Garvan, Garven, Garvyn, Garwan, Garwen, Garwin, Garwon, Garwyn, Garwynn, Gervon

Garwood (English) evergreen forest. See also Wood, Woody.
Garrwood

Gary (German) mighty spearman. (English) a familiar form of Gerald. See also Kali.
Gare, Garey, Gari, Garie

Gaspar (French) a form of Casper.
Gáspár, Gasparas, Gaspard, Gaspare, Gaspari, Gasparo, Gasper, Gazsi

Gaston (French) from Gascony, France.
Gascon, Gastan, Gastaun, Gasten, Gastin, Gastyn

Gastón (French) a form of Gaston.

Gaudencio, Gaudioso (Latin) he who is happy and content.

Gauge (French) a form of Gage.

Gausberto (Germanic) the Gothic brightness.

Gautam (Indian) another name for Buddha.

Gaute (Norwegian) great.
Gaut, Gauta

Gautier (French) a form of Walter.
Galtero, Gatier, Gatyer, Gaulterio, Gaultier, Gaultiero, Gauthier

Gaven, Gavyn (Welsh) forms of Gavin.
Gavynn

Gavin ⭐ (Welsh) white hawk.
Gav, Gavan, Gavinn, Gavn, Gavohn, Gavon, Gavun

Gavino (Italian) a form of Gavin.

Gavriel (Hebrew) man of God.
Gav, Gavi, Gavrel, Gavryel, Gavryele, Gavryell, Gavryelle, Gavy

Gavril (Russian) a form of Gavriel. (Hebrew) a form of Gabriel.
Ganya, Gavrilla, Gavrilo, Gavryl, Gavryle, Gavryll, Gavrylle

Gavrilovich (Russian) a form of Gavril.

Gawain (Welsh) a form of Gavin.
Gauvain, Gawaine, Gawayn, Gawayne, Gawen, Gwayne

Gaylen, Gaylon (Greek) forms of Galen.
Gaylin, Gaylinn, Gaylyn

Gaylord (French) merry lord; jailer.
Gaelor, Gaelord, Gailard, Gaillard, Gailor, Gailord, Gallard, Gay, Gayelord, Gayler, Gaylor

Gaynor (Irish) son of the fair-skinned man.
Gaenor, Gainer, Gainor, Gay, Gayner, Gaynnor

Geary (English) variable, changeable.
Gearee, Gearey, Geari, Gearie, Gery

Geb (Egyptian) land of God.

Gedeon (Bulgarian, French) a form of Gideon.

Gedeón (Hebrew) a form of Gedeon.

Geet (Indian) song.

Geffrey (English) a form of Geoffrey. See also Jeffrey.
Gefaree, Gefarey, Gefari, Gefarie, Gefary, Geferi, Geferie, Gefery, Geffaree, Geffarey, Geffari, Geffarie, Geffary, Gefferee, Gefferey, Gefferi, Gefferie, Geffery, Geffree, Geffri, Geffrie, Geffry

Gelasio (Greek) cheerful and happy.

Gellert (Hungarian) a form of Gerald.

Gemelo (Latin) fraternal twin.

Geminiano (Latin) identical twin.

Gena GB (Russian) a short form of Yevgenyi.
Genya, Gine

Genadio (Greek) lineage.

Genardo (German) of strong lineage.

Genaro (Latin) consecrated to God.
Genereo, Genero, Gennaro

Genciano (Latin) family.

Gencio (Latin) he who loves family.

Gene (Greek) a short form of Eugene.

Genek (Polish) a form of Gene.

Gener (Catalan) January.

Generos, Generoso (Spanish) generous.

Genesis GB (Greek) beginning, origin.

Geno (Italian) a form of John. A short form of Genovese.
Genio, Jeno

Genovese (Italian) from Genoa, Italy.
Genovis

Gent (English) gentleman.
Gental, Gentel, Gentil, Gentle, Gentyl, Gentyle

Gentry BG (English) a form of Gent.

Genty (Irish, English) snow.
Genti, Gentie

Geoff (English) a short form of Geoffrey.
Gef, Geff, Geof

Geoffery (English) a form of Geoffrey.
Geofery

Geoffrey (English) a form of Jeffrey. See also Giotto, Godfrey, Gottfried, Jeff.
Geoffre, Geoffri, Geoffrie, Geoffroi, Geoffroy, Geoffry, Geofrey, Geofri, Gofery

Geordan (Scottish) a form of Gordon.
Geordann, Geordian, Geordin, Geordon

Geordie (Scottish) a form of George.
Geordi, Geordy

Georg (Scandinavian) a form of George.

George (Greek) farmer. See also Durko, Egor, Iorgos, Jerzy, Jiri, Joji, Jörg, Jorge, Jorgen, Joris, Jorrín, Jur, Jurgis, Keoki, Semer, Yegor, Yorgos, Yorick, Yoyi, Yrjo, Yuri, Zhora.
Georgas, Georget, Gheorghe, Giorgos, Goerge, Gordios, Gorje, Gorya, Grzegorz

Georges (French) a form of George.
Geórges

Georgio (Italian) a form of George.

Georgios (Greek) a form of George.
Georgious, Georgius

Georgy (Greek) a familiar form of George.
Georgi, Georgie, Georgii, Georgij, Georgiy

Geovani, Geovanni, Geovanny, Geovany (Italian) forms of Giovanni.
Geovan, Geovanne, Geovannee, Geovannhi

Geraint (English) old.
Geraynt

Gerald (German) mighty spearman. See also Fitzgerald, Jarel, Jarrell, Jerald, Jerry, Kharald.
Garald, Garold, Garolds, Gearalt, Gellert, Gérald, Geralde, Gerale, Gerold, Gerrald, Gerrell, Gerrild, Gerrin, Gerrold, Geryld, Giraldo, Giraud, Girauld

Geraldo (Italian, Spanish) a form of Gerald.

Gerard (English) brave spearman. See also Jerard, Jerry.
Garrat, Garratt, Gearard, Gerad, Gerar, Gérard, Geraro, Gerd, Gerrard, Girard

Gerardo (Spanish) a form of Gerard.
Gherardo

Gerasimo (Greek) award, recompense.

Géraud (French) a form of Gerard.
Geraud, Gerrad, Gerraud

Gerbrando (Germanic) sword.

Gerek (Polish) a form of Gerald, Gerard.

Geremia (Hebrew) exalted by God. (Italian) a form of Jeremiah.
Geremya

Geremiah (Italian) a form of Jeremiah.
Gerimiah, Geromiah

Geremy (English) a form of Jeremy.

Gerhard (German) a form of Gerard.
Garhard, Gerhardi, Gerhardt, Gerhart, Gerhort

Gerik (Polish) a form of Edgar.
Gerek, Geric, Gerick, Gérrick

Gerino (German) lance.

Germain (French) from Germany. (English) sprout, bud. See also Jermaine.
Germane, Germano, Germayn, Germayne, Germin, Germon, Germyn

Germaine **BG** (French, English) a form of Germain.

German (French, English) a form of Germain.

Germán (French) a form of German.

Germana (Latin) ready for action.

Germinal (Latin) he who sprouts.

Geroldo (Germanic) the commander of the lance.

Gerome (English) a form of Jerome.

Geroncio (Greek) little old man.

Geronimo (Greek, Italian) a form of Jerome. History: a famous Apache chief.
Geronemo, Geronymo

Gerónimo (Greek) a form of Geronimo.

Gerrit (Irish) a form of Garrett. (Dutch) a form of Gerald. (English) a form of Gerard.

Gerrod (English) a form of Garrad.
Gerred, Gerrid

Gerry (English) a familiar form of Gerald, Gerard. See also Jerry.
Geri, Gerre, Gerri, Gerrie, Gerryson

Gershom (Hebrew) exiled. (Yiddish) stranger in exile.
Gersham, Gersho, Gershon, Geurson, Gursham, Gurshan

Gershón (Hebrew) a form of Gershom.

Gerson (English) son of Gar. (Hebrew, Yiddish) a form of Gershom.
Gersan, Gershawn

Gert (German, Danish) fighter.

Gervaise **BG** (French) honorable. See also Jervis.
Garvais, Garvaise, Garvas, Garvase, Gerivas, Gervais, Gervas, Gervase, Gervasio, Gervaso, Gervasy, Gervayse, Gervis, Gerwazy

Gerwin (Welsh) fair love.
Gerwen, Gerwyn

Gesualdo (Germanic) the prisoner of the king.

Getachew (African) your teacher.

Geteye (African) his teacher.

Gethin (Welsh) dusky.
Geth, Gethyn

Getulio (Latin) he who came from Getulia.

Gevork (Armenian) a form of George.

Ghalib (Indian) excellent.

Ghâlib (Arabic) a form of Victor.

Ghanashyam, Giridari, Giridhar (Indian) other names for the Hindu god Krishna.

Ghazi (Arabic) conqueror.

Ghedi (Somali) traveler.

Ghilchrist (Irish) servant of Christ. See also Gil.
Ghylchrist

Ghislain (French) pledge.

Gi (Korean) brave.

Gia 🇬🇧 (Vietnamese) family.
Giah, Gya, Gyah

Giacinto (Portuguese, Spanish) a form of Jacinto.
Giacintho, Gyacinto, Gyacynto

Giacomo (Italian) a form of Jacob.
Gaimo, Giacamo, Giaco, Giacobbe, Giacobo, Giacopo, Gyacomo

Gian (Italian) a form of Giovanni, John.
Ghian, Ghyan, Gianetto, Giann, Gianne, Giannes, Giannis, Giannos, Gyan

Giancarlo (Italian) a combination of Gian + Carlo.
Giancarlos, Gianncarlo, Gyancarlo

Gianfranco (Italian) a combination of Gian + Franco.

Gianluca (Italian) a combination of Gian + Luca.

Gianmarco (Italian) a combination of Gian + Marco.

Gianni (Italian) a form of Johnie.
Giani, Gionni

Gianpaolo (Italian) a combination of Gian + Paolo.
Gianpaulo

Gib (English) a short form of Gilbert.
Gibb, Gibbie, Gibby

Gibert (Catalan) a form of Gilberto.

Gibor (Hebrew) powerful.
Gibbor

Gibson (English) son of Gilbert.
Gibbon, Gibbons, Gibbs, Gibbson, Gilson

Gideon (Hebrew) tree cutter. Bible: the judge who defeated the Midianites.
Gedeon, Gideone, Gydeon, Hedeon

Gidon (Hebrew) a form of Gideon.

Gifford (English) bold giver.
Giff, Giffard, Gifferd, Giffie, Giffy, Gyfford, Gyford

Gig (English) horse-drawn carriage.

Gil (Greek) shield bearer. (Hebrew) happy. (English) a short form of Ghilchrist, Gilbert.
Gili, Gilie, Gill, Gilley, Gilli, Gillie, Gillis, Gilly, Gyl, Gyll

Gilad (Arabic) camel hump; from Giladi, Saudi Arabia.
Giladi, Giladie, Gilead, Gylad, Gylead

Gilamu (Basque) a form of William.
Gillen, Gylamu

Gilbert (English) brilliant pledge; trustworthy. See also Gil, Gillett.
Gib, Gilburt, Gilibeirt, Gillbert, Gillburt, Gilleabert, Giselbert, Giselberto, Giselbertus, Guilbert, Gylbert, Gylbirt, Gylburt, Gylbyrt

Gilberto (Spanish) a form of Gilbert.
Gilburto

Gilby (Scandinavian) hostage's estate. (Irish) blond boy.
Gilbee, Gilbey, Gilbi, Gilbie, Gillbee, Gillbey, Gillbi, Gillbie, Gillby, Gylbee, Gylbey, Gylbi, Gylbie, Gylby, Gyllbee, Gyllbey, Gyllbi, Gyllbie, Gyllby

Gilchrist (Irish) a form of Ghilchrist.
Gilcrist

Gildardo (German) good.

Gildo (Spanish) a form of Hermenegildo.

Gilen (Basque, German) illustrious pledge.
Gilenn, Gylen

Giles (French) goatskin shield.
Gide, Gyles, Gylles

Gillean (Irish) Bible: Saint John's servant.
Gillan, Gillen, Gillian, Gillyan

Gillermo (Spanish) resolute protector.

Gilles (French) a form of Giles.

Gillespie (Irish) son of the bishop's servant.
Gillis, Gyllespie, Gyllespy

Gillett (French) young Gilbert.
Gelett, Gelette, Gilet, Gilett, Gilette, Gillette, Gillit, Gylet, Gylett, Gylit, Gylitt, Gylyt, Gylytt

Gilmer (English) famous hostage.
Gilmar, Gylmar, Gylmer

Gilmore (Irish) devoted to the Virgin Mary.
*Gillmoor, Gillmoore, Gillmor, Gillmore,
Gillmour, Gilmoor, Gilmoore, Gilmor,
Gilmour, Gylmoor, Gylmoore, Gylmor,
Gylmore*

Gilon (Hebrew) circle.
Gylon

Gilroy (Irish) devoted to the king.
*Gilderoi, Gilderoy, Gildray, Gildroi, Gildroy,
Gillroi, Gillroy, Gyllroi, Gyllroy, Gylroi,
Gylroy, Roy*

Gines (Greek) he who produces life.

Ginés (Greek) a form of Genesis.

Gino (Greek) a familiar form of Eugene.
(Italian) a short form of names ending in
"gene," "gino."
Ghino, Gyno

Giona (Italian) a form of Jonah.
Gionah, Gyona, Gyonah

Giordano (Italian) a form of Jordan.
Giordan, Giordana, Giordin, Guordan

Giorgio (Italian) a form of George.

Giorgos (Greek) a form of George.
Georgos, Giorgios

Giosia (Italian) a form of Joshua.
Giosiah, Giosya, Gyosia, Gyosya, Gyosyah

Giotto (Italian) a form of Geoffrey.

Giovani, Giovanny, Giovany (Italian) forms
of Giovanni.
*Giavani, Giovan, Giovane, Giovanie,
Giovonny, Gyovani, Gyovanie, Gyovany*

Giovanni BG (Italian) a form of John. See
also Jeovanni, Jiovanni.
*Giannino, Giovann, Giovannie, Giovanno,
Giovon, Giovonathon, Giovonni, Giovonnia,
Giovonnie, Givonni*

Gipsy (English) wanderer.
Gipson, Gypsy

Giri (Indian) mountain.

Girik, Girilal, Girindra, Girish (Indian)
other names for the Hindu god Shiva.

Giriraj (Indian) lord of the mountains.

Girvin (Irish) small; tough.
Girvan, Girven, Girvon, Girvyn, Gyrvyn

Gisberto (Germanic) he who shines in battle with his sword.

Gitano (Spanish) gypsy.
Gytano

Giuliano (Italian) a form of Julius.
Giulano, Giulino, Giullliano

Giulio (Italian) a form of Julius.
Gyulio, Gyulyo

Giuseppe (Italian) a form of Joseph.
*Giuseppi, Giuseppino, Giusseppe, Guiseppe,
Guiseppi, Guiseppie, Guisseppe*

Giustino (Italian) a form of Justin.
Giusto, Giustyno, Gyustino, Gyusto, Gyustyno

Givon (Hebrew) hill; heights.
Givan, Givawn, Given, Givyn

Gladwin (English) cheerful. See also Win.
*Glad, Gladdie, Gladdy, Gladwen, Gladwenn,
Gladwinn, Gladwyn, Gladwynn, Gladwynne*

Glanville (English) village with oak trees.
*Glannville, Glanvil, Glanvill, Glanvyl,
Glanvyll, Glanvylle*

Glasson (Scottish) from Glasgow, Scotland.
Glason, Glassan, Glassen, Glassin, Glassyn

Glen, Glenn (Irish) short forms of Glendon.
*Glean, Gleann, Glennie, Glennis, Glennon,
Glenny*

Glendon (Scottish) fortress in the glen.
*Glandan, Glandun, Glenden, Glendin,
Glendyn, Glenndan, Glennden, Glenndin,
Glenndon, Glenndyn, Glennton, Glenton,
Glyndan, Glynden, Glyndin, Glyndon,
Glyndyn, Glynndan, Glynnden, Glynndin,
Glynndon, Glynndun, Glynndyn*

Glendower (Welsh) from Glyndwr, Wales.

Glenrowan (Irish) valley with rowan trees.
*Glennrowan, Glenrowen, Glenrowin,
Glenrowyn, Glynnrowan, Glynnrowen,
Glynnrowin, Glynnrowon, Glynnrowyn,
Glynrowan, Glynrowen, Glynrowin,
Glynrowon, Glynrowyn*

Glenton (Scottish) valley town.
Glennton, Glynnton, Glynton

Glenville (Irish) village in the glen.
*Glenvyl, Glenvyle, Glenvyll, Glenvylle,
Glynnville, Glynville*

Glyn, Glynn (Welsh) forms of Glen.
Glin, Glinn

Godardo (German) a form of Goddard.

Goddard (German) divinely firm.
*Godard, Godart, Goddart, Godhardt,
Godhart, Gothart, Gotthard, Gotthardt,
Gotthart*

Godeardo (German) a form of Gotardo.

Godfredo (Spanish) friend of God.

Godfrey (Irish) God's peace. (German) a
form of Jeffrey. See also Geoffrey, Gottfried.
*Goddfree, Goddfrey, Godefroi, Godfree,
Godfry, Godofredo, Godoired, Godrey,
Goffredo, Gofraidh, Gofredo, Gorry*

Godwin (English) friend of God. See also
Win.
*Godewyn, Godwen, Godwinn, Godwyn,
Godwynn, Goodwin, Goodwyn, Goodwynn,
Goodwynne*

Goel (Hebrew) redeemer.

Gogo (African) like a grandfather.

Gokul (Indian) place where the Hindu god
Krishna was brought up.

Golden (English) a form of Goldwin.

Goldwin (English) golden friend. See also
Win.
*Goldewin, Goldewinn, Goldewyn, Goldwinn,
Goldwinne, Goldwyn, Goldwyne, Goldwynn,
Goldwynne*

Goliard (Spanish) the rebel.

Goliat (Hebrew) he who lives his life making pilgrimages.

Goliath (Hebrew) exiled. Bible: the giant
Philistine whom David slew with a sling-
shot.
Golliath, Golyath

Gomda (Kiowa) wind.
Gomdah

Gomer (Hebrew) completed, finished.
(English) famous battle.

Gomez (Spanish) man.
Gomaz

Gontrán (German, Spanish) famous warrior.

Gonza (Rutooro) love.
Gonzah

Gonzalo (Spanish) wolf.
*Goncalve, Gonsalo, Gonsalve, Gonsalvo,
Gonzales, Gonzalos, Gonzalous, Gonzelee,
Gonzolo*

Gopal (Indian) protector of cows; another
name for the Hindu god Krishna.

Gopesh (Indian) another name for the
Hindu god Krishna.

Gopichand (Indian) name of a king.

Gorakh (Indian) cowherd.

Goran (Greek) a form of George.

Gordon (English) triangular-shaped hill.
*Gord, Gordain, Gordan, Gorden, Gordin,
Gordonn, Gordun, Gordyn*

Gordy (English) a familiar form of Gordon.
Gordie

Gore (English) triangular-shaped land;
wedge-shaped land.

Gorge (Latin) gorge. (Greek) a form of
George.

Gorgonio (Greek) the violent one.

Gorman (Irish) small; blue eyed.
Gormen

Goro (Japanese) fifth.

Gosheven (Native American) great leaper.

Gosvino (Teutonic) friend of God.

Gotardo (Germanic) he who is valiant
because of the strength God gives him.

Gottfried (German) a form of Geoffrey,
Godfrey.
Gotfrid, Gotfrids, Gottfrid

Gotzon (German) a form of Angel.

Govert (Dutch) heavenly peace.

Gower (Welsh) pure.

Gowon (Tiv) rainmaker.
Gowan, Gowen, Gowin, Gowyn

Goyo (Spanish) a form of Gerardo.

Gozol (Hebrew) soaring bird.
Gozal

Gracia (Latin) nice; welcome.

Gracián (Latin) the possessor of grace.

Graciano (Latin) the one recognized by God.

Grady (Irish) noble; illustrious.
Gradea, Gradee, Gradey, Gradi, Gradie, Gradleigh, Graidee, Graidey, Graidi, Graidie, Graidy, Graydee, Graydey, Graydi, Graydie, Graydy

Graeme (Scottish) a form of Graham.
Graem, Graiam, Gram, Grame, Gramm, Grayeme

Graham (English) grand home.
Graeham, Graehame, Graehme, Grahame, Grahamme, Grahem, Graheme, Grahim, Grahime, Grahm, Grahme, Grahym, Graiham, Graihame, Grayham, Grayhame, Grayhim, Grayhym, Greyham, Greyhame, Greyhem, Greyheme

Granger (French) farmer.
Grainger, Grange, Graynger

Grant **Bɢ** (English) a short form of Grantland.
Grand, Grandt, Grantham, Granthem

Grantland (English) great plains.
Granlan, Granland, Grantlan

Grantley (English) great meadow.
Grantlea, Grantlee, Grantleigh, Grantli, Grantlie, Grantly

Granville (French) large village.
Gran, Granvel, Granvil, Granvile, Granvill, Granvyl, Granvyll, Granvylle, Grenville, Greville

Grato (Latin) the one recognized by God.

Grau (Spanish) a form of Gerardo.

Gray (English) gray haired.
Grae, Grai, Graye, Greye

Grayden (English) gray haired.
Graden, Graedan, Graeden, Graedin,

Graedyn, Graidan, Graiden, Graidin, Graidyn, Graydan, Graydin, Graydyn, Greyden, Greydin, Greydyn

Graydon (English) gray hill.
Gradon, Graedon, Graidon, Grayton, Greydon

Grayson **Bɢ** (English) bailiff's son. See also Sonny.
Graeson, Graison, Graysen

Greeley (English) gray meadow.
Greelea, Greeleigh, Greeli, Greelie, Greely

Greenwood (English) green forest.
Green, Greener, Greenerwood, Greenewood

Greg, Gregg (Latin) short forms of Gregory.
Graig, Gregson, Greig, Greigg

Greggory (Latin) a form of Gregory.
Greggery, Greggori, Greggorie

Gregor (Scottish) a form of Gregory.
Gregoor, Grégor, Gregore

Gregorio (Italian, Portuguese) a form of Gregory.
Gregorios

Gregory (Latin) vigilant watchman. See also Jörn, Krikor.
Gergely, Gergo, Greagoir, Greagory, Greer, Gregary, Greger, Gregery, Grégoire, Gregorey, Gregori, Grégorie, Gregorius, Gregors, Gregos, Gregrey, Gregroy, Gregry, Greigoor, Greigor, Greigore, Greogry, Gries, Grisha, Grzegorz

Gresham (English) village in the pasture.

Grey (English) a form of Gray.

Greyson (English) a form of Grayson.
Greysen, Greysten, Greyston

Griffen (Latin) a form of Griffin.
Grifen

Griffin (Latin) hooked nose.
Griff, Griffie, Griffon, Griffy, Griffyn, Griffynn, Gryffin, Gryffyn, Gryphon

Griffith (Welsh) fierce chief; ruddy.
Griff, Griffeth, Griffie, Griffy, Gryffith

Grigor (Bulgarian) a form of Gregory.

Grigori (Bulgarian) a form of Gregory.
Grigoi, Grigore, Grigorij, Grigorios, Grigorov, Grigory

Grigorii (Russian) a form of Gregory.

Grimoaldo (Spanish) confessor.

Grimshaw (English) dark woods.
Grymshaw

Grisha (Russian) a form of Gregory.
Grysha

Griswold (German, French) gray forest.
Gris, Griswald, Griswaldo, Griswoldo, Griz, Grizwald, Gryswald, Gryswaldo

Grosvener (French) big hunter.

Grosvenor (French) great hunter.

Grover (English) grove.
Grove

Guacraya (Quechua) strong and brave like a bull.

Guadalberto (Germanic) he is all powerful.

Guadalupe GB (Arabic) river of black stones.
Guadalope

Guaina (Quechua) young.

Guala (German) governor.

Gualberto (Spanish) a form of Walter.

Gualtiero (Italian) a form of Walter.
Gualterio

Guaman (Quechua) falcon.

Guamanachachi (Quechua) he who has valorous ancestors like the falcon.

Guamancapac (Quechua) lord falcon.

Guamancaranca (Quechua) he who fights like a thousand falcons.

Guamanchaua (Quechua) cruel as a falcon.

Guamanchuri (Quechua) son of the falcon.

Guamanpuma (Quechua) strong and powerful as a puma and a falcon.

Guamantiupac (Quechua) glorious falcon.

Guamanyana (Quechua) black falcon.

Guamanyurac (Quechua) white falcon.

Guamay (Quechua) young, fresh.

Guanca, Guancar (Quechua) rock; summit.

Guanpú (Aymara) born in a festive time.

Guari (Quechua) savage, untamable.

Guarino (Teutonic) he who defends well.

Guariruna (Quechua) untamed and wild man.

Guarititu, Guartito (Quechua) untamed and difficult to handle.

Guascar (Quechua) he of the chain, rope, or bindweed.

Guaual (Quechua) myrtle.

Guayasamin (Quechua) happy white bird in flight.

Guayau (Quechua) royal willow.

Guaynacapac (Quechua) young master.

Guaynarimac (Quechua) young speaker.

Guaynay (Quechua) my youngster.

Guaypa, Guaypaya (Quechua) rooster; creator.

Guayra (Quechua) fast as the wind.

Guayua (Aymara) restless; mischievous.

Guglielmo (Italian) a form of William.

Guido (Italian) a form of Guy.

Guifford (French) chubby cheeks.

Guifré (Catalan) a form of Wilfredo.

Guilford (English) ford with yellow flowers.
Guildford

Guilherme (Portuguese) a form of William.

Güillac (Quechua) he who warns.

Guillaume (French) a form of William.
Guilem, Guillaums, Guilleaume, Guyllaume

Guillerme (German) a form of William.

Guillermo (Spanish) a form of William.
Guillerrmo

Guir (Irish) beige.

Güiracocha, Güiracucha (Quechua) sea foam.

Güisa (Quechua) prophet.

Güiuyac (Quechua) brilliant, luminous.

Güiyca (Quechua) sacred.

Güiycauaman (Quechua) sacred falcon.

Gumaro (Germanic) army of men; disciplined man.

Gumersindo (Germanic) the excellent man.

Gundelberto (Teutonic) he who shines in battle.

Gundislavo (German) joy; strength.

Gunnar (Scandinavian) a form of Gunther.

Gunner (English) soldier with a gun. (Scandinavian) a form of Gunther.
Guner

Gunter (Scandinavian) a form of Gunther.
Guenter, Guntar, Guntero

Gunther (Scandinavian) battle army; warrior.
Guenther, Gun, Gunthar, Günther

Guotin (Chinese) polite; strong leader.

Gurdeep (Sikh) lamp of the guru.

Gurion (Hebrew) young lion.
Gur, Guri, Guriel, Guryon

Gurjot (Sikh) light of the guru.

Gurpreet BG (Sikh) devoted to the guru; devoted to the Prophet.
Gurjeet, Gurmeet, Guruprit

Gurveer (Sikh) guru's warrior.

Gurvir (Sikh) a form of Gurveer.

Gus (Scandinavian) a short form of Angus, Augustine, Gustave.
Guss, Gussie, Gussy, Gusti, Gustry, Gusty

Gustaf (Swedish) a form of Gustave.
Gustaaf, Gustaff

Gustave (Scandinavian) staff of the Goths. History: Gustavus Adolphus was a king of Sweden. See also Kosti, Tabo, Tavo.
Gustaof, Gustav, Gustáv, Gustava, Gustaves, Gustavius, Gustavs, Gustavus, Gustik, Gustus, Gusztav

Gustavo (Italian, Spanish) a form of Gustave.
Gustabo

Guthrie (German) war hero. (Irish) windy place.
Guthre, Guthree, Guthrey, Guthri, Guthry

Gutierre (Spanish) a form of Walter.

Guy (Hebrew) valley. (German) warrior. (French) guide. See also Guido.
Guie, Guyon

Guyapi (Native American) candid.

Guyllaume (French) a form of William.

Guzman, Guzmán (Gothic) good man; man of God.

Gwayne (Welsh) a form of Gawain.
Gwaine, Gwayn

Gwidon (Polish) life.
Gwydon

Gwilym (Welsh) a form of William.
Gwillym

Gwyn GB (Welsh) fair; blessed.
Gwinn, Gwinne, Gwynn, Gwynne

Gyasi (Akan) marvelous baby.

Gyorgy (Russian) a form of George.
Gyoergy, György, Gyuri, Gyurka

Gyula (Hungarian) youth.
Gyala, Gyuszi

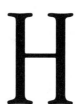

Habacuc (Hebrew) embrace.

Habib (Arabic) beloved.
Habyb

Habîb (Hebrew) a form of Habib.

Habid (Arabic) the appreciated one.

Hacan (Quechua) brilliant, splendorous.

Hacanpoma, Hacanpuma (Quechua) brilliant puma.

Hackett (German, French) little wood cutter.
Hacket, Hackit, Hackitt, Hackyt, Hackytt

Hackman (German, French) wood cutter.
Hackmen

Hadar (Hebrew) glory.

Haddad (Arabic) blacksmith.
Hadad

Haddâd (Arabic) a form of Haddad.

Hadden (English) heather-covered hill.
Haddan, Haddin, Haddon, Haddyn

Haden (English) a form of Hadden.
*Hadan, Hadin, Hadon, Hadun, Hadyn,
Haeden*

Hadi (Arabic) guiding to the right.
Haddi, Hadee, Hady

Hadley GB (English) heather-covered
meadow.
Had, Hadlea, Hadlee, Hadleigh, Hadly, Leigh

Hadrian (Latin, Swedish) dark.
*Adrian, Hadrien, Hadrion, Hadryan,
Hadryen, Hadryin, Hadryn, Hadryon*

Hadrián (Latin) a form of Hadrian.

Hadulfo (Germanic) the combat wolf.

Hadwin (English) friend in a time of war.
*Hadwen, Hadwinn, Hadwyn, Hadwynn,
Hadwynne*

Hafiz (Indian) protected.

Hagan (German) strong defense.
Haggan

Hagar GB (Hebrew) forsaken; stranger.
Hager, Hagir, Hagor, Hagyr

Hagen (Irish) young, youthful.
Hagin, Hagon, Hagun, Hagyn

Hagley (English) enclosed meadow.
*Haglea, Haglee, Hagleigh, Hagli, Haglie,
Hagly*

Hagop (Armenian) a form of James.

Hagos (Ethiopian) happy.

Hahnee (Native American) beggar.

Hai (Vietnamese) sea.

Haidar (Arabic) lion.

Haiden BG (English) a form of Hayden.
*Haidan, Haidin, Haidn, Haidon, Haidun,
Haidyn*

Haider (Arabic) a form of Haidar.

Haig (English) enclosed with hedges.
Hayg

Hailama (Hawaiian) famous brother.
*Hailamah, Hailaman, Hairama, Hilama,
Hilamah*

Hailey GB (Irish) a form of Haley.
*Haile, Hailea, Hailee, Haileigh, Haille, Haily,
Halee*

Haines (English) from the vine-covered cottage.
Hanes, Haynes

Haji (Swahili) born during the pilgrimage to
Mecca.

Hajjâj (Arabic) traveler.

Hakan (Native American) fiery.
Haken, Hakin, Hakon, Hakyn

Hakeem (Arabic) a form of Hakim.
Hakam, Hakem

Hakim (Arabic) wise. (Ethiopian) doctor.
Hackeem, Hackim, Hakiem, Hakym

Hakîm (Arabic) a form of Hakim.

Hakizimana (Egyptian) salvation of God.

Hakon (Scandinavian) of Nordic ancestry.
*Haaken, Haakin, Haakon, Haeo, Hak,
Hakan, Hakin, Hako, Hakyn*

Hal (English) a short form of Halden, Hall,
Harold.

Halbert (English) shining hero.
Bert, Halbirt, Halburt, Halbyrt

Halcyon (Greek) tranquil, peaceful; kingfisher. Mythology: the kingfisher bird was
supposed to have the power to calm the
wind and the waves while nesting near the
sea.
Halcion

Halden (Scandinavian) half-Danish. See also
Dane.
*Hal, Haldan, Haldane, Haldin, Haldon,
Haldyn, Halfdan, Halvdan*

Hale (English) a short form of Haley.
(Hawaiian) a form of Harry.
Hael, Haele, Hail, Hayl, Hayle, Heall

Halen (Swedish) hall.
Hailen, Hailin, Hailon, Hailyn, Hallen, Hallene, Haylen

Haley GB (Irish) ingenious.
Haleigh, Halley, Hayleigh, Hayley, Hayli

Halford (English) valley ford.
Haleford

Hali GB (Greek) sea.
Halea, Halee, Halie

Halian (Zuni) young.
Halyan

Halifax (English) holy field.
Halyfax

Halil (Turkish) dear friend.
Halill, Halyl

Halim (Arabic) mild, gentle.
Haleem, Halym

Hall (English) manor, hall.

Hallam (English) valley.
Halam

Hallan (English) dweller at the hall; dweller
at the manor.
*Hailan, Halan, Halin, Hallin, Hallon,
Hallyn, Halon, Halyn, Haylan*

Halley GB (English) meadow near the hall;
holy.
Hallee, Halleigh, Halli, Hallie, Hally

Halliwell (English) holy well.
*Haliwel, Haliwell, Hallewell, Halliwel,
Hallywel, Hallywell, Halywel, Halywell,
Hellewell, Helliwell*

Hallward (English) hall guard.
Halward

Halsey GB (English) Hal's island.
Hallsea, Hallsey, Hallsy, Halsea, Halsy

Halstead (English) manor grounds.
Halsted

Halton (English) estate on the hill.
Haltan, Halten, Haltin, Haltyn

Halvor (Norwegian) rock; protector.
Hallvar, Hallvard, Halvar, Halvard

Ham (Hebrew) hot. Bible: one of Noah's
sons.

Hamal (Arabic) lamb. Astronomy: a bright
star in the constellation of Aries.
Hamel, Hamol

Hamar (Scandinavian) hammer.
Hamer, Hammar, Hammer

Hamdân (Arabic) praised.

Hamed (Arabic) a form of Hamid.
Hamedo, Hameed, Hammed

Hamid (Arabic) praised. See also
Muhammad.
*Haamid, Hamaad, Hamadi, Hamd,
Hamdrem, Hammad, Hammyd, Hammydd,
Humayd*

Hamîd (Arabic) a form of Hamid.

Hamidi (Kenyan) admired.
Hamidie, Hamidy

Hamill (English) scarred.
*Hamel, Hamell, Hamil, Hammil, Hammill,
Hamyl, Hamyll*

Hamilton (English) proud estate.
*Hamelton, Hamiltan, Hamilten, Hamiltun,
Hamiltyn, Hamylton, Tony*

Hamir (Indian) a raga, an ancient form of
Hindu devotional music.

Hamish (Scottish) a form of Jacob, James.
Hamysh

Hamisi (Swahili) born on Thursday.
Hamisie, Hamisy

Hamlet (German, French) little village;
home. Literature: one of Shakespeare's
tragic heroes.
Hamlit, Hamlot

Hamlin (German, French) loves his home.
*Hamblin, Hamelen, Hamelin, Hamlan,
Hamlen, Hamlon, Hamlyn, Lin*

Hammet (English, Scandinavian) village.
Hammett, Hamnet, Hamnett

Hammond (English) village.
Hammon, Hammund, Hamond, Hamund

Hampton (English) Geography: a town in England.
Hamp, Hampden, Hamptan, Hampten, Hamptin, Hamptyn

Hamza (Arabic) powerful.
Hamze, Hamzia

Hamzah (Arabic) a form of Hamza.
Hamzeh

Hanale (Hawaiian) a form of Henry.
Haneke

Hanan 🇬🇧 (Hebrew) grace.
Hananel, Hananiah, Johanan

Hanbal (Arabic) pure. History: Ahmad Ibn Hanbal founded an Islamic school of thought.
Hanbel, Hanbil, Hanbyn

Handel (German, English) a form of John. Music: George Frideric Handel was a German composer whose works include *Messiah* and *Water Music*.
Handal, Handil, Handol, Handyl

Hanford (English) high ford.

Hani (Lebanese) happy.

Hâni (Arabic) happy, satisfied.

Hanif (Arabic) true believer.
Haneef, Hanef, Hanyf

Hanisi (Swahili) born on Thursday.

Hank (American) a familiar form of Henry.

Hanley (English) high meadow.
Handlea, Handlee, Handleigh, Handley, Handli, Handlie, Handly, Hanlea, Hanlee, Hanleigh, Hanly

Hanna 🇬🇧 (German) a form of Johann.

Hannah 🇬🇧 (German) a form of Johann.

Hannes (Finnish) a form of John.
Hanes, Hannus

Hannibal (Phoenician) grace of God. History: a famous Carthaginian general who fought the Romans.
Anibal, Hanibal, Hannybal, Hanybal

Hanno (German) a short form of Johann.
Hannon, Hannu, Hano, Hanon

Hans (Scandinavian) a form of John.
Hants, Hanz

Hansel (Scandinavian) a form of Hans.
Haensel, Hannsel, Hansal, Hansell, Hansil, Hansl, Hansol, Hansyl, Hanzel

Hansen (Scandinavian) son of Hans.
Hansan, Hansin, Hanssen, Hansun, Hansyn

Hansh (Hindi) god; godlike.

Hanson (Scandinavian) a form of Hansen.
Hansson

Hanuman, Hanumant (Indian) the Hindu monkey god.

Hanus (Czech) a form of John.

Haoa (Hawaiian) a form of Howard.

Hapi (Egyptian) god of the Nile.

Hapu (Egyptian) pharaoh.

Hara 🇬🇧 (Hindi) seizer. Religion: another name for the Hindu god Shiva.

Harald (Scandinavian) a form of Harold.
Haraldas, Haralds, Haralpos

Harb (Arabic) warrior.

Harbin (German, French) little bright warrior.
Harban, Harben, Harbon, Harbyn

Harcourt (French) fortified dwelling.
Court, Harcort

Hardeep (Punjabi) a form of Harpreet.

Harden (English) valley of the hares.
Hardan, Hardian, Hardin, Hardon, Hardun, Hardyn

Hardik (Indian) heartfelt.

Harding (English) brave; hardy.
Hardyng

Hardwin (English) brave friend.
Hardinn, Hardwen, Hardwenn, Hardwyn, Hardwynn

Hardy (German) bold, daring.
Harde, Hardee, Hardey, Hardi, Hardie

Harekrishna, Haresh, Harigopal, Harkrishna (Indian) other names for the Hindu god Krishna.

Harel (Hebrew) mountain of God.
Haral, Harell, Hariel, Harrel, Harrell, Haryel, Haryell

Harendra, Harishankar (Indian) other names for the Hindu god Shiva.

Harford (English) ford of the hares.
Hareford

Hargrove (English) grove of the hares.
Haregrove, Hargreave, Hargreaves

Hari (Hindi) tawny.
Harin

Haridas (Indian) servant of the Hindu god Krishna.

Harihar, Harinarayan, Hariom (Indian) other names for the Hindu god Vishnu.

Hariprasad (Indian) blessed by the Hindu god Krishna.

Hariram (Indian) another name for the Hindu god Rama.

Haris (English) a form of Harris.
Hariss, Harys, Heris, Herys

Harishchandra (Indian) charitable; a king of the Surya dynasty, 1435–1523.

Haritbaran (Indian) green.

Harith (Arabic) cultivator.
Haryth

Harjot BG (Sikh) light of God.
Harjeet, Harjit, Harjodh

Harkin (Irish) dark red.
Harkan, Harken, Harkon, Harkyn

Harlan (English) hare's land; army land.
Harlen, Harlenn, Harlin, Harlon, Harlyn, Harlynn

Harland (English) a form of Harlan.
Harlend

Harley BG (English) hare's meadow; army meadow.
Arley, Harle, Harlea, Harlee, Harleigh, Harly

Harlow (English) hare's hill; army hill. See also Arlo.
Harlo

Harman, Harmon (English) forms of Herman.
Harm, Harmann, Harmen, Harmin, Harmond, Harms, Harmyn

Harmendra (Indian) moon.

Harmodio (Greek) convenient.

Harold (Scandinavian) army ruler. See also Jindra.
Araldo, Garald, Garold, Harald, Hareld, Harild, Haryld, Herald, Hereld, Herold, Heronim, Heryld

Haroon (Arabic) a form of Haroun.

Haroun (Arabic) lofty; exalted.
Haaroun, Haarun, Harin, Haron, Harron, Harrun, Harun

Harper GB (English) harp player.
Harp, Harpo

Harpreet GB (Punjabi) loves God, devoted to God.

Harrington (English) Harry's town.
Harringtown

Harris (English) a short form of Harrison.
Harrys, Herris, Herrys

Harrison (English) son of Harry.
Harison, Harreson, Harrisen, Harrisson, Harryson, Haryson

Harrod (Hebrew) hero; conqueror.
Harod

Harry (English) a familiar form of Harold, Henry. See also Arrigo, Hale, Parry.
Harray, Harrey, Harri, Harrie, Hary

Harsh (Indian) happiness.

Harshad (Indian) giver of joy.

Harshavardhan (Indian) creator of joy.

Harshil, Harshit, Harshita (Indian) joyful.

Hart (English) a short form of Hartley.
Harte, Heart

Hartley (English) deer meadow.
Hartlea, Hartlee, Hartleigh, Hartly, Heartlea, Heartlee, Heartleigh, Heartley, Heartli, Heartlie, Heartly

Hartman (German) hard; strong.
Hartmen

Hartwell (English) deer well.
Hartwel, Hartwil, Hartwill, Hartwyl,
Hartwyll, Harwel, Harwell, Harwil, Harwill

Hartwig (German) strong advisor.
Hartwyg

Hartwood (English) deer forest.
Harwood

Hârûn (Arabic) a form of Aaron.

Harvey (German) army warrior.
Harv, Harvee, Harvi, Harvie, Harvy, Herve

Harvir (Sikh) God's warrior.
Harvier

Hasaan, Hasan (Arabic) forms of Hassan.
Hasain, Hasaun, Hashaan, Hason

Hasad (Turkish) reaper, harvester.
Hassad

Hasani (Swahili) handsome.
Hasanni, Hassani, Hassian, Heseny, Husani

Hashim (Arabic) destroyer of evil.
Haashim, Hasham, Hasheem, Hashem,
Hashym

Hashîm (Arabic) a form of Hashim.

Hasin (Hindi) laughing.
Haseen, Hasen, Hassin, Hassyn, Hasyn,
Hesen

Haskel (Hebrew) a form of Ezekiel.
Haskell

Haslett (English) hazel-tree land.
Haslet, Haze, Hazel, Hazlet, Hazlett, Hazlitt

Hassan (Arabic) handsome.
Hassen, Hasson

Hassân (Arabic) a form of Hassan.

Hassel (German, English) witches' corner.
Hasel, Hasell, Hassal, Hassall, Hassell,
Hazael, Hazell

Hastin (Hindi) elephant.
Hastan, Hasten, Haston, Hastyn

Hastings (Latin) spear. (English) house
council.
Hastie, Hasting, Hasty

Hastu (Quechua) bird of the Andes.

Hatim (Arabic) judge.
Hateem, Hatem

Hatuntupac (Quechua) magnificent, great
and majestic.

Hauk (Norwegian) hawk.
Haukeye

Havelock (Norwegian) sea battler.
Haveloc, Haveloch, Havloche, Havlocke

Haven GB (Dutch, English) harbor, port; safe
place.
Haeven, Havan, Havin, Havon, Havyn,
Hevin, Hevon, Hovan

Havgan (Irish) white.
Havgen, Havgin, Havgon, Havgun, Havgyn

Havika (Hawaiian) a form of David.
Havyka

Hawk (English) hawk.
Hawke, Hawkin, Hawkins

Hawley (English) hedged meadow.
Hawlea, Hawlee, Hawleigh, Hawli, Hawlie,
Hawly

Hawthorne (English) hawthorn tree.
Hawthorn

Hayden ☀ BG (English) hedged valley.
Haydan, Haydenn, Haydin, Haydun,
Haydyn, Heydan, Heyden, Heydin, Heydn,
Heydon, Heydun, Heydyn

Haydn, Haydon (English) forms of Hayden.

Hayes (English) hedged valley.
Hais, Haise, Haiz, Haize, Hays, Hayse, Hayz

Hayward (English) guardian of the hedged
area.
Haiward, Haward, Heiward, Heyvard,
Heyward

Haywood (English) hedged forest.
Heiwood, Heywood, Woody

Hazen (Hindi) a form of Hasin.

Haziel (Hebrew) vision of God.

Hearn (Scottish, English) a short form of
Ahearn.
Hearne, Herin, Hern, Herne

Heath (English) heath.
Heaf, Heaff, Heathe, Heith

Heathcliff (English) cliff near the heath. Literature: the hero of Emily Brontë's novel *Wuthering Heights.*
Heafcliff, Heafcliff, Heaffclif, Heaffcliff, Heaffcliffe, Heaffclyffe, Heathclif, Heathcliffe, Heathclyffe

Heaton (English) high place.
Heatan, Heaten, Heatin, Heatyn

Heber (Hebrew) ally, partner.
Hebar

Hector (Greek) steadfast. Mythology: the greatest hero of the Trojan War in Homer's epic poem *Iliad.*
Ector, Heckter, Hecktir, Hecktore, Hecktur, Hectar, Hektar, Hekter, Hektir, Hektor, Hektore, Hektur

Héctor (Greek) a form of Hector.

Hedley (English) heather-filled meadow.
Headley, Headly, Heddlea, Heddlee, Heddleigh, Heddley, Heddli, Heddlie, Heddly, Hedlea, Hedlee, Hedleigh, Hedli, Hedlie, Hedly

Hedwig BG (German) fighter.
Heddwig, Heddwyg, Hedwyg

Hedwyn (Welsh) friend of peace and blessings. (English) a form of Hadwin.
Heddwin, Heddwyn, Hedwen, Hedwin

Hegesipo (Greek) horse rider.

Heh (Egyptian) god of the immeasurable.

Heinrich (German) a form of Henry.
Heiner, Heinreich, Heinric, Heinriche, Heinrick, Heinrik, Heynric, Heynrich, Heynrick, Heynrik, Hinric, Hinrich, Hinrick, Hynric, Hynrich, Hynrick, Hynrik

Heinz (German) a familiar form of Henry.

Héitor (Spanish) a form of Hector.

Helaku BG (Native American) sunny day.

Heldrado (Germanic) counselor of warriors.

Helge (Russian) holy.
Helg

Heli (Hebrew) he who offers himself to God.

Helio (Greek) Mythology: Helios was the sun god.

Heliodoro (Greek) gift of the sun god.

Heliogabalo (Syrian) he who adores the sun.

Helki BG (Moquelumnan) touching.

Helmer (German) warrior's wrath.

Helmut (German) courageous.
Hellmut, Helmuth

Helué (Arabic) sweet.

Heman (Hebrew) faithful.
Hemen

Henderson (Scottish, English) son of Henry.
Hendrie, Hendries, Hendron, Henryson

Hendrick (Dutch) a form of Henry.
Hedric, Hedrick, Heindric, Heindrick, Hendric, Hendricks, Hendrickson, Hendrik, Hendriks, Hendrikus, Hendrix, Hendryc, Hendryck, Hendrycks, Hendryx

Heniek (Polish) a form of Henry.
Henier

Henley (English) high meadow.
Henlea, Henlee, Henleigh, Henli, Henlie, Henly

Henning (German) a form of Hendrick, Henry.
Hennings

Henoch (Yiddish) initiator.
Enoch, Henock, Henok

Henri (French) a form of Henry.
Henrico, Henrri

Henrick (Dutch) a form of Henry.
Heinrick, Henerik, Henric, Henrich, Henrik, Henryc, Henryck, Henryk

Henrique (Portuguese) a form of Henry.

Henry (German) ruler of the household. See also Arrigo, Enric, Enrico, Enrikos, Enrique, Hanale, Honok, Kiki.
Harro, Heike, Henery, Henraoi, Henrim, Henrry, Heromin

Heracleos, Heraclio (Greek) belonging to Hercules.

Heracles, Hércules (Greek) forms of Hercules.

Heraclito, Heráclito (Greek) he who is drawn to the sacred.

Heraldo (Spanish) a form of Harold.
Haraldo, Haroldo, Haryldo, Heryldo, Hiraldo, Hyraldo

Herb (German) a short form of Herbert.
Herbe, Herbee, Herbi, Herbie, Herby

Herbert (German) glorious soldier.
Bert, Erbert, Eriberto, Harbert, Hebert, Hébert, Heberto, Herberte, Herbirt, Herburt, Herbyrt, Hirbert, Hirbirt, Hirburt, Hirbyrt, Hurbert, Hyrbert, Hyrbirt, Hyrburt, Hyrbyrt

Herculano (Latin) belonging to Hercules.

Hercules (Latin) glorious gift. Mythology: a Greek hero of fabulous strength, renowned for his twelve labors.
Herakles, Herc, Hercule, Herculie

Heriberto (Spanish) a form of Herbert.
Heribert

Hermagoras (Greek) disciple of Hermes.

Hermalindo, Hermelindo (German) he who is like a shield of strength.

Herman (Latin) noble. (German) soldier. See also Armand, Ermanno, Ermano, Mandek.
Hermaan, Hermann, Hermano, Hermie, Herminio, Hermino, Hermon, Hermy, Hermyn, Heromin

Hermán (Germanic) a form of Herman.

Hermenegildo (Germanic) he who offers sacrifices to God.

Hermes (Greek) messenger. Mythology: the divine herald of Greek mythology.

Hermilo (Greek) little Hermes.

Hermócrates (Greek) powerful like Hermes.

Hermógenes (Greek) sent from Hermes.

Hermolao (Greek) messenger of God.

Hermoso (Latin) with shape.

Hernan (German) peacemaker.

Hernán (Spanish) a form of Hernan.

Hernández (Spanish) a form of Ferdinand.

Hernando (Spanish) a form of Ferdinand.
Hernandes, Hernandez

Herodes (Greek) the fire dragon.

Herodías (Greek) leader.

Herodoto (Greek) the sacred talent.

Heródoto (Greek) the divine talent.

Herón, Heros (Latin) hero.

Herrick (German) war ruler.
Herick, Herik, Herrik, Herryc, Herryck, Herryk

Herschel (Hebrew) a form of Hershel.
Herchel, Herschell, Hirschel, Hyrschel

Hersh (Hebrew) a short form of Hershel.
Hersch, Hirsch

Hershel (Hebrew) deer.
Hershal, Hershall, Hershell, Herzl, Hirshel, Hyrshel

Hertz (Yiddish) my strife.
Herts, Herzel

Heru (Egyptian) god of the sun.

Hervé (French) a form of Harvey.
Herv, Hervee, Hervey, Hervi, Hervie, Hervy

Hesiquio (Greek) tranquil.

Hesperia (Greek) one who follows the star of the first evening performance.

Hesperos (Greek) evening star.
Hespero

Hesutu (Moquelumnan) picking up a yellow jacket's nest.

Hew (Welsh) a form of Hugh.
Hewe, Huw

Hewitt (German, French) little smart one.
Hewet, Hewett, Hewie, Hewit, Hewlett, Hewlitt, Hughet, Hughett, Hughit, Hughitt, Hughyt, Hughytt

Hewson (English) son of Hugh.
Hueson, Hughson

Hezekiah (Hebrew) God gives strength.
Hazikiah, Hezekia, Hezekyah, Hezikyah

Hiamovi (Cheyenne) high chief.
Hyamovi

Hiawatha BG (Iraquoian) river maker. History: the Onondagan leader credited with organizing the Iroquois confederacy.

Hibah GB (Arabic) gift.
Hibah, Hyba, Hybah

Hidalgo (Spanish) noble one.

Hideaki (Japanese) smart, clever.
Hideo, Hydeaki

Hieremias (Greek) God will uplift.

Hieronymos (Greek) a form of Jerome. Art: Hieronymus Bosch was a fifteenth-century Dutch painter.
Hierome, Hieronim, Hieronimo, Hieronimos, Hieronymo, Hieronymus

Hieu (Vietnamese) respectful.
Hyew

Higinio (Greek) he who has good health.

Hilal (Arabic) new moon.
Hylal

Hilâl (Arabic) a form of Hilal.

Hilaria, Hilarión (Latin) happy, content.

Hilario (Spanish) a form of Hilary.

Hilary GB (Latin) cheerful. See also Ilari.
Hi, Hil, Hilair, Hilaire, Hilare, Hilarie, Hilarion, Hilarius, Hilery, Hill, Hillary, Hillery, Hilliary, Hillie, Hilly, Hylarie, Hylary

Hildebrand (German) battle sword.
Hildebrando, Hildo

Hildemaro (Germanic) famous in combat.

Hilderic (German) warrior; fortress.
Hilderich, Hilderiche, Hylderic, Hylderych, Hylderyche

Hillel (Hebrew) greatly praised. Religion: Rabbi Hillel originated the Talmud.
Hilel, Hylel, Hyllel

Hilliard (German) brave warrior.
Hiliard, Hillard, Hiller, Hillier, Hillierd, Hillyard, Hillyer, Hillyerd, Hyliard, Hylliar

Hilmar (Swedish) famous noble.
Hillmar, Hilmer, Hylmar, Hylmer

Hilton (English) town on a hill.
Hillton, Hylton

Hinto (Dakota) blue.
Hynto

Hinun (Native American) spirit of the storm.
Hynun

Hipacio (Spanish) confessor.

Hipócrates (Greek) powerful because of his cavalry.

Hipolito (Spanish) a form of Hippolyte.

Hipólito (Greek) a form of Hipolito.

Hippolyte (Greek) horseman.
Hippolit, Hippolitos, Hippolytus, Ippolito

Hiram (Hebrew) noblest; exalted.
Hi, Hirom, Huram

Hiromasa (Japanese) fair, just.

Hiroshi (Japanese) generous.
Hyroshi

Hishâm (Arabic) generosity.

Hisoka (Japanese) secretive, reserved.
Hysoka

Hiu (Hawaiian) a form of Hugh.
Hyu

Hixinio (Greek) vigorous.

Ho (Chinese) good.

Hoang (Vietnamese) finished.

Hobart (German) Bart's hill. A form of Hubert.
Hobard, Hobarte, Hoebard, Hoebart

Hobert (German) Bert's hill.
Hobirt, Hoburt, Hobyrt

Hobie (German) a short form of Hobart, Hobert.
Hobbie, Hobby, Hobey

Hobson (English) son of Robert.
Hobbs, Hobs, Hobsan, Hobsen, Hobsin, Hobsyn

Hoc (Vietnamese) studious.
Hock, Hok

Hod (Hebrew) a short form of Hodgson.

Hodgson (English) son of Roger.
Hod

Hoffman (German) influential.
Hoffmen, Hofman, Hofmen

Hogan (Irish) youth.
Hogen, Hogin, Hogun, Hogyn

Holbrook (English) brook in the hollow.
Brook, Holbrooke

Holden (English) hollow in the valley.
Holdan, Holdin, Holdon, Holdun, Holdyn

Holic (Czech) barber.
Holick, Holik, Holyc, Holyck, Holyk

Holland GB (French) Geography: a former province of the Netherlands.
Holand, Hollan

Holleb (Polish) dove.
Hollub, Holub

Hollis BG (English) grove of holly trees.
Hollie, Holliss, Holly, Hollys, Hollyss

Holmes (English) river islands.

Holt (English) forest.
Holtan, Holten, Holtin, Holton, Holtyn

Homar (Greek) a form of Homer.

Homer (Greek) hostage; pledge; security. Literature: a renowned Greek epic poet.
Homere, Homère, Homeros, Homerus, Omero

Homero (Spanish) a form of Homer.

Hondo (Shona) warrior.

Honesto (Filipino) honest.

Honi (Hebrew) gracious.
Choni, Honie, Hony

Honok (Polish) a form of Henry.

Honon (Moquelumnan) bear.

Honorato (Spanish) honorable.

Honoré (Latin) honored.
Honor, Honoratus, Honoray, Honorio, Honorius

Honovi BG (Native American) strong.

Honza (Czech) a form of John.

Hop (Chinese) agreeable.

Horace (Latin) keeper of the hours. Literature: a famous Roman lyric poet and satirist.
Horaz

Horacio (Latin) a form of Horace.
Horazio, Orazio

Horado (Spanish) timekeeper.

Horangel (Greek) the messenger from the mountain.

Horatio (Latin) clan name. See also Orris.
Horatius, Oratio

Hormisdas (Persian) the great wise one.

Horst (German) dense grove, thicket.

Hortencio, Hortensio (Latin) he who has a garden and loves it.

Horton (English) garden estate.
Hort, Hortan, Horten, Hortin, Hortun, Hortyn, Orton

Horus (Egyptian) god of the sky.

Hosa (Arapaho) young crow.
Hosah

Hosea (Hebrew) salvation. Bible: a Hebrew prophet.
Hose, Hoseia, Hoshea, Hosheah

Hospicio (Spanish) he who is accommodating.

Hotah (Lakota) white.
Hota

Hototo (Native American) whistler.
Hoto

Houghton (English) settlement on the headland.
Houghtan, Houghten, Houghtin, Huetan, Hueten, Huetin, Hueton, Hughtan, Hughten, Hughtin, Hughton

Houston (English) hill town. Geography: a city in Texas.
Houstan, Housten, Houstin, Houstun, Houstyn

Howard (English) watchman. See also Haoa.
Howerd, Ward

Howe (German) high.

Howell (Welsh) remarkable.
Hoell, Howal, Howall, Howel, Huell, Hywel, Hywell

Howi BG (Moquelumnan) turtledove.

Howie (English) a familiar form of Howard, Howland.
Howee, Howey, Howy

Howin (Chinese) loyal swallow.
Howyn

Howland (English) hilly land.
Howie, Howlan, Howlande, Howlen

Hoyt (Irish) mind; spirit.
Hoit, Hoyts

Hu (Chinese) tiger.

Huaiquilaf (Mapuche) good, straight lance.

Huapi (Mapuche) island.

Hubbard (German) a form of Hubert.

Hubert (German) bright mind; bright spirit. See also Beredei, Uberto.
Bert, Hubbert, Huber, Hubertek, Hubertson, Hubirt, Huburt, Hubyrt, Hugibert, Huibert

Huberto (Spanish) a form of Hubert.

Hubie (English) a familiar form of Hubert.
Hube, Hubi

Hucsuncu (Quechua) he who has only one love.

Hud (Arabic) Religion: a Muslim prophet.

Hudson (English) son of Hud.
Hudsan, Hudsen, Hudsin, Hudsyn

Huechacura (Mapuche) sharp rock; peak.

Huemac (Nahuatl) name of a Toltec king.

Huenchulaf (Mapuche) healthy man.

Huenchuleo (Mapuche) brave, handsome river.

Huenchuman (Mapuche) proud, male condor.

Huenchumilla (Mapuche) ascending light.

Huenchuñir (Mapuche) male fox.

Huentemil (Mapuche) light from above.

Huenu (Araucanian) heaven.

Huenuhueque (Mapuche) lamb from heaven.

Huenullan (Mapuche) heavenly altar.

Huenuman (Mapuche) condor from the sky.

Huenupan (Mapuche) branch from heaven.

Huey (English) a familiar form of Hugh.
Hughee, Hughey, Hughi, Hughie, Hughy, Hui

Hueypín (Mapuche) broken, odd land.

Hugh (English) a short form of Hubert. See also Ea, Hewitt, Huxley, Maccoy, Ugo.
Fitzhugh, Hew, Hiu, Hue, Hughe, Hughes, Huw, Huwe

Hugo (Latin) a form of Hugh.
Huego, Ugo

Hugolino (Germanic) he who has spirit and intelligence.

Hugues (French) a form of Hugh.

Huichacura (Mapuche) rock with just one ridge.

Huichahue (Mapuche) battlefield.

Huichalef (Mapuche) he who runs on just one side.

Huichañir (Mapuche) fox from another region.

Huidaleo (Mapuche) branch in the river.

Huinculche (Mapuche) people that live on the hill.

Huircalaf (Mapuche) cry of joy.

Huircaleo (Mapuche) whisper of the river.

Huitzilli (Nahuatl) hummingbird.

Hulbert (German) brilliant grace.
Bert, Holbard, Holbert, Holberte, Holbirt, Holburt, Holbyrt, Hulbard, Hulberte, Hulbirt, Hulburd, Hulburt, Hulbyrt, Hull

Huldá (Hebrew) valiant.

Hullen (Mapuche) spring.

Humam (Arabic) courageous; generous.

Humbaldo (Germanic) daring as a lion cub.

Humbert (German) brilliant strength. See also Umberto.
Hum, Humbirt, Humburt, Humbyrt

Humberto (Portuguese) a form of Humbert.

Humphrey (German) peaceful strength. See also Onofrio, Onufry.
Homfree, Homfrey, Homphree, Homphrey, Homphry, Hum, Humfredo, Humfree, Humfrey, Humfri, Humfrid, Humfrie, Humfried, Humfry, Hump, Humph, Humphery, Humphree, Humphry, Humphrys, Hunfredo

Hung (Vietnamese) brave.

Hunt (English) a short form of names beginning with "Hunt."
Hunta

Hunter ☀ BG (English) hunter.
Huntar, Huntur

Huntington (English) hunting estate.
Huntingdon

Huntley (English) hunter's meadow.
Huntlea, Huntlee, Huntleigh, Huntli, Huntlie, Huntly

Hurley (Irish) sea tide.
Hurlea, Hurlee, Hurleigh, Hurli, Hurlie, Hurly

Hurst (English) a form of Horst.
Hearst, Hirst, Hyrst

Husai (Hebrew) the hurried one.

Husam (Arabic) sword.

Husamettin (Turkish) sharp sword.

Huslu (Native American) hairy bear.

Hussain, Hussien (Arabic) forms of Hussein.
Hossain, Husain, Husani, Husayn, Husian, Hussan, Hussayn, Hussin

Hussein (Arabic) little; handsome.
Hossein, Houssein, Houssin, Huissien, Huossein, Husein, Husien

Huston (English) a form of Houston.
Hustin

Hutchinson (English) son of the hutch dweller.
Hutcheson

Hute (Native American) star.

Hutton (English) house on the jutting ledge.
Hut, Hutan, Huten, Hutin, Huton, Hutt, Huttan, Hutten, Huttin, Huttun, Huttyn, Hutun, Hutyn

Huxley (English) Hugh's meadow.
Hux, Huxlea, Huxlee, Huxleigh, Huxli, Huxlie, Huxly, Lee

Huy (Vietnamese) glorious.

Hy (Vietnamese) hopeful. (English) a short form of Hyman.

Hyacinthe (French) hyacinth.

Hyatt (English) high gate.
Hiat, Hiatt, Hiatte, Hyat, Hyatte

Hyde (English) cache; measure of land equal to 120 acres; animal hide.

Hyder (English) tanner, preparer of animal hides for tanning.

Hyman (English) a form of Chaim.
Haim, Hayim, Hayvim, Hayyim, Hy, Hyam, Hymie

Hyrum (Hebrew) a form of Hiram.
Hyram

Hyun-Ki (Korean) wise.

Hyun-Shik (Korean) clever.

I

'Imâd, 'Imad Al-Dîn (Arabic) support; pillar.

'Isà-Eisà (Arabic) a form of Jesus.

'Issâm (Arabic) shelter.

Iadón (Hebrew) thankful.

Iago (Spanish, Welsh) a form of Jacob, James. Literature: the villain in Shakespeare's *Othello*.
Jago

Iain (Scottish) a form of Ian.

Iajín (Hebrew) God establishes.

Iakobos (Greek) a form of Jacob.
Iakov, Iakovos, Iakovs

Iakona (Hawaiian) healer.
Iakonah

Ialeel (Hebrew) waiting for God.

Iamín (Hebrew) right hand.

Ian ☀ BG (Scottish) a form of John. See also Ean, Eian.
Iane, Iann, Iin, Ion

Ianos (Czech) a form of John.
Iannis

Iazeel (Hebrew) contributions of God.

Ib (Phoenician, Danish) oath of Baal.

Iban (Basque) a form of John.

Ibán (German) glorious.

Iber, Ibérico, Iberio, Ibero, Ibi (Latin) native of Iberia.

Ibon (Basque) a form of Ivor.

Ibrahim (Hausa) my father is exalted. (Arabic) a form of Abraham.
Ibrahaim, Ibraham, Ibraheem, Ibrahem, Ibrahiem, Ibrahiim, Ibrahmim

Ibrahîm (Arabic) a form of Ibrahim.

Ibsen (German) archer's son. Literature: Henrik Ibsen was a nineteenth-century Norwegian poet and playwright whose works influenced the development of modern drama.
Ibsan, Ibsin, Ibson, Ibsyn

Icabod (Hebrew) without glory.

Ícaro (Greek) image.

Iccauhtli (Nahuatl) younger brother.

Ichabod (Hebrew) glory is gone. Literature: Ichabod Crane is the main character of Washington Irving's story "The Legend of Sleepy Hollow."

Ichiro (Japanese) born first.

Ichtaca (Nahuatl) secret.

Icnoyotl (Nahuatl) friendship.

Iden (English) pasture in the wood.
Idan, Idin, Idon, Idun, Idyn

Idi (Swahili) born during the Idd festival.

Idogbe (Egyptian) brother of twins.

Idris (Welsh) eager lord. (Arabic) Religion: a Muslim prophet.
Idrease, Idrees, Idres, Idress, Idreus, Idriece, Idriss, Idrissa, Idriys, Idrys, Idryss

Idrîs (Arabic) a form of Idris.

Idumeo (Latin) red.

Iedidiá (Hebrew) loved by God.

Iejiel (Hebrew) God lives.

Iestyn (Welsh) a form of Justin.

Igashu (Native American) wanderer; seeker.
Igasho

Iggy (Latin) a familiar form of Ignatius.
Iggie

Ignacio (Italian) a form of Ignatius.
Ignazio

Ignado (Spanish) fiery or ardent.

Ignatius (Latin) fiery, ardent. Religion: Saint Ignatius of Loyola founded the Jesuit order. See also Inigo, Neci.
Ignaas, Ignac, Ignác, Ignace, Ignacey, Ignacius, Ignas, Ignatas, Ignatios, Ignatious, Ignatus, Ignatys, Ignatz, Ignaz

Igor (Russian) a form of Inger, Ingvar. See also Egor, Yegor.
Igoryok

Iham (Indian) expected.

Ihit (Indian) prize; honor.

Ihsan (Turkish) compassionate.

Ihsân (Turkish) a form of Ihsan.

Ihuicatl (Nahuatl) sky.

Ike (Hebrew) a familiar form of Isaac. History: the nickname of the thirty-fourth U.S. president Dwight D. Eisenhower.
Ikee, Ikey, Ikke

Iker (Basque) visitation.

Ilan (Hebrew) tree. (Basque) youth.

Ilari (Basque) a form of Hilary.
Ilario, Ilaryo

Ilbert (German) distinguished fighter.
Ilbirt, Ilburt, Ilbyrt

Ildefonso (German) totally prepared for combat.

Ilhicamina (Nahuatl) he shoots arrows at the sky.

Ilhuitl (Nahuatl) day.

Ilias (Greek) a form of Elijah.
Illias

Ilidio (Latin) troop.

Illan (Basque, Latin) youth.

Illayuc (Quechua) luminous.

Ilom (Ibo) my enemies are many.

Iluminado (Latin) he who receives the inspiration of God.

Ilya (Russian) a form of Elijah.
Ilia, Ilie, Ilija, Iliya, Ilja, Illia, Illya, Ilyah

Ilyas (Greek) a form of Elijah.
Illyas, Ilyes

Imad (Arabic) supportive; mainstay.

Iman GB (Hebrew) a short form of Immanuel.

Imani GB (Hebrew) a short form of Immanuel.
Imanni

Imaran (Indian) strong.

Imbert (German) poet.
Imbirt, Imburt, Imbyrt

Immanuel (Hebrew) a form of Emmanuel.
Imanol, Imanual, Imanuel, Imanuele, Immanual, Immanuele, Immuneal

Imran (Arabic) host.
Imraan, Imren, Imrin, Imryn

Imre (Hungarian) a form of Emery.
Imri

Imrich (Czech) a form of Emery.
Imric, Imrick, Imrie, Imrus

Imtiaz (Indian) power of discrimination.

Inalef (Mapuche) the swift reinforcement.

Inay (Hindi) god; godlike.

Inca (Quechua) prince.

Incaurco, Incaurcu (Quechua) hill; Inca god.

Ince (Hungarian) innocent.

Incencio (Spanish) white.

Incendio (Spanish) fire.

Indalecio (Arabic) the same as the master.

Inder (Hindi) god; godlike.
Inderbir, Inderdeep, Inderjeet, Inderjit, Inderpal, Inderpreet, Inderveer, Indervir, Indra, Indrajit

Indiana BG (Hindi) from India.
Indi, Indy

Indíbil (Spanish) he who is very black.

Indivar (Indian) blue lotus.

Indrajeet (Indian) conqueror.

Indrakanta (Indian) another name for the Hindu god Indra.

Indraneel (Indian) sapphire.

Indro (Spanish) the victor.

Indubhushan (Indian) the moon

Induhasan, Indukanta, Indushekhar (Indian) like a moon.

Indulal (Indian) moon's luster.

Inek (Welsh) a form of Irvin.

Inés (Greek) pure.

Ing (Scandinavian) a short form of Ingmar.
Inge

Ingelbert (German) a form of Engelbert.
Ingelberte, Ingelbirt, Ingelburt, Ingelburte, Ingelbyrt, Inglebert, Ingleberte

Inger (Scandinavian) son's army.
Ingar

Inglis (Scottish) English.
Ingliss, Inglys, Inglyss

Ingmar (Scandinavian) famous son.
Ingamar, Ingamur, Ingemar

Ingram (English) angel.
Ingra, Ingraham, Ingrem, Ingrim, Ingrym

Ingvar (Scandinavian) Ing's soldier.
Ingevar

Ini-Herit (Egyptian) he who returns from far away.

Inigo (Basque) a form of Ignatius.
Iñaki, Iniego, Iñigo

Íñigo (Basque) a form of Inigo.

Iniko (Ibo) born during bad times.

Inir (Welsh) honorable.
Inyr

Innis (Irish) island.
Inis, Iniss, Innes, Inness, Inniss, Innys, Innyss

Innocenzio (Italian) innocent.
Innocenty, Innocentz, Innocenz, Innocenzyo, Inocenci, Inocencio, Inocente, Inocenzio, Inocenzyo, Inosente

Intekhab (Indian) chosen.

Inteus (Native American) proud; unashamed.

Inti (Aymara) he who is bold.

Intiauqui (Quechua) sun prince.

Intichurin (Quechua) child of the sun.

Intiguaman (Quechua) sun falcon.

Intiyafa (Quechua) ray of sunlight.

Ioakim (Russian) a form of Joachim.
Ioachime, Ioakimo, Iov

Ioan (Greek, Bulgarian, Romanian) a form of John.
Ioane, Ioann, Ioannikios, Ionel

Ioannis (Greek, Bulgarian, Romanian) a form of Ioan.
Ioannes

Iojanán (Hebrew) God is merciful.

Iokepa (Hawaiian) a form of Joseph.
Keo

Iokia (Hawaiian) healed by God.
Iokiah, Iokya, Iokyah

Iolo (Welsh) the Lord is worthy.
Iorwerth

Ionakana (Hawaiian) a form of Jonathan.

Iorgos (Greek) a form of George.

Iosef (Hebrew) a form of Iosif.

Iosif (Greek, Russian) a form of Joseph.

Iosua (Romanian) a form of Joshua.

Ipyana (Nyakyusa) graceful.
Ipyanah

Iqbal (Indian) desire.

Ira BG (Hebrew) watchful.
Irah

Iram (English) bright.

Ireneo, Irineo (Greek) the lover of peace.

Irfan (Arabic) thankfulness.

Irmin (German) strong.
Irman, Irmen, Irmun, Irmyn

Irshaad (Indian) signal.

Irumba (Rutooro) born after twins.

Irv (Irish, Welsh, English) a short form of Irvin, Irving.

Irvin (Irish, Welsh, English) a short form of Irving. See also Ervine.
Irven, Irvine, Irvinn, Irvon, Irvyn, Irvyne

Irving (Irish) handsome. (Welsh) white river. (English) sea friend. See also Ervin, Ervine.
Irvington, Irvyng

Irwin (English) a form of Irving. See also Ervin.
Irwing, Irwinn, Irwyn

Isa BG (Hebrew) a form of Isaiah. (Arabic) a form of Jesus.
Isaah, Isah

Isaac ☆ (Hebrew) he will laugh. Bible: the son of Abraham and Sarah. See also Itzak, Izak, Yitzchak.
Aizik, Icek, Ikey, Ikie, Isaack, Isaakios, Isacco, Isaic, Ishaq, Isiac, Isiacc, Issca

Isaak (Hebrew) a form of Isaac.
Isack, Isak, Isik, Issak

Isac, Isacc, Issac (Hebrew) forms of Isaac.
Issacc, Issaic, Issiac

Isacar (Hebrew) he was given for a favor.

Isacio (Greek) equality.

Isadoro (Spanish) gift of Isis.

Isai, Isaih (Hebrew) forms of Isaiah.

Isaiah ☆ (Hebrew) God is my salvation. Bible: a Hebrew prophet.
Essaiah, Isaia, Isaid, Isaish, Isaya, Isayah, Isia, Isiash, Issia, Izaiah, Izaiha, Izaya, Izayah, Izayaih, Izayiah, Izeyah, Izeyha

Isaias (Hebrew) a form of Isaiah.
Isaiahs, Isais, Izayus

Isaías (Hebrew) a form of Isaias.

Isam (Arabic) safeguard.

Isamu (Japanese) courageous.

Isar (Indian) eminent; another name for the Hindu god Shiva.

Isarno (Germanic) eagle of iron.

Isas (Japanese) meritorious.

Iscay (Quechua) second child.

Iscaycuari (Quechua) doubly savage and untamable.

Isekemu (Native American) slow-moving creek.

Isham (English) home of the iron one.

Ishan (Hindi) direction.
Ishaan, Ishaun

Ishaq (Arabic) a form of Isaac.
Ishaac, Ishak

Ishâq (Arabic) a form of Ishaq.

Ishboshet (Hebrew) man of shame.

Ishmael (Hebrew) God will hear. Literature: the narrator of Herman Melville's novel *Moby-Dick*.
Isamael, Isamail, Ishma, Ishmail, Ishmale, Ishmeal, Ishmeil, Ishmel, Ishmil

Ishmerai (Hebrew) God takes care.

Ishrat (Indian) affection.

Ishwar (Indian) God.

Isiah, Issiah (Hebrew) forms of Isaiah.
Issaiah, Issia

Isidore (Greek) gift of Isis. See also Dorian, Esidore, Ysidro.
Isador, Isadore, Isadorios, Isidor, Issy, Ixidor, Izador, Izadore, Izidor, Izidore, Izydor

Isidoro (Greek) a form of Isidore.
Isidoros

Isidro (Greek) a form of Isidore.

Iskander (Afghan) a form of Alexander.

Iskinder (Ethiopian) a form of Alexander.

Islam (Arabic) submission; the religion of Muhammad.

Isma'il (Arabic) a form of Ismael.

Ismael, Ismail (Arabic) forms of Ishmael.
Ismal, Ismale, Ismeil, Ismiel

Isocrates (Greek) he who can do as much as the next man.

Isócrates (Greek) one who shares power with the same legal authority.

Isod (Hebrew) God fights and prevails.

Isra'îl (Arabic) a form of Israel.

Israel (Hebrew) prince of God; wrestled with God. History: the nation of Israel took its name from the name given Jacob after he wrestled with the angel of the Lord. See also Yisrael.
Iser, Israele, Israhel, Isrell, Isrrael, Isser, Izrael

Isreal (Hebrew) a form of Israel.
Isrieal

Issa (Swahili) God is our salvation.
Issah

Issmat (Lebanese) infallible.

Istu (Native American) sugar pine.

István (Hungarian) a form of Stephen.
Isti, Istvan, Pista

Itaete (Guarani) blade.

Italo (Latin) he came from the land that is between the seas.

Ithamat (Hebrew) a form of Ittamar.

Ithel (Welsh) generous lord.
Ithell

Itotia (Nahuatl) dance.

Ittamar (Hebrew) island of palms.
Itamar

Ittmar (Hebrew) a form of Ittamar.

Itzak (Hebrew) a form of Isaac, Yitzchak.
Itzik

Itzjac (Hebrew) reason for joy.

Itztli (Nahuatl) obsidian knife.

Iuitl (Nahuatl) feather.

Iukini (Hawaiian) a form of Eugene.
Kini

Iustin (Bulgarian, Russian) a form of Justin.

Ivan, Ivann (Russian) forms of John. See also Vanya.
Iván, Ivano, Ivas, Iven, Ivin, Ivon, Ivun, Ivyn, Yvan, Yvann

Ivana (Catalan) a form of Ivo.

Ivanhoe (Hebrew) God's tiller. Literature: *Ivanhoe* is a historical romance by Sir Walter Scott.
Ivanho, Ivanhow

Ivar (Scandinavian) a form of Ivor. See also Yves, Yvon.
Iv, Iva, Iver

Ives (English) young archer.
Ive, Iven, Ivey, Yves

Ivo (German) yew wood; bow wood.
Ivon, Ivonnie, Yvo

Ivor (Scandinavian) a form of Ivo.
Ibon, Ifor, Ivar, Ivry, Yvor

Ivory GB (Latin) made of ivory.
Ivoree, Ivorey, Ivori, Ivorie

Ivy GB (English) ivy tree.
Ivi, Ivie, Ivye

Iwan (Polish) a form of John.

Ixtli (Nahuatl) face.

Iyafa, Iyapa (Quechua) lightning.

Iyapo (Yoruba) many trials; many obstacles.

Iyapoma, Iyapuma, Iyaticsi (Quechua) puma of light.

Iyapu (Quechua) lightning.

Iyatecsi (Quechua) eternal light.

Iye (Native American) smoke.

Izaac (Czech) a form of Izak.
Izaack, Izaak

Izak (Czech) a form of Isaac.
Itzhak, Ixaka, Izac, Izaic, Izec, Izeke, Izick, Izik, Izsak, Izsák, Izzak

Izar (Basque) star.

Izhar (Indian) submission.

Izod (Irish) light haired.
Izad, Ized, Izid, Izud, Izyd

Izzy (Hebrew) a familiar form of Isaac, Isidore, Israel.
Isi, Isie, Issi, Issie, Issy, Izi, Izie, Izy, Izzi, Izzie

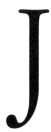

J (American) an initial used as a first name.

J. (American) a form of J.

J'quan (American) a form of Jaquan.

Ja BG (Korean) attractive, magnetic.

Ja'far (Sanskrit) little stream.
Jafari, Jaffar, Jaffer, Jafur

Ja'juan (American) a form of Jajuan.

Ja'marcus (American) a form of Jamarcus.

Ja'quan (American) a form of Jaquan.

Ja'von (American) a form of Javan.

Jaali (Swahili) powerful.
Jali

Jaan (Estonian) a form of Christian. (Dutch, Slavic) a form of Jan.

Jaap (Dutch) a form of Jim.
Jape

Jabari (Swahili) fearless, brave.
Jabahri, Jabarae, Jabare, Jabaree, Jabarei, Jabarie, Jabarri, Jabarrie, Jabary, Jabbaree, Jabbari, Jabiari, Jabier, Jabori, Jaborie

Jabbar (Arabic) fixer.
Jabaar, Jabar, Jaber

Jabel (Hebrew) like the arrow that flies.

Jâber (Arabic) comforter.

Jabez (Hebrew) born in pain.
Jabe, Jabes, Jabesh

Jabin (Hebrew) God has created.
Jabain, Jabien, Jabon, Jabyn

Jabín (Hebrew) a form of Jabin.

Jabir (Arabic) consoler, comforter.
Jabiri, Jabori, Jabyr

Jabril (Arabic) a form of Jibril.
Jabrail, Jabree, Jabreel, Jabrel, Jabrell, Jabrelle, Jabri, Jabrial, Jabrie, Jabriel, Jabrielle, Jabrille

Jabulani (Shona) happy.

Jacan (Hebrew) trouble.
Jachin

Jacari (American) a form of Jacorey.
Jacarey, Jacaris, Jacarius, Jacarre, Jacarri, Jacarrus, Jacarus, Jacary, Jacaure, Jacauri, Jaccar, Jaccari

Jaccob (Hebrew) a form of Jacob.

Jace (American) a combination of the initials J. + C. See also Jayce.
J.C., Jacee, Jaci, Jacie, Jaece, Jaecee, Jaecey, Jaeci, Jaice, Jaicee, Jaicey, Jaici, Jaicie, Jaicy, JC

Jacek (American) a form of Jace.

Jacen (Greek) a form of Jason.
Jaceon, Jacin, Jacon, Jacyn

Jacey GB (American) a form of Jace.

Jacinto (Portuguese, Spanish) hyacinth. See also Giacinto.
Jacindo, Jacint, Jacinta, Jacynto

Jack ☀ (American) a familiar form of Jacob, John. See also Keaka.
Jaac, Jaack, Jaak, Jac, Jacke, Jacko, Jackub, Jak, Jakk, Jax

Jackie BG (American) a familiar form of Jack.
Jackey, Jacki

Jackson ☀ BG (English) son of Jack.
Jacksen, Jacksin, Jacson, Jakson

Jacky (American) a familiar form of Jack.

Jaco (Portuguese) a form of Jacob.

Jacob ☀ BG (Hebrew) supplanter, substitute. Bible: son of Isaac, brother of Esau. See also Akiva, Chago, Checha, Cobi, Diego, Giacomo, Hamish, Iago, Iakobos, Kiva, Kobi, Kuba, Tiago, Yakov, Yasha, Yoakim.
Jachob, Jaco, Jacobb, Jacub, Jaecob, Jaicob, Jalu, Jecis, Jeks, Jeska, Jocek, Jock, Jocob, Jocobb, Jokubas

Jacobe, Jacoby (Hebrew) forms of Jacob.
Jachobi, Jacobbe, Jacobee, Jacobey, Jacobie, Jacobii, Jacobis, Jocoby

Jacoberto (Germanic) famous.

Jacobi BG (Hebrew) a form of Jacob.

Jacobo (Hebrew) a form of Jacob.
Jacobos

Jacobson (English) son of Jacob.
Jacobs, Jacobsen, Jacobsin, Jacobus

Jacolby (Hebrew) a form of Jacob.
Jacolbi, Jocolby

Jacorey (American) a combination of Jacob + Corey.
Jacori, Jacoria, Jacorie, Jacoris, Jacorius, Jacorrey, Jacorrien, Jacorry, Jacouri, Jacourie

Jacory (American) a form of Jacorey.

Jacquan (French) a form of Jacques.

Jacque (French) a form of Jacob.
Jackque, Jacquay, Jacqui

Jacquel (French) a form of Jacques.

Jacques (French) a form of Jacob, James. See also Coco.
Jackques, Jackquise, Jacot, Jacquees, Jacquese, Jacquess, Jacquet, Jacquett, Jacquis, Jacquise, Jarques, Jarquis

Jacquez, Jaquez (French) forms of Jacques.
Jaques, Jaquese, Jaqueus, Jaqueze, Jaquis, Jaquise, Jaquze

Jacy GB (Tupi-Guarani) moon. (American) a form of Jace.
Jaicy, Jaycee

Jad (Hebrew) a short form of Jadon. (American) a short form of Jadrien.
Jada, Jadd

Jadarius (American) a combination of the prefix Ja + Darius.

Jade GB (Spanish) jade, precious stone.
Jaed, Jaeid, Jaid, Jaide, Jayd

Jaden ☀ BG (Hebrew) a form of Jadon.
Jadee, Jadeen, Jadenn, Jadeon, Jadyne

Jadon (Hebrew) God has heard.
Jadan, Jadin, Jaiden

Jadrien (American) a combination of Jay + Adrien.
Jader, Jadrian, Jadryen, Jaedrian, Jaedrien, Jaidrian, Jaidrien, Jaidrion, Jaidryon, Jaydrian, Jaydrien, Jaydrion, Jaydryan

Jadyn GB (Hebrew) a form of Jadon.

Jae BG (French, English) a form of Jay.

Jae-Hwa (Korean) rich, prosperous.

Jaeden, Jaedon (Hebrew) forms of Jadon.
Jaedan, Jaedin, Jaedyn

Jaegar (German) hunter.
Jaager, Jaeger, Jagur, Jaigar, Jaygar

Jael GB (Hebrew) mountain goat.
Jayl, Yael

Jaelen, Jaelin, Jaelon (American) forms of Jalen.
Jaelan, Jaelaun, Jaelyn

Jafar (Sanskrit) a form of Ja'far.

Jafet (Hebrew) enlargement.

Jag, Jagat (Indian) the universe.

Jagadbandu (Indian) another name for the Hindu god Krishna.

Jagadish (Indian) lord of the universe.

Jaganmay (Indian) spread over the universe.

Jagannath (Indian) another name for the Hindu god Vishnu.

Jagdeep (Sikh) the lamp of the world.

Jagger (English) carter.
Gagger, Jagar, Jager, Jaggar

Jagjeevan (Indian) worldly life.

Jagmeet (Sikh) friend of the world.

Jago (English) a form of Jacob, James.
Jaego, Jaigo, Jaygo

Jaguar (Spanish) jaguar.
Jagguar

Jahan (Indian) the world.

Jahi (Swahili) dignified.

Jahleel (Hindi) a form of Jalil.
Jahlal, Jahlee, Jahliel

Jahlil (Hindi) a form of Jalil.

Jahmal (Arabic) a form of Jamal.
Jahmall, Jahmalle, Jahmeal, Jahmeel, Jahmeil, Jahmel, Jahmelle, Jahmil, Jahmile, Jahmill, Jahmille

Jahmar (American) a form of Jamar.
Jahmare, Jahmari, Jahmarr, Jahmer

Jahvon (Hebrew) a form of Javan.
Jahvan, Jahvaughn, Jahvine, Jahwaan, Jahwon

Jai BG (Tai) heart.
Jaie, Jaii

Jaichand (Indian) victory of the moon.

Jaidayal (Indian) victory of kindness.

Jaiden BG (Hebrew) a form of Jadon.
Jaidan, Jaidin, Jaidon, Jaidyn

Jaidev (Indian) victory of God.

Jaigopal, Jaikrishna (Indian) victory of the Hindu god Krishna.

Jailen (American) a form of Jalen.
Jailan, Jailani, Jaileen, Jailen, Jailon, Jailyn, Jailynn

Jaime BG (Spanish) a form of Jacob, James.
Jaimee, Jaimey, Jaimie, Jaimito, Jaimy

Jaimini (Indian) an ancient Hindu philosopher.

Jainarayan, Jaiwant (Indian) victory.

Jaipal (Indian) another name for the Hindu god Brahma.

Jaiquan (American) a form of Jaquan.
Jaiqaun

Jair (Spanish) a form of Jairo.

Jaír (Spanish) a form of Jair.

Jairaj (Indian) lord of victory.

Jairo (Spanish) God enlightens.
Jairay, Jaire, Jayrus

Jairus (American) a form of Jairo.

Jaisal (Indian) famous folk.

Jaison (Greek) a form of Jason.
Jaisan, Jaisen, Jaishon, Jaishun, Jaisin, Jaisun, Jaisyn

Jaisukh (Indian) joy of winning.

Jaivon (Hebrew) a form of Javan.
Jaiven, Jaivion, Jaiwon

Jaja (Ibo) honored.
Jajah

Jajuan (American) a combination of the prefix Ja + Juan.
Ja Juan, Jaejuan, Jaijuan, Jauan, Jayjuan, Jejuan

Jakari (American) a form of Jacorey.
Jakaire, Jakar, Jakaray, Jakarie, Jakarious, Jakarius, Jakarre, Jakarri, Jakarus

Jake ☀ (Hebrew) a short form of Jacob.
Jaik, Jakie, Jayck, Jayk, Jayke

Jakeb, Jakeob, Jakob, Jakub (Hebrew) forms of Jacob.
Jaekob, Jaikab, Jaikob, Jakab, Jakeub, Jakib, Jakiv, Jakobe, Jakobi, Jakobus, Jakoby, Jakov, Jakovian, Jakubek, Jekebs

Jakeem (Arabic) uplifted.
Jakeam, Jakim, Jakym

Jakome (Basque) a form of James.
Jakom

Jal (Gypsy) wanderer.
Jall

Jalâl (Arabic) glorious.

Jalan, Jalin, Jalon (American) forms of Jalen.
Jalaan, Jalaen, Jalain, Jaland, Jalane, Jalani, Jalanie, Jalann, Jalaun, Jalean, Jalian, Jaline, Jallan, Jalone, Jaloni, Jalun, Jalynn, Jalynne

Jaleel (Hindi) a form of Jalil.
Jaleell, Jaleil, Jalel

Jaleen (American) a form of Jalen.

Jalen BG (American) a combination of the prefix Ja + Len.
Jalend, Jallen

Jalendu (Indian) moon in the water.

Jalene BG (American) a form of Jalen.

Jalil (Hindi) revered.
Jalaal, Jalal

Jalisat (Arabic) he who receives little, gives more.

Jalyn GB (American) a form of Jalen.

Jam (American) a short form of Jamal, Jamar.
Jama

Jamaal, Jamahl, Jamall, Jamaul (Arabic) forms of Jamal.
Jammaal

Jamaine (Arabic) a form of Germain.
Jamain, Jamayn, Jamayne

Jamal (Arabic) handsome. See also Gamal.
Jaimal, Jamael, Jamail, Jamaile, Jamala, Jamarl, Jammal, Jamual, Jaumal, Jomal, Jomall

Jamâl (Arabic) a form of Jamal.

Jamale (Arabic) a form of Jamal.
Jamalle

Jamar (American) a form of Jamal.
Jamaar, Jamaari, Jamaarie, Jamahrae, Jamair, Jamara, Jamaras, Jamaraus, Jamarr, Jamarre, Jamarrea, Jamarree, Jamarri, Jamarvis, Jamaur, Jammar, Jarmar, Jarmarr, Jaumar, Jemaar, Jemar, Jimar

Jamarcus (American) a combination of the prefix Ja + Marcus.
Jamarco, Jemarcus, Jimarcus, Jymarcus

Jamare (American) a form of Jamario.
Jamareh

Jamaree, Jamari (American) forms of Jamario.
Jamarea, Jamaria, Jamarie

Jamario (American) a combination of the prefix Ja + Mario.
Jamareo, Jamariel, Jamariya, Jamaryo, Jemario

Jamarious, Jamarius (American) forms of Jamario.

Jamaris (American) a form of Jamario.
Jemarus

Jamarkus (American) a combination of the prefix Ja + Markus.
Jamark

Jamarquis (American) a combination of the prefix Ja + Marquis.
Jamarkees, Jamarkeus, Jamarkis, Jamarqese, Jamarqueis, Jamarques, Jamarquez, Jamarquios, Jamarqus

Jameel (Arabic) a form of Jamal.
Jameal, Jamele, Jamyl, Jamyle, Jarmil

Jamel, Jamell (Arabic) forms of Jamal.
Jamelle, Jammel, Jamuel, Jamul, Jarmel, Jaumell, Je-Mell, Jimell

Jamen, Jamon (Hebrew) forms of Jamin.
Jaemon, Jaimon, Jamohn, Jamone, Jamoni

James ⭐ BG (Hebrew) supplanter, substitute. (English) a form of Jacob. Bible: James the Great and James the Less were two of the Twelve Apostles. See also Diego, Hamish, Iago, Kimo, Santiago, Seamus, Seumas, Yago, Yasha.
Jaemes, Jaimes, Jamesie, Jamesy, Jamies, Jamse, Jamyes, Jemes

Jameson (English) son of James.
Jaemeson, Jaimeson, Jamerson, Jamesian, Jamesyn, Jaymeson

Jamey GB (English) a familiar form of James.
Jaeme, Jaemee, Jaemey, Jaemi, Jaemie, Jaemy, Jaimee, Jaimey, Jaimie, Jame, Jamee, Jameyel, Jami, Jamia, Jamiah, Jamian, Jamiee, Jamme, Jammey, Jammie, Jammy, Jamy, Jamye

Jamez (Hebrew) a form of James.
Jameze, Jamze

Jamie GB (English) a familiar form of James.

Jamieson (English) a form of Jamison.
Jamiesen

Jamil (Arabic) a form of Jamal.
Jamiel, Jamiell, Jamielle, Jamile, Jamill, Jamille

Jamin (Hebrew) favored.
Jaman, Jamian, Jamien, Jamion, Jamionn, Jamun, Jamyn, Jarmin, Jarmon, Jaymin, Jaymon

Jamir (American) a form of Jamar.
Jamire, Jamiree

Jamison BG (English) son of James.
Jaemison, Jaemyson, Jaimison, Jaimyson, Jamis, Jamisen, Jamyson, Jaymison, Jaymyson

Jamond (American) a combination of James + Raymond.
Jaemond, Jaemund, Jaimond, Jaimund, Jamod, Jamont, Jamonta, Jamontae, Jamontay, Jamonte, Jamund, Jarmond, Jarmund, Jaymond, Jaymund

Jamor (American) a form of Jamal.
Jamoree, Jamori, Jamorie, Jamorius, Jamorrio, Jamorris, Jamory, Jamour

Jamsheed (Persian) from Persia.
Jamshaid, Jamshead, Jamshed

Jan BG (Dutch, Slavic) a form of John.
Jahn, Jana, Janae, Jann, Jano, Jenda, Jhan, Yan

Janco (Czech) a form of John.
Jancsi, Janke, Janko

Jando (Spanish) a form of Alexander.
Jandino

Janeil (American) a combination of the prefix Ja + Neil.
Janal, Janel, Janell, Janelle, Janiel, Janielle, Janile, Janille, Jarnail, Jarneil, Jarnell

Janek (Polish) a form of John.
Janak, Janik, Janika, Janka, Jankiel, Janko, Jhanick

Janina (Hebrew) grace.

Janis GB (Latvian) a form of John. See also Zanis.
Ansis, Jancis, Janyc, Janyce, Janys

Janne (Finnish) a form of John.
Jann, Jannes

János (Hungarian) a form of John.
Jancsi, Jani, Jankia, Jano

Jansen (Scandinavian) a form of Janson.
Janssen

Janson (Scandinavian) son of Jan.
Jansan, Janse, Jansin, Janssan, Janssin, Jansson, Jansun, Jansyn

Jantzen (Scandinavian) a form of Janson.
Janten, Jantsen, Jantson, Janzen

Janus (Latin) gate, passageway; born in January. Mythology: the Roman god of beginnings and endings.
Jannese, Jannus, Januario, Janusz

Janvier (French) a form of Jenaro.

Japa (Indian) chanting.

Japendra, Japesh (Indian) lord of chants; other names for the Hindu god Shiva.

Japheth (Hebrew) handsome. (Arabic) abundant. Bible: a son of Noah. See also Yaphet.
Japeth, Japhet

Jaquan (American) a combination of the prefix Ja + Quan.
Jacquin, Jacquyn, Jaequan, Jaqaun, Jaquaan, Jaquain, Jaquane, Jaquann, Jaquanne, Jaquin, Jaquyn

Jaquarius (American) a combination of Jaquan + Darius.
Jaquari, Jaquarious, Jaquaris

Jaquavious, Jaquavius (American) forms of Jaquavis.
Jaquaveis, Jaquaveius, Jaquaveon, Jaquaveous, Jaquavias

Jaquavis (American) a form of Jaquan.
Jaquavas, Jaquavus

Jaquawn, Jaquon (American) forms of Jaquan.
Jaequon, Jaqawan, Jaqoun, Jaquinn, Jaqune, Jaquoin, Jaquone, Jaqwan, Jaqwon

Jarad, Jarid, Jarod, Jarrad, Jarred, Jarrid, Jarrod, Jarryd, Jaryd (Hebrew) forms of Jared.
Jaraad, Jarodd, Jaroid, Jarrayd

Jarah (Hebrew) sweet as honey.
Jara, Jarra, Jarrah, Jera, Jerah, Jerra, Jerrah

Jaran, Jaren, Jarin, Jarren, Jarron, Jaryn (Hebrew) forms of Jaron.
Jarian, Jarien, Jarion, Jarrain, Jarran, Jarrian, Jarrin, Jarryn, Jarynn, Jaryon

Jardan (French) garden. (Hebrew) a form of Jordan.
Jarden, Jardin, Jardon, Jardyn, Jardyne

Jareb (Hebrew) contending.
Jarib, Jaryb

Jared (Hebrew) a form of Jordan.
Ja'red, Jahred, Jaired, Jaraed, Jaredd, Jareid, Jerred

Jarek (Slavic) born in January.
Januarius, Januisz, Jarec, Jareck, Jaric, Jarick, Jarik, Jarrek, Jarric, Jarrick, Jaryc, Jaryck, Jaryk

Jarel, Jarell (Scandinavian) forms of Gerald.
Jaerel, Jaerell, Jaeril, Jaerill, Jaeryl, Jaeryll, Jairel, Jairell, Jarael, Jareil, Jarelle, Jariel, Jarryl, Jarryll, Jayryl, Jayryll, Jharell

Jaret, Jarett, Jarret (English) forms of Jarrett.

Jareth (American) a combination of Jared + Gareth.
Jaref, Jareff, Jarif, Jariff, Jarith, Jaryf, Jaryff, Jaryth, Jereth

Jarius, Jarrius (American) forms of Jairo.

Jarl (Scandinavian) earl, nobleman.
Jarlee, Jarleigh, Jarley, Jarli, Jarlie, Jarly

Jarlath (Latin) in control.
Jarlaf, Jarlen

Jarmal (Arabic) a form of Jamal.

Jarman (German) from Germany.
Jarmen, Jarmin, Jarmon, Jarmyn, Jerman, Jermen, Jermin, Jermon, Jermyn

Jarmarcus (American) a form of Jamarcus.

Jarom (Latin) a form of Jerome.
Jarome, Jarrom, Jarrome

Jaron (Hebrew) he will sing; he will cry out.
J'ron, Jaaron, Jaeron, Jairon, Jarone, Jayron, Jayrone, Jayronn, Je Ronn

Jaroslav (Czech) glory of spring.

Jarrell (English) a form of Gerald.
Jarrel, Jerall, Jerrell

Jarreth (American) a form of Jareth.
Jarref, Jarreff, Jarrif, Jarriff, Jarrith, Jarryf, Jarryff, Jarryth

Jarrett (English) a form of Garrett, Jared.
Jairet, Jairett, Jarat, Jarette, Jarhett, Jarit, Jarrat, Jarratt, Jarrette, Jarrit, Jarritt, Jarrot, Jarrote, Jarrott, Jarrotte, Jaryt, Jarytt

Jarvis (German) skilled with a spear.
Jaravis, Jarv, Jarvaris, Jarvas, Jarvaska, Jarvey, Jarvez, Jarvice, Jarvie, Jarvios, Jarvious, Jarvise, Jarvius, Jarvorice, Jarvoris, Jarvous, Jarvus, Jarvyc, Jarvyce, Jarvys, Jarvyse, Jervey

Jas BG (English) a familiar form of James. (Polish) a form of John.
Jasio

Jasbeer (Indian) victorious hero.

Jasdeep (Sikh) the lamp radiating God's glories.

Jase (Greek) a short form of Jason.

Jasen, Jasson (Greek) forms of Jason.
Jassen, Jassin, Jassyn

Jasha (Russian) a familiar form of Jacob, James.
Jascha

Jashawn (American) a combination of the prefix Ja + Shawn.
Jasean, Jashan, Jashaun, Jashion, Jashon

Jashua (Hebrew) a form of Joshua.

Jaskaran (Sikh) sings praises to the Lord.
Jaskaren, Jaskiran

Jaskarn (Sikh) a form of Jaskaran.

Jasmeet **BG** (Sikh) friend of the Lord.
(Persian) a form of Jasmin.

Jasmin **GB** (Persian) jasmine flower.
Jasman, Jasmanie, Jasmine, Jasmon, Jasmond

Jason ✻ (Greek) healer. Mythology: the
hero who led the Argonauts in search of
the Golden Fleece.
*Jaasan, Jaasen, Jaasin, Jaason, Jaasun, Jaasyn,
Jaesan, Jaesen, Jaesin, Jaeson, Jaesun, Jaesyn,
Jahsan, Jahsen, Jahson, Jasan, Jasaun, Jasin,
Jasten, Jasun, Jasyn*

Jasón (Greek) a form of Jason.

Jaspal (Punjabi) living a virtuous lifestyle.
Jaspel

Jasper **BG** (French) brown, red, or yellow
ornamental stone. (English) a form of
Casper. See also Kasper.
Jaspar, Jazper, Jespar, Jesper

Jaspreet **BG** (Punjabi) virtuous.

Jaswant (Indian) famous.

Jathan (Greek) a form of Jason.
Jathon

Jatinra (Hindi) great Brahmin sage.
Jatinrah

Jaume (Catalan) a form of Jaime.

Javan (Hebrew) Bible: son of Japheth.
Jaavan, Jaewan, Javyn, Jayvin, Jayvine

Javante (American) a form of Javan.
Javantae, Javantai, Javantée, Javanti

Javar (American) a form of Jarvis.

Javari (American) a form of Jarvis.
Javarri

Javarious, Javarius (American) forms of Javar.
*Javarias, Javarreis, Javarrious, Javorious, Javorius,
Javouris*

Javaris (English) a form of Javar.
*Javaor, Javaras, Javare, Javares, Javaries, Javario,
Javarios, Javaro, Javaron, Javarous, Javarre,
Javarris, Javarro, Javarros, Javarte, Javarus,
Javarys, Javoris*

Javas (Sanskrit) quick, swift.
Jayvas, Jayvis

Javaughn (American) a form of Javan.
Jahvaughan, JaVaughn

Javen, Javin (Hebrew) forms of Javan.
Jaevin, Javine

Javeon (American) a form of Javan.

Javian, Javion (American) forms of Javan.
Javien, Javionne

Javier (Spanish) owner of a new house. See
also Xavier.
Jabier, Javer, Javere, Javiar, Javyer

Javiero (Spanish) a form of Javier.

Javilá (Hebrew) strip of sand.

Javon **BG** (Hebrew) a form of Javan.
*Jaavon, Jaevon, Jaewon, Jahvon, Javaon,
Javohn, Javoni, Javonn, Javonni, Javonnie,
Javoun*

Javone (Hebrew) a form of Javan.
Javoney, Javonne

Javonta (American) a form of Javan.
Javona, Javonteh

Javontae, Javontay, Javonte, Javonté
(American) forms of Javan.
*Javonnte, Javontai, Javontaye, Javontee,
Javontey*

Jawad (Arabic) openhanded, generous.

Jawan, Jawaun, Jawon, Jawuan (American)
forms of Jajuan.
Jawaan, Jawann, Jawn

Jawara (African) peace and love.

Jawhar (Arabic) jewel; essence.

Jaxon, Jaxson (English) forms of Jackson.
Jaxen, Jaxsen, Jaxsun, Jaxun

Jay (French) blue jay. (English) a short form
of James, Jason.
Jai, Jave, Jeays, Jeyes

Jayanti (Hindi) sacred anniversary.

Jayce **BG** (American) a combination of the
initials J. + C. See also Jace.
*J.C., Jay Cee, Jayc, Jaycee, Jaycey, Jayci, Jaycie,
Jaycy, JC, Jecie*

Jaycob (Hebrew) a form of Jacob.
Jaycobb, Jaycub, Jaykob, Jaykobb

Jayde GB (American) a combination of the initials J. + D.
J.D., Jayd, Jaydee, JD

Jayden ★ BG (Hebrew) a form of Jadon. (American) a form of Jayde.

Jaydon BG (Hebrew) a form of Jadon.
Jaydan, Jaydin, Jaydn, Jaydyn

Jaye BG (French, English) a form of Jay.

Jaylan, Jayln, Jaylon (American) forms of Jaylen.
Jaylaan, Jayleon, Jaylian, Jayline, Jaylynn, Jaylynne

Jayland (American) a form of Jaylen.
Jaylend, Jaylund, Jaylynd

Jaylee GB (American) a combination of Jay + Lee.
Jaelea, Jaelee, Jaeleigh, Jaeley, Jaeli, Jaelie, Jaely, Jailea, Jailee, Jaileigh, Jailey, Jaili, Jailie, Jaily, Jayla, Jayle, Jaylea, Jayleigh, Jayley, Jayli, Jaylie, Jayly

Jaylen BG (American) a combination of Jay + Len. A form of Jaylee.
Jayleen, Jaylun

Jaylin BG (American) a form of Jaylen.

Jaylyn BG (American) a form of Jaylen.

Jayme GB (English) a form of Jamey.
Jaymee, Jaymey, Jaymi, Jaymie, Jaymy

Jaymes, Jaymz (English) forms of James.
Jaymis, Jayms

Jayquan (American) a combination of Jay + Quan.
Jaykwan, Jaykwon, Jayqon, Jayquawn, Jayqunn

Jayro (Spanish) a form of Jairo.

Jaysen, Jayson (Greek) forms of Jason.
Jaycent, Jaysan, Jaysin, Jaysn, Jayssen, Jaysson, Jaysun, Jaysyn

Jayshawn (American) a combination of Jay + Shawn. A form of Jaysen.
Jaysean, Jayshaun, Jayshon, Jayshun

Jayvon (American) a form of Javon.
Jayvion, Jayvohn, Jayvone, Jayvonn, Jayvontay, Jayvonte, Jaywan, Jaywaun, Jaywin

Jaz (American) a form of Jazz.

Jazael (Hebrew) perceives God.

Jazz BG (American) jazz.
Jaze, Jazze, Jazzlee, Jazzman, Jazzmen, Jazzmin, Jazzmon, Jazztin, Jazzton, Jazzy

Jean BG (French) a form of John.
Jéan, Jeane, Jeannah, Jeannie, Jeannot, Jeano, Jeanot, Jeanty, Jeen, Jene

Jean Benoit (French) a combination of Jean + Benoit.

Jean Christoph (French) a combination of Jean + Christoph.

Jean Daniel (French) a combination of Jean + Daniel.

Jean David (French) a combination of Jean + David.

Jean Denis (French) a combination of Jean + Denis.

Jean Felix (French) a combination of Jean + Felix.

Jean Francois, Jean-Francois (French) combinations of Jean + Francois.

Jean Gabriel (French) a combination of Jean + Gabriel.

Jean Luc, Jean-Luc, Jeanluc (French) combinations of Jean + Luc.

Jean Marc, Jean-Marc (French) combinations of Jean + Marc.

Jean Michel (French) a combination of Jean + Michel.

Jean Nicholas (French) a combination of Jean + Nicholas.

Jean Pascal (French) a combination of Jean + Pascal.

Jean Philip, Jean Philippe, Jean-Philippe (French) combinations of Jean + Philip.

Jean Samuel (French) a combination of Jean + Samuel.

Jean Sebastien (French) a combination of Jean + Sebastien.

Jean Simon (French) a combination of Jean +Simon.

Jean-Claude (French) a combination of Jean + Claude.

Jean-Paul, Jeanpaul (French) combinations of Jean + Paul.

Jean-Pierre, Jeanpierre (French) combinations of Jean + Pierre.

Jeb (Hebrew) a short form of Jebediah.
Jebb, Jebi, Jeby

Jebediah (Hebrew) a form of Jedidiah.
Jebadia, Jebadiah, Jebadieh, Jebidia, Jebidiah, Jebidya, Jebydia, Jebydiah, Jebydya, Jebydyah

Jed (Hebrew) a short form of Jedidiah. (Arabic) hand.
Jedd, Jeddy, Jedi

Jediah (Hebrew) hand of God.
Jadaya, Jedaia, Jedaiah, Jedayah, Jedeiah, Jedi, Yedaya

Jedidiah (Hebrew) friend of God, beloved of God. See also Didi.
Jedadiah, Jeddediah, Jededia, Jedidia, Jedidiyah, Yedidya

Jedrek (Polish) strong; manly.
Jedrec, Jedreck, Jedric, Jedrick, Jedrik, Jedryc, Jedryck, Jedryk

Jeff (English) a short form of Jefferson, Jeffrey. A familiar form of Geoffrey.
Jef, Jefe, Jeffe, Jeffey, Jeffie, Jeffy, Jeph, Jhef

Jefferey, Jeffery (English) forms of Jeffrey.
Jefaree, Jefarey, Jefari, Jefarie, Jefary, Jeferee, Jeferey, Jeferi, Jeferie, Jefery, Jeffaree, Jeffarey, Jeffari, Jeffarie, Jeffary, Jeffeory, Jefferay, Jefferee, Jeffereoy, Jefferi, Jefferie, Jefferies, Jeffory

Jefferson (English) son of Jeff. History: Thomas Jefferson was the third U.S. president.
Gefferson, Jeferson, Jeffers

Jefford (English) Jeff's ford.
Jeford

Jeffrey (English) divinely peaceful. See also Geffrey, Geoffrey, Godfrey.
Jeffre, Jeffree, Jeffri, Jeffrie, Jeffries, Jefre, Jefri, Jeoffroi, Joffre, Joffrey

Jeffry (English) a form of Jeffrey.
Jefry

Jehan (French) a form of John.
Jehann

Jehová (Hebrew) I am what I am.

Jehu (Hebrew) God lives. Bible: a military commander and king of Israel.
Yehu

Jela (Swahili) father that has suffered during birth.

Jelani BG (Swahili) mighty.
Jel, Jelan, Jelanee, Jelaney, Jelanie, Jelany, Jelaun

Jem GB (English) a short form of James, Jeremiah.
Jemi, Jemie, Jemmi, Jemmie, Jemmy, Jemy

Jemal (Arabic) a form of Jamal.
Jemaal, Jemael, Jemale

Jemel (Arabic) a form of Jamal.
Jemeal, Jemehl, Jemehyl, Jemell, Jemelle, Jemello, Jemeyle, Jemile

Jemond (French) worldly.
Jemon, Jémond, Jemonde, Jemone, Jemun, Jemund

Jenaro (Latin) born in January.

Jenkin (Flemish) little John.
Jenkins, Jenkyn, Jenkyns, Jennings

Jennifer GB (Welsh) white wave; white phantom. A form of Guinevere (see Girls' Names).

Jenö (Hungarian) a form of Eugene.
Jenoe

Jenofonte (Greek) he who comes from another country and is eloquent.

Jens (Danish) a form of John.
Jense, Jentz

Jensen GB (Scandinavian) a form of Janson.
Jensan, Jensin, Jenson, Jenssen, Jensyn

Jensi (Hungarian) born to nobility. (Danish) a familiar form of Jens.
Jenci, Jency, Jensee, Jensie, Jensy

Jeovanni (Italian) a form of Giovanni.
Jeovahny, Jeovan, Jeovani, Jeovanie, Jeovanny, Jeovany

Jequan (American) a combination of the prefix Je + Quan.
Jeqaun, Jequann, Jequon

Jerad, Jered, Jerid, Jerod, Jerrad, Jerred, Jerrid, Jerrod (Hebrew) forms of Jared.
Jeread, Jeredd, Jereed, Jerode, Jeroid, Jerryd, Jeryd

Jerahmy (Hebrew) a form of Jeremy.
Jerahmeel, Jerahmeil, Jerahmey

Jerald, Jerold, Jerrold (English) forms of Gerald.
Jeraldo, Jeroldo, Jerrald, Jerraldo, Jerroldo, Jerryld, Jeryld

Jerall (English) a form of Gerald.
Jerael, Jerai, Jerail, Jeraile, Jeral, Jerale, Jerall, Jerrail, Jerral, Jerrall

Jeramey, Jeramie, Jeramy (Hebrew) forms of Jeremy.
Jerame, Jeramee, Jerami, Jerammie

Jeramiah (Hebrew) a form of Jeremiah.

Jerard (French) a form of Gerard.
Jarard, Jarrard, Jeraude, Jerrard

Jerardo (Spanish) a form of Gerard.

Jere (Hebrew) a short form of Jeremiah, Jeremy.
Jeré, Jeree

Jerel, Jerell, Jerrell (English) forms of Gerald.
Jerelle, Jeriel, Jeril, Jerrail, Jerrel, Jerrelle, Jerrill, Jerrol, Jerroll, Jerryl, Jerryll, Jeryl, Jeryle

Jereme, Jeremey, Jeremi, Jeremie, Jérémie (English) forms of Jeremy.
Jarame, Jaremi, Jeremee, Jérémie, Jeremii

Jeremiah ☀ (Hebrew) God will uplift. Bible: a Hebrew prophet. See also Dermot, Yeremey, Yirmaya.
Geremiah, Jaramia, Jemeriah, Jemiah, Jeramiha, Jereias, Jeremaya, Jeremia, Jeremial, Jeremija, Jeremya, Jeremyah

Jeremias (Hebrew) a form of Jeremiah.
Jeremyas

Jeremías (Hebrew) a form of Jeremias.

Jeremiel (Hebrew) God lifts me up.

Jeremy (English) a form of Jeremiah.
Jaremay, Jaremy, Jere, Jereamy, Jeremry, Jérémy, Jeremye, Jereomy, Jeriemy, Jerime, Jerimy, Jerremy

Jeriah (Hebrew) Jehovah has seen.
Jeria, Jerya, Jeryah

Jeric, Jerick (Arabic) short forms of Jericho. (American) forms of Jerrick.
Jerric

Jericho (Arabic) city of the moon. Bible: a city conquered by Joshua.
Jericko, Jeriko, Jerricko, Jerricoh, Jerriko, Jerrycko, Jerryko

Jerico (Arabic) a short form of Jericho.
Jerrico, Jerryco

Jérico (Spanish) a form of Jericho.

Jerimiah (Hebrew) a form of Jeremiah.
Jerimiha, Jerimya

Jermain (French, English) a form of Jermaine.

Jermaine 🅱🅶 (French) a form of Germain. (English) sprout, bud.
Jarman, Jer-Mon, Jeremaine, Jeremane, Jerimane, Jerman, Jermane, Jermanie, Jermanne, Jermany, Jermayn, Jermayne, Jermiane, Jermine, Jermoney, Jhirmaine

Jermal (Arabic) a form of Jamal.
Jermaal, Jermael, Jermail, Jermall, Jermaul, Jermil, Jermol, Jermyll

Jérme (French) a form of Jerome.

Jermel, Jermell (Arabic) forms of Jamal.

Jermey (English) a form of Jeremy.
Jerme, Jermee, Jermere, Jermery, Jermie, Jermy, Jhermie

Jermiah (Hebrew) a form of Jeremiah.
Jermiha, Jermija, Jermiya

Jerney (Slavic) a form of Bartholomew.

Jerolin (Basque, Latin) holy.
Jerolyn

Jerome (Latin) holy. See also Geronimo, Hieronymos.
Gerome, Jere, Jeroen, Jerom, Jérome, Jérôme, Jeromo, Jerrome

Jeromy (Latin) a form of Jerome.
Jeromee, Jeromey, Jeromie, Jerromy

Jeron, Jerrin, Jerron (English) forms of Jerome.
J'ron, Jéron, Jerone, Jerrion, Jerrone

Jeronimo (Greek, Italian) a form of Jerome.

Jerónimo (Spanish) a form of Jeronimo.

Jerret, Jerrett (Hebrew) forms of Jarrett.
Jeret, Jerett, Jeritt, Jerrete, Jerrette, Jerriot, Jerritt, Jerrot, Jerrott

Jerrick (American) a combination of Jerry + Derric.
Jaric, Jarrick, Jerik, Jerrik, Jerryc, Jerryck, Jerryk

Jerry (German) mighty spearman. (English) a familiar form of Gerald, Gerard. See also Gerry, Kele.
Jehri, Jere, Jeree, Jeri, Jerie, Jeris, Jerison, Jerree, Jerri, Jerrie, Jery

Jerusalén (Hebrew) peaceful place.

Jervis (English) a form of Gervaise, Jarvis.
Jervice, Jervise, Jervys

Jerzy (Polish) a form of George.
Jersey, Jerzey, Jerzi, Jurek

Jesabel (Hebrew) oath of God.

Jesé (Hebrew) riches.

Jeshua (Hebrew) a form of Joshua.
Jeshuah

Jess (Hebrew) a short form of Jesse.

Jesse ★ **BG** (Hebrew) wealthy. Bible: the father of David. See also Yishai.
Jescee, Jese, Jesee, Jesi, Jessé, Jezze, Jezzee

Jessee, Jessey (Hebrew) forms of Jesse.
Jescey, Jesie, Jessye, Jessyie, Jesy, Jezzey, Jezzi, Jezzie, Jezzy

Jessi **GB** (Hebrew) a form of Jesse.

Jessica **GB** (Hebrew) a form of Jesse. Literature: a name perhaps invented by Shakespeare for a character in his play *The Merchant of Venice*.

Jessie **BG** (Hebrew) a form of Jesse.

Jessy **BG** (Hebrew) a form of Jesse.

Jestin (Welsh) a form of Justin.
Jessten, Jesstin, Jesston, Jesten, Jeston

Jesualdo (Germanic) he who takes the lead.

Jesus ★ **BG** (Hebrew) a form of Joshua. Bible: son of Mary and Joseph, believed by Christians to be the Son of God. See also Chucho, Isa, Yosu.
Jecho, Jessus, Jesu, Jezus, Josu

Jesús (Hispanic) a form of Jesus.

Jethro (Hebrew) abundant. Bible: the father-in-law of Moses. See also Yitro.
Jeth, Jethroe, Jetro, Jetrow, Jettro

Jethró (Hebrew) a form of Jethro.

Jett (English) hard, black mineral. (Hebrew) a short form of Jethro.
Jet, Jetson, Jette, Jetter, Jetty

Jevan (Hebrew) a form of Javan.
Jevaun, Jeven, Jevyn, Jevynn

Jevin (Hebrew) a form of Javan.

Jevon (Hebrew) a form of Javan.
Jevion, Jevohn, Jevone, Jevonn, Jevonne, Jevonnie

Jevonte (American) a form of Jevon.
Jevonta, Jevontae, Jevontaye, Jevonté

Jezabel (Hebrew) oath of God.

Jhon (Hebrew) a form of John.

Jhonathan (Hebrew) a form of Jonathan.

Jhonny (Hebrew) a form of Johnie.

Jiang (Chinese) fire.

Jibade (Yoruba) born close to royalty.
Jibad, Jybad, Jybade

Jibben (Gypsy) life.
Jibin

Jibril (Arabic) archangel of Allah.
Jibreel, Jibriel

Jibrîl (Arabic) a form of Jibril.

Jihad (Arabic) struggle; holy war.

Jilt (Dutch) money.
Jylt

Jim (Hebrew, English) a short form of James. See also Jaap.
Jimbo, Jimm, Jym, Jymm

Jimbo (American) a familiar form of Jim.
Jimboo

Jimell (Arabic) a form of Jamel.
Jimel, Jimelle, Jimill, Jimmell, Jimmelle, Jimmiel, Jimmil, Jimmill, Jimmyl, Jimmyll, Jymel, Jymell, Jymil, Jymill, Jymmel, Jymmell, Jymmil, Jymmill, Jymmyl, Jymmyll, Jymyl, Jymyll

Jimeno (Spanish) a form of Simeón.

Jimi BG (English) a form of Jimmy.
Jimie, Jimmi

Jimiyu (Abaluhya) born in the dry season.

Jimmie (English) a form of Jimmy.

Jimmy (English) a familiar form of Jim.
Jimee, Jimey, Jimme, Jimmee, Jimmey, Jimmye, Jimmyjo, Jimy, Jyme, Jymee, Jymey, Jymi, Jymie, Jymme, Jymmee, Jymmey, Jymmi, Jymmie, Jymy

Jimmy Lee (American) a combination of Jimmy + Lee.

Jimoh (Swahili) born on Friday.
Jimo, Jymo, Jymoh

Jin BG (Chinese) gold.
Jinn, Jyn, Jynn

Jina GB (Swahili) name.

Jinan (Arabic) garden.
Jinen, Jinon, Jinyn

Jindra (Czech) a form of Harold.
Jindrah

Jing-Quo (Chinese) ruler of the country.

Jiovanni (Italian) a form of Giovanni.
Jio, Jiovani, Jiovanie, Jiovann, Jiovannie, Jiovanny, Jiovany, Jiovoni, Jivan, Jyovani, Jyovanie, Jyovany

Jirair (Armenian) strong; hard working.
Jyrair

Jiri (Czech) a form of George.
Jirka

Jiro (Japanese) second son.

Jivin (Hindi) life giver.
Jivan, Jivanta, Jiven, Jivon, Jivyn, Jyvan, Jyven, Jyvin, Jyvon, Jyvyn

Jjiri (Zimbabwe) wild fruits of the jungle.

Jo GB (Hebrew, Japanese) a form of Joe.

Joab (Hebrew) God is father. See also Yoav.
Joabe, Joaby

Joachim (Hebrew) God will establish. See also Akeem, Ioakim, Yehoyakem.
Joacheim, Joakim, Joaquim, Jokim, Jov

Joan GB (German) a form of Johann.

Joao, João (Portuguese) forms of John.
Joáo

Joaquim (Portuguese) a form of Joachim.

Joaquin, Joaquín (Spanish) forms of Joachim.
Jehoichin, Joaquyn, Joaquynn, Joquin, Juaquyn

Job (Hebrew) afflicted. Bible: a righteous man whose faith in God survived the test of many afflictions.
Jobe, Jobert

Joben (Japanese) enjoys cleanliness.
Joban, Jobin, Jobon, Jobyn

Jobo (Spanish) a familiar form of Joseph.

Joby BG (Hebrew) a familiar form of Job.
Jobee, Jobey, Jobi, Jobie

Jocelyn GB (Latin) joyous.

Jock (American) a familiar form of Jacob. A form of Jack.
Jocko, Joco, Jocoby, Jocolby

Jocquez (French) a form of Jacquez.
Jocques, Jocquis, Jocquise

Jocqui (French) a form of Jacque.
Jocque

Jocundo (Latin) pleasant, festive.

Jodan (Hebrew) a combination of Jo + Dan.
Jodahn, Joden, Jodhan, Jodian, Jodin, Jodon, Jodonnis, Jodyn

Jody BG (Hebrew) a familiar form of Joseph.
Jodee, Jodey, Jodi, Jodie, Jodiha, Joedee, Joedey, Joedi, Joedie, Joedy

Joe (Hebrew) a short form of Joseph.
Jow

Joel (Hebrew) God is willing. Bible: an Old Testament Hebrew prophet.
Joël, Jóel, Joell, Joelle, Joely, Jole, Yoel

Joeseph, Joesph (Hebrew) forms of Joseph.

Joey BG (Hebrew) a familiar form of Joe, Joseph.

Johan (German) a form of Johann.

Johann (German) a form of John. See also Anno, Hanno, Yoan, Yohan.
Joahan, Johahn, Johanan, Johane, Johannan, Johaun, Johon

Johannes (German) a form of Johann.
Joannes, Johanes, Johannas, Johannus, Johansen, Johanson, Johonson

Johathan (Hebrew) a form of Jonathan.
Johanthan, Johatan, Johathe, Johathon

John ☆ (Hebrew) God is gracious. Bible: the name honoring John the Baptist and John the Evangelist. See also Elchanan, Evan, Geno, Gian, Giovanni, Handel, Hannes, Hans, Hanus, Honza, Ian, Ianos, Iban, Ioan, Ivan, Iwan, Keoni, Kwam, Ohannes, Sean, Ugutz, Yan, Yanka, Yanni, Yochanan, Yohance, Zane.
Jaenda, Janco, Jantje, Jen, Jian, Joen, Johne, Jone

John Paul, John-Paul, Johnpaul (American) combinations of John + Paul.

John-Michael, Johnmichael (American) combinations of John + Michael.

John-Robert (American) a combination of John + Robert.

Johnathan, Johnathen, Johnathon (Hebrew) forms of Jonathan. See also Yanton.
Johnatan, Johnathann, Johnathaon, Johnathyne, Johnaton, Johnatten, Johniathin, Johnothan

Johnie, Johnny, Johny (Hebrew) familiar forms of John. See also Gianni.
Johnee, Johney, Johni, Johnier, Johnney, Johnni

Johnnie BG (Hebrew) a familiar form of John.

Johnpatrick (American) a combination of John + Patick.

Johnson (English) son of John.
Johnston, Jonson

Johntavius (American) a form of John.

Johnthan (Hebrew) a form of Jonathan.

Joji (Japanese) a form of George.

Jojo (Fante) born on Monday.

Jokim (Basque) a form of Joachim.
Jokeam, Jokeem, Jokin, Jokym

Jolon (Native American) valley of the dead oaks.
Jolyon

Jomar (American) a form of Jamar.
Jomari, Jomarie, Jomarri

Jomei (Japanese) spreads light.
Jomey

Jomo (African) farmer.

Jon (Hebrew) a form of John. A short form of Jonathan.
J'on, Jonn

Jon-Michael (American) a combination of Jon + Michael.

Jon-Pierre (American) a combination of Jon + Pierre.

Jonah (Hebrew) dove. Bible: an Old Testament prophet who was swallowed by a large fish.
Giona, Jona, Yonah, Yunus

Jonas (Hebrew) he accomplishes. (Lithuanian) a form of John.
Jonahs, Jonass, Jonaus, Jonelis, Jonukas, Jonus, Jonutis, Jonys, Joonas

Jonás (Hebrew) a form of Jonas.

Jonatan (Hebrew) a form of Jonathan.
Jonatane, Jonate, Jonattan, Jonnattan

Jonathan ☆ BG (Hebrew) gift of God. Bible: the son of King Saul who became a loyal friend of David. See also Ionakana, Yanton, Yonatan.
Janathan, Jonatha, Jonathin, Jonathun, Jonathyn, Jonethen, Jonnatha, Jonnathun

Jonathen, Jonathon, Jonnathan (Hebrew)
forms of Jonathan.
Joanathon, Jonaton, Jonnathon, Jonthon, Jounathon, Yanaton

Jones (Welsh) son of John.
Joenes, Joennes, Joenns, Johnsie, Joness, Jonesy

Jonny (Hebrew) a familiar form of John.
Jonhy, Joni, Jonnee, Jonni, Jonnie, Jony

Jonothan (Hebrew) a form of Jonathan.
Jonothon

Jontae (French) a combination of Jon + the
suffix Tae.
Johntae, Jontea, Jonteau

Jontavious (American) a form of Jon.

Jontay, Jonte (American) forms of Jontae.
Johntay, Johnte, Johntez, Jontai, Jonté, Jontez

Jonthan (Hebrew) a form of Jonathan.

Joop (Dutch) a familiar form of Joseph.
Jopie

Joost (Dutch) just.

Joquin (Spanish) a form of Joaquin.
Jocquin, Jocquinn, Jocquyn, Jocquynn, Joquan, Joquawn, Joqunn, Joquon

Jora 🅶🅱 (Hebrew) teacher.
Jorah, Yora, Yorah

Joram (Hebrew) Jehovah is exalted.
Joran, Jorim

Jordan ⭐ 🅱🅶 (Hebrew) descending. See
also Giordano, Yarden.
Jardan, Jordaan, Jordae, Jordain, Jordaine, Jordane, Jordani, Jordanio, Jordann, Jordanny, Jordano, Jordany, Jordáo, Jordayne, Jordian, Jordun, Jorrdan

Jordán (Hebrew) a form of Jordan.

Jorden 🅱🅶 (Hebrew) a form of Jordan.
Jeordon, Johordan, Jordenn

Jordi, Jordie, Jordy (Hebrew) familiar
forms of Jordan.

Jordin, Jordyn 🅶🅱 (Hebrew) forms of
Jordan.

Jordon 🅱🅶 (Hebrew) a form of Jordan.

Jorell (American) he saves. Literature: a
name inspired by the fictional character

Jor-El, Superman's father.
Jor-El, Jorel, Jorelle, Jorl, Jorrel, Jorrell, Jorrelle

Jorey (Hebrew) a familiar form of Jordan.
Joar, Joary, Jori, Jorie, Jorrie

Jörg (German) a form of George.
Jeorg, Juergen, Jungen, Jürgen

Jorge, Jorje (Spanish) forms of George.

Jorgeluis (Spanish) a combination of Jorge
+ Luis.

Jorgen (Danish) a form of George.
Joergen, Jorgan, Jörgen

Joris (Dutch) a form of George.

Jörn (German) a familiar form of Gregory.

Jorrín (Spanish) a form of George.
Jorian

Jory 🅱🅶 (Hebrew) a familiar form of Jordan.

Josafat (Hebrew) God's judgment.

Jose ⚡ 🅱🅶 (Spanish) a form of Joseph. See
also Che, Pepe.
Josean, Josecito, Josee, Joseito, Joselito

José (Spanish) a form of Joseph.

Josealfredo (Spanish) a combination of Jose
+ Alfredo.

Joseantonio (Spanish) a combination of
Jose + Antonio.

Josef (German, Portuguese, Czech,
Scandinavian) a form of Joseph.
Joosef, Joseff, Josif, Jossif, Juzef, Juzuf

Joseguadalup (Spanish) a combination of
Jose + Guadalupe.

Joseluis (Spanish) a combination of Jose +
Luis.

Josemanuel (Spanish) a combination of Jose
+ Manuel.

Joseph ⚡ 🅱🅶 (Hebrew) God will add, God
will increase. Bible: in the Old Testament,
the son of Jacob who came to rule Egypt;
in the New Testament, the husband of
Mary. See also Beppe, Cheche, Chepe,
Giuseppe, Iokepa, Iosif, Osip, Pepa, Peppe,
Pino, Sepp, Yeska, Yosef, Yousef, Youssel,
Yusef, Yusif, Zeusef.
Jazeps, Jooseppi, Joseba, Josep, Josephat,

Josephe, Josephie, Josephus, Josheph, Josip, Jóska, Joza, Joze, Jozeph, Jozhe, Jozio, Jozka, Jozsi, Jozzepi, Jupp, Jusepe, Juziu

Josey **GB** (Spanish) a form of Joseph.

Josh (Hebrew) a short form of Joshua.
Joshe

Josha (Hindi) satisfied.
Joshah

Joshawa (Hebrew) a form of Joshua.

Joshi (Swahili) galloping.
Joshee, Joshey, Joshie, Joshy

Joshua ⭐ **BG** (Hebrew) God is my salvation. Bible: led the Israelites into the Promised Land. See also Giosia, Iosua, Jesus, Yehoshua.
Johsua, Johusa, Joshau, Joshaua, Joshauh, Joshawah, Joshia, Joshuaa, Joshuea, Joshuia, Joshula, Joshus, Joshusa, Joshuwa, Joshwa, Jousha, Jozshua, Jozsua, Jozua, Jushua

Joshuah (Hebrew) a form of Joshua.

Joshue (Hebrew) a form of Joshua.

Josiah (Hebrew) fire of the Lord. See also Yoshiyahu.
Joshiah, Josia, Josiahs, Josian, Josie, Josya, Josyah

Josias (Hebrew) a form of Josiah.

Josías (Spanish) a form of Josias.

Joss (Chinese) luck; fate.
Jos, Josse, Jossy

Josue (Hebrew) a form of Joshua.
Joshu, Jossue, Josu, Josua, Josuha, Jozus

Josué (Spanish) a form of Josue.

Jotham (Hebrew) may God complete. Bible: a king of Judah.
Jothem, Jothim, Jothom, Jothym

Jourdan **GB** (Hebrew) a form of Jordan.
Jourdain, Jourden, Jourdin, Jourdon, Jourdyn

Jovan (Latin) Jove-like, majestic. (Slavic) a form of John. Mythology: Jove, also known as Jupiter, was the supreme Roman deity.
Johvan, Johvon, Jovaan, Jovaann, Jovane, Jovanic, Jovann, Jovannis, Jovaughn, Jovaun, Joven, Jovenal, Jovenel, Jovi, Jovian, Jovin, Jovito, Jowan, Jowaun, Yovan, Yovani

Jovani, Jovanni, Jovanny, Jovany (Latin) forms of Jovan.
Jovanie, Jovannie, Jovoni, Jovonie, Jovonni, Jovony

Jovante (American) a combination of Jovan + the suffix Te.

Jovon (Latin) a form of Jovan.
Jovoan, Jovone, Jovonn, Jovonne

Jovonté (American) a combination of Jovon + the suffix Te.

Jozef (German, Portuguese, Czech, Scandinavian) a form of Josef.
Jozeff, József

Jr (Latin) a short form of Junior.
Jr.

Juan ⭐ (Spanish) a form of John. See also Chan.
Juanch, Juanchito, Juane, Juann, Juaun

Juan Carlos, Juancarlos (Spanish) combinations of Juan + Carlos.

Juanantonio (Spanish) a combination of Juan + Antonio.

Juandaniel (Spanish) a combination of Juan + Daniel.

Juanelo (Spanish) a form of Juan.

Juanito (Spanish) a form of Juan.

Juanjo (Spanish) a combination of Juan and José.

Juanjose (Spanish) a combination of Juan + Jose.

Juanma (Spanish) a combination of Juan and Manuel.

Juanmanuel (Spanish) a combination of Juan + Manuel.

Juaquin (Spanish) a form of Joaquin.
Juaqin, Juaqine, Juaquine

Jubal (Hebrew) ram's horn. Bible: a musician and a descendant of Cain.

Jucundo (Latin) happy, joyous one.

Judah (Hebrew) praised. Bible: the fourth of Jacob's sons. See also Yehudi.
Juda, Judda, Juddah

Judas (Latin) a form of Judah. Bible: Judas Iscariot was the disciple who betrayed Jesus.
Juddas

Judás (Hebrew) a form of Judas.

Judd (Hebrew) a short form of Judah.
Jud

Jude (Latin) a short form of Judah, Judas. Bible: one of the Twelve Apostles, author of "The Epistle of Jude."

Judson (English) son of Judd.
Juddson

Juhana (Finnish) a form of John.
Juha, Juhanah, Juhanna, Juhannah, Juho

Jujuan (American) a form of Jajuan.

Juku (Estonian) a form of Richard.
Jukka

Jules (French) a form of Julius.
Joles, Julas, Jule

Julian ☆ BG (Greek, Latin) a form of Julius.
Jolyon, Julean, Juliaan, Julianne, Julion, Julyan, Julyin, Julyon

Julián (Spanish) a form of Julian.

Juliano (Spanish) a form of Julian.

Julien (Latin) a form of Julian.
Julen, Juliene, Julienn, Julienne, Jullien, Jullin, Julyen

Julio (Hispanic) a form of Julius.
Juleo, Juliyo, Julyo

Juliocesar (Hispanic) a combination of Julio + Cesar.

Julis (Spanish) a form of Julius.

Julius (Greek, Latin) youthful, downy bearded. History: Julius Caesar was a great Roman dictator. See also Giuliano.
Julias, Julious, Juliusz, Jullius, Juluis

Jullian BG (Greek, Latin) a form of Julius.

Jumaane (Swahili) born on Tuesday.
Jumane

Jumah (Arabic, Swahili) born on Friday, a holy day in the Islamic religion.
Jimoh, Juma

Jumoke (Yoruba) loved by everyone.
Jumok

Jun BG (Chinese) truthful. (Japanese) obedient; pure.
Joon, Junnie

Junior (Latin) young.
Junious, Junius, Junor, Junyor

Júpiter (Latin) origin of light.

Jupp (German) a form of Joseph.
Jup

Juquan (Spanish) a form of Juaquin.

Jur (Czech) a form of George.
Juraz, Jurek, Jurik, Jurko

Jurgis (Lithuanian) a form of George.
Jurgi, Juri

Juro (Japanese) best wishes; long life.

Jurrien (Dutch) God will uplift.
Jore, Jurian, Jurion, Jurre, Juryan, Juryen, Juryin, Juryon

Justan, Justen, Juston, Justyn (Latin) forms of Justin.
Jasten, Jaston, Justyne, Justynn

Justice GB (Latin) a form of Justis.
Justic, Justiz, Justyc, Justyce

Justin ☆ BG (Latin) just, righteous. See also Giustino, Iestyn, Iustin, Tutu, Ustin, Yustyn.
Jastin, Jobst, Jost, Jusa, Just, Justain, Justek, Justian, Justinas, Justinian, Justinius, Justinn, Justins, Justinus, Justn, Justo, Justton, Justukas, Justun

Justine GB (Latin) a form of Justin.

Justiniano (Spanish) a form of Justino.

Justino (Spanish) a form of Justin.

Justis BG (French) just.
Justas, Justise, Justs, Justyse

Justus BG (French) a form of Justis.

Jutta (Germanic) fair.

Juven, Juvencio, Juventino (Latin) one that represents youth.

Juvenal (Latin) young. Literature: a Roman satirist.
Juventin, Juventyn, Juvon, Juvone

Juwan, Juwon (American) forms of Jajuan.
*Juvaun, Juvon, Juvone, Juwaan, Juwain,
Juwane, Juwann, Juwaun, Juwonn, Juwuan,
Juwuane, Juwvan, Jwan, Jwon*

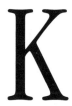

Ka'eo (Hawaiian) victorious.

Kabiito (Rutooro) born while foreigners are visiting.
Kabito, Kabyto

Kabil (Turkish) a form of Cain.
Kabel, Kabyl

Kabir (Hindi) History: an Indian mystic poet.
Kabar, Kabeer, Kabier, Kabyr, Khabir

Kabonero (Runyankore) sign.

Kabonesa (Rutooro) difficult birth.
Kabonesah

Kacey GB (Irish) a form of Casey. (American) a combination of the initials K. + C. See also Kasey, KC.
*Kace, Kacee, Kaci, Kaecee, Kaecey, Kaeci,
Kaecie, Kaecy, Kaicee, Kaicey, Kaici, Kaicie,
Kaicy, Kaycee*

Kacy GB (Irish, American) a form of Kacey.

Kadar (Arabic) powerful.
Kader, Kador

Kadarius (American) a combination of Kade + Darius.
*Kadairious, Kadarious, Kadaris, Kadarrius,
Kadarus, Kaddarrius, Kaderious, Kaderius*

Kade (Scottish) wetlands. (American) a combination of the initials K. + D.
Kadee, Kady, Kaed, Kayde, Kaydee

Kadeem (Arabic) servant.
Kadim, Kadym, Khadeem

Kaden (Arabic) a form of Kadin.
Caden, Kadeen, Kadein

Kadin (Arabic) friend, companion.
Kadan, Kadon, Kadyn

Kadîn (Arabic) a form of Kadin.

Kadir (Arabic) spring greening.
Kadeer, Kadyr

Kado (Japanese) gateway.

Kaeden (Arabic) a form of Kadin.
Kaedin, Kaedon, Kaedyn

Kaelan, Kaelon (Irish) forms of Kellen.
Kael, Kaelyn

Kaeleb (Hebrew) a form of Kaleb.
Kaelib, Kaelob, Kaelyb, Kailab, Kaileb

Kaelen BG (Irish) a form of Kellen.

Kaelin BG (Irish) a form of Kellen.

Kaemon (Japanese) joyful; right-handed.
Kaeman, Kaemen, Kaemin, Kaimon, Kaymon

Kaenan (Irish) a form of Keenan.
Kaenen, Kaenin, Kaenyn

Kafele (Nguni) worth dying for.

Kaga (Native American) writer.
Kagah

Kagan (Irish) a form of Keegan.
Kage, Kagen, Kaghen, Kaigan

Kahale (Hawaiian) home.
Kahail, Kahayl

Kahana (Hawaiian) priest.
Kahanah, Kahanna, Kahannah

Kahil (Turkish) young; inexperienced; naive. See also Cahil.
Kaheel, Kaheil, Kahill, Kahyl, Kahyll

Kahlil (Arabic) a form of Khalil.
*Kahleal, Kahlee, Kahleel, Kahleil, Kahli,
Kahliel, Kahlill*

Kaholo (Hawaiian) runner.

Kahraman (Turkish) hero.

Kai BG (Welsh) keeper of the keys. (Hawaiian) sea. (German) a form of Kay. (Danish) a form of Kaj.
Kae, Kaie, Kaii

Kaid (Scottish, American) a form of Kade.
Kaide

Kaiden (Arabic) a form of Kadin.
Kaidan

Kailas (Indian) abode of the Hindu god Shiva.

Kailashchandra, Kailashnath (Indian) other names for the Hindu god Shiva.

Kailen GB (Irish) a form of Kellen.
Kail, Kailan, Kailey, Kailin, Kaillan, Kailon, Kailyn

Kaili GB (Hawaiian) Religion: a Hawaiian god.
Kaelea, Kaelee, Kaeleigh, Kaeley, Kaeli, Kaelie, Kaely, Kailea, Kailee, Kaileigh, Kailey, Kailie, Kailli, Kaily, Kaylea, Kaylee, Kayleigh, Kayley, Kayli, Kaylie, Kayly

Kain, Kaine (Welsh, Irish) forms of Kane.
Kainan, Kainen, Kainin, Kainon

Kainoa (Hawaiian) name.

Kaipo (Hawaiian) sweetheart.
Kaypo

Kairo (Arabic) a form of Cairo.
Kaire, Kairee, Kairi, Kayro

Kaiser (German) a form of Caesar.
Kaesar, Kaisar, Kaizer, Kayser

Kaiven (American) a form of Kevin.
Kaivan, Kaivon, Kaiwan

Kaj (Danish) earth.
Kaje

Kajuan (American) a combination of the prefix Ka + Juan.

Kakar (Hindi) grass.

Kala GB (Hindi) black; phase. (Hawaiian) sun.
Kalah

Kalama BG (Hawaiian) torch.
Kalam, Kalamah

Kalameli (Tongan) caramel.
Kalamelie, Kalamely

Kalan BG (Hawaiian) a form of Kalani. (Irish) a form of Kalen.
Kalane, Kallan

Kalani GB (Hawaiian) sky; chief.
Kalanee, Kalaney, Kalanie, Kalany

Kalash (Indian) sacred pot.

Kale (Arabic) a short form of Kahlil. (Hawaiian) a familiar form of Carl.
Kael, Kaell, Kail, Kaill, Kaleu, Kayl

Kalea GB (Hawaiian) happy; joy.
Kaleah, Kalei, Kaleigh, Kaley

Kaleb, Kalib, Kalob (Hebrew) forms of Caleb.
Kaelab, Kailab, Kal, Kalab, Kalabe, Kalb, Kaleob, Kalev, Kalieb, Kallb, Kalleb, Kaloeb, Kalub, Kalyb, Kaylab, Kilab, Kylab

Kaled, Kalid (Arabic) immortal.

Kaleel (Arabic) a form of Khalíl.
Kalel, Kalell

Kalen BG (Arabic, Hawaiian) a form of Kale. (Irish) a form of Kellen.
Kallin

Kalevi (Finnish) hero.
Kalevee, Kalevey, Kalevie, Kalevy

Kali GB (Arabic) a short form of Kalil. (Hawaiian) a form of Gary.
Kalee, Kalie, Kaly

Kalicharan, Kalidas, Kalimohan, Kalipada, Kaliranjan (Indian) devoted to the Hindu goddess Kali.

Kalil (Arabic) a form of Khalíl.
Kaliel, Kaliil

Kalin BG (Arabic, Hawaiian) a form of Kale. (Irish) a form of Kellen.

Kaliq (Arabic) a form of Khaliq.
Kalic, Kaliqu, Kalique

Kalkin (Hindi) tenth. Religion: Kalki is the final incarnation of the Hindu god Vishnu.
Kalki, Kalkyn

Kalle BG (Scandinavian) a form of Carl. (Arabic, Hawaiian) a form of Kale.

Kallen, Kalon (Irish) forms of Kellen.
Kallan, Kallin, Kallion, Kallon, Kallun, Kallyn, Kalone, Kalonn, Kalun, Kalyen, Kalyne, Kalynn

Kalmin (Scandinavian) manly, strong.
Kalman, Kalmen, Kalmon, Kalmyn

Kaloosh (Armenian) blessed event.

Kalvin (Latin) a form of Calvin.
Kal, Kalv, Kalvan, Kalven, Kalvon, Kalvun, Kalvyn, Vinny

Kalyan (Indian) welfare.

Kalyn **GB** (Irish) a form of Kellen.

Kamaka (Hawaiian) face.
Kamakah

Kamakani (Hawaiian) wind.
Kamakanee, Kamakaney, Kamakanie, Kamakany

Kamal (Hindi) lotus. (Arabic) perfect, perfection.
Kamaal, Kamyl

Kamâl, Kamîl (Arabic) forms of Kamal.

Kamalakar, Kamalapati (Indian) other names for the Hindu god Vishnu.

Kamalesh (Indian) one with eyes like a lotus; another name for the Hindu god Vishnu.

Kamalnayan (Indian) one with eyes like a lotus.

Kamari **BG** (Swahili) a short form of Kamaria (see Girls' Names).

Kamau (Kikuyu) quiet warrior.

Kambod, Kambodi, Kamod (Indian) a raga, an ancient form of Hindu devotional music.

Kamden (Scottish) a form of Camden.
Kamdan, Kamdin, Kamdon, Kamdyn

Kamel (Hindi, Arabic) a form of Kamal.
Kameel

Kameron **BG** (Scottish) a form of Cameron.
Kam, Kamaren, Kamaron, Kameran, Kameren, Kamerin, Kamerion, Kamerron, Kamerun, Kameryn, Kamey, Kammeren, Kammeron, Kammy, Kamoryn

Kamesh, Kameshwar, Kamraj, Kandarpa (Indian) the Hindu god of love.

Kami **GB** (Hindi) loving.
Kamee, Kamey, Kamie, Kamy

Kamil (Arabic) a form of Kamal.
Kameel

Kamilo (Latin) a form of Camilo.
Kamillo, Kamillow, Kamyllo, Kamylo

Kampbell (Scottish) a form of Campbell.
Kambel, Kambell, Kamp

Kamran, Kamren, Kamron (Scottish) forms of Kameron.
Kammron, Kamrein, Kamrin, Kamrun

Kamryn **GB** (Scottish) a form of Kameron.

Kamuela (Hawaiian) a form of Samuel.
Kamuelah, Kamuele

Kamuhanda (Runyankore) born on the way to the hospital.

Kamukama (Runyankore) protected by God.

Kamuzu (Nguni) medicine.

Kamya (Luganda) born after twin brothers.

Kana (Japanese) powerful; capable. (Hawaiian) Mythology: a demigod.
Kanah

Kanaan (Hindi) a form of Kannan.

Kanad (Indian) an ancient Indian sage.

Kanaiela (Hawaiian) a form of Daniel.
Kana, Kaneii

Kanchan (Indian) gold.

Kane **BG** (Welsh) beautiful. (Irish) tribute. (Japanese) golden. (Hawaiian) eastern sky. (English) a form of Keene. See also Cain.
Kaen, Kahan, Kaney

Kanen (Hindi) a form of Kannan.

Kange (Lakota) raven.
Kang, Kanga, Kangee, Kangi, Kangie, Kangy

Kanhaiya, Kanhaiyalal (Indian) other names for the Hindu god Krishna.

Kaniel (Hebrew) stalk, reed.
Kan, Kani, Kaniell, Kannie, Kanny, Kannyel, Kanyel

Kanishka (Indian) name of a king.

Kannan (Hindi) Religion: another name for the Hindu god Krishna.
Kanan, Kanin, Kanine, Kannen

Kannon (Polynesian) free. (French) a form of Cannon.
Kanon

Kanoa BG (Hawaiian) free.
Kanoah

Kantu (Hindi) happy.

Kanu (Swahili) wildcat.

Kanya GB (Australian) rock. (Hindi) virgin.
Kania, Kaniah, Kanyah

Kanyon (Latin) a form of Canyon.

Kaori (Japanese) strong.
Kaoru

Kapali (Hawaiian) cliff.
Kapalee, Kapalie, Kapaly

Kapeni (Malawian) knife.
Kapenee, Kapenie, Kapeny

Kaphiri (Egyptian) hill.

Kapila (Hindi) ancient prophet.
Kapil, Kapill, Kapilla, Kapyla, Kapylla

Kapono (Hawaiian) righteous.
Kapena

Kappi (Gypsy) a form of Cappi.
Kappee, Kappey, Kappie, Kappy

Karan (Greek) a form of Karen (see Girls' Names).

Kardal (Arabic) mustard seed.
Karandal, Kardel, Kardell

Kare (Norwegian) enormous.

Kareb (Danish) pure; immaculate.

Kareem (Arabic) noble; distinguished.
Karem, Kareme, Karreem, Karriem, Karrym, Karym

Karel BG (Czech) a form of Carl.
Karell, Karil, Karrell

Karey GB (Greek) a form of Carey.
Karee, Kari, Karie, Karree, Karrey, Karri, Karrie, Karry, Kary

Karif (Arabic) born in autumn.
Kareef, Kariff

Kariisa (Runyankore) herdsman.

Karim (Arabic) a form of Kareem.

Karl (German) a form of Carl.
Kaarle, Kaarlo, Karcsi, Karlitis, Karlo, Kjell

Karlen (Latvian, Russian) a form of Carl.
Karlan, Karlens, Karlik, Karlin, Karlis, Karlon, Karlyn

Karlos (Spanish) a form of Carlos.
Karlus

Karlton (English) a form of Carlton.

Karmel BG (Hebrew) a form of Carmel.
Karmeli, Karmelo, Karmiel, Karmilo

Karney (Irish) a form of Carney.
Karnee, Karni, Karnie, Karny

Karol BG (Czech, Polish) a form of Carl.
Karal, Karalos, Karolek, Karolis, Károly, Karrel, Karrol, Karroll

Karoly (French) strong and masculine.

Karon BG (Greek) a form of Karen.

Karr (Scandinavian) a form of Carr.

Karsen BG (English) a form of Carson.
Karrson, Karsan, Karsin, Karsyn

Karson BG (English) a form of Carson.

Karsten (Greek) anointed.
Carsten, Karstan, Karstein, Karstin, Karston, Karstyn

Karu (Hindi) cousin.
Karun

Karutunda (Runyankore) little.

Karwana (Rutooro) born during wartime.

Kaseem (Arabic) divided.
Kasceem, Kaseam, Kaseym, Kazeem

Kaseko (Rhodesian) mocked, ridiculed.

Kasem (Tai) happiness.
Kaseme

Kasen BG (Basque) protected with a helmet.
Kasan, Kasean, Kasene, Kaseon, Kasin, Kassen, Kasyn

Kasey GB (Irish) a form of Casey.
Kaese, Kaesee, Kaesey, Kaesi, Kaesie, Kaesy, Kasay, Kase, Kasee, Kasi, Kasie, Kassee, Kassey, Kassi, Kassie, Kassy, Kasy, Kazee, Kazey, Kazy, Kazzee, Kazzey, Kazzi, Kazzie, Kazzy

Kashawn (American) a combination of the prefix Ka + Shawn.
Kashain, Kashan, Kashaun, Kashen, Kashon

Kasib (Arabic) fertile.
Kasyb

Kasîb (Arabic) a form of Kasib.

Kasim (Arabic) a form of Kaseem.
Kassim, Kasym

Kasimir (Arabic) peace. (Slavic) a form of Casimir.
Kashmir, Kasimyr, Kasymyr, Kazimier, Kazimir, Kazmer, Kazmér, Kázmér

Kasiya (Nguni) separate.
Kasiyah

Kason (Basque) a form of Kasen.

Kasper (Persian) treasurer. (German) a form of Casper.
Jasper, Kaspar, Kaspero, Kaspir, Kaspor, Kaspyr

Kass (German) blackbird.
Kaese, Kasch, Kase

Kasseem (Arabic) a form of Kaseem.
Kassem

Kassidy GB (Irish) a form of Cassidy.
Kassadee, Kassadey, Kassadi, Kassadie, Kassady, Kassedee, Kassedey, Kassedi, Kassedie, Kassedy, Kassidee, Kassidey, Kassidi, Kassidie, Kassie, Kassy, Kassydee, Kassydey, Kassydi, Kassydie, Kassydy

Kateb (Arabic) writer.

Kato (Runyankore) second of twins.

Katriel GB (Hebrew) crowned with God's glory. (Arabic) peace.
Katryel

Katungi (Runyankore) rich.
Katungie, Katungy

Kaufman (German) merchant.
Kaufmann

Kauri (Polynesian) tree.
Kaeree, Kaurie, Kaury

Kavan (Irish) a form of Kevin. See also Cavan.
Kavaugn, Kavyn

Kavanagh (Irish) Kavan's follower.
Cavanagh, Kavenagh, Kavenaugh

Kaveh (Persian) ancient hero.
Kavah

Kaven, Kavin, Kavon (Irish) forms of Kavan.
Kaveon, Kavion, Kavone, Kaywon

Kavi (Hindi) poet.
Kavee, Kavey, Kavie, Kavy

Kawika (Hawaiian) a form of David.
Kawyka

Kay GB (Greek) rejoicing. (German) fortified place. Literature: one of King Arthur's knights of the Round Table.
Kaye, Kayson

Kayden BG (Arabic) a form of Kadin.
Kaydin, Kaydn, Kaydon

Kayin (Nigerian) celebrated. (Yoruba) long-hoped-for child.
Kaiyan, Kaiyen, Kaiyin, Kaiyon, Kayan, Kayen, Kayin, Kayon

Kaylan GB (Irish) a form of Kellen.
Kaylyn, Kaylynn

Kayle GB (Hebrew) faithful dog. (Arabic) a short form of Kahlil. (Arabic, Hawaiian) a form of Kale.
Kaile, Kayl, Kayla

Kayleb (Hebrew) a form of Caleb.
Kaylib, Kaylob, Kaylub

Kaylen GB (Irish) a form of Kellen.

Kaylin GB (Irish) a form of Kellen.

Kaylon BG (Irish) a form of Kellen.

Kayne (Hebrew) a form of Cain.
Kaynan, Kaynen, Kaynon

Kayode (Yoruba) he brought joy.

Kayonga (Runyankore) ash.

Kayvan, Kayvon (Irish) forms of Kavan.

Kazemde (Egyptian) ambassador.

Kazio (Polish) a form of Casimir, Kasimir. See also Cassidy.

Kazuo (Japanese) man of peace.

Kc BG (American) a form of KC.

KC BG (American) a combination of the initials K. + C. See also Kacey.
K.C., Kcee, Kcey

Keagan BG (Irish) a form of Keegan.
Keagean, Keagen, Keaghan, Keagyn

Keahi (Hawaiian) flames.

Keaka (Hawaiian) a form of Jack.

Kealoha (Hawaiian) fragrant.
Ke'ala, Kealohah

Kean (German, Irish, English) a form of
Keane.

Keanan (Irish) a form of Keenan.
Keanen, Keanna, Keannan, Keannen, Keanon

Keandre (American) a combination of the
prefix Ke + Andre.
*Keandra, Keandray, Keandré, Keandree,
Keandrell*

Kéandre (American) a form of Keandre.

Keane (German) bold; sharp. (Irish) handsome. (English) a form of Keene.

Keano (Irish) a form of Keanu.
Keanno, Keeno

Keanu BG (Hawaiian) cool breeze over the
mountains (Irish) a form of Keenan.
*Keaneu, Keani, Keanie, Keanue, Keany,
Keenu, Kianu*

Kearn (Irish) a short form of Kearney.
Kearne

Kearney (Irish) a form of Carney.
Kearny

Keary (Irish) a form of Kerry.
Kearie

Keaton BG (English) where hawks fly.
*Keatan, Keaten, Keatin, Keatton, Keatun,
Keatyn, Keetan, Keeten, Keetin, Keeton, Keetun,
Keetyn, Keitan, Keiten, Keiton, Keitun, Keityn*

Keaven (Irish) a form of Kevin.
Keavan, Keavin, Keavon, Keavun, Keavyn

Keawe (Hawaiian) strand.

Keb (Egyptian) earth. Mythology: an ancient
earth god, also known as Geb.
Kebb

Kedar (Hindi) mountain lord. (Arabic) pow-
erful. Religion: another name for the
Hindu god Shiva.
Kadar, Kedaar, Keder

Keddy (Scottish) a form of Adam.
Keddi, Keddie

Kedem (Hebrew) ancient.
Kedeam, Kedeem, Kedim, Kedym

Kedric, Kedrick (English) forms of Cedric.
*Keddric, Keddrick, Keddrik, Keddryc,
Keddryck, Keddryk, Kederick, Kedrek, Kedrik,
Kedryc, Kedryck, Kedryk, Kiedric, Kiedrick*

Keefe (Irish) handsome; loved.
*Keaf, Keafe, Keaff, Keaffe, Keef, Keeff, Keif,
Keife, Keiff, Keiffe, Keyf, Keyfe, Keyff, Keyffe*

Keegan BG (Irish) little; fiery.
*Kaegan, Keagen, Keegen, Keeghan, Keegin,
Keegon, Keegun*

Keelan (Irish) little; slender. A form of
Kellen.
*Kealan, Kealen, Kealin, Kealon, Kealyn,
Keelen, Keelin, Keelon, Keelun, Keelyn*

Keeley GB (Irish) handsome.
*Kealee, Kealeigh, Kealey, Keali, Kealie, Kealy,
Keelea, Keelee, Keeleigh, Keeli, Keelian,
Keelie, Keelli, Keellie, Keelly, Keely*

Keenan (Irish) little Keene.
Kaenan, Keennan

Keene (German) bold; sharp. (English)
smart. See also Kane.
Kaene, Keen, Kein, Keine, Keyn, Keyne

Keenen, Keenon (Irish) forms of Keenan.
Keenin, Keynen, Kienen

Kees (Dutch) a form of Kornelius.
Keas, Kease, Keese, Keesee, Keis, Keyes, Keys

Keevon (Irish) a form of Kevin.
*Keevan, Keeven, Keevin, Keevun, Keevyn,
Keewan, Keewin*

Kegan (Irish) a form of Keegan.
*Kegen, Keghan, Keghen, Kegin, Kegon,
Kegun, Kegyn*

Kehind (Yoruba) second-born twin.
Kehinde, Kehynd

Keifer, Keiffer (German) forms of Cooper.
Keefer, Keyfer, Keyffer

Keigan (Irish) a form of Keegan.
*Keigen, Keighan, Keighen, Keigin, Keigon,
Keigun, Keigyn, Keygan, Keygen, Keygin,
Keygon, Keygyn*

Keiji (Japanese) cautious ruler.
Keyjiy

Keilan (Irish) a form of Keelan.
Keilen, Keilin, Keillene, Keillyn, Keilon, Keilyn, Keilynn, Keylan, Keylen, Keylin, Keylon, Keylyn

Keiley (Irish) a form of Keeley.
Keilea, Keilee, Keileigh, Keili, Keilie, Keily, Keylea, Keylee, Keyleigh, Keyley, Keyli, Keylie, Keyly

Keion (Irish) a form of Keon.
Keionne

Keir (Irish) a short form of Kieran.
Keyr

Keiran (Irish) a form of Kieran.
Keiren, Keirin, Keiron

Keitaro (Japanese) blessed.
Keataro, Keita, Keytaro

Keith (Welsh) forest. (Scottish) battle place. See also Kika.
Keath, Keeth, Keithe, Keyth

Keithen (Welsh, Scottish) a form of Keith.
Keithan, Keitheon, Keithon

Keivan (Irish) a form of Kevin.
Keiven, Keivin, Keivn, Keivon, Keivone, Keivyn

Kejuan (American) a combination of the prefix Ke + Juan.

Kek (Egyptian) god of the darkness.

Kekapa (Hawaiian) tapa cloth.
Kekapah

Kekipi (Hawaiian) rebel.

Kekoa (Hawaiian) bold, courageous.
Kekoah

Kelan (Irish) a form of Keelan.

Kelby BG (German) farm by the spring. (English) a form of Kolby.
Keelby, Kelbee, Kelbey, Kelbi, Kelbie, Kellbee, Kellbey, Kellbi, Kellbie, Kellby

Kelcey GB (Scandinavian) a form of Kelsey.
Kelci, Kelcie, Kelcy, Kellci, Kellcie, Kellcy

Keldon (English) a form of Kelton.
Keldan, Kelden, Keldin

Kele BG (Hopi) sparrow hawk. (Hawaiian) a form of Jerry.
Kelle

Kelemen (Hungarian) gentle; kind.
Kelleman, Kellemen, Kellieman, Kelliemen, Kelliman, Kellimen, Kellyman, Kellymen, Kelyman, Kelymen

Kelevi (Finnish) hero.
Kelevee, Kelevey, Kelevie, Kelevy

Keli GB (Hawaiian) a form of Terry.
Kelee, Keleigh, Kelie, Kely

Keli'i (Hawaiian) chief.

Kelile (Ethiopian) protected.
Kelyle

Kell (Scandinavian) spring.
Kel

Kellan BG (Irish) a form of Kellen.
Keillan

Kellen BG (Irish) mighty warrior. A form of Kelly.
Kelden, Kelin, Kelle, Kellin, Kellyn, Kelyn, Kelynn

Keller (Irish) little companion.
Keler

Kelley GB (Irish) a form of Kelly.

Kelly GB (Irish) warrior.
Keallea, Keallee, Kealleigh, Kealley, Kealli, Keallie, Keally, Keilee, Keileigh, Keiley, Keili, Keilie, Keillea, Keillee, Keilleigh, Keilley, Keilli, Keillie, Keilly, Keily, Kelle, Kellee, Kelli, Kellie, Kely, Keylee, Keyleigh, Keyley, Keyli, Keylie, Keyllee, Keylleigh, Keylley, Keyly

Kelmen (Basque) merciful.
Kellman, Kellmen, Kelman, Kelmin

Kelsey GB (Scandinavian) island of ships.
Kelse, Kelsea, Kelsi, Kelsie, Kelso, Kelsy, Kesley, Kesly

Kelson (English) a form of Kelton.
Kelston

Kelton (English) keel town; port.
Keltan, Kelten, Keltin, Keltonn, Keltyn

Kelvin (Irish, English) narrow river. Geography: a river in Scotland.
Kelvan, Kelven, Kelvon, Kelvyn

Kelwin (English) friend from the ridge.
Kelwen, Kelwinn, Kelwyn, Kelwynn,
Kelwynne

Kemal (Turkish) highest honor.
Kemel

Kemen (Basque) strong.
Keaman, Keamen, Keeman, Keemen, Keiman,
Keimen, Keman, Keyman, Keymen

Kemp (English) fighter; champion.
Kempe

Kempton (English) military town.
Kemptan, Kempten, Kemptin, Kemptyn

Ken (Japanese) one's own kind. (Scottish) a
short form of Kendall, Kendrick, Kenneth.
Kena, Kenn, Keno

Kenan (Irish) a form of Keenan.
Kenen, Kenin, Kenon, Kenyn

Kenán (Hebrew) to acquire.

Kenaniá (Hebrew) God stabilizes.

Kenard (Irish) a form of Kennard.
Kenerd

Kenaz (Hebrew) bright.

Kendal 🇬🇧 (English) a form of Kendall.
Kendali, Kendelle, Kendul, Kendyl

Kendale (English) a form of Kendall.

Kendall 🇬🇧 (English) valley of the river Kent.
Kendell, Kendyll, Kyndall

Kendarius (American) a combination of
Ken + Darius.
Kendarious, Kendarrious, Kendarrius,
Kenderious, Kenderius, Kenderyious

Kendel 🇧🇬 (English) a form of Kendall.

Kendell 🇧🇬 (English) a form of Kendall.

Kendrell (English) a form of Kendall.
Kendrall, Kendrel, Kendryll

Kendrew (Scottish) a form of Andrew.
Kandrew

Kendric (Irish, Scottish) a form of Kendrick.
Kendryc

Kendrick (Irish) son of Henry. (Scottish)
royal chieftain.
Kenderrick, Kendrich, Kendricks, Kendrik,

Kendrix, Kendryck, Kendryk, Kenedrick,
Kenndrick, Keondric, Keondrick, Keondryc,
Keondryck, Keondryk

Kenji (Japanese) intelligent second son.

Kenley 🇧🇬 (English) royal meadow.
Kenlea, Kenlee, Kenleigh, Kenli, Kenlie,
Kenly, Kennlea, Kennlee, Kennleigh, Kennley,
Kennli, Kennlie, Kennly

Kenn (Scottish) a form of Ken.

Kennan (Scottish) little Ken.
Kenna, Kennen, Kennin, Kennyn

Kennard (Irish) brave chieftain.
Kenner, Kennerd

Kennedy 🇬🇧 (Irish) helmeted chief. History:
John F. Kennedy was the thirty-fifth U.S.
president.
Kenedy, Kenidy, Kennadie, Kennady,
Kennedey, Kennedi, Kennedie

Kenneth (Irish) handsome. (English) royal
oath.
Keneth, Kenneith, Kennet, Kennethen,
Kennett, Kennieth, Kennth, Kennyth, Kenyth

Kennith (Irish, English) a form of Kenneth.

Kennon (Scottish) a form of Kennan.

Kenny (Scottish) a familiar form of Kenneth.
Keni, Kenney, Kenni, Kennie, Kinnie

Kenric (English) a form of Kenrick.

Kenrick (English) bold ruler; royal ruler.
Kennric, Kennrick, Kennrik, Kennryc,
Kennryck, Kennryk, Kenricks, Kenrik,
Kenryc, Kenryck, Kenryk, Kenryks

Kent (Welsh) white; bright. (English) a short
form of Kenton. Geography: a region in
England.

Kentaro (Japanese) big boy.

Kenton (English) from Kent, England.
Kentan, Kenten, Kentin, Kentonn, Kentyn

Kentrell (English) king's estate.
Kenreal, Kentrel, Kentrelle

Kenward (English) brave; royal guardian.

Kenya 🇬🇧 (Hebrew) animal horn. (Russian)
a form of Kenneth. Geography: a country

in east-central Africa.
Kenia, Keniah, Kenja

Kenyan (Irish) a form of Kenyon.

Kenyatta GB (American) a form of Kenya.
Kenyat, Kenyata, Kenyatae, Kenyatee,
Kenyatt, Kenyatter, Kenyatti, Kenyotta

Kenyon (Irish) white haired, blond.
Kenyen, Kenyin, Kenynn, Keonyon

Kenzie GB (Scottish) wise leader. See also
Mackenzie.
Kensi, Kensie, Kensy, Kenzi, Kenzy

Keoki (Hawaiian) a form of George.

Keola (Hawaiian) life.

Keon (Irish) a form of Ewan.
Keaon, Keeon, Keone, Keonne, Kyon

Keondre (American) a form of Keandre.

Keoni BG (Hawaiian) a form of John.
Keonee, Keonie, Keony

Keonta (American) a form of Keon.

Keontae, Keonte, Keonté (American)
forms of Keon.
Keonntay, Keontay, Keontaye, Keontez,
Keontia, Keontis, Keontrae, Keontre, Keontrey,
Keontrye

Kerbasi (Basque) warrior.

Kerel (Afrikaans) young.
Kerell

Kerem (Turkish) noble; kind.
Kereem

Kerey (Gypsy) homeward bound.
Ker, Keree, Keri, Kerie, Kery

Kerman (Basque) from Germany.
Kermen, Kerrman, Kerrmen

Kermit (Irish) a form of Dermot.
Kermey, Kermie, Kermitt, Kermy, Kermyt,
Kermytt

Kern (Irish) a short form of Kieran.
Keirn, Keirne, Kerne, Kerrn, Kerrne, Keyrn,
Keyrne

Keron (Hebrew) a form of Keren (see Girls'
Names).

Kerr (Scandinavian) a form of Carr.
Karr

Kerrick (English) king's rule.
Keric, Kerick, Kerik, Kerric, Kerrik, Kerryc,
Kerryck, Kerryk, Keryc, Keryck, Keryk

Kerry GB (Irish) dark; dark haired.
Kerree, Kerrey, Kerri, Kerrie, Kery

Kers (Todas) Botany: an Indian plant.

Kersen (Indonesian) cherry.
Kersan, Kersin, Kerson, Kersyn

Kerstan (Dutch) a form of Christian.
Kersten, Kerstin, Kerston, Kerstyn

Kervin (Irish, English) a form of Kerwin.
Kervyn

Kerwin (Irish) little; dark. (English) friend of
the marshlands.
Kerwain, Kerwaine, Kerwan, Kerwane,
Kerwinn, Kerwon, Kerwyn, Kerwynn,
Kerwynne, Kirwin, Kirwyn

Kesar (Russian) a form of Caesar.
Kesare

Keshaun, Késhawn, Keshon (American)
forms of Keshawn.

Keshawn (American) a combination of the
prefix Ke + Shawn.
Keeshaun, Keeshawn, Keeshon, Kesean,
Keshan, Keshane, Keshayne, Keshion,
Keshone

Keshun (American) a form of Keshawn.

Kesin (Hindi) long-haired beggar.
Kesyn

Kesse (Ashanti, Fante) chubby baby.
Kesse, Kessi, Kessie, Kessy, Kezi, Kezie,
Kezy, Kezzi, Kezzie, Kezzy

Kester (English) a form of Christopher.

Kestrel (English) falcon.
Kes, Kestrell

Keung (Chinese) universe.

Kevan, Keven, Kevon (Irish) forms of
Kevin.
Keve, Keveen, Kevone, Kevonne, Kevoyn,
Kevron, Keyvan, Keyven, Keyvon, Keyvyn,
Kiven, Kivon

Kevin ⚝ (Irish) handsome. See also Cavan.
Kaiven, Keaven, Keivan, Kev, Keverne,
Kevian, Kevien, Kévin, Kevinn, Kevins,
Kevis, Kevn, Kevun, Kevvy, Keyvin

Kevion (Irish) a form of Kevin.
Keveon

Kevontae, Kevonte (American) forms of
Kevin.

Kevyn 🅱️🅶 (Irish) a form of Kevin.

Kewan, Kewon (American) forms of Kevin.
Kewane, Kewaun, Kewone, Kiwan, Kiwane

Key (English) key; protected.
Kei, Keye

Keyan, Keyon (Irish) forms of Keon.
Keyen, Keyin, Keyion

Keynan (Irish) a form of Keenan.
Keynin, Keynon, Keynyn

Keyonta (American) a form of Keon.

Keyshawn (American) a combination of
Key + Shawn.
Keyshan, Keyshaun, Keyshon, Keyshun

Keyton (English) a form of Keaton.
Keytan, Keyten, Keytin, Keytun, Keytyn

Khachig (Armenian) small cross.

Khachik (Armenian) a form of Khachig.

Khaim (Russian) a form of Chaim.

Khaldun (Arabic) forever.
Khaldoon, Khaldoun

Khaldûn (Arabic) a form of Khaldun.

Khaled, Khalid, Khallid (Arabic) forms of
Khälid.

Khaleel (Arabic) a form of Khalíl.

Khalfani (Swahili) born to lead.
Khalfan

Khalîd (Arabic) a form of Khälid.

Khälid (Arabic) eternal.
Khalyd

Khalil (Arabic) a form of Khalíl.

Khalíl (Arabic) friend.
Khahlil, Khailil, Khailyl, Khalee, Khaleil, Khali,
Khalial, Khaliel, Khalihl, Khalill, Khaliyl

Khalîl (Arabic) a form of Khalil.

Khaliq (Arabic) creative.
Khaliqu, Khalique, Khalyq, Khalyqu, Khalyque

Khâliq (Arabic) a form of Khaliq.

Khamisi (Swahili) born on Thursday.
Kham, Khamisy, Khamysi, Khamysy

Khan (Turkish) prince.
Chan, Kahn, Khanh

Kharald (Russian) a form of Gerald.

Khayrî (Arabic) charitable.

Khayru (Arabic) benevolent.

Khentimentiu (Egyptian) god of death.

Khiry (Arabic) a form of Khayru.
Khiri, Kiry

Khnum (Egyptian) rising sun.

Khons (Egyptian) god of the moon.

Khoury (Arabic) priest.
Khori, Khorie, Khory, Khouri, Khourie

Khrisna (Indian) the black one.

Khristian (Greek) a form of Christian,
Kristian.
Khris, Khristan, Khristin, Khriston,
Khrystian, Khrystiyan

Khristopher (Greek) a form of Kristopher.
Khristofer, Khristoffer, Khristoph, Khristophar,
Khristophe, Khrystopher

Khristos (Greek) a form of Christos.
Khrystos, Krystous

Khûrî (Arabic) priest.

Ki 🅱️🅶 (Korean) arisen.

Kian, Kion (Irish) forms of Keon.
Kione, Kionie, Kionne

Kibuuka (Luganda) brave warrior.
Mythology: a Ganda warrior deity.
Kybuuka

Kidd (English) child; young goat.
Kid, Kyd

Kiefer, Kieffer (German) forms of Keifer.
Kief, Kiefor, Kiffer, Kiiefer

Kiel (Irish) a form of Kyle.
Kiell

Kiele GB (Hawaiian) gardenia.
Kyele

Kienan (Irish) a form of Keenan.
Kienon

Kier (Irish) a short form of Kieran.
Kierr, Kierre

Kieran BG (Irish) little and dark; little Keir.
*Keeran, Keeren, Keerin, Keeron, Kiaron,
Kiarron, Kierian, Kierien, Kierin*

Kieren, Kieron (Irish) forms of Kieran.
Kierron

Kiernan (Irish) a form of Kieran.
Kern, Kernan, Kiernen

Kiet (Tai) honor.
Kyet

Kifeda (Luo) only boy among girls.
Kyfeda

Kiho (Rutooro) born on a foggy day.
Kyho

Kijika (Native American) quiet walker.
Kijyka, Kyjika, Kyjyka

Kika (Hawaiian) a form of Keith.
Kikah, Kyka, Kykah

Kiki GB (Spanish) a form of Henry.

Kile (Irish) a form of Kyle.
*Kilee, Kilei, Kileigh, Kilen, Kili, Kilie, Kily,
Kiyl, Kiyle*

Kiley GB (Irish) a form of Kyle.
Kylee, Kyley, Kylie

Killian (Irish) little Kelly.
*Kilean, Kilian, Kiliane, Kilien, Killie,
Killiean, Killien, Killienn, Killion, Killy,
Kylia, Kylien, Kyllian, Kyllien*

Kim GB (English) a short form of Kimball.
Kimie, Kimmy, Kym

Kimani BG (Shoshone) a form of Kimana
(see Girls' Names).

Kimball (Greek) hollow vessel. (English)
warrior chief.
*Kimbal, Kimbel, Kimbele, Kimbell, Kimble,
Kymbal, Kymbel, Kymbele, Kymbell*

Kimo (Hawaiian) a form of James.

Kimokeo (Hawaiian) a form of Timothy.

Kin (Japanese) golden.
Kyn

Kincaid (Scottish) battle chief.
*Kincade, Kincaide, Kincayd, Kincayde,
Kinkaid, Kyncaid, Kyncayd, Kyncayde*

Kindin (Basque) fifth.
Kindyn, Kyndin, Kyndyn

King (English) king. A short form of names
beginning with "King."
Kyng

Kingsley (English) king's meadow.
*Kings, Kingslea, Kingslee, Kingsleigh, Kingsli,
Kingslie, Kingsly, Kingzlee, Kinslea, Kinslee,
Kinsleigh, Kinsley, Kinsli, Kinslie, Kinsly,
Kyngs, Kyngslea, Kyngslee, Kyngsleigh,
Kyngsley, Kyngsli, Kyngslie, Kyngsly*

Kingston (English) king's estate.
Kinston, Kyngston, Kynston

Kingswell (English) king's well.
Kingswel, Kyngswel, Kyngswell

Kini GB (Hawaiian) a short form of Iukini.

Kinnard (Irish) tall slope.
Kinard, Kynard, Kynnard

Kinsey GB (English) victorious royalty.
*Kinsee, Kinsi, Kinsie, Kinze, Kinzie, Kynsee,
Kynsey, Kynsi, Kynsie, Kynsy*

Kinton (Hindi) crowned.
Kynton

Kioshi (Japanese) quiet.

Kip BG (English) a form of Kipp.
Kyp

Kipp (English) pointed hill.
Kippar, Kipper, Kippie, Kippy, Kypp

Kir (Bulgarian) a familiar form of Cyrus.

Kiral (Turkish) king; supreme leader.
Kyral

Kiran GB (Sanskrit) beam of light.
Kiren, Kirin, Kiron, Kirun, Kiryn

Kirby 🅱🅖 (Scandinavian) church village.
(English) cottage by the water.
Kerbbee, Kerbbey, Kerbbi, Kerbbie, Kerbby,
Kerbee, Kerbey, Kerbi, Kerbie, Kerby, Kirbee,
Kirbey, Kirbie, Kirkby, Kyrbbee, Kyrbbey,
Kyrbbi, Kyrbbie, Kyrbby, Kyrbee, Kyrbey,
Kyrbi, Kyrbie, Kyrby

Kiri (Cambodian) mountain.
Kiry, Kyri, Kyry

Kirian (Irish) he who was born in a dark
place.

Kiril (Slavic) a form of Cyril.
Kirill, Kiryl, Kiryll, Kyril, Kyrill, Kyrillos,
Kyryl, Kyryll

Kirios (Greek) the supreme being.

Kiritan (Hindi) wearing a crown.
Kiriten, Kiritin, Kiriton, Kirityn

Kirk (Scandinavian) church.
Kerc, Kerck, Kerk, Kirc, Kirck, Kurc, Kurck,
Kurk, Kyrc, Kyrck, Kyrk

Kirkland (English) church land.
Kerkland, Kirklind, Kirklynd, Kurkland,
Kyrkland

Kirkley (English) church meadow.
Kerklea, Kerklee, Kerkleigh, Kerkley, Kerkli,
Kerklie, Kerkly, Kirklea, Kirklee, Kirkleigh,
Kirkli, Kirklie, Kirkly, Kurklea, Kurklee,
Kurkleigh, Kurkley, Kurkli, Kurklie, Kurkly,
Kyrklea, Kyrklee, Kyrkleigh, Kyrkley, Kyrkli,
Kyrklie, Kyrkly

Kirklin (English) a form of Kirkland.
Kerklan, Kirklan, Kirklen, Kirkline, Kirkloun,
Kirklun, Kirklyn, Kirklynn, Kurklan, Kyrklan

Kirkwell (English) church well; church
spring.
Kerkwel, Kerkwell, Kirkwel, Kurkwel,
Kurkwell, Kyrkwel, Kyrkwell

Kirkwood (English) church forest.
Kerkwood, Kurkwood, Kyrkwood

Kirt (Latin, German, French) a form of Kurt.

Kirton (English) church town.
Kerston, Kirston, Kurston, Kyrston

Kishan (American) a form of Keshawn.
Kishaun, Kishawn, Kishen, Kishon, Kyshon,
Kyshun

Kistna (Hindi) sacred, holy. Geography: a
sacred river in India.
Kisstna, Kysstna, Kystna

Kistur (Gypsy) skillful rider.

Kit (Greek) a familiar form of Christian,
Christopher, Kristopher.
Kitt, Kitts

Kito (Swahili) jewel; precious child.
Kitto, Kyto, Kytto

Kitwana (Swahili) pledged to live.
Kitwanah

Kiva (Hebrew) a short form of Akiva, Jacob.
Kiba, Kivah, Kivi, Kiwa, Kyva, Kyvah

Kiyoshi (Japanese) quiet; peaceful.

Kizza (Luganda) born after twins.
Kiza, Kizah, Kizzi, Kizzie, Kizzy, Kyza,
Kyzah, Kyzza, Kyzzah, Kyzzi, Kyzzie,
Kyzzy

Kjell (Swedish) a form of Karl.
Kjel

Klaus (German) a short form of Nicholas. A
form of Claus.
Klaas, Klaes, Klas, Klause

Klay (English) a form of Clay.

Klayton (English) a form of Clayton.

Kleef (Dutch) cliff.

Klement (Czech) a form of Clement.
Klema, Klemenis, Klemens, Klemet, Klemo,
Klim, Klimek, Kliment, Klimka

Kleng (Norwegian) claw.

Knight (English) armored knight.
Knightleigh, Knightly, Knyght

Knoton (Native American) a form of
Nodin.

Knowles (English) grassy slope.
Knolls, Nowles

Knox (English) hill.

Knute (Scandinavian) a form of Canute.
Kanut, Kanute, Knud, Knut

Kobi, Koby (Polish) familiar forms of Jacob.
Kobby, Kobe, Kobee, Kobey, Kobia, Kobie

Kodey (English) a form of Cody.
Kode, Kodee, Kodi, Kodye

Kodi BG (English) a form of Cody.

Kodie BG (English) a form of Cody.

Kody BG (English) a form of Cody.

Kofi (Twi) born on Friday.

Kohana (Lakota) swift.
Kohanah

Kohl (English) a form of Cole.
Kohle

Koi (Choctaw) panther. (Hawaiian) a form of Troy.

Kojo (Akan) born on Monday.

Koka (Hawaiian) Scotsman.
Kokah

Kokayi (Shona) gathered together.

Kolby BG (English) a form of Colby.
Koalby, Koelby, Kohlbe, Kohlby, Kolbe, Kolbey, Kolbi, Kolbie, Kolebe, Koleby, Kollby

Kole (English) a form of Cole.

Koleman (English) a form of Coleman.
Kolemann, Kolemen

Kolin, Kollin (English) forms of Colin.
Kolen, Kollen, Kollyn, Kolyn

Kolt (English) a short form of Koltan. A form of Colt.
Kolte

Koltan, Kolten, Koltin, Kolton, Koltyn (English) forms of Colton.
Koltn

Kolya (Russian) a familiar form of Nikolai, Nikolos.
Kola, Kolenka, Kolia, Koliah, Kolja

Kona BG (Hawaiian) a form of Don.
Konah, Konala

Konane (Hawaiian) bright moonlight.
Konan

Kondo (Swahili) war.

Kong (Chinese) glorious; sky.

Konner, Konnor (Irish) forms of Connar, Connor.
Kohner, Kohnor, Konar, Koner, Konor

Kono (Moquelumnan) squirrel eating a pine nut.

Konrad (German) a form of Conrad.
Khonrad, Koen, Koenraad, Kon, Konn, Konney, Konni, Konnie, Konny, Konrád, Konrade, Konrado, Kord, Kunz

Konstantin (German, Russian) a form of Constantine. See also Dinos.
Konstadine, Konstadino, Konstancji, Konstandinos, Konstantinas, Konstantine, Konstantio, Konstanty, Konstantyn, Konstantyne, Konstanz, Konstatino, Kostadino, Kostadinos, Kostandino, Kostandinos, Kostantin, Kostantino, Kostenka, Kostya, Kotsos

Konstantinos (Greek) a form of Constantine.

Kontar (Akan) only child.

Korb (German) basket.

Korbin (English) a form of Corbin.
Korban, Korben, Korbyn

Kordell (English) a form of Cordell.
Kordel

Korey BG (Irish) a form of Corey, Kory.
Korrey, Korri, Korrie

Kori, Korie GB (Irish) forms of Corey, Kory.

Kornel (Latin) a form of Cornelius, Kornelius.
Korneil, Kornél, Korneli, Kornelisz, Kornell, Krelis, Soma

Kornelius (Latin) a form of Cornelius. See also Kees, Kornel.
Karnelius, Korneilius, Korneliaus, Kornelious, Kornellius

Korrigan (Irish) a form of Corrigan.
Korigan, Korrigon, Korrigun

Kort (German, Dutch) a form of Cort, Kurt. (German) a form of Konrad.
Kourt

Kortney GB (English) a form of Courtney.
Kortni, Kourtney

Korudon (Greek) helmeted one.

Kory BG (Irish) a form of Corey.
Kore, Koree, Korei, Korio, Korre, Korree, Korria, Korry, Korrye

Korydon (Greek) a form of Corydon.
Koridan, Koriden, Koridin, Koridon, Koridyn, Korydan, Koryden, Korydin, Korydyn

Kosey (African) lion.
Kosse, Kossee, Kossey

Kosmo (Greek) a form of Cosmo.
Kosmas, Kosmos, Kosmy, Kozmo

Kostas (Greek) a short form of Konstantin.

Kosti (Finnish) a form of Gustave.

Kosumi (Moquelumnan) spear fisher.

Koty (English) a form of Cody.

Koukalaka (Hawaiian) a form of Douglas.

Kourtland (English) a form of Courtland.
Kortlan, Kortland, Kortlend, Kortlon, Kourtlin

Kovit (Tai) expert.
Kovyt

Kraig (Irish, Scottish) a form of Craig.
Kraggie, Kraggy, Krayg, Kreg, Kreig, Kreigh

Kramer (English) a form of Cramer.
Krammer

Krikor (Armenian) a form of Gregory.

Kris BG (Greek) a form of Chris. A short form of Kristian, Kristofer, Kristopher.
Kriss, Krys

Krischan, Krishan (German) forms of Christian.
Krishaun, Krishawn, Krishon, Krishun

Krishna BG (Hindi) delightful, pleasurable. Religion: the eighth and principal avatar of the Hindu god Vishnu.
Kistna, Kistnah, Krisha, Krishnah, Kryshanh, Kryshna

Krisiant (Welsh) a form of Crisiant.
Krisient, Krysient, Krysyent

Krispin (Latin) a form of Crispin.
Krispian, Krispino, Krispo, Kryspyn

Kristen GB (Greek) a form of Kristian.
Kristan, Kristin, Kristinn

Krister (Swedish) a form of Christian.
Krist, Kristar

Kristian BG (Greek) a form of Christian, Khristian.
Kristek, Kristien, Kristine, Kristion

Kristjan (Estonian) a form of Christian, Khristian.

Kristo (Greek) a short form of Khristopher.
Khristo, Khrysto

Kristofer, Kristoffer (Swedish) forms of Kristopher.
Kristafer, Kristef, Kristfer, Kristfor, Kristifer, Kristofo, Kristofor, Kristoforo, Kristofyr, Kristufer, Kristus

Kristoff (Greek) a short form of Kristofer, Kristopher.
Khristof, Khristoff, Khrystof, Khrystoff, Kristof, Kristóf, Krystof, Krystoff

Kriston BG (Greek) a form of Kristian.

Kristophe (French) a form of Kristopher.
Khristoph, Khrystoph, Kristoph, Krystoph

Kristopher (Greek) a form of Christopher. See also Topher.
Krisstopher, Kristapher, Kristepher, Kristophor, Krisus, Krystupas

Kruz (Spanish) a form of Cruz.
Kruise, Kruize, Kruse, Kruze, Kruzz

Krystian BG (Polish) a form of Christian.
Krys, Krystek, Krystien, Krystin

Krystopher (Greek) a form of Christopher.
Krystofer

Krzysztof (Polish) a form of Kristoff.

Kuba (Czech) a form of Jacob.
Kubo, Kubus

Kueng (Chinese) universe.

Kugonza (Rutooro) love.

Kuiril (Basque) lord.

Kullen (Irish) a form of Cullen.

Kumar (Sanskrit) prince.

Kunle (Yoruba) home filled with honors.

Kuper (Yiddish) copper.
Kopper, Kupor, Kupper

Kurt (Latin, German, French) a short form of Kurtis. A form of Curt.
Kuno, Kurtt

Kurtis (Latin, French) a form of Curtis.
Kirtis, Kirtus, Kurtes, Kurtez, Kurtice, Kurties, Kurtiss, Kurtus, Kurtys, Kurtyss

Kuruk (Pawnee) bear.

Kuzih (Carrier) good speaker.

Kwabena (Akan) born on Tuesday.

Kwacha (Nguni) morning.

Kwako (Akan) born on Wednesday.
Kwaka, Kwakou, Kwaku

Kwam (Zuni) a form of John.

Kwame (Akan) born on Saturday.
Kwamen, Kwami, Kwamin

Kwamé (Akan) a form of Kwame.

Kwan (Korean) strong.
Kwane

Kwasi (Akan) born on Sunday. (Swahili) wealthy.
Kwasie, Kwazzi, Kwesi

Kwayera (Nguni) dawn.

Kwende (Nguni) let's go.

Ky, Kye (Irish, Yiddish) short forms of Kyle.

Kyele (Irish) a form of Kyle.

Kylan, Kylen (Irish) forms of Kyle.
Kyelen, Kyleen, Kylin, Kyline, Kylon, Kylun

Kylar, Kylor (English) forms of Kyle.

Kyle ✰ BG (Irish) narrow piece of land; place where cattle graze. (Yiddish) crowned with laurels.
Cyle, Kilan, Kilen, Kyel, Kyll, Kyrell

Kyler BG (English) a form of Kyle.

Kylle (Irish) a form of Kyle.

Kynan (Welsh) chief.
Kinan

Kyndall GB (English) a form of Kendall.
Kyndal, Kyndel, Kyndell, Kyndle

Kyne (English) royal.

Kyran, Kyren, Kyron (Irish) forms of Kieran. (Sanskrit) forms of Kiran.
Kyrin, Kyrone, Kyrun, Kyryn

Kyree (Cambodian, Maori, Greek) a form of Kyrie (see Girls' Names).

Kyrios (Greek) sir.

Kyros (Greek) master.
Kiros

Kyven (American) a form of Kevin.
Kyvan, Kyvaun, Kyvon, Kywon, Kywynn

La'darius, Ladarrius (American) forms of Ladarius.
Ladarrias, Ladarries, Ladarrious

Laban (Hawaiian) white.
Laben, Labin, Labon, Labyn, Lebaan, Leban

Labán (Hebrew) a form of Laban.

Labaron (American) a combination of the prefix La + Baron.
Labaren, Labarren, Labarron, Labearon, Labron

Labib (Arabic) sensible; intelligent.
Labyb

Labîb (Arabic) a form of Labib.

Labrentsis (Russian) a form of Lawrence.
Labhras, Labhruinn, Labrencis

Lachlan (Scottish) land of lakes.
Lache, Lachlann, Lachlun, Lachlunn, Lachunn, Lakelan, Lakeland

Lacy GB (Greek, Latin) cheerful.

Ladarian (American) a combination of the prefix La + Darian.
Ladarien, Ladarin, Ladarion, Ladarren, Ladarrian, Ladarrien, Ladarrin, Ladarrion, Laderion, Laderrian, Laderrion

Ladarius (American) a combination of the prefix La + Darius.
Ladarious, Ladaris, Ladauris, Laderius, Laderrious, Laderris, Ladirus

Ladd (English) attendant.
Lad, Laddey, Laddie, Laddy

Laderrick (American) a combination of the prefix La + Derric.
Ladarrick, Ladereck, Laderic, Laderricks

Ladio (Slavic) he who governs with glory.

Ladislav (Czech) a form of Walter.
Laco, Lada, Ladislao, Ladislas, Ladislaus, Ladyslas, Ladyslaus, Ladyslav

Lado (Fante) second-born son.

Ladolfo, Landolf, Landolfo (Germanic) skillful as a wolf in the city.

Laertes (Greek) the rock-picker.

Lafayette (French) History: Marquis de Lafayette was a French soldier and politician who aided the American Revolution.
Lafaiete, Lafayett, Lafette, Laffyette

Lagan (Indian) appropriate time.

Lahual (Araucanian) larch tree.

Laidley (English) path along the marshy meadow.
Laedlea, Laedlee, Laedleigh, Laedley, Laedli, Laedlie, Laedly, Laidlea, Laidlee, Laidleigh, Laidli, Laidlie, Laidly, Laydlea, Laydlee, Laydleigh, Laydley, Laydli, Laydlie, Laydly

Lain (English) a form of Lane.

Laine BG (English) a form of Lane.

Laird (Scottish) wealthy landowner.
Layrd

Lais (Arabic) lion.
Lays

Laith (Scandinavian, English) a form of Latham.
Lathe

Lajos (Hungarian) famous; holy.
Lajcsi, Laji, Lali

Lajuan (American) a combination of the prefix La + Juan.

Lake (English) lake.
Laek, Laik, Lakan, Lakane, Lakee, Laken, Lakin, Layk

Lakeith (American) a combination of the prefix La + Keith.

Lakota BG (Dakota) a tribal name.
Lakoda

Lakshman (Indian) younger brother of the Hindu god Rama.

Lakshmibanta (Indian) fortunate.

Lakshmidhar, Lakshmigopal, Lakshmikanta, Lohitaksha, Loknath, Lokranjan (Indian) other names for the Hindu god Vishnu.

Lal (Hindi) beloved.

Lalit, Lalitkishore, Lalitkumar, Lalitmohan (Indian) beautiful.

Lalla (Spanish) well spoken.

Lamani BG (Tongan) lemon.
Lamanee, Lamaney, Lamanie, Lamany

Lamar (German) famous throughout the land. (French) sea, ocean.
Lamair, Lamaris, Lamarre, Larmar, Lemar

Lamarcus (American) a combination of the prefix La + Marcus.

Lamario (American) a form of Lamar.

Lamarr (German, French) a form of Lamar.

Lambert (German) bright land.
Bert, Lambard, Lamberto, Lamberts, Lambirt, Lambirto, Lamburt, Lamburto, Lambyrt, Lambyrto, Lampard, Landbert, Landberto, Landbirt, Landbirto, Landburt, Landburto, Landbyrt, Landbyrto, Landebirt, Landeburt, Landebyrt

Lambodar (Indian) another name for the Hindu god Ganesh.

Lami (Tongan) hidden.
Lamee, Lamey, Lamie, Lamy

Lamon (French) a form of Lamond.

Lamond (French) world.
Lammond, Lamonde, Lamondo, Lamondre, Lamund, Lemond, Lemund

Lamont (Scandinavian) lawyer.
Lamaunt, Lamonta, Lamontie, Lamonto, Lamount, Lemmont, Lemont, Lemonte

Lamonte (Scandinavian) a form of Lamont.

Lance (German) a short form of Lancelot.
Lancey, Lancy, Lanse, Lantz, Lanz, Launce

Lancelin (French) servant.

Lancelot (French) attendant. Literature: the knight who loved King Arthur's wife, Queen Guinevere.
Lancelott, Lancilot, Lancilott, Lancilotte, Lancilotto, Lancylot, Lancylott, Lancylotte, Launcelet, Launcelot, Launcelott, Launcelotte

Landan, Landen, Landin (English) forms of Landon.
Landenn

Landelino (Teutonic) he who is a friend of the earth.

Lander (Basque) lion man. (English) landowner.
Landar, Landers, Landor, Landors, Launder, Launders

Landerico (Teutonic) powerful in the region.

Landis (French) one who comes from the prairie.

Lando (Portuguese, Spanish) a short form of Orlando, Rolando.
Londow

Landon ⭐ BG (English) open, grassy meadow. A form of Langdon.
Landun, Landyn

Landrada (Teutonic) counselor in his village.

Landric (German) ruler of the land.
Landrick, Landrik, Landryc, Landryck, Landryk

Landry (French, English) ruler.
Landre, Landré, Landri, Landrie, Landrue

Lane BG (English) narrow road.
Laney, Lani, Lanie, Layne

Lang (Scandinavian) tall man.
Laing, Lange

Langdon (English) long hill.
Langdan, Langden, Langdin, Langdun, Langdyn

Langford (English) long ford.
Laingford, Lanford, Lankford

Langi (Tongan) heaven.
Langee, Langey, Langie, Langy

Langley GB (English) long meadow.
Lainglea, Lainglee, Laingleigh, Laingley, Laingli, Lainglie, Laingly, Langlea, Langlee, Langleigh, Langli, Langlie, Langly

Langston (English) long, narrow town.
Laingston, Langsden, Langsdon, Langstone

Langundo (Native American) peaceful.
Langund

Lani GB (Hawaiian) heaven.
Lanee, Laney, Lanie, Lany

Lankesh (Indian) another name for the Hindu demon king Ravana.

Lanny (American) a familiar form of Laurence, Lawrence.
Lannee, Lanney, Lanni, Lannie

Lanu (Moquelumnan) running around the pole.

Lanz (Italian) a form of Lance.
Lanzo, Lonzo

Lao (Spanish) a short form of Stanislaus.

Lap (Vietnamese) independent.

Lapidos (Hebrew) torches.
Lapidoth

Laquan (American) a combination of the prefix La + Quan.
Laquain, Laquann, Laquanta, Laquantae, Laquante, Laquawn, Laquawne, Laquin, Laquinn, Laqun, Laquon, Laquone, Laqwan, Laqwon

Laquintin (American) a combination of the prefix La + Quinten.
Laquentin, Laquenton, Laquintas, Laquinten, Laquintiss, Laquinton, Laquyntan, Laquynten, Laquyntin, Laquynton, Laquyntun, Laquyntyn

Laramie GB (French) tears of love. Geography: a town in Wyoming on the Overland Trail.
Laramee, Laramey, Larami, Laramy, Laremy

Larenz (Italian, Spanish) a short form of Larenzo.

Larenzo (Italian, Spanish) a form of Lorenzo.
Larenza, Larinzo, Laurenzo

Larkin (Irish) rough; fierce.
Larkan, Larken, Larklin, Larklyn, Larkyn

Larnell (American) a combination of Larry + Darnell.
Larnel

Laron (French) thief.
La Ron, La Ruan, La'ron, Laran, Laraun, Laren, Larin, Larone, Laronn, Larron, Larun, Laryn

Larrimore (French) armorer.
Larimore, Larmer, Larmor

Larry (Latin) a familiar form of Lawrence.
Lari, Larie, Larri, Larrie, Lary

Lars (Scandinavian) a form of Lawrence.
Laris, Larris, Larse, Larz, Laurans, Laurits, Lavrans, Lorens

Larson (Scandinavian) son of Lars.
Larsen, Larsson, Larzon

LaSalle (French) hall.
Lasal, Lasale, Lasalle, Lascell, Lascelles

Lash (Gypsy) a form of Louis.
Lashi, Lasho

Lashaun BG (American) a form of Lashawn.

Lashawn BG (American) a combination of the prefix La + Shawn.
Lasaun, Lasean, Lashajaun, Lashan, Lashane, Lashun

Lashon GB (American) a form of Lashawn.

Lashone (American) a form of Lashawn.
Lashonne

Lasse (Finnish) a form of Nicholas.
Lase

László (Hungarian) famous ruler.
Laci, Lacko, Laslo, Lazlo

Latafat (Indian) elegance.

Lateef (Arabic) gentle; pleasant.
Latif, Latyf, Letif, Letyf

Latham (Scandinavian) barn. (English) district.
Lathe, Lay

Lathan (American) a combination of the prefix La + Nathan.
Lathaniel, Lathen, Lathin, Lathyn, Leathan

Lathrop (English) barn, farmstead.
Lathe, Lathrope, Lay

Latîf (Arabic) friendly; pleasant.

Latimer (English) interpreter.
Lat, Latimor, Lattie, Latty, Latymer

Latravis (American) a combination of the prefix La + Travis.
Latavious, Latavius, Lataveus, Latraviaus, Latravious, Latravius, Latravys, Latrayvious, Latrayvous, Latrivis

Latrell (American) a combination of the prefix La + Kentrell.
Latreal, Latreil, Latrel, Latrelle, Letreal, Letrel, Letrell, Letrelle

Laudalino (Portuguese) praised.
Laudalin, Laudalyn, Laudalyno

Laughlin (Irish) servant of Saint Secundinus.
Lanty, Lauchlin, Laughlyn, Leachlain, Leachlainn

Laura GB (Latin) a form of Laurence.

Laurelino, Laurelito, Laurentino (Latin) winner.

Lauren GB (Latin) a form of Laurence.
Lauran

Laurence GB (Latin) crowned with laurel. A form of Lawrence. See also Rance, Raulas, Raulo, Renzo.
Larance, Larrance, Laurance, Laurans, Laureano, Laurencho, Laurentij, Laurentios, Laurentiu, Laurentius, Laurentz, Laurentzi, Laurenz, Laurin, Laurits, Lauritz, Laurnet, Laurus, Lurance

Laurencio (Spanish) a form of Laurence.
Lorencio

Laurens (Dutch) a form of Laurence.
Laurenz

Laurent (French) a form of Laurence.
Laurente

Laurie GB (English) a familiar form of Laurence.
Lauree, Laurey, Lauri, Laurri, Laurrie, Laurry, Laury, Lorry

Lauris (Swedish) a form of Laurence.

Lauro (Filipino) a form of Laurence.

Lautaro (Araucanian) daring and enterprising.

Lav, Luv (Indian) son of the Hindu god Rama.

LaValle (French) valley.
Lavail, Laval, Lavalei, Lavall, Lavalle

Lavan (Hebrew) white.
Lavane, Lavaughan, Laven, Lavin, Lavyn, Levan, Leven

Lavaughan (American) a form of Lavan.
Lavaughn, Levaughan, Levaughn

Lave BG (Italian) lava. (English) lord.
Laev, Laeve, Laiv, Laive, Layv, Layve

Lavell (French) a form of LaValle.
Lavel, Lavele, Levele, Levell, Levelle

Lavelle BG (French) a form of LaValle.

Lavi (Hebrew) lion.
Lavee, Lavey, Lavie, Lavy

Lavon (American) a form of Lavan.
Lavion, Lavone, Lavonn, Lavonne, Lavont

Lavonte, Lavonté (American) forms of Lavon.

Lavrenti (Russian) a form of Lawrence.
Laiurenty, Larenti, Lavrentij, Lavrenty, Lavrik, Lavro, Lavrusha

Lawerence (Latin) a form of Lawrence.
Lawerance

Lawford (English) ford on the hill.

Lawler (Irish) soft-spoken.
Lawlor, Lollar, Loller

Lawley (English) low meadow on a hill.
Lawlea, Lawlee, Lawleigh, Lawli, Lawlie, Lawly

Lawrance (Latin) a form of Lawrence.

Lawrence (Latin) crowned with laurel. See also Brencis, Chencho.
Lanty, Larian, Larien, Larka, Larrance, Larrence, Larya, Law, Lawren, Lawron, Loreca, Lorenis, Lourenco, Lowrance, Lowrence

Lawry (English) a familiar form of Lawrence.
Lawree, Lawrey, Lawri, Lawrie, Lowree, Lowrey, Lowri, Lowrie, Lowry

Lawson (English) son of Lawrence.
Lawsen, Layson

Lawton (English) town on the hill.
Laughton, Law

Layne BG (English) a form of Lane.
Layn, Laynee, Layni, Laynie, Layny

Layton (English) a form of Leighton.
Laydon, Layten, Layth, Laythan, Laython

Lazar (Greek) a short form of Lazarus.
Lázár, Lazare

Lazaro (Italian) a form of Lazarus.
Lazarillo, Lazarito, Lazzaro

Lázaro (Italian) a form of Lazaro.

Lazarus (Greek) a form of Eleazar. Bible: Lazarus was raised from the dead by Jesus.
Lazarius, Lazaros, Lazorus

Le BG (Vietnamese) pearl.

Leal (Spanish) loyal and faithful worker.

Leander (Greek) lion-man; brave as a lion.
Ander

Leandre (French) a form of Leander.
Léandre

Leandro (Spanish) a form of Leander.
Leandra, Leandrew, Leandros

Learco (Greek) judge of his village.

Leben (Yiddish) life.
Laben, Lebon

Lebna (Ethiopian) spirit; heart.

Ledarius (American) a combination of the prefix Le + Darius.
Ledarrious, Ledarrius, Lederious, Lederris

Lee BG (English) a short form of Farley, Leonard, and names containing "lee."
Leigh

Legget (French) a form of Leggett.

Leggett (French) one who is sent; delegate.
Legat, Legate, Legette, Leggitt, Liggett, Lyggett

Lei BG (Chinese) thunder. (Hawaiian) a form of Ray.
Ley

Leib (Yiddish) roaring lion.
Leibel

Leif BC (Scandinavian) beloved.
Laif, Leaf, Leef, Leife, Leiff, Leyf, Lief

Leigh GB (English) a form of Lee.

Leighton (English) meadow farm.
Laeton, Laiton, Lay, Leeton, Leiton, Leyton

Leith (Scottish) broad river.

Leixandre (Galician) a form of Alejandro.

Lek (Tai) small.

Lekeke (Hawaiian) powerful ruler.

Leks (Estonian) a familiar form of Alexander.
Leksik, Lekso

Lel (Gypsy) taker.

Leland (English) meadowland; protected land.
Layland, Lealan, Lealand, Leelan, Leeland, Leighlan, Leighland, Lelan, Lelann, Lelend, Lelund, Leylan, Leyland

Lelio (Latin) he who is talkative.

Lemar (French) a form of Lamar.
Lemario, Lemarr, Limar, Limarr, Lymar, Lymarr

Lemuel (Hebrew) devoted to God.
Lem, Lemmie, Lemmy

Len (Hopi) flute. (German) a short form of Leonard.
Lenn

Lenard (German) a form of Leonard.
Lennard

Lencho (Spanish) a form of Lawrence.
Lenci, Lenzy

Lenin (Russian) one who belongs to the river Lena.

Lennart (Swedish) a form of Leonard.
Lennerd

Lennie, Lenny (German) familiar forms of Leonard. (American) forms of Lanny.
Lenee, Leney, Leni, Lenie, Lennee, Lenney, Lenni, Leny

Lenno (Native American) man.
Leno

Lennon (Irish) small cloak; cape.
Lennan, Lennen, Lennin, Lennyn, Lenon

Lennor (Gypsy) spring; summer.
Lenor

Lennox (Scottish) with many elms.
Lennix, Lenox

Lenya (Russian) lion.

Leo (Latin) lion. (German) a short form of Leon, Leopold.
Lavi, Leão, Leeo, Leio, Léo, Léocadie, Leos, Leosko, Leosoko, Nardek

Leobardo (Italian) a form of Leonard.

Leocadie (French) lion.

Leocadio (Greek) he who shines because of his whiteness.

Leodegrance (French) lion.

Leodoualdo, Leodovaldo (Teutonic) he who governs his village.

Leofrido (Teutonic) he who brings peace to his village.

Leon (Greek, German) a short form of Leonard, Napoleon.
Leahon, Leaon, Léon, Leonas, Léonce, Leoncio, Leondris, Leone, Leonek, Leonetti, Leoni, Leonirez, Leonizio, Leonon, Leons, Leontes, Leontios, Leontrae, Leyon, Lion, Liutas, Lyon

León (Greek) a form of Leon.

Leonard (German) brave as a lion.
Leanard, Leanardas, Leanardus, Lena, Lennart, Léonard, Leonardis, Leonart, Leonerd, Leonhard, Leonidas, Leonnard, Leontes, Lernard, Lienard, Linek, Lionard, Lnard, Londard, Lonnard, Lonya, Lynnard, Lyonard

Leonardo (Italian) a form of Leonard.
Leonaldo, Lionardo, Lonnardo

Leonce (French) lion.

Leondre (American) a form of Leon.

Leonel (English) little lion. See also Lionel.
Leaonal, Leaonall, Leaonel, Leaonell, Leional, Leionall, Leionel, Leionell, Leonell

Leonelo (Spanish) a form of Leonel.

Leonhard (German) a form of Leonard.
Leanhard, Leonhards, Lienhardt

Leonid (Russian) a form of Leonard.
Leonide, Lyonya

Leonidas (Greek) a form of Leonard.
Leonida, Leonides

Leónidas (Spanish) a form of León.

Leontino (German) strong as a lion.

Leopold (German) brave people.
Leorad, Lipót, Lopolda, Luepold, Luitpold,
Poldi

Leopoldo (Italian) a form of Leopold.

Leor (Hebrew) my light.
Leory, Lior

Leovixildo (German) armed warrior.

Lequinton (American) a combination of the
prefix Le + Quinten.
Lequentin, Lequenton, Lequinn

Lerenzo (Italian, Spanish) a form of
Lorenzo.
Leranzo, Lerinzo, Leronzo, Lerynzo

Leron (French) round, circle. (American) a
combination of the prefix Le + Ron.
Le Ron, Leeron, Lerin, Lerone, Lerrin, Leryn,
Liron, Lyron

Leroy (French) king. See also Delroy, Elroy.
Learoi, Learoy, Leeroy, LeeRoy, Leighroi,
Leighroy, Leiroi, Leiroy, Lerai, Leroi, LeRoi,
LeRoy, Leyroi, Leyroy, Roy

Les (Scottish, English) a short form of Leslie,
Lester.
Less, Lessie

Lesharo (Pawnee) chief.

Leshawn (American) a combination of the
prefix Le + Shawn.
Lashan, Lesean, Leshaun, Leshon, Leshonne,
Leshun

Leslie **GB** (Scottish) gray fortress.
Leslea, Leslee, Leslei, Lesleigh, Lesley, Lesli,
Lesly, Lezlea, Lezlee, Lezlei, Lezleigh, Lezley,
Lezli, Lezlie, Lezly

Lesmes (Teutonic) he whose nobility protects him.

Lester (Latin) chosen camp. (English) from
Leicester, England.
Leicester

Let (Catalan) a form of Leto.

Leto (Latin) he who is always happy.

Leuco (Greek) the luminous one.

Leuter (Galician) a form of Eleuterio.

Lev (Hebrew) heart. (Russian) a form of
Leo. A short form of Leverett, Levi.
Leb, Leva, Levko

Levant (Latin) rising.
Lavant, Lavante, Levante

Leveni (Tongan) raven.
Levenee, Leveney, Levenie, Leveny

Leverett (French) young hare.
Leveret, Leverette, Leverit, Leveritt, Leveryt,
Leverytt

Levi (Hebrew) joined in harmony. Bible: the
third son of Jacob; Levites are the priestly
tribe of the Israelites.
Leavi, Leevi, Leevie, Levey, Levie, Levitis,
Levy, Lewi, Leyvi

Levin (Hebrew) a form of Levi.
Levine, Levion, Levyn, Levynn

Levina (Hebrew) one who unites.

Levka, Levushka (Russian) lion.

Levon (American) a form of Lavon.
Leevon, Levone, Levonn, Levonne, Lyvon,
Lyvonn, Lyvonne

Levonte (American) a form of Levon.

Lew (English) a short form of Lewis.

Lewin (English) beloved friend.
Lewan, Lewen, Lewon, Lewyn

Lewis (Welsh) a form of Llewellyn. (English)
a form of Louis.
Lew, Lewes, Lewie, Lewy, Lewys

Lex (English) a short form of Alexander.
Lexi, Lexie, Lexin

Lexus **GB** (Greek) a short form of
Alexander.
Lexis, Lexius, Lexxus

Leyati (Moquelumnan) shape of an abalone
shell.
Leyatie, Leyaty

Lí (Chinese) strong.

Lía (Spanish) an abbreviation of names that end with the suffix Lia.

Liam (Irish) a form of William.
Lliam, Lyam

Lian GB (Irish) guardian. (Chinese) graceful willow.
Lyan

Liang (Chinese) good, excellent.
Lyang

Liban (Hawaiian) a form of Laban.
Libaan, Lieban

Libanio (Latin) tree of incense.

Líbano (Latin) white.

Liber (Latin) he who spreads abundance.

Liberal (Latin) the lover of liberty.

Liberato (Latin) the liberated one.

Liberio (Portuguese) liberation.
Liberaratore, Libero, Liborio, Lyberio, Lyberyo

Libiac, Llipiac (Quechua) ray of light.

Libio, Livio (Latin) born in a dry place.

Licas (Greek) wolf.

Licerio (Greek) pertaining to light.

Licurgo (Greek) he who frightens off wolves.

Lidia (Greek) one who comes from Lidia.

Lidio (Greek, Portuguese) ancient.

Liem (Irish) a form of Liam.

Ligongo (Yao) who is this?
Lygongo

Lihue, Lihuel (Araucanian) life; existence.

Likeke (Hawaiian) a form of Richard.

Liko (Chinese) protected by Buddha. (Hawaiian) bud.
Like, Lyko

Lin GB (Burmese) bright. (English) a short form of Lyndon.
Linh, Linn, Linny

Linc (English) a short form of Lincoln.
Link, Lynk

Lincoln (English) settlement by the pool. History: Abraham Lincoln was the sixteenth U.S. president.
Lincon, Lincoyn, Lyncoln

Lindberg (German) mountain where linden grow.
Lindbergh, Lindbert, Lindburg, Lindy, Lyndberg, Lyndbergh, Lyndburg

Lindbert (German) a form of Lindberg.
Linbert, Linbirt, Linburt, Linbyrt, Lindbirt, Lindburt, Lynbert, Lynbirt, Lynburt, Lynbyrt, Lyndbert, Lyndbirt, Lyndburt, Lyndbyrt

Lindell (English) valley of the linden. See also Lyndal.
Lendall, Lendel, Lendell, Lindal, Lindall, Lindel

Linden BG (English) a form of Lyndon.
Lindan, Lindin, Lindyn

Lindley (English) linden field.
Lindlea, Lindlee, Lindleigh, Lindli, Lindlie, Lindly, Lyndlea, Lyndlee, Lyndleigh, Lyndley, Lyndli, Lyndlie, Lyndly

Lindon (English) a form of Lyndon.

Lindor (Latin) he who seduces.

Lindsay GB (English) a form of Lindsey.
Linsay, Lyndsay

Lindsey GB (English) linden island.
Lind, Lindsee, Lindsie, Lindsy, Lindzy, Linsey, Linzie, Linzy, Lyndsey, Lyndsie, Lynzie

Linford (English) linden ford.
Lynford

Linfred (German) peaceful, calm.
Linfrid, Linfryd, Lynfrid, Lynfryd

Linley GB (English) flax meadow.
Linlea, Linlee, Linleigh, Linli, Linlie, Linly, Lynlea, Lynlee, Lynleigh, Lynley, Lynli, Lynlie, Lynly

Lino (Portuguese) a short form of Laudalino.

Linton (English) flax town.
Lintonn, Lynton, Lyntonn

Linu (Hindi) lily.
Lynu

Linus (Greek) flaxen haired.
Linas, Linis, Liniss, Linous, Linux, Lynis, Lyniss, Lynus

Linwood (English) flax wood.

Lio (Hawaiian) a form of Leo.
Lyo

Lionel (French) lion cub. See also Leonel.
Lional, Lionall, Lionell, Lionello, Lynel, Lynell, Lyonal, Lyonall, Lyonel, Lyonell, Lyonello

Liron **BG** (Hebrew) my song.
Lyron

Lisandro (Spanish) liberator.

Lisardo (Hebrew) defender of the faith.

Lise **GB** (Moquelumnan) salmon's head coming out of the water.
Lyse

Lisias, Lisístrato (Greek) liberator.

Lisimba (Yao) lion.
Lasimba, Lasimbah, Lisimbah, Lysimba, Lysymba, Simba

Lister (English) dyer.
Lyster

Litton (English) town on the hill.
Liton, Lyton, Lytten, Lytton

Liu (African) voice.

Liuz (Polish) light.
Lius, Lyus

Livingston (English) Leif's town.
Livingstone, Livinston, Livinstone

Liwanu (Moquelumnan) growling bear.
Lywanu

Llacsa (Quechua) he who is the color of bronze.

Llallaua (Aymara) magnificent.

Llancamil (Mapuche) shining stone.

Llancañir (Mapuche) fox that is pearl-colored.

Llanqui (Quechua) potter's clay.

Llarico, Llaricu (Aymara) indomitable.

Llashapoma, Llashapuma (Quechua) heavy puma; slow.

Llewellyn (Welsh) lionlike.
Lewelan, Lewelen, Llewelin, Llewellen, Llewelleyn, Llewellin, Llewelyn, Llywellyn, Llywellynn, Llywelyn

Lleyton (English) a form of Leighton.

Llipiac, Lloque, Lluqui (Quechua) left-handed, from the left side.

Lloqueyupanqui, Lluquiyupanqui (Quechua) left-handed; memorable.

Lloyd (Welsh) gray haired; holy. See also Floyd.
Loy, Loyd, Loyde, Loydie

Lobo (Spanish) wolf.

Lochan (Indian) eye.

Lochlain (Irish, Scottish) land of lakes.
Loche, Lochee, Lochlan, Lochlann, Lochlen, Lochlin, Lochlon, Lochlyn, Locklynn

Locke (English) forest.
Loc, Lock, Lockwood

Loe (Hawaiian) a form of Roy.

Logan ⭐ **BG** (Irish) meadow.
Llogan, Loagan, Loagen, Loagon, Logann, Loggan, Loghan, Login, Logn, Logon, Logun, Logunn, Logyn

Logen (Irish) a form of Logan.

Lois (German) famous in battle.

Lok (Chinese) happy.

Lokela (Hawaiian) a form of Roger.
Lokelah

Lokesh (Indian) another name for the Hindu god Brahma.

Lokni (Moquelumnan) raining through the roof.

Lomán (Irish) bare. (Slavic) sensitive.
Lomen

Lombard (Latin) long bearded.
Bard, Barr, Lombarda, Lombardi, Lombardo

Lon (Irish) fierce. (Spanish) a short form of Alonso, Leonard, Lonnie.
Lonn

Lonan (Zuni) cloud.
Lonen, Lonin, Lonon, Lonyn

Lonato (Native American) flint stone.

Loncopan (Mapuche) puma's head.

London BG (English) fortress of the moon. Geography: the capital of the United Kingdom.
Londen, Londyn, Lunden, Lundon

Long (Chinese) dragon. (Vietnamese) hair.

Longinos (Latin) long.

Lonnie, Lonny (German, Spanish) familiar forms of Alonso.
Loni, Lonie, Lonnell, Lonney, Lonni, Lonniel, Lony

Lono (Hawaiian) Mythology: the god of learning and intellect.

Lonzo (German, Spanish) a short form of Alonso.
Lonso

Lootah (Lakota) red.
Loota

Lopaka (Hawaiian) a form of Robert.

Lope (Latin) wolf.

Loran (American) a form of Lauren.

Loránd (Hungarian) a form of Roland.

Lóránt (Hungarian) a form of Lawrence.
Lorant

Lorcan (Irish) little; fierce.
Lorcen, Lorcin, Lorcon, Lorcyn

Lord (English) noble title.

Loren GB (Latin) a short form of Lawrence.
Lorren, Lorrin, Loryn

Lorenza BG (Italian, Spanish) a form of Lorenzo.
Larinza

Lorenzo (Italian, Spanish) a form of Lawrence.
Laurenzo, Laurinzo, Laurynzo, Lewrenzo, Lorantzo, Lorenc, Lorence, Lorenco, Lorencz, Lorenczo, Lorens, Lorenso, Lorentz, Lorentzo, Lorenz, Loretto, Lorinc, Lörinc, Lorinzo, Loritz, Lorrenzo, Lorrynzo, Lorynzo, Lourenza, Lourenzo, Lowrenzo, Zo

Loretto (Italian) a form of Lawrence.
Loreto

Lorién (Aragonese) a form of Lorenzo.

Lorimer (Latin) harness maker.
Lorrimer, Lorrymer, Lorymer

Lorin GB (Latin) a short form of Lawrence.

Loring (German) son of the famous warrior.
Lorring, Lorryng, Loryng

Loris BG (Dutch) clown.
Lorys

Loritz (Latin, Danish) laurel.
Lauritz, Laurytz, Lorytz

Lorne (Latin) a short form of Lawrence.
Lorn, Lornie, Lorny

Lorry (English) a form of Laurie. (Latin) a form of Lorimer.
Lori, Lorie, Lorri, Lorrie, Lory

Lot (Hebrew) hidden, covered. Bible: Lot fled from Sodom, but his wife glanced back upon its destruction and was transformed into a pillar of salt.
Lott

Lotario (Germanic) the distinguished warrior.

Lothar (German) a form of Luther.
Lotair, Lotaire, Lotarrio, Lothair, Lothaire, Lothario, Lotharrio, Lottario

Lou BG (German) a short form of Louis.

Loudon (German) low valley.
Lewdan, Lewden, Lewdin, Lewdon, Lewdyn, Loudan, Louden, Loudin, Loudyn, Lowdan, Lowden, Lowdin, Lowdon, Lowdyn

Louie (German) a familiar form of Louis.

Louis (German) famous warrior. See also Aloisio, Aloysius, Clovis, Luigi.
Loudovicus, Louies, Louise, Lucho, Lude, Ludek, Ludirk, Ludis, Ludko, Lughaidh, Lutek

Louis Alexander (French) a combination of Louis + Alexander.

Louis Charles (French) a combination of Louis + Charles.

Louis David (French) a combination of Louis + David.

Louis Mathieu (French) a combination of Louis + Mathieu.

Louis Philipp (French) a combination of Louis + Philip.

Louis Xavier (French) a combination of Louis + Xavier.

Lourdes **GB** (French) from Lourdes, France. Religion: a place where the Virgin Mary was said to have appeared.
Lordes

Louvain (English) Lou's vanity. Geography: a city in Belgium.
Louvayn, Louvin

Lovell (English) a form of Lowell.
Louvell, Lovel, Lovelle, Lovey

Lowell (French) young wolf. (English) beloved.
Lowe, Lowel, Lowelle

Loyal (English) faithful, loyal.
Loial, Loy, Loyall, Loye, Lyall, Lyell

Loyola (Latin) has a wolf on his shield.

Luano (Latin) fountain.

Lubomir (Polish) lover of peace.
Lubomyr

Luboslaw (Polish) lover of glory.
Lubs, Lubz

Luc (French) a form of Luke.
Luce

Luca **BG** (Italian) a form of Lucius.
Lucah, Lucca, Luka

Lucas ⭐ (German, Irish, Danish, Dutch) a form of Lucius.
Lucais, Lucassie, Lucaus, Luccas, Luccus, Luckas, Lucys

Lucero, Lucío (Spanish) bringer of light.

Lucian (Latin) a form of Lucius.
Liuz, Lucan, Lucanus, Lucianus, Lucias, Lucjan, Lucyan, Lukianos, Lukyan, Luzian

Luciano (Italian) a form of Lucian.
Lucino

Lucien (French) a form of Lucius.
Lucyen, Luzien

Lucífero, Lucila (Latin) he who gives light.

Lucio (Italian) a form of Lucius.
Luzio

Lucius (Latin) light; bringer of light.
Lucanus, Luce, Lucious, Lucis, Lucyas, Lucyus, Lusio, Luzius

Lucky **BG** (American) fortunate. (Latin) a familiar form of Luke.
Luckee, Lucki, Luckie, Luckson, Lucson, Luki, Lukie, Luky

Lucrecio (Latin) twilight of dawn.

Lucus (German, Irish, Danish, Dutch) a form of Lucas.

Ludlow (English) prince's hill.

Ludovic, Ludovick (German) forms of Ludwig.
Ludovico

Ludwig (German) a form of Louis. Music: Ludwig van Beethoven was a famous nineteenth-century German composer.
Ludvig, Ludvik, Ludwik, Lutz

Luftî (Arabic) friendly.

Lui (Hawaiian) a form of Louis.

Luigi (Italian) a form of Louis.
Lui, Luiggi, Luigino, Luigy

Luis ⭐ (Spanish) a form of Louis.
Luise

Luís, Luiz (Spanish) forms of Louis.

Luisalberto (Spanish) a combination of Luis + Alberto.

Luisangel (Spanish) a combination of Luis + Angel.

Luisantonio (Spanish) a combination of Luis + Antonio.

Luisenrique (Spanish) a combination of Luis + Enrique.

Luka (Italian) a form of Luke.

Lukas, Lukasz, Lukus (Greek, Czech, Swedish) forms of Luke.
Loukas, Lukais, Lukash, Lukasha, Lukass, Lukaus, Lukkas, Lukys

Luke ⚝ (Latin) a form of Lucius. Bible: companion of Saint Paul and author of the third Gospel of the New Testament.
Luchok, Luck, Luk, Lúkács, Luken, Lukes, Lukyan, Lusio

Lukela (Hawaiian) a form of Russell.

Luken (Basque) bringer of light.
Lucan, Lucane, Lucano, Luk

Luki (Basque) famous warrior.

Lukman (Arabic) prophet.
Luqman

Lulani BG (Hawaiian) highest point in heaven.
Lulanee, Lulaney, Lulanie, Lulany

Lumo (Ewe) born facedown.

Lundy GB (Scottish) grove by the island.
Lundee, Lundey, Lundi, Lundie

Lunn (Irish) warlike.
Lonn, Lunni, Lunnie, Lunny

Lunt (Swedish) grove.
Lont

Lupercio (Latin) name given to people from Lupercus.

Luperco (Latin) he who frightens off wolves.

Luqmân (Arabic) prophet.

Lusila (Hindi) leader.
Lusyla

Lusio (Zuni) a form of Lucius.
Lusyo

Lusorio (Latin) he enjoys games.

Lutalo (Luganda) warrior.

Lutardo (Teutonic) he who is valiant in his village.

Lutfi (Arabic) kind, friendly.

Luther (German) famous warrior. History: Martin Luther was one of the central figures of the Reformation.
Lothar, Lother, Lothur, Lutero, Luthor

Lutherum (Gypsy) slumber.

Luyu BG (Moquelumnan) head shaker.

Luzige (Egyptian) lobster.

Lyall, Lyell (Scottish) loyal.
Lyal, Lyel

Lyle (French) island.
Lisle, Ly, Lysle

Lyman (English) meadow.
Leaman, Leamen, Leeman, Leemen, Leiman, Leimen, Leyman, Liman, Limen, Limin, Limon, Limyn, Lymen, Lymin, Lymon, Lymyn

Lynch (Irish) mariner.
Linch

Lyndal (English) valley of lime trees. See also Lindell.
Lyndale, Lyndall, Lyndel, Lyndell

Lynden (English) a form of Lyndon.

Lyndon (English) linden hill. History: Lyndon B. Johnson was the thirty-sixth U.S. president.
Lyden, Lydon, Lyndan, Lyndin, Lyndyn

Lynn GB (English) waterfall; brook. A short form of Lyndon. (Burmese, English) a form of Lin.
Lyn, Lynell, Lynette, Lynnard, Lynoll

Lyonechka (Russian) lion.

Lyron (Hebrew) a form of Leron, Liron.

Lysander (Greek) liberator.
Lyzander, Sander

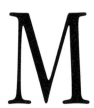

Ma'an (Arabic) benefit.

Ma'mûn (Arabic) reliable.

Maalik (Punjabi) a form of Málik.
Maalek, Maaliek

Mac (Scottish) son.
Macs, Mak

Macabee (Hebrew) hammer.
Maccabee, Mackabee, Makabee

Macadam (Scottish) son of Adam.
MacAdam, Mackadam, Makadam, McAdam

Macaire (French) a form of Macario.

Macalla (Australian) full moon.
Macala, Macalah, Macallah

Macallister (Irish) son of Alistair.
*Macalaster, MacAlistair, Macalister, MacAlister,
Mackalistair, Mackalister, Makalistair,
Makalister, McAlister, McAllister*

Macario (Spanish) a form of Makarios.
Macarios, Macaryo, Maccario, Maccarios

Macarthur (Irish) son of Arthur.
MacArthur, Mackarthur, Makarthur, McArthur

Macaulay (Scottish) son of righteousness.
*Macaulea, Macaulee, Macaulei, Macauleigh,
Macauley, Macauli, Macaulie, Macaully,
Macauly, Maccauley, Mackaulea, Mackaulee,
Mackaulei, Mackauleigh, Mackauley,
Mackauli, Mackaulie, Mackauly, Macaualay,
McCaulea, McCaulee, McCaulei,
McCauleigh, McCauley, McCauli, McCaulie,
McCauly*

Macbride (Scottish) son of a follower of
Saint Brigid.
*Macbryde, Mackbride, Mackbryde, Makbride,
Makbryde, Mcbride, McBride, McBryde*

Maccoy (Irish) son of Hugh, Coy.
*MacCoi, MacCoy, Mackoi, Mackoy, Makoi,
Makoy*

Maccrea (Irish) son of grace.
*MacCrae, MacCrai, MacCray, MacCrea,
Mackrea, Macrae, Macray, Makcrea, Makray,
Makrea, Mccrea, McCrea*

Macdonald (Scottish) son of Donald.
*MacDonald, Mackdonald, MackDonald,
Makdonald, MakDonald, Mcdonald,
McDonald, Mcdonna, Mcdonnell, McDonnell*

Macdougal (Scottish) son of Dougal.
*MacDougal, MacDougall, Mackdougal,
Makdougal, MakDougal, Makdougall,
MakDougall, Mcdougal, McDougal,
McDougall*

Mace (French) club. (English) a short form
of Macy, Mason.
Macean, Macer, Macey, Macie

Macedonio (Greek) he who triumphs and
grows in stature.

Maceo (Spanish) a form of Mace.

Macèo (Italian) gift of God.

Macerio (Spanish) blessed.

Macfarlane (English) son of Farlane.
*Macfarlan, Mackfarlan, Mackfarlane,
Macpharlan, Macpharlane, Makfarlan,
Makfarlane, Makpharlan, Makpharlane,
Mcfarlan, Mcfarlane, Mcpharlan, Mcpharlane*

Macgregor (Scottish) son of Gregor.
Macgreggor

Macharios (Greek) blessed.
Macarius, Macharyos, Makarius

Machas (Polish) a form of Michael.

Macián, Macías (Hebrew) forms of Matias.

Maciel (Latin) very slender.

Mack (Scottish) a short form of names
beginning with "Mac" and "Mc."
Macke, Mackey, Mackie, Macks, Macky, Mak

Mackenzie GB (Irish) son of Kenzie.
*Mackensy, Mackenze, Mackenzee, Mackenzey,
Mackenzi, MacKenzie, Mackenzly,
Mackienzie, Mackinsey, Mackinzie, Mickenzie*

Mackenzy BG (Irish) a form of Mackenzie.

Mackinley (Irish) a form of Mackinnley.

Mackinnley (Irish) son of the learned ruler.
*Mackinlea, Mackinlee, Mackinlei,
Mackinleigh, Mackinli, Mackinlie, Mackinly,
MacKinnley, Mackinnly, Mackynlea,
Mackynlee, Mackynlei, Mackynleigh,
Mackynley, Mackynli, Mackynlie, Mackynly,
Makinlea, Makinlee, Makinlei, Makinleigh,
Makinley, Makinli, Makinlie, Makinly,
Makynlea, Makynlee, Makynlei, Makynleigh,
Makynley, Makynli, Makynlie, Makynly*

Macklain (Irish) a form of Maclean.
Macklaine, Macklane

Macklin (Scottish) a form of Mack.

Maclean (Irish) son of Leander.
*Machlin, Macklain, Macklean, MacKlean,
MacLain, MacLean, Maclin, Maclyn,
Maklean, Makleen, McClean, McLaine,
McLean*

Macmahon (Irish) son of Mahon.
Mackmahon, MacMahon, Makmahon,
McMahon

Macmurray (Irish) son of Murray.
Mackmuray, Mackmurray, Macmuray,
Macmurry, Makmuray, Makmurray, McMurray,
Mcmurry

Macnair (Scottish) son of the heir.
Macknair, Macknayr, Maknair, Maknayr,
McMayr, McNair

Maco (Hungarian) a form of Emmanuel.
Macko, Mako

Macon (German, English) maker.
Macan, Macen, Macin, Macun, Macyn

Macrobio (Greek) he who enjoys a long
life.

Macy GB (French) Matthew's estate.
Macey, Maci, Macie

Madangopal, Madhav, Madhusudan
(Indian) other names for the Hindu god
Krishna.

Maddock (Welsh) generous.
Maddoc, Maddoch, Maddok, Madoc, Madoch,
Madock, Madog

Maddox BG (Welsh, English) benefactor's
son.
Maddux, Madox

Madhar (Hindi) full of intoxication; relating
to spring.

Madhavdas (Indian) servant of the Hindu
god Krishna.

Madhu (Indian) honey.

Madhuk, Madhukar, Madhup (Indian)
honeybee.

Madhukanta (Indian) moon.

Madhur (Indian) sweet.

Madison GB (English) son of Maude; good
son.
Maddie, Maddison, Maddy, Maddyson,
Madisen, Madisson, Madisyn, Madsen,
Madyson, Son, Sonny

Madon (Irish) charitable.
Madan, Maddan, Madden, Maddin, Maddon,
Maddyn, Maden, Madin, Madyn

Madongo (Luganda) uncircumcised.

Madu (Ibo) people.

Mael (Celtic) prince.

Magan (Indian) engrossed.

Magar (Armenian) groom's attendant.
Magarious

Magee (Irish) son of Hugh.
MacGee, MacGhee, McGee

Magen GB (Hebrew) protector.

Magín (Latin) he who is imaginative.

Magina (Latin) sage; charmer.

Magnar (Norwegian) strong; warrior.
Magne

Magno (Latin) great.

Magnus (Latin) great.
Maghnus, Magnes, Magnuss, Manius

Magomu (Luganda) younger of twins.

Maguire (Irish) son of the beige one.
MacGuire, Macguyre, McGuire, McGwire

Mahabahu (Indian) another name for
Arjuna, a warrior prince in the Indian epic
poem *Mahabharata*.

Mahadev, Mahesh, Maheshwar (Indian)
other names for the Hindu god Shiva.

Mahammed (Arabic) a form of
Muhammad.
Mahamad, Mahamed, Mahammad

Mahaniya (Indian) worthy of honor.

Mahavir (Indian) the twenty-fourth and last
Tirthankar, a type of Jain god; very courageous.

Mahdi (Arabic) guided to the right path.
Mahde, Mahdee, Mahdy

Mahendra (Indian) another name for the
Hindu god Vishnu.

Maher (Arabic, Hebrew) a form of Mahir.

Mâher (Arabic) a form of Maher.

Mahesa BG (Hindi) great lord. Religion:
another name for the Hindu god Shiva.

Mahi'ai (Hawaiian) a form of George.

Mahieu (French) gift of God.

Mahin (Indian) the earth.

Mahindra, Mahipal, Mahish (Indian) king.

Mahir (Arabic, Hebrew) excellent; industrious.
Mair

Mahkah (Lakota) earth.
Maka, Makah

Mahlí (Hebrew) astute; shrewd.

Mahmoud, Mahmúd (Arabic) forms of Muhammad.
Mahamoud, Mahmed, Mahmmoud, Mahmood, Mahmuod, Mahmut

Mahmud (Indian) another name for Muhammad, the founder of Islam.

Mahmûd (Arabic) a form of Mahmoud.

Mahoma (Arabic) worthy of being praised.

Mahomet (Arabic) a form of Muhammad.

Mahon (Irish) bear.

Mahpee (Lakota) sky.

Mahtab (Indian) moon.

Mahuizoh (Nahuatl) glorious person.

Maicu (Quechua) eagle.

Maidoc (Welsh) fortunate.
Maedoc, Maedock, Maedok, Maidoc, Maidock, Maidok, Maydoc, Maydock, Maydok

Mailhairer (French) unfortunate.

Maimun (Arabic) lucky.
Maimon, Maymon

Mainak (Indian) a mountain in the Himalayas.

Mainque (Mapuche) condor.

Maiqui (Quechua) tree.

Mairtin (Irish) a form of Martin.

Maison **BG** (French) house. A form of Mason.
Maisan, Maisen, Maisin, Maisun, Maisyn

Maitias (Irish) a form of Mathias.
Maithias

Maitiú (Irish) a form of Matthew.

Maitland **GB** (English) meadowland.
Maitlan, Maytlan, Maytland

Majed (Arabic) a form of Majid.

Majencio (Latin) he who becomes more famous.

Majid (Arabic) great, glorious.
Majd, Majde, Majdi, Majdy, Majeed, Majyd

Mâjid (Arabic) a form of Majid.

Major (Latin) greater; military rank.
Majar, Maje, Majer

Makaio (Hawaiian) a form of Matthew.
Makayo

Makalani (Mwera) writer.
Makalanee, Makalaney, Makalanie, Makalany

Makani **BG** (Hawaiian) wind.
Makanie, Makany

Makarios (Greek) happy; blessed.
Makari, Makarie, Makaryos

Makenzie **GB** (Irish) a form of Mackenzie.
Makensie, Makenzee, Makenzey, Makenzi, Makenzy

Makin (Arabic) strong.
Makeen, Makyn

Makis (Greek) a form of Michael.
Makys

Makoto (Japanese) sincere.

Maks (Hungarian) a form of Max.
Makszi

Maksim (Russian) a form of Maximilian.

Maksym (Polish) a form of Maximilian.
Makimus, Maksymilian

Makyah (Hopi) eagle hunter.
Makia, Makiah, Makyah

Mal (Irish) a short form of names beginning with "Mal."

Malachi (Hebrew) angel of God. Bible: the last canonical Hebrew prophet.
Maeleachlainn, Malachai, Malachia, Malachie, Malchija

Malachy (Irish) a form of Malachi.
Malechy

Malají (Hebrew) my messenger.

Malajitm (Sanskrit) garland of victory.

Malakai (Hebrew) a form of Malachi.
Malake, Malaki

Malaquias, Malaquías (Hebrew) God's messenger.

Malco, Malcon (Hebrew) he who is like a king.

Malcolm (Scottish) follower of Saint Columba, who Christianized North Scotland. (Arabic) dove.
Malcalm, Malcohm, Malcolum, Malkolm

Malcom (Scottish) a form of Malcolm.
Malcome, Malcum, Malkom, Malkum

Malden (English) meeting place in a pasture.
Mal, Maldan, Maldin, Maldon, Maldun, Maldyn

Maleek, Maliek, Malique (Arabic) forms of Málik.

Malek, Malik (Arabic) forms of Málik.
Maleak, Maleik, Maleka, Maleke, Mallek

Maleko (Hawaiian) a form of Mark.

Málik (Punjabi) lord, master. (Arabic) a form of Malachi.
Mailik, Malak, Malic, Malick, Malicke, Maliik, Malike, Malikh, Maliq, Mallik, Malyc, Malyck, Malyk, Malyq

Mâlik (Arabic) a form of Malik.

Malin (English) strong, little warrior.
Malen, Mallen, Mallin, Mallon, Mallyn, Malon, Malyn

Malleville (French) comes from Malleville.

Mallory GB (German) army counselor. (French) wild duck.
Lory, Mallery, Mallorey, Mallori, Mallorie, Malorey, Malori, Malorie, Malory

Maloney (Irish) church going.
Malone, Malonee, Maloni, Malonie, Malony

Malvern (Welsh) bare hill.
Malverne, Malvirn, Malvirne, Malvyrn, Malvyrne

Malvin (Irish, English) a form of Melvin.
Malvan, Malven, Malvinn, Malvon, Malvyn, Malvynn

Mamani (Aymara) falcon.

Mamés (Greek) mother.

Mamo BG (Hawaiian) yellow flower; yellow bird.

Mampu (Araucanian) caress.

Man-Shik (Korean) deeply rooted.

Man-Young (Korean) ten thousand years of prosperity.

Manases, Manasés (Hebrew) he who forgets everything.

Manauia (Nahuatl) defend.

Manchu (Chinese) pure.

Mancio (Latin) he who foretells the future.

Manco (Peruvian) supreme leader. History: a sixteenth-century Incan king.

Mandala (Yao) flowers.
Manda, Mandela, Mandelah

Mandeep BG (Punjabi) mind full of light.
Mandieep

Mandek (Polish) a form of Herman.
Mandie

Mandel (German) almond.
Mandell

Mander (Gypsy) from me.
Mandar, Mandir, Mandor, Mandyr

Manés (Greek) craziness.

Manesio (Greek) a form of Manés.

Manford (English) small ford.
Manforde, Menford, Menforde

Manfred (English) man of peace. See also Fred.
Manfredo, Manfret, Manfrid, Manfried, Manfryd, Maniferd, Manifrid, Manifryd, Mannfred, Mannfryd, Manyfred, Manyfrid, Manyfryd

Manger (French) stable.
Mangar, Mangor

Mango (Spanish) a familiar form of Emmanuel, Manuel.

Manheim (German) servant's home.

Manipi (Native American) living marvel.

Manius (Scottish) a form of Magnus.
Manus, Manyus

Manjot **BG** (Indian) light of the mind.

Manley (English) hero's meadow.
Manlea, Manlee, Manleigh, Manli, Manlie, Manly

Manlio (Latin) he who was born in the morning.

Mann (German) man.
Man, Manin

Manneville (French) one who comes from the great state.

Manning (English) son of the hero.
Maning

Mannix (Irish) monk.
Mainchin, Mannox, Mannyx, Manox, Manyx

Manny (German, Spanish) a familiar form of Manuel.
Mani, Manni, Mannie, Many

Mano (Hawaiian) shark. (Spanish) a short form of Manuel.
Manno, Manolo

Manoj (Sanskrit) cupid.

Manolito (Spanish) God is with us.

Manpreet **GB** (Punjabi) mind full of love.

Manque (Mapuche) condor.

Manquecura (Mapuche) refuge from the condor; two-colored rock.

Manquepan (Mapuche) the condor's branch.

Manric (Catalan) a form of Manrique.

Manrico (American) a combination of Mann + Enrico.
Manricko, Manriko, Manrycko, Manryco, Manryko

Manrique (Germanic) powerful leader.

Mansa (Swahili) king. History: a fourteenth-century king of Mali.
Mansah

Mansel (English) manse; house occupied by a clergyman.
Mansell

Mansfield (English) field by the river; hero's field.
Mansfyld

Manso (Latin) the delivered, trusted one.

Mansueto (Latin) he who is peaceful, docile.

Mansûr (Arabic) a form of Mansur.

Mansür (Arabic) divinely aided.
Mansoor, Mansour

Mantel (French) designer.

Manton (English) man's town; hero's town.
Mannton, Mantan, Manten, Mantin, Mantyn

Manu (Hindi) lawmaker. History: the reputed writer of the Hindi compendium of sacred laws and customs. (Hawaiian) bird. (Ghanaian) second-born son.

Manuel (Hebrew) a short form of Emmanuel.
Mannuel, Mano, Manolón, Manual, Manuale, Manue, Manuell, Manuelli, Manuelo, Manuil, Manyuil, Minel

Manville (French) worker's village. (English) hero's village.
Mandeville, Manvel, Manvil, Manvill, Manvyl, Manvyle, Manvyll, Manvylle

Manzo (Japanese) third son.

Manzur (Arabic) the winner.

Maona (Winnebago) creator, earth maker.

Mapira (Yao) millet.
Mapirah

Marat (Indian) life-death-birth-giving cycle.

Marc (French) a form of Mark. (Latin) a short form of Marcus.

Marc Alexander (French) a combination of Marc + Alexander.

Marc Andre, Marc-Andre (French) combinations of Marc + Andre.

Marc Antoine, Marc-Antoine (French) combinations of Marc + Antoine.

Marc Etienne (French) a combination of Marc + Etienne.

Marc Olivier, Marc-Olivier (French) combinations of Marc + Olivier.

Marcanthony (American) a combination of Marc + Anthony.

Marcel, Marcell (French) forms of Marcellus.
Marcele, Marcelle, Marsale, Marsel, Marzel, Marzell

Marceliano (Spanish) a form of Marcello.

Marcelino (Italian) a form of Marcellus.
Marceleno, Marcelin, Marcellin, Marcellino

Marcellis, Marcellous (Latin) forms of Marcellus.
Marcelis

Marcello, Marcelo (Italian) forms of Marcellus.
Marchello, Marsello, Marselo

Marcellus (Latin) a familiar form of Marcus.
Marceau, Marceles, Marcelias, Marcelius, Marcellas, Marcelleous, Marcelluas, Marcelus, Marcely, Marciano, Marcilka, Marcsseau, Marzellos, Marzellous, Marzellus

March (English) dweller by a boundary.

Marciano (Italian) a form of Martin.
Marci, Marcio

Marcilka (Hungarian) a form of Marcellus.
Marci, Marcilki

Marcin (Polish) a form of Martin.

Marco (Italian) a form of Marcus. History: Marco Polo was a thirteenth-century Venetian traveler who explored Asia.
Marcko, Marko

Marcoantonio (Italian) a combination of Marco + Antonio.

Marcos (Spanish) a form of Marcus.
Marckos, Marcous, Markose

Marcus (Latin) martial, warlike.
Marcas, Marcio, Marckus, Marcuss, Marcuus, Marcux, Markov

Marden BG (English) valley with a pool.
Madrin, Mardan, Mardon, Mardun, Mardyn

Mardonio (Persian) the male warrior.

Mardoqueo (Hebrew) he who adores the god of war.

Mâred (Arabic) rebel.

Marek (Slavic) a form of Marcus.

Maren GB (Basque) sea.
Maran, Maron

Mareo (Japanese) uncommon.

Margarito (Latin) pearl.

Marian GB (Polish) a form of Mark.
Maryan

Mariano (Italian) a form of Mark. A form of Marion.
Maryano

Marid (Arabic) rebellious.
Maryd

Marin GB (French) sailor.
Marine, Mariner, Marriner, Marryner, Maryn, Maryner

Marino (Italian) a form of Marin.
Marinos, Marinus, Mariono, Marynos, Marynus

Mario (Italian) a form of Marino.
Mareo, Marios, Marrio, Maryon

Marion GB (French) bitter; sea of bitterness.
Mareon, Maryon

Marius (Latin) a form of Marin.
Marious

Mark (Latin) a form of Marcus. Bible: author of the second Gospel in the New Testament. See also Maleko.
Marck, Marian, Marke, Markee, Markey, Markk, Markusha, Marx

Mark Anthony, Markanthony (Italian) combinations of Mark + Anthony.

Marke (Polish) a form of Mark.

Markel (Latin) a form of Mark.
Markelle, Markelo

Markell BG (Latin) a form of Mark.

Markes (Portuguese) a form of Marques.
Markess, Markest

Markese (French) a form of Marquis.
Markease, Markeece, Markees, Markeese, Markei, Markeice, Markeis, Markeise, Markes, Markice

Markez (French) a form of Marquis.
Markeze

Markham (English) homestead on the boundary.

Markis (French) a form of Marquis.
Markies, Markiese, Markise, Markiss, Markist

Marko (Latin) a form of Marco, Mark.
Markco

Markos (Spanish) a form of Marcos. (Latin) a form of Mark, Markus.

Markus (Latin) a form of Marcus.
Markas, Markcus, Markcuss, Markous, Márkus, Markys

Marland (English) lake land.
Mahland, Mahlend, Mahlind, Marlend, Marlind, Marlond, Marlynd

Marley GB (English) lake meadow.
Marlea, Marlee, Marleigh, Marli, Marlie, Marly, Marrley

Marlin BG (English) deep-sea fish.
Marlen, Marlion, Marlyn

Marlo BG (English) a form of Marlow.

Marlon (French) a form of Merlin.
Marlan

Marlow (English) hill by the lake.
Mar, Marlowe

Marmion (French) small.
Marmien, Marmyon

Marnin (Hebrew) singer; bringer of joy.
Marnyn

Maro (Japanese) myself.
Marow

Marón (Arabic) the male saint.

Marquan (American) a combination of Mark + Quan.
Marquane, Marquante

Marque (American) a form of Mark.

Marquel, Marquell (American) forms of Marcellus.
Marqueal, Marquelis, Marquelle, Marquellis, Marquiel, Marquil, Marquiles, Marquill, Marquille, Marquillus, Marqwel, Marqwell

Marques (Portuguese) nobleman.
Markes, Markqes, Markques, Markqueus, Marquees, Marquess, Marquest

Marqués (Portuguese) a form of Marques.

Marquese (Portuguese) a form of Marques.
Markquese, Marqese, Marqesse, Marquesse

Marquez (Portuguese) a form of Marques.
Marqez, Marqeze, Marqueze, Marquiez

Marquice (American) a form of Marquis.
Marquaice, Marquece

Marquies (American) a form of Marquis.

Marquis BG (French) nobleman.
Marcquis, Marcuis, Markquis, Markquise, Markuis, Marqise, Marquee, Marqui, Marquie, Marquiss, Marquist, Marquiz, Marquize

Marquise BG (French) nobleman.

Marquon (American) a combination of Mark + Quon.
Marquin, Marquinn, Marqwan, Marqwon, Marqwyn

Marqus (American) a form of Markus. (Portuguese) a form of Marques.

Marr (Spanish) divine. (Arabic) forbidden.

Mars (Latin) bold warrior. Mythology: the Roman god of war.

Marsalis (Italian) a form of Marcellus.
Marsalius, Marsallis, Marsellis, Marsellius, Marsellus

Marsden (English) marsh valley.
Marsdan, Marsdin, Marsdon, Marsdyn

Marsh (English) swamp land. (French) a short form of Marshall.

Marshal (French) a form of Marshall.
Marschal, Marshel

Marshall (French) caretaker of the horses; military title.
Marshell

Marshaun, Marshon (American) forms of Marshawn.

Marshawn (American) a combination of Mark + Shawn.
Marshaine, Marshauwn, Marshean, Marshun

Marston (English) town by the marsh.
Marstan, Marsten, Marstin, Marstyn

Martel (English) a form of Martell.
Martal, Martele

Martell (English) hammerer.
Martall, Martellis

Marten (Dutch) a form of Martin.
Maarten, Martein, Merten

Martese (Spanish) a form of Martez.

Martez (Spanish) a form of Martin.
Martaz, Martaze, Martes, Marteze, Marties, Martiese, Martiez, Martis, Martise, Martize

Marti GB (Spanish) a form of Martin.
Marte, Martee, Martie

Martial (French) a form of Mark.

Martice (Spanish) a form of Martez.
Martiece

Martin (Latin, French) a form of Martinus. History: Martin Luther King, Jr. led the Civil Rights movement and won the Nobel Peace Prize. See also Tynek.
Maartan, Maartin, Maarton, Maartyn, Mart, Martain, Martainn, Martan, Martijn, Martine, Martinien, Marto, Marton, Márton, Marts, Mattin, Mertin, Mertyn

Martín (Latin) a form of Martin.

Martinez (Spanish) a form of Martin.
Martines

Martínez (Spanish) a form of Martinez.

Martinho (Portuguese) a form of Martin.

Martino (Italian) a form of Martin.
Martiniano

Martiño (Spanish) a form of Martino.

Martins (Latvian) a form of Martin.

Martinus (Latin) martial, warlike.
Martinas, Martinos, Martinous, Martynas, Martynis, Martynos, Martynus, Martynys

Martir (Greek) he who gives a testament of faith.

Martirio (Latin) testimony.

Marty BG (Latin) a familiar form of Martin.
Martey

Martyn (Latin, French) a form of Martin.
Martyne

Marut (Hindi) Religion: the Hindu god of the wind.

Marv (English) a short form of Marvin.
Marve, Marvi, Marvis

Marvel (Latin) marvel.

Marvell (Latin) a form of Marvel.

Marvin (English) lover of the sea.
Marvein, Marven, Marvion, Marvn, Marvon, Marvyn, Marvyne, Murvan, Murven, Murvin, Murvine, Murvon, Murvyn, Murvyne, Murwin, Murwyn

Marwan (Arabic) history personage.
Marwen, Marwin, Marwon, Marwyn, Marwynn, Marwynne

Marwood (English) forest pond.

Marzûq (Arabic) blessed by God.

Mas'ûd (Arabic) a form of Masud.

Masaccio (Italian) twin.
Masaki

Masahiro (Japanese) broad-minded.
Masahyro

Masamba (Yao) leaves.
Masambah

Masao (Japanese) righteous.

Masato (Japanese) just.

Mashama (Shona) surprising.
Mashamah

Maska (Native American) powerful. (Russian) mask.
Maskah

Maskini (Egyptian) poor.

Maslin (French) little Thomas.
Maslan, Maslen, Masling, Maslon, Maslyn

Mason ☀ BG (French) stone worker.
Masan, Masen, Masin, Masson, Masun, Masyn, Sonny

Masou (Native American) fire god.

Massey (English) twin.
Massi, Massie, Masy

Massimo (Italian) greatest.
Massymo

Masud (Arabic, Swahili) fortunate.
Masood, Masoud, Mhasood

Matai (Basque, Bulgarian) a form of Matthew.
Máté, Matei

Matalino (Filipino) bright.

Matán (Hebrew) gift.

Matatías (Hebrew) gift of God.

Mateo, Matteo (Spanish) forms of Matthew.

Mateos (Hebrew) offered up to God.

Mateusz (Polish) a form of Matthew.
Matejs, Mateus

Mathe (German) a short form of Matthew.

Mather (English) powerful army.

Matheu (German) a form of Matthew.
Matheau, Matheus, Mathu

Mathew (Hebrew) a form of Matthew.

Mathias, Matthias (German, Swedish) forms of Matthew.
Mathi, Mathia, Matthia, Matthieus, Matus

Mathías (German) a form of Mathias.

Mathieu **BG** (French) a form of Matthew.
Mathie, Mathieux, Mathiew, Matthiew, Mattieu, Mattieux

Mathis (German, Swedish) a form of Mathias.

Matias, Matías, Mattias (Spanish) forms of Mathias.
Mattia

Matitiahu (Hebrew) given by God.

Matlal (Nahuatl) dark green; net.

Matlalihuitl (Nahuatl) blue-green feather.

Mato (Native American) brave.

Matope (Rhodesian) our last child.
Matop

Matoskah (Lakota) white bear.

Mats (Swedish) a familiar form of Matthew.
Matts, Matz

Matsimela (Egyptian) roots.

Matson (Hebrew) son of Matt.
Matsen, Mattson

Matt (Hebrew) a short form of Matthew.
Mat

Matteen (Afghan) disciplined; polite.
Mateen, Matin, Matyn

Matteus (Scandinavian) a form of Matthew.
Matthaeus, Matthaios, Matthews

Mattew (Hebrew) a form of Matthew.

Mattheus (Scandinavian) a form of Matthew.

Matthew ⭐ **BG** (Hebrew) gift of God. Bible: author of the first Gospel of the New Testament.
Maitiú, Makaio, Mata, Matai, Matek, Matfei, Mathe, Mathian, Mathieson, Matro, Matthaus, Matthäus, Mattmias, Maztheson

Matthieu (French) a form of Matthew.

Mattison **BG** (Hebrew) a form of Matson.
Matison

Matty **BG** (Hebrew) a familiar form of Matthew.
Mattie

Matus (Czech) a form of Mathias.

Matusalén (Hebrew) symbol of longevity.

Matvey (Russian) a form of Matthew.
Matviy, Matviyko, Matyash, Motka, Motya

Matyas (Polish) a form of Matthew.
Mátyás

Mauli **BG** (Hawaiian) a form of Maurice.

Maurice (Latin) dark skinned; moor; marsh-land. See also Seymour.
Maur, Maurance, Maureo, Mauri, Maurids, Mauriece, Maurikas, Maurin, Maurino, Maurise, Mauritius, Maurius, Maurrel, Maurtel, Mauryc, Mauryce, Maurycy, Maurys, Mauryse, Meurig, Meurisse, Morice, Moritz, Morrice

Mauricio (Spanish) a form of Maurice.
Mauriccio, Mauriceo, Maurico, Maurisio

Mauritz (German) a form of Maurice.
Maurits

Maurizio (Italian) a form of Maurice.

Mauro (Latin) a short form of Maurice.
Maur, Maurio

Maury (Latin) a familiar form of Maurice.
Maurey, Maurie

Maverick BG (American) independent.
*Maveric, Maverik, Maveryc, Maveryck,
Maveryk, Maveryke, Mavric, Mavrick,
Mavrik, Mavryc, Mavryck, Mavryk*

Mavilo (Latin) to not want.

Mawuli (Ewe) there is a God.

Max, Maxx (Latin) short forms of
Maximilian, Maxwell.
Maks, Maxe

Maxfield (English) Mack's field.
*Macfield, Mackfield, Mackfyld, Makfield,
Makfyld*

Maxi (Czech, Hungarian, Spanish) a familiar
form of Maximilian, Maximo.
Makszi, Maxie, Maxis

Maxim (Russian) a form of Maxime.
Maixim, Maxem

Maxime BG (French) most excellent.

Maximilian (Latin) greatest.
*Maksimilian, Maksimillian, Maksymilian,
Maxamilian, Maxamillion, Maxemilian,
Maxemilion, Maximalian, Maximili,
Maximilia, Maximilianos, Maximilianus,
Maximillion, Maxmilian, Maxmillion,
Maxon, Maxximillion, Maxymilian*

Maximiliano (Italian) a form of Maximilian.
Massimiliano, Maximiano

Maximilien, Maximillian (Latin) forms of
Maximilian.
*Maximillan, Maximillano, Maximillien,
Maxmillian, Maxximillian, Maxymillian*

Maximino (Italian) a form of Maximilian.

Maximo, Máximo (Spanish) forms of
Maximilian.
Maxi

Maximos (Greek) a form of Maximilian.
Maxymos, Maxymus

Maxwell (English) great spring.
Maxwel, Maxwill, Maxxwell

Maxy (English) a familiar form of Max,
Maxwell.
Maxey

Maxyme (French) a form of Maxime.

Mayer (Latin) a form of Magnus, Major.
(Hebrew) a form of Meir.
*Mahyar, Maier, Mayar, Mayeer, Mayir, Mayor,
Mayur*

Mayes (English) field.
Maies, Mays

Mayhew (English) a form of Matthew.
(Latin) a form of Maximilian.
Maehew, Maihew

Maymûm (Arabic) fortunate.

Maynard (English) powerful; brave. See also
Meinhard.
Mainard, May, Mayne, Maynhard, Ménard

Maynor (English) a form of Maynard.

Mayo (Irish) yew-tree plain. (English) a form
of Mayes. Geography: a county in Ireland.
Maio

Mayon (Indian) person of black complexion. Religion: another name for the Indian
god Mal.
Maion

Mayonga (Luganda) lake sailor.

Mayson (French) a form of Mason.

Mayta (Quechua) where are you?

Maytacuapac (Quechua) Oh, Lord, where
are you?

Mayua (Quechua) violet, purple.

Mazatl (Nahuatl) deer.

Mazi (Ibo) sir.
Mazzi

Mazin (Arabic) proper.
*Mazan, Mazen, Mazinn, Mazon, Mazyn,
Mazzin*

Mbita (Swahili) born on a cold night.

Mbizi (Egyptian) water.

Mbwana (Swahili) master.

Mc Kenzie, McKenzie BG (Irish) forms of
Mackenzie.

Mccoy (Irish) a form of Maccoy.
McCoi, McCoy

McGeorge (Scottish) son of George.
MacGeorge

Mckade (Scottish) son of Kade.
Mccade

Mckay (Scottish) son of Kay.
Macai, Macay, Mackai, Mackay, MacKay, Mackaye, Makkai, Makkay, Makkaye, Mckae, Mckai, McKay

Mckenna GB (American) a form of Mackenzie.

Mckenzie GB (Irish) a form of Mackenzie.
Mccenzie, Mckennzie, Mckensey, Mckensie, Mckenson, Mckensson, Mckenzee, Mckenzi, Mckenzy, Mckinzie

Mckinley BG (Irish) a form of Mackinnley.
Mckinely, Mckinnely, Mckinnlee, Mckinnley, McKinnley

Mead BG (English) meadow.
Meade, Meed

Mecatl (Nahuatl) rope; lineage.

Medardo (Germanic) boldly powerful.

Medarno (Saxon) he who deserves to be honored.

Medgar (German) a form of Edgar.
Medger

Medín (Greek) rejecter, defender.

Medir (Greek) a form of Medín.

Medric (English) flourishing meadow.
Medrick, Medrik, Medryc, Medryck, Medryk

Medwin (German) faithful friend.
Medwyn

Megan GB (Greek) pearl; great. (Irish) a form of Margaret (see Girls' Names).

Meginardo (Teutonic) he who is a strong leader.

Mehetabel (Hebrew) who God benefits.

Mehmet (Arabic) a form of Mahomet, Mohamet.
Mehemet

Mehrdad (Persian) gift of the sun.

Mehtar (Sanskrit) prince.
Mehta

Meinhard (German) strong, firm. See also Maynard.
Meinhardt, Meinke, Meino, Mendar, Meynhard

Meinrad (German) strong counsel.
Meynrad

Meir (Hebrew) one who brightens, shines; enlightener. History: Golda Meir was the prime minister of Israel.
Mayer, Meyer, Meyr, Muki, Myer

Meka GB (Hawaiian) eyes.
Mekah

Mel BG (English, Irish) a familiar form of Melvin.
Mell

Melanio (Greek) having black skin.

Melbourne (English) mill stream.
Melborn, Melborne, Melburn, Melburne, Melby

Melchior (Hebrew) king.
Meilseoir, Melker, Melkior

Melchor (Hebrew) a form of Melchior.

Meldon (English) mill hill.
Meldan, Melden, Meldin, Meldyn

Meldrick (English) strong mill.
Meldric, Meldrik, Meldryc, Meldryck, Meldryk

Melecio (Greek) careful and attentive.

Melibeo (Greek) he who takes care of the mentally handicapped.

Melino (Tongan) peace.
Melin, Melinos, Melyn, Melyno, Melynos

Meliso (Greek) bee.

Melito (Greek) sugary sweet; pleasant.

Meliton, Melitón (Greek) from the island of Malta.

Melivilu (Mapuche) four snakes.

Melquiades, Melquíades (Hebrew) Yahweh is my God.

Melrone (Irish) servant of Saint Ruadhan.

Melvern (Native American) great chief.
Melverne, Melvirn, Melvirne, Melvyrn, Melvyrne

Melville (French) mill town. Literature:
Herman Melville was a well-known
nineteenth-century American writer.
*Malvil, Malvill, Malville, Melvil, Melvill,
Milville*

Melvin (Irish) armored chief. (English) mill
friend; council friend. See also Vinny.
*Melvan, Melven, Melvine, Melvino, Melvon,
Melvyn, Melwin, Melwyn, Melwynn*

Memphis (Egyptian) one who comes from
Memphis.

Menachem (Hebrew) comforter.
Menahem, Nachman

Menajem (Hebrew) comforting.

Menandro (Greek) he who remains a man.

Menas (Greek) related to the months.

Menassah (Hebrew) cause to forget.
*Manasseh, Menashe, Menashi, Menashia,
Menashiah, Menashya*

Mendel (English) repairman.
*Mendal, Mendeley, Mendell, Mendie, Mendil,
Mendy, Mendyl*

Mendo (Spanish) a form of Hermenegildo.

Menelao (Greek) he who goes to the village to fight.

Menes (Egyptian) name of the king.

Mengesha (Ethiopian) kingdom.

Menico (Spanish) a short form of
Domenico.

Mensah (Ewe) third son.
Mensa

Mentor (Greek) the teacher.

Menz (German) a short form of Clement.

Mercer (English) storekeeper.
Merce

Mercurio (Latin) he who pays attention to
business.

Mered (Hebrew) revolter.

Meredith GB (Welsh) guardian from the sea.
*Meredeth, Meredyth, Merideth, Meridith,
Merry, Merydeth, Merydith, Merydyth*

Merion (Welsh) from Merion, Wales.
Merrion

Merivale (English) pleasant valley.
Merival, Meryval, Meryvale

Merle BG (French) a short form of Merlin,
Merrill.
Merl, Meryl, Murl, Murle

Merlin (English) falcon. Literature: the magi-
cian who served as counselor in King
Arthur's court.
Merlen, Merlinn, Merlyn, Merlynn

Merlín (French) a form of Merlin.

Merlino (Spanish) a form of Merlín.

Merrick (English) ruler of the sea.
*Merek, Meric, Merick, Merik, Merric, Merrik,
Merryc, Merryck, Merryk, Meryk, Meyrick,
Myrucj*

Merrill (Irish) bright sea. (French) famous.
*Meril, Merill, Merrel, Merrell, Merril, Meryl,
Meryll*

Merritt BG (Latin, Irish) valuable; deserving.
Merit, Meritt, Merrett, Merrit, Merryt

Merton (English) sea town.
Mertan, Merten, Mertin, Mertyn, Murton

Merulo (Latin) he who is fine as a blackbird.

Merv (Irish) a short form of Mervin.
Merve

Merville (French) sea village.

Mervin (Irish) a form of Marvin.
*Merv, Mervan, Merven, Mervine, Mervon,
Mervyn, Mervyne, Mervynn, Merwin,
Merwinn, Merwyn, Murvin, Murvyn,
Myrvyn, Myrvynn, Myrwyn*

Meshach (Hebrew) artist. Bible: one of
Daniel's three friends who emerged
unharmed from the fiery furnace of
Babylon.

Meshulam (Hebrew) paid.

Mesut (Turkish) happy.

Metikla (Moquelumnan) reaching a hand
underwater to catch a fish.

Metrenco (Mapuche) still water.

Metrofanes (Greek) he who resembles his mother.

Mette (Greek, Danish) pearl.
Almeta, Mete

Meulén (Mapuche) whirlwind.

Meurig (Welsh) a form of Maurice.

Meyer (German) farmer. (Hebrew) a form of Meir.
Mayeer, Mayer, Meier, Myer

Meztli (Nahuatl) moon.

Mhina (Swahili) delightful.
Mhinah

Micael (Hebrew) a form of Michael.

Micah BG (Hebrew) a form of Michael. Bible: a Hebrew prophet.
Mic, Mica, Myca, Mycah

Micaiah BG (Hebrew) a form of Micah.
Michiah

Micha GB (Hebrew) a short form of Michael.
Micha, Michah

Michael ☆ BG (Hebrew) who is like God? See also Micah, Miguel, Mika, Miles.
Machael, Machas, Maikal, Makael, Makal, Makel, Makell, Makis, Meikil, Meikyl, Mekil, Mekyl, Mhichael, Micahel, Mical, Michaele, Michaell, Michalel, Michau, Michelet, Michiel, Micho, Michoel, Miekil, Miekyl, Mihail, Mihalje, Mihkel, Mikáele

Michaelangel (American) a form of Michael + Angel.

Michail (Russian) a form of Michael.
Mihas, Mikale

Michal BG (Polish) a form of Michael.
Michak, Michalek, Michall

Michale (Polish) a form of Michal.

Micheal (Irish) a form of Michael.

Michel BG (French) a form of Michael.
Michaud, Miche, Michee, Micheil, Michell, Michelle, Michon

Michelangelo (Italian) a combination of Michael + Angelo. Art: Michelangelo Buonarroti was one of the greatest Renaissance painters.
Michelange

Michele GB (Italian) a form of Michael.

Michio (Japanese) man with the strength of three thousand.

Mick (English) a short form of Michael, Mickey.
Myc, Myck

Mickael, Mickel (English) forms of Michael.
Mickaele, Mickal, Mickale, Mickeal, Mickell, Mickelle, Mickle, Myckael, Myckaele, Myckaell

Mickenzie GB (Irish) a form of Mackenzie.
Mickenze, Mickenzy, Mikenzie

Mickey (Irish) a familiar form of Michael.
Mickee, Micki, Mickie, Micky, Miki, Mikie, Miky, Mycke, Myckee, Myckey, Mycki, Myckie, Mycky, Mykee, Mykey, Myki, Mykie, Myky

Micu (Hungarian) a form of Nick.

Midas (Greek) the fleeting and admirable business.

Migel (Portuguese, Spanish) a form of Miguel.

Miguel ☆ (Portuguese, Spanish) a form of Michael.
Migeal, Migeel, Miguelly, Miguil, Myguel, Myguele, Myguell, Myguelle

Miguelangel (Spanish) a combination of Miguel + Angel.
Miguelangelo

Mihail (Greek, Bulgarian, Romanian) a form of Mikhail.
Mahail, Maichail, Mekhail, Micheil, Mihailo, Mihal, Mihalis

Mijael, Mijaiá (Hebrew) who but God?

Mijaíl (Russian) a form of Miguel.

Mika GB (Ponca) raccoon. (Hebrew) a form of Micah. (Russian) a familiar form of Michael.
Miika, Myka, Mykah

Mikael (Swedish) a form of Michael.
Mikaeel, Mikaele, Mykael, Mykaele, Mykaell

Mikáele (Hawaiian) a form of Michael.
Mikele

Mikah BG (Hebrew) a form of Micah.
(Hebrew, Russian, Ponca) a form of Mika.

Mikail (Greek, Russian) a form of Mikhail.

Mikal BG (Hebrew) a form of Michael.
Meikal, Mekal, Miekal, Mikahl, Mikale

Mikasi (Omaha) coyote.
Mykasi

Mike (Hebrew) a short form of Michael.
Myk, Myke

Mikeal (Irish) a form of Michael.

Mikel BG (Basque) a form of Michael.
*Meikel, Mekel, Mekell, Miekel, Mikele,
Mikelle*

Mikelis (Latvian) a form of Michael.
Mikus, Milkins

Mikell (Basque) a form of Michael.

Mikey (Hebrew) a short form of Michael.

Mikhael (Greek, Russian) a form of
Mikhail.

Mikhail (Greek, Russian) a form of Michael.
*Mekhail, Mihály, Mikhale, Mikhalis,
Mikhalka, Mikhall, Mikhel, Mikhial, Mikhos*

Miki GB (Japanese) tree.
Mikio

Mikizli (Nahuatl) rest after hard work.

Mikkel (Norwegian) a form of Michael.
Mikkael, Mikle

Mikko (Finnish) a form of Michael.
Mikk, Mikka, Mikkohl, Mikkol, Miko, Mikol

Mikolaj (Polish) a form of Nicholas.
Mikolai

Mikolas (Greek) a form of Nicholas.
Miklós

Miksa (Hungarian) a form of Max.
Miks, Myksa

Milagro (Spanish) miracle.

Milan BG (Italian) northerner. Geography: a
city in northern Italy.
Milaan, Milano, Milen, Millan, Millen

Milap (Native American) giving.

Milborough (English) middle borough.
Milbrough, Mylborough, Mylbrough

Milburn (English) stream by the mill. A
form of Melbourne.
*Milborn, Milborne, Milbourn, Milbourne,
Milburne, Millborn, Millborne, Millbourn,
Millbourne, Millburn, Millburne*

Milcíades (Greek) he of reddish complexion.

Milek (Polish) a familiar form of Nicholas.
Mylek

Miles (Greek) millstone. (Latin) soldier.
(German) merciful. (English) a short form
of Michael.
Milas, Milles, Milson

Milford (English) mill by the ford.
Millford, Mylford, Myllford

Mililani BG (Hawaiian) heavenly caress.
Mililanee, Mililaney, Mililanie, Mililany

Milintica (Nahuatl) he is waving; fire.

Milko (German) a familiar form of Emil.
(Czech) a form of Michael.
Milkins

Millán (Latin) belonging to the Emilia family.

Millañir (Mapuche) silver fox.

Millard (Latin) caretaker of the mill.
Mill, Millward, Milward, Mylard, Myllard

Miller (English) miller; grain grinder.
*Mellar, Meller, Mellor, Milar, Miler, Millar,
Millen, Milor, Mylar, Myler, Myllar, Myller,
Mylor*

Mills (English) mills.
Mils, Mylls, Myls

Milo (German) a form of Miles. A familiar
form of Emil.
Millo, Mylo

Milos (Greek, Slavic) pleasant.
Mylos

Miloslav (Czech) lover of glory.
Myloslav

Milt (English) a short form of Milton.

Milton (English) mill town.
Millton, Miltie, Milty, Myllton, Mylton

Mimis (Greek) a familiar form of Demetrius.

Min (Burmese) king.
Mina, Myn

Mincho (Spanish) a form of Benjamin.

Minel (Spanish) a form of Manuel.

Miner (English) miner.
Myner

Minervino (Greek) a form of Minervo.

Minervo (Greek) power; young.

Mingan (Native American) gray wolf.
Myngan

Mingo (Spanish) a short form of Domingo.

Minh (Vietnamese) bright.
Minhao, Minhduc, Minhkhan, Minhtong, Minhy, Mynh

Minkah (Akan) just, fair.
Minka, Mynka, Mynkah

Minor (Latin) junior; younger.

Minoru (Japanese) fruitful.

Mío (Spanish) mine.

Mique (Spanish) a form of Mickey.

Miquel (Spanish) a form of Mique.
Mequel, Mequelin

Miracle GB (Latin) miracle.

Mirco (Spanish) he who assures the peace.

Mirko (Slavic) glorious for having assured peace.

Miron (Polish) peace.

Miroslav (Czech) peace; glory.
Mirek, Miroslaw, Miroslawy, Myroslav

Miroslavo (Slavic) a form of Miroslav.

Mirwais (Afghan) noble ruler.

Mirza (Persian) sir.

Misael, Missael (Hebrew) forms of Michael.
Mischael, Mishael

Misha GB (Russian) a short form of Michail.
Misa, Mischa, Mishael, Mishal, Mishe, Mishenka, Mishka

Miska (Hungarian) a form of Michael.
Misi, Misik, Misko, Miso

Mister (English) mister.
Mistar, Mistur, Mystar, Myster, Mystur

Misu (Moquelumnan) rippling water.
Mysu

Mitch (English) a short form of Mitchell.
Mytch

Mitchel (English) a form of Mitchell.
Mitchael, Mitchal, Mitcheal, Mitchele, Mitchil, Mytchel

Mitchell (English) a form of Michael.
Mitchall, Mitchelle, Mitchem, Mytchell

Mitsos (Greek) a familiar form of Demetrius.

Mixel (Catalan) a form of Miguel.

Moctezuma (Nahuatl) prince of the austere gesture.

Modesto (Latin) modest.
Modesti, Modestie, Modesty

Moe (English) a short form of Moses.
Mo

Mogens (Dutch) powerful.
Mogen

Mohamad, Mohamed, Mohammad, Mohammed (Arabic) forms of Muhammad.
Mohamd, Mohameed, Mohamid, Mohammadi, Mohammd, Mohammid, Mohanad, Mohaned, Mohmad

Mohamet (Arabic) a form of Muhammad.

Mohamud (Arabic) a form of Muhammad.
Mohammud, Mohamoud

Mohan (Hindi) delightful.

Moise (Portuguese, Spanish) a form of Moises.

Moises (Portuguese, Spanish) a form of Moses.
Moices, Moisei, Moisés, Moisey, Moisis

Moishe (Yiddish) a form of Moses.

Mojag (Native American) crying baby.

Moki (Australian) cloudy.
Mokee, Mokey, Mokie, Moky

Molimo (Moquelumnan) bear going under shady trees.

Momoztli (Nahuatl) altar.

Momuso (Moquelumnan) yellow jackets crowded in their nests for the winter.

Mona GB (Moquelumnan) gathering jimsonweed seed.
Monah

Monahan (Irish) monk.
Monaghan, Monoghan

Mongo (Yoruba) famous.

Mónico (Latin) solitary.

Monitor (Latin) he who counsels.

Monolo (Spanish) a familiar form of Manuel.

Monroe (Irish) from the mount on the river Roe.
Monro, Monrow, Munro, Munroe, Munrow

Montague (French) pointed mountain.
Montagne, Montagu

Montaigu (French) one who comes from the hill.

Montana GB (Spanish) mountain.
Geography: a U.S. state.
Montaine, Montanah, Montanna

Montaro (Japanese) big boy.
Montero

Monte (French) a form of Montague. (Spanish) a short form of Montgomery.
Montae, Montaé, Montay, Montea, Montee, Monti, Montie, Montoya

Montego (Spanish) mountainous.

Montel, Montell (American) forms of Montreal.
Montele, Montelle

Montenegro (Spanish) black mountain.

Monterio (Japanese) a form of Montaro.
Montario

Montes, Móntez (Spanish) forms of Montez.

Montez (Spanish) dweller in the mountains.
Monteiz, Monteze, Montezz, Montise, Montisze, Montiz, Montize, Montyz, Montyze

Montgomery BG (English) rich man's mountain.
Montgomerie, Mountgomery

Month (Egyptian) god of Thebes.

Montre (French) show.
Montra, Montrae, Montrai, Montray, Montrey

Montreal (French) royal mountain.
Geography: a city in Quebec.
Montel, Monterial, Monterrell, Montrail, Montreall, Montrial

Montrel, Montrell (French) forms of Montreal.
Montral, Montrale, Montrall, Montrele, Montrelle

Montrez (French) a form of Montre.
Montraz, Montres, Montreze

Montserrat (Catalan) upon the mountain range.

Montsho (Tswana) black.

Monty (English) a familiar form of Montgomery.
Montey

Moore (French) dark; moor; marshland.
Moar, Moare, Moor, Mooro, More, Morre

Mordecai (Hebrew) martial, warlike. Bible: wise counselor to Queen Esther.
Mord, Mordie, Mordy

Mordechai (Hebrew) a form of Mordecai.
Mordachai

Mordred (Latin) painful. Literature: the bastard son of King Arthur.
Modred, Mordryd

Morel (French) an edible mushroom.
Morell, Morrel

Moreland (English) moor; marshland.
Moarlan, Moarland, Moorelan, Mooreland, Moorlan, Moorland, Morelan, Morlan, Morland

Morell (French) dark; from Morocco.
Morelle, Morelli, Morill, Morrell, Morrill, Murrel, Murrell

Morey (Greek) a familiar form of Moris. (Latin) a form of Morrie.
Moree, Morree, Morrey, Morry, Mory, Morye

Morfeo (Greek) he who makes you see beautiful figures.

Morgan GB (Scottish) sea warrior.
Morghan, Morgin, Morgon, Morgun, Morgunn, Morgwn, Morgyn, Morrgan

Morgen GB (Scottish) a form of Morgan.

Morio (Japanese) forest.
Moryo

Moris (Greek) son of the dark one. (English) a form of Morris.
Morey, Morisz, Moriz, Morys

Moritz (German) a form of Maurice, Morris.
Morisz

Morley (English) meadow by the moor.
Moorley, Moorly, Morlea, Morlee, Morleigh, Morli, Morlie, Morlon, Morly, Morlyn, Morrley

Morrie (Latin) a familiar form of Maurice, Morse.
Morey, Mori, Morie, Morri

Morris (Latin) dark skinned; moor; marshland. (English) a form of Maurice.
Moris, Moriss, Moritz, Morrese, Morrise, Morriss, Morrys, Moss

Morse (English) son of Maurice.
Morresse, Morrison, Morrisson

Mort (French, English) a short form of Mordecai, Morten, Mortimer, Morton.
Morte, Mortey, Mortie, Mortty, Morty

Morten (Norwegian) a form of Martin.
Mortan, Mortin, Mortyn

Mortimer (French) still water.
Mortymer

Morton (English) town near the moor.

Morven (Scottish) mariner.
Morvan, Morvien, Morvin

Mose (Hebrew) a short form of Moses.
Moyse

Mosegi (Egyptian) tailor.

Moses (Hebrew) drawn out of the water. (Egyptian) son, child. Bible: the Hebrew lawgiver who brought the Ten Commandments down from Mount Sinai.
Mosese, Mosiah, Mosie, Mosses, Mosya, Mosze, Moszek, Moyses, Moze, Mozes

Moshe (Hebrew, Polish) a form of Moses.
Mosheh

Moshé (Hebrew) a form of Moshe.

Mosi BG (Swahili) first-born.
Mosee, Mosey, Mosie, Mosy

Moss (Irish) a short form of Maurice, Morris. (English) a short form of Moses.
Mos

Moswen BG (African) light in color.
Moswin, Moswyn

Motega (Native American) new arrow.
Motegah

Mouhamed (Arabic) a form of Muhammad.
Mouhamad, Mouhamadou, Mouhammed, Mouhamoin

Mousa (Arabic) a form of Moses.
Moussa

Moyolehuani (Nahuatl) enamored one.

Mozart (Italian) breathless. Music: Wolfgang Amadeus Mozart was a famous eighteenth-century Austrian composer.
Mozar

Moze (Lithuanian) a form of Moses.
Mózes

Mpasa (Nguni) mat.
Mpasah

Mposi (Nyakyusa) blacksmith.

Mpoza (Luganda) tax collector.

Msamaki (Egyptian) fish.

Msrah (Akan) sixth-born.

Mtima (Nguni) heart.

Mu'âdh (Arabic) protected.

Mû'awîyya (Arabic) young fox.

Mu'tassim (Arabic) adhered to faith.

Mu'tazz (Arabic) proud.

Muata (Moquelumnan) yellow jackets in
their nest.
Mutah

Mubârak (Arabic) blessed.

Mucio (Latin) he who endures silence.

Mufid (Arabic) useful.

Mugamba (Runyoro) talks too much.

Mugisa (Rutooro) lucky.
Mugisha, Mukisa

Muhammad (Arabic) praised. History: the
founder of the Islamic religion. See also
Ahmad, Hamid, Yasin.
*Mahmúd, Muhamad, Muhamed, Muhamet,
Muhammadali*

Muhammed (Arabic) a form of
Muhammad.

Muhannad (Arabic) sword.
Muhanad

Muhsin (Arabic) beneficent; charitable.

Muhtadi (Arabic) rightly guided.

Muir (Scottish) moor; marshland.
Muire, Muyr, Muyre

Mujahid (Arabic) fighter in the way of
Allah.

Mujâhid (Arabic) a form of Mujahid.

Mukasa (Luganda) God's chief administrator.
Mukasah

Mukhtar (Arabic) chosen.
Mukhtaar

Mukhwana (Egyptian) twins.

Mukul (Sanskrit) bud, blossom; soul.

Mullu (Quechua) coral, jewel.

Mulogo (Musoga) wizard.

Mun-Hee (Korean) literate; shiny.

Mundan (Rhodesian) garden.

Mundo (Spanish) a short form of Edmundo.

Mundy (Irish) from Reamonn.
Munde, Mundee, Mundey, Mundi, Mundie

Mungo (Scottish) amiable.

Munir (Arabic) brilliant; shining.
Munyr

Munny (Cambodian) wise.
*Munee, Muney, Muni, Munie, Munnee,
Munney, Munni, Munnie, Muny*

Muntassir (Arabic) victorious.

Muraco (Native American) white moon.
Muracco

Murali (Hindi) flute. Religion: the instrument the Hindu god Krishna is usually
depicted as playing.

Murat (Turkish) wish come true.

Murdock (Scottish) wealthy sailor.
Murdo, Murdoc, Murdoch, Murtagh

Murphy 🅱🅶 (Irish) sea warrior.
*Murffee, Murffey, Murffi, Murffie, Murffy,
Murfy, Murphee, Murphey, Murphi, Murphie*

Murray (Scottish) sailor.
*Moray, Murae, Murai, Muray, Murrae, Murrai,
Murree, Murrey, Murri, Murrie, Murry*

Murtadi (Arabic) satisfied.

Murtagh (Irish) a form of Murdock.
Murtaugh

Musa (Swahili) child.

Mûsà (Arabic) a form of Moises.

Musád (Arabic) untied camel.

Mushin (Arabic) charitable.

Muslim (Egyptian) believer.

Musoke (Rukonjo) born while a rainbow
was in the sky.

Mustafa (Arabic) chosen; royal.
*Mostafa, Mostafah, Mostaffa, Mostaffah,
Moustafa, Mustafaa, Mustafah, Mustafe,
Mustaffa, Mustafo, Mustoffa, Mustofo*

Mustafá, Mustafà (Arabic) forms of
Mustafa.

Mustapha (Arabic) a form of Mustafa.
Mostapha, Moustapha

Muti (Arabic) obedient.

Muwaffaq (Arabic) successful.

Mwaka (Luganda) born on New Year's Eve.

Mwamba (Nyakyusa) strong.

Mwanje (Luganda) leopard.

Mwinyi (Swahili) king.

Mwita (Swahili) summoner.

Mychael (American) a form of Michael.

Mychajlo (Latvian) a form of Michael.
Mykhaltso, Mykhas

Mychal (American) a form of Michael.
Mychall, Mychalo, Mycheal

Myer (English) a form of Meir.
Myers, Myur

Mykal (American) a form of Michael.
Mykall, Mykell, Mykil, Mykill, Mykyl,
Mykyle, Mykyll, Mykylle

Mykel BG (American) a form of Michael.

Myles (Latin) soldier. (German) a form of
Miles.
Myels, Mylez, Mylles, Mylz

Mylon (Italian) a form of Milan.
Mylan, Mylen, Mylyn, Mylynn

Mynor (Latin) a form of Minor.

Myo (Burmese) city.

Myriam GB (American) a form of Miriam
(see Girls' Names).

Myron (Greek) fragrant ointment. (Polish) a
form of Miron.
Mehran, Mehrayan, My, Myran, Myrone, Ron

Myung-Dae (Korean) right; great.

Mzuzi (Swahili) inventive.

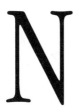

N'namdi (Ibo) his father's name lives on.

Naaman (Hebrew) pleasant.
Naman

Nabarun (Indian) morning sun.

Nabeel (Arabic) a form of Nabil.

Nabendu (Indian) new moon.

Nabhân, Nabîh (Arabic) worthy.

Nabhi (Indian) focus; the best.

Nabiha (Arabic) intelligent.
Nabihah

Nabil (Arabic) noble.
Nabiel, Nabill, Nabyl, Nabyll

Nabor (Hebrew) the prophet's light.

Nabucodonosor (Chaldean) God protects
my reign.

Nachiketa (Indian) an ancient Rishi, or
Hindu sage; fire.

Nachman (Hebrew) a short form of
Menachem.
Nachum

Nada GB (Arabic) generous.
Nadah

Nadav (Hebrew) generous; noble.
Nadiv

Nader (Afghan, Arabic) a form of Nadir.

Nadidah (Arabic) equal to anyone else.

Nadim (Arabic) friend.
Nadeem, Nadym

Nadîm (Arabic) a form of Nadim.

Nadir (Afghan, Arabic) dear, rare.
Nadar, Nadyr

Nadisu (Hindi) beautiful river.
Nadysu

Naeem (Arabic) benevolent.
Naem, Naim, Naiym, Naym, Nieem

Naftali (Hebrew) wreath.
Naftalie

Naftalí (Hebrew) a form of Naftali.

Nagendra, Nagesh (Indian) other names
for the Hindu serpent god Sesh.

Nagid (Hebrew) ruler; prince.
Nagyd

Nahele (Hawaiian) forest.

Nahma (Native American) sturgeon.
Nahmah

Nahuatl (Nahuatl) four waters.

Nahuel (Araucanian) tiger.

Nahum (Hebrew) a form of Nachman.

Nahusha (Indian) a mythological king.

Naiara (Spanish) of the Virgin Mary.

Nailah GB (Arabic) successful.
Naila, Nayla, Naylah

Nairit (Indian) southwest.

Nairn (Scottish) river with alder trees.
Nairne, Nayrn, Nayrne

Naishadh (Indian) another name for King
Nala, a hero from the Indian epic poem
Mahabharata.

Najee BG (Arabic) a form of Naji.
Najae, Najée, Najei, Najiee

Naji (Arabic) safe.
Najie, Najih, Najy

Nâji (Arabic) a form of Naji.

Najíb (Arabic) born to nobility.
Najeeb, Najib, Najyb, Nejeeb, Nejib, Nejyb

Najjâr (Arabic) carpenter.

Najm Al-Dîn (Arabic) star of faith.

Nakia GB (Arabic) pure.
Nakai, Nakee, Nakeia, Naki, Nakiah, Nakii

Nakos (Arapaho) sage, wise.

Nakshatra (Indian) star.

Nakul (Indian) one of the Pandavas, descendents of King Pandu in the Indian epic
poem *Mahabharata.*

Naldo (Spanish) a familiar form of
Reginald.

Nalin (Indian) lotus.

Nalinaksha (Indian) one with eyes like a
lotus.

Nalren (Dene) thawed out.

Nam (Vietnamese) scrape off.

Namacuix (Nahuatl) king.

Namaka (Hawaiian) eyes.
Namakah

Namdev, Narahari (Indian) other names for
the Hindu god Vishnu.

Namid (Ojibwa) star dancer.
Namyd

Namir (Hebrew) leopard.
Namer, Namyr

Namuncura, Namuncurá (Mapuche) foot
of stone, strong foot.

Nana BG (Hawaiian) spring.

Nanak (Indian) Sikh guru.

Ñancuvilu (Mapuche) snake that is the color
of lead.

Nand (Indian) joyful.

Nandi (Indian) another name for the Hindu
god Shiva; the bull of Shiva.

Nandin (Hindi) Religion: a servant of the
Hindu god Shiva.
Nandan, Nandyn

Nando (German) a familiar form of
Ferdinand.
Nandor

Nangila (Abaluhya) born while parents traveled.
Nangilah, Nangyla, Nangylah

Nangwaya (Mwera) don't mess with me.

Nansen (Swedish) son of Nancy.
Nansan, Nansin, Nanson, Nansyn

Nantai (Navajo) chief.
Nantay

Nantan (Apache) spokesman.
Nanten, Nantin, Nanton, Nantyn

Naoko (Japanese) straight, honest.

Naolin (Spanish) sun god of the Mexican
people.

Naotau (Indian) new.

Napayshni (Lakota) he does not flee; courageous.

Napier (Spanish) new city.
Napyer, Neper, Nepier, Nepyer

Napoleon (Greek) lion of the woodland. (Italian) from Naples, Italy. History: Napoleon Bonaparte was a famous nineteenth-century French emperor.
Leon, Nap, Napolean, Napoléon, Napoleone, Nappie, Nappy

Napoleón (Greek) a form of Napoleon.

Naquan (American) a combination of the prefix Na + Quan.
Naqawn, Naquain, Naquen, Naquon

Narain (Hindi) protector. Religion: another name for the Hindu god Vishnu.
Narayan

Narasimha (Indian) an incarnation of the Hindu god Vishnu.

Narcisse (French) a form of Narcissus.
Narcis, Narciso, Narcisso, Narcyso, Narcyss, Narcysse, Narkis

Narcissus (Greek) daffodil. Mythology: the youth who fell in love with his own reflection.
Narcisse, Narcyssus, Narkissos

Nard (Persian) chess player.

Nardo (German) strong, hardy. (Spanish) a short form of Bernardo.

Narendra (Indian) king.

Naresh (Hindi) the king.

Narmer (Egyptian) name of the king.

Narno (Latin) he who was born in the Italian city of Narnia.

Narrie (Australian) bush fire.
Narree, Narrey, Narri, Narry

Narses (Persian) what the two martyrs brought from Persia.

Narve (Dutch) healthy, strong.
Narv

Nashashuk (Fox, Sauk) loud thunder.

Nâshe (Arabic) counselor.

Nashoba (Choctaw) wolf.

Nasim (Persian) breeze; fresh air.
Naseem, Nassim, Nasym

Nasîm (Persian) a form of Nasim.

Nasir (Arabic) a form of Nasser.
Nassir

Nassar (Arabic) protector.

Nasser (Arabic) victorious.
Naseer, Naser, Nasier, Nasr, Nassor, Nassyr

Nat (English) a short form of Nathan, Nathaniel.
Natt, Natty

Natal (Spanish) a form of Noël.
Natale, Natalie, Natalino, Natalio, Nataly

Natalicio (Latin) day of birth.

Natan (Hebrew, Hungarian, Polish, Russian, Spanish) God has given.
Natain, Nataine, Natayn, Natayne, Naten

Natán (Hebrew) a form of Natan.

Natanael (Hebrew) a form of Nathaniel.
Nataneal, Natanel, Nataniel, Nataniello

Nate (Hebrew) a short form of Nathan, Nathaniel.
Nait, Naite, Nayt, Nayte

Natesh (Hindi) destroyer. Religion: another name for the Hindu god Shiva.

Nathan ☆ (Hebrew) a short form of Nathaniel. Bible: a prophet during the reigns of David and Solomon.
Naethan, Naethin, Naethun, Naethyn, Naithan, Naithin, Naithon, Naithun, Naithyn, Nathann, Nathean, Nathian, Nathin, Nathun, Nathyn, Natthan, Naythan, Naythun, Naythyn, Nethan

Nathanael (Hebrew) gift of God. Bible: one of the Twelve Apostles, also known as Bartholomew.
Naethanael, Naethanial, Nafanael, Nafanail, Nafanyl, Nafanyle, Naithanael, Naithanyael, Naithanyal, Nathanae, Nathanal, Nathaneil, Nathanel, Nathaneol, Nathanual, Nathanyal Natthanial, Natthanyal, Nayfanial, Naythaneal, Naythanial, Nithanial, Nithanyal, Nothanial, Nothanyal

Nathaneal, Nathanial (Hebrew) forms of Nathanael.
Naithanyel, Nathanielle, Nathanil, Nathanile, Nathanuel, Nathanyel, Nathanyl, Natheal, Nathel, Nathinel, Natthaniel, Natthanielle, Natthaniuel, Natthanyel, Naythaniel, Naythanielle, Nethaniel, Nithaniel, Nithanyel, Nothaniel, Nothanielle, Nothanyel, Thaniel

Nathanie (Hebrew) a familiar form of Nathaniel.
Nathania, Nathanni

Nathaniel ☀ (Hebrew) a form of Nathanael.

Nathen, Nathon (Hebrew) forms of Nathan.
Naethen, Naethon, Naithen, Naythen, Naython

Natividad (Spanish) nativity.

Natlalihuitl (Nahuatl) blue-green feather or purple feather.

Natwar (Indian) another name for the Hindu god Krishna.

Ñaupac, Ñaupari (Quechua) firstborn.

Ñauque, Ñauqui (Quechua) before everyone.

Nav (Gypsy) name.

Naval (Latin) god of the sailing vessels.

Navaneet (Indian) butter.

Navarro (Spanish) plains.
Navara, Navaro, Navarra, Navarre

Navdeep BG (Sikh) new light.
Navdip

Naveen BG (Hindi) a form of Navin.

Navin (Hindi) new, novel.
Naven, Navyn

Navrang (Indian) beautiful.

Navroz (Indian) Parsi festival to celebrate the new year.

Nawat (Native American) left-handed.

Nawkaw (Winnebago) wood.

Nayan (Indian) eye.

Nayati (Native American) wrestler.
Nayaty

Nayi (Lebanese) saved.

Nayland (English) island dweller.
Nailan, Nailand, Naylan

Nazareno (Hebrew) he who has separated himself from the rest.

Nazareth (Hebrew) born in Nazareth, Israel.
Nazaire, Nazaret, Nazarie, Nazario, Nazaryo, Nazerene, Nazerine

Nâzeh (Arabic) chaste.

Nazih (Arabic) pure, chaste.
Nazeeh, Nazeem, Nazeer, Nazieh, Nazim, Nazir, Nazyh, Nazz

Ndale (Nguni) trick.

Neal, Neel (Irish) forms of Neil.
Neale, Neall, Nealle, Nealon, Nealy, Nealye, Neele, Neell, Neelle

Neandro (Greek) young and manly.

Neb-Er-Tcher (Egyptian) god of the universe.

Nebrido (Greek) graceful like the fawn.

Necalli (Nahuatl) battle.

Neci BG (Latin) a familiar form of Ignatius.

Nectario (Greek) he who sweetens life with nectar.

Nectarios (Greek) Religion: a saint in the Greek Orthodox Church.

Necuamatl (Nahuatl) king.

Neculman (Mapuche) swift condor.

Neculqueo (Mapuche) rapid speaker.

Ned (English) a familiar form of Edward, Edwin.
Nedd, Neddie, Neddym, Nedrick

Neeladri (Indian) the Nilgiris, a mountainous region in India.

Neelambar (Indian) blue sky.

Neema BG (Swahili) born during prosperous times.

Nefertum (Egyptian) cultured in Memphis.

Neftalí (Hebrew) one who helps in the struggle.

Neguib (Arabic) famous.

Nehemiah (Hebrew) compassion of Jehovah. Bible: a Jewish leader.
Nahemia, Nahemiah, Nechemia, Nechemya, Nehemia, Nehemias, Nehemie, Nehemyah, Nehimiah, Nehmia, Nehmiah, Nemo, Neyamia, Neyamiah, Neyamya, Neyamyah

Nehru (Hindi) canal.

Nehuén (Araucanian) strong.

Neil (Irish) champion.
Neihl, Neile, Neill, Neille

Neka (Native American) wild goose.
Nekah

Nekiron (Japanese) unsure.

Nelek (Polish) a form of Cornelius.
Nelik

Nelius (Latin) a short form of Cornelius.

Nelli (Nahuatl) truth.

Nellie GB (English) a familiar form of Cornelius, Cornell, Nelson.
Nell, Nelly

Nelo (Spanish) a form of Daniel.
Nello, Nilo

Nels (Scandinavian) a form of Neil, Nelson.
Nelse

Nelson (English) son of Neil.
Nealsan, Nealsen, Nealson, Nealsun, Nealsyn, Neelsan, Neelsen, Neelsin, Neelsun, Neelsyn, Neilsan, Neilsen, Neilsin, Neilson, Neilsun, Neilsyn, Nellie, Nels, Nelsen, Nelsin, Nelsun, Nelsyn, Neylsan, Neylsen, Neylsin, Neylson, Neylsun, Neylsyn, Nilsan, Nilsen, Nilsin, Nilson, Nilsson, Nilsun, Nilsyn, Nylsan, Nylsen, Nylsin, Nylson, Nylsun, Nylsyn

Nemesia (Latin) punishment of the gods.

Nemesio (Spanish) just.
Nemesyo, Nemi

Nemo (Greek) glen, glade. (Hebrew) a short form of Nehemiah.
Nimo, Nymo

Nemorio (Latin) belongs to the sacred forest.

Nemuel (Hebrew) God's sea.
Nemuele, Nemuell, Nemuelle

Nen (Egyptian) ancient waters.

Neo (Greek) new. (African) gift.

Neofito (Greek) he who began recently.

Neon (Greek) he who is strong.

Neopolo (Spanish) a form of Napoleon.

Nepomuceno (Slavic) he who gives his help.

Neptune (Latin) sea ruler. Mythology: the Roman god of the sea.

Neptuno (Latin) a form of Neptune.

Nereo (Greek) he who is the captain at sea.

Nereu (Catalan) a form of Nereo.

Neriá (Hebrew) light of God.

Nerio (Greek) sea traveler.

Nero (Latin, Spanish) stern. History: a cruel Roman emperor.
Niro, Nyro

Neron (Spanish) strong.
Nerone, Nerron

Nerón (Spanish) a form of Neron.

Nerville (French, Irish) village by the sea.
Nervil, Nervile, Nervill, Nervyl, Nervyle, Nervyll, Nervylle

Nery (Hebrew, Arabic) a form of Nuri.
Neri

Nesbit (English) nose-shaped bend in a river.
Naisbit, Naisbitt, Naisbyt, Naisbytt, Nesbitt, Nesbyt, Nesbytt, Nisbet, Nisbett, Nysbet, Nysbett, Nysbit, Nysbitt, Nysbyt, Nysbytt

Nesto (Spanish) serious.

Nestor (Greek) traveler; wise.
Nestar, Nester, Nestyr

Néstor (Greek) a form of Nestor.

Nestorio (Greek) a form of Nestor.

Nethaniel (Hebrew) a form of Nathaniel.
Netanel, Netania, Netaniah, Netaniel,
Netanya, Nethanel, Nethanial, Nethaniel,
Nethanuel, Nethanyal, Nethanyel

Neto (Spanish) a short form of Ernesto.

Netzahualcoyotl (Nahuatl) hungry coyote.

Neuveville (French) one who comes from
the new city.

Nevada 🇬🇧 (Spanish) covered in snow.
Geography: a U.S. state.
Navada, Nevadah, Nevade, Nevadia, Nevadya

Nevan (Irish) holy.
Nefan, Nefen, Nevean, Neven, Nevon,
Nevun, Nivan, Niven, Nivon, Nyvan, Nyven,
Nyvon

Neville (French) new town.
Nev, Neval, Nevall, Nevel, Nevele, Nevell,
Nevil, Nevile, Nevill, Nevyl, Nevyle, Nevyll,
Nevylle

Nevin (Irish) worshiper of the saint.
(English) middle; herb.
Nefin, Nev, Nevins, Nevyn, Nivyn, Nyvin,
Nyvyn

Newbold (English) new tree.

Newell (English) new hall.
Newall, Newel, Newyle

Newland (English) new land.
Newlan

Newlin (Welsh) new lake.
Newlyn

Newman (English) newcomer.
Neiman, Neimann, Neimon, Neuman,
Neumann, Newmann, Newmen, Numan,
Numen

Newton (English) new town.
Nauton, Newt, Newtown

Neyén (Araucanian) a smooth breath.

Nezahualcoyotl (Nahuatl) fasting coyote.

Nezahualpilli (Nahuatl) a prince who fasts.

Ngai (Vietnamese) herb.

Nghia (Vietnamese) forever.

Ngozi (Ibo) blessing.

Ngu (Vietnamese) sleep.

Nguyen 🇧🇬 (Vietnamese) a form of Ngu.

Nhean (Cambodian) self-knowledge.

Niall (Irish) a form of Neil. History: Niall of
the Nine Hostages was a famous Irish
king.
Nial, Niale, Nialle, Niel, Niele, Niell, Nielle,
Nyal, Nyale, Nyall, Nyalle, Nyeal, Nyeale,
Nyeall, Nyealle

Nibal (Arabic) arrows.
Nibel, Nybal

Nibaw (Native American) standing tall.
Nybaw

Nicabar (Gypsy) stealthy.
Nycabar

Nicandro (Greek) he who is victorious
among men.

Nicasio (Greek) the victorious one.

Nicco, Nico (Greek) short forms of
Nicholas.

Niccolo, Nicolo (Italian) forms of Nicholas.
Niccolò, Nicholo, Nicol, Nicolao, Nicoll,
Nicollo

Níceas (Greek) he of the great victory.

Nicéforo (Greek) he who brings victory.

Nicetas, Niceto (Greek) victorious.

Nicho (Spanish) a form of Dennis.
Nycho

Nicholai (Norwegian, Russian) a form of
Nicholas.

Nicholas ☀ 🇧🇬 (Greek) victorious people.
Religion: Nicholas of Myra is a patron
saint of children. See also Caelan, Claus,
Cola, Colar, Cole, Colin, Colson, Klaus,
Lasse, Mikolaj, Mikolas, Milek.
Niccolas, Nichalas, Nichelas, Nichele, Nichlas,
Nichlos, Nichola, Nicholaas, Nicholaes,
Nicholase, Nichole, Nicholias, Nicholl,
Nichollas, Nicholus, Nioclás, Niocol, Nycholas

Nicholaus (Greek) a form of Nicholas.
Nichalaus, Nichalous, Nichaolas, Nichlaus,
Nichloas, Nichlous, Nicholaos, Nicholous,
Nicolaus

Nicholes, Nichols (English) son of
Nicholas.
Nickoles, Nicolls

Nicholis (English) a form of Nicholes.

Nicholos (Greek) a form of Nicholas.

Nicholson (English) son of Nicholas.
*Nickelson, Nickoleson, Nycholson, Nyckolson,
Nykolson*

Nick (English) a short form of Dominic,
Nicholas. See also Micu.
Nic, Nicc, Nik, Nyck, Nyk

Nickalas, Nickalus (Greek) forms of
Nicholas.
*Nickalaus, Nickalis, Nickalos, Nickalous,
Nickelas, Nickelous, Nickelus, Nickolau*

Nicklaus, Nicklas (Greek) forms of
Nicholas.
*Nicklauss, Nicklos, Nicklous, Nicklus, Niclas,
Niclasse, Niklaus*

Nickolas, Nickolaus, Nickolis, Nickolus
(Greek) forms of Nicholas.
Nickolaos, Nickolos, Nickolys, Nickoulas

Nicky BG (Greek) a familiar form of
Nicholas.
Nickey, Nicki, Nickie

Nicodemo (Greek) a form of Nicodemus.

Nicodemus (Greek) conqueror of the peo-
ple.
*Nicodem, Nicodemius, Nikodem, Nikodema,
Nikodemious, Nikodim*

Nicola GB (Italian) a form of Nicholas. See
also Cola.
Nickola, Nicolá, Nikolah

Nicolaas, Nicolaus (Italian) forms of
Nicolas.
Nicolás, Nicoles, Nicolis, Nicolus

Nicolai (Norwegian, Russian) a form of
Nicholas.
*Nickolai, Nicolaj, Nicolau, Nicolay, Nicoly,
Nikalai*

Nicolas BG (Italian) a form of Nicolas.

Nicole GB (French) a form of Nicholas.

Nicomedes (Greek) he who prepares the
victories.

Nicón (Greek) the victorious one.

Nicostrato (Greek) the general who leads
to victory.

Ñielol (Mapuche) eye of the cave.

Niels (Danish) a form of Neil.
Niel, Nielsen, Nielson

Nien (Vietnamese) year.
Nyen

Nigan (Native American) ahead.
Nigen

Nigel (Latin) dark night.
*Niegal, Niegel, Nigal, Nigale, Nigele, Nigell,
Nigiel, Nigil, Nigle, Nijel, Nygal, Nygel,
Nyigel, Nyjil*

Niguel (Spanish) champion.

Nika GB (Yoruba) ferocious.
*Nica, Nicah, Nicka, Nickah, Nikah, Nikka,
Nyca, Nycah, Nycka, Nyckah, Nyka, Nykah*

Nike BG (Greek) victorious.
*Nikee, Nikey, Nikie, Nykee, Nykei, Nykey,
Nykie*

Nikhil (Indian) a form of Nicholas.

Niki GB (Hungarian) a familiar form of
Nicholas.
Nikia, Nikiah, Nikkie, Niky, Nyki, Nyky

Nikita GB (Russian) a form of Nicholas.
*Nakita, Nakitah, Nykita, Nykitah, Nykyta,
Nykytah*

Nikiti (Native American) round and smooth
like an abalone shell.
*Nikity, Nikyti, Nityty, Nykiti, Nykity,
Nykyty*

Nikki GB (Hungarian) a familiar form of
Nicholas.

Nikko, Niko (Hungarian) forms of
Nicholas.
Nikoe, Nyko

Niklas (Latvian, Swedish) a form of
Nicholas.
Niklaas, Niklaus

Nikola (Greek) a short form of Nicholas.
Nikolao, Nikolay, Nykola

Nikolai (Estonian, Russian) a form of Nicholas.
Kolya, Nikolais, Nikolaj, Nikolajs, Nikolay, Nikoli, Nikolia, Nikula

Nikolaos (Greek) a form of Nicholas.

Nikolas, Nikolaus (Greek) forms of Nicholas.
Nicanor, Nikalas, Nikalis, Nikalous, Nikalus, Nikholas, Nikolaas, Nikolis, Nikos, Nikulas, Nilos, Nykolas, Nykolus

Nikolos (Greek) a form of Nicholas. See also Kolya.
Niklos, Nikolaos, Nikolò, Nikolous, Nikolus

Nil (Russian) a form of Neil.
Nill, Nille, Nilya

Nila GB (Hindi) blue.
Nilah, Nyla, Nylah

Nile (Russian) a form of Nil.

Niles (English) son of Neil.
Nilese, Nilesh, Nyles, Nylles

Nilo (Finnish) a form of Neil.
Niilo

Nils (Swedish) a short form of Nicholas. (Danish) a form of Niels.

Nima BG (Hebrew) thread. (Arabic) blessing.

Nimrod (Hebrew) rebel. Bible: a great-grandson of Noah.
Nymrod

Ninacolla (Quechua) flame of fire.

Ninacuyuchi, Ninan (Quechua) he who stokes the fire.

Ninauari (Quechua) llama-like animal of fire.

Ninauíca (Quechua) sacred fire.

Nino (Spanish) a form of Niño.

Niño (Spanish) young child.
Neño, Nyño

Niran (Tai) eternal.
Niren, Nirin, Niron, Niryn, Nyran, Nyren, Nyrin, Nyron, Nyryn

Nishan (Armenian) cross, sign, mark.
Nishon, Nyshan

Nissan (Hebrew) sign, omen; miracle.
Nisan, Nissim, Nissin, Nisson, Nyssan

Nitgardo (Germanic) fighter who maintains combative fire.

Nitis (Native American) friend.
Netis, Nytis, Nytys

Nixon (English) son of Nick.
Nixan, Nixen, Nixin, Nixson, Nixun, Nixyn, Nyxen, Nyxin, Nyxon, Nyxyx

Nizam (Arabic) leader.
Nyzam

Nkosi (Egyptian) rule.

Nkrumah (Egyptian) ninth born.

Nkunda (Runyankore) loves those who hate him.
Nkundah

Noach (Hebrew) a form of Noah.

Noah ⚝ BG (Hebrew) peaceful, restful. Bible: the patriarch who built the ark to survive the Flood.
Noach, Noak

Noaj (Hebrew) a rest.

Noam (Hebrew) sweet; friend.

Noble (Latin) born to nobility.
Nobe, Nobel, Nobie, Noby

Nochehuatl (Nahuatl) consistent.

Nochtli (Nahuatl) prickly pear fruit.

Nodin (Native American) wind.
Knoton, Nodyn, Noton

Noe (Czech, French) a form of Noah.
Noé, Noi

Noé (Hebrew, Spanish) quiet, peaceful. See also Noah.

Noel BG (French) a form of Noël.

Noël (French) day of Christ's birth. See also Natal.
Noél, Noell, Nole, Noli, Nowel, Nowele, Nowell

Noelino (Spanish) a form of Natal.

Nohea (Hawaiian) handsome.
Noha, Nohe

Nokonyu (Native American) katydid's nose.
Noko, Nokoni

Nolan (Irish) famous; noble.
Noland, Nolande, Nolane, Nolin, Nollan, Nolon, Nolyn

Nolasco (Hebrew) he who departs and forgets about promises.

Nolberto (Teutonic) a form of Norberto.

Nolen (Irish) a form of Nolan.

Nollie BG (Latin, Scandinavian) a familiar form of Oliver.
Noll, Nolly

Nono (Latin) ninth born.

Noor GB (Sikh) divine light. (Aramaic) a form of Nura (see Girls' Names).

Nopaltzin (Nahuatl) cactus; king.

Norbert (Scandinavian) brilliant hero.
Bert, Norbie, Norburt, Norby, Norbyrt, Northbert, Northburt, Northbyrt

Norberto (Spanish) a form of Norbert.
Norburto, Norbyrto, Northberto, Northburto, Northbyrto

Norman (French) Norseman. History: a name for the Scandinavians who settled in northern France in the tenth century, and who later conquered England in 1066.
Norm, Normand, Normen, Normie, Normin, Normon, Normy, Normyn

Normando (Spanish) man of the north.

Norris (French) northerner. (English) Norman's horse.
Norice, Norie, Noris, Norreys, Norrie, Norry, Norrys

Northcliff (English) northern cliff.
Northclif, Northcliffe, Northclyf, Northclyfe, Northclyff, Northclyffe

Northrop (English) north farm.
North, Northup

Norton (English) northern town.
Northton

Norville (French, English) northern town.
Norval, Norvel, Norvell, Norvil, Norvile, Norvill, Norvylle

Norvin (English) northern friend.
Norvyn, Norwin, Norwinn, Norwyn, Norwynn

Norward (English) protector of the north.
Norwerd

Norwood (English) northern woods.
Northwood

Nostriano (Latin) he who is from our homeland.

Notaku (Moquelumnan) growing bear.

Notelmo (Teutonic) he who protects himself in combat with the helmet.

Nouel (French) almond.

Nour GB (Aramaic) a short form of Nura (see Girls' Names).

Nowles (English) a short form of Knowles.
Nowl, Nowle

Nsoah (Akan) seventh-born.
Nsoa

Numa (Arabic) pleasant.
Numah

Numair (Arabic) panther.
Numayr

Nun (Egyptian) god of the ocean.

Nuncio (Italian) messenger.
Nunzi, Nunzio

Nuno (Basque) monk.

Nuri (Hebrew, Arabic) my fire.
Noori, Nur, Nuris, Nurism, Nury

Nuriel (Hebrew, Arabic) fire of the Lord.
Nuria, Nuriah, Nuriya, Nuryel

Nuru BG (Swahili) born in daylight.

Nusair (Arabic) bird of prey.
Nusayr

Nwa (Nigerian) son.

Nwake (Nigerian) born on market day.

Nye (English) a familiar form of Aneurin, Nigel.

Nyle (English) island. (Irish) a form of Neil.
Nyal, Nyl, Nyll, Nylle

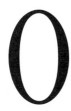

O'shea BG (Irish) a form of O'Shea.

O'neil (Irish) son of Neil.
*O'neal, O'neel, O'neele, O'neile, O'neill,
O'niel, O'niele, O'nil, O'nile, O'nyel,
O'nyele, O'nyl, O'nyle, Oneal, Oneil, Onel,
Oniel, Onil*

O'shay, Oshay, Oshea (Irish) forms of
O'Shea.

O'Shea BG (Irish) son of Shea.
*O'Shane, Oshae, Oshai, Oshane, Oshaun,
Oshaye, Oshe, Osheon*

Oakes (English) oak trees.
Oak, Oake, Oaks, Ochs

Oakley (English) oak-tree field.
*Oak, Oakie, Oaklea, Oaklee, Oakleigh,
Oakli, Oaklie, Oakly, Oaky*

Oalo (Spanish) a form of Paul.

Oba BG (Yoruba) king.
Obah

Obadele (Yoruba) king arrives at the house.
Obadel

Obadiah (Hebrew) servant of God.
*Obadia, Obadias, Obadya, Obadyah,
Obadyas, Obediah, Obedias, Obedya,
Obedyah, Obedyas, Ovadiach, Ovadiah,
Ovadya*

Obdulio (Latin) he who calms in sorrowful
moments.

Obed (English) a short form of Obadiah.
Obad

Oberon (German) noble; bearlike.
Literature: the king of the fairies in the
Shakespearean play *A Midsummer Night's
Dream.* See also Auberon, Aubrey.
*Oberan, Oberen, Oberin, Oberron, Oberun,
Oberyn, Oeberon*

Obert (German) wealthy; bright.
Obirt, Oburt, Obyrt

Oberto (Germanic) a form of Adalberto.

Obie (English) a familiar form of Obadiah.
Obbie, Obe, Obee, Obey, Obi, Oby

Ocan (Luo) hard times.

Ocean BG (Greek) a short form of Oceanus.
Oceane

Oceanus (Greek) Mythology: a Titan who
rules over the outer sea encircling the
earth.
Oceanis, Oceanos, Oceanous, Oceanys

Ocotlán (Nahuatl) pine.

Octavio (Latin) eighth. See also Tavey,
Tavian.
*Octave, Octavee, Octavey, Octavia, Octavian,
Octaviano, Octavien, Octavo, Octavyo, Ottavio*

Octavious, Octavius (Latin) forms of
Octavio.
*Octavaius, Octaveous, Octaveus, Octavias,
Octaviaus, Octavous, Octavyos, Octavyous,
Octavyus, Ottavios, Ottavious, Ottavius*

Octavis (Latin) a form of Octavio.
Octavus

Odakota (Lakota) friendly.
Oda, Odakotah

Odd (Norwegian) point.
Oddvar

Ode BG (Benin) born along the road. (Irish,
English) a short form of Odell.
Odee, Odey, Odi, Odie, Ody

Odeberto (Teutonic) he who shines
because of his possessions.

Oded (Hebrew) encouraging.

Odell (Greek) ode, melody. (Irish) otter.
(English) forested hill.
Dell, Odall, Odel, Odele

Oderico (Germanic) powerful in riches.

Odilón (Teutonic) owner of a bountiful
inheritance.

Odin (Scandinavian) ruler. Mythology: the
Norse god of wisdom and war.
Oden, Odyn

Odín (Scandinavian) a form of Odin.

Odion (Benin) first of twins.
Odyon

Odo (Norwegian) a form of Otto.
Audo, Oddo, Odoh

Odoacro (German) he who watches over his inheritance.

Odolf (German) prosperous wolf.
Odolfe, Odolff, Odolph, Odolphe, Odulf

Odom (Ghanaian) oak tree.

Odon (Hungarian) wealthy protector.

Odón (Hungarian) a form of Odon.

Odran (Irish) pale green.
Odhrán, Odren, Odrin, Odron, Odryn

Odwin (German) noble friend.
Odwinn, Odwyn, Odwynn

Odysseus (Greek) wrathful. Literature: the hero of Homer's epic poem *Odyssey*.
Odeseus

Ofer (Hebrew) young deer.
Opher

Ofir (Hebrew) ferocious.

Og (Aramaic) king. Bible: the king of Basham.

Ogaleesha (Lakota) red shirt.

Ogbay (Ethiopian) don't take him from me.
Ogbae, Ogbai

Ogbonna (Ibo) image of his father.
Ogbonnah, Ogbonnia

Ogden (English) oak valley. Literature: Ogden Nash was a twentieth-century American writer of light verse.
Ogdan, Ogdin, Ogdon, Ogdyn

Ogilvie (Welsh) high.
Ogil, Ogyl, Ogylvie

Ogima (Ojibwa) chief.
Ogimah, Ogyma, Ogymah

Ogun (Nigerian) Mythology: the god of war.
Ogunkeye, Ogunsanwo, Ogunsheye

Ohanko (Native American) restless.

Ohannes (Turkish) a form of John.
Ohan, Ohane, Ohanes, Ohann, Ohanne

Ohanzee (Lakota) comforting shadow.
Ohanze

Ohin (African) chief.
Ohan, Ohyn

Ohitekah (Lakota) brave.
Ohiteka

Ohtli (Nahuatl) road.

Oisin (Irish) small deer.
Oisyn, Oysin, Oysyn

Oistin (Irish) a form of Austin.
Oistan, Oisten, Oistyn

OJ (American) a combination of the initials O. + J.
O.J., Ojay

Ojas (Indian) luster.

Ojo (Yoruba) difficult delivery.

Okapi (Swahili) an African animal related to the giraffe but having a short neck.
Okapie, Okapy

Oke (Hawaiian) a form of Oscar.

Okechuku (Ibo) God's gift.

Okeke (Ibo) born on market day.
Okorie

Okie (American) from Oklahoma.
Okee, Okey, Oki, Oky

Oko (Ghanaian) older twin. (Yoruba) god of war.

Okorie (Ibo) a form of Okeke.

Okpara (Ibo) first son.
Okparah

Okuth (Luo) born in a rain shower.

Ola GB (Yoruba) wealthy, rich.
Olah, Olla, Ollah

Olaf (Scandinavian) ancestor. History: a patron saint and king of Norway.
Olaff, Olafur, Olaph, Ole, Olef, Olof, Oluf

Olaguer (Catalan) a form of Olegario.

Olajuwon (Yoruba) wealth and honor are God's gifts.
Olajawon, Olajawun, Olajowuan, Olajuan, Olajuanne, Olajuawon, Olajuwa, Olajuwan, Olaujawon, Oljuwoun

Olamina (Yoruba) this is my wealth.
Olaminah, Olamyna, Olamynah

Olatunji (Yoruba) honor reawakens.

Olav (Scandinavian) a form of Olaf.
Ola, Olave, Olavus, Olov, Olyn

Ole (Scandinavian) a familiar form of Olaf, Olav.
Olay, Oleh, Olle

Oleg (Latvian, Russian) holy.

Olegario (Germanic) he who dominates with his strength and his lance.

Oleguer (Catalan) a form of Olegario.

Oleksandr (Russian) a form of Alexander.
Olek, Olesandr, Olesko

Olen BG (Scandinavian) a form of Olaf. (Scandinavian, English) a form of Olin.

Oleos (Spanish) holy oil used in church.

Olés (Polish) a familiar form of Alexander.

Olezka (Russian) saint.

Olimpíades (Greek) a form of Olympia (see Girls' Names).

Olimpio (Greek) Mount Olympus.

Olimpo (Greek) sky.

Olin (English) holly. (Scandinavian) a form of Olaf.
Olney, Olyn

Olindo (Italian) from Olinthos, Greece.
Olind, Olynd, Olyndo

Oliver (Latin) olive tree. (Scandinavian) kind; affectionate.
Nollie, Oilibhéar, Olivar, Ollivar, Olliver, Ollivor, Ollyvar, Ollyver, Ollyvir, Ollyvyr, Olvan, Olven, Olvin, Olyvar

Olivero, Oliveros (Italian, Spanish) forms of Oliver.
Oliveras, Oliverio, Oliverios, Olivieras, Oliviero

Olivier (French) a form of Oliver.
Olier

Olivo (Latin) olive branch.

Oliwa (Hawaiian) a form of Oliver.
Olliva, Ollyva

Ollanta (Aymara) the warrior who sees everything from his watchtower.

Ollantay (Aymara) one who sees all.

Ollie BG (English) a familiar form of Oliver.
Olea, Olee, Oleigh, Oley, Oli, Olie, Olle, Ollee, Olleigh, Olley, Olli, Olly, Oly

Ollin (Nahuatl) movement.

Olo (Spanish) a short form of Orlando, Rolando.

Olric (German) a form of Ulric.
Oldrech, Oldrich, Olrick, Olrik, Olryc, Olryck, Olryk

Olubayo (Yoruba) highest joy.

Olufemi (Yoruba) wealth and honor favors me.

Olujimi (Yoruba) God gave me this.

Olushola (Yoruba) God has blessed me.

Om (Indian) the sacred syllable.

Omair (Arabic) a form of Omar.

Omar (Arabic) highest; follower of the Prophet. (Hebrew) reverent. See also Umar.
Omir, Omyr

Omari (Swahili) a form of Omar.
Omare, Omaree, Omarey, Omarie, Omary

Omarr (Arabic) a form of Omar.

Omer (Arabic) a form of Omar.
Omeer, Omero

Omja (Indian) born of cosmic unity.

Omkar (Indian) the sound of the sacred syllable.

Omolara (Benin) child born at the right time.
Omolarah

Omprakash (Indian) light of God.

Omrao (Indian) king.

Omswaroop (Indian) manifestation of divinity.

On (Burmese) coconut. (Chinese) peace.

Onan (Turkish) prosperous.
Onen, Onin, Onon, Onyn

Onani (African) quick look.
Onanee, Onanie, Onany

Onaona (Hawaiian) pleasant fragrance.
Onaonah

Ondro (Czech) a form of Andrew.
Ondra, Ondre, Ondrea, Ondrey

Onesíforo (Greek) he who bears much fruit.

Onésimo (Greek) he who is useful and worthwhile.

Onfroi (French) calm.

Onkar (Hindi) God in his entirety.

Onofrio (German) a form of Humphrey.
Oinfre, Onfre, Onfrio, Onofre, Onofredo

Onslow (English) enthusiast's hill.
Ounslow

Ontario BG (Native American) beautiful lake. Geography: a province and a lake in Canada.

Onufry (Polish) a form of Humphrey.

Onur (Turkish) honor.

Ophir (Hebrew) faithful. Bible: an Old Testament people and country.
Ophyr

Opio (Ateso) first of twin boys.
Opyo

Optato (Latin) desired.

Oral (Latin) verbal; speaker.

Oran BG (Irish) green.
Ora, Orane, Orran, Orron

Orangel (Greek) the messenger from the mountain.

Oratio (Latin) a form of Horatio.
Oratyo, Orazio, Orazyo

Orbán (Hungarian) born in the city.
Orben, Orbin, Orbon, Orbyn

Ordell (Latin) beginning.
Orde, Ordel, Ordele, Ordelle

Orel (Latin) listener. (Russian) eagle.
Oreel, Orele, Orell, Oriel, Oriele, Oriell, Orrel, Orrele, Orrell

Oren (Hebrew) pine tree. (Irish) light skinned, white.
Orono, Orren

Orencio (Greek) examining judge.

Orestes (Greek) mountain man. Mythology: the son of the Greek leader Agamemnon.
Aresty, Orest, Oreste

Orfeo (Greek) he who has a good voice.

Ori (Hebrew) my light.
Oree, Orey, Orie, Orri, Ory

Orien (Latin) visitor from the east.
Orian, Orie, Oris, Oron, Orono, Oryan, Oryen, Oryin

Orígenes (Greek) born into caring arms.

Orin (English) a form of Orrin.

Oriol (Latin) golden oriole.

Orion (Greek) son of fire. Mythology: a giant hunter who was killed by Artemis. See also Zorion.
Orryon, Oryon

Orión (Greek) a form of Orion.

Orji (Ibo) mighty tree.

Orlán, Orlín (Spanish) renowned in the land. Forms of Roland.

Orlando (German) famous throughout the land. (Spanish) a form of Roland.
Lando, Olando, Orlan, Orland, Orlanda, Orlandas, Orlande, Orlandes, Orlandis, Orlandos, Orlandous, Orlandus, Orlo, Orlondo, Orlondon

Orleans (Latin) golden.
Orlean, Orlin

Orman (German) mariner, seaman. (Scandinavian) serpent, worm.
Ormand, Ormen

Ormond (English) bear mountain; spear protector.
Ormande, Ormon, Ormonde, Ormondo

Oro (Spanish) golden.

Oroncio (Persian) runner.

Orono (Latin) a form of Oren.
Oron, Orun

Orosco (Greek) he who lives in the mountains.

Orpheus (Greek) Mythology: a fabulous musician.
Orfeus

Orrick (English) old oak tree.
Oric, Orick, Orik, Orric, Orrik, Orryc, Orryck, Orryk, Oryc, Oryck, Oryk

Orrin (English) river.
Orryn, Oryn, Orynn

Orris (Latin) a form of Horatio.
Oris, Orriss, Orrys, Orryss

Orry (Latin) from the Orient.
Oarri, Oarrie, Orrey, Orri, Orrie, Ory

Orsino (Italian) a form of Orson.
Orscino, Orsine, Orsyne, Orsyno

Orson (Latin) bearlike. See also Urson.
Orsen, Orsin, Orsini, Orsino, Orsyn, Son, Sonny

Orton (English) shore town.
Ortan, Orten, Ortin, Ortyn

Ortzi (Basque) sky.
Ortzy

Orunjan (Yoruba) born under the midday sun.

Orval (English) a form of Orville.
Orvel

Orville (French) golden village. History: Orville Wright and his brother Wilbur were the first men to fly an airplane.
Orv, Orvell, Orvie, Orvil, Orvile, Orvill, Orvyl, Orvyle, Orvyll

Orvin (English) spear friend.
Orvan, Orven, Orvon, Orvyn, Orwin, Orwyn, Owynn

Osahar (Benin) God hears.

Osayaba (Benin) God forgives.

Osaze (Benin) whom God likes.
Osaz

Osbaldo (Spanish) a form of Oswald.
Osbalto

Osbert (English) divine; bright.
Osbirt, Osbyrt

Osborn (Scandinavian) divine bear. (English) warrior of God.
Osbern, Osbon, Osborne, Osbourn, Osbourne, Osburn, Osburne, Ozborn, Ozborne, Ozbourn, Ozbourne

Oscar (Scandinavian) divine spearman.
Oszkar

Óscar (Scandinavian) a form of Oscar.

Oseas, Osías (Hebrew) the Lord sustains me.

Osei (Fante) noble.
Osee, Osey, Osi, Osie, Osy

Osgood (English) divinely good.

Osip (Russian, Ukrainian) a form of Joseph, Yosef. See also Osya.

Osiris (Egyptian) he who possesses a powerful vision.

Oskar (Scandinavian) a form of Oscar.
Osker, Ozker

Osman (Turkish) ruler. (English) servant of God. A form of Osmond.
Osmanek, Osmen, Osmin, Osmon, Osmyn

Osmán (Turkish) a form of Osman.

Osmar (English) divine; wonderful.
Osmer, Osmir, Osmor, Osmyr

Osmara, Osmaro (Germanic) he who shines like the glory of God.

Osmond (English) divine protector.
Osmand, Osmonde, Osmondo, Osmont, Osmonte, Osmund, Osmunde, Osmundo, Osmunt, Osmunte

Osorio (Slavic) the killer of wolves.

Osric (English) divine ruler.
Osrick, Osrig, Osrik, Osryc, Osryck, Osryg, Osryk

Ostiano (Spanish) confessor.

Ostin (Latin) a form of Austin.
Ostan, Osten, Oston, Ostun, Ostyn, Ostynn

Osvaldo (Spanish) a form of Oswald.
Osvald, Osvalda

Oswald (English) God's power; God's crest. See also Waldo.
Oswal, Oswall, Oswel, Osweld, Oswell, Oswold

Oswaldo (Spanish) a form of Oswald.
Osweldo

Oswin (English) divine friend.
Osvin, Oswinn, Oswyn, Oswynn

Osya (Russian) a familiar form of Osip.

Ota (Czech) prosperous.
Otah

Otadan (Native American) plentiful.

Otaktay (Lakota) kills many; strikes many.

Otek (Polish) a form of Otto.
Otik

Otello (Italian) a form of Othello.

Otelo (Spanish) a form of Otello.

Otem (Luo) born away from home.

Othello (Spanish) a form of Otto. Literature: the title character in the Shakespearean tragedy *Othello*.
Otello

Othman (German) wealthy.
Othmen, Ottoman

Othmân (Arabic) name of one of the prophet's companions.

Othniel (Hebrew) strength of God.

Otilde (Teutonic) owner of a bountiful inheritance.

Otis (Greek) keen of hearing. (German) son of Otto.
Oates, Odis, Otes, Otess, Otez, Otise, Ottis, Ottys, Otys

Otniel, Otoniel (Hebrew) God is my strength.

Otoronco (Quechua) jaguar.

Ottah (Nigerian) thin baby.
Otta

Ottar (Norwegian) point warrior; fright warrior.
Otar

Ottmar (Turkish) a form of Osman.
Otman, Otmen, Otomar, Otomars, Otthmor, Ottmar, Ottmen, Ottmer, Ottmor, Ottomar

Otto (German) rich.
Odo, Otek, Otello, Otfried, Otho, Othon,

Otilio, Otman, Oto, Otoe, Otón, Otow, Otton, Ottone

Ottokar (German) happy warrior.
Otokar, Otokars, Ottocar

Otu (Native American) collecting seashells in a basket.
Ottu

Oubastet (Egyptian) cat.

Ouray (Ute) arrow. Astrology: born under the sign of Sagittarius.

Ourson (French) small bear.

Oved (Hebrew) worshiper, follower.
Ovid, Ovyd

Overton (English) high town.
Overtan, Overten, Overtin, Overtyn

Ovidio (Spanish) shepherd.

Owen ☆ (Irish) born to nobility; young warrior. (Welsh) a form of Evan. See also Uaine, Ywain.
Owain, Owaine, Owan, Owayn, Owayne, Owens, Owin, Owine, Owon, Owone, Owyn, Owyne

Owney (Irish) elderly.
Onee, Oney, Oni, Onie, Ony, Ownee, Owni, Ownie, Owny

Oxford (English) place where oxen cross the river.
Ford, Oxforde

Oxley (English) ox meadow.
Oxlea, Oxlee, Oxleigh, Oxli, Oxlie, Oxly

Oxton (English) ox town.
Oxtan, Oxten, Oxtin, Oxtyn

Oya BG (Moquelumnan) speaking of the jacksnipe.
Oyah

Oystein (Norwegian) rock of happiness.
Ostein, Osten, Ostin, Øystein

Oz BG (Hebrew) a short form of Osborn, Oswald.
Ozz

Ozias (Hebrew) God's strength.
Ozia, Oziah, Ozya, Ozyah, Ozyas

Oziel (Hebrew) he who has divine strength.

Ozturk (Turkish) pure; genuine Turk.

Ozuru (Japanese) stork.
Ozuro, Ozuroo

Ozzie, Ozzy (English) familiar forms of Osborn, Oswald.
Osi, Osie, Ossi, Ossie, Ossy, Osy, Ozee, Ozi, Ozie, Ozy, Ozzi

P

Paavan (Indian) purifier.

Paavo (Finnish) a form of Paul.
Paav, Paaveli

Pabel (Russian) a form of Paul.

Pabla (Spanish) a form of Paul.

Pablo (Spanish) a form of Paul.
Pable, Paublo

Pace (English) a form of Pascal.
Paice, Payce

Pacey (English) a form of Pace.

Pachacutec, Pachacutic (Quechua) he who changes the world.

Pacho (Spanish) free.

Paciano (Latin) he who belongs to the peace.

Paciente (Latin) he who knows how to be patient.

Pacifico (Filipino) peaceful.
Pacific, Pacifyc, Pacyfyc

Pacífico (Filipino) a form of Pacifico.

Paco (Italian) pack. (Spanish) a familiar form of Francisco. (Native American) bald eagle. See also Quico.
Packo, Pacorro, Pako, Panchito, Paquito

Pacomio (Greek) he who is robust.

Paddy (Irish) a familiar form of Padraic, Patrick.
Paddee, Paddey, Paddi, Paddie, Padi, Padie, Pady

Paden (English) a form of Patton.

Padget BG (English) a form of Page.
Padgett, Paget, Pagett, Paiget, Paigett, Payget, Paygett

Padman, Pankaj (Indian) lotus.

Padmanabha, Padmapati (Indian) other names for the Hindu god Vishnu.

Padraic (Irish) a form of Patrick.
Paddrick, Padhraig, Padrai, Pádraig, Padraigh, Padreic, Padriac, Padric, Padron, Padruig

Pafnucio (Greek) rich in merits.

Pagan GB (Latin) from the country.
Paegan, Paegen, Paegin, Paegon, Paegyn, Pagen, Pagin, Pagon, Pagun, Pagyn, Paigan, Paigen, Paigin, Paigon, Paigyn

Page GB (French) youthful assistant.
Paggio, Payg, Payge

Pagiel (Hebrew) worshiping God.
Paegel, Paegell, Pagiell, Paigel, Paigell, Paygel, Paygell

Paien (French) name of the noble ones.

Paige GB (English) a form of Page.
Paeg, Paege, Paig

Paillalef (Mapuche) return quickly.

Painecura (Mapuche) iridescent stone.

Painevilu (Mapuche) iridescent snake.

Painter (Latin) artist, painter.
Paintar, Paintor, Payntar, Paynter, Payntor

Paio (Latin) belonging to the sea.

Pakelika (Hawaiian) a form of Patrick.

Paki (African) witness.

Pakile (Hawaiian) royal.
Pakil, Pakill, Pakyl, Pakyll

Pal (Swedish) a form of Paul.
Paal, Pall

Pál (Hungarian) a form of Paul.
Pali, Palika

Palaina (Hawaiian) a form of Brian.
Palainah

Palak (Indian) eyelash.

Palaki (Polynesian) black.
Palakee, Palakey, Palakie, Palaky

Palani (Hawaiian) a form of Frank.
Palanee, Palaney, Palanie, Palany

Palash (Hindi) flowery tree.

Palashkusum (Indian) the flower of a Palash tree.

Palashranjan (Indian) beautiful like a Palash tree.

Palatino (Latin) he who comes from Mount Palatine.

Palban, Palbán, Palbén (Basque) blond.

Palben (Basque) blond.

Pallab (Indian) new leaves.

Palladin (Native American) fighter.
Palladyn, Pallaton, Palleten

Palmacio (Latin) adorned with bordered palm leaves.

Palmer BG (English) palm-bearing pilgrim.
Pallmer, Palmar

Palmiro (Latin) born on Palm Sunday.
Palmira, Palmirow, Palmyro

Palti (Hebrew) God liberates.
Palti-el

Pampín (Latin) he who has the vigor of a sprouting plant.

Panas (Russian) immortal.

Panayiotis (Greek) a form of Peter.
Panagiotis, Panajotis, Panayioti, Panayoti, Panayotis

Panchanan (Indian) another name for the Hindu god Shiva.

Pancho (Spanish) a familiar form of Francisco, Frank.
Panchito

Pancracio (Greek) all powerful.

Pandhari, Panduranga (Indian) other names for Vithobha, an incarnation of the Hindu god Krishna.

Panfilo, Pánfilo (Greek) friend of all.

Panini (Indian) a great Sanskrit scholar-grammarian of ancient India.

Pannalal (Indian) emerald.

Panos (Greek) a form of Peter.
Pano

Pantaleón (Greek) all merciful.

Panteno (Greek) he who is worthy of all praise.

Panti (Quechua) species of brush.

Paolo (Italian) a form of Paul.

Papias (Greek) the venerable father.

Paquito (Spanish) a familiar form of Paco.

Parag (Indian) pollen.

Parakram (Indian) strength.

Param (Indian) the best.

Paramananda (Indian) superlative joy.

Paramesh (Hindi) greatest. Religion: another name for the Hindu god Shiva.

Paramhansa (Indian) supreme soul.

Paranjay (Indian) another name for the Hindu god Varun, lord of the waters.

Parantapa (Indian) conqueror; another name for Arjuna, a warrior prince in the Indian epic poem *Mahabharata*.

Parashar (Indian) an ancient Indian sage.

Parashuram (Indian) sixth incarnation of the Hindu god Vishnu.

Parasmani (Indian) touchstone.

Paravasu (Indian) an ancient Indian sage.

Pardeep (Sikh) mystic light.
Pardip

Pardulfo (Germanic) brave warrior.

Paresh (Indian) supreme lord.

Parfait (French) perfect.

Paris GB (Greek) lover. Geography: the capital of France. Mythology: the prince of Troy who started the Trojan War by abducting Helen.
Paras, Paree, Pares, Parese, Parie, Parys

París (Greek) a form of Paris.

Parish (English) a form of Parrish.

Parisio (Spanish) a form of Paris.

Pariuana (Quechua) Andean flamingo.

Park (Chinese) cypress tree. (English) a short form of Parker.
Parc, Parke, Parkes, Parkey, Parks

Parker BG (English) park keeper.
Park

Parkin (English) little Peter.
Parkyn

Parlan (Scottish) a form of Bartholomew. See also Parthalán.
Parlen, Parlin, Parlon, Parlyn

Parménides, Parmenio (Greek) he who is a constant presence.

Parnell (French) little Peter. History: Charles Stewart Parnell was a famous Irish politician.
Nell, Parle, Parnel, Parnele, Parnelle, Parrnell

Parodio (Greek) he who imitates the singing.

Parr (English) cattle enclosure, barn.

Parris GB (Greek) a form of Paris.

Parrish (English) church district.
Parrie, Parrisch, Parrysh, Parysh

Parry (Welsh) son of Harry.
Paree, Parey, Pari, Parie, Parree, Parrey, Parri, Parrie, Pary

Partemio (Greek) having a pure and virginal appearance.

Parth (Irish) a short form of Parthalán.
Partha, Parthey

Parthalán (Irish) plowman. See also Bartholomew.

Parthenios (Greek) virgin. Religion: a Greek Orthodox saint.

Pascal (French) born on Easter or Passover.
Pascale, Pascall, Pascalle, Paschal, Paschalis, Pascoe, Pascoli, Pascow

Pascua (Hebrew) in reference to Easter.

Pascual (Spanish) a form of Pascal.
Pascul

Pasha BG (Russian) a form of Paul.
Pashah, Pashka

Pashenka (Russian) small.

Pasicrates (Greek) he who dominates everyone.

Pasquale (Italian) a form of Pascal.
Pascuale, Pasqual, Pasquali, Pasquel

Pastor (Latin) spiritual leader.
Pastar, Paster, Pastir, Pastyr

Pastora (Latin) a form of Pastor.

Pat BG (Native American) fish. (English) a short form of Patrick.
Pati, Patie, Patt, Patti, Pattie, Patty, Paty

Patakusu (Moquelumnan) ant biting a person.

Patamon BG (Native American) raging.
Pataman, Patamen, Patamin, Patamyn

Patek (Polish) a form of Patrick.
Patick

Paterio (Greek) he who was born in Pateria.

Paterno (Latin) belonging to the father.

Patli (Nahuatl) medicine.

Patric, Patrik, Patryk (Latin) forms of Patrick.
Patryc, Patryck

Patrice GB (French) a form of Patrick.

Patricio (Spanish) a form of Patrick.
Patricius, Patrizio

Patrick ☀ (Latin) nobleman. Religion: the patron saint of Ireland. See also Fitzpatrick, Ticho.
Pakelika, Patrickk, Patrique, Patrizius, Pats, Patsy, Pattrick

Patrido (Latin) noble.

Patrin (Gypsy) leaf trail.

Patrocinio (Latin) patronage.

Patterson (Irish) son of Pat.
Paterson, Patteson

Pattin (Gypsy) leaf. (English) a form of Patton.
Patin, Pattyn, Patyn

Patton (English) warrior's town.
Patan, Paten, Paton, Pattan, Patten, Pattun, Patty, Peton

Patwin (Native American) man.
Patwyn

Patxi (Basque, Teutonic) free.

Paucar (Quechua) very refined, excellent.

Paucartupac (Quechua) majestic and excellent.

Paul (Latin) small. Bible: Saul, later renamed Paul, was the first to bring the teachings of Christ to the Gentiles.
Oalo, Pasko, Paulia, Paulis, Paull, Paulle, Paulot, Pauls, Paulus, Pavlos

Paúl (Latin) a form of Paul.

Pauli (Latin) a familiar form of Paul.
Pauley, Paulie, Pauly

Paulin (German, Polish) a form of Paul.

Paulino (Spanish) a form of Paul.

Pauliño (Spanish) a form of Paul.

Paulinus (Lithuanian) a form of Paul.
Paulinas

Paulo (Portuguese, Swedish, Hawaiian) a form of Paul.

Pausidio (Greek) deliberate, calm man.

Pauyu (Aymara) he who finishes.

Pavel (Russian) a form of Paul.
Paavel, Paval, Pavil, Pavils, Pavlik, Pavlo, Pavol

Pavit (Hindi) pious, pure.
Pavitt, Pavyt, Pavytt

Pavla, Pavlov, Pavlusha, Pavlushka, Pavlushshenka, Pavlya (Russian) small.

Pawel (Polish) a form of Paul.
Pawelek, Pawell, Pawl

Pax (Latin) peaceful.
Paxx

Paxton BG (Latin) peaceful town.
Packston, Paxon, Paxtan, Paxten, Paxtin, Paxtun, Paxtyn

Payat (Native American) he is on his way.
Pay, Payatt

Payden (English) a form of Payton.
Paydon

Payne (Latin) from the country.
Paine, Pane, Payn, Paynn

Payo (Galician) a short form of Pelayo.

Paytah (Lakota) fire.
Pay, Payta

Payton GB (English) a form of Patton.
Paiton, Pate, Peaton

Paz GB (Spanish) a form of Pax.

Pearce (English) a form of Pierce.
Pears, Pearse

Pearson (English) son of Peter. See also Pierson.
Pearsson, Pehrson, Peirson

Peder (Scandinavian) a form of Peter.
Peadair, Peadar, Peader, Pedey

Pedro (Spanish) a form of Peter.
Pedrin, Pedrín, Petronio

Peerless (American) incomparable, without a peer.

Peers (English) a form of Peter.
Peerus

Peeter (Estonian) a form of Peter.
Peet

Pegaso (Greek) born next to the fountain.

Pehuen (Mapuche) nut.

Peirce (English) a form of Peter.
Peirs

Pekelo (Hawaiian) a form of Peter.
Pekeio, Pekka

Pelagio, Pelayo (Greek) excellent sailor.

Peleke (Hawaiian) a form of Frederick.

Pelham (English) tannery town.
Pelhem, Pelhim, Pelhom, Pelhym

Pelí (Latin, Basque) happy.
Pelie, Pely

Pell (English) parchment.
Pall, Pel

Pello (Greek, Basque) stone.
Peru, Piarres

Pelope (Greek) having a brown complexion.

Pelton (English) town by a pool.
Peltan, Pelten, Peltin, Peltyn

Pembroke (Welsh) headland. (French) wine dealer. (English) broken fence.
Pembrock, Pembrok, Pembrook

Pendle (English) hill.
Pendal, Pendel, Penndal, Penndel, Penndle

Peniamina (Hawaiian) a form of Benjamin.
Peni, Penmina, Penminah, Penmyna, Penmynah

Penley (English) enclosed meadow.
Penlea, Penlee, Penleigh, Penli, Penlie, Penly

Penn (Latin) pen, quill. (English) enclosure. (German) a short form of Penrod.
Pen, Penna

Penrod (German) famous commander.
Penn, Pennrod, Rod

Pepa (Czech) a familiar form of Joseph.
Pepek, Pepik

Pepe (Spanish) a familiar form of Jose.
Pepee, Pepey, Pepi, Pepie, Pepillo, Pepito, Pepy, Pequin, Pipo

Pepin (German) determined; petitioner. History: Pepin the Short was an eighth-century king of the Franks.
Pepan, Pepen, Pepon, Peppie, Peppy, Pepyn

Peppe (Italian) a familiar form of Joseph.
Peppee, Peppey, Peppi, Peppie, Peppo, Peppy

Peppin (French) a form of Pepin.

Per (Swedish) a form of Peter.

Perben (Greek, Danish) stone.
Perban, Perbin, Perbon, Perbyn

Percival (French) pierce the valley. Literature: a knight of the Round Table who first appears in Chrétien de Troyes's poem about the quest for the Holy Grail.
Parsafal, Parsefal, Parsifal, Parzival, Perc, Perce, Perceval, Percevall, Percivale, Percivall, Percyval, Peredur, Purcell

Percy (French) a familiar form of Percival.
Pearcey, Pearcy, Percee, Percey, Perci, Percie, Piercey, Piercy

Pere (Catalan) a form of Pedro.

Peregrine (Latin) traveler; pilgrim; falcon.
Pelgrim, Pellegrino, Peregrin, Peregryn, Peregryne, Perergrin, Perergryn

Peregrino (Latin) a form of Peregrine.

Perfecto (Latin) without any defects.

Periandro (Greek) worries about men.

Pericles (Greek) just leader. History: an Athenian statesman.
Perycles

Perico (Spanish) a form of Peter.
Pequin, Perequin

Perine (Latin) a short form of Peregrine.
Perino, Perion

Perkin (English) little Peter.
Perka, Perkins, Perkyn, Perkyns

Pernell (French) a form of Parnell.
Perren, Perrnall

Perpetuo (Latin) having an unchanging goal.

Perrin (Latin) a short form of Peregrine.
Perryn

Perry BG (English) a familiar form of Peregrine, Peter.
Peree, Perey, Peri, Perie, Perree, Perrey, Perri, Perrie, Perrye, Pery

Perseo (Greek) the destroyer.

Perth (Scottish) thorn-bush thicket. Geography: a burgh in Scotland; a city in Australia.
Pirth, Pyrth

Pervis (Latin) passage.
Pervez, Pervys

Pesach (Hebrew) spared. Religion: another name for Passover.
Pesac, Pessach

Petar (Greek) a form of Peter.

Pete (English) a short form of Peter.
Peat, Peate, Peet, Peete, Peit, Peite, Petey, Peti, Petie, Peyt, Piet, Pit, Pyete

Petenka (Russian) stone.

Peter (Greek, Latin) small rock. Bible: Simon, renamed Peter, was the leader of

the Twelve Apostles. See also Boutros, Ferris, Takis.
Peater, Peiter, Péter, Peterke, Peterus, Piaras, Piero, Piter, Piti, Pjeter, Pyeter

Peterson (English) son of Peter.
Peteris, Petersen

Petiri (Shona) where we are.
Petri, Petyri, Petyry

Peton (English) a form of Patton.
Peaten, Peatin, Peaton, Peatun, Peatyn, Peighton, Peiton, Petan, Peten, Petin, Petun, Petyn

Petr (Bulgarian) a form of Peter.
Pedr

Petras (Lithuanian) a form of Peter.
Petra, Petrelis

Petros (Greek) a form of Peter.
Petro

Petru (Romanian) a form of Peter.
Petrukas, Petruno, Petrus, Petruso

Petruos (Latin) firm as a rock.

Petter (Norwegian) a form of Peter.

Peverell (French) piper.
Peverall, Peverel, Peveril, Peveryl

Peyo (Spanish) a form of Peter.

Peyton BG (English) a form of Patton, Payton.
Peyt, Peyten, Peython, Peytonn

Phalguni (Indian) born in the Hindu month of Falgun.

Pharaoh (Latin) ruler. History: a title for the ancient kings of Egypt.
Faro, Faroh, Pharo, Pharoah, Pharoh

Phelan (Irish) wolf.
Felan, Pheland

Phelipe (Spanish) a form of Philip.
Phelippe

Phelix (Latin) a form of Felix.
Phelyx

Phelps (English) son of Phillip.
Felps, Phelp

Phil (Greek) a short form of Philip, Phillip.
Fil, Phill

Philander (Greek) lover of mankind.
Filander, Fylander, Phylander

Philart (Greek) lover of virtue.
Filart, Filarte, Fylart, Fylarte, Phylart, Phylarte

Philbert (English) a form of Filbert.
Philberte, Philberti, Philberto, Philbirt, Philbirte, Philburt, Philburte, Philibert, Philiberte, Philibirt, Philibirte, Philiburt, Philiburte, Phillbert, Phillberte, Phillbirt, Phillbirte, Phillburt, Phillburte, Phillibert, Philliberte, Phillibirt, Phillibirte, Philliburt, Philliburte, Phylbert, Phylberte, Phylbirt, Phylbirte, Phylburt, Phylburte, Phylibert, Phyliberte, Phylibirt, Phylibirte, Phyliburt, Phyliburte, Phyllbert, Phyllberte, Phyllbirt, Phyllbirte, Phyllburt, Phyllburte, Phyllibert, Phylliberte, Phyllibirt, Phyllibirte, Phylliburt, Phylliburte

Philemon (Greek) kiss.
Phila, Philamin, Philamina, Philamine, Philamyn, Phileman, Philémon, Philmon, Philmyn, Philmyne, Phylmin, Phylmine, Phylmon, Phylmyn

Philip (Greek) lover of horses. Bible: one of the Twelve Apostles. See also Felipe, Felippo, Filip, Fillipp, Filya, Fischel, Flip.
Philippo, Phillp, Philp, Phyleap, Phyleep, Phylip, Phylyp, Pilib, Pippo

Philipe, Philippe (French) forms of Philip.
Phillepe, Phillipe, Phillippe, Phillippee, Phyllipe

Philipp (German) a form of Philip.
Phillipp

Phillip (Greek) a form of Philip.
Phillipp, Phillips, Phylleap, Phylleep, Phyllip, Phyllyp

Phillipos (Greek) a form of Phillip.
Philippos

Philly (American) a familiar form of Philip, Phillip.
Phillie

Philo (Greek) love.
Filo, Fylo, Phylo

Phinean (Irish) a form of Finian.
Phinian, Phinyan, Phynian, Phynyan

Phineas (English) a form of Pinchas. See also Fineas.
Phinehas, Phinny, Phyneas

Phirun (Cambodian) rain.

Phoenix BG (Latin) phoenix, a legendary bird.
Phenix, Pheonix, Phynix

Phuok (Vietnamese) good.
Phuoc

Pias (Gypsy) fun.

Pichi (Araucanian) small.

Pichiu (Quechua) baby bird.

Pichulman (Mapuche) the condor's feather.

Pichunlaf (Mapuche) lucky feather.

Pickford (English) ford at the peak.

Pickworth (English) wood cutter's estate.

Picton (English) town on the hill's peak.
Picktown, Picktun, Picktyn, Pictan, Picten, Piktan, Pikten, Piktin, Pikton, Piktown, Piktun, Piktyn, Pyckton, Pyctin, Pycton, Pyctyn, Pyktin, Pykton, Pyktyn

Pier Alexander (French) a combination of Pierre + Alexander.

Pier Luc, Pierre Luc, Pierre-Luc (French) combinations of Pierre + Luc.
Piere Luc

Pier Olivier, Pierre Olivier (French) combinations of Pierre + Olivier.

Pierce BG (English) a form of Peter.
Peerce, Peirce, Piercy

Piero (Italian) a form of Peter.
Pero, Pierro

Pierpont, Pierrepont (French) living underneath the stone bridge.

Pierre (French) a form of Peter.
Peirre, Piere, Pierrot

Pierre Alexan (French) a combination of Pierre + Alexander.

Pierre Andre (French) a combination of Pierre + Andre.

Pierre Antoin (French) a combination of Pierre + Antoine.

Pierre Etienn (French) a combination of Pierre + Etienne.

Pierre Marc (French) a combination of Pierre + Marc.

Pierre Yves (French) a combination of Pierre + Yves.

Piers (English) a form of Peter. A form of Peers.

Pierson (English) son of Peter. See also Pearson.
Pierrson, Piersen, Piersson, Piersun, Pyerson

Pieter (Dutch) a form of Peter.
Pietr, Pietrek

Pietro (Italian) a form of Peter.

Pigmalion (Spanish) sculptor.

Pilar GB (Spanish) pillar.
Pillar, Pylar, Pyllar

Pilato (Latin) soldier armed with a lance.

Pilatos (Latin) he who is armed with a pick.

Pili (Swahili) second born.
Pyli, Pyly

Pilipo (Hawaiian) a form of Philip.

Pillan (Native American) supreme essence.
Pilan, Pylan, Pyllan

Pin (Vietnamese) faithful boy.
Pyn

Pinchas (Hebrew) oracle. (Egyptian) dark skinned.
Phineas, Pincas, Pinchos, Pincus, Pinkas, Pinkus, Pynchas

Pinito (Greek) inspired; very wise.

Pinjás (Hebrew) mouth of the serpent.

Pinky (American) a familiar form of Pinchas.
Pink

Pino (Italian) a form of Joseph.

Piñon (Tupi-Guarani) Mythology: the hunter who became the constellation Orion.

Pio (Latin) pious.
Pyo

Pío (Latin) a form of Pio.

Piotr (Bulgarian) a form of Peter.
Piotrek

Pipino (German) a form of Pippin.

Pippin (German) father.
Pippyn

Piquichaqui (Quechua) light footed.

Piran (Irish) prayer. Religion: the patron saint of miners.
Peran, Pieran, Pieren, Pieryn, Pyran

Pirrin (Australian) cave.
Pirryn, Pyrrin, Pyrryn

Pirro (Greek, Spanish) flaming hair.
Piro, Pyro, Pyrro

Pista (Hungarian) a familiar form of István.
Pisti

Pitágoras (Greek) he who is like a divine oracle.

Piti (Spanish) a form of Peter.

Pitin (Spanish) a form of Felix.
Pito

Pitney (English) island of the strong-willed man.
Pitnee, Pitni, Pitnie, Pitny, Pittney, Pytnee, Pytney, Pytni, Pytnie, Pytny

Pitt (English) pit, ditch.
Pit

Piuque (Araucanian) heart.

Piyco, Piycomayu, Piycu, Piycumayu (Quechua) red bird.

Placido (Spanish) serene.
Placide, Placidio, Placidus, Placyd, Placydius, Placydo

Plácido (Spanish) a form of Placido.

Plato (Greek) broad shouldered. History: a famous Greek philosopher.
Platan, Platen, Platin, Platon, Platun, Platyn

Platón (Greek) a form of Plato.

Platt (French) flatland.
Platte

Plauto, Plotino (Greek) he who has flat feet.

Plaxico (American) a form of Placido.

Plinio (Latin) he who has many skills.

Plubio (Greek) man of the sea.

Plutarco (Greek) rich prince.

Plutón (Greek) owner of many riches.

Po Sin (Chinese) grandfather elephant.

Pol (Swedish) a form of Paul.
Pól, Pola, Poll, Poul

Poldi (German) a familiar form of Leopold.
Poldo

Poliano (Greek) he who suffers.

Policarpo (Greek) he who produces abundant fruit.

Policeto (Greek) he who caused much sorrow.

Polidoro (Greek) having virtues.

Poliecto (Greek) he who is very desired.

Polifemo (Greek) he who is spoken about a lot.

Polión (Greek) the powerful Lord who protects.

Pollard (German) close-cropped head.
Polard, Polerd, Pollerd, Pollyrd

Pollock (English) a form of Pollux. Art: American artist Jackson Pollock was a leader of abstract expressionism.
Polick, Pollack, Pollick, Polloch, Pollok, Polock, Polok

Pollux (Greek) crown. Astronomy: one of the stars in the constellation Gemini.
Pollock, Polux

Polo (Tibetan) brave wanderer. (Greek) a short form of Apollo. Culture: a game played on horseback. History: Marco Polo was a thirteenth-century Venetian explorer who traveled throughout Asia.
Pollo

Poma, Pomacana, Puma, Pumacana (Quechua) strong and powerful puma.

Pomacaua, Pumacaua (Quechua) he who guards with the quietness of a puma.

Pomagüiyca, Pumagüiyca (Quechua) sacred like the puma.

Pomalloque, Pumalluqui (Quechua) left-handed puma.

Pomauari, Pumauari (Quechua) indomitable as a vicuna and strong as a puma.

Pomayauri, Pumayauri (Quechua) copper-colored puma.

Pomeroy (French) apple orchard.
Pomaroi, Pomaroy, Pomeroi, Pommeray, Pommeroy

Pommeraie (French) a form of Pomeroy.

Pompeo (Greek) a form of Pompeyo.

Pompeyo (Greek) he who heads the procession.

Pomponio (Latin) the lover of grandeur and the open plains.

Ponce (Spanish) fifth. History: Juan Ponce de León of Spain searched for the Fountain of Youth in Florida.

Poncio (Greek) having come from the sea.

Ponpey (English) a form of Pompeyo.

Pony (Scottish) small horse.
Poni

Porcio (Latin) he who earns his living raising pigs.

Porfirio (Greek, Spanish) purple stone.
Porfiryo, Porfryio, Porfryo, Porphirios, Prophyrios

Porfiro (Greek) a form of Porfirio.

Porter 🅱🅶 (Latin) gatekeeper.
Port, Portie, Porty

Poseidón (Greek) the owner of the waters.

Poshita (Sanskrit) cherished.

Posidio (Greek) he who is devoted to Poseidon.

Potenciano (Latin) he who dominates with his empire.

Poul (Danish) a form of Paul.
Poulos, Poulus

Pov (Gypsy) earth.

Powa (Native American) wealthy.
Powah

Powell (English) alert.
Powal, Powall, Powel, Powil, Powill, Powyl, Powyll

Prabhjot (Sikh) the light of God.

Prácido (Latin) tranquil, calm.

Pragnacio (Greek) he who is skillful and practical in business.

Pramad (Hindi) rejoicing.

Pravat (Tai) history.

Pravin (Hindi) capable.
Pravyn

Prem (Hindi) love.

Prentice (English) apprentice.
Prent, Prentis, Prentise, Prentiss, Prentyc, Prentyce, Prentys, Prentyse, Printes, Printiss

Prescott (English) priest's cottage. See also Scott.
Prescot, Prestcot, Prestcott

Presidio (Latin) he who gives pleasant shelter.

Presley 🅶🅱 (English) priest's meadow. Music: Elvis Presley was an influential American rock 'n' roll singer.
Preslea, Preslee, Presleigh, Presli, Preslie, Presly, Presslee, Pressley, Prestley, Priestley, Priestly

Preston (English) priest's estate.
Prestan, Presten, Prestin, Prestyn

Pretextato (Latin) covered by a toga.

Prewitt (French) brave little one.
Preuet, Prewet, Prewett, Prewit, Prewyt, Prewytt, Pruit, Pruitt, Pruyt, Pruytt

Priamo, Príamo (Greek) the rescued one.

Price (Welsh) son of the ardent one.
Pryce

Pricha (Tai) clever.

Priest (English) holy man. A short form of Preston.

Prilidiano, Prilidíano (Greek) he who remembers things from the past.

Primael (Latin) chosen first.

Primeiro (Italian) born first.

Primitivo (Latin) original.

Primo (Italian) first; premier quality.
Preemo, Premo, Prymo

Prince (Latin) chief; prince.
Prence, Prins, Prinse, Prinz, Prinze, Prynce,
Pryns, Prynse

Princeton (English) princely town.
Prenston, Princeston, Princton

Prisco (Latin) old; from another time.

Probo (Latin) having moral conduct.

Proceso (Latin) he who moves forward.

Procopio (Greek) he who progresses.

Procoro (Greek) he who prospers.

Proctor (Latin) official, administrator.
Prockter, Proctar, Procter

Proculo (Latin) he who was born far from
home.

Prokopios (Greek) declared leader.

Promaco (Greek) he who prepares for battle.

Prometeo (Greek) he who resembles God.

Prosper (Latin) fortunate.
Prospero, Próspero

Protasio, Protólico (Greek) preferred one.

Proteo (Greek) lord of the waves of the sea.

Proterio, Proto (Greek) he who precedes
all the rest.

Prudenciano (Spanish) humble and honest.

Prudencio (Latin) he who works with sen-
sitivity and modesty.

Prudens (German) a form of Prudencio.

Pryor (Latin) head of the monastery; prior.
Prior, Pry

Ptah (Egyptian) cultured by God in
Memphis.

Publio (Latin) he who is popular.

Puchac (Quechua) leader.

Pueblo (Spanish) from the city.

Pulqueria (Latin) the beautiful one.

Pulqui (Araucanian) arrow.

Pumasonjo, Pumasuncu (Quechua) heart
of a puma.

Pumeet (Sanskrit) pure.

Pupulo (Latin) the little boy.

Purdy (Hindi) recluse.

Puric (Quechua) walker.

Purvis (French, English) providing food.
Pervis, Purves, Purvise, Purviss, Purvys,
Purvyss

Pusaki (Indigenous) fire.

Putnam (English) dweller by the pond.
Putnem, Putnum

Pyotr (Russian) a form of Peter.
Petya, Pyatr

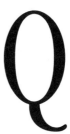

Qabic (Arabic) able.
Quabic, Quabick, Quabik, Quabyc, Quabyck,
Quabyk

Qabil (Arabic) able.
Qabill, Qabyl, Qabyll

Qadim (Arabic) ancient.
Quadym

Qadir (Arabic) powerful.
Qaadir, Qadeer, Quaadir, Quadeer, Quadir

Qamar (Arabic) moon.
Quamar, Quamir

Qasim (Arabic) divider.
Qasym, Quasim

Qeb (Egyptian) father of the earth.

Qimat (Hindi) valuable.
Qymat

Quaashie BG (Ewe) born on Sunday.
Quaashi, Quashi, Quashie

Quadarius (American) a combination of Quan + Darius.
Quadara, Quadarious, Quadaris, Quandarious, Quandarius, Quandarrius, Qudarius, Qudaruis

Quade (Latin) fourth.
Quadell, Quaden, Quadon, Quadre, Quadrie, Quadrine, Quadrion, Quaid, Quayd, Quayde, Qwade

Quain (French) clever.
Quayn

Quamaine (American) a combination of Quan + Jermaine.
Quamain, Quaman, Quamane, Quamayne, Quarmaine

Quan (Comanche) a short form of Quanah.

Quanah (Comanche) fragrant.

Quandre (American) a combination of Quan + Andre.
Quandrae, Quandré

Quant (Greek) how much?
Quanta, Quantae, Quantah, Quantai, Quantas, Quantay, Quante, Quantea, Quantey, Quantu

Quantavious (American) a form of Quantavius.

Quantavius (American) a combination of Quan + Octavius.
Quantavian, Quantavin, Quantavion, Quantavis, Quantavous, Quatavious, Quatavius

Quantez (American) a form of Quant.

Quashawn (American) a combination of Quan + Shawn.
Quasean, Quashaan, Quashan, Quashaun, Quashaunn, Quashon, Quashone, Quashun, Queshan, Queshon, Qweshawn, Qyshawn

Quauhtli (Nahuatl) eagle.

Qudamah (Arabic) courage.
Qudam, Qudama

Quenán (Hebrew) fixed.

Quenby BG (Scandinavian) a form of Quimby.
Quenbee, Quenbey, Quenbi, Quenbie, Quinbee, Quinby, Quynbee, Quynbey, Quynbi, Quynbie, Quynby

Quennell (French) small oak.
Quenal, Quenall, Quenel, Quenell, Quennal, Quennall, Quennel

Quenten, Quenton (Latin) forms of Quentin.
Quienten, Quienton

Quenti, Quinti (Quechua) hummingbird.

Quentin (Latin) fifth. (English) queen's town.
Qeuntin, Quantin, Queintin, Quent, Quentan, Quentine, Quentyn, Quentynn, Quientin, Quintan, Quyntan, Quyntyn, Qwentan, Qwentin, Qwentyn, Qwyntan, Qwyntyn

Querubín (Hebrew) swift, young bull.

Quesnel (French) one who comes from the oak tree.

Quespi (Quechua) jewel, shiny like a diamond.

Quest (Latin) quest.

Queupulicán (Mapuche) white stone with a black stripe.

Queupumil (Mapuche) shining stone.

Quichuasamin (Quechua) he who brings fortune and happiness to the Quechua village.

Quico (Spanish) a familiar form of many names.

Quidequeo (Mapuche) brilliant.

Quigley (Irish) maternal side.
Quiglea, Quiglee, Quigleigh, Quigli, Quiglie, Quigly

Quillan (Irish) cub.
Quilan, Quilen, Quilin, Quill, Quille, Quillen, Quillin, Quillyn, Quilyn

Quillén (Araucanian) tear.

Quillinchu, Quilliyicu (Quechua) sparrow hawk.

Quillon (Latin) sword.
Quilon, Quyllon, Quylon

Quimby (Scandinavian) woman's estate.
Quembee, Quembey, Quemby, Quenby,
Quymbee, Quymbey, Quymbi, Quymbie,
Quymby

Quimey (Araucanian) pretty; beautiful.

Quin (Irish) a form of Quinn.

Quincey BG (French) a form of Quincy.

Quincy BG (French) fifth son's estate.
Quenci, Quency, Quince, Quincee, Quinci,
Quinncy, Quinnsey, Quinnsy, Quinsey,
Quinzy, Quyncee, Quyncey, Quynnsey,
Quynnsy, Quynsy

Quindarius (American) a combination of
Quinn + Darius.
Quindarious, Quindarrius, Quinderious,
Quinderus, Quindrius

Quiñelef (Mapuche) quick race.

Quinlan (Irish) strong; well shaped.
Quindlen, Quinlen, Quinlin, Quinnlan,
Quinnlin, Quynlan, Quynlen, Quynlin,
Quynlon, Quynlyn

Quinn BG (Irish) a short form of Quincy,
Quinlan, Quinten.
Quyn, Quynn

Quintavious (American) a form of
Quintavius.

Quintavis (American) a form of Quintavius.

Quintavius (American) a combination of
Quinn + Octavius.
Quintavus, Quintayvious

Quinten, Quintin, Quinton (Latin) forms
of Quentin.
Quinneton, Quinnten, Quinntin, Quinnton,
Quint, Quintan, Quintann, Quintine,
Quintion, Quintus, Quintyn, Quiton,
Qunton, Quynten, Quyntin, Quynton,
Qwenten, Qwentin, Qwenton, Qwinton,
Qwynten, Qwyntin, Qwynton

Quintilian (French) a form of Quintiliano.

Quintiliano (Spanish) a form of Quintilio.

Quintilio (Latin) he who was born in the
fifth month.

Quintrilpe (Mapuche) place of organiza-
tion.

Quintuillan (Mapuche) searching for the
altar.

Quiqui (Spanish) a familiar form of Enrique.
Quinto, Quiquin, Quyquy

Quiríaco (Greek) a form of Ciriaco.

Quirino (Latin) he who carries a lance.

Quispe, Quispi (Quechua) jewel.

Quispiyupanqui (Quechua) he who honors
his liberty.

Quisu (Aymara) he who appreciates the
value of things.

Quitin (Latin) a short form of Quinten.
Quiten, Quito, Quiton

Quito (Spanish) a short form of Quinten.

Quoc (Vietnamese) nation.

Quon (Chinese) bright.

Qutub (Indian) tall.

R

Ra (Egyptian) sunshine.

Ra`Id (Arabic) leader.

Ra`Is (Arabic) boss.

Ra'shawn, Rashaan, Rashaun, Rashon
(American) forms of Rashawn.
Rasaun, Rashann, Rashion, Rashone,
Rashonn, Rashuan, Rashun, Rhashaun

Raamah (Hebrew) thunder.
Raama, Rama, Ramah

Raanan (Hebrew) fresh; luxuriant.
Ranan

Rabah (Arabic) winner.

Rabel (Catalan) a form of Rafael.

Rabi BG (Arabic) breeze. (Scottish) famous.
Rabbi, Rabby, Rabee, Rabeeh, Rabey, Rabiah,
Rabie, Rabih, Raby

Race (English) race.
Racee, Racel

Racham (Hebrew) compassionate.
Rachaman, Rachamim, Rachamin, Rachamyn, Rachim, Rachman, Rachmiel, Rachmyel, Rachum, Raham, Rahamim, Rahamym

Rachel 🇬🇧 (Hebrew) sheep.

Rachid (Lebanese) prudent.

Rad (English) advisor. (Slavic) happy.
Raad, Radd, Raddie, Raddy, Rade, Radee, Radell, Radey, Radi

Radbert (English) brilliant advisor.
Radbirt, Radburt, Radbyrt, Raddbert, Raddbirt, Raddburt, Raddbyrt

Radburn (English) red brook; brook with reeds.
Radbern, Radborn, Radborne, Radbourn, Radbourne, Radburne, Radbyrn, Radbyrne

Radcliff (English) red cliff; cliff with reeds.
Radclif, Radcliffe, Radclith, Radclithe, Radclyffe, Radclyth, Redclif, Redcliff, Redcliffe, Redclyth

Radek (Czech) famous ruler.
Radec, Radeque

Radford (English) red ford; ford with reeds.

Radhakanta (Indian) another name for the Hindu god Krishna.

Radhakrishna (Indian) the Hindu god Krishna and Radha, lover of Krishna.

Radhavallabh (Indian) beloved of Radha; another name for the Hindu god Krishna.

Radheshyam (Indian) another name for the Hindu god Krishna.

Radheya (Indian) another name for Karna, a hero in the Indian epic poem *Mahabharata*.

Radley (English) red meadow; meadow of reeds. See also Redley.
Radlea, Radlee, Radleigh, Radly

Radman (Slavic) joyful.
Raddman, Radmen, Radmon, Reddman, Redman

Radnor (English) red shore; shore with reeds.
Radnore, Rednor, Rednore

Radomil (Slavic) happy peace.
Radomyl

Radoslaw (Polish) happy glory.
Rado, Radoslav, Radzmir, Slawek

Radwan (Arabic) pleasant, delightful.
Radwen, Radwin, Radwon, Radwyn

Raekwon, Raequan (American) forms of Raquan.
Raekwan, Raequon, Raeqwon, Raikwan, Raiqoun, Raiquan, Raiquen, Rakwane, Rakwon

Raeshawn (American) a form of Rashawn.
Raesean, Raeshaun, Raeshon, Raeshun

Rafa (Hebrew) the giant.

Rafael (Spanish) a form of Raphael. See also Falito.
Rafaell, Rafaello, Rafaelo, Rafeal, Rafeé, Rafello, Raffaell, Raffaello, Raffaelo, Raffeal, Raffel, Raffiel, Rafiel

Rafaele, Raffaele (Italian) forms of Raphael.
Raffael

Rafaelle 🇬🇧 (French) a form of Raphael.
Rafelle

Rafal (Polish) a form of Raphael.
Rafel

Rafat (Indian) elevation.

Rafe (English) a short form of Rafferty, Ralph.
Raff, Raffe

Rafer (Irish) a short form of Rafferty.
Raffer

Rafferty (Irish) rich, prosperous.
Rafe, Rafer, Rafertee, Rafertey, Raferti, Rafertie, Raferty, Raffarty

Raffi (Hebrew, Arabic) a form of Rafi.
Raffee, Raffey, Raffie, Raffy

Rafi (Arabic) exalted. (Hebrew) a familiar form of Raphael.
Rafee, Rafey, Rafie, Rafy

Rafiq (Arabic) friend.
Raafiq, Rafeeq, Rafic, Rafique, Rafyq, Rafyque

Rafiq (Arabic) a form of Rafiq.

Raghav, Raghavendra, Raghunandan, Raghunath, Raghupati, Raghuvir
(Indian) other names for the Hindu god Rama.

Raghib (Arabic) desirous.
Raghyb, Raquib, Raquyb

Raghîb (Arabic) a form of Raghib.

Raghnall (Irish) wise power.
Raghnal, Ragnal, Ragnall

Raghu (Indian) family of the Hindu god Rama.

Ragnar (Norwegian) powerful army.
Ragner, Ragnir, Ragnor, Ragnyr, Ranieri

Rago (Hausa) ram.

Raguel (Hebrew) everybody's friend.

Rahas (Indian) secret.

Raheem BG (Punjabi) compassionate God.

Raheim (Punjabi) a form of Raheem.

Rahim (Arabic) merciful.
Raaheim, Rahaeim, Raheam, Rahiem, Rahiim, Rahime, Rahium

Rahman (Arabic) compassionate.
Rahmatt, Rahmen, Rahmet, Rahmin, Rahmon, Rahmyn

Rahsaan (American) a form of Rashean.

Rahul (Arabic) traveler.

Raíd (Arabic) leader.
Rayd

Raiden (Japanese) Mythology: the thunder god.
Raedan, Raeden, Raedin, Raedon, Raedyn, Raidan, Raidin, Raidon, Raidyn, Reidan, Reiden, Reidin, Reidon, Reidyn

Railef (Mapuche) a flower that is bedraggled because of a strong wind.

Raimi (Quechua) party, celebration.

Raimondo (Italian) a form of Raymond.
Raymondo, Reimundo

Raimund (German) a form of Raymond.
Rajmund

Raimundo (Portuguese, Spanish) a form of Raymond.
Mundo, Raimon, Raimond, Raimonds

Raine GB (English) lord; wise.
Raen, Raene, Rain, Raines

Rainer (German) counselor.
Rainar, Raineier, Rainey, Rainier, Rainieri, Rayner, Reinar

Rainerio, Rainero, Rainiero (German) forms of Rainer.

Rainey GB (German) a familiar form of Rainer.
Rainee, Rainie, Rainney, Rainy, Raynee, Rayney, Rayni, Raynie, Rayny, Reiny

Raini GB (Tupi-Guarani) Religion: the god who created the world.

Rainier (French) a form of Rainer.
Ranier, Raynier, Reignier, Reinier

Rainieri (Italian) a form of Rainer.
Rainierie

Raishawn (American) a form of Rashawn.
Raishon, Raishun

Raj (Hindi) a short form of Rajah.

Raja GB (Hindi) a form of Rajah.

Rajabu (Swahili) born in the seventh month of the Islamic calendar.

Rajah (Hindi) prince; chief.
Rajaah, Rajae, Rajahe, Raje, Rajeh, Raji

Rajak (Hindi) cleansing.

Rajam (Indian) another name for the Hindu goddess Lakshmi.

Rajan (Hindi) a form of Rajah.
Rajaahn, Rajain, Rajen, Rajin

Rajarshi, Rajrishi (Indian) king's sage.

Rajas (Indian) mastery; fame; pride.

Rajat (Indian) silver.

Rajatshubhra (Indian) white as silver.

Rajdulari (Indian) dear princess.

Rajendra, Rajendrakumar, Rajendramohan, Rajesh (Indian) king.

Rajit (Indian) decorated.

Rakeem (Punjabi) a form of Raheem.
Rakeeme, Rakeim, Rakem

Rakim (Arabic) a form of Rahim.
Rakiim

Rakin (Arabic) respectable.
Rakeen, Rakyn

Raktim (Hindi) bright red.
Raktym

Raleigh BG (English) a form of Rawleigh.
*Raelea, Raelee, Raeleigh, Raeley, Railea,
Railee, Raileigh, Railey, Ralegh, Raylea,
Raylee, Rayleigh, Rayley*

Ralph (English) wolf counselor.
*Radolphus, Radulf, Rafe, Ralf, Ralpheal,
Ralphel*

Ralphie (English) a familiar form of Ralph.
Ralphy

Ralston (English) Ralph's settlement.
*Ralfston, Ralfstone, Ralfton, Ralftone,
Ralphstone, Ralphton, Ralphtone, Ralstone,
Ralstyn*

Ram (Hindi) god; godlike. Religion: another
name for the Hindu god Rama. (English)
male sheep. A short form of Ramsey.
Ramie

Ramadan (Arabic) ninth month in the
Islamic calendar.
Rama

Ramanan (Hindi) god; godlike.
Raman, Ramanjit, Ramanjot

Ramandeep GB (Hindi) a form of
Ramanan.

Rambert (German) strong; brilliant.
Rambirt, Ramburt, Rambyrt

Rami (Hindi, English) a form of Ram.
(Spanish) a short form of Ramiro.
Rame, Ramee, Ramey, Ramih

Ramírez (Spanish) judicious.

Ramiro (Portuguese, Spanish) supreme
judge.
*Ramario, Rameer, Rameir, Ramere, Rameriz,
Ramero, Ramires, Ramirez, Ramos, Ramyro*

Ramlal (Hindi) son of the god Ram.

Ramon, Ramón (Spanish) forms of
Raymond.
*Raman, Ramin, Ramyn, Remon, Remone,
Romon, Romone*

Ramond (Dutch) a form of Raymond.

Ramone (Dutch) a form of Raymond.
Raemon, Raemonn, Ramonte, Remone

Ramsden (English) valley of rams.
Ramsdan, Ramsdin, Ramsdon, Ramsdyn

Ramsey BG (English) ram's island.
Ramsay, Ramsee, Ramsi, Ramsie, Ramsy

Ramy (Hindi, English) a form of Ram.

Ramzi (American) a form of Ramsey.
Ramzee, Ramzey, Ramzy

Rance (American) a familiar form of
Laurence. (English) a short form of
Ransom.
*Rancel, Rancell, Rances, Rancey, Rancie,
Rancy, Ransel, Ransell*

Rancul (Araucanian) plant from the grass-
lands whose leaves are used to make roofs
for huts.

Rand (English) shield; warrior.

Randal, Randell (English) forms of
Randall.
Randahl, Randale, Randel, Randl, Randle

Randall BG (English) a form of Randolph.
Randyll

Randeep (Sikh) battle lamp.

Randolph (English) shield wolf.
*Randol, Randolf, Randolfe, Randolfo,
Randolphe, Randolpho, Randolphus, Randulf,
Randulfe, Randulph, Randulphe, Ranolph*

Randy BG (English) a familiar form of
Rand, Randall, Randolph.
*Randdy, Randee, Randey, Randi, Randie,
Ranndy*

Ranen (Hebrew) joyful.
Ranan, Ranin, Ranon, Ranun, Ranyn

Ranger (French) forest keeper.
Rainger, Range, Raynger, Reinger, Reynger

Rangle (American) cowboy. See also
Wrangle.
Ranglar, Rangler

Rangsey (Cambodian) seven kinds of colors.
Rangsea, Rangsee, Rangseigh, Rangsi,
Rangsie, Rangsy

Rangvald (Scandinavian) a form of Reynold.

Rani GB (Hebrew) my song; my joy.
Ranee, Raney, Ranie, Rany, Roni

Ranieri (Italian) a form of Ragnar.
Raneir, Ranier, Rannier

Ranjan (Hindi) delighted; gladdened.

Rankin (English) small shield.
Randkin, Rankyn

Ransford (English) raven's ford.
Ransforde, Rensford, Rensforde

Ransley (English) raven's field.
Ranslea, Ranslee, Ransleigh, Ransli, Ranslie,
Ransly, Renslee, Rensleigh, Rensley, Rensli,
Renslie, Rensly

Ransom (Latin) redeemer. (English) son of
the shield.
Randsom, Randsome, Ransome, Ranson

Raoul (French) a form of Ralph, Rudolph.
Raol, Reuel

Raphael (Hebrew) God has healed. Bible:
one of the archangels. Art: a prominent
painter of the Renaissance. See also Falito,
Rafi.
Raphaél, Raphaello, Raphale, Raphel,
Raphello, Raphiel, Rephael

Rapheal (Hebrew) a form of Raphael.
Rafel, Raphiel

Rapier (French) blade-sharp.
Rapyer

Rapiman (Mapuche) the condor's vomit;
indigestion.

Raquan (American) a combination of the
prefix Ra + Quan.
Raaquan, Rackwon, Racquan, Rahquan,
Raquané, Raquon, Raquwan, Raquwn,
Raquwon, Raqwan, Raqwann

Rashaad, Rashaud, Rashod (Arabic) forms
of Rashad.
Rachaud, Rashaude, Rashoda, Rashodd,
Rashoud, Rayshod, Reyshaad, Reyshod,
Rhashod

Rashad (Arabic) wise counselor.
Raashad, Rachad, Rachard, Raeshad,
Raishard, Rashaad, Rashadd, Rashade,
Rashaud, Rasheed, Rashod, Reshad, Rhashad

Rashâd (Arabic) a form of Rashad.

Rashan (American) a form of Rashawn.

Rashard (American) a form of Richard.
Rasharrd

Rashawn BG (American) a combination of
the prefix Ra + Shawn.
Raashawn, Raashen, Raeshawn, Rahshawn,
Raishawn, Rasaan, Rasawn, Rashaughn,
Rashaw, Rashun, Rashunn, Raushan,
Raushawn, Rhashan, Rhashawn

Rashean (American) a combination of the
prefix Ra + Sean.
Rahsean, Rahseen, Rasean, Rashane,
Rashien, Rashiena

Rasheed (Arabic) a form of Rashad.
Rashead, Rashed, Rasheid, Rasheyd,
Rhasheed

Rasheen (American) a form of Rashean.

Rashid (Arabic) a form of Rashad.
Rasheyd, Rashied, Rashyd, Raushaid

Rashîd (Arabic) a form of Rashid.

Rashida GB (Swahili) righteous.
Rashidah, Rashieda

Rashidi (Swahili) wise counselor.

Rasmus (Greek, Danish) a short form of
Erasmus.

Râteb (Arabic) administrator.

Rauel (Hebrew) friend of God.

Raul (French) a form of Ralph.
Raúl

Raulas (Lithuanian) a form of Laurence.

Raulo (Lithuanian) a form of Laurence.

Raurac (Quechua) burning, ardent.

Raven GB (English) a short form of
Ravenel.
Ravan, Ravean, Raveen, Ravin, Ravine,
Ravyn, Ravynn, Reven, Rhaven

Ravenel (English) raven.
Ravenell, Revenel

Ravi (Hindi) sun.
Ravee, Ravijot, Ravy

Ravid (Hebrew) a form of Arvid.
Ravyd

Raviv (Hebrew) rain, dew.
Ravyv

Ravon BG (English) a form of Raven.
Raveon, Ravion, Ravone, Ravonn, Ravonne, Revon

Rawdon (English) rough hill.
Rawdan, Rawden, Rawdin, Rawdyn

Rawleigh (English) deer meadow.
Rawle, Rawlea, Rawlee, Rawley, Rawli, Rawlie, Rawly

Rawlins (French) a form of Roland.
Rawlin, Rawling, Rawlings, Rawlinson, Rawlyn, Rawlyng, Rawlyngs, Rawson

Ray (French) kingly, royal. (English) a short form of Rayburn, Raymond. See also Lei.
Rae, Rai, Raie, Raye

Rayan BG (Irish) a form of Ryan.
Rayaun

Rayburn (English) deer brook.
Burney, Raeborn, Raeborne, Raebourn, Raebourne, Raeburn, Raeburne, Raibourn, Raibourne, Raiburn, Raiburne, Raybourn, Raybourne, Rayburne, Reibourn, Reibourne, Reiburn, Reiburne, Reybourn, Reybourne, Reyburn, Reyburne

Rayce (English) a form of Race.

Rayden (Japanese) a form of Raiden.
Raydun, Rayedon, Reydan, Reyden, Reydin, Reydon, Reydyn

Rayfield (English) stream in the field.
Raefield, Raifield, Reifield, Reyfield

Rayford (English) stream ford.
Raeford, Raeforde, Raiford, Raiforde, Reiford, Reiforde, Reyford, Reyforde

Rayhan (Arabic) favored by God.
Raehan, Raihan, Rayhaan

Rayi (Hebrew) my friend, my companion.

Raymán (Spanish) a form of Raymond.

Raymon (English) a form of Raymond.
Raeman, Raemen, Raemin, Raemon, Raemyn, Raiman, Raimen, Raimin, Raimon, Raimyn, Rayman, Raymann, Raymen, Raymin, Raymone, Raymun, Raymyn, Reaman, Reamon, Reamonn, Reamyn, Reymon, Reymun

Raymón (Spanish) a form of Raymon.

Raymond (English) mighty; wise protector. See also Ayman.
Radmond, Raemond, Ramonde, Raymand, Rayment, Raymont, Raymund, Raymunde, Redmond, Reimond, Reimund

Raymundo (Spanish) a form of Raymond. (Portuguese, Spanish) a form of Raimundo.
Raemondo, Raimondo, Raymondo

Raynaldo (Spanish) a form of Reynold.
Raynal, Raynald, Raynold

Raynard (French) a form of Renard, Reynard.
Raynarde

Rayne GB (English) a form of Raine.
Rayn, Rayno

Rayner (German) a form of Rainer.
Raynar, Reynar, Reyner, Reynir

Raynor (Scandinavian) a form of Ragnar.
Rainor, Reynor

Rayquan (American) a combination of Ray + Quan.

Raysean, Rayshaun, Rayshon (American) forms of Rayshawn.
Rayshonn

Rayshawn (American) a combination of Ray + Shawn.
Rayshaan, Rayshan, Raysheen, Rayshone, Rayshun, Rayshunn

Rayshod (American) a form of Rashad.
Raeshod, Raishod, Raychard, Rayshad, Rayshard, Rayshaud

Rayvon (American) a form of Ravon.
Rayvan, Rayvaun, Rayven, Rayvone, Reyven, Reyvon

Razi BG (Aramaic) my secret.
Raz, Razee, Razey, Razie, Raziq, Razy

Raziel (Aramaic) a form of Razi.

Re (Egyptian) half day.

Read (English) a form of Reed, Reid.
Raed, Raede, Raeed, Reaad, Reade

Reading (English) son of the red wanderer.
Redding, Reeding, Reiding

Reagan GB (Irish) little king. History: Ronald Wilson Reagan was the fortieth U.S. president.
Raegan, Raegin, Raegon, Raegyn, Raigan, Raigen, Raigin, Raigon, Raigyn, Raygan, Raygen, Raygin, Raygon, Raygyn, Reagen, Reaghan, Reegan, Reegen, Reegin, Reegon, Reegyn, Reigan, Reigen, Reighan, Reigin, Reign, Reigon, Reigyn, Reygan, Reygen, Reygin, Reygon, Reygyn, Rheagan

Real (Latin) real.

Rebel (American) rebel.
Reb, Rebell, Rebil, Rebill, Rebyl, Rebyll

Recaredo (Teutonic) counsels his superiors.

Red (American) red, redhead.
Redd

Reda (Arabic) satisfied.
Redah, Rida, Ridah, Ridha

Redempto, Redento (Latin) redeemed.

Redford (English) red river crossing.
Ford, Radford, Reaford, Red, Redd

Redley (English) red meadow; meadow with reeds. See also Radley.
Redlea, Redlee, Redleigh, Redli, Redlie, Redly

Redmond (German) protecting counselor. (English) a form of Raymond.
Radmond, Radmondo, Radmun, Radmund, Radmundo, Reddin, Redmon, Redmondo, Redmun, Redmund, Redmundo

Redpath (English) red path.
Raddpath, Radpath, Reddpath

Reece (Welsh) a form of Rhys.
Reace, Rece, Reice, Reyce, Ryese

Reed BG (English) a form of Reid.
Raeed, Reyde, Rheed

Rees, Reese (Welsh) forms of Rhys.
Rease, Reis, Reise, Reiss, Reyse, Riese, Riess

Reeve (English) steward.
Reav, Reave, Reaves, Reeves, Reive, Reyve, Rhyve

Reg (English) a short form of Reginald.
Regg

Regan GB (Irish) a form of Reagan.
Regen, Regin, Regon, Regyn

Reggie BG (English) a familiar form of Reginald.
Reggi, Reggy, Regi, Regie, Regy

Reginal (English) a form of Reginald.
Reginale, Reginel

Reginald (English) king's advisor. A form of Reynold. See also Naldo.
Regginald, Reginaldo, Reginalt, Reginauld, Reginault, Reginold, Reginuld, Regnauld, Ryginald, Ryginaldo

Regis (Latin) regal.
Reggis, Regiss, Regys, Regyss

Regulo, Régulo (Latin) forms of Rex.

Rehema (Swahili) second-born.
Rehemah

Rei GB (Japanese) rule, law.

Reid BG (English) redhead.
Reide, Reyd, Reyde, Ried

Reidar (Norwegian) nest warrior.
Reydar

Reilly BG (Irish) a form of Riley.
Reilea, Reilee, Reileigh, Reiley, Reili, Reilie, Reillea, Reillee, Reilleigh, Reilley, Reilli, Reillie, Reily

Reimunde (German) counselor and protector.

Reinaldo (Spanish) a form of Reynold.
Reinaldos

Reinardo (Teutonic) valiant counselor.

Reinhart (German) a form of Reynard. (English) a form of Reynold.
Rainart, Rainert, Rainhard, Rainhardt, Rainhart, Reinart, Reinhard, Reinhardt, Renke, Reynart, Reynhard, Reynhardt

Reinhold (Swedish) a form of Ragnar. (English) a form of Reynold.
Reinold

Reku (Finnish) a form of Richard.

Remedio (Latin) medicine.

Remi 🅱🅶 (French) a form of Remy.
Remie, Remmi, Remmie

Rémi (French) a form of Remy.

Remigio (Latin) he who mans the oars.

Remington 🅱🅶 (English) raven estate.
Rem, Reminton, Tony

Remo (Greek) the strong one.

Remus (Latin) speedy, quick. Mythology:
Remus and his twin brother, Romulus,
founded Rome.
Remas, Remos

Remy 🅱🅶 (French) from Rheims, France.
*Ramey, Remee, Remey, Remmee, Remmey,
Remmy*

Renaldo (Spanish) a form of Reynold.
*Rainaldo, Ranaldo, Raynaldo, Reynoldo,
Rinaldo, Rynaldo*

Renán (Irish) seal.

Renard (French) a form of Reynard.
Ranard, Reinard, Rennard

Renardo (Italian) a form of Reynard.

Renato (Italian) reborn.
Renat, Renatis, Renatus, Renatys

Renaud (French) a form of Reynard,
Reynold.
Renauld, Renauldo, Renault, Renould

Rendor (Hungarian) policeman.
Rendar, Render, Rendir, Rendyr

Rene 🅱🅶 (French) a form of René.

René (French) reborn.
Renay, Renne

Renee 🅶🅱 (French) a form of René. (Irish,
French) a form of Renny.

Renfred (English) lasting peace.
*Ranfred, Ranfrid, Ranfryd, Rinfred, Rinfryd,
Ronfred, Ronfryd, Rynfred, Rynfryd*

Renfrew (Welsh) raven woods.
Ranfrew

Renjiro (Japanese) virtuous.
Renjyro

Renny (Irish) small but strong. (French) a
familiar form of René.
*Ren, Reney, Reni, Renie, Renn, Rennee,
Renney, Renni, Rennie, Reny*

Reno (American) gambler. Geography: a city
in Nevada known for gambling.
Renos, Rino, Ryno

Renshaw (English) raven woods.
Ranshaw, Renishaw, Renshore

Renton (English) settlement of the roe deer.
Rentown

Renzo (Latin) a familiar form of Laurence.
(Italian) a short form of Lorenzo.
Renz, Renzy, Renzzo

Repucura (Mapuche) jagged rock; rocky
road.

Reshad (American) a form of Rashad.
*Reshade, Reshard, Resharrd, Reshaud,
Reshawd, Reshead, Reshod*

Reshawn (American) a combination of the
prefix Re + Shawn.
Reshaun, Reshaw, Reshon, Reshun

Reshean (American) a combination of the
prefix Re + Sean.
*Resean, Reshae, Reshane, Reshay, Reshayne,
Reshea, Resheen, Reshey*

Respicio (Latin) I look behind.

Restituto (Latin) he who returns to God.

Reuben (Hebrew) behold a son.
Reuban, Reubin, Rheuben, Rhuben

Reule (French) famous wolf.

Reuquén (Araucanian) tempestuous.

Reuven (Hebrew) a form of Reuben.
Reuvin, Rouvin, Ruvim

Rex (Latin) king.
Rexx

Rexford (English) king's ford.
Rexforde

Rexton (English) king's town.

Rey (Spanish) a short form of Reynaldo,
Reynard, Reynold. (French) a form of
Roy.

Reyes (English) a form of Reece.
Reyce

Reyhan BG (Arabic) favored by God.
Reihan, Reyham

Reymond (English) a form of Raymond.
Reymon, Reymound, Reymund

Reymundo (Spanish) a form of Raymond.
Reimonde, Reimundo, Reymondo

Reynaldo (Spanish) a form of Reynold.
Reynaldos, Reynauldo

Reynard (French) wise; bold, courageous.
Raenard, Rainard, Reinhard, Reinhardt,
Reinhart, Reiyard, Rennard, Reynardo,
Reynaud

Reynold (English) king's advisor. See also
Reginald.
Raenold, Rainault, Rainhold, Rainold,
Ranald, Raynaldo, Raynold, Reinald,
Reinwald, Renald, Renaldi, Renauld,
Rennold, Renold, Reynald, Reynol, Reynolds,
Rinaldo

Réz BG (Hungarian) copper; redhead.
Rezsö

Reza BG (German) a form of Resi (see
Girls' Names).

Rezin (Hebrew) pleasant, delightful.
Rezan, Rezen, Rezi, Rezie, Rezon, Rezy,
Rezyn

Rhett (Welsh) a form of Rhys. Literature:
Rhett Butler was the hero of Margaret
Mitchell's novel *Gone with the Wind*.
Rhet

Rhodes (Greek) where roses grow.
Geography: an island of southeast Greece.
Rhoads, Rhodas, Rodas

Rhyan BG (Irish) a form of Ryan.
Rhian

Rhys (Welsh) enthusiastic; stream.
Rhyce, Rhyse

Rian GB (Irish) little king. See also Ryan.
Rhian, Rhien, Rhion, Rhiun, Rhiyn, Rien,
Rion, Riun, Riyn

Riberto (German) brilliant because of his
power.

Ric (Italian, Spanish) a short form of Rico.
(German, English) a form of Rick.
Ricca

Ricardo, Riccardo (Portuguese, Spanish)
forms of Richard.
Racardo, Recard, Recardo, Ricaldo, Ricard,
Ricardoe, Ricardos, Riccard, Riccarrdo,
Ricciardo, Richardo, Rickardo, Rikardo,
Rychardo, Ryckardo, Rykardo

Ricco, Rico (Italian) short forms of Enrico.
(Spanish) familiar forms of Richard.
Rycco, Ryco

Rice (English) rich, noble. (Welsh) a form of
Reece.
Ryce

Rich (English) a short form of Richard.
Ritch, Rych

Richard ☆ (English) a form of Richart. See
also Aric, Dick, Juku, Likeke.
Richar, Richards, Richardson, Richaud, Richer,
Richerd, Richird, Richshard, Rickert, Rihardos,
Rihards, Riocard, Riócard, Risa, Risardas,
Rishard, Ristéard, Rostik, Rychard, Rychardt,
Rychird, Rychyrd, Rysio, Ryszard

Richart (German) rich and powerful ruler.

Richie (English) a familiar form of Richard.
Richee, Richey, Richi, Richy, Rychee, Rychey,
Rychi, Rychie, Rychy

Richman (English) powerful.
Richmen, Richmun, Rychman, Rychmen,
Rychmon, Rychmun

Richmond (German) powerful protector.
Richmand, Richmando, Richmon, Richmondo,
Richmondt, Richmound, Richmund,
Richmundo, Rychmand, Rychmond,
Rychmondo, Rychmont, Rychmund,
Rychmundo, Rychmunt

Rick (German, English) a short form of
Cedric, Frederick, Richard.
Ricke, Ricks, Rik, Riki, Ryc, Ryck, Ryk,
Rykk

Rickard (Swedish) a form of Richard.
Ryckard

Ricker (English) powerful army.
Rickar, Rikar, Ryckar, Rykar

Rickey, Ricky (English) familiar forms of Richard, Rick.
Ricci, Rickee, Riczi

Ricki GB (English) a familiar form of Richard, Rick.

Rickie BG (English) a familiar form of Richard, Rick.

Rickward (English) mighty guardian.
Rickwerd, Rickwood, Ricward, Ryckward, Rycward

Rida BG (Arabic) favor.
Ridah, Ryda, Rydah

Riddock (Irish) smooth field.
Riddick, Riddoc, Riddok, Ridoc, Ridock, Ridok, Rydoc, Rydock, Rydok

Rider (English) horseman.
Ridar, Ridder, Rydar

Ridge (English) ridge of a cliff.
Ridgy, Rig, Rydge

Ridgeley (English) meadow near the ridge.
Ridgeleigh, Ridglea, Ridglee, Ridgleigh, Ridgley, Ridgli, Ridglie, Ridgly, Rydglea, Rydglee, Rydgleigh, Rydgley, Rydgli, Rydglie, Rydgly

Ridgeway (English) path along the ridge.
Rydgeway

Ridley (English) meadow of reeds.
Rhidley, Riddley, Ridlea, Ridlee, Ridleigh, Ridli, Ridlie, Ridly

Riel (Spanish) a short form of Gabriel.
Reil, Reill, Riell, Rielle, Ryel, Ryell, Ryelle

Rigby (English) ruler's valley.
Rigbee, Rigbey, Rigbi, Rigbie, Rygbee, Rygbey, Rygbi, Rygbie, Rygby

Rigel (Arabic) foot. Astronomy: one of the stars in the constellation Orion.
Rygel

Rigg (English) ridge.
Rig, Riggs, Ryg, Rygg, Ryggs, Rygs

Rigo (Italian) a form of Rigg.

Rigoberto (German) splendid; wealthy.
Rigobert

Rikard (Scandinavian) a form of Richard.
Rikárd, Rykard

Riker (American) a form of Ryker.

Riki GB (Estonian) a form of Rick.
Rikkey, Rikky, Riks, Riky

Rikki GB (Estonian) a form of Rick.

Riley BG (Irish) valiant.
Rhiley, Rhylee, Rhyley, Rieley, Rielly, Riely, Rilee, Rilley, Rily, Rilye

Rimac (Quechua) speaker, eloquent.

Rimachi (Quechua) he who makes us speak.

Rinaldo (Italian) a form of Reynold.
Rinald, Rinaldi

Ring (English) ring.
Ryng

Ringo (Japanese) apple. (English) a familiar form of Ring.
Ryngo

Rio BG (Spanish) river. Geography: Rio de Janeiro is a city in Brazil.

Río (Spanish) a form of Rio.

Riordan (Irish) bard, royal poet.
Rearden, Reardin, Reardon, Ryordan

Rip (Dutch) ripe; full grown. (English) a short form of Ripley.
Ripp, Ryp, Rypp

Ripley (English) meadow near the river.
Rip, Riplea, Riplee, Ripleigh, Ripli, Riplie, Riply, Ripplee, Rippleigh, Rippley, Rippli, Ripplie, Ripply, Ryplea, Ryplee, Rypleigh, Rypley, Rypli, Ryplie, Ryply, Rypplea, Rypplee, Ryppleigh, Ryppley, Ryppli, Rypplie, Rypply

Riqui (Spanish) a form of Rickey.

Rishad (American) a form of Rashad.
Rishaad

Rishawn (American) a combination of the prefix Ri + Shawn.
Rishan, Rishaun, Rishon, Rishone

Rishi (Hindi) sage. (English) a form of Richie.
Ryshi

Risley (English) meadow with shrubs. See also Wrisley.
Rislea, Rislee, Risleigh, Risli, Rislie, Risly,

*Ryslea, Ryslee, Rysleigh, Rysley, Rysli,
Ryslie, Rysly*

Risto (Finnish) a short form of Christopher.
Rysto

Riston (English) settlement near the shrubs.
See also Wriston.
Ryston

Ritchard (English) a form of Richard.
*Ritchardt, Ritcherd, Ritchyrd, Ritshard,
Ritsherd*

Ritchie (English) a form of Richie.
Ritchee, Ritchey, Ritchi, Ritchy

Rithisak (Cambodian) powerful.

Ritter (German) knight; chivalrous.
Rittar, Rittner, Ryttar, Rytter

River BG (English) river; riverbank.
Rivar, Rive, Rivers, Riviera, Rivor, Ryv, Ryver

Riyad (Arabic) gardens.
Riad, Riyaad, Riyadh, Riyaz, Riyod

Riyâd (Arabic) a form of Riyad.

Rizieri (Germanic) army of the leader.

Roald (Norwegian) famous ruler.

Roan (English) a short form of Rowan.
Rhoan, Roen

Roano (Spanish) reddish brown skin.

Roar (Norwegian) praised warrior.
Roary

Roarke (Irish) famous ruler.
Roark, Rork, Rorke, Rourk, Rourke, Ruark

Rob (English) a short form of Robert.
Rab, Robb, Robe

Robbie BG (English) a familiar form of
Robert.
*Rabbie, Raby, Rhobbie, Robbee, Robbey,
Robbi, Robee, Robey, Robhy, Robi, Robie,
Roby*

Robby (English) a familiar form of Robert.

Robert ☆ BG (English) famous brilliance.
See also Bobek, Dob, Lopaka.
*Bob, Bobby, Riobard, Riobart, Robars, Robart,
Rober, Roberd, Robers, Roberte, Robirt,
Robyrt, Roibeárd, Rosertas, Rudbert*

Roberto (Italian, Portuguese, Spanish) a
form of Robert.
Robertino, Ruberto

Roberts, Robertson (English) son of
Robert.
*Roberson, Robertas, Robirtson, Roburtson,
Robyrtson*

Robin GB (English) a short form of Robert.
*Roban, Robban, Robben, Robbin, Robbon,
Roben, Robinet, Robinn, Robon, Roibín*

Robinson (English) a form of Roberts.
*Robbins, Robbinson, Robens, Robenson,
Robeson, Robins, Robson, Robynson*

Robustiano (Latin) strong as the wood of
an oak tree.

Robyn GB (English) a form of Robin.
Robbyn

Roca, Ruca (Aymara) principal; chief.

Rocco (Italian) rock.
Rocca, Rocio, Rocko, Rokko, Roko

Roch (English) a form of Rock.

Rochester (English) rocky fortress.
Chester, Chet

Rock (English) a short form of Rockwell.
Roc, Rok

Rockford (English) rocky ford.

Rockland (English) rocky land.
Rocklan

Rockledge (English) rocky ledge.

Rockley (English) rocky field.
*Rockle, Rocklea, Rocklee, Rockleigh, Rockli,
Rocklie, Rockly*

Rockwell (English) rocky spring. Art:
Norman Rockwell was a well-known
twentieth-century American illustrator.
Rockwel, Rocwel, Rocwell, Rokwel, Rokwell

Rocky (American) a familiar form of
Rocco, Rock.
*Rockee, Rockey, Rocki, Rockie, Rokee, Rokey,
Roki, Rokie, Roky*

Rod (English) a short form of Penrod,
Roderick, Rodney.
Rodd

Rodas (Greek, Spanish) a form of Rhodes.

Roddy (English) a familiar form of Roderick.
Roddie, Rody

Rode (Greek) pink.

Roden (English) red valley. Art: Auguste Rodin was an innovative French sculptor.
Rodan, Rodden, Rodin, Rodon, Rodyn, Roedan, Roeddan, Roedden, Roeddin, Roeddon, Roeddyn, Roeden, Roedin, Roedon, Roedyn

Roderich (German) a form of Roderick.

Roderick (German) famous ruler. See also Broderick, Rodrik.
Rhoderic, Rhoderick, Rhoderik, Rhoderyc, Rhoderyck, Rhoderyk, Rodaric, Rodarick, Rodarik, Rodderick, Roderic, Roderik, Roderikus, Roderrick, Roderyc, Roderyck, Roderyk, Rodgrick, Rodrugue, Roodney, Rurik, Ruy

Rodger (German) a form of Roger.
Rodge, Rodgir, Rodgy, Rodgyr

Rodman (German) famous man, hero.
Rodmann, Rodmond

Rodney (English) island clearing.
Rhodney, Roddnee, Roddney, Roddni, Roddnie, Roddny, Rodnee, Rodnei, Rodni, Rodnie, Rodnne, Rodny

Rodolfo (Spanish) a form of Rudolph, Rudolpho.
Rodolpho, Rodulfo

Rodrick (German) a form of Rodrik.
Roddrick, Rodric, Rodrich, Rodrique, Rodryc, Rodryck

Rodrigo (Italian, Spanish) a form of Roderick.
Roderigo, Rodrigue

Rodriguez (Spanish) son of Rodrigo.
Roddrigues, Rodrigues

Rodrik (German) famous ruler. See also Roderick.
Rodricki, Rodryk

Rodriquez (Spanish) a form of Rodriguez.
Rodrigquez, Rodriques, Rodriquiez

Roe (English) roe deer.
Row, Rowe

Rogan (Irish) redhead.
Rogein, Rogen, Rogin, Rogon, Rogun, Rogyn

Rogelio (Spanish) famous warrior. A form of Roger.
Rogelyo

Roger (German) famous spearman. See also Lokela.
Rog, Rogerick, Rogers, Rogier, Rogir, Rogyer, Rüdiger

Rogerio (Portuguese, Spanish) a form of Roger.
Rogerios, Rogerius, Rogero, Rogiero

Rohan (Hindi) sandalwood.

Rohin (Hindi) upward path.
Rohyn

Rohit (Hindi) big and beautiful fish.
Rohyt

Roi (French) a form of Roy.

Roja (Spanish) red.
Rojay

Rojelio (Spanish) a form of Rogelio.

Rolán (Spanish) a form of Rolando.

Roland (German) famous throughout the land.
Loránd, Roelan, Roeland, Rolan, Rolanda, Rolek, Rowe

Rolando (Portuguese, Spanish) a form of Roland.
Lando, Olo, Roldan, Roldán, Rollando, Rolondo

Rolf (German) a form of Ralph. A short form of Rudolph.
Rolfe, Rolph, Rolphe

Rolland (German) a form of Roland.

Rolle (Swedish) a familiar form of Roland, Rolf.

Rollie (English) a familiar form of Roland.
Roley, Rolle, Rolli, Rolly

Rollin (English) a form of Roland.
Rolin, Rollins

Rollo (English) a familiar form of Roland.
Rolla, Rolo

Rolon (Spanish) famous wolf.
Rollon

Romain (French) a form of Roman.
Romaine, Romane, Romanne, Romayn,
Romayne, Romin, Romyn

Roman (Latin) from Rome, Italy. (Gypsy)
gypsy; wanderer.
Roma, Romann, Romman

Román (Latin) a form of Roman.

Romanos (Greek) a form of Roman.
Romano

Romany (Gypsy) a form of Roman.
Romanee, Romaney, Romani, Romanie

Romario (Italian) a form of Romeo,
Romero.
Romar, Romarius, Romaro, Romarrio

Romea (Latin) pilgrim.

Romel, Romell, Rommel (Latin) short
forms of Romulus.
Romele

Romelio (Hebrew) God's very beloved one.

Romelo, Romello (Italian) forms of Romel.
Rommello

Romeo (Italian) pilgrim to Rome; Roman.
Literature: the title character of the
Shakespearean play *Romeo and Juliet.*
Roméo, Romio, Romyo

Romero (Latin) a form of Romeo.
Romeiro, Romer, Romere, Romerio, Romeris,
Romeryo

Romildo (Germanic) the glorious hero.

Romney (Welsh) winding river.
Romni, Romnie, Romny, Romoney

Romochka (Russian) from Rome.

Romualdo (Germanic) the glorious king.

Rómulo (Greek) he who is full of strength.

Romulus (Latin) citizen of Rome.
Mythology: Romulus and his twin brother,
Remus, founded Rome.
Romolo, Romono, Romulo

Romy GB (Italian) a familiar form of
Roman.
Romee, Romey, Romi, Romie, Rommie,
Rommy

Ron (Hebrew) a short form of Aaron,
Ronald.
Ronn

Ronald (Scottish) a form of Reginald.
(English) a form of Reynold.
Ranald, Ronal, Ronnald, Ronnold, Rynald

Ronaldo (Portuguese) a form of Ronald.
Ronoldo, Rynaldo

Ronan (Irish) a form of Rónán.

Rónán (Irish) seal.
Renan, Ronat

Rondel (French) short poem.
Rondal, Rondale, Rondeal, Rondey, Rondie,
Rondy

Rondell (French) a form of Rondel.
Rondall, Rondrell

Ronel, Ronell, Ronnell (American) forms
of Rondel.
Ronal, Ronelle, Ronil, Ronnel, Ronyell,
Ronyl

Roni GB (Hebrew) my song; my joy.
(Scottish) a form of Ronnie.
Rani, Roneet, Roney, Ronit, Ronli

Ronnie BG (Scottish) a familiar form of
Ronald.
Ronee, Roney, Ronie, Ronnee, Ronney, Ronni

Ronny BG (Scottish) a familiar form of
Ronald.

Ronson (Scottish) son of Ronald.
Ronaldson, Ronsen, Ronsin, Ronsun, Ronsyn

Ronté (American) a combination of Ron +
the suffix Te.
Rontae, Rontay, Ronte, Rontez

Rony (Hebrew) a form of Roni. (Scottish) a
form of Ronnie.

Rooney (Irish) redhead.
Roonee, Rooni, Roonie, Roony, Rowney

Roosevelt (Dutch) rose field. History: Theodore and Franklin D. Roosevelt were the twenty-sixth and thirty-second U.S. presidents, respectively.
Roosvelt, Rosevelt

Roper (English) rope maker.

Roque (Italian) a form of Rocco.

Rory BG (German) a familiar form of Roderick. (Irish) red king.
Roree, Rorey, Rori, Rorie, Rorrie, Rorry

Rosalio (Spanish) rose.
Rosalino

Rosario GB (Portuguese) rosary.
Rosaryo, Rozario, Rozaryo

Roscoe (Scandinavian) deer forest.
Rosco, Roscow

Rosendo (Germanic) the excellent master.

Roshad (American) a form of Rashad.
Roshard

Roshan BG (American) a form of Roshean.

Roshean (American) a combination of the prefix Ro + Sean.
Roshain, Roshane, Roshaun, Roshawn, Roshay, Rosheen, Roshene

Rosito (Filipino) rose.
Rosyto

Ross (Latin) rose. (Scottish) peninsula. (French) red. (English) a short form of Roswald.
Ros, Rosse, Rossell, Rossi, Rossie, Rossy

Rosswell (English) springtime of roses.
Rosswel, Rosvel, Roswel, Roswell

Rostislav (Czech) growing glory.
Rosta, Rostya

Roswald (English) field of roses.

Roth (German) redhead.

Rothwell (Scandinavian) red spring.
Rothwel

Rover (English) traveler.
Rovar, Rovir, Rovor

Rowan BG (English) tree with red berries.
Roan, Rowe, Rowen, Rowin, Rowney, Rowon, Rowyn

Rowdy (American) rowdy.

Rowell (English) roe-deer well.
Roewel, Roewell, Rowel

Rowland (English) rough land. (German) a form of Roland.
Rowlan, Rowlando, Rowlands, Rowlandson

Rowley (English) rough meadow.
Rowlea, Rowlee, Rowleigh, Rowli, Rowlie, Rowly

Rowson (English) son of the redhead.
Rawson

Roxbury (English) rook's town or fortress.
Roxburg, Roxburge, Roxburghe

Roxelio (German) a form of Rogelio.

Roy (French) king. A short form of Royal, Royce. See also Conroy, Delroy, Fitzroy, Leroy, Loe.
Roye, Ruy

Royal (French) kingly, royal.
Roial, Royale, Royall, Royell

Royce (English) son of Roy.
Roice, Roise, Royse, Royz

Royden (English) rye hill.
Roidan, Roiden, Roidin, Roidon, Roidyn, Royd, Roydan, Roydin, Roydon, Roydyn

Ruben, Rubin (Hebrew) forms of Reuben.
Ruban, Rube, Rubean, Rubens, Rubon, Rubyn

Rubén (Hebrew) a form of Ruben.

Rubert (Czech) a form of Robert.

Ruby GB (Hebrew) a familiar form of Reuben, Ruben.
Rube, Rubey

Rucahue (Mapuche) place of construction.

Rucalaf (Mapuche) house of joy.

Ruda (Czech) a form of Rudolph.
Rude, Rudek

Rudd (English) a short form of Rudyard.

Rudecindo (Spanish) a form of Rosendo.

Rudesindo (Teutonic) excellent gentleman.

Rudi (Spanish) a familiar form of Rudolph. (English) a form of Rudy.
Ruedi

Rudiger (German) a form of Rogelio.

Rudo (Shona) love.

Rudolf (German) a form of Rudolph.
Rodolf, Rudolfe, Ruedolf

Rudolph (German) famous wolf. See also Dolf.
Rezsó, Rodolph, Rodolphe, Rudek, Rudolphus

Rudolpho (Italian) a form of Rudolph.
Ridolfo, Rudolfo

Rudy (English) a familiar form of Rudolph.
Roody, Ruddey, Ruddi, Ruddie, Ruddy, Rudey, Rudie

Rudyard (English) red enclosure.

Rueben (Hebrew) a form of Reuben.
Rueban, Ruebin

Ruelle, Rule (French) famous wolf.

Rufay (Quechua) warm.

Ruff (French) redhead.
Ruf

Rufin (Polish) redhead.
Ruffin, Ruffyn, Rufyn

Rufino (Spanish) a form of Rufin, Rufus.

Rufio (Latin) a form of Rufus.

Ruford (English) red ford; ford with reeds.
Rufford

Rufus (Latin) redhead.
Rayfus, Ruefus, Rufe, Ruffis, Ruffus, Rufo, Rufous

Rugby (English) rook fortress. History: a famous British school after which the sport of Rugby was named.
Rugbee, Rugbey, Rugbi, Rugbie

Ruggerio (Italian) a form of Roger.
Rogero, Ruggero, Ruggiero

Ruhakana (Rukiga) argumentative.

Ruland (German) a form of Roland.
Rulan, Rulon, Rulondo

Rumford (English) wide river crossing.

Rumi (Quechua) stone, rock.

Rumimaqui, Rumiñaui (Quechua) he who has strong hands.

Rumisonjo, Rumisuncu (Quechua) hard hearted.

Runacatu, Runacoto (Quechua) short man.

Runako (Shona) handsome.

Rune (German, Swedish) secret.

Runihura (Egyptian) destructor.

Runrot (Tai) prosperous.

Runto, Runtu (Quechua) hailstone.

Rupert (German) a form of Robert.
Ruepert, Rueperth, Ruperth, Rupirt, Rupyrt

Ruperto (Italian) a form of Rupert.
Ruberto

Ruprecht (German) a form of Rupert.
Rupprecht

Rush (French) redhead. (English) a short form of Russell.
Rushi

Rushford (English) ford with rushes.
Rushforde

Rusk (Spanish) twisted bread.

Ruskin (French) redhead.
Ruskyn

Russ (French) a short form of Russell.

Russel (French) a form of Russell.
Rusal, Rusel, Russal, Russil, Russyl

Russell (French) redhead; fox colored. See also Lukela.
Roussell, Rusell, Russall, Russelle, Russill, Russyll

Rustin (French) a form of Rusty.
Ruston, Rustyn

Rusty (French) a familiar form of Russell.
Ruste, Rustee, Rusten, Rustey, Rusti, Rustie

Rutger (Scandinavian) a form of Roger.
Ruttger

Rutherford (English) cattle ford.
Rutherfurd, Ruverford

Rutland (Scandinavian) red land.
Rutlan

Rutledge (English) red ledge.

Rutley (English) red meadow.
Rutlea, Rutlee, Rutleigh, Rutli, Rutlie, Rutly

Ruy (Spanish) a short form of Roderick.
Rui

Ruyan (Spanish) a form of Ryan.

Ryan ☆ BG (Irish) little king. See also Rian.
Rhyne, Ryane, Ryian, Ryiann, Ryin, Ryuan, Ryun, Ryyan

Ryann GB (Irish) a form of Ryan.
Ryein, Ryien

Rycroft (English) rye field.
Ricroft, Ryecroft

Ryder (English) a form of Rider.
Rydder

Rye (English) a grain used in cereal and whiskey. A short form of Richard, Ryder. (Gypsy) gentleman.
Rie, Ry

Ryen, Ryon (Irish) forms of Ryan.

Ryerson (English) son of Rider, Ryder.

Ryese (English) a form of Reece.
Reyse, Ryez, Ryse

Ryker (American) a surname used as a first name.
Ryk

Rylan (English) land where rye is grown.
Rilan, Rylean, Rylen, Rylin, Rylon, Rylyn, Rylynn

Ryland (English) a form of Rylan.
Riland, Ryeland, Rylund

Ryle (English) rye hill.
Riel, Riell, Ryal, Ryel, Ryele, Ryell, Ryelle

Rylee GB (Irish) a form of Riley.
Rillie, Ryeleigh, Ryely, Ryleigh, Ryli, Ryly

Ryley BG (Irish) a form of Riley.

Rylie GB (Irish) a form of Riley.

Ryman (English) rye seller.
Riman

Ryne (Irish) a form of Ryan.
Rine, Rynn

Ryo BG (Spanish) a form of Rio.

S

Sa'id (Arabic) happy.
Sa'ad, Sa'eed, Sa'ied, Saaid, Saed, Saeed, Sahid, Saide, Saied, Saiyed, Saiyeed, Sajid, Sajjid, Sayed, Sayeed, Sayid, Sayyid, Seyed

Saa (Egyptian) God's nature.

Saad (Arabic) fortunate, lucky.
Sad, Sadd

Sabas (Hebrew) conversion.

Sabastian (Greek) a form of Sebastian.
Sabastain, Sabastiano, Sabastin, Sabastion, Sabaston, Sabbastiun, Sabestian

Sabastien (French) a form of Sebastian.

Sabatino (Latin) festive day.

Sabelio (Spanish) a form of Sabino.

Saber (French) sword.
Sabar, Sabir, Sabor, Sabre, Sabyr

Sabin (Basque) a form of Sabine (see Girls' Names).
Saban, Saben, Sabian, Sabien, Sabyn

Sabino (Basque) a form of Sabin.

Sabiti (Rutooro) born on Sunday.
Sabit, Sabyti

Sabola (Nguni) pepper.
Sabol, Sabolah

Sabrina GB (Latin) boundary line. (English) royal child. (Hebrew) a familiar form of Sabra (see Girls' Names).

Saburo (Japanese) third-born son.
Saburow

Sacchidananda (Indian) total bliss.

Sacha BG (Russian) a form of Sasha.
Sascha

Sachar (Russian) a form of Zachary.

Sachet, Sachit (Indian) consciousness.

Sachetan (Indian) animated.

Sachin (Indian) another name for the Hindu god Indra.

Sadashiva (Indian) eternally pure.

Saddam (Arabic) powerful ruler.
Sadam

Sadeepan (Indian) lit up.

Sadiki (Swahili) faithful.
Saadiq, Sadeek, Sadek, Sadik, Sadiq, Sadique, Sadyki, Sadyky

Sadler (English) saddle maker.
Saddler

Sadoc (Hebrew) sacred.
Sadock, Sadok

Sadurní (Catalan) a form of Satordi.

Sadurniño (Spanish) pertaining to the god Saturn.

Safari (Swahili) born while traveling.
Safa, Safarian

Safford (English) willow river crossing.
Saford

Sagar (Indian) ocean.

Sage BG (English) wise. Botany: an herb.
Sagen, Sager, Saig, Saje, Sayg, Sayge

Sagun (Indian) possessed of divine qualities.

Sahaj (Indian) natural.

Sahale (Native American) falcon.
Sael, Sahal, Sahel

Sahas (Indian) bravery.

Sahdev (Indian) one of the Pandava princes, descendents of King Pandu in the Indian epic poem *Mahabharata*.

Sahen (Hindi) above.
Sahan, Sahin, Sahon, Sahyn

Sahib (Indian) lord.

Sahil (Native American) a form of Sahale.
Saheel, Sahel, Sahyl

Sahir (Hindi) friend.
Sahyr

Sahúl (Hebrew) requested.

Said (Arabic) a form of Sa'id.

Saîd (Arabic) a form of Said.

Saige GB (English) a form of Sage.

Sainath (Indian) another name for Saibaba, a Hindu guru.

Saipraasad (Indian) blessing.

Saipratap (Indian) blessing of Saibaba.

Sajag (Hindi) watchful.

Sajal (Indian) moist.

Sajan (Indian) beloved.

Saka (Swahili) hunter.
Sakah

Sakeri (Danish) a form of Zachary.
Sakarai, Sakaree, Sakarey, Sakari, Sakaria, Sakarie, Sakary

Saket (Indian) another name for the Hindu god Krishna.

Sakima (Native American) king.
Sakimah, Sakyma, Sakymah

Sakuruta (Pawnee) coming sun.

Sal (Italian) a short form of Salvatore.
Sall

Saladin (Arabic) good; faithful.
Saladine, Saladyn, Saladyne

Salah (Arabic) righteousness. (Hindi) a form of Sala (see Girls' Names).

Salâh (Arabic) a form of Salah.

Salam (Arabic) lamb.
Salaam

Salamon (Spanish) a form of Solomon.
Salaman, Salamen, Salamun, Saloman, Salomón

Salamón (Spanish) a form of Salamon.

Salarjung (Indian) beautiful.

Salaun (French) a form of Solomon.

Saleem (Arabic) a form of Salím.

Saleh (Arabic) a form of Sálih.

Sâleh (Arabic) a form of Saleh.

Salem GB (Arabic) a form of Salím.

Salene (Swahili) good.
Salin, Saline, Salyn, Salyne

Salih (Egyptian) respectable.

Sálih (Arabic) right, good.
Saleeh, Salehe

Salil (Indian) water.

Salim (Swahili) peaceful.

Salím (Arabic) peaceful, safe.
Saliym, Salom, Salym

Salîm (Arabic) a form of Salim.

Salisbury (English) fort at the willow pool.
Salisberi, Salisberie, Salisberri, Salisberrie,
Salisberry, Salisbery, Salisburi, Salisburie,
Salisburri, Salisburrie, Salisburry, Salysberry,
Salysbery, Salysburry, Salysbury

Salmalin (Hindi) taloned.

Salman (Czech) a form of Salím, Solomon.
Salmaan, Salmaine, Salmin, Salmon, Salmun,
Salmyn

Salmân (Czech) a form of Salman.

Salomé (Hebrew) complete; perfect.

Salomon (French) a form of Solomon.
Saloman, Salomo, Salomone

Salton (English) manor town; willow town.
Saltan, Salten, Saltin, Saltyn

Salustiano (German) he who enjoys good health.

Salustio (Latin) he who offers salvation.

Salvador (Spanish) savior.
Salvadore

Salvatore (Italian) savior. See also Xavier.
Salbatore, Sallie, Sally, Salvator, Salvattore,
Salvidor, Sauveur

Salviano (Spanish) a form of Salvo.

Salvino (Spanish) a short form of Salvador.

Salvio, Salvo (Latin) cured, healthy.

Sam (Hebrew) a short form of Samuel.
Samm, Sem, Shmuel

Samantha GB (Aramaic) listener. (Hebrew) told by God.

Samar (Indian) war.

Samarendra, Samarendu, Samarjit
(Indian) other names for the Hindu god Vishnu.

Samarth (Indian) powerful.

Sambo (American) a familiar form of Samuel.
Sambou

Sameer (Arabic) a form of Samír.

Sami BG (Hebrew) a form of Sammie.
Saamy, Samee, Sameeh, Sameh, Samey,
Samie, Samih, Sammi

Sâmî (Arabic) tall.

Samín (Quechua) fortunate, lucky.

Samir (Arabic) a form of Samír.

Samír (Arabic) entertaining companion.
Samyr

Samîr (Arabic) a form of Samír.

Samman (Arabic) grocer.
Saman, Samen, Samin, Sammen, Sammin,
Sammon, Sammun, Sammyn, Samon, Samun,
Samyn

Sammie BG (Hebrew) a familiar form of Samuel.
Sammee, Sammey

Sammy BG (Hebrew) a familiar form of Samuel.

Samo (Czech) a form of Samuel.
Samho, Samko, Samu

Sampson (Hebrew) a form of Samson.
Sampsan, Sampsen, Sampsin, Sampsun,
Sampsyn

Samson (Hebrew) like the sun. Bible: a judge and powerful warrior betrayed by Delilah.
Sansao, Sansim, Sansom, Sansome, Sansum,
Shymson

Samual (Hebrew) a form of Samuel.
Samuael, Samuail

Samuel ☀ BG (Hebrew) heard God; asked of God. Bible: a famous Old Testament prophet and judge. See also Kamuela, Zamiel, Zanvil.
Samael, Samaru, Samauel, Samaul, Samel,

Sameul, Samiel, Sammail, Sammel, Sammuel,
Samouel, Samuelis, Samuell, Samuello,
Samuil, Samuka, Samule, Samvel, Sanko,
Saumel, Simuel, Somhairle, Zamuel

Samuele (Italian) a form of Samuel.
Samulle

Samuru (Japanese) a form of Samuel.

Samy (Hebrew) a form of Sammie.

Sanat (Hindi) ancient.

Sanborn (English) sandy brook.
Sanborne, Sanbourn, Sanbourne, Sanburn,
Sanburne, Sandborn, Sandborne, Sandbourn,
Sandbourne

Sanchez (Latin) a form of Sancho.
Sanchaz, Sancheze

Sancho (Latin) sanctified; sincere. Literature:
Sancho Panza was Don Quixote's squire.
Sauncho

Sandeep BG (Punjabi) enlightened.
Sandip

Sander (English) a short form of Alexander,
Lysander.
Sandir, Sandyr, Saunder

Sanders (English) son of Sander.
Sanderson, Saunders, Saunderson

Sándor (Hungarian) a short form of
Alexander.
Sandar, Sandor, Sandur, Sanyi

Sandro (Greek, Italian) a short form of
Alexander.
Sandero, Sandor, Sandre, Saundro, Shandro

Sandy GB (English) a familiar form of
Alexander, Sanford.
Sande, Sandee, Sandey, Sandi, Sandie

Sanford (English) sandy river crossing.
Sandford, Sanforde

Sani (Hindi) the planet Saturn. (Navajo) old.
Sanee, Saney, Sanie, Sany

Sanjay (American) a combination of
Sanford + Jay.
Sanjai, Sanjaya, Sanjaye, Sanje, Sanjey, Sanjo,
Sanjy, Sanjye

Sanjiv (Hindi) long-lived.
Sanjeev, Sanjyv

Sankar (Hindi) another name for the Hindu
god Shiva.

Sansón (Spanish) a form of Samson.
Sanson, Sansone, Sansun

Santana GB (Spanish) History: Antonio
López de Santa Anna was a Mexican gen-
eral and political leader.
Santanah, Santanio, Santanna, Santanyo

Santiago (Spanish) a form of James.
Santyago

Santino (Spanish) a form of Santonio.
Santion

Santo (Italian, Spanish) holy.

Santon (English) sandy town.
Santan, Santen, Santin, Santun, Santyn

Santonio (Spanish) Geography: a short form
of San Antonio, a city in Texas.
Santon, Santoni, Santonino, Santonyo

Santos (Spanish) saint.

Santosh (Hindi) satisfied.

Sanya (Russian) defender of men.

Sanyu BG (Luganda) happy.

Sapay (Quechua) unique.

Saqr (Arabic) falcon.

Saquan (American) a combination of the
prefix Sa + Quan.
Saquané, Saquin, Saquon, Saqwan, Saqwone

Sarad (Hindi) born in the autumn.
Saradd

Sarah GB (Hebrew) royal child.

Sargent (French) army officer.
Sargant, Sarge, Sarjant, Sergeant, Sergent,
Serjeant

Sargon (Persian) sun prince.
Sargan, Sargen, Sargin, Sargyn

Sarik (Hindi) bird.
Saarik

Sarito (Spanish) a form of Caesar.
Sarit

Saritupac (Quechua) glorious prince.

Sariyah (Arabic) clouds at night.
Sariya

Sarngin (Hindi) archer; protector.
Sarngyn

Sarojin (Hindi) like a lotus.
Sarojun, Sarojyn

Sasha GB (Russian) a short form of Alexander.
Sash, Sausha

Sasson (Hebrew) joyful.
Sason

Satchel (French) small bag.
Satch

Satordi (French) Saturn.
Satordie, Satordy, Satori, Saturno

Saturio (Latin) protector of the sown fields.

Saturnín (Spanish) gift of Saturn.

Sáturno (Italian) mythological god of planting and harvesting.

Saul (Hebrew) asked for, borrowed. Bible: in the Old Testament, a king of Israel and the father of Jonathan; in the New Testament, Saint Paul's original name was Saul.
Saül, Shaul

Saúl (Hebrew) a form of Saul.

Saulo (Greek) he who is tender and delicate.

Saverio (Italian) a form of Xavier.

Saville (French) willow town.
Savelle, Savil, Savile, Savill, Savyl, Savyle, Savyll, Savylle, Seville, Siville

Savion (American, Spanish) a form of Savon.

Savon (American) a form of Savannah (see Girls' Names).
Savan, Savaughn, Saveion, Saveon, Savhon, Saviahn, Savian, Savino, Savo, Savone, Sayvon, Sayvone

Saw (Burmese) early.

Sawyer BG (English) wood worker.
Sawer, Sawier, Sawyere, Soier

Sax (English) a short form of Saxon.
Saxe

Saxby (Scandinavian) Saxon farm.
Saxbee, Saxbey, Saxbi, Saxbie

Saxon (English) swordsman. History: the Roman name for the Teutonic raiders who ravaged the Roman British coasts.
Sax, Saxan, Saxen, Saxin, Saxsin, Saxun, Saxxon, Saxyn

Saxton (English) Saxon town.
Saxtan, Saxten, Saxtin, Saxtyn

Sayani (Quechua) I stay on foot.

Sayarumi (Quechua) strong as stone.

Sayer (Welsh) carpenter.
Say, Saye, Sayers, Sayr, Sayre, Sayres

Sayri (Quechua) prince.

Sayyid (Arabic) master.
Sayed, Sayid, Sayyad, Sayyed

Scanlon (Irish) little trapper.
Scanlan, Scanlen, Scanlin, Scanlyn

Schafer (German) shepherd.
Schaefer, Schaffer, Schiffer, Shaffar, Shäffer

Schmidt (German) blacksmith.
Schmid, Schmit, Schmitt, Schmydt, Schmyt, Schmytt

Schneider (German) tailor.
Schnieder, Snider, Snyder

Schön (German) handsome.
Schoen, Schönn

Schuman (German) shoemaker.
Schumann, Schumen, Schumenn, Shoeman, Shoemann, Shoemen, Shoemenn, Shooman, Shoomann, Shoomen, Shoomenn, Shueman, Shuemann, Shuemen, Shuemenn, Shuman, Shumann, Shumen, Shumenn, Shumyn, Shumynn, Shyman, Shymann

Schuyler (Dutch) sheltering.
Schuylar, Scoy, Scy

Schyler GB (Dutch) a form of Schuyler.
Schylar, Schylor, Schylre, Schylur

Scipion (Latin) staff; stick.
Scipio, Scipione, Scipyo, Scypion, Scypyo

Scoey (French) a short form of Scoville.
Scoee, Scoi, Scoie, Scowi, Scowie, Scowy, Scoy

Scorpio (Latin) dangerous, deadly. Astronomy: a southern constellation near Libra and Sagittarius. Astrology: the eighth sign of the zodiac.
Scorpeo, Scorpyo

Scot (English) a form of Scott.

Scott (English) from Scotland. A familiar form of Prescott.
Scotto, Skot, Skott

Scottie, Scotty (English) familiar forms of Scott.
Scotie, Scottey, Scotti

Scoville (French) Scott's town.
Scovil, Scovile, Scovill, Scovyl, Scovyle, Scovyll, Scovylle

Scribe (Latin) keeper of accounts; writer.
Scribner, Scryb, Scrybe

Scully (Irish) town crier.
Scullea, Scullee, Sculleigh, Sculley, Sculli, Scullie

Seabert (English) shining sea.
Seabirt, Seabright, Seaburt, Seabyrt, Sebert, Seebert, Seebirt, Seeburt, Seebyrt, Seibert, Seibirt, Seiburt, Seibyrt, Seybert, Seybirt, Seyburt, Seybyrt

Seabrook (English) brook near the sea.
Seabrooke, Seebrook, Seebrooke, Seibrook, Seibrooke, Seybrook, Seybrooke

Seamus (Irish) a form of James.
Seamas, Seumas

Sean ✰ BG (Irish) a form of John.
Seaghan, Seain, Seaine, Seán, Séan, Seane, Seann, Seayn, Seayne, Sión

Seanan (Irish) wise.
Seanán, Seanen, Seannan, Seannen, Seannon, Senan, Sinan, Sinon

Searlas (Irish, French) a form of Charles.
Séarlas, Searles, Searlus

Searle (English) armor.
Searl, Serl, Serle

Seasar (Latin) a form of Caesar.
Seasare, Seazar, Sesar, Sesear, Sezar

Seaton (English) town near the sea.
Seatan, Seaten, Seatin, Seatun, Seatyn, Seeton, Setan, Seten, Setin, Seton, Setun, Setyn

Seb (Egyptian) God of earth.

Sebastian ✰ (Greek) venerable. (Latin) revered. See also Bastien.
Sebashtian, Sebastain, Sebastao, Sebastiane, Sebastiao, Sebastin, Sebastine, Sebastyn, Sebbie, Sebo, Sepasetiano

Sebastián (Greek) a form of Sebastian.

Sebastiano (Italian) a form of Sebastian.

Sebastien, Sébastien (French) forms of Sebastian.
Sebaste, Sebasten, Sebastyen, Sebestyén

Sebastion (Greek) a form of Sebastian.

Secundino (Latin) second.

Secundus (Latin) second-born.
Secondas, Secondus, Secondys

Sedgely (English) sword meadow.
Sedgeley, Sedglea, Sedglee, Sedgleigh, Sedgley, Sedgli, Sedglie, Sedgly

Sedgwick (English) sword grass.
Sedgwic, Sedgwik, Sedgwyc, Sedgwyck, Sedgwyk

Sedric, Sedrick (Irish) forms of Cedric.
Seddrick, Sederick, Sedrik, Sedriq

Seeley (English) blessed.
Sealea, Sealee, Sealeigh, Sealey, Seali, Sealie, Sealy, Seelea, Seelee, Seeleigh, Seeli, Seelie, Seely, Seilea, Seilee, Seileigh, Seiley, Seili, Seilie, Seily, Seylea, Seylee, Seyleigh, Seyley, Seyli, Seylie, Seyly

Sef (Egyptian) yesterday. Mythology: one of the two lions that make up the Akeru, guardian of the gates of morning and night.
Seff

Sefonías (Hebrew) God protects.

Sefton (English) village of rushes.
Seftan, Seften, Seftin, Seftun, Seftyn

Sefu (Swahili) sword.

Segada (Gaelic) admirable.

Seger (English) sea spear; sea warrior.
Seagar, Seager, Seegar, Seeger, Segar

Segismundo (Germanic) the victorious protector.

Segun (Yoruba) conqueror.
Segan, Segen, Segin, Segon, Segyn

Segundino (Latin) the family's second son.

Segundo (Spanish) second.

Seibert (English) bright sea.
Sebert

Seif (Arabic) religion's sword.
Seyf

Seifert (German) a form of Siegfried.
Seifried

Sein (Basque) innocent.
Seyn

Sekani (Egyptian) to laugh.

Sekaye (Shona) laughter.
Sekai, Sekay

Sekou (Guinean) learned.

Selby (English) village by the mansion.
Selbee, Selbey, Selbi, Selbie

Seldon (English) willow tree valley.
Seldan, Selden, Seldin, Seldun, Seldyn, Sellden

Selemías (Hebrew) God rewards.

Selesio (Latin) select.

Selig (German) a form of Seeley. See also Zelig.
Seligg, Seligman, Seligmann, Selyg, Selygg

Selwyn (English) friend from the palace. See also Wyn.
Selvin, Selwin, Selwinn, Selwynn, Selwynne

Semaj 🅱🅶 (Turkish) a form of Sema (see Girls' Names).

Semanda (Luganda) cow clan.
Semandah

Semarias (Hebrew) God guarded him.

Semer (Ethiopian) a form of George.
Semere, Semier

Semi (Polynesian) character.
Semee, Semey, Semie, Semy

Semon (Greek) a form of Simon.
Semion

Sempala (Luganda) born in prosperous times.
Sempalah

Sempronio (Latin) name of a Roman family based on male descent.

Sen (Japanese) wood fairy.
Senh

Seneca, Séneca (Latin) an honorable elder.

Sener (Turkish) bringer of joy.

Senior (French) lord.
Senyor

Sennett (French) elderly.
Senet, Senett, Senit, Senitt, Sennet, Sennit, Sennyt, Senyt

Senon (Spanish) living.
Senan, Senen, Senin, Senyn

Senón (Spanish) a form of Senon.

Senwe (African) dry as a grain stalk.

Sepp (German) a form of Joseph.
Sep, Sepee, Sepey, Sepi, Sepie, Seppee, Seppey, Seppi, Seppie, Seppy, Sepy

Septimio, Septimo, Séptimo (Latin) the seventh child.

Septimus (Latin) seventh.
Septimous

Serafin (Hebrew) a form of Seraphim.
Seraphin

Serafín (Hebrew) a form of Serafin.

Serafino (Portuguese) a form of Seraphim.
Seraphino

Seraphim (Hebrew) fiery, burning. Bible: the highest order of angels, known for their zeal and love.
Saraf, Saraph, Serafim, Seraphimus

Serapión (Greek) a form of Serapio.

Sereno (Latin) calm, tranquil.
Sereen, Serene, Serino, Seryno

Serge (Latin) attendant.
Seargeoh, Serg, Sergios, Sergius, Sergiusz, Serguel, Sirgio, Sirgios

Sergei, Sergey (Russian) forms of Serge.
Serghey, Sergi, Sergie, Sergo, Seryozha, Serzh

Sergio, Serjio (Italian) forms of Serge.
Serginio, Serigo

Serni (Catalan) a form of Saturno.

Serug (Hebrew) interwoven.

Servacio (Latin) he who observes and guards the law.

Servando (Spanish) to serve.
Servan, Servio

Seth ☆ (Hebrew) appointed. Bible: the third son of Adam.
Set, Sethan, Sethe, Shet

Sethos (Egyptian) prince.

Setimba (Luganda) river dweller. Geography: a river in Uganda.
Setimbah

Seumas (Scottish) a form of James.
Seaumus

Severiano (Italian) a form of Séverin.

Séverin (French) severe.
Seve, Sevé, Severan, Severen, Severian, Severo, Severyn, Sevien, Sevrin

Severino (Spanish) a form of Séverin.

Severn (English) boundary.
Sevearn, Sevirn, Sevren, Sevrnn, Sevyrn

Sevilen (Turkish) beloved.
Sevilan, Sevilin, Sevilon, Sevilyn

Seward (English) sea guardian.
Seaward, Seawrd, Seeward, Seiward, Sewerd, Seyward, Siward

Sewati (Moquelumnan) curved bear claws.
Sewatee, Sewatey

Sewell (English) sea wall.
Seawal, Seawall, Seawel, Seawell, Seewal, Seewall, Seewel, Seewell, Seiwal, Seiwall, Seiwel, Seiwell, Sewal, Sewall, Sewel, Seywal, Seywall, Seywel, Seywell

Sexton (English) church offical; sexton.
Sextan, Sexten, Sextin, Sextyn

Sextus (Latin) sixth.
Sextis, Sextys, Sixtus

Seymour (French) prayer. Religion: name honoring Saint Maur. See also Maurice.
Seamoor, Seamoore, Seamor, Seamore, Seamour, Seamoure, See, Seemoor, Seemoore, Seemor, Seemore, Seemour, Seemoure, Seimoor, Seimoore, Seimor, Seimore, Seimour, Seymoor, Seymore, Seymoure

Shaan (Hebrew, Irish) a form of Sean.

Shabaka (Egyptian) king.

Shabouh (Armenian) king, noble. History: a fourth-century Persian king.

Shad (Punjabi) happy-go-lucky.
Shadd

Shade BG (English) shade.
Shaed, Shaede, Shaid, Shaide, Shayd, Shayde

Shadi (Arabic) singer.
Shadde, Shaddi, Shaddy, Shadee, Shadeed, Shadey, Shadie, Shydee, Shydi

Shadow BG (English) shadow.

Shadrach (Babylonian) god; godlike. Bible: one of three companions who emerged unharmed from the fiery furnace of Babylon.
Shadrac, Shadrack, Shadrak

Shadrick (Babylonian) a form of Shadrach.
Shadriq

Shadwell (English) shed by a well.
Shadwal, Shadwall, Shadwel, Shedwal, Shedwall, Shedwel, Shedwell

Shady (Arabic) a form of Shadi.

Shae GB (Hebrew) a form of Shai. (Irish) a form of Shea.

Shafiq (Arabic) compassionate.

Shah (Persian) king. History: a title for rulers of Iran.

Shaheed (Arabic) a form of Sa'id.
Shahed, Shahyd

Shaheem (American) a combination of Shah + Raheem.
Shaheim, Shahiem, Shahm

Shahid (Arabic) a form of Sa'id.

Shai BG (Irish) a form of Shea. (Hebrew) a short form of Yeshaya.
Shaie

Shaiming (Chinese) life; sunshine.
Shaimin, Shayming

Shain, Shaine (Irish) forms of Sean.

Shaka BG (Zulu) founder, first. History: Shaka Zulu was the founder of the Zulu empire.
Shakah

Shakeel (Arabic) a form of Shaquille.
Shakeil, Shakel, Shakell, Shakiel, Shakil, Shakille, Shakyle

Shakir (Arabic) thankful.
Shaakir, Shakeer, Shakeir, Shakyr

Shakîr (Arabic) a form of Shakir.

Shakur (Arabic) a form of Shakir.
Shakuur

Shalom (Hebrew) peace.
Shalum, Shlomo, Sholem, Sholom

Shalya (Hindi) throne.

Shaman (Sanskrit) holy man, mystic, medicine man.
Shaiman, Shaimen, Shamaine, Shamaun, Shamen, Shamin, Shamine, Shammon, Shamon, Shamone, Shayman, Shaymen

Shamar (Hebrew) a form of Shamir.
Shamaar, Shamare

Shamari BG (Hebrew) a form of Shamir.

Shamir (Hebrew) precious stone.
Shahmeer, Shahmir, Shameer, Shamyr

Shamus (American) slang for detective. (Irish) a form of Seamus.
Shaimis, Shaimus, Shamas, Shames, Shamis, Shamos, Shaymis, Shaymus, Shemus

Shan (Irish) a form of Shane.
Shann, Shanne

Shanahan (Irish) wise, clever.
Seanahan, Shaunahan, Shawnahan

Shandy (English) rambunctious.
Shande, Shandea, Shandey, Shandi, Shandie

Shane BG (Irish) a form of Sean.
Shaen, Shaene

Shangobunni (Yoruba) gift from Shango.

Shani GB (Hebrew) red. (Swahili) marvelous.
Shanee, Shaney, Shanie, Shany

Shanley GB (Irish) small; ancient.
Shaneley, Shanlea, Shanlee, Shanleigh, Shanli, Shanlie, Shanly, Shannley

Shannon GB (Irish) small and wise.
Shanan, Shanen, Shanin, Shannan, Shannen, Shannin, Shannone, Shannyn, Shanon, Shanyn

Shant (French) a short form of Shantae.

Shantae GB (French) a form of Chante.
Shanta, Shantai, Shantay, Shante, Shantell, Shantelle, Shanti, Shantia, Shantie, Shanton, Shanty

Shap (English) a form of Shep.

Shaq (American) a short form of Shaquan, Shaquille.

Shaquan BG (American) a combination of the prefix Sha + Quan.
Shaqaun, Shaquand, Shaquane, Shaquann, Shaquaunn, Shaquawn, Shaquen, Shaquian, Shaquin, Shaqwan

Shaquell (American) a form of Shaquille.
Shaqueal, Shaqueil, Shaquel, Shaquelle, Shaquiel, Shaquiell, Shaquielle

Shaquile (Arabic) a form of Shaquille.

Shaquill (Arabic) a form of Shaquille.

Shaquille BG (Arabic) handsome.
Shaquell, Shaquil, Shaqul, Shaquyl, Shaquyle, Shaquyll, Shaquylle

Shaquon (American) a combination of the prefix Sha + Quon.
Shaikwon, Shaqon, Shaquoin, Shaquoné

Sharad (Pakistani) autumn.
Sharid, Sharyd

Shareef (Arabic) a form of Sharíf.

Sharif (Arabic) a form of Sharíf.

Sharíf (Arabic) honest; noble.
Sharef, Shareff, Shareif, Sharief, Sharife, Shariff, Shariyf, Sharrif, Sharyf, Sharyff, Sharyif

Sharîf (Arabic) a form of Sharíf.

Sharod (Pakistani) a form of Sharad.
Sharrod

Sharón (Hebrew) a form of Sharron.

Sharron GB (Hebrew) flat area, plain.
Sharan, Sharen, Sharin, Sharon, Sharone, Sharonn, Sharonne, Sharran, Sharren, Sharrin, Sharryn, Sharyn

Shashenka (Russian) defender of humanity.

Shattuck (English) little shad fish.
Shatuck

Shaun BG (Irish) a form of Sean.
Schaun, Schaune, Shaughan, Shaughn,
Shaugn, Shauna, Shaunahan, Shaune,
Shaunn, Shaunne

Shavar (Hebrew) comet.
Shaver, Shavir, Shavyr

Shavon GB (American) a combination of
the prefix Sha + Yvon.
Shauvan, Shauvon, Shavan, Shavaughn,
Shaven, Shavin, Shavone, Shawan, Shawon,
Shawun

Shaw (English) grove.
Shawe

Shawn BG (Irish) a form of Sean.
Schawn, Schawne, Shawen, Shawne, Shawnee,
Shawnn, Shawon

Shawnta GB (American) a combination of
Shawn + the suffix Ta.
Seanta, Seantah, Shaunta, Shawntae,
Shawntah, Shawntel, Shawnti

Shay BG (Irish) a form of Shea.
Shaya, Shey

Shayan (Cheyenne) a form of Cheyenne.
Shayaan, Shayann, Shayon

Shaye GB (Irish) a form of Shea.

Shayn (Hebrew) a form of Sean.
Shaynne, Shean

Shayne BG (Hebrew) a form of Sean.

Shea GB (Irish) courteous.
Sheah

Sheary (Irish) peaceful.
Shearee, Shearey, Sheari, Shearie

Sheba (Hebrew) promise.

Shedrick (Babylonian) a form of Shadrach.
Sheddrach, Shederick, Shedrach, Shedric,
Shedrik, Shedrique, Shedryc, Shedryck,
Shedryk

Sheehan (Irish) little; peaceful.
Shean, Sheehen

Sheffield (English) crooked field.
Field, Shef, Sheff, Sheffie, Sheffy, Sheffyeld,
Shefield, Shefyeld

Shel (English) a short form of Shelby,
Sheldon, Shelton.
Shell

Shelby GB (English) ledge estate. A form of
Selby.
Shelbe, Shelbea, Shelbee, Shelbey, Shelbi,
Shelbie, Shellby

Sheldon BG (English) farm on the ledge.
Sheldan, Shelden, Sheldin, Sheldun, Sheldyn

Shelley GB (English) a familiar form of
Shelby, Sheldon, Shelton. Literature: Percy
Bysshe Shelley was a nineteenth-century
British poet.
Shell, Shellea, Shellee, Shelleigh, Shelli,
Shellie, Shelly

Shelomó (Hebrew) of peace.

Shelton (English) town on a ledge.
Sheltan, Shelten, Sheltin, Sheltyn

Shem (Hebrew) name; reputation. A form of
Samson. (English) a short form of Samuel.
Bible: Noah's oldest son.

Shen (Egyptian) sacred amulet. (Chinese)
meditation.

Shep (English) a short form of Shepherd.
Shepp, Ship, Shipp

Shepherd (English) shepherd.
Shepard, Shephard, Sheppard, Shepperd

Shepley (English) sheep meadow.
Sheplea, Sheplee, Shepleigh, Shepli, Sheplie,
Sheply, Shepply, Shipley

Sherborn (English) clear brook.
Sherborne, Sherbourn, Sherburn, Sherburne

Sheridan GB (Irish) wild.
Sheredan, Sheriden, Sheridon, Sheridyn,
Sherridan, Sherydan, Sheryden, Sherydin,
Sherydon, Sherydyn

Sherill (English) shire on a hill.
Sheril, Sherril, Sherrill, Sheryl, Sheryll

Sherlock (English) light haired. Literature:
Sherlock Holmes is a famous British detec-
tive character, created by Sir Arthur Conan
Doyle.
Sherloc, Sherloch, Sherloche, Sherlocke,
Sherlok, Shurlock, Shurlocke

Sherma (English) one who shears sheep.

Sherman (English) sheep shearer; resident of a shire.
Scherman, Schermann, Sherm, Shermain, Shermaine, Shermann, Shermen, Shermie, Shermon, Shermy, Shirman, Shirmann, Shyrman, Shyrmann

Sherrod (English) clearer of the land.
Sherod, Sherrad, Sherrard, Sherrodd

Sherwin (English) swift runner, one who cuts the wind.
Sherveen, Shervin, Sherwan, Sherwind, Sherwinn, Sherwyn, Sherwynd, Sherwynn, Sherwynne, Win

Sherwood (English) bright forest.
Sharwood, Sherwoode, Shurwood, Woody

Shihab (Arabic) blaze.
Shyhab

Shihâb (Arabic) a form of Shihab.

Shìlín (Chinese) intellectual.
Shilan, Shilyn, Shylin, Shylyn

Shilo BG (Hebrew) a form of Shiloh.

Shiloh GB (Hebrew) God's gift.
Shi, Shile, Shiley, Shiloe, Shy, Shyle, Shylo, Shyloh

Shimeón (Hebrew) he heard.

Shimon (Hebrew) a form of Simon.
Shymon

Shimshon (Hebrew) a form of Samson.
Shimson

Shing (Chinese) victory.
Shingae, Shingo, Shyng

Shipley (English) sheep meadow.
Shiplea, Shiplee, Shipleigh, Shipli, Shiplie, Shiply, Shyplea, Shyplee, Shypleigh, Shypley, Shypli, Shyplie, Shyply

Shipton (English) sheep village; ship village.
Shiptan, Shipten, Shiptin, Shiptun, Shiptyn, Shyptan, Shypten, Shyptin, Shypton, Shyptun, Shyptyn

Shiquan (American) a combination of the prefix Shi + Quan.
Shiquane, Shiquann, Shiquawn, Shiquoin, Shiqwan

Shiro (Japanese) fourth-born son.
Shirow, Shyro, Shyrow

Shiva (Hindi) life and death. Religion: the most common name for the Hindu god of destruction and reproduction.
Shiv, Shivah, Shivan, Shyva, Shyvah, Siva

Shlomo (Hebrew) a form of Solomon.
Shelmu, Shelomo, Shelomoh, Shlomi, Shlomot

Shmuel (Hebrew) a form of Samuel.
Schmuel, Shemuel, Shmiel

Shneur (Yiddish) senior.
Shneiur

Shomer (Hebrew) protector.
Shomar, Shomir, Shomor, Shomyr

Shon (German) a form of Schön. (American) a form of Sean.
Shoan, Shoen, Shondae, Shondale, Shondel, Shone, Shonn, Shonntay, Shontae, Shontarious, Shouan, Shoun

Shoni (Hebrew) changing.
Shonee, Shoney, Shonie, Shony

Shu (Egyptian) air.

Shunnar (Arabic) pheasant.
Shunar

Si (Hebrew) a short form of Silas, Simon.

Siañu (Quechua) brown like the color of coffee.

Sid (French) a short form of Sidney.
Sidd, Siddie, Siddy, Sidey, Syd, Sydd

Siddel (English) wide valley.
Siddell, Sidel, Sidell, Sydel, Sydell

Siddhartha (Hindi) History: Siddhartha Gautama was the original name of Buddha, the founder of Buddhism.
Sida, Siddartha, Siddhaarth, Siddhart, Siddharth, Sidh, Sidharth, Sidhartha, Sidhdharth, Sydartha, Syddhartha

Sidney GB (French) from Saint-Denis, France.
Cydney, Sidnee, Sidni, Sidnie, Sidny

Sidonio (Spanish) a form of Sidney.
Sidon

Sidwell (English) wide stream.
Siddwal, Siddwall, Siddwel, Siddwell, Sidwal,

Sidwall, Sidwel, Syddwal, Syddwall, Syddwel,
Syddwell, Sydwal, Sydwall, Sydwel, Sydwell

Siegfried (German) victorious peace. See
also Zigfrid, Ziggy.
Siegfred, Sigfrid, Sigfried, Sigfroi, Sigfryd,
Sigvard, Singefrid, Sygfred, Sygfreid, Sygfreyd,
Sygfrid, Sygfried, Sygfryd

Sierra GB (Irish) black. (Spanish) saw-
toothed.
Siera, Sierah, Sierrah, Syera, Syerah, Syerra,
Syerrah

Siervo (Spanish) a man who serves God.

Siffre (French) a form of Siegfried.

Siffredo (Italian) a form of Siegfried.
Sifredo, Syffredo

Sig (German) a short form of Siegfried,
Sigmund.

Siggy (German) a familiar form of Siegfried,
Sigmund.

Sigifredo (German) a form of Siegfried.
Sigefredo, Sigefriedo, Sigfrido, Siguefredo

Sigismond (French) a form of Sigmund.
Sygismond, Sygismund, Sygysmon,
Sygysmond, Sygysmun, Sygysmund

Sigismundo (Italian, Spanish) a form of
Sigmund.
Sigismondo, Sygismondo, Sygismundo,
Sygysmondo, Sygysmundo

Sigmund (German) victorious protector.
See also Ziggy, Zsigmond, Zygmunt.
Saegmond, Saegmund, Siegmund, Sigismund,
Sigismundus, Sigmond, Sigmundo, Sigsmond,
Sygmond, Sygmondo, Sygmund, Sygmundo,
Szygmond

Sigurd (German, Scandinavian) victorious
guardian.
Sigord, Sjure, Sygurd, Syver

Sigwald (German) victorious leader.
Sigwaldo, Sygwald, Sygwaldo

Silas (Latin) a short form of Silvan.
Sias

Silburn (English) blessed.
Silborn, Silborne, Silbourn, Silbourne, Silburn,
Silburne, Sylborn, Sylborne, Sylbourn,
Sylbourne, Sylburn, Sylburne

Silvan (Latin) forest dweller.
Silvaon, Silvie, Sylvanus

Silvano (Italian) a form of Silvan.
Silvanos

Silverio (Spanish) Greek god of trees.

Silvester (Latin) a form of Sylvester.
Silvestr, Silvy

Silvestre (Spanish) a form of Sylvester.

Silvestro (Italian) a form of Sylvester.

Silvino (Italian) a form of Silvan.

Silvio (Italian) a form of Silvan.
Sylvio

Simão (Portuguese) a form of Samuel.
Simao

Simba (Swahili) lion. (Yao) a short form of
Lisimba.
Sim, Simbah, Symba, Symbah

Simcha BG (Hebrew) joyful.
Simmy

Simeon (French) a form of Simon.
Seameon, Seemeon, Simion, Simione, Simone,
Symeon, Symyan

Simeón (Spanish) a form of Simón.

Simms (Hebrew) son of Simon.
Simm, Sims, Symms, Syms

Simmy (Hebrew) a familiar form of Simcha,
Simon.
Simmey, Simmi, Simmie, Symmy

Simon (Hebrew) he heard. Bible: one of the
Twelve Disciples. See also Symington,
Ximenes, Zimon.
Saimon, Samien, Seimein, Semein, Seymeon,
Seymon, Sim, Simen, Simmon, Simmonds,
Simmons, Simonas, Simone, Simons, Simyon,
Siomon, Síomón, Siomonn, Symonn, Symonns

Simón (Hebrew) he who has listened to me.

Simon Pierre (French) a combination of
Simon + Pierre.

Simplicio (Latin) simple.

Simpson (Hebrew) son of Simon.
Simonson, Simpsan, Simpsen, Simpsin,
Simpsyn, Simson, Sympsan, Sympsen,
Sympsin, Sympson, Sympsyn

Simran GB (Sikh) absorbed in God.

Sina BG (Irish) a form of Seana (see Girls' Names).

Sinbad (German) prince; sparkling.
Sinbald, Synbad, Synbald

Sinche, Sinchi (Quechua) boss, leader; strong; valorous; hard working.

Sinchipuma (Quechua) strong leader and as valuable as a puma.

Sinchiroca (Quechua) strongest prince among the strong ones.

Sinclair GB (French) prayer. Religion: name honoring Saint Clair.
Sinclaire, Sinclar, Sinclare, Synclair, Synclaire, Synclar, Synclare, Synclayr

Sinesio (Greek) the intelligent one.

Sinforiano (Spanish) a form of Sinforoso.

Sinforoso (Greek) he who is full of misfortune.

Singh (Hindi) lion.
Sing

Sinjin (English) a form of Sinjon.

Sinjon (English) saint, holy man. Religion: name honoring Saint John.
Sinjun, Sjohn, Syngen, Synjen, Synjon

Sione (Tongan) God is gracious.
Sionee, Sioney, Sioni, Sionie, Soane, Sone

Sipatu (Moquelumnan) pulled out.
Sypatu

Sipho (Zulu) present.
Sypho

Sir (English) sir, sire.

Siraj (Arabic) lamp, light.
Syraj

Sirâj (Arabic) a form of Siraj.

Sirio, Siro (Latin) native of Syria.

Sirviente (Latin) God's servant.

Siseal (Irish) a form of Cecil.

Sisebuto (Teutonic) he who fulfills his leadership role whole-heartedly.

Sisi (Fante) born on Sunday.
Sysi, Sysy

Sitric (Scandinavian) conqueror.
Sitrick, Sitrik, Sytric, Sytrick, Sytrik, Sytryc, Sytryck, Sytryk

Siuca (Quechua) youngest son.

Siva (Hindi) a form of Shiva.
Siv

Sivan (Hebrew) ninth month of the Jewish year.
Syvan

Siwatu (Swahili) born during a time of conflict.
Siwazuri

Siwili (Native American) long fox's tail.
Siwilie, Siwily, Siwyli, Siwylie, Siwyly, Sywili, Sywilie, Sywily, Sywyly

Sixto (Greek) the courteous one.

Skah (Lakota) white.
Skai

Skee (Scandinavian) projectile.
Ski, Skie

Skeeter (English) swift.
Skeat, Skeet, Skeets

Skelly (Irish) storyteller.
Shell, Skelea, Skelee, Skeleigh, Skeley, Skeli, Skelie, Skellea, Skellee, Skelleigh, Skelley, Skelli, Skellie, Skely

Skelton (Dutch) shell town.

Skerry (Scandinavian) stony island.
Skery

Skip (Scandinavian) a short form of Skipper.
Skipp, Skyp, Skypp

Skipper (Scandinavian) shipmaster.

Skippie (Scandinavian) a familiar form of Skipper.
Skipi, Skipie, Skippi, Skippy, Skipy, Skypi, Skypie, Skyppi, Skyppie, Skyppy, Skypy

Skipton (English) ship town.
Skippton, Skyppton, Skypton

Skiriki (Pawnee) coyote.

Skule (Norwegian) hidden.
Skul, Skull

Sky BG (Dutch) a short form of Skylar.

Skye GB (Dutch) a short form of Skylar.

Skylar BG (Dutch) a form of Schuyler.
Skieler, Skilar, Skiler, Skkylar, Skuylar,
Skuyler, Skyelar, Skyeler, Skyelor, Skylaar,
Skylare, Skylarr, Skylayr, Skylee, Skyller,
Skyloer, Skylore, Skylour, Skylur, Skylyr

Skyler BG (Dutch) a form of Schuyler.

Skylor (Dutch) a form of Schuyler.

Slade (English) a short form of Sladen.
Slaid, Slaide, Slayd, Slayde

Sladen (English) child of the valley.
Sladan, Sladein, Sladon, Sladyn, Slaidan,
Slaiden, Slaidin, Slaidon, Slaidyn, Slaydan,
Slayden, Slaydin, Slaydon, Slaydyn

Slane (Czech) salty.
Slain, Slaine, Slan, Slayn, Slayne

Slater (English) roof slater.
Slader, Slaiter, Slate, Slayter

Slava (Russian) a short form of Stanislav,
Vladislav, Vyacheslav.
Slavah, Slavik

Slawek (Polish) a short form of Radoslaw.

Slevin (Irish) mountaineer.
Slavan, Slaven, Slavin, Slavon, Slavyn,
Slawin, Slevan, Sleven, Slevon, Slevyn

Sloan BG (Irish) warrior.
Sloane, Slone

Smedley (English) flat meadow.
Smedlea, Smedlee, Smedleigh, Smedli,
Smedlie, Smedly

Smith (English) blacksmith.
Schmidt, Smid, Smidt, Smithe, Smithey,
Smithi, Smithie, Smithy, Smitt, Smitth,
Smitty, Smyth, Smythe

Snowden (English) snowy hill.
Snowdan, Snowdin, Snowdon, Snowdyn

Sobhî (Arabic) sunrise.

Socorro (Spanish) helper.

Socrates (Greek) wise, learned. History: a
famous ancient Greek philosopher.
Socratis, Sokrates, Sokratis

Sócrates (Greek) a form of Socrates.

Socso, Sucsu (Quechua) blackbird.

Sofanor (Greek) the wise man.

Sofian (Arabic) devoted.
Sofyan

Sofiân (Arabic) a form of Sofian.

Sofoclés, Sófocles (Greek) famous for his
wisdom.

Sofronio (Greek) prudent; healthy in spirit.

Sohail (Arabic) a form of Suhail.
Sohayl, Souhail

Sohar (Russian) farmer.

Sohrab (Persian) ancient hero.

Soja (Yoruba) soldier.
Sojah

Sol (Hebrew) a short form of Saul, Solomon.
Soll

Solano (Latin) like the eastern wind.

Solly (Hebrew) a familiar form of Saul,
Solomon. See also Zollie.
Sollie

Solomon BG (Hebrew) peaceful. Bible: a
king of Israel famous for his wisdom. See
also Zalman.
Salaun, Selim, Shelomah, Solaman, Solamh,
Solmon, Soloman, Solomo, Solomonas, Solomyn

Solon (Greek) wise. History: a noted ancient
Athenian lawmaker.
Solan, Solen, Solin, Solyn

Solón (Greek) a form of Solon.

Somac (Quechua) beautiful.

Somer (French) born in summer.

Somerset (English) place of the summer set-
tlers. Literature: William Somerset Maugham
was a well-known British writer.
Sommerset, Sumerset, Summerset

Somerton (English) summer town.
Summerton

Somerville (English) summer village.
Somervil, Somervill, Somervyl, Somervyll,
Somervylle, Sumervil, Sumervill, Sumerville,
Sumervyl, Sumervyll, Sumervylle, Summervil,
Summervill, Summerville, Summervyl,
Summervyll, Summervylle

Son (Vietnamese) mountain. (Native
American) star. (English) son, boy. A short
form of Madison, Orson.

Sonco, Soncoyoc, Sonjoc, Sonjoyoc
(Quechua) he who has a good and noble
heart.

Songan (Native American) strong.
Song

Sonny (English) a familiar form of Grayson,
Madison, Orson, Son.
Sonee, Soney, Soni, Sonie, Sonnee, Sonney,
Sonni, Sonnie, Sony

Sono (Akan) elephant.

Sonu (Hindi) handsome.

Soren (Danish) a form of Sören.

Sören (Danish) thunder; war.
Sorren

Sorley (Scandinavian) summer traveler;
Viking.
Sorlea, Sorlee, Sorleigh, Sorli, Sorlie, Sorly

Soroush (Persian) happy.

Sorrel GB (French) reddish brown.
Sorel, Sorell, Soril, Sorill, Sorrell, Sorril,
Sorrill, Soryl, Soryll

Soterios (Greek) savior.
Soteris, Sotero

Southwell (English) south well.
Southwal, Southwall, Southwel

Sovann (Cambodian) gold.
Sovan

Sowande (Yoruba) wise healer sought me
out.
Sowand

Spalding (English) divided field.
Spaulding

Spangler (German) tinsmith.
Spengler

Spark (English) happy.
Sparke, Sparkee, Sparkey, Sparki, Sparkie,
Sparky

Spear (English) spear carrier.
Speare, Spears, Speer, Speers, Speir, Speyr,
Spiers

Speedy (English) quick; successful.
Speed, Speedee, Speedey, Speedi, Speedie

Spence (English) a short form of Spencer.
Spense

Spencer BG (English) dispenser of provisions.
Spencre

Spenser BG (English) a form of Spencer.
Literature: Edmund Spenser was the British
poet who wrote *The Faerie Queene.*
Spanser

Spike (English) ear of grain; long nail.
Spyke

Spiridone (Italian) a form of Spiro.
Spiridion, Spiridon, Spyridion, Spyridon,
Spyridone

Spiro (Greek) round basket; breath.
Spyro, Spyros

Spoor (English) spur maker.
Spoors

Spreckley (English) twigs.
Sprecklea, Sprecklee, Spreckleigh, Spreckli,
Sprecklie, Spreckly

Springsteen (English) stream by the rocks.
Springstein, Springsteyn, Spryngsteen,
Spryngstein, Spryngsteyn

Sproule (English) energetic.
Sprowle

Spurgeon (English) shrub.

Spyros (Greek) a form of Spiro.
Spiros

Squire (English) knight's assistant; large
landholder.
Squyre

Stacey GB (English) a familiar form of
Eustace.
Stace, Stacee, Staci, Stacie

Stacy GB (English) a familiar form of
Eustace.

Stafford (English) riverbank landing.
Staffard, Stafforde, Staford

Stamford (English) a form of Stanford.
Stemford

Stamos (Greek) a form of Stephen.
Stamatis, Stamatos

Stan (Latin, English) a short form of Stanley.
Stann

Stanbury (English) stone fortification.
Stanberi, Stanberie, Stanberri, Stanberrie,
Stanberry, Stanbery, Stanburghe, Stanburi,
Stanburie, Stanburri, Stanburrie, Stanburry,
Stanbury, Stansbury

Stancil (English) beam.
Stancile, Stancyl, Stancyle

Stancio (Spanish) a form of Constantine.
Stancy

Stancliff (English) stony cliff.
Stanclif, Stanclife, Stancliffe, Stanclyf, Stanclyff

Standish (English) stony parkland. History:
Miles Standish was a leader in colonial
America.
Standysh

Stane (Slavic) a short form of Stanislaus.

Stanfield (English) stony field.
Stanfyld, Stansfield

Stanford (English) rocky ford.
Stamford, Standforde

Stanislaus (Latin) stand of glory. See also
Lao, Tano.
Slavik, Stana, Standa, Stane, Stanislao,
Stanislas, Stanislau, Stanislus, Stannes, Stano,
Stanyslaus

Stanislav (Slavic) a form of Stanislaus. See
also Slava.
Stanislaw

Stanislov (Russian) a form of Stanislaus.

Stanley (English) stony meadow.
Stanely, Stanlea, Stanlee, Stanleigh, Stanli,
Stanlie, Stanly

Stanmore (English) stony lake.
Stanmoar, Stanmoare, Stanmoor, Stanmoore,
Stanmor

Stannard (English) hard as stone.
Stanard

Stanton (English) stony farm.
Stanten, Staunton

Stanway (English) stony road.
Stanwai, Stenwai, Stenway

Stanwick (English) stony village.
Stanwic, Stanwicke, Stanwik, Stanwyc,
Stanwyck, Stanwyk

Stanwood (English) stony woods.
Stenwood

Starbuck (English) challenger of fate.
Literature: a character in Herman Melville's
novel *Moby-Dick*.
Starrbuck

Stark (German) strong, vigorous.
Starke, Stärke, Starkie

Starling BG (English) bird.
Starlin, Starlyn, Starlyng

Starr GB (English) star.
Star, Staret, Starlight, Starlon, Starwin

Stasik (Russian) a familiar form of
Stanislaus.
Stas, Stash, Stashka, Stashko, Stasiek

Stasio (Polish) a form of Stanislaus.
Stas, Stasiek, Stasiu, Staska, Stasko

Stavros (Greek) a form of Stephen.
Stavro

Steadman (English) owner of a farmstead.
Steadmann, Steed

Stedman (English) a form of Steadman.
Stedmen

Steel (English) like steel.

Steele (English) a form of Steel.
Steale

Steen (German, Danish) stone.
Stean, Steane, Steene, Steenn

Steenie (Scottish) a form of Stephen.
Steeni, Steeny, Steinee, Steiney, Steini, Steinie,
Steiny, Steynee, Steyney, Steyni, Steynie,
Steyny

Steeve (Greek) a short form of Steeven.

Steeven (Greek) a form of Steven.
Steaven, Steavin, Steavon, Steevan, Steevn

Stefan (German, Polish, Swedish) a form of Stephen.
Steafan, Steafeán, Stefaan, Stefanson, Stefaun, Stefawn

Stefano (Italian) a form of Stephen.
Steffano

Stefanos (Greek) a form of Stephen.
Stefans, Stefos, Stephano, Stephanos

Stefen, Steffen (Norwegian) forms of Stephen.
Steffin, Stefin

Steffan (Swedish) a form of Stefan.
Staffan

Steffon, Stefon (Polish) forms of Stephon.
Staffon, Steffone, Stefone, Stefonne

Stein (German) a form of Steen.
Steine, Steyn, Steyne

Steinar (Norwegian) rock warrior.
Steanar, Steaner, Steenar, Steener, Steiner, Steynar, Steyner

Stepan (Russian) a form of Stephen.
Stepa, Stepane, Stepanya, Stepka, Stipan

Steph (English) a short form of Stephen.

Stephan (Greek) a form of Stephen.
Stepfan, Stephanas, Stephano, Stephanos, Stephanus

Stephane, Stéphane (French) forms of Stephen.
Stefane, Stepháne, Stephanne

Stephanie GB (Greek) a form of Stephen.

Stephaun (Greek) a form of Stephen.

Stephen (Greek) crowned. See also Esteban, Estebe, Estevan, Estevao, Etienne, István, Szczepan, Tapani, Teb, Teppo, Tiennot.
Stenya, Stepanos, Stephanas, Stephens, Stephfan, Stephin, Stepven

Stephenson (English) son of Stephen.

Stephon (Greek) a form of Stephen.
Stepfon, Stepfone, Stephfon, Stephion, Stephonn, Stephonne

Stephone (Greek) a form of Stephon.

Sterlin (English) a form of Sterling.
Sterlen, Styrlin, Styrlyn

Sterling BG (English) valuable; silver penny. A form of Starling.
Styrling, Styrlyng

Stern (German) star.
Sturn

Sterne (English) austere.
Stearn, Stearne, Stearns, Sturne

Stetson (Danish) stepson.
Steston, Steton, Stetsen, Stetzon

Stevan (Greek) a form of Steven.
Stevano, Stevanoe, Stevaughn, Stevean

Steve (Greek) a short form of Stephen, Steven.
Steave, Stevy

Steven ⚝ (Greek) a form of Stephen.
Steiven, Stiven

Stevens (English) son of Steven.
Stevenson, Stevinson

Stevie GB (English) a familiar form of Stephen, Steven.
Stevey, Stevy

Stevin, Stevon (Greek) forms of Steven.
Stevieon, Stevion, Stevyn

Stewart (English) a form of Stuart.
Steward, Stu

Stian (Norwegian) quick on his feet.

Stig (Swedish) mount.

Stiggur (Gypsy) gate.

Stillman (English) quiet.
Stillmann, Stillmon, Stilman, Styllman, Stylman

Sting (English) spike of grain.
Styng

Stirling (English) a form of Sterling.
Stirlin

Stockley (English) tree-stump meadow.
Stocklea, Stocklee, Stockleigh, Stockli, Stocklie, Stockly

Stockman (English) tree-stump remover.
Stockmen

Stockton (English) tree-stump town.

Stockwell (English) tree-stump well.
Stockwal, Stockwall, Stockwel

Stoddard (English) horse keeper.
Stodard

Stoffel (German) a short form of Christopher.

Stoker (English) furnace tender.
Stoke, Stokes, Stroker

Stone (English) stone.
Stoen, Stonee, Stoner

Stoney (English) a form of Stone.
Stoni, Stonie, Stoniy, Stony

Storm BG (English) tempest, storm.
Storme

Stormy GB (English) a form of Storm.
Stormee, Stormey, Stormi, Stormie, Stormmie

Storr (Norwegian) great.
Story

Stover (English) stove tender.

Stowe (English) hidden; packed away.
Stow

Strahan (Irish) minstrel.
Strachan

Stratford (English) bridge over the river. Literature: Stratford-upon-Avon was Shakespeare's birthplace.
Stradford, Strattford

Stratton (Scottish) river valley town.
Straten, Straton

Strephon (Greek) one who turns.

Strom (Greek) bed, mattress. (German) stream.

Strong (English) powerful.
Stronge

Stroud (English) thicket.

Struthers (Irish) brook.

Stu (English) a short form of Stewart, Stuart.
Stew

Stuart (English) caretaker, steward. History: a Scottish and English royal family.
Stuarrt

Studs (English) rounded nail heads; shirt ornaments; male horses used for breeding. History: Louis "Studs" Terkel is a famous American journalist.
Stud, Studd

Styles (English) stairs put over a wall to help cross it.
Stiles, Style, Stylz

Subhi (Arabic) early morning.

Subhî (Arabic) a form of Subhi.

Suck Chin (Korean) unshakable rock.

Sudi (Swahili) lucky.
Su'ud

Sued (Arabic) master, chief.

Suede (Arabic) a form of Sued.

Suelita (Spanish) little lily.

Suffield (English) southern field.
Sufield

Sufiân (Arabic) consecrated.

Sugden (English) valley of sows.
Sugdan, Sugdin, Sugdon, Sugdyn

Suhail (Arabic) gentle.
Suhael, Sujal

Suhay (Quechua) he who is like yellow corn: fine and abundant.

Suhuba (Swahili) friend.
Suhubah

Sukhpreet (Sikh) one who values inner peace and joy.

Sukru (Turkish) grateful.
Sukroo

Sulaiman (Arabic) a form of Solomon.
Sulaman, Sulay, Sulaymaan, Sulayman, Suleiman, Suleman, Suleyman, Sulieman, Sulman, Sulomon, Sulyman

Sullivan BG (Irish) black eyed.
Sullavan, Sullevan, Syllyvan

Sully (French) stain, tarnish. (English) south meadow. (Irish) a familiar form of Sullivan.
Sullea, Sullee, Sulleigh, Sulley, Sulli, Sullie

Sultan (Swahili) ruler.
Sultaan, Sulten, Sultin, Sulton, Sultyn

Sum (Tai) appropriate.

Sumainca (Quechua) beautiful Inca.

Sumarville (French) one who comes from summertime.

Sumeet (English) a form of Summit.

Sumit (English) a form of Summit.

Summit (English) peak, top.
Sumet, Summet, Summitt, Summyt, Sumyt

Sumner (English) church officer; summoner.
Summner

Suncu, Suncuyuc (Quechua) he who has a good and noble heart.

Sundeep (Punjabi) light; enlightened.
Sundip

Sunny BG (English) sunny, sunshine.
Sun, Suni, Sunie, Sunni, Sunnie, Suny

Sunreep (Hindi) pure.
Sunrip

Suri (Quechua) fast like an ostrich.

Surya BG (Sanskrit) sun.
Suria, Suriah, Suryah

Susumu (Japanese) move forward.

Sutcliff (English) southern cliff.
Sutclif, Sutcliffe, Sutclyf, Sutclyff, Suttclif, Suttcliff

Sutherland (Scandinavian) southern land.
Southerland, Sutherlan

Sutton (English) southern town.
Suton

Suyai, Suyay (Quechua) hope.

Suycauaman (Quechua) the youngest son of the falcons.

Sven (Scandinavian) youth.
Svein, Svend, Svenn, Swen, Swenson

Swaggart (English) one who sways and staggers.
Swaggert

Swain (English) herdsman; knight's attendant.
Swaine, Swane, Swanson, Swayn, Swayne

Swaley (English) winding stream.
Swail, Swailey, Swale, Swalea, Swalee, Swaleigh, Swales, Swali, Swalie, Swaly

Swannee (English) swan.
Swanee, Swaney, Swani, Swanie, Swanney, Swanni, Swannie, Swanny, Swany

Sweeney (Irish) small hero.
Sweanee, Sweaney, Sweani, Sweanie, Sweany, Sweenee, Sweeni, Sweenie, Sweeny

Swinbourne (English) stream used by swine.
Swinborn, Swinborne, Swinburn, Swinburne, Swinbyrn, Swynborn

Swindel (English) valley of the swine.
Swindell, Swyndel, Swyndell

Swinfen (English) swine's mud.
Swynfen

Swinford (English) swine's crossing.
Swynford

Swinton (English) swine town.
Swynton

Swithbert (English) strong and bright.
Swithbirt, Swithburt, Swithbyrt, Swythbert, Swythbirt, Swythburt, Swythbyrt

Swithin (German) strong.
Swithan, Swithen, Swithon, Swithun, Swithyn, Swythan, Swythen, Swythin, Swython, Swythun, Swythyn

Sy (Latin) a short form of Sylas, Symon.

Sydney GB (French) a form of Sidney.
Syd, Sydne, Sydnee, Sydni, Sydnie, Sydny, Syndey

Syed (Arabic) happy.
Syeed, Syid

Sying BG (Chinese) star.

Sylas (Latin) a form of Silas.
Syles, Sylus

Sylvain (French) a form of Silvan, Sylvester.
Silvain, Sylvian

Sylvan (Latin) a form of Silvan.
Silvanus

Sylvester (Latin) forest dweller.
Sly, Syl, Sylverster, Sylvestre

Symington (English) Simon's town, Simon's estate.
Simington

Symon (Greek) a form of Simon.
Syman, Symeon, Symion, Symms, Symone, Symonn, Symonns

Szczepan (Polish) a form of Stephen.

Szygfrid (Hungarian) a form of Siegfried.
Szigfrid

Szymon (Polish) a form of Simon.
Szimon

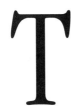

Taaveti (Finnish) a form of David.
Taavetie, Taavety, Taavi, Taavo, Taveti, Tavetie, Tavety

Tab (English) a short form of Tabner.
Tabb, Tabbie, Tabby, Tabi, Tabie, Taby

Tabare (Tupi) one who lives apart from the rest.

Tabaré (Tupi) man of the village.

Tabari (Arabic) he remembers.
Tabahri, Tabares, Tabarious, Tabarius, Tabarus, Tabary, Tabur

Tabib (Turkish) physician.
Tabeeb, Tabyb

Tabner (German) shining, brilliant; spring. (English) drummer.
Tab, Tabbener, Tabener

Tabo (Spanish) a short form of Gustave.

Tabor (Persian) drummer. (Hungarian) encampment.
Tabber, Taber, Taboras, Taibor, Taver, Tayber, Taybor

Taciano (Spanish) a form of Tacio.

Tacio (Latin) he who is quiet.

Tácito (Spanish) a form of Tacio.

Tad (Welsh) father. (Greek, Latin) a short form of Thaddeus.
Tadd, Taddy, Tade, Tadek, Tadey

Tadan (Native American) plentiful.
Taden

Tadarius (American) a combination of the prefix Ta + Darius.
Tadar, Tadarious, Tadaris, Tadarrius

Tadashi (Japanese) faithful servant.
Tadashee, Tadashie, Tadashy

Taddeo (Italian) a form of Thaddeus.
Tadeo

Taddeus (Greek, Latin) a form of Thaddeus.
Taddeous, Taddius, Tadeas, Tades, Tadio, Tadious

Tadi (Omaha) wind.
Tadee, Tadey, Tadie, Tady

Tadleigh (English) poet from a meadow.
Tadlea, Tadlee, Tadley, Tadli, Tadlie, Tadly

Tadzi (Carrier) loon.
Tadzie, Tadzy

Tadzio (Polish, Spanish) a form of Thaddeus.
Taddeusz, Tadeusz

Taffy GB (Welsh) a form of David. (English) a familiar form of Taft.
Taffee, Taffey, Taffi, Taffie, Tafy

Taft (English) river.
Tafte, Tafton

Tage (Danish) day.
Tag, Taig, Taige, Tayg, Tayge

Taggart (Irish) son of the priest.
Tagart, Tagert, Taggert, Taggirt, Taggurt, Taggyrt, Tagirt, Tagurt, Tagyrt

Tãher (Arabic) pure; clean.

Tahir (Indian) holy.

Tahír (Arabic) innocent, pure.
Taheer, Taher, Tahyr

Tai BG (Vietnamese) weather; prosperous; talented.

Taillefer (French) works with iron.

Taima GB (Native American) born during a storm.
Taimah, Tayma, Taymah

Tain (Irish) stream. (Native American) new moon.
Taine, Tainn, Tayn, Tayne

Taishawn (American) a combination of Tai + Shawn.
Taisen, Taishaun, Taishon

Tait (Scandinavian) a form of Tate.
Taite, Taitt, Tayt, Tayte

Taiwan (Chinese) island; island dweller. Geography: a country off the coast of China.
Taewon, Tahwan, Taivon, Taiwain, Tawain, Tawan, Tawann, Tawaun, Tawon, Taywan

Taiwo (Yoruba) first-born of twins.
Taywo

Taizeen (Indian) encouragement.

Taj (Urdu) crown.
Taje, Tajee, Tajeh, Tajh, Taji

Tajdar (Indian) crowned.

Tajo (Spanish) day.
Taio

Tajuan (American) a combination of the prefix Ta + Juan.
Taijuan, Taijun, Taijuon, Tájuan, Tajwan, Tayjuan

Takeo (Japanese) strong as bamboo.
Takeyo

Takeshi (Japanese) strong.

Takis (Greek) a familiar form of Peter.
Takias, Takius

Takoda (Lakota) friend to everyone.
Takodah, Takota, Takotah

Tal (Hebrew) dew; rain. (Tswana) a form of Tale.
Talia, Tall, Talya

Talâl (Arabic) pleasant; admirable.

Talat (Indian) prayer.

Talbert (German) bright valley.
Talberte, Talbirt, Talburt, Talburte, Talbyrt

Talbot (French) boot maker.
Talbott, Talibot, Talibott, Tallbot, Tallbott, Tallie, Tally, Talybot, Talybott

Talcott (English) cottage near the lake.
Talcot

Tale (Tswana) green.
Tael, Tail, Tayl

Tâleb (Arabic) a form of Talib.

Talen (English) a form of Talon.
Tallen

Talib (Arabic) seeker.
Taleb, Talyb

Taliesin (Welsh) radiant brow.
Taliesen, Talieson, Taliesyn, Talisan, Tallas, Talyersyn, Talyesin, Tayliesin, Tayliesyn

Taliki (Hausa) fellow.

Talleen (Indian) absorbed.

Talli (Delaware) legendary hero.
Talee, Taley, Tali, Tallee Talley, Tallie, Tally, Taly

Tallis BG (Persian) wise.
Talis, Tallys, Talys

Tallon (English, French) a form of Talon.

Talmadge (English) lake between two towns.
Talmage

Talmai (Aramaic) mound; furrow.
Talmay, Talmie, Telem

Talman BG (Aramaic) injured; oppressed.
Talmen, Talmin, Talmon, Talmyn

Talon BG (French, English) claw, nail.
Taelon, Taelyn, Talin, Tallin, Talyn

Talor GB (English) a form of Tal, Taylor.
Taelor, Taelur

Tam BG (Vietnamese) number eight. (Hebrew) honest. (English) a short form of Thomas.
Tamlane, Tamm

Tamal (Indian) a tree with very dark bark.

Taman (Slavic) dark, black.
Tama, Tamann, Tamen, Tamin, Tammen, Tamon, Tamone, Tamyn

Tamar GB (Hebrew) date; palm tree.
Tamarie, Tamario, Tamarr, Tamer, Tamor

Tamas (Hungarian) a form of Thomas.
Tamás, Tameas, Tammas

Tambo (Swahili) vigorous.
Tambow

Tamir (Arabic) tall as a palm tree.
Tameer, Tamirr, Tamyr, Tamyrr, Timir, Tymir, Tymyr

Tamkinat (Indian) pomp.

Tammâm (Arabic) generous.

Tammany (Delaware) friendly.
Tamany

Tammy GB (English) a familiar form of Thomas.
Tammie

Tamonash (Indian) destroyer of ignorance.

Tamson (Scandinavian) son of Thomas.
Tamsan, Tamsen, Tamsin, Tamson, Tamsun, Tamsyn

Tan (Burmese) million. (Vietnamese) new.
Than

Tanay, Tanuj (Indian) son.

Tancredo (Germanic) he who shrewdly gives advice.

Tandie (English) team.
Tandee, Tandey, Tandi, Tandy

Tane (Maori) husband.
Tain, Taine, Tainn, Tayn, Tayne, Taynn

Tanek (Greek) immortal. See also Atek.

Taneli (Finnish) God is my judge.
Taneil, Tanel, Tanelie, Tanell, Tanella, Tanelle, Tanely

Taner (English) a form of Tanner.
Tanar, Tanery

Tanguy (French) warrior.
Tangui

Tani GB (Japanese) valley.
Tanee, Taney, Tanie, Tany

Taniel GB (Estonian) a form of Daniel.
Taniell, Tanyel, Tanyell

Tanis GB (Slavic) a form of Tania, Tanya (see Girls' Names).

Tanmay (Sanskrit) engrossed.

Tanner BG (English) leather worker; tanner.
Tann, Tannar, Tannery, Tannir, Tannor

Tannin (English) tan colored; dark.
Tanin, Tannen, Tannon, Tanyen, Tanyon

Tannis GB (Slavic) a form of Tania, Tanya (see Girls' Names).

Tanny (English) a familiar form of Tanner.
Tana, Tannee, Tanney, Tanni, Tannie, Tany

Tano (Spanish) camp glory. (Ghanaian) Geography: a river in Ghana. (Russian) a short form of Stanislaus.
Tanno

Tanton (English) town by the still river.
Tantan, Tantin, Tantun, Tantyn

Tanveer (Indian) enlightened.

Tapan (Sanskrit) sun; summer.

Tapani (Finnish) a form of Stephen.
Tapamn, Tapanee, Tapaney, Tapanie, Tapany

Tapas (Indian) ascetic.

Tapasendra, Tarakeshwar, Taraknath (Indian) other names for the Hindu god Shiva.

Tapasranjan (Indian) another name for the Hindu god Vishnu.

Täpko (Kiowa) antelope.

Tapomay (Indian) full of moral virtue.

Taquan (American) a combination of the prefix Ta + Quan.
Taquann, Taquawn, Taquon, Taqwan

Taquiri (Quechua) he who creates much music and dance.

Tarachand, Taraprashad (Indian) star.

Tarak (Sanskrit) star; protector.

Taral (Indian) honeybee.

Taran BG (Sanskrit) heaven. A form of Tarun.
Tarran

Taranga (Indian) wave.

Taree GB (Australian) fig tree.
Tarey, Tari, Tarie, Tary

Tarek, Tarik, Tariq (Arabic) forms of Táriq.
Tareck, Tareek, Tareke, Taric, Tarick, Tariek, Tarikh, Tarreq, Tarrick, Tarrik, Taryc, Taryck, Taryk, Teryc, Teryck, Teryk

Tarell, Tarrell (German) forms of Terrell.
Tarelle, Tarrel, Taryl

Taren, Tarren (American) forms of Taron.
Tarrin, Tarryn, Taryon

Tàreq (Arabic) name of a star.

Tareton (English) a form of Tarleton.
Taretan, Tareten, Taretin, Taretyn, Tartan, Tarten, Tartin, Tarton, Tartyn

Tarif (Arabic) uncommon.
Tareef, Taryf

Táriq (Arabic) conqueror. History: Tariq bin Ziyad was the Muslim general who conquered Spain.
Tareck, Tarique, Tarreq, Tereik

Tarit (Indian) lightning.

Tarleton (English) Thor's settlement.
Tareton, Tarletan, Tarleten, Tarletin, Tarletyn, Tarlton

Taro (Japanese) first-born male.

Taron (American) a combination of Tad + Ron.
Taeron, Tahron, Tarone, Tarrion, Tarron, Tarrun

Tarquino (Latin) he who was born in Tarquinia.

Tarrance (Latin) a form of Terrence.
Tarance, Tarence, Tarince, Tarrence, Tarrince, Tarrynce, Tarynce

Tarrant (Welsh) thunder.
Tarant, Tarent, Tarrent, Terrant, Torant, Torent, Torrant, Torrent

Tarsicio (Latin) he who belongs to Tarso.

Tarun (Sanskrit) young, youth.

Taruntapan (Indian) morning sun.

Tarver (English) tower; hill; leader.
Terver

Taryn GB (American) a form of Taron.

Tas (Gypsy) bird's nest.

Tashawn (American) a combination of the prefix Ta + Shawn.
Tashaan, Tashan, Tashaun, Tashon, Tashun

Tass (Hungarian) ancient mythology name.

Tasunke (Dakota) horse.

Tate BG (Scandinavian, English) cheerful. (Native American) long-winded talker.

Tathagata (Indian) the Buddha.

Tatiano (Latin) he who is quiet.

Tatius (Latin) king, ruler. History: a Sabine king.
Tatianus, Tazio, Tytius, Tytyus

Tatum GB (English) cheerful.
Taitam, Taitem, Taitim, Taitom, Taitum, Taitym, Tatam, Tatem, Tatim, Tatom, Taytam, Taytem, Taytim, Taytom, Taytum, Taytym

Tau (Tswana) lion.

Taua (Quechua) the fourth child.

Tauacapac (Quechua) the fourth lord.

Tauno (Finnish) a form of Donald.

Taurean (Latin) strong; forceful. Astrology: born under the sign of Taurus.
Tauraun, Taurein, Taurin, Taurino, Taurion, Taurone, Tauryan, Tauryen, Tauryon

Tauro (Spanish) a form of Toro.

Taurus (Latin) Astrology: the second sign of the zodiac.
Taurice, Tauris

Tausiq (Indian) reinforcement.

Tavares (Aramaic) a form of Tavor.
Tarvarres, Tavar, Tavaras, Taveress

Tavaris, Tavarus (Aramaic) forms of Tavor.
Tarvaris, Tavari, Tavarian, Tavarous, Tavarri, Tavarris, Tavars, Tavarse, Tavarys, Tevaris, Tevarus, Tevarys, Teverus, Teverys

Tavarius (Aramaic) a form of Tavor.
Tavarious, Tevarius

Taved (Estonian) a form of David.
Tavad, Tavid, Tavod, Tavyd

Tavey (Latin) a familiar form of Octavio.
Tavy

Tavi (Aramaic) good.
Tavee, Tavie

Tavian (Latin) a form of Octavio.
Taveon, Taviann, Tavien, Tavieon, Tavio, Tavionne

Tavin, Tavon (American) forms of Tavian.
Tavonn, Tavonne, Tavonni

Tavion (Latin) a form of Tavian.

Tavis (Scottish) a form of Tavish.
Taviss, Tavys, Tavyss

Tavish (Scottish) a form of Thomas.
Tav, Tavysh

Tavo (Slavic) a short form of Gustave.

Tavor (Aramaic) misfortune.
Tarvoris, Tavores, Tavorious, Tavoris, Tavorise, Tavorres, Tavorris, Tavorrys, Tavorys, Tavuris, Tavurys

Tawfiq (Arabic) success.

Tawno (Gypsy) little one.
Tawn

Tayib (Hindi) good; delicate.

Tayler GB (English) a form of Taylor.
Tailar, Tailer, Taylar, Tayller, Teyler

Taylor GB (English) tailor.
Taelor, Tailor, Talor, Tayllor, Taylour, Taylr, Teylor

Taymullah (Arabic) servant of God.

Tayshawn (American) a combination of Taylor + Shawn.
Taysean, Tayshan, Tayshun, Tayson

Tayvon (American) a form of Tavian.
Tayvan, Tayvaughn, Tayven, Tayveon, Tayvin, Tayvohn, Taywon

Tayyeb (Arabic) good.

Taz (Arabic) shallow ornamental cup.
Tazz

Tazio (Italian) a form of Tatius.

Teagan GB (Irish) a form of Teague.
Teagen, Teagun, Teegan

Teague (Irish) bard, poet.
Teag, Teage, Teak, Teeg, Teegue, Teig, Teige, Teigue, Tyg, Tygue

Teale (English) small freshwater duck.
Teal, Teel, Teele, Teil, Teile, Teyl, Teyle

Tearence (Latin) a form of Terrence.
Tearance, Tearnce, Tearrance

Tearlach (Scottish) a form of Charles.
Tearlache, Tearloc, Tearloch, Tearloche, Tearlock, Tearlok

Tearle (English) stern, severe.
Tearl

Teasdale (English) river dweller. Geography: a river in England.
Tedale

Teb (Spanish) a short form of Stephen.

Ted (English) a short form of Edward, Edwin, Theodore.
Tedd, Tedek, Tedik, Tedson

Teddy (English) a familiar form of Edward, Theodore.
Teddee, Teddey, Teddi, Teddie, Tedee, Tedey, Tedi, Tedie, Tedy

Tedmund (English) protector of the land.
Tedman, Tedmand, Tedmon, Tedmond, Tedmondo, Tedmun

Tedorik (Polish) a form of Theodore.
Tedorek, Tedoric, Tedorick, Tedoryc, Tedoryck, Tedoryk, Teodoor, Teodor, Teodorek

Tedrick (American) a combination of Ted + Rick.
Teddrick, Tederick, Tedric, Tedrik, Tedryc, Tedryck, Tedryk

Teerthankar (Indian) another form of Tirthankar, a type of Jain god.

Teetonka (Lakota) big lodge.

Tefere (Ethiopian) seed.
Tefer

Tegan GB (Irish) a form of Teague.
Teghan, Teigan, Teigen, Tiegan

Tehuti (Egyptian) god of earth, air, and sea.

Tej (Sanskrit) light; lustrous.

Tejano (Spanish) Texan man.

Tejas (Sanskrit) sharp. (American) a form of Tex.

Tekle (Ethiopian) plant.

Telek (Polish) a form of Telford.

Telem (Hebrew) mound; furrow.
Talmai, Tel, Tellem

Telémaco (Greek) he who prepares for battle.

Telesforo (Greek) man from the countryside.

Telford (French) iron cutter.
Telfer, Telfor, Telforde, Telfour, Tellford, Tellforde

Teller (English) storyteller.
Tell

Telly (Greek) a familiar form of Teller, Theodore.
Telli, Tellie, Tely

Telmo (English) tiller, cultivator.

Telutci (Moquelumnan) bear making dust as it runs.

Telvin (American) a combination of the prefix Te + Melvin.
Tellvin, Telvan

Tem (Gypsy) country.

Teman (Hebrew) on the right side; southward.
Temani, Temanie, Temany, Temen, Temin, Temon, Temyn

Temán (Hebrew) a form of Teman.

Tembo (Swahili) elephant.
Tembeau

Temotzin (Nahuatl) one who descends.

Tempest GB (French) storm.
Tempes, Tempess

Temple (Latin) sanctuary.

Templeton (English) town near the temple.
Temp, Templeten, Templetown

Tennant (English) tenant, renter.
Tenant, Tennent

Tenner (Irish) Religion: a small form of a rosary.

Tennessee (Cherokee) mighty warrior. Geography: a southern U.S. state.
Tennesy, Tennysee

Tennyson (English) a form of Dennison. Literature: Alfred, Lord Tennyson was a nineteenth-century British poet.
Tenney, Tenneyson, Tennie, Tennis, Tennison, Tenny, Tenson, Tenyson

Tenyoa (Nahuatl) of a good family name.

Teo (Vietnamese) a form of Tom.
Tio, Tyo

Teobaldo (Italian, Spanish) a form of Theobald.

Teócrito (Greek) God's chosen one.

Teodoro (Italian, Spanish) a form of Theodore.
Teodore, Teodorico

Teodosio (Greek) a form of Theodore.

Teófano, Teófilo (Greek) loved by God.

Teon (Greek) a form of Teona (see Girls' Names).

Teotetl (Nahuatl) divine stone.

Teoxihuitl (Nahuatl) turquoise; precious, divine.

Tepiltzin (Nahuatl) privileged son.

Teppo (French) a familiar form of Stephen. (Finnish) a form of Tapani.

Tequan (American) a combination of the prefix Te + Quan.
Tequinn, Tequon

Teraj (Hebrew) wild goat.

Teran, Terran, Terren (Latin) short forms of Terrence.
Teren, Terin, Terone, Terrien, Terrone, Terryn, Teryn, Tiren

Terance, Terence, Terrance (Latin) forms of Terrence.
Terince, Terriance, Terrince, Terrynce, Terynce

Terciero (Spanish) born third.

Tercio, Tertulio (Greek) the third child.

Terel, Terell, Terelle (German) forms of Terrell.
Tereall

Teremun (Tiv) father's acceptance.

Terencio (Spanish) a form of Terrence.

Terez (Greek) a form of Teresa (see Girls' Names).

Teron (Latin) a form of Teran. (American) a form of Tyrone.

Terrell (German) thunder ruler.
Terrail, Terral, Terrale, Terrall, Terreal, Terryal, Terryel, Turrell

Terrelle BG (German) a form of Terrell.

Terrence (Latin) smooth.

Terrick (American) a combination of the prefix Te + Derric.
Teric, Terick, Terik, Teriq, Terric, Terrik, Tirek, Tirik

Terrill (German) a form of Terrell.
Teriel, Teriell, Terril, Terryl, Terryll, Teryl, Teryll, Tyrill

Terrin BG (Latin) a short form of Terrence.

Terrion (American) a form of Terron.
Tereon, Terion, Terione, Terrione, Terriyon, Terryon

Terris (Latin) son of Terry.
Teris, Terrys, Terys

Terron (American) a form of Tyrone.
Terone, Terrone, Terronn, Tiron

Terry BG (English) a familiar form of Terrence. See also Keli.
Tarry, Teree, Terey, Teri, Terie, Terree, Terrey, Terri, Terrie, Tery

Tertius (Latin) third.

Teseo (Greek) the founder.

Teshawn (American) a combination of the prefix Te + Shawn.
Tesean, Teshaun, Teshon

Tetley (English) Tate's meadow.
Tatlea, Tatlee, Tatleigh, Tetli, Tetlie, Tetly

Tetsuya (Japanese) smart.

Teva (Hebrew) nature.
Tevah

Tevan, Tevon, Tevyn (American) forms of Tevin.
Tevion, Tevohn, Tevone, Tevonne, Tevoun, Tevvan, Teyvon

Tevel (Yiddish) a form of David.
Tevell, Tevil, Tevill, Tevyl, Tevyll

Tevin (American) a combination of the prefix Te + Kevin.
Teavin, Teivon, Tevaughan, Tevaughn, Teven, Tevien, Tevinn, Tevvin

Tevis (Scottish) a form of Thomas.
Tevish, Teviss, Tevys, Tevyss

Tewdor (German) a form of Theodore.

Tex (American) from Texas.
Texx

Teyo (Spanish) God.

Tezcacoatl (Nahuatl) reflecting serpent; king.

Thâbet (Arabic) a form of Thabit.

Thabit (Arabic) firm, strong.
Thabyt

Thad (Greek, Latin) a short form of Thaddeus.
Thadd, Thade

Thaddeus (Greek) courageous. (Latin) praiser. Bible: one of the Twelve Apostles. See also Fadey.
Thaddaeus, Thaddaus, Thaddeau, Thaddeaus, Thaddeo, Thaddeos, Thaddeous, Thaddeys, Thaddiaus, Thaddis, Thaddius, Thadeaou, Thadeys, Thadia, Thadus

Thadeus (Greek, Latin) a form of Thaddeus.
Thadeas, Thadeaus, Thadeis, Thadeos, Thadeous, Thadieus, Thadios, Thadious, Thadius, Thadiys, Thadyas, Thadyos, Thadyus

Thady (Irish) praise.
Thaddy, Thadee, Thady

Thai (Vietnamese) many, multiple.

Thalmus (Greek) flowering.
Thalmas, Thalmis, Thalmos, Thalmous, Thalmys

Thaman (Hindi) god; godlike.
Thamane, Thamen

Than (Burmese) million.
Tan

Thandie BG (Zulu) beloved.
Thandee, Thandey, Thandi, Thandiwe, Thandy

Thane (English) attendant warrior.
Thain, Thaine, Thayn, Thayne

Thang (Vietnamese) victorious.

Thanh BG (Vietnamese) finished.

Thaniel (Hebrew) a short form of Nathaniel.
Thaneal, Thaneel, Thaneil, Thaneyl, Thaniell, Thanielle, Thanyel, Thanyell, Thanyelle

Thanos (Greek) nobleman; bear–man.
Athanasios, Thanasis, Thanus

Thatcher (English) roof thatcher, repairer of roofs.
Thacher, Thatch, Thaxter

Thaw (English) melting ice.

Thayer (French) nation's army.
Thay

Thebault (French) a form of Theobald.
Teobaud, Theòbault

Thel (English) upper story.

Thenga (Yao) bring him.
Thengah

Theo (English) a short form of Theodore.
Teo, Thio, Thyo

Theobald (German) people's prince. See also Dietbald.
Tebaldo, Teobald, Teobaldo, Teobalt, Theballd, Theobaldo, Theobalt, Thibault, Thyobald, Thyobaldo, Thyobalt, Tibald, Tibalt, Tibold, Tiebold, Tiebout, Toiboid, Tybald, Tybalt

Theodore (Greek) gift of God. See also Feodor, Fyodor.
Téadóir, Teodomiro, Teodus, Teos, Theodor, Theódor, Theodors, Theodorus, Theodosios, Theodrekr, Tivadar, Tolek

Theodoric (German) ruler of the people. See also Dedrick, Derek, Dirk.
Teodorico, Thedric, Thedrick, Thedrik, Theodorick, Theodorik, Theodrick, Theodryc, Theodryck, Theodryk

Theophilus (Greek) loved by God.
Teofil, Théophile, Theophlous, Theopolis

Theron (Greek) hunter.
Theran, Theren, Thereon, Therin, Therion, Therrin, Therron, Theryn, Theryon

Theros (Greek) summer.
Theross

Thian (Vietnamese) smooth.

Thibault (French) a form of Theobald.
Thibaud, Thibaut, Tybault

Thien (Vietnamese) a form of Thian.

Thierry (French) a form of Theodoric.
Theirry, Theory

Thiery (French) a form of Thierry.

Thom (English) a short form of Thomas.
Thomy

Thoma (German) a form of Thomas.

Thomas ☀ (Greek, Aramaic) twin. Bible: one of the Twelve Apostles. See also Chuma, Foma, Maslin.
Thomason, Thomaz, Thommas, Thumas, Tomcy

Thommy (Hebrew) a familiar form of Thomas.
Thomee, Thomey, Thomi, Thomie, Thommee, Thommey, Thommi, Thommie, Thomy

Thompson (English) son of Thomas.
Thomasin, Thomason, Thomeson, Thomison, Thomsen, Thomson, Tompson, Tomson

Thor (Scandinavian) thunder. Mythology: the Norse god of thunder.
Thore, Thorin, Thorr, Tor

Thorald (Scandinavian) Thor's follower.
Thorold, Torald

Thorbert (Scandinavian) Thor's brightness.
Thorbirt, Thorburt, Thorbyrt, Torbert, Torbirt, Torburt, Torbyrt

Thorbjorn (Scandinavian) Thor's bear.
Thorborn, Thorborne, Thorburn, Thorburne, Thorbyrn, Thorbyrne, Thurborn, Thurborne, Thurburn, Thurburne

Thorgood (English) Thor is good.

Thorleif (Scandinavian) Thor's beloved.
Thorleyf, Thorlief

Thorley (English) Thor's meadow.
Thorlea, Thorlee, Thorleigh, Thorli, Thorlie, Thorly, Torlee, Torleigh, Torley, Torli, Torlie, Torly

Thormond (English) Thor's protection.
Thormon, Thormondo, Thormun, Thormund, Thormundo

Thorndike (English) thorny embankment.
Thordike, Thordyke, Thorndyck, Thorndyke, Thorne, Thornedike, Thornedyke

Thorne (English) a short form of names beginning with "Thorn."
Thorn, Thornie, Thorny

Thornley (English) thorny meadow.
Thorley, Thorne, Thornlea, Thornlee, Thornleigh, Thornli, Thornlie, Thornly

Thornton (English) thorny town.
Thorne, Thornetan, Thorneten, Thornetin, Thorneton, Thornetown, Thornetyn, Thortan, Thorten, Thortin, Thorton, Thortyn

Thorpe (English) village.
Thorp

Thorwald (Scandinavian) Thor's forest.
Thorvald, Thorvaldo, Thorwaldo, Torvald

Thuc (Vietnamese) aware.

Thunder (English) thunder.

Thurlow (English) Thor's hill.
Thurlo

Thurman (English) Thor's servant.
Thirman, Thirmen, Thorman, Thurmen, Thurmun, Thurnman, Thurnmen

Thurmond (English) defended by Thor.
Thormond, Thurmondo, Thurmund, Thurmundo

Thurston (Scandinavian) Thor's stone.
Thirstan, Thirstein, Thirsten, Thirstin, Thirston, Thirstyn, Thorstan, Thorsteen, Thorstein, Thorsten, Thorstin, Thorstine, Thorston, Thorstyn, Thurstain, Thurstan, Thursteen, Thurstein, Thursten, Thurstin, Thurstine, Thurstyn, Torsten, Torston

Tiago (Spanish) a form of Jacob.

Tiba (Navajo) gray.
Tibah, Tibba, Tibbah, Tyba, Tybah, Tybba, Tybbah

Tibault (French) rules of humankind.

Tibbot (Irish) bold.
Tibbott, Tibot, Tibott, Tibout, Tybbot, Tybot

Tiberio (Italian) from the Tiber River region.
Tiberias, Tiberious, Tiberiu, Tiberius, Tibius, Tyberious, Tyberius, Tyberrius

Tibor (Hungarian) holy place.
Tiburcio, Tybor

Tiburón (Spanish) shark.

Tichawanna (Shona) we shall see.

Ticho (Spanish) a short form of Patrick.
Ticcho, Ticco, Tycco, Tycho, Tyco

Ticiano (Spanish) a form of Tito.

Tico (Greek) adventurous; fortunate.

Tieler (English) a form of Tyler.
Tielar, Tielor, Tielyr

Tien (Chinese) heaven.
Tyen

Tiennan (French) a form of Stephen.
Tyennan

Tiennot (French) a form of Stephen.
Tien

Tiernan (Irish) lord.
Tiarnach, Tiernan

Tierney GB (Irish) lordly.
Tyrney

Tige (English) a short form of Tiger.
Ti, Tig, Tyg, Tyge, Tygh

Tiger (American) tiger; powerful and energetic.
Tiga, Tige, Tigger, Tyger

Tighe (Irish) a form of Teague. (English) a short form of Tiger.

Tigrio (Latin) tiger.

Tiimu (Moquelumnan) caterpillar coming out of the ground.
Timu, Tymu

Tiktu (Moquelumnan) bird digging up potatoes.

Tilden (English) tilled valley; tiller of the valley.
Tildan, Tildin, Tildon, Tildyn

Tilford (English) prosperous ford.
Tilforde, Tillford, Tillforde

Till (German) a short form of Theodoric.
Thilo, Til, Tillman, Tillmann, Tilman, Tilson, Tyl, Tyll

Tilo (Teutonic) skillful and praises God.

Tilton (English) prosperous town.
Tiltown, Tylton, Tyltown

Tim (Greek) a short form of Timothy.
Timm, Tym, Tymm

Timin (Arabic) born near the sea.
Timyn, Tymin, Tymyn

Timmie, Timmy (Greek) familiar forms of Timothy.
Timee, Timey, Timi, Timie, Timmee, Timmey, Timmi, Tymee, Tymey, Tymi, Tymie, Tymmee, Tymmey, Tymmi, Tymmie, Tymmy, Tymy

Timmothy (Greek) a form of Timothy.
Timmathy, Timmithy, Timmothee, Timmothey, Timmoty, Timmthy

Timo (Finnish) a form of Timothy.
Timio, Timmo, Tymmo, Tymo

Timofey (Russian) a form of Timothy.
Timofee, Timofei, Timofej, Timofeo

Timon (Greek) honorable.
Timan, Timen, Timin, Timyn

Timoteo (Italian, Portuguese, Spanish) a form of Timothy.
Timotao, Timotei

Timoteu (Greek) a form of Timothy.

Timothe, Timothee (Greek) forms of Timothy.
Timothé, Timothée

Timothy ☀ (Greek) honoring God. See also Kimokeo.
Tadhg, Taidgh, Tiege, Tima, Timathee, Timathey, Timathy, Timithy, Timka, Timkin, Timok, Timontheo, Timonthy, Timót, Timote, Timoteus, Timotheo, Timotheos, Timotheus, Timothey, Timothie, Timthie, Tiomóid, Tomothy

Timur (Russian) conqueror. (Hebrew) a form of Tamar.
Timar, Timarr, Timer, Timor, Timour, Tymar, Tymarr, Tymer, Tymur

Tin (Vietnamese) thinker.
Tyn

Tincupuma, Tinquipoma (Quechua) he who creates much music and dance.

Tino (Spanish) venerable, majestic. (Italian) small. A familiar form of Antonio. (Greek) a short form of Augustine.
Tion, Tyno

Tinsley (English) fortified field.
Tinslea, Tinslee, Tinsleigh, Tinsli, Tinslie, Tinsly, Tynslea, Tynslee, Tynsleigh, Tynsley, Tynsli, Tynslie, Tynsly

Tiquan (American) a combination of the prefix Ti + Quan.
Tiquawn, Tiquine, Tiquon, Tiquwan, Tiqwan

Tíquico (Greek) very fortunate person.

Tirrell (German) a form of Terrell.
Tirel, Tirrel

Tirso (Greek) crowned with fig leaves.

Tisha GB (Russian) a form of Timothy.

Tishawn (American) a combination of the prefix Ti + Shawn.
Tisean, Tishaan, Tishaun, Tishean, Tishon, Tishun

Tite (French) a form of Titus.
Tyte

Tito (Italian) a form of Titus.
Titos, Tyto

Titoatauchi, Tituatauchi (Quechua) he who brings luck in trying times.

Titu (Quechua) difficult, complicated.

Titus (Greek) giant. (Latin) hero. A form of Tatius. History: a Roman emperor.
Titan, Titas, Titek, Titis

Tivon (Hebrew) nature lover.

Tiziano (Latin) the giant.

Tj BG (American) a form of TJ.

TJ BG (American) a combination of the initials T. + J.
T Jae, T.J., Teejay, Tjayda

Tlacaelel (Nahuatl) diligent person.

Tlacelel (Nahuatl) greatest of our heroes.

Tlachinolli (Nahuatl) fire.

Tláloc (Nahuatl) wine of the earth.

Tlanextic (Nahuatl) the light of dawn.

Tlanextli (Nahuatl) radiance, brilliance; majesty, splendor.

Tlatecuhtli (Nahuatl) gentleman of the earth.

Tlazohtlaloni (Nahuatl) one who is loved.

Tlazopilli (Nahuatl) precious noble.

Tlexictli (Nahuatl) fire navel.

Tlilpotonqui (Nahuatl) feathered in black.

Toan (Vietnamese) complete; mathematics.

Tobal (Spanish) a short form of Christopher.
Tabalito

Tobar (Gypsy) road.
Tobbar

Tobi GB (Yoruba) great.
Tobbi

Tobias (Hebrew) God is good.
Tebes, Tobia, Tobiah, Tobiás, Tobiasz, Tobiath, Tobies, Tobyas

Tobías (Hebrew) a form of Tobias.

Tobin (Hebrew) a form of Tobias.
Toben, Tobian, Tobyn, Tovin

Tobit (Hebrew) son of Tobias.
Tobyt

Toby (Hebrew) a familiar form of Tobias.
Tobbee, Tobbey, Tobbie, Tobby, Tobe, Tobee, Tobey, Tobie, Tobye

Tochtli (Nahuatl) rabbit.

Tod (English) a form of Todd.

Todd (English) fox.
Todde, Toddie, Toddy

Todor (Basque, Russian) a form of Theodore.
Teador, Tedor, Teodor, Todar, Todas, Todos

Toft (English) small farm.

Togar (Australian) smoke.
Tager, Togir, Togor, Togyr

Tohías (Spanish) God is good.

Tohon (Native American) cougar.

Tokala (Dakota) fox.
Tokalah

Tokoni BG (Tongan) assistant, helper.
Tokonee, Tokonie, Tokony

Toland (English) owner of taxed land.
Tolan, Tolen, Tolin, Tolland, Tolon, Tolun, Tolyn

Tolbert (English) bright tax collector.
Tolberte, Tolbirt, Tolburt, Tolburte, Tolbyrt

Tolenka, Tolya (Russian) one who comes from the east.

Toli (Spanish) plowman.

Toller (English) tax collector.
Toler

Tolman (English) tax man.
Tollman, Tollmen, Tolmen

Tolomeo (Greek) powerful in battle.

Toltecatl, Toltecatli (Nahuatl) artist.

Tom (English) a short form of Thomas, Tomas.
Teo, Teom, Tome, Tomm

Toma (Romanian) a form of Thomas.
Tomah

Tomas (German) a form of Thomas.
Tomaisin, Tomaz, Tomcio, Tomek, Tomelis, Tomico, Tomik, Tomislaw, Tommas, Tomo

Tomás (Irish, Spanish) a form of Thomas.
Tómas

Tomasso (Italian) a form of Thomas.
Tomaso, Tommaso

Tomasz (Polish) a form of Thomas.

Tombe (Kakwa) northerners.
Tomba

Tomé (Hebrew) the identical twin brother.

Tomer (Hebrew) tall.
Tomar, Tomir, Tomyr

Tomey, Tomy (Irish) familiar forms of Thomas.
Tome, Tomi, Tomie

Tomi GB (Japanese) rich. (Hungarian) a form of Thomas.
Tomee

Tomkin (English) little Tom.
Thomkin, Thomkyn, Tomkyn

Tomlin (English) little Tom.
Thomllin, Thomlyn, Tomlinson, Tomlyn

Tommie BG (Hebrew) a familiar form of Thomas.
Tommee, Tommey, Tommi

Tommy (Hebrew) a familiar form of Thomas.

Tonatiuh (Nahuatl) sunshine.

Tonatiúh (Nahuatl) the highest heaven and greatest honor for the revolutionaries.

Tonauac (Nahuatl) the one who possesses light.

Tonda (Czech) a form of Tony.
Tondah, Toneek, Tonek, Tonik

Toney, Toni, Tonny (Greek, Latin, English) forms of Tony.

Tong (Vietnamese) fragrant.

Toni GB (Greek, German, Slavic) a form of Tony.
Tonee, Tonie, Tonis, Tonnie

Tonio (Italian) a short form of Antonio. (Portuguese) a form of Tony.
Tono, Tonyo

Tony (Greek) flourishing. (Latin) praiseworthy. (English) a short form of Anthony. A familiar form of Remington.
Tonye

Tooantuh (Cherokee) spring frog.

Toomas (Estonian) a form of Thomas.
Toomis, Tuomas, Tuomo

Topa, Tupa (Quechua) title of honor.

Topher (Greek) a short form of Christopher, Kristopher.
Tofer, Tophor

Topo (Spanish) gopher.

Topper (English) hill.
Toper

Tor (Norwegian) thunder. (Tiv) royalty, king.
Tore, Torre

Torcuato (Latin) adorned with a collar or garland.

Toren, Torren (Irish) short forms of Torrence.
Torehn, Torreon, Torrin

Torey BG (English) a familiar form of Torr, Torrence.
Toree, Toreey, Torie, Torre, Torri

Tori GB (English) a familiar form of Torr, Torrence.

Torian (Irish) a form of Torin.
Toran, Torean, Toriano, Toriaun, Torien, Torion, Torrian, Torrien, Torryan

Toribio (Greek) he who makes bows.

Torin (Irish) chief. (Latin, Irish) a form of Torrence.
Thorfin, Thorin, Thorstein, Thoryn, Torine, Torrine, Torryn, Torryne, Toryn

Torio (Japanese) tail of a bird.
Torrio, Torryo, Toryo

Torkel (Swedish) Thor's cauldron.

Tormey (Irish) thunder spirit.
Tormé, Tormee, Tormi, Tormie, Tormy

Tormod (Scottish) north.
Tormed, Tormon, Tormond, Tormondo, Tormun, Tormund, Tormundo

Torn (Irish) a short form of Torrence.
Toran, Torne

Toro (Spanish) bull.

Torquil (Danish) Thor's kettle.
Torkel

Torr (English) tower.

Torrance (Irish) a form of Torrence.
Torance, Turance

Torrence (Irish) knolls. (Latin) a form of Terrence.
Tawrence, Toreence, Torence, Torenze, Torynce, Tuarence

Torrey BG (English) a familiar form of Torr, Torrence.

Torrie GB (English) a familiar form of Torr, Torrence.

Torrin (Irish, Latin, Irish) a form of Torin.

Torry (English) a familiar form of Torr, Torrence.

Torsten (Scandinavian) thunderstone.
Torstan, Torstin, Torston

Toru (Japanese) sea.

Toruato (Latin) adorned with a necklace.

Tory BG (English) a familiar form of Torr, Torrence.

Toshi-Shita (Japanese) junior.

Tosya (Russian) further than what is expected.

Tototl (Nahuatl) bird.

Toufic (Lebanese) success.

Toussaint (French) all the saints.

Tovi (Hebrew) good.
Tov, Tovee, Tovie, Tovy

Townley (English) town meadow.
Tonlea, Tonlee, Tonleigh, Tonley, Tonli, Tonlie, Tonly, Townlea, Townlee, Townleigh, Townli, Townlie, Townly

Townsend (English) town's end.
Town, Townes, Towney, Townie, Townsen, Townshend, Towny

Tra'von (American) a form of Travon.

Trabunco (Mapuche) meeting at the marsh.

Trace (Irish) a form of Tracy.
Trayce

Tracey GB (Irish) a form of Tracy.
Traci, Tracie, Treacey, Treaci, Treacie

Tracy GB (Greek) harvester. (Latin) courageous. (Irish) battler.
Tracee, Tracie, Treacy

Trader (English) well-trodden path; skilled worker.
Trade

Trae (English) a form of Trey.
Traey, Traie

Traevon (American) a form of Trevon.

Traful (Araucanian) union.

Trahern (Welsh) strong as iron.
Traherne, Trayhern, Trayherne

Trai (English) a form of Trey.

Tramaine (Scottish) a form of Tremaine.
Tramain, Traman, Tramane, Tramayn, Tramayne, Traymain, Traymon

Tranamil (Mapuche) low, scattered light

Tranquilino (Roman) tranquil, serene.

Tránsito (Latin) one who goes on to another life.

Traquan (American) a combination of Travis + Quan.
Traequan, Traqon, Traquon, Traqwan, Traqwaun, Trayquan, Trayquane, Trayqwon

Trashawn BG (American) a combination of Travis + Shawn.
Trasean, Trasen, Trashaun, Trashon, Trashone, Trashun, Trayshaun, Trayshawn

Trasíbulo (Greek) daring counselor.

Traugott (German) God's truth.
Traugot

Travaris (French) a form of Travers.
Travares, Travaress, Travarious, Travarius, Travarous,

Travarus, Travauris, Traveress, Traverez, Traverus, Travoris, Travorus, Trevares, Trevarious, Trevaris, Trevarius, Trevaros, Trevarus, Trevores, Trevoris, Trevorus

Travell (English) traveler.
Travail, Travale, Travel, Traveler, Travelis, Travelle, Travil, Travill, Traville, Travyl, Travyll, Travylle

Traven (American) a form of Trevon.
Travan, Trayven

Traveon (American) a form of Trevon.

Travers (French) crossroads.
Traver

Travion (American) a form of Trevon.
Travian, Travien, Travione, Travioun

Travis (English) a form of Travers.
Travais, Travees, Traves, Traveus, Travious, Traviss, Travius, Travous, Travus, Travys, Travyss, Trayvis

Travon (American) a form of Trevon.
Traivon, Travone, Travonn, Travonne

Travonte (American) a combination of Travon + the suffix Te.

Tray (English) a form of Trey.
Traye

Trayton (English) town full of trees.
Traiton, Trayten

Trayvion (American) a form of Trayvon.
Trayveon

Trayvon (American) a combination of Tray + Von.
Trayvin, Trayvone, Trayvonne, Trayvyon

Trayvond (American) a form of Trayvon.

Tre, Tré (American) forms of Trevon. (English) forms of Trey.

Tre Von (American) a form of Trevon.

Trea (English) a form of Trey.

Treat (English) delight.
Treet, Treit, Treyt

Treavon (American) a form of Trevon.
Treavan, Treavin, Treavion

Treavor (Irish, Welsh) a form of Trevor.

Trebor (Irish, Welsh) a form of Trevor.

Trecaman (Mapuche) majestic steps of the condor.

Tredway (English) well-worn road.
Treadway

Tremaine, Tremayne (Scottish) house of stone.
Tremain, Tremane, Tremayn, Treymain, Treymaine, Treymayn, Treymayne, Trimaine

Trent (Latin) torrent, rapid stream. (French) thirty. Geography: a city in northern Italy.
Trant, Trante, Trente, Trentino, Trento, Trentonio

Trenten (Latin) a form of Trenton.

Trenton (Latin) town by the rapid stream. Geography: the capital of New Jersey.
Trendon, Trendun, Trentan, Trentin, Trentine, Trentton, Trentyn, Trinten, Trintin, Trinton

Trequan (American) a combination of Trey + Quan.
Trequanne, Trequaun, Trequian, Trequon, Trequon, Treyquane

Treshaun (American) a form of Treshawn.

Treshawn (American) a combination of Trey + Shawn.
Treshon, Treshun, Treysean, Treyshawn, Treyshon

Treston (Welsh) a form of Tristan.
Trestan, Trestin, Trestton, Trestyn

Trev (Irish, Welsh) a short form of Trevor.

Trevar (Irish, Welsh) a form of Trevor.

Trevaughn (American) a combination of Trey + Vaughn.
Trevaughan, Trevaugn, Trevaun, Trevaune, Trevaunn, Treyvaughn

Trevell (English) a form of Travell.
Trevel, Trevelle, Trevil, Trevill, Treville, Trevyl, Trevyll, Trevylle

Trevelyan (English) Elian's homestead.
Trevelian

Treven, Trevin (American) forms of Trevon.
Trevien, Trevine, Trevinne, Trevyn, Treyvin

Treveon (American) a form of Trevon.
Treveyon, Treyveon

Trever (Irish, Welsh) a form of Trevor.

Trevion, Trévion (American) forms of Trevon.
Trevian, Trevione, Trevionne, Trevyon, Treyvion

Trevis (English) a form of Travis.
Trevais, Treves, Trevez, Treveze, Trevius, Trevus, Trevys, Trevyss

Trevon (American) a combination of Trey + Von.
Trevohn, Trevoine, Trevone, Trevonn

Trévon, Trevonne (American) forms of Trevon.
Trévan

Trevond (American) a form of Trevon.

Trevonte (American) a combination of Trevon + the suffix Te.

Trevor (Irish) prudent. (Welsh) homestead.
Travar, Traver, Travir, Travor, Trefor, Trevore, Trevour, Trevyr, Treyvor

Trey (English) three; third.
Trei, Treye

Treyton (English) a form of Trayton.
Treiton

Treyvon (American) a form of Trevon.
Treyvan, Treyven, Treyvenn, Treyvone, Treyvonn, Treyvun

Tri (English) a form of Trey.
Trie

Trifón (Greek) having a sumptuous, free-spirited life.

Trigg (Scandinavian) trusty.
Trig

Trini GB (Latin) a short form of Trinity.
Triny, Tryny

Trinidad (Latin) a form of Trinity.

Trinity GB (Latin) holy trinity.
Trenedy, Trinidy, Trinitee, Trinitey, Triniti, Trinitie, Trynyty

Trip, Tripp (English) traveler.
Tryp, Trypp

Tristan BG (Welsh) bold. Literature: a knight in the Arthurian legends who fell in love with his uncle's wife.
Tris, Trisan, Tristain, Tristann

Tristán (Welsh) a form of Tristan.

Tristano (Italian) a form of Tristan.

Tristen BG (Welsh) a form of Tristan.
Trisden, Trissten, Tristinn

Tristian BG (Welsh) a form of Tristan.

Tristin BG (Welsh) a form of Tristan.

Triston BG (Welsh) a form of Tristan.

Tristram (Welsh) sorrowful. Literature: the title character in Laurence Sterne's eighteenth-century novel *Tristram Shandy*.
Tristam, Trystram, Trystran

Tristyn BG (Welsh) a form of Tristan.

Trófimo (Greek) fed.

Troilo (Egyptian) he who was born in Troy.

Trot (English) trickling stream.

Trowbridge (English) bridge by the tree.
Throwbridge

Troy BG (Irish) foot soldier. (French) curly haired. (English) water. See also Koi.
Troi, Troye, Troyton

True (English) faithful, loyal.
Tru

Truesdale (English) faithful one's homestead.
Trudail, Trudale, Trudayl, Trudayle

Truitt (English) little and honest.
Truet, Truett, Truit, Truyt, Truytt

Truman (English) honest. History: Harry S. Truman was the thirty-third U.S. president.
Trueman, Trumain, Trumaine, Trumann

Trumble (English) strong; bold.
Trumbal, Trumball, Trumbel, Trumbell, Trumbul, Trumbull

Trung (Vietnamese) central; loyalty.

Trustin (English) trustworthy.
Trustan, Trusten, Truston

Trygve (Norwegian) brave victor.

Trystan BG (Welsh) a form of Tristan.
Tristynne, Tryistan, Trystann, Trystian, Trystin, Trystion, Trystn, Trystyn

Trysten, Tryston (Welsh) forms of Tristan.

Tsalani (Nguni) good-bye.

Tse (Ewe) younger of twins.

Tsekani (Egyptian) closed.

Tu BG (Vietnamese) tree.

Tuaco (Ghanaian) eleventh-born.

Tuan (Vietnamese) goes smoothly.
Tuane

Tuari (Laguna) young eagle.
Tuarie, Tuary

Tubal (Hebrew) he who tills the soil.

Tubau (Catalan) a form of Teobaldo.

Tucker (English) fuller, tucker of cloth.
Tuck, Tuckar, Tuckie, Tucky, Tuckyr

Tudor (Welsh) a form of Theodore. History: an English ruling dynasty.
Todor, Tudore

Tufic (Lebanese) success.

Tug (Scandinavian) draw, pull.
Tugg

Tuketu (Moquelumnan) bear making dust as it runs.

Tukuli (Moquelumnan) caterpillar crawling down a tree.

Tulio (Italian, Spanish) lively.
Tullio

Tullis (Latin) title, rank.
Tullius, Tullos, Tully, Tullys

Tully BG (Irish) at peace with God. (Latin) a familiar form of Tullis.
Tulea, Tulee, Tuley, Tuli, Tulie, Tull, Tullea, Tullee, Tulley, Tulli, Tullie, Tuly

Tumaini (Mwera) hope.

Tumu (Moquelumnan) deer thinking about eating wild onions.

Tung (Vietnamese) stately, dignified. (Chinese) everyone.

Tungar (Sanskrit) high; lofty.

Tupac (Quechua) the Lord.

Tupacamaru (Quechua) glorious Amaru.

Tupacapac (Quechua) glorious and kind-hearted lord.

Tupacusi (Quechua) happy and majestic.

Tupaquiupanqui, Tupayupanqui
(Quechua) memorable and glorious lord.

Tupi (Moquelumnan) pulled up.
Tupe, Tupee, Tupie, Tupy

Tupper (English) ram raiser.

Turi (Spanish) a short form of Arthur.
Ture

Turk (English) from Turkey.

Turlough (Irish) thunder shaped.
Thorlough, Torlough

Turner (Latin) lathe worker; wood worker.
Terner

Turpin (Scandinavian) Finn named after Thor.
Thorpin, Torpin

Tusya (Russian) surpassing expectations.

Tut (Arabic) strong and courageous. History: a
short form of Tutankhamen, an Egyptian king.
Tutt

Tutu (Spanish) a familiar form of Justin.

Tuvya (Hebrew) a form of Tobias.
Tevya, Tuvia, Tuviah

Tuwile (Mwera) death is inevitable.

Tuxford (Scandinavian) shallow river crossing.
Tuxforde

Tuyen GB (Vietnamese) angel.

Twain (English) divided in two. Literature:
Mark Twain (whose real name was Samuel
Langhorne Clemens) was one of the most
prominent nineteenth-century American
writers.
Tawine, Twaine, Twan, Twane, Tway, Twayn, Twayne

Twia (Fante) born after twins.
Twiah

Twitchell (English) narrow passage.
Twitchel, Twytchel, Twytchell

Twyford (English) double river crossing.
Twiford, Twiforde, Twyforde

Txomin (Basque) like the Lord.

Ty BG (English) a short form of Tyler,
Tyrone, Tyrus.
Ti, Tie

Tybalt (Greek) people's prince.
Tibalt, Tybolt

Tyce (French) a form of Tyson.

Tye (English) a form of Ty.

Tyee (Native American) chief.

Tyger (English) a form of Tiger.
Tige, Tyg, Tygar, Tygger

Tyjuan (American) a form of Tajuan.

Tylar BG (English) a form of Tyler.
Tilar, Tilor, Tyelar, Tylarr, Tylour

Tyler ✵ BG (English) tile maker.
*Tiler, Tyel, Tyeler, Tyelor, Tyhler, Tyle, Tylee,
Tylere, Tyller, Tylyr*

Tylor BG (English) a form of Tyler.

Tymon (Polish) a form of Timothy. (Greek)
a form of Timon.
*Tymain, Tymaine, Tyman, Tymane, Tymeik,
Tymek, Tymen, Tymin, Tymyn*

Tymothy (English) a form of Timothy.
*Tymithy, Tymmothee, Tymmothey, Tymmothi,
Tymmothie, Tymmothy, Tymoteusz, Tymothee,
Tymothi, Tymothie*

Tynan (Irish) dark.
Tinan, Tinane, Tynane

Tynek (Czech) a form of Martin.
Tynko

Tyquan (American) a combination of Ty +
Quan.
*Tykwan, Tykwane, Tykwon, Tyquaan, Tyquane,
Tyquann, Tyquine, Tyquinn, Tyquon, Tyquone,
Tyquwon, Tyqwan*

Tyran, Tyren, Tyrin, Tyron (American)
forms of Tyrone.
*Teiron, Tiron, Tirown, Tyraine, Tyrane, Tyrinn,
Tyrion, Tyrohn, Tyronn, Tyronna, Tyroon,
Tyroun, Tyrown, Tyrrin, Tyryn*

Tyre (Scottish) a form of Tyree.

Tyrece, Tyrese, Tyrice (American) forms of
Tyreese.
Tyreas, Tyresse

Tyree BG (Scottish) island dweller.
Geography: Tiree is an island off the west
coast of Scotland.
Tyra, Tyrae, Tyrai, Tyray, Tyrea, Tyrey, Tyry

Tyrée (Scottish) a form of Tyree.

Tyreek (American) a form of Tyrick.
Tyreik

Tyreese (American) a form of Terrence.
Tyrease, Tyreece, Tyreice, Tyres, Tyriece, Tyriese

Tyrek, Tyrik, Tyriq (American) forms of Tyrick.
Tyreck, Tyreke

Tyrel, Tyrell, Tyrelle (American) forms of Terrell.
Tyrrel, Tyrrell

Tyrez (American) a form of Tyreese.
Tyreze

Tyrick (American) a combination of Ty + Rick.
Tyric, Tyriek, Tyrique

Tyrone (Greek) sovereign. (Irish) land of Owen.
Tayron, Tayrone, Teirone, Tirone, Tirowne, Tyerone, Tyhrone, Tyroney, Tyronne, Tyrowne

Tyrus (English) a form of Thor.
Tirus, Tiruss, Tyruss, Tyryss

Tysen (French) a form of Tyson.

Tyshaun, Tyshon (American) forms of Tyshawn.

Tyshawn (American) a combination of Ty + Shawn.
Tysean, Tyshan, Tyshauwn, Tyshian, Tyshinn, Tyshion, Tyshone, Tyshonne, Tyshun, Tyshunn, Tyshyn

Tyson (French) son of Ty.
Tison, Tiszon, Tycen, Tyesn, Tyeson, Tysie, Tysin, Tysne, Tysone

Tytus (Polish) a form of Titus.
Tytan

Tyus (Polish) a form of Tytus.

Tyvon (American) a combination of Ty + Von. (Hebrew) a form of Tivon.
Tyvan, Tyvin, Tyvinn, Tyvone, Tyvonne

Tywan, Tywon (Chinese) forms of Taiwan.
Tywain, Tywaine, Tywane, Tywann, Tywaun, Tywen, Tywone, Tywonne

Tzadok (Hebrew) righteous. See also Zadok.
Tzadik

Tzion (Hebrew) sign from God. See also Zion.

Tzuriel (Hebrew) God is my rock.
Tzuriya

Tzvi (Hebrew) deer. See also Zevi.
Tzevi

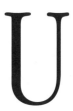

Uaine (Irish) a form of Owen.

Ualtar (Irish) a form of Walter.
Uailtar, Ualteir, Ualter

Ualusi (Tongan) walrus.
Ualusee, Ualusey, Ualusie, Ualusy

Ubadah (Arabic) serves God.
Ubada

Ubaid (Arabic) faithful.

Ubalde (French) a form of Ubaldus.
Ubald, Ubold

Ubaldo (Italian) a form of Ubaldus.
Uboldo

Ubaldus (Teutonic) peace of mind.
Ubaldas, Uboldas, Uboldus

Ubayd (Arabic) faithful.

Ubayda (Arabic) servant of God.

Ubayy (Arabic) boy.

Uberto (Italian) a form of Hubert.

Ucello (Italian) bird.
Uccelo, Ucelo, Uzelo

Uche (Ibo) thought.

Uchu (Quechua) hot like pepper.

Ucumari (Quechua) he who has the strength of a bear.

Udar (Indian) generous.

Uday (Sanskrit) to rise.
Udae, Udai

Udayachal (Indian) eastern horizon.

Udayan (Indian) rising; king of the city of Avanti.

Uddhar (Indian) liberation.

Uddhav (Indian) friend of the Hindu god Krishna.

Udell (English) yew-tree valley. See also Dell, Yudell.
Eudel, Udale, Udall, Udalle, Udel, Udele, Udelle

Udit (Sanskrit) grown; shining.

Udo (Japanese) ginseng plant. (German) a short form of Udolf.

Udolf (English) prosperous wolf.
Udolfe, Udolff, Udolfo, Udolph, Udolphe

Udyam (Indian) effort.

Udyan (Indian) garden.

Ueli (Swiss) noble ruler.
Uelie, Uely

Ueman (Nahuatl) venerable time.

Uetzcayotl (Nahuatl) the essence of light.

Ufa (Egyptian) flower.

Uffo (German) wild bear.
Ufo

Ugo (Italian) a form of Hugh, Hugo.
Ugon

Ugutz (Basque) a form of John.

Uhila (Tongan) lightning.
Uhilah, Uhyla, Uhylah

Uilliam (Irish) a form of William.
Uileog, Uilleam, Ulick

Uinseann (Irish) a form of Vincent.

Uistean (Irish) intelligent.
Uisdean

Uja (Sanskrit) growing.

Ujagar, Ujala, Ujjala, Ujwal (Indian) bright.

Uku (Hawaiian) flea, insect; skilled ukulele player.

Ulan (African) first-born twin.
Ulen, Ulin, Ulon, Ulyn

Ulbrecht (German) a form of Albert.
Ulbright, Ulbryght

Uldric (Lettish) a form of Aldrich.
Uldrick, Uldrics, Uldrik, Uldryc, Uldryck, Uldryk

Uleki (Hawaiian) wrathful.
Ulekee, Ulekie, Uleky

Ulf (German) wolf.
Ulph

Ulfer (German) warrior fierce as a wolf.
Ulpher

Ulfred (German) peaceful wolf.
Ulfrid, Ulfryd, Ulphrid, Ulphryd

Ulfrido (Teutonic) he imposes peace through force.

Ulger (German) warring wolf.
Ulga, Ulgar

Ulhas (Indian) happiness.

Ulices (Latin) a form of Ulysses.

Ulick (Scandinavian) bright, rewarding mind.
Ulic, Ulik, Ulyc, Ulyck, Ulyk

Ulises, Ulisses (Latin) forms of Ulysses.
Ulishes, Ulisse

Ullanta, Ullantay (Aymara) the warrior who sees everything from his watchtower.

Ullivieri (Italian) olive tree.
Ulivieri

Ullock (German) sporting wolf.
Ulloc, Ulloch, Ulloche, Ullok, Ulloke, Uloc, Uloch, Uloche, Ulock, Ulok, Uloke

Ulmer (English) famous wolf.
Ullmar, Ulmar, Ulmor, Ulmore

Ulmo (German) from Ulm, Germany.

Ulpiano, Ulpio (Latin) sly as a fox.

Ulric (German) a form of Ulrich.
Ullric, Ullryc, Ulryc

Ulrich (German) wolf ruler; ruler of all. See also Alaric, Olric.
Uli, Ull, Ullrich, Ullrick, Ullrik, Ullrych, Ullryck, Ullryk, Ulrech, Ulrick, Ulrico, Ulrik, Ulrike, Ulrych, Ulryck, Ulryk, Ulu, Ulz, Uwe

Ultan (German) noble stone.
Ulten, Ultin, Ulton, Ultyn

Ultman (Hindi) god; godlike.

Ulyses (Latin) a form of Ulysses.
Ulysee, Ulysees

Ulysses (Latin) wrathful. A form of Odysseus.
Eulises, Ulysse, Ulyssees, Ulyssius

Umanant, Umakant, Umanand, Umashankar, Umesh (Indian) other names for the Hindu god Shiva.

Umang (Sanskrit) enthusiastic.
Umanga

Umaprasad (Indian) blessing of the Hindu goddess Parvati.

Umar (Arabic) a form of Omar.
Umair, Umarr, Umayr, Umer

Umara (Arabic) a form of Umar.

Umberto (Italian) a form of Humbert.
Umbirto, Umburto, Umbyrto

Umed (Indian) hope.

Umi (Yao) life.
Umee, Umie, Umy

Umit (Turkish) hope.

Umrao (Indian) noble; king.

Unai (Basque) shepherd.
Una

Unay (Quechua) remote, underlying.

Uner (Turkish) famous.

Unika GB (Lomwe) brighten.
Unikah

Unique GB (Latin) only, unique.
Uneek, Unek, Unikque, Uniqué, Unyque

Unity GB (English) unity.
Unitee, Unitey, Uniti, Unitie

Unmesh (Indian) revelation.

Unnat, Urjita (Indian) energized.

Uno (Latin) one; first-born.
Unno

Unwin (English) nonfriend.
Unwinn, Unwyn

Upagupta (Indian) Buddhist monk.

Upamanyu (Indian) devoted pupil.

Upendra (Indian) another name for the Hindu god Vishnu.

Upshaw (English) upper wooded area.

Upton (English) upper town.
Uptown

Upwood (English) upper forest.

Ur, Uratum (Egyptian) great.

Urania (Greek) blind.

Urban (Latin) city dweller; courteous.
Urbain, Urbaine, Urbanus, Urvan, Urvane

Urbane (English) a form of Urban.

Urbano (Italian) a form of Urban.

Urcucolla (Quechua) hill.

Uri BG (Hebrew) a short form of Uriah.
Urie

Uriá (Hebrew) a form of Uriah.

Uriah (Hebrew) my light. Bible: a soldier and the husband of Bathsheba. See also Yuri.
Uria, Urias, Urijah

Urian (Greek) heaven.
Urien, Urihaan, Uryan, Uryen

Urías (Greek) light of the Lord.

Uriel (Hebrew) God is my light.
Yuriel, Yuryel

Urso (Latin) a form of Urson.

Urson (French) a form of Orson.
Ursan, Ursen, Ursin, Ursine, Ursus, Ursyn

Urtzi (Basque) sky.

Urvil (Hindi) sea.
Ervil, Ervyl, Urvyl

Usama (Arabic) a form of Usamah.

Usamah (Arabic) like a lion.

Usco, Uscouiyca, Uscu, Uscuiyca (Quechua) wild cat.

Useni (Yao) tell me.
Usene, Usenet, Usenie, Useny

Usher (English) doorkeeper.
Usha

Usi (Yao) smoke.

Usman (Arabic) a form of Uthman.

Ustin (Russian) a form of Justin.
Ustan, Usten, Uston, Ustyn

Usuy (Quechua) he who brings abundances.

Utatci (Moquelumnan) bear scratching itself.
Utatch

Utba (Arabic) boy.

Uthman (Arabic) companion of the Prophet.
Uthmaan, Uthmen

Uttam (Sanskrit) best.

Uturuncu (Quechua) jaguar.

Uturuncu Achachi (Quechua) he who has brave ancestors.

Uwe (German) a familiar form of Ulrich.

Uxío (Greek) born into nobility.

Uzair (Arabic) helpful.
Uzaire, Uzayr, Uzayre

Uzi (Hebrew) my strength.
Uzee, Uzey, Uzie, Uzy

Uziel (Hebrew) God is my strength; mighty force.
Uzia, Uzyel, Uzzia, Uzziah, Uzziel, Uzzyel

Uzoma (Nigerian) born during a journey.
Uzomah

Uzumati (Moquelumnan) grizzly bear.

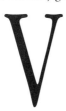

Vachan (Indian) speech.

Vachel (French) small cow.
Vache, Vachell, Vachelle

Vaclav (Czech) wreath of glory.
Vasek

Vadin (Hindi) speaker.
Vaden

Vaibhav (Indian) riches.

Vaijnath (Indian) another name for the Hindu god Shiva.

Vail 🅱🄶 (English) valley. See also Bail.
Vael, Vaiel, Vaile, Vaill, Vale, Valle, Vayel, Vayl, Vayle

Vaina (Finnish) river's mouth.
Vainah, Vaino, Vayna, Vaynah, Vayno

Vajra (Indian) great-grandson of the Hindu god Krishna; diamond.

Vajradhar, Vajrapani (Indian) other names of the Hindu god Indra.

Val 🅱🄶 (Latin) a short form of Valentin.
Vaal

Valarico (Germanic) leader of the battle.

Valborg (Swedish) mighty mountain.
Valbor

Valdemar (Swedish) famous ruler.
Valdimar, Valdymar, Vlademar

Valdo (Teutonic) he who governs.

Valdus (German) powerful.
Valdis, Valdys

Valente (Italian) a form of Valentin.
Valenté

Valentin (Latin) strong; healthy.
Valentijn, Valentine, Valenton, Valenty, Valentyn, Valentyne

Valentín (Latin) a form of Valentin.

Valentino (Italian) a form of Valentin.
Valencio, Valentyno, Velentino

Valere (French) a form of Valerian.

Valerian (Latin) strong; healthy.
Valeriano, Valerio, Valerius, Valerya, Valeryan, Valeryn

Valerii (Russian) a form of Valerian.
Valera, Valerie, Valerij, Valerik, Valeriy, Valery

Valero (Latin) valiant.

Valfredo (Germanic) the peaceful king.

Valfrid (Swedish) strong peace.

Valgard (Scandinavian) foreign spear.
Valgarde, Valguard

Vali (Tongan) paint.
Valea, Valee, Valeigh, Valey, Valie, Valy

Valiant (French) valiant.

Valin (Hindi) a form of Balin.
Valan, Valen, Valon, Valyn

Vallabh (Indian) beloved.

Vallis (French) from Wales.
Valis, Vallys, Valys

Valmik, Valmiki (Indian) author of the Indian epic poem *Ramayana*.

Valter (Lithuanian, Swedish) a form of Walter.
Valters, Valther, Valtr

Vaman (Indian) fifth incarnation of the Hindu god Vishnu.

Vamana (Sanskrit) praiseworthy.
Vamanah

Vamsi (Indian) name of a raga, an ancient form of Hindu devotional music.

Van BG (Dutch) a short form of Vandyke.
Vane, Vanno

Vanajit (Indian) lord of the forest.

Vance (English) thresher.
Vanse

Vanda GB (Lithuanian) a form of Walter.
Vandah, Venda

Vandan (Hindi) saved.
Vanden, Vandin, Vandon, Vandyn

Vander (Dutch) belongs.
Vandar, Vandir, Vandor, Vandyr, Vendar, Vender, Vendir, Vendor, Vendyr

Vandyke (Dutch) dyke.
Vandike

Vann (Dutch) a short form of Vandyke.

Vanya BG (Russian) a familiar form of Ivan.
Vanechka, Vanek, Vania, Vanja, Vanka, Vanusha, Vanyah, Wanya

Vanyusha (Russian) gift from God.

Varad (Hungarian) from the fortress.
Vared, Varid, Varod, Varyd

Vardhaman (Indian) another name for Mahavir, the twenty-fourth and last Tirthankar, a type of Jain god.

Vardon (French) green knoll.
Vardaan, Vardan, Varden, Vardin, Vardon, Vardyn, Verdan, Verden, Verdin, Verdon, Verdun, Verdyn

Varen (Hindi) better.
Varan, Varin, Varon, Varyn

Varian (Latin) variable.
Varien, Varion, Varyan

Varick (German) protecting ruler.
Varak, Varek, Varic, Varik, Varyc, Varyck, Varyk, Warrick

Varij (Indian) lotus.

Varil (Hindi) water.
Varal, Varel, Varol, Varyl

Varindra (Indian) another name for the Hindu god Varun, lord of the waters.

Vartan (Armenian) rose producer; rose giver.
Varten, Vartin, Varton, Vartyn

Varun (Hindi) rain god.
Varan, Varen, Varin, Varon, Varron, Varyn

Vasant (Sanskrit) spring.
Vasan, Vasanth

Vashawn (American) a combination of the prefix Va + Shawn.
Vashae, Vashan, Vashann, Vashaun, Vashawnn, Vashun

Vashon (American) a form of Vashawn.
Vishon

Vasilios (Italian) a form of Vasilis.
Vasileios, Vasilos, Vassilios

Vasilis (Greek) a form of Basil.
Vas, Vasaya, Vaselios, Vasil, Vasile, Vasileior, Vasilius, Vasilus, Vasily, Vasilys, Vasylis, Vasylko, Vasyltso, Vasylys, Vazul

Vasily (Russian) a form of Vasilis.
Vasilea, Vasilee, Vasileigh, Vasiley, Vasili, Vasilie, Vasilii, Vasilije, Vasilik, Vasiliy, Vassilea, Vassilee, Vassileigh, Vassiley, Vassili, Vassilie, Vassilij, Vassily, Vasya

Vasin (Hindi) ruler, lord.
Vasan, Vasen, Vason, Vasun, Vasyn

Vasishtha, Vasistha (Indian) an ancient Indian sage.

Vasu (Sanskrit) wealth.

Vasudev (Indian) father of the Hindu god Krishna.

Vasudha (Indian) earth.

Vasyl (German, Slavic) a form of William.
Vasos, Vassos

Vatsal (Indian) affectionate.

Vaughan (Welsh) a form of Vaughn.
Vaughen

Vaughn (Welsh) small.
Vaun, Vaune, Vawn, Vawne, Voughn

Veasna (Cambodian) lucky.
Veasnah

Ved (Sanskrit) sacred knowledge.

Vedanga (Indian) meaning of Vedas, Hindu scriptures.

Vedavrata (Indian) vow of the Vedas, Hindu scriptures.

Vedie (Latin) sight.
Vedi, Vedy

Vedmohan (Indian) another name for the Hindu god Krishna.

Vedprakash (Indian) light of the Vedas, Hindu scriptures.

Veer (Sanskrit) brave.
Vear, Veere

Veera (Indian) brave.

Vegard (Norwegian) sanctuary; protection.

Veiko (Finnish) brother.
Veyko

Veit (Swedish) wide.
Veyt

Velvel (Yiddish) wolf.

Venancio (Latin) a fan of hunting.

Vencel (Hungarian) a short form of Wenceslaus.
Vencal, Venci, Vencie, Vencil, Vencyl

Venceslao (Slavic) crowned with glory.

Venedictos (Greek) a form of Benedict.
Venedict, Venediktos, Venedyct

Veni (Indian) another name for the Hindu god Krishna.

Veniamin (Bulgarian) a form of Benjamin.
Venyamin, Verniamin

Venkat (Hindi) god; godlike. Religion: another name for the Hindu god Vishnu.

Ventura (Latin) he who will be happy.

Venturo (Spanish) good fortune.

Venya (Russian) a familiar form of Benedict.
Venka

Verdun (French) fort on a hill. Geography: a city in France and in Quebec, Canada.
Virdun, Vyrdun

Vere (Latin, French) true.
Veir, Ver, Vir, Vyr

Vered (Hebrew) rose.
Verad, Verid, Verod, Veryd

Vergil (Latin) a form of Virgil. Literature: a Roman poet best known for his epic poem *Aenid*.
Verge, Vergel, Vergill, Vergille

Verlin (Latin) blooming.
Verlain, Verlan, Verlinn, Verlion, Verlon, Verlyn, Verlynn

Vermundo (Spanish) protective bear.
Vermond, Vermondo, Vermund

Vern (Latin) a short form of Vernon.
Verna, Vernal, Verne, Vernine, Vernis, Vernol, Virn, Virne, Vyrn, Vyrne

Vernados (German) courage of the bear.

Vernell (Latin) a form of Vernon.
Verneal, Vernel, Vernelle, Vernial

Verner (German) defending army.
Varner

Verney (French) alder grove.
Varney, Vernee, Verni, Vernie, Verny, Virnee, Virney, Virni, Virnie, Virny, Vurnee, Vurney, Vurni, Vurnie, Vurny, Vyrnee, Vyrney, Vyrni, Vyrnie, Vyrny

Vernon (Latin) springlike; youthful.
Varnan, Vernen, Vernin, Vernun, Vernyn

Vero (Latin) truthful, credible.

Verrill (German) masculine. (French) loyal.
Veral, Verall, Veril, Verill, Verral, Verrall, Verrell, Verroll, Veryl, Veryll

Vespasiano (Latin) the name of a Roman emperor.

Veston (English) church town.
Vestan, Vesten, Vestin, Vestun, Vestyn

Veto (Spanish) intelligent.

Vian (English) a short form of Vivian (see Girls' Names).

Vibert (American) a combination of Vic + Bert.
Viberte, Vybert, Vyberte

Vic (Latin) a short form of Victor.
Vick, Vicken, Vickenson, Vik, Vyc, Vyck, Vyk, Vykk

Vicar (Latin) priest, cleric.
Vickar, Vicker, Vickor, Vikar, Vycar, Vyckar, Vykar

Vicente (Spanish) a form of Vincent.
Vicent, Visente

Vicenzo (Italian) a form of Vincent.

Victoir (French) a form of Victor.

Victor (Latin) victor, conqueror. See also Wikoli, Wiktor, Witek.
Victa, Victer, Victorien, Victorin, Vitin, Vyctor

Víctor (Spanish) a form of Victor.

Victoriano (Spanish) a form of Victor.

Victorio (Spanish) a form of Victor.
Victorino

Victormanuel (Spanish) a combination of Victor + Manuel.

Victoro (Latin) a form of Victor.

Vidal BG (Spanish) a form of Vitas.
Vida, Vidale, Vidall, Videll, Vydal, Vydall

Vidar (Norwegian) tree warrior.

Videl (Spanish) a form of Vidal.

Vidor (Hungarian) cheerful.
Vidoor, Vidore, Vydor

Vidur (Hindi) wise.

Vidya (Sanskrit) wise.
Vidyah, Vydya, Vydyah

Viet (Vietnamese) Vietnamese.

Vigberto (Germanic) one who shines in battle.

Viho (Cheyenne) chief.

Vijai (Hindi) a form of Vijay.

Vijay (Hindi) victorious.

Vikas (Hindi) growing.
Vikash, Vikesh

Viking (Scandinavian) Viking; Scandinavian.
Vikin, Vykin, Vyking, Vykyn, Vykyng

Vikram (Hindi) valorous.
Vikrum

Vikrant (Hindi) powerful.
Vikran

Viktor (German, Hungarian, Russian) a form of Victor.
Viktoras, Viktors, Vyktor

Vilfredo (Germanic) the peaceful king.

Vilhelm (German) a form of William.
Vilhelms, Vilho, Vilis, Viljo, Villem

Vili (Hungarian) a short form of William.
Villy, Vilmos

Viliam (Czech) a form of William.
Vila, Vilek, Vilém, Viliami, Viliamu, Vilko, Vilous

Viljo (Finnish) a form of William.

Ville (Swedish) a short form of William.

Vimal (Hindi) pure.
Vylmal

Vin (Latin) a short form of Vincent.
Vinn

Vinay (Hindi) polite.
Vynah

Vince (English) a short form of Vincent.
Vence, Vinse, Vint, Vynce, Vynse

Vincens (German) a form of Vincent.
Vincents, Vincentz, Vincenz

Vincent BG (Latin) victor, conqueror. See also Binkentios, Binky, Wincent.
Uinseann, Vencent, Vicenzo, Vikent, Vikenti, Vikesha, Vincence, Vincentij, Vincentius, Vincenty, Vincien, Vincient, Vincint, Vinicent, Vinsent, Vinsint, Vinsynt, Vyncent, Vyncynt, Vyncynte, Vynsynt

Vincente (Spanish) a form of Vincent.
Vencente, Vinciente, Vinsynte, Vyncente

Vincenzo (Italian) a form of Vincent.
Vincencio, Vincenza, Vincenzio, Vinchenzo, Vinezio, Vinzenz

Vinci (Hungarian, Italian) a familiar form of Vincent.
Vinci, Vinco, Vincze

Vinny (English) a familiar form of Calvin, Melvin, Vincent.
Vinnee, Vinney, Vinni, Vinnie, Vynni, Vynnie, Vynny, Vyny

Vinod (Hindi) happy, joyful.
Vinodh, Vinood

Vinson (English) son of Vincent.
Vinnis, Vinsan, Vinsen, Vinsin, Vinsun, Vinsyn, Vyncen, Vyncyn, Vynsan, Vynsen, Vynsin, Vynson, Vynsun, Vynsyn

Vipul (Hindi) plentiful.

Viraj (Hindi) resplendent.

Virat (Hindi) very big.

Virgil (Latin) rod bearer, staff bearer.
Virge, Virgial, Virgie, Virgille, Virgilo, Vurgil, Vurgyl, Vyrge, Vyrgil, Vyrgyl

Virgilio (Spanish) a form of Virgil.
Virjilio

Virginio (Latin) he is pure and simple.

Virote (Tai) strong, powerful.

Virxilio (Latin) a form of Virgil.

Vishal (Hindi) huge; great.
Vishaal

Vishnu (Hindi) protector.

Vitaliano, Vitalicio (Latin) young and strong.

Vitalis (Latin) life; alive.
Vital, Vitale, Vitaliss, Vitalys, Vitalyss, Vytal, Vytalis, Vytalys

Vitas (Latin) alive, vital.
Vitis, Vitus, Vytas, Vytus

Vito (Latin) a short form of Vittorio.
Veit, Vitin, Vitto, Vyto, Vytto

Vítor (Latin) a form of Victor.

Vitoriano (Latin) the victor.

Vittorio (Italian) a form of Victor.
Vitor, Vitorio, Vittore, Vittorios

Vitya (Russian) a form of Victor.
Vitia, Vitja

Vivek (Hindi) wisdom.
Vivekinan

Viviano (Spanish) small man.

Vlad (Russian) a short form of Vladimir, Vladislav.
Vladd, Vladik, Vladko

Vladimir (Russian) famous prince. See also Dima, Waldemar, Walter.
Bladimir, Vimka, Vladamar, Vladamir, Vladimar, Vladimeer, Vladimer, Vladimere, Vladimire, Vladimyr, Vladjimir, Vladlen, Vladmir, Vladymar, Vladymer, Vladymir, Vladymyr, Volodimir, Volodya, Volya, Wladimir

Vladimiro (Spanish) a form of Vladimir.

Vladislav (Slavic) glorious ruler. See also Slava.
Vladya, Vladyslau, Vladyslav, Vlasislava, Wladislav

Vlas (Russian) a short form of Vladislav.

Vogel (German) bird.
Vogal, Vogil, Vogol, Vogyl

Volker (German) people's guard.
Folke

Volley (Latin) flying.
Volea, Volee, Voleigh, Voley, Voli, Volie, Vollea, Vollee, Volleigh, Volli, Vollie, Volly, Voly

Volney (German) national spirit.
Volnee, Volni, Volnie, Volny

Von (German) a short form of many German names. (Welsh) a form of Vaughn.
Vonn

Vova (Russian) a form of Walter.
Vovah, Vovka

Vuai (Swahili) savior.

Vulpiano (Latin) sly as a fox.

Vyacheslav (Russian) a form of Vladislav. See also Slava.

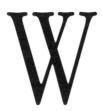

Wa`El (Arabic) one who goes toward salvation.

Waban (Ojibwa) white.
Waben, Wabin, Wabon, Wabyn

Wade (English) ford; river crossing.
Wad, Wadi, Wadie, Waed, Waede, Waid, Waide, Whaid

Wâdî (Arabic) calm, peaceful.

Wadih (Lebanese) alone.

Wadley (English) ford meadow.
Wadlea, Wadlee, Wadlei, Wadleigh, Wadli, Wadlie, Wadly

Wadsworth (English) village near the ford.
Waddsworth, Wadesworth

Wael (English) a form of Wales.

Wafic (Lebanese) arbitrator.

Wafîq (Arabic) successful.

Wagner (German) wagoner, wagon maker. Music: Richard Wagner was a famous nineteenth-century German composer.
Waggoner, Wagnar, Wagnor, Wagoner

Wahab (Indian) large-hearted.

Wâhed (Arabic) a form of Wahid.

Wahid (Arabic) single; exclusively unequaled.
Waheed, Wahyd

Wahkan (Lakota) sacred.

Wahkoowah (Lakota) charging.

Wain (English) a short form of Wainwright. A form of Wayne.
Waine, Wane

Wainwright (English) wagon maker.
Wainright, Wainryght, Wayneright, Waynewright, Waynright, Waynryght

Waite (English) watchman.
Wait, Waitman, Waiton, Waits, Wayt, Wayte

Wajidali (Indian) obsessed.

Wake (English) awake, alert.
Waik, Waike, Wayk, Wayke

Wakefield (English) wet field.
Field, Waikfield, Waykfield

Wakely (English) wet meadow.
Wakelea, Wakelee, Wakelei, Wakeleigh, Wakeli, Wakelie, Wakely

Wakeman (English) watchman.

Wakîl (Arabic) lawyer.

Wakiza (Native American) determined warrior.
Wakyza

Walberto (Germanic) one who remains in power.

Walby (English) house near a wall.
Walbee, Walbey, Walbi, Walbie

Walcott (English) cottage by the wall.
Walcot, Wallcot, Wallcott, Wolcott

Waldemar (German) powerful; famous. See also Valdemar, Vladimir.
Waldermar

Walden (English) wooded valley. Literature: Henry David Thoreau made Walden Pond famous with his book *Walden*.
Waldan, Waldin, Waldon, Waldyn, Welti

Waldino (Teutonic) having an open and bold spirit.

Waldo (German) a familiar form of Oswald, Waldemar, Walden.
Wald, Waldy

Waldron (English) ruler.
Waldran, Waldren, Waldrin, Waldryn

Waleed (Arabic) newborn.
Walead, Waled, Waleyd, Walyd

Walerian (Polish) strong; brave.
Waleryan

Wales (English) from Wales.
Wail, Whales

Walford (English) Welshman's ford.

Walfred (German) peaceful ruler.
Walfredd, Walfredo, Walfrid, Walfridd, Walfried, Walfryd, Walfrydd

Wali (Arabic) all-governing.

Walid (Arabic) a form of Waleed.

Walîd (Arabic) a form of Walid.

Walker BG (English) cloth walker; cloth cleaner.

Wallace (English) from Wales.
Wallas

Wallach (German) a form of Wallace.
Wallache, Walloch, Waloch

Waller (German) powerful. (English) wall maker.
Waler

Wallis GB (English) a form of Wallace.
Walice, Walise, Wallice, Wallise, Wallyce, Wallyse, Walyce, Walyse

Wally (English) a familiar form of Walter.
Walea, Walee, Waleigh, Waley, Wali, Walie, Wallea, Wallee, Walleigh, Walley, Walli, Wallie, Waly

Walmond (German) mighty ruler.

Walsh (English) a form of Wallace.
Walshi, Walshie, Walshy, Welch

Walt (English) a short form of Walter, Walton.
Waltey, Waltli, Walty

Walter (German) army ruler, general. (English) woodsman. See also Gautier, Gualberto, Gualtiero, Gutierre, Ladislav, Ualtar, Vladimir.
Valter, Vanda, Vova, Walder, Waltir, Waltli, Waltor, Waltyr, Wat, Wualter

Walther (German) a form of Walter.

Waltier (French) a form of Walter.
Waltyer

Walton (English) walled town.
Waltan, Walten, Waltin, Waltyn

Waltr (Czech) a form of Walter.

Walworth (English) fenced-in farm.
Wallsworth, Wallworth, Walsworth

Walwyn (English) Welsh friend.
Walwin, Walwinn, Walwynn, Walwynne, Welwyn

Wamblee (Lakota) eagle.
Wamblea, Wambleigh, Wambley, Wambli, Wamblie, Wambly

Wanbi (Australian) wild dingo.
Wanbee, Wanbey, Wanbie, Wanby

Wanda (Germanic) boss of the hoodlums.

Wang (Chinese) hope; wish.

Wanikiya (Lakota) savior.
Wanikiyah

Wanya (Russian) a form of Vanya.
Wanyai

Wapi (Native American) lucky.
Wapie, Wapy

Warburton (English) fortified town.

Ward (English) watchman, guardian.
Warde

Wardell (English) watchman's hill.
Wardel

Warden (English) valley guardian.
Wardan, Wardin, Wardon, Wardun, Wardyn, Worden

Wardley (English) watchman's meadow.
Wardlea, Wardlee, Wardleigh, Wardli, Wardlie, Wardly

Ware (English) wary, cautious. (German) a form of Warren.
Warey

Warfield (English) field near the weir or fish trap.
Warfyeld

Warford (English) ford near the weir or fish trap.

Warick (English) town hero.
Waric, Warik, Warric, Warrick, Warrik, Warryc, Warryck, Warryk, Waryc, Waryck, Waryk

Warley (English) meadow near the weir or fish trap.
Warlea, Warlee, Warlei, Warleigh, Warli, Warlie, Warly

Warmond (English) true guardian.
Warmon, Warmondo, Warmun, Warmund, Warmundo

Warner (German) armed defender. (French) park keeper.
Warnor

Warren (German) general; warden; rabbit hutch.
Waran, Waren, Waring, Warran, Warrenson, Warrin, Warriner, Warron, Warrun, Warryn, Worrin

Warton (English) town near the weir or fish trap.
Wartan, Warten, Wartin, Wartyn

Warwick (English) buildings near the weir or fish trap.
Warick, Warrick, Warwic, Warwik, Warwyc, Warwyck, Warwyk

Waseem (Arabic) a form of Wasim.
Wasseem

Washburn (English) overflowing river.
Washbern, Washberne, Washbirn, Washbirne, Washborn, Washborne, Washbourn, Washbourne, Washburne, Washbyrn, Washbyrne

Washington (English) town near water. History: George Washington was the first U.S. president.
Wash, Washingtan, Washingten, Washingtin, Washingyn

Wasili (Russian) a form of Basil.
Wasily, Wassily, Wassyly, Wasyl, Wasyly

Wasim (Arabic) graceful; good-looking.
Wassim, Wasym

Wâsim (Arabic) a form of Wasim.

Watende (Nyakyusa) there will be revenge.
Watend

Waterio (Spanish) a form of Walter.
Gualtiero

Watford (English) wattle ford; dam made of twigs and sticks.
Wattford

Watkins (English) son of Walter.
Watkin, Watkyn, Watkyns, Wattkin, Wattkins, Wattkyn, Wattkyns

Watson (English) son of Walter.
Wathson, Wattson, Whatson

Waverly GB (English) quaking aspen-tree meadow.
Waverlea, Waverlee, Waverleigh, Waverley, Waverli, Waverlie

Wayde (English) a form of Wade.
Wayd, Waydell

Wayland (English) a form of Waylon.
Wailand, Waland, Weiland, Weyland

Waylon (English) land by the road.
Wailan, Wailon, Walan, Wallen, Walon, Way, Waylan, Waylen, Waylin, Waylyn, Whalan, Whalen, Whalin, Whalon, Whalyn

Wayman (English) road man; traveler.
Waymon

Wayne (English) wagon maker. A short form of Wainwright.
Wanye, Wayn, Waynell, Waynne, Whayne

Wazir (Arabic) minister.
Wazyr

Wazîr (Arabic) a form of Wazir.

Webb (English) weaver.
Web, Weeb

Weber (German) weaver.
Webber, Webner

Webley (English) weaver's meadow.
Webblea, Webblee, Webbleigh, Webbley, Webbli, Webblie, Webbly, Weblea, Weblee, Webleigh, Webli, Weblie, Webly

Webster (English) weaver.
Webstar

Weddel (English) valley near the ford.
Weddell, Wedel, Wedell

Wei-Quo (Chinese) ruler of the country.
Wei

Weiss (German) white.
Weis, Weise, Weisse, Weys, Weyse, Weyss, Weysse

Welborne (English) spring-fed stream.
Welbern, Welberne, Welbirn, Welbirne, Welborn, Welbourne, Welburn, Welburne, Welbyrn, Welbyrne, Wellbern, Wellberne, Wellbirn, Wellbirne, Wellborn, Wellborne, Wellbourn, Wellbourne, Wellburn, Wellbyrn, Wellbyrne

Welby (German) farm near the well.
Welbee, Welbey, Welbi, Welbie, Wellbey, Wellby

Weldon (English) hill near the well.
Weldan, Welden, Weldin, Weldyn

Welfel (Yiddish) a form of William.
Welvel

Welford (English) ford near the well.
Wellford

Wellington (English) rich man's town.
History: the Duke of Wellington was the
British general who defeated Napoleon at
Waterloo.
Wellinton

Wells (English) springs.
Welles, Wels

Welsh (English) a form of Wallace, Walsh.
Welch

Welton (English) town near the well.
*Welltan, Wellten, Welltin, Wellton, Welltyn,
Weltan, Welten, Weltin, Weltyn*

Wemilat (Native American) all give to him.

Wemilo (Native American) all speak to him.

Wen (Gypsy) born in winter.

Wenceslaus (Slavic) wreath of honor.
Vencel, Wenceslao, Wenceslas, Wiencyslaw

Wendel (German, English) a form of
Wendell.

Wendell (German) wanderer. (English) good
dale, good valley.
*Wandale, Wendall, Wendil, Wendill, Wendle,
Wendyl, Wendyll*

Wene (Hawaiian) a form of Wayne.

Wenford (English) white ford.
Wynford

Wenlock (Welsh) monastery lake.
Wenloc, Wenloch, Wenlok

Wensley (English) clearing in a meadow.
*Wenslea, Wenslee, Wensleigh, Wensli, Wenslie,
Wensly*

Wentworth (English) pale man's settlement.

Wenutu (Native American) clear sky.

Wenzel (Slavic) knowing. A form of
Wenceslaus.
Wensel, Wensyl, Wenzell, Wenzil

Werner (English) a form of Warner.
Wernhar, Wernher

Wes (English) a short form of Wesley.
Wess

Wesh (Gypsy) woods.

Wesley ☆⚹ (English) western meadow.
*Weseley, Wesle, Weslea, Weslee, Wesleigh,
Wesleyan, Wesli, Weslie, Wessley, Wezley*

Wesly (English) a form of Wesley.

West (English) west. A short form of
Weston.

Westbrook (English) western brook.
Brook, Wesbrook, Wesbrooke, Westbrooke

Westby (English) western farmstead.
*Wesbee, Wesbey, Wesbi, Wesbie, Westbee,
Westbey, Westbi, Westbie*

Westcott (English) western cottage.
Wescot, Wescott, Westcot

Westin (English) a form of Weston.

Westley (English) a form of Wesley.
Westlee, Westleigh, Westly

Weston (English) western town.
Westan, Westen, Westyn

Wetherby (English) wether-sheep farm.
*Weatherbey, Weatherbie, Weatherby, Wetherbey,
Wetherbi, Wetherbie*

Wetherell (English) wether-sheep corner.
*Wetheral, Wetherall, Wetherel, Wetheril,
Wetherill, Wetheryl, Wetheryll*

Wetherly (English) wether-sheep meadow.
*Wetherlea, Wetherlee, Wetherleigh, Wetherley,
Wetherli, Wetherlie*

Weylin (English) a form of Waylon.
*Weilin, Weilyn, Weylan, Weylen, Weylon,
Weylyn*

Whalley (English) woods near a hill.
*Whalea, Whalee, Whaleigh, Whaley, Whali,
Whalie, Whallea, Whallee, Whalleigh, Whalli,
Whallie, Whally, Whaly*

Wharton (English) town on the bank of a lake.
Warton

Wheatley (English) wheat field.
Whatlea, Whatlee, Whatleigh, Whatley, Whatli, Whatlie, Whatly, Wheatlea, Wheatlee, Wheatleigh, Wheatli, Wheatlie, Wheatly

Wheaton (English) wheat town.
Wheatan, Wheaten, Wheatin, Wheatyn

Wheeler (English) wheel maker; wagon driver.
Wheelar

Whistler (English) whistler, piper.

Whit (English) a short form of Whitman, Whitney.
Whitt, Whyt, Whyte, Wit, Witt

Whitby (English) white house.
Whitbea, Whitbee, Whitbey, Whitbi, Whitbie

Whitcomb (English) white valley.
Whitcombe, Whitcumb, Whytcomb, Whytcombe

Whitelaw (English) small hill.
Whitlaw, Whytlaw

Whitey (English) white skinned; white haired.
Whitee, Whiti, Whitie, Whity

Whitfield (English) white field.
Whytfield

Whitford (English) white ford.
Whytford

Whitley GB (English) white meadow.
Whitlea, Whitlee, Whitleigh, Whitli, Whitlie, Whitly

Whitlock (English) white lock of hair.
Whitloc, Whitloch, Whitlok, Whytloc, Whytloch, Whytlock, Whytlok

Whitman (English) white-haired man.
Whit, Whitmen, Whytman, Whytmen

Whitmore (English) white moor.
Whitmoor, Whitmoore, Whittemoor, Whittemoore, Whittemore, Whytmoor, Whytmoore, Whytmore, Whyttmoor, Whyttmoore, Witmoor, Witmoore, Witmore, Wittemore, Wittmoor, Wittmoore, Wittmore, Wytmoor, Wytmoore, Wytmore, Wyttmoor, Wyttmoore, Wyttmore

Whitney GB (English) white island; white water.
Whittney, Whytnew, Whyttney, Widney, Widny

Whittaker (English) white field.
Whitacker, Whitaker, Whitmaker, Whytaker, Whyttaker

Wicasa (Dakota) man.
Wicasah

Wicent (Polish) a form of Vincent.
Wicek, Wicus

Wichado (Native American) willing.

Wickham (English) village enclosure.
Wick, Wikham, Wyckham, Wykham

Wickley (English) village meadow.
Wicklea, Wicklee, Wickleigh, Wickli, Wicklie, Wickly, Wilcley, Wycklea, Wycklee, Wyckleigh, Wyckley, Wyckli, Wycklie, Wyckly, Wyklea, Wyklee, Wykleigh, Wykley, Wykli, Wyklie, Wykly

Wid (English) wide.
Wido, Wyd, Wydo

Wies (German) renowned warrior.
Wiess, Wyes, Wyess

Wikoli (Hawaiian) a form of Victor.

Wiktor (Polish) a form of Victor.
Wyktor

Wil, Will (English) short forms of Wilfred, William.
Wilm, Wim, Wyl, Wyll

Wilanu (Moquelumnan) pouring water on flour.
Wylanu

Wilber (English) a form of Wilbur.

Wilbert (German) brilliant; resolute.
Wilberto, Wilbirt, Wilburt, Wilbyrt, Wylbert, Wylbirt, Wylburt, Wylbyrt

Wilbur (English) wall fortification; bright willows.
Wilburn, Wilburne, Willber, Willbur, Wilver, Wylber, Wylbir, Wylbur, Wylbyr, Wyllber, Wyllbir, Wyllbur

Wilder (English) wilderness, wild.
Wilde, Wylde, Wylder

Wildon (English) wooded hill.
Wildan, Wilden, Wildin, Wildyn, Willdan, Willden, Willdin, Willdon, Willdyn, Wyldan, Wylden, Wyldin, Wyldon, Wyldyn, Wylldan, Wyllden, Wylldin, Wylldon, Wylldyn

Wile (Hawaiian) a form of Willie.

Wiley (English) willow meadow; Will's meadow. See also Wylie.
Whiley, Wildy, Wilea, Wilee, Wileigh, Wili, Wilie, Willey, Wily

Wilford (English) willow-tree ford.
Wilferd, Willford, Wylford, Wyllford

Wilfred (German) determined peacemaker.
Wilferd, Wilfrid, Wilfride, Wilfried, Wilfryd, Willfred, Willfrid, Willfried, Willfryd

Wilfredo, Wilfrido (Spanish) forms of Wilfred.
Fredo, Wifredo, Willfredo

Wilhelm (German) determined guardian.
Wilhelmus, Wylhelm, Wyllhelm

Wiliama (Hawaiian) a form of William.
Pila

Wilkie (English) a familiar form of Wilkins.
Wikie, Wilke

Wilkins (English) William's kin.
Wilken, Wilkens, Wilkes, Wilkin, Wilks, Willkes, Willkins, Wylkin, Wylkins, Wylkyn, Wylkyns

Wilkinson (English) son of little William.
Wilkenson, Willkinson, Wylkenson, Wylkinson, Wylkynson

Willard (German) determined and brave.
Wilard, Williard, Wylard, Wyllard

Willem (German) a form of Wilhelm, William.
Willim

William ☀ 🅱🅶 (English) a form of Wilhelm. See also Gilamu, Guglielmo, Guilherme, Guillaume, Guillermo, Gwilym, Liam, Uilliam.
Bill, Billy, Vasyl, Vilhelm, Vili, Viliam, Viljo, Ville, Villiam, Wilek, Wiliam, Wiliame, Willaim, Willam, Willeam, Willil, Willium, Williw, Willyam, Wyliam, Wylliam, Wyllyam, Wylyam

Williams (German) son of William.
Wilams, Wiliamson, Willaims, Williamson, Wuliams, Wyliams, Wyliamson, Wylliams, Wylliamson, Wyllyams, Wylyams

Willie 🅱🅶 (German) a familiar form of William.
Wille, Willea, Willee, Willeigh, Willey, Willi, Willia, Wily, Wyllea, Wyllee, Wylleigh, Wylley, Wylli, Wyllie, Wylly

Willis (German) son of Willie.
Wilis, Willice, Williss, Willus, Wylis, Wyliss, Wyllis, Wylys, Wylyss

Willoughby (English) willow farm.
Willobee, Willobey, Willoughbey, Willoughbie, Willowbee, Willowbey, Willowbie, Willowby, Wyllowbee, Wyllowbey, Wyllowbi, Wyllowbie, Wyllowby, Wylobee, Wylobey, Wylobi, Wylobie, Wyloby

Wills (English) son of Will.

Willy (German) a familiar form of William.

Wilmer (German) determined and famous.
Willimar, Willmer, Wilm, Wilmar, Wylmar, Wylmer

Wilmot (Teutonic) resolute spirit.
Willmont, Willmot, Wilm, Wilmont, Wilmott, Wylmot, Wylmott

Wilny (Native American) eagle singing while flying.
Wilni, Wilnie, Wylni, Wylnie, Wylny

Wilson (English) son of Will.
Willsan, Willsen, Willsin, Willson, Willsyn, Wilsan, Wilsen, Wilsin, Wilsyn, Wolson, Wyllsan, Wyllsen, Wyllsin, Wyllson, Wyllsyn, Wylsan, Wylsen, Wylsin, Wylson, Wylsyn

Wilstan (German) wolf stone.
Wilsten, Wilstin, Wilstyn, Wylstan, Wylsten, Wylstin, Wylstyn

Wilt (English) a short form of Wilton.

Wilton (English) farm by the spring.
Willtan, Willten, Willtin, Willton, Willtyn, Wiltan, Wilten, Wiltin, Wiltyn, Wylltan, Wyllten, Wylltin, Wyllton, Wylltyn, Wyltan, Wylten, Wyltin, Wylton, Wyltyn

Wilu (Moquelumnan) chicken hawk squawking.

Win 🅱🅶 (Cambodian) bright. (English) a short form of Winston and names ending in "win."
Winn, Winnie, Winny

Wincent (Polish) a form of Vincent.
Wicek, Wicenty, Wicus, Wince, Wincenty

Winchell (English) bend in the road; bend in the land.
Winchel, Wynchel, Wynchell

Windell (English) windy valley.
Windel, Wyndel, Wyndell

Windsor (English) riverbank with a winch. History: the surname of the British royal family.
Wincer, Windsar, Windser, Winsor, Wyndsar, Wyndser, Wyndsor

Winfield (English) friendly field.
Field, Winfrey, Winifield, Winnfield, Wynfield, Wynnfield

Winfred (English) a form of Winfield. (German) a form of Winfried.
Winfredd, Wynfred, Wynfredd

Winfried (German) friend of peace.
Winfrid, Winfryd, Wynfrid, Wynfryd

Wing 🅶🅱 (Chinese) glory.
Wing-Chiu, Wing-Kit

Wingate (English) winding gate.
Wyngate

Wingi (Native American) willing.
Wingee, Wingie, Wingy, Wyngi, Wyngie, Wyngy

Winslow (English) friend's hill.
Winslowe, Wynslow, Wynslowe

Winston (English) friendly town; victory town.
Winstan, Winsten, Winstin, Winstonn, Winstyn, Wynstan, Wynsten, Wynstin, Wynston, Wynstyn

Winter 🅶🅱 (English) born in winter.
Winterford, Winters, Wynter, Wynters

Winthrop (English) victory at the crossroads.
Wynthrop

Winton (English) a form of Winston.

Winward (English) friend's guardian; friend's forest.
Wynward

Wit (Polish) life. (English) a form of Whit. (Flemish) a short form of DeWitt.
Witt, Wittie, Witty, Wyt, Wytt

Witek (Polish) a form of Victor.
Wytek

Witha (Arabic) handsome.
Wytha

Witter (English) wise warrior.
Whiter, Whitter, Whyter, Whytter, Wytter

Witton (English) wise man's estate.
Whiton, Whyton, Wyton, Wytton

Wladislav (Polish) a form of Vladislav.
Wladislaw, Wladyslav, Wladyslaw

Wolcott (English) cottage in the woods.

Wolf (German, English) a short form of Wolfe, Wolfgang.
Wolff, Wolfie, Wolfy

Wolfe (English) wolf.
Woolf

Wolfgang (German) wolf quarrel. Music: Wolfgang Amadeus Mozart was a famous eighteenth-century Austrian composer.
Wolfegang, Wolfgans

Wood (English) a short form of Elwood, Garwood, Woodrow.

Woodfield (English) forest meadow.
Woodfyeld

Woodford (English) ford through the forest.
Woodforde

Woodley (English) wooded meadow.
Woodlea, Woodlee, Woodleigh, Woodli, Woodlie, Woodly

Woodrow (English) passage in the woods. History: Thomas Woodrow Wilson was the twenty–eighth U.S. president.
Woodman, Woodroe

Woodruff (English) forest ranger.
Woodruf

Woodson (English) son of Wood.
Woods, Woodsan, Woodsen, Woodsin, Woodsyn

Woodville (English) town at the edge of the woods.
Woodvil, Woodvill, Woodvyl, Woodvyll, Woodvylle

Woodward (English) forest warden.
Woodard

Woody (American) a familiar form of Elwood, Garwood, Wood, Woodrow.
Wooddy, Woodi, Woodie

Woolsey (English) victorious wolf.
Woolsee, Woolsi, Woolsie, Woolsy

Worcester (English) forest army camp.

Wordsworth (English) wolf-guardian's farm. Literature: William Wordsworth was a famous British poet.
Wordworth

Worie (Ibo) born on market day.

Worrell (English) lives at the manor of the loyal one.
Worel, Worell, Woril, Worill, Worrel, Worril, Worryl

Worth (English) a short form of Wordsworth.
Worthey, Worthi, Worthie, Worthington, Worthy

Worton (English) farm town.
Wortan, Worten, Wortin, Wortyn

Wouter (German) powerful warrior.

Wrangle (American) a form of Rangle.
Wrangla, Wrangler

Wray (Scandinavian) corner property. (English) crooked.
Wrae, Wrai, Wreh

Wren BG (Welsh) chief, ruler. (English) wren.
Ren

Wright (English) a short form of Wainwright.
Right, Wryght

Wrisley (English) a form of Risley.
Wrisee, Wrislie, Wrisly

Wriston (English) a form of Riston.
Wryston

Wuliton (Native American) will do well.
Wulitan, Wuliten, Wulitin, Wulityn

Wunand (Native American) God is good.
Wunan

Wuyi (Moquelumnan) turkey vulture flying.

Wyatt ☀ (French) little warrior.
Whiat, Whyatt, Wiat, Wiatt, Wyat, Wyatte, Wye, Wyeth, Wyett, Wyitt, Wytt

Wybert (English) battle bright.
Wibert, Wibirt, Wiburt, Wibyrt, Wybirt, Wyburt, Wybyrt

Wyborn (Scandinavian) war bear.
Wibjorn, Wiborn, Wybjorn

Wyck (Scandinavian) village.
Wic, Wick, Wik, Wyc, Wyk

Wycliff (English) white cliff; village near the cliff.
Wiclif, Wicliff, Wicliffe, Wyckliffe, Wycliffe

Wylie (English) charming. See also Wiley.
Wye, Wylea, Wylee, Wyleigh, Wyley, Wyli, Wyllie, Wyly

Wyman (English) fighter, warrior.
Waiman, Waimen, Wayman, Waymen, Wiman, Wimen

Wymer (English) famous in battle.
Wimer

Wyn (Welsh) light skinned; white. (English) friend. A short form of Selwyn.
Wyne, Wynn, Wynne

Wyndham (Scottish) village near the winding road.
Windham, Winham, Wynndham

Wynono (Native American) first-born son.

Wynton (English) a form of Winston.
Wynten

Wythe (English) willow tree.
Withe, Wyth

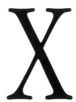

X

Xabat (Basque) savior.

Xacinto (Greek) the hyacinth flower.

Xacob (Galician) a form of Jacob.

Xacobo, Xaime (Hebrew) second son.

Xaiver (Basque) a form of Xavier.
Xajavier, Xzaiver

Xalbador, Xalvador (Spanish) savior.

Xan (Greek) a short form of Alexander.
Xane

Xander (Greek) a short form of Alexander.
Xande, Xzander

Xanthippus (Greek) light-colored horse.
See also Zanthippus.
Xanthyppus

Xanthus (Latin) golden haired. See also
Zanthus.
Xanthius, Xanthos, Xanthyas

Xarles (Basque) a form of Charles.

Xaver (Spanish) a form of Xavier.
Xever, Zever

Xavier ⭐ BG (Arabic) bright. (Basque)
owner of the new house. See also Exavier,
Javier, Salvatore, Saverio, Zavier.
*Xabier, Xavaeir, Xaver, Xavery, Xavian,
Xaviar, Xaviero, Xavior, Xavon, Xavyer,
Xizavier, Xxavier*

Xenaro (Latin) porter.

Xeneroso (Latin) generous.

Xenophon (Greek) strange voice.
Xeno, Zennie, Zenophon

Xenos (Greek) stranger; guest.
Zenos

Xenxo (Greek) protector of the family.

Xerardo (German) a form of Gerardo.

Xerman (Galician) a form of German.

Xerome, Xerónimo, Xes (Greek) saintly
name.

Xerxes (Persian) ruler. History: a king of
Persia.
Xeres, Xerus, Zerk, Zerzes

Xesús (Hebrew) savior.

Xeven (Slavic) lively.
Xyven

Xian (Galician) a form of Julian.

Xián, Xiao, Xillao, Xulio (Latin) from the
Lulia family.

Xicohtencatl (Nahuatl) angry bumblebee.

Xicoténcatl (Nahuatl) from the place of the
reefs.

Xihuitl (Nahuatl) year; comet.

Xil (Greek) young goat.

Xilberte, Xilberto (German) forms of
Gilbert.

Xildas (German) taxes.

Ximén (Spanish) obedient.

Ximenes (Spanish) a form of Simon.
*Ximen, Ximene, Ximenez, Ximon, Ximun,
Xymen, Xymenes, Xymon, Zimenes, Zymenes*

Xipil (Nahuatl) noble of the fire.

Xipilli (Nahuatl) jeweled prince.

Xiuhcoatl (Nahuatl) fire serpent; weapon of
destruction.

Xiutecuhtli (Nahuatl) gentleman of the fire.

Xoan (Hebrew) God is good.

Xoaquín (Hebrew) a form of Joaquín.

Xob (Hebrew) persecuted, afflicted.

Xochiel, Xochitl, Xochtiel (Nahuatl)
flower.

Xochipepe (Nahuatl) flower gatherer.

Xólotl (Nahuatl) precious twin.

Xorxe, Xurxo (Greek) tiller of the soil.

Xose (Galician) a form of Jose.

Xosé (Hebrew) seated on the right-hand
side of God.

Xudas (Hebrew) a form of Judas.

Xusto (Latin) fair, just.

Xylon (Greek) forest.
Xilon, Zilon, Zylon

Xzavier (Basque) a form of Xavier.
Xzavaier, Xzaver, Xzavion, Xzavior, Xzvaier

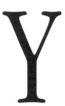

Yaaseen (Indian) another name for Muhammad, the founder of Islam.

Yabarak (Australian) sea.
Yabarac, Yabarack

Yacu (Quechua) water.

Yad (Lebanese) jade.

Yadav, Yadavendra, Yadunandan, Yadunath, Yaduraj, Yaduvir, Yajnarup (Indian) other names for the Hindu god Krishna.

Yadid (Hebrew) friend; beloved.
Yadyd, Yedid

Yadon (Hebrew) he will judge.
Yadean, Yadin, Yadun

Yael GB (Hebrew) a form of Jael.
Yaell

Yafeu (Ibo) bold.

Yagil (Hebrew) he will rejoice.
Yagel, Yagyl, Yogil, Yogyl

Yagna (Indian) ceremonial rites to God.

Yago (Spanish) a form of James.

Yaguatí (Guarani) leopard.

Yahto (Lakota) blue.

Yahya (Arabic) living.

Yahyaa (Indian) prophet.

Yahye (Arabic) a form of Yahya.

Yair (Hebrew) he will enlighten.
Yahir, Yayr

Yaj (Indian) a sage.

Yajat, Yamajit (Indian) other names for the Hindu god Shiva.

Yajnadhar, Yajnesh, Yamahil (Indian) other names for the Hindu god Vishnu.

Yakecen (Dene) sky song.

Yakez (Carrier) heaven.

Yakir (Hebrew) honored.
Yakire, Yakyr, Yakyre

Yakov (Russian) a form of Jacob.
Yaacob, Yaacov, Yaakov, Yachov, Yacoub, Yacov, Yakob, Yashko

Yale (German) productive. (English) old.
Yail, Yaill, Yayl, Yayll

Yaman (Indian) another name for Yama, the Hindu god of death.

Yamil (Arabic) a form of Yamila (see Girls' Names).

Yamir (Indian) moon.

Yamqui (Aymara) title of nobility.

Yan, Yann (Russian) forms of John.

Yana BG (Native American) bear.

Yanamayu (Quechua) black river.

Yancey (Native American) a form of Yancy.
Yansey, Yantsey, Yauncey

Yancy (Native American) Englishman, Yankee.
Yance, Yanci, Yansy, Yauncy, Yency

Yang (Chinese) people of goat tongue.

Yanick, Yanik, Yannick (Russian) familiar forms of Yan.
Yanic, Yannic, Yannik, Yonic, Yonnik

Yanka (Russian) a familiar form of John.

Yanni (Greek) a form of John.
Ioannis, Yani, Yannakis, Yannis, Yanny, Yiannis

Yanton (Hebrew) a form of Johnathon, Jonathen.

Yanuario (Latin) voyage.

Yao (Ewe) born on Thursday.

Yaotl (Nahuatl) war; warrior.

Yaphet (Hebrew) a form of Japheth.
Yapheth, Yefat, Yephat

Yarb (Gypsy) herb.

Yardan (Arabic) king.

Yarden (Hebrew) a form of Jordan.

Yardley (English) enclosed meadow.
Lee, Yard, Yardlea, Yardlee, Yardleigh, Yardli, Yardlie, Yardly

Yarom (Hebrew) he will raise up.
Yarum

Yaron (Hebrew) he will sing; he will cry out.
Jaron, Yairon

Yasaar (Indian) ease; wealth.

Yasâr, Yassêr (Arabic) forms of Yasir.

Yasashiku (Japanese) gentle; polite.

Yash (Hindi) victorious; glory.

Yasha (Russian) a form of Jacob, James.
Yascha, Yashka, Yashko

Yashas (Indian) fame.

Yashodev (Indian) lord of fame.

Yashodhan (Indian) rich in fame.

Yashodhara (Indian) one who has achieved fame.

Yashpal (Indian) protector of fame.

Yashwant (Hindi) glorious.

Yasin (Arabic) prophet.
Yasine, Yasseen, Yassin, Yassine, Yazen

Yasir (Afghan) humble; takes it easy. (Arabic) wealthy.
Yasar, Yaser, Yashar, Yasser

Yasuo (Japanese) restful.

Yates (English) gates.
Yaits, Yayts, Yeats

Yatin (Hindi) ascetic.

Yatindra (Indian) another name for the Hindu god Indra.

Yatish (Indian) lord of devotees.

Yauar (Quechua) blood.

Yauarguacac (Quechua) he sheds tears of blood.

Yauarpuma (Quechua) puma blood.

Yauri (Quechua) lance, needle.

Yavin (Hebrew) he will understand.
Jabin

Yawo (Akan) born on Thursday.

Yayauhqui (Nahuatl) black smoking mirror.

Yazid (Arabic) his power will increase.
Yazeed, Yazide, Yazyd

Yâzid (Arabic) a form of Yazid.

Yechiel (Hebrew) God lives.

Yedidya (Hebrew) a form of Jedidiah. See also Didi.
Yadai, Yedidia, Yedidiah, Yido

Yegor (Russian) a form of George. See also Egor, Igor.
Ygor

Yehoshua (Hebrew) a form of Joshua.
Y'shua, Yeshua, Yeshuah, Yoshua, Yushua

Yehoyakem (Hebrew) a form of Joachim.
Yakim, Yehayakim, Yokim, Yoyakim

Yehuda, Yehudah (Hebrew) forms of Yehudi.

Yehudi (Hebrew) a form of Judah.
Yechudi, Yechudit, Yehudie, Yehudit, Yehudy

Yelutci (Moquelumnan) bear walking silently.

Yeoman (English) attendant; retainer.
Yeomen, Yoeman, Yoman, Youman

Yeremey (Russian) a form of Jeremiah.
Yarema, Yaremka, Yeremy, Yerik

Yervant (Armenian) king, ruler. History: an Armenian king.

Yeshaya (Hebrew) gift. See also Shai.

Yeshurun (Hebrew) right way.

Yeska (Russian) a form of Joseph.
Yesya

Yestin (Welsh) just.
Yestan, Yesten, Yeston, Yestyn

Yeudiel (Hebrew) I give thanks to God.

Yevgeny (Russian) a form of Yevgenyi.

Yevgenyi (Russian) a form of Eugene.
Gena, Yevgeni, Yevgenij, Yevgeniy, Yevgeny

Yigal (Hebrew) he will redeem.
Yagel, Yigael

Yihad (Lebanese) struggle.

Yirmaya (Hebrew) a form of Jeremiah.
Yirmayahu

Yishai (Hebrew) a form of Jesse.

Yisrael (Hebrew) a form of Israel.
Yesarel, Ysrael

Yisroel (Hebrew) a form of Yisrael.

Yitro (Hebrew) a form of Jethro.

Yitzchak (Hebrew) a form of Isaac. See also Itzak.
Yitzaac, Yitzaack, Yitzaak, Yitzac, Yitzack, Yitzak, Yitzchok, Yitzhak

Yngve (Swedish) ancestor; lord, master.

Yo (Cambodian) honest.

Yoakim (Slavic) a form of Jacob.
Yoackim

Yoan, Yoann (German) forms of Johann.

Yoav (Hebrew) a form of Joab.

Yobanis (Spanish) percussionist.

Yochanan (Hebrew) a form of John.
Yohanan

Yoel (Hebrew) a form of Joel.

Yogesh (Hindi) ascetic. Religion: another name for the Hindu god Shiva.

Yogi (Sanskrit) union; person who practices yoga.
Yogee, Yogey, Yogie, Yogy

Yohan, Yohann (German) forms of Johann.
Yohane, Yohanes, Yohanne, Yohannes, Yohans, Yohn

Yohance (Hausa) a form of John.

Yolotli (Nahuatl) heart.

Yoltic (Nahuatl) he who is alive.

Yolyamanitzin (Nahuatl) just; tender and considerate person.

Yonah (Hebrew) a form of Jonah.
Yona, Yonas

Yonatan (Hebrew) a form of Jonathan.
Yonathon, Yonaton, Yonattan

Yonathan (Hebrew) a form of Yonatan.

Yong (Chinese) courageous.
Yonge

Yong-Sun (Korean) dragon in the first position; courageous.

Yoni (Greek) a form of Yanni.
Yonny, Yony

Yonis (Hebrew) a form of Yonus.

Yonus (Hebrew) dove.
Yonas, Yonnas, Yonos, Yonys

Yoofi (Akan) born on Friday.

Yooku (Fante) born on Wednesday.

Yoram (Hebrew) God is high.
Joram

Yorgos (Greek) a form of George.
Yiorgos, Yorgo

Yorick (English) farmer. (Scandinavian) a form of George.
Yoric, Yorik, Yorrick, Yoryc, Yoryck, Yoryk

York (English) boar estate; yew-tree estate.
Yorke, Yorker, Yorkie

Yorkoo (Fante) born on Thursday.

Yosef (Hebrew) a form of Joseph. See also Osip.
Yoceph, Yoosuf, Yoseff, Yoseph, Yosief, Yosif, Yosuf, Yosyf

Yóshi (Japanese) adopted son.
Yoshee, Yoshie, Yoshiki, Yoshiuki

Yoshiyahu (Hebrew) a form of Josiah.
Yoshia, Yoshiah, Yoshiya, Yoshiyah, Yosiah

Yoskolo (Moquelumnan) breaking off pine cones.

Yosu (Hebrew) a form of Jesus.

Yotimo (Moquelumnan) yellow jacket carrying food to its hive.

Yottoko (Native American) mud at the water's edge.

Younes (Lebanese) prophet.

Young (English) young.
Yung

Young-Jae (Korean) pile of prosperity.

Young-Soo (Korean) keeping the prosperity.

Youri (Russian) a form of Yuri.

Youseef, Yousef (Yiddish) forms of Joseph.
Yousaf, Youseph, Yousif, Youssef, Yousseff, Yousuf

Youssel (Yiddish) a familiar form of Joseph.
Yussel

Yov (Russian) a short form of Yoakim.

Yovani (Slavic) a form of Jovan.
Yovan, Yovanni, Yovanny, Yovany, Yovni

Yoyi (Hebrew) a form of George.

Yrjo (Finnish) a form of George.

Ysidro (Greek) a short form of Isidore.

Yu BG (Chinese) universe.
Yue

Yuçef (Arabic) a form of José.

Yudan (Hebrew) judgment.
Yuden, Yudin, Yudon, Yudyn

Yudell (English) a form of Udell.
Yudale, Yudel

Yuhannà (Arabic) a form of Juan.

Yuki BG (Japanese) snow.
Yukiko, Yukio

Yul (Mongolian) beyond the horizon.

Yule (English) born at Christmas.
Yull

Yuli (Basque) youthful.

Yuma (Native American) son of a chief.
Yumah

Yunes (Lebanese) prophet.

Yunus (Turkish) a form of Jonah.
Younis, Younys, Yunis, Yunys

Yupanqui (Quechua) he who honors his ancestors.

Yurac (Quechua) white.

Yurcel (Turkish) sublime.

Yuri GB (Russian, Ukrainian) a form of George. (Hebrew) a familiar form of Uriah.
Yehor, Yura, Yure, Yuria, Yuric, Yurii, Yurij, Yurik, Yurko, Yurri, Yury, Yurya, Yusha

Yurochka (Russian) farmer.

Yusef, Yusuf (Arabic, Swahili) forms of Joseph.
Yussef, Yusuff

Yusif (Russian) a form of Joseph.
Yuseph, Yusof, Yussof, Yusup, Yuzef, Yuzep

Yustyn (Russian) a form of Justin.
Yusts

Yutu (Moquelumnan) coyote out hunting.

Yuuki (Japanese) a form of Yuki.

Yuval (Hebrew) rejoicing.

Yves (French) a form of Ivar, Ives.
Yvens, Yyves

Yvet (French) archer.

Yvon (French) a form of Ivar, Yves.
Ivon, Yuvon, Yvan, Yven, Yvin, Yvonne, Yvyn

Ywain (Irish) a form of Owen.
Ywaine, Ywayn, Ywayne, Ywyn

Z

Zabdi (Hebrew) a short form of Zabdiel.
Zabad, Zabdy, Zabi, Zavdi, Zebdy

Zabdiel (Hebrew) present, gift.
Zabdil, Zabdyl, Zavdiel, Zebdiel

Zabulón (Hebrew) purple house.

Zac (Hebrew) a short form of Zachariah, Zachary.
Zacc

Zacarias (Portuguese, Spanish) a form of Zachariah.
Zacaria, Zacariah, Zacarious, Zacarius, Zaccaria, Zaccariah

Zacarías (Spanish) a form of Zacarias.

Zacary, Zaccary (Hebrew) forms of Zachary.
Zacaras, Zacari, Zacarie, Zaccari, Zaccary, Zaccea, Zaccury, Zacery, Zacrye

Zacchaeus (Hebrew) a form of Zaccheus.

Zaccheus (Hebrew) innocent, pure.
Zacceus, Zacchious, Zachaios

Zach (Hebrew) a short form of Zachariah, Zachary.

Zacharey, Zachari (Hebrew) forms of Zachary.
Zaccharie, Zachare, Zacharee, Zacheri, Zachurie, Zecharie

Zacharia (Hebrew) a form of Zachariah.
Zacharya

Zachariah (Hebrew) God remembered.
Zacharyah, Zackeria, Zackoriah, Zaquero, Zeggery, Zhachory

Zacharias (German) a form of Zachariah.
Zacharais, Zachariaus, Zacharius, Zackarias, Zakarias, Zakarius, Zecharias, Zekarias

Zacharie BG (Hebrew) a form of Zachary.

Zachary ☀ BG (Hebrew) a familiar form of Zachariah. History: Zachary Taylor was the twelfth U.S. president. See also Sachar, Sakeri.
Xachary, Zacchary, Zacha, Zachaery, Zacharay, Zacharry, Zachaury, Zechary

Zacheriah (Hebrew) a form of Zachariah.
Zacheria, Zacherias, Zacherius, Zackeriah

Zachery (Hebrew) a form of Zachary.
Zacchery, Zacheray, Zacherey, Zacherie, Zechery

Zachory (Hebrew) a form of Zachary.
Zachuery, Zachury

Zachrey, Zachry (Hebrew) forms of Zachary.
Zachre, Zachri, Zackree, Zackrey, Zackry, Zakree, Zakri, Zakris, Zakry

Zack (Hebrew) a short form of Zachariah, Zachary.

Zackariah (Hebrew) a form of Zachariah.

Zackary (Hebrew) a form of Zachary.
Zackare, Zackaree, Zackari, Zackarie, Zackhary, Zackie

Zackery (Hebrew) a form of Zachary.
Zackere, Zackeree, Zackerey, Zackeri, Zackerie, Zackerry

Zackory (Hebrew) a form of Zachary.
Zackorie, Zacorey, Zacori, Zacory, Zacry, Zakory

Zadok (Hebrew) a short form of Tzadok.
Zadak, Zaddik, Zadik, Zadoc, Zadock, Zaydok

Zadornin (Basque) Saturn.

Zafir (Arabic) victorious.
Zafar, Zafeer, Zafer, Zaffar

Zah (Lebanese) bright, luminous.

Zahid (Arabic) self-denying, ascetic.
Zaheed, Zahyd

Zâhid (Arabic) a form of Zahid.

Zahir (Arabic) shining, bright.
Zahair, Zahar, Zaheer, Zahi, Zahyr, Zair, Zayyir

Zahîr (Arabic) a form of Zahir.

Zahur (Swahili) flower.

Zaid (Arabic) increase, growth.
Zaied, Zaiid, Zayd

Zaide (Hebrew) older.
Zayde

Zaim (Arabic) brigadier general.
Zaym

Zain (English) a form of Zane.
Zaine

Zaire BG (Arabic) a form of Zahir. Geography: a country of central Africa.

Zak (Hebrew) a short form of Zachariah, Zachary.
Zaks

Zakari, Zakary, Zakkary (Hebrew) forms of Zachary.
Zakarai, Zakare, Zakaree, Zakarie, Zakariye, Zake, Zakhar, Zakir, Zakkai, Zakkari, Zakkyre, Zakqary

Zakaria, Zakariya (Hebrew) forms of Zachariah.
Zakaraiya, Zakareeya, Zakareeyah, Zakariah, Zakeria, Zakeriah

Zakariyya (Arabic) prophet. Religion: an Islamic prophet.

Zakery (Hebrew) a form of Zachary.
Zakeri, Zakerie, Zakiry, Zakkery

Zaki (Arabic) bright; pure. (Hausa) lion.
Zakee, Zakie, Zakiy, Zakki, Zaky